Bone and Soft Tissue Pathology

Other books in this series:

Prayson: Neuropathology

Iacobuzio-Donahue & Montgomery: Gastrointestinal and Liver Pathology

Thompson: Head and Neck Pathology

O'Malley & Pinder: Breast Pathology

Thompson: Endocrine Pathology

Zhou & Magi-Galluzzi: Genitourinary Pathology

Hsi: Hematopathology

Sidawy & Ali: Fine Needle Aspiration Cytology

Zander & Farver: Pulmonary Pathology

Busam: Dermatopathology

Nucci & Oliva: Gynecologic Pathology

Tubbs & Stoler: Cell and Tissue Based Molecular Pathology

Bone and Soft Tissue Pathology

A Volume in the Series
Foundations in Diagnostic Pathology

Edited by

Andrew L. Folpe, MD
Consultant
Division of Anatomic Pathology
Professor of Laboratory Medicine and Pathology
Mayo Clinic
Rochester, Minnesota

Carrie Y. Inwards, MD
Consultant
Division of Anatomic Pathology
Associate Professor of Laboratory Medicine and Pathology
Mayo Clinic
Rochester, Minnesota

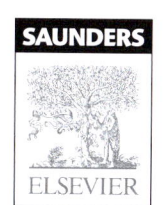

SAUNDERS
ELSEVIER

SAUNDERS
ELSEVIER

1600 John F. Kennedy Blvd.
Ste 1800
Philadelphia, PA 19103-2899

BONE AND SOFT TISSUE PATHOLOGY
(A VOLUME IN THE SERIES FOUNDATIONS IN DIAGNOSTIC PATHOLOGY)

ISBN: 978-0-443-06688-7

Copyright © 2010 by Saunders, an imprint of Elsevier, Inc.
Drawings copyright © Mayo Foundation for Medical Education and Research

All rights reserved. No part of this publication may be reproduced or transmitted in any form or by any means, electronic or mechanical, including photocopying, recording, or any information storage and retrieval system, without permission in writing from the publisher. Permissions may be sought directly from Elsevier's Rights Department: phone: (+1) 215 239 3804 (US) or (+44) 1865 843830 (UK); fax: (+44) 1865 853333; e-mail: healthpermissions@elsevier.com. You may also complete your request on-line via the Elsevier website at http://www.elsevier.com/permissions.

NOTICE

Knowledge and best practice in this field are constantly changing. As new research and experience broaden our knowledge, changes in practice, treatment and drug therapy may become necessary or appropriate. Readers are advised to check the most current information provided (i) on procedures featured or (ii) by the manufacturer of each product to be administered, to verify the recommended dose or formula, the method and duration of administration, and contraindications. It is the responsibility of the practitioner, relying on their own experience and knowledge of the patient, to make diagnoses, to determine dosages and the best treatment for each individual patient, and to take all appropriate safety precautions. To the fullest extent of the law, neither the Publisher nor the Editors assume any liability for any injury and/or damage to persons or property arising out of or related to any use of the material contained in this book.

The Publisher

Library of Congress Cataloging-in-Publication Data
Bone and soft tissue pathology / edited by Andrew L. Folpe, Carrie Y. Inwards. -- 1st ed.
p. ; cm. -- (Foundations in diagnostic pathology)
Includes bibliographical references and index.
ISBN 978-0-443-06688-7
1. Musculoskeletal system--Tumors--Pathophysiology. I. Folpe, Andrew L. II. Inwards, Carrie Y.
III. Title. IV. Series.
[DNLM: 1. Bone Neoplasms--pathology. 2. Soft Tissue Neoplasms--pathology. WE 258 B71043 2010]
RC280.M83.B66 2010
616.99'47--dc22

2008047217

Acquisitions Editor: William Schmitt
Developmental Editor: Barbara Cicalese
Project Manager: Bryan Hayward
Design Direction: Lou Forgione

Printed in China

Last digit is the print number: 9 8 7 6 5 4 3 2 1

Working together to grow
libraries in developing countries

www.elsevier.com | www.bookaid.org | www.sabre.org

ELSEVIER | BOOK AID International | Sabre Foundation

To our families who patiently endured the creation of this book.
To my wife Anastasia, and children Leah, Elizabeth, and Benjamin—ALF
To my husband David, and children Ryan and Sarah—CYI

Contributors

Patrizia Bacchini, MD
Pathology Consultant, Villa Erbosa Hospital, Bologna, Italy
Giant Cell Tumor of Bone

Franco Bertoni, MD
Professor of Pathology, University of Bologna, Bologna, Italy
Giant Cell Tumor of Bone

S. Fiona Bonar, MD
Adjunct Professor, Anatomical Pathology, Douglass Hanly Moir Pathology and Notre Dame University; Consultant, Orthopaedic Pathology, Royal Prince Alfred Hospital; Douglass Hanly Moir Pathology, Mater Misericordiae Hospital, Sydney, New South Wales, Australia
Bone Tumors of Miscellaneous Type or Uncertain Lineage

Enrique de Alava, MD, PhD
Research Professor of Pathology and Head of the Molecular Pathology Program, Centro de Investigación del Cáncer-IBMCC, Salamanca, Spain
Adjuvant Techniques—Immunohistochemistry, Cytogenetics, and Molecular Genetics

Angelo Paolo Dei Tos, MD
Chair of the Pathology Department, General Hospital, Treviso, Italy
Adipocytic Tumors

Andrea T. Deyrup, MD, PhD
Assistant Professor of Pathology, Emory University, Atlanta, Georgia, United States
Smooth Muscle Tumors

Julie C. Fanburg-Smith, MD
Deputy Chair and Director of Education, Department of Orthopaedic and Soft Tissue Pathology, Armed Forces Institute of Pathology, Washington, DC, United States
Nerve Sheath and Neuroectodermal Tumors

Andrew L. Folpe, MD
Consultant, Division of Anatomic Pathology, and Professor of Laboratory Medicine and Pathology, Mayo Clinic, Rochester, Minnesota, United States
Adjuvant Techniques—Immunohistochemistry, Cytogenetics, and Molecular Genetics; Fibroblastic and Fibrohistiocytic Tumors; Tumor of Perivascular Cells; Vascular Tumors of Soft Tissue; Tumors of Miscellaneous Type or Uncertain Lineage

Louis Guillou, MD
Professor of Pathology, University Institute of Pathology, Centre Hospitalier Universitaire Vaudois and University of Lausanne, Lausanne, Switzerland
Fibroblastic and Fibrohistiocytic Tumors; Tumor of Perivascular Cells

Andrew Horvai, MD, PhD
Associate Clinical Professor of Pathology, University of California, San Francisco, California, United States
Cartilage-Forming Tumors; Vascular Tumors of Bone; Notochordal Tumors

Carrie Y. Inwards, MD
Consultant, Division of Anatomic Pathology, and Associate Professor of Laboratory Medicine and Pathology, Mayo Clinic, Rochester, Minnesota, United States

Leonard B. Kahn, MBBCh, FRCP, MMedPath
Professor of Pathology, Albert Einstein College of Medicine, New York, New York; Pathology Chair, Long Island Jewish Medical Center, New Hyde Park, New York, United States
Adamantinoma

Michael J. Klein, MD
Director, Department of Pathology and Laboratory Medicine, Hospital for Special Surgery, New York, New York, United States
Ewing Sarcoma

Edward F. McCarthy, MD
Professor of Pathology and Orthopaedic Surgery, Johns Hopkins University, Baltimore, Maryland, United States
Fibroblastic and Fibrohistiocytic Tumors; Hematopoietic Tumors

Yasuaki Nakashima, MD
Laboratory of Anatomic Pathology, Kyoto University Hospital, Kyoto, Japan
Metastases Involving Bone

G. Petur Nielsen, MD
Associate Professor, Harvard Medical School; Associate Pathologist, Massachusetts General Hospital, Boston, Massachusetts, United States
Tumors of Synovial Tissue; Bone-Forming Tumors

John X. O'Connell, MBBCh, FRCPC
Clinical Associate Professor of Laboratory Medicine, University of British Columbia, Vancouver; Pathologist, CJ Coady Associates, Surrey, British Columbia, Canada
Osteocartilaginous Tumors; Tumors of Synovial Tissue

R. Lor Randall, MD, FACS
Associate Professor of Orthopaedics, University of Utah School of Medicine; Medical Director, Orthopaedics Department, Huntsman Cancer Hospital; Orthopaedic Surgery Department, Primary Children's Medical Center; Director of Sarcoma Services, Huntsman Cancer Institute, Salt Lake City, Utah, United States
Approach to the Diagnosis of Bone and Soft Tissue Tumors—Clinical, Radiologic, and Classification Aspects

Andrew E. Rosenberg, MD
Professor of Pathology, Harvard Medical School; Pathologist, Massachusetts General Hospital, Boston, Massachusetts, United States
Bone-Forming Tumors

Brian P. Rubin, MD, PhD
Associate Professor of Anatomic Pathology, Cleveland Clinic Taussig Cancer Institute; Director of Soft Tissue Pathology, Cleveland Clinic Lerner Research Institute, Cleveland, Ohio, United States
Gastrointestinal Stromal Tumor

Raf Sciot, MD, PhD
Professor of Pathology, Department of Morphology and Molecular Pathology, Catholic University of Leuven; Chair of Pathology Department, University Hospital Gasthuisberg, Leuven, Belgium
Skeletal Muscle Tumors

Foreword

The study and practice of anatomic pathology is both exciting and overwhelming. Surgical pathology, with all of the subspecialties it encompasses, and cytopathology have become increasingly complex and sophisticated, and it is not possible for any individual to master the skills and knowledge required to perform all of these tasks at the highest level. Simply being able to make a correct diagnosis is challenging enough, but the standard of care has far surpassed merely providing a diagnosis. Pathologists are now asked to provide large amounts of ancillary information, both diagnostic and prognostic, often on small amounts of tissue, a task that can be daunting even to the most experienced pathologist.

Although large general surgical pathology textbooks are useful resources, they by necessity could not possibly cover many of the aspects that pathologists need to know and include in their reports. As such, the concept behind *Foundations in Diagnostic Pathology* was born. This series is designed to cover the major areas of surgical and cytopathology, and each edition is focused on one major topic. The goal of every book in this series is to provide the essential information that any pathologist, whether general or subspecialized, in training or in practice, would find useful in the evaluation of virtually any type of specimen encountered.

Dr. Andrew Folpe and Dr. Carrie Inwards, both from the Mayo Clinic, have combined their expertise in soft tissue and orthopedic pathology, respectively, to edit an outstanding book covering the essential aspects of this discipline, an area of pathology that I have a particular love for. It has been my experience that many pathologists are intimidated by sarcomas, a field which has evolved rapidly over the past 10 years. However, this book efficiently communicates the essential knowledge that surgical pathologists require to effectively handle these sometimes complex specimens. The list of contributors is truly an impressive one, and includes renowned pathologists from the United States and around the world. The content in each chapter is extremely practical, well-organized, and concisely written, focusing on the thorough evaluation of both biopsy and resection specimens. As with all other editions in the *Foundations in Diagnostic Pathology* series, this information is presented in an accessible manner, including numerous practical tables and high-quality photomicrographs. Where appropriate, the authors seamlessly integrate the use of ancillary diagnostic techniques, including immunohistochemistry and molecular diagnostics, which, of course, are an essential part of the diagnostic armamentarium.

This edition is organized into three major areas, including general aspects (clinical and radiologic approach to the diagnosis of bone and soft tissue tumors and the use of adjuvant diagnostic techniques) and 11 chapters each on specific entities in soft tissue and bone pathology. All of the chapters incorporate up-to-date nomenclature and the newest entities, some of which have been described only within the past 5 years.

I wish to extend my sincerest gratitude to Drs. Folpe and Inwards for pouring their hearts and souls into this edition of the *Foundation in Diagnostic Pathology* series. I would also like to extend my heartfelt appreciation to the many authors who took time from their busy schedules to contribute their knowledge and expertise. I sincerely hope you enjoy this volume of *Foundations in Diagnostic Pathology*.

JOHN R. GOLDBLUM, MD

Preface

Several textbooks on bone and soft tissue pathologies are available. What makes this book different? First, this book has *Disease Fact* and *Pathologic Feature* boxes for each major disease entity of bone and soft tissues so that the essential clinical, radiographic, and pathologic features of each entity can be easily appreciated and understood and thus serve as a quick reference during routine sign-out. Second, emphasis has been placed throughout on practical diagnostic issues while maintaining sufficient clinical information to allow the pathologist to participate fully in the multidisciplinary care of patients with tumors of the musculoskeletal system.

This book is primarily intended to be a day-to-day supplement to larger and more comprehensive bone and soft tissue pathology textbooks. It provides up-to-date information on the surgical pathology of bone and soft tissue and emphasizes practical diagnostic aspects. These are addressed with more than 600 high-quality, full-color illustrations, as well as numerous boxes and tables to enhance and facilitate the presentation of information. Additionally, this book employs a novel format that allows easy use and learning.

We are very fortunate to have many world-renowned bone and soft tissue pathologists contribute to this book. We are greatly appreciative of their time, efforts, and expertise.

ANDREW L. FOLPE, MD
CARRIE Y. INWARDS, MD

Contents

Section I—General Aspects

Chapter 1
Approach to the Diagnosis of Bone and Soft Tissue Tumors—Clinical, Radiologic, and Classification Aspects   3
R. Lor Randall

Chapter 2
Adjuvant Techniques—Immunohistochemistry, Cytogenetics, and Molecular Genetics   18
Andrew L. Folpe and Enrique de Alava

Section II—Soft Tissue Pathology

Chapter 3
Fibroblastic and Fibrohistiocytic Tumors   43
Louis Guillou and Andrew L. Folpe

Chapter 4
Adipocytic Tumors   97
Angelo Paolo Dei Tos

Chapter 5
Smooth Muscle Tumors   119
Andrea T. Deyrup

Chapter 6
Skeletal Muscle Tumors   131
Raf Sciot

Chapter 7
Tumor of Perivascular Cells   146
Andrew L. Folpe and Louis Guillou

Chapter 8
Gastrointestinal Stromal Tumor   158
Brian P. Rubin

Chapter 9
Vascular Tumors of Soft Tissue   164
Andrew L. Folpe

Chapter 10
Nerve Sheath and Neuroectodermal Tumors   193
Julie C. Fanburg-Smith

Chapter 11
Osteocartilaginous Tumors   239
John X. O'Connell

Chapter 12
Tumors of Synovial Tissue   255
G. Petur Nielsen and John X. O'Connell

Chapter 13
Tumors of Miscellaneous Type or Uncertain Lineage   276
Andrew L. Folpe

Section III—Bone Pathology

Chapter 14
Bone-Forming Tumors   309
G. Petur Nielsen and Andrew E. Rosenberg

Chapter 15
Cartilage-Forming Tumors   330
Andrew Horvai

Chapter 16
Fibroblastic and Fibrohistiocytic Tumors   355
Edward F. McCarthy

Chapter 17
Ewing Sarcoma   367
Michael J. Klein

Chapter 18
Hematopoietic Tumors   379
Edward F. McCarthy

Chapter 19
Vascular Tumors of Bone   389
Andrew Horvai

Chapter 20
Giant Cell Tumor of Bone   401
Patrizia Bacchini and Franco Bertoni

Chapter 21
Notochordal Tumors   408
Andrew Horvai

Chapter 22
Adamantinoma 414
Leonard B. Kahn

Chapter 23
Bone Tumors of Miscellaneous Type or Uncertain Lineage 419
S. Fiona Bonar

Chapter 24
Metastases Involving Bone 446
Yasuaki Nakashima

Index 455

Section I

General Aspects

1 Approach to the Diagnosis of Bone and Soft Tissue Tumors—Clinical, Radiologic, and Classification Aspects
R. Lor Randall

2 Adjuvant Techniques—Immunohistochemistry, Cytogenetics, and Molecular Genetics
Andrew L. Folpe · Enrique De Alava

1

Approach to the Diagnosis of Bone and Soft Tissue Tumors – Clinical, Radiologic, and Classification Aspects

R. Lor Randall

- Overview
- Evaluation of Tumors
- Grading of Soft Tissue and Bone Sarcomas
- Staging Systems
- General Classification of Mesenchymal Tumors

OVERVIEW

Tumors of the musculoskeletal system are an extremely heterogeneous group of neoplasms consisting of well greater than 200 benign types of neoplasms and approximately 90 malignant conditions. The relative incidence of benign to malignant disease is 200:1. They are categorized according to their differentiated or adult histology with current classification schemes being essentially descriptive. Each histologic type of tumor expresses individual, distinct behaviors with great variation between tumor types. Benign disease, by definition, behaves in a nonaggressive fashion with little tendency to recur locally or to metastasize. Malignant tumors or sarcomas, such as osteosarcoma and synovial sarcoma, are capable of invasive, locally destructive growth with a tendency to recur and to metastasize.

Neoplastic processes arise in tissues of mesenchymal origin far less frequently compared with those of ectodermal and endodermal origin. Soft tissue and bone sarcomas have an annual incidence in the United States of more than 6000 and 3000 new cases, respectively. When compared with the overall average cancer mortality of 550,000 cases per year, sarcomas are a small fraction of the problem. However, although a relatively uncommon form of cancer, these mesenchymal tumors behave in an aggressive fashion with reported current mortality rates in some series greater than 50%. According to the National Cancer Institute's Surveillance, Epidemiology, and End Results (SEER) Program, approximately 5700 new soft tissue sarcomas developed in the United States in 1990, with 3100 sarcoma-related deaths. More recent epidemiologic studies support this. The associated morbidity rate is much greater. These tumors inflict a tremendous emotional and financial toll on individuals and society alike. Furthermore, sarcomas are more common in older patients, with 15% affecting patients younger than 15 years and 40% affecting persons older than 55 years. Accordingly, as the population ages, as it is doing at a rapid rate, the incidence of these tumors will increase.

EVALUATION OF TUMORS

HISTORY AND PHYSICAL EXAMINATION

When evaluating a new patient with a possible tumor, the workup must commence with a careful and thorough history and physical. Before ordering any diagnostic studies, particular questions must be answered, as well as an assessment of the physical characteristics of the mass in question. This will prevent the ordering of unnecessary tests and better enable the physician to determine which tests will be most helpful in diagnosing the condition and facilitating therapeutic interventions if needed.

The clinical history is of paramount importance (Box 1-1). The age of the patient will permit the generation of a list of potential diagnoses that, when combined with the history and a few additional studies, should permit establishing a diagnosis. The duration of symptoms, rate of growth, presence of pain, and a history of trauma can help to elucidate the diagnosis. A careful medical history, family history, and review of systems must not be overlooked either.

A thorough physical examination is also critical (Box 1-2). The clinician must assess the location and size of the mass, the quality of the overlying skin, the presence of warmth, any associated swelling, the presence of tenderness, and the firmness of the lesion. Range of motion of all joints in proximity to the tumor, above and below, must be recorded, as well as a complete

> **Box 1-1: QUESTIONS THAT MUST BE ASKED IN THE WORKUP OF A POSSIBLE TUMOR**
>
> 1. The patient's age: Certain tumors are relatively specific to particular age groups.
> 2. Duration of complaint: Benign lesions generally have been present for an extended period (years). Malignant tumors usually have been noticed for only weeks to months.
> 3. Rate of growth: A rapidly growing mass, as in weeks to months, is more likely to be malignant. Growth may be difficult to assess by the patient if it is deep seated, as can be the case with bone. Deep lesions may be much larger than the patient thought ("tip-of-the-iceberg" phenomenon).
> 4. Pain associated with the mass: Benign processes are usually asymptomatic. Osteochondromas may cause secondary symptoms because of encroachment on surrounding structures. Malignant lesions may cause pain.
> 5. History of trauma: With a history of penetrating trauma, one must rule out osteomyelitis. With a history of blunt trauma, healing fracture must be entertained.
> 6. Personal or family history of cancer: Adults with a history of prostate, renal, lung, breast, or thyroid tumors are at risk for development of metastatic bone disease. Children with neuroblastoma are prone to bony metastases. Patients with retinoblastoma are at an increased risk for osteosarcoma. Secondary osteosarcomas and other malignancies can result from treatment of other childhood cancers. Family history of conditions such as Li–Fraumeni syndrome must raise suspicion of any bone lesion. Furthermore, certain benign bone tumors can run in families (e.g., multiple hereditary exostoses).
> 7. Systemic signs or symptoms: Generally, no significant findings should exist on the review of systems with benign tumors. Fevers, chills, night sweats, malaise, change in appetite, weight loss, and so forth should alert the physician that an infectious or neoplastic process may be involved.

> **Box 1-2: ASPECTS OF PHYSICAL EXAMINATION THAT SHOULD BE DOCUMENTED WHEN EVALUATING A PATIENT WITH A MASS**
>
> 1. Skin color
> 2. Warmth
> 3. Location
> 4. Swelling: swelling, in addition to the primary mass effect, may reflect a more aggressive process
> 5. Neurovascular examination: changes may reflect a more aggressive process
> 6. Joint range of motion of all joints in proximity to the region in question, above and below
> 7. Size: a mass greater than 5 cm should raise the suspicion of malignancy
> 8. Tenderness: tenderness may reflect a more rapidly growing process
> 9. Firmness: malignant tumors tend to be more firm on examination than benign processes; this applies more to soft tissue tumors than to osseous ones
> 10. Lymph nodes: certain sarcomas (e.g., rhabdomyosarcoma, synovial sarcoma, epithelioid, and clear cell sarcomas all have increased rates of lymph node involvement)
>
> Note these findings assume the absence of trauma.

neurovascular examination. An assessment of the related lymph node chains and an examination for an enlarged liver or spleen should be performed.

The clinician must consider pseudotumors in addition to true neoplastic conditions. A history of trauma suggests a possible stress fracture or myositis ossificans as a diagnosis. The history of stress-related physical activity and the exact timing of symptom presentation and variations of symptoms with the passage of time are important considerations in establishing a differential diagnosis.

IMAGING STUDIES

CONVENTIONAL RADIOGRAPHY

Initial evaluation should begin with plain radiography irrespective of whether a bone or soft tissue lesion is suspected. In every patient with a palpable mass, orthogonal anteroposterior and lateral views of the affected area should be taken. Low-kilovolt radiographs may facilitate viewing soft tissue planes. In many cases for bone lesions, radiographic examination will be diagnostic, and no further imaging studies will be indicated. However, in the case of a more aggressive process, the diagnosis may be able to be determined on the plain radiographs, but further evaluation with advanced studies is usually indicated to determine the extent of local soft tissue involvement and to assess the extent of disseminated disease (staging).

The initial radiographic images must be scrutinized because a great deal of information can be gleaned from this simple imaging modality (Figure 1-1). In addition to evaluating lesions arising from the bone, one must inspect whether a mass arising from the soft tissue is involving and possibly eroding the bone cortex. For bone lesions, the location within the bone (e.g., epiphyseal, metaphyseal, or diaphyseal) must be considered and will facilitate the diagnosis (Figure 1-2, Table 1-1). Epiphyseal tumors are usually benign. The more malignant primary sarcomas, such as osteosarcoma, are typically seen in a metaphyseal location (Figure 1-3). Round cell tumors, such as Ewing sarcoma, multiple myeloma, and lymphomas, are usually medullary diaphyseal lesions but can be seen in the metaphysis as well. A tumor arising from the surface of a long bone may be a benign lesion, such as an osteochondroma, or may be a low-grade sarcoma, such as a parosteal osteosarcoma.

Terms such as *geographic, well circumscribed, permeative,* and *moth-eaten* are used to describe the appearance of radiographic abnormalities associated with bone tumors (Table 1-2). "Geographic" or "well circumscribed" implies that the lesion has a distinct boundary

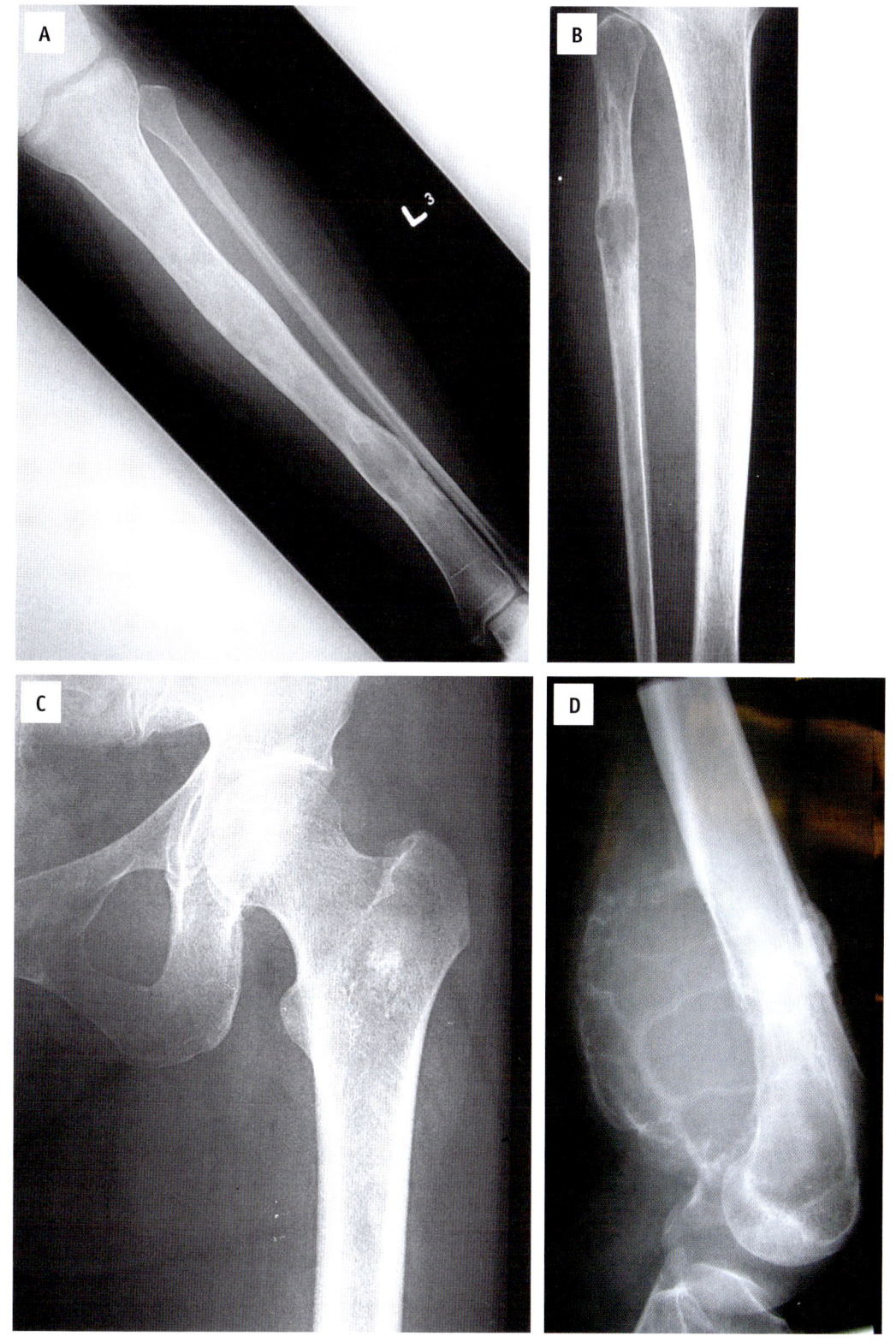

FIGURE 1-1

A, Anteroposterior (AP) radiograph of the tibia and fibula demonstrates the permeative, "ground-glass" appearance of fibrous dysplasia in the distal half of the tibia. **B,** Another AP radiograph of the tibia and fibula demonstrates the more aggressive permeative pattern of adamantinoma involving the proximal fibula. **C,** AP radiograph of the hip demonstrates the central calcifications of a cartilage-based tumor in the intertrochanteric region. The differential would include enchondroma versus low-grade chondrosarcoma. **D,** Lateral radiograph of the distal femur reveals a large expansile mass. The aneurysmal features suggest a diagnosis of aneurysmal bone cyst; however, the irregular cortical involvement must raise a suspicion for telangiectatic osteosarcoma.

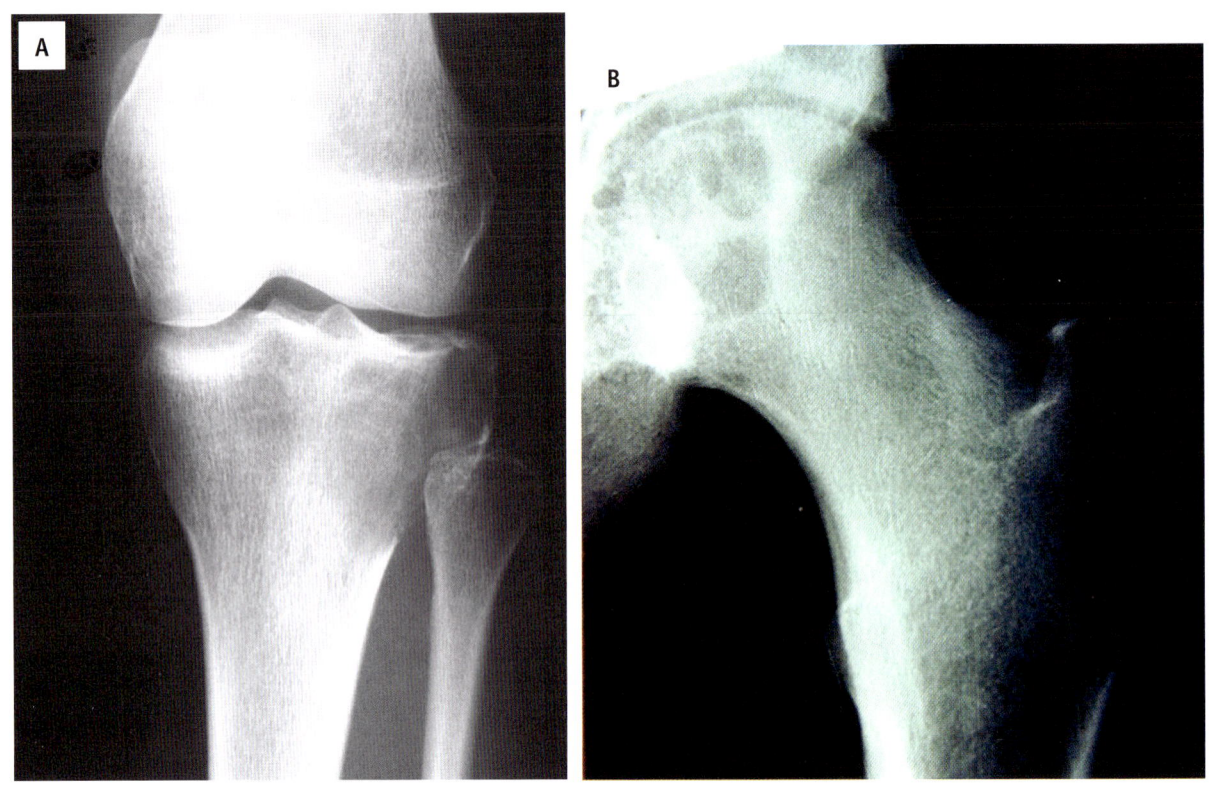

FIGURE 1-2
A, Anteroposterior (AP) radiograph of the proximal tibia and fibula reveals an epiphyseal equivalent lesion of the proximal tibia highly suggestive of giant cell tumor of bone. **B**, AP radiograph of the hip demonstrates a radiolucent lesion of the epiphyseal equivalent. Although the physis is closed, this proved to be a chondroblastoma.

and is sharply marginated, suggesting a benign tumor (Figure 1-4). A poorly defined, infiltrative process is described as "permeative" or "moth-eaten" and is sometimes characterized by a periosteal reaction (Figure 1-5). These features reflect a more aggressive process suggesting a possible malignancy. An exception to this rule is multiple myeloma, which frequently demonstrates a punched-out, well-demarcated appearance but in multiple locations.

With a careful history, physical examination, and appropriate radiographs, the physician can reach a working diagnosis of the lesion. Although benign and malignant tumors can mimic each other, some tumors can be ruled out on the basis of the history, the age of the patient, the location of the tumor (if a bone tumor, in which bone and where in the bone), and the radiographic appearance of the tumor. For example, a 20-year-old man with a 3-month history of pain in the knee is found to have an epiphyseal lesion in the distal femur. The lesion has a benign, geographic appearance. If the tumor is benign, the criteria of the patient's age eliminate only solitary bone cyst and osteofibrous dysplasia, but all other benign tumors remain possibilities. If the tumor is malignant, it is likely to be an osteosarcoma (various types), Ewing sarcoma, fibrosarcoma, vascular sarcoma, or possibly, chondrosarcoma, according to the age criterion. The most common site for bone tumors is about the knee, especially the distal femur. The likely benign tumors are giant cell tumor, nonossifying fibroma, chondroma, osteochondroma, and chondroblastoma. Most malignant tumors are metaphyseal. Based on location in the bone (see Table 1-1), the most likely benign tumors are chondroblastoma and giant cell tumor. The geographic appearance implies a benign radiographic appearance. Thus, the working diagnosis would be chondroblastoma or, possibly, giant cell tumor if the lesion were benign, whereas it would be osteosarcoma or chondrosarcoma if the lesion were malignant, which is less likely. In this age group, metastatic disease is unlikely, but low-grade infection may mimic a tumor, particularly if the patient is immunocompromised, which can be determined from the patient's history.

Ultrasound

Ultrasound has a limited practical role in evaluating soft tissue masses. Its use in workup for bone lesions is essentially nonexistent. If the clinician has a high index of suspicion that the mass may be a ganglion, hematoma, or other fluid collection, ultrasound may be used to confirm this. Otherwise, magnetic resonance

TABLE 1-1
Location of a Tumor within a Bone May Facilitate Diagnosis

Diaphyseal

Ewing sarcoma
(Osteo)fibrous dysplasia
Adamantinoma
Langerhans cell histiocytosis
Lymphoma
Metaphyseal

Eccentric

Osteosarcoma
Nonossifying fibroma (fibrous cortical defect)
Osteochondroma
Aneurysmal bone cyst
Osteomyelitis
Central
Enchondroma
Chondrosarcoma
Solitary bone cyst
Osteomyelitis

Epiphyseal

Giant cell tumor
Chondroblastoma
Osteomyelitis
Degenerative cyst
Dysplasia epiphysealis hemimelica
Pigmented villonodular synovitis

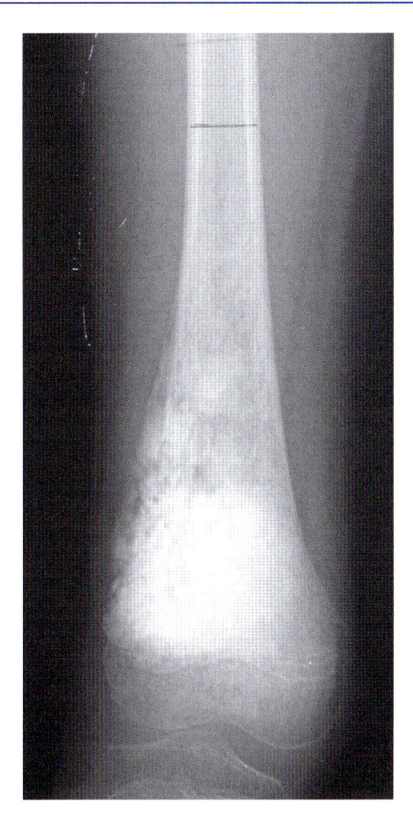

FIGURE 1-3
Anteroposterior radiograph of the distal femur reveals a destructive, bone-forming tumor of the metaphysis diagnostic of osteosarcoma.

TABLE 1-2
Radiographic Features Associated with Benign and Malignant Tumors of Bone

Benign

Well circumscribed
Geographic
Sclerosis

Malignant

Ill-defined
Loss of cortical integrity
"Moth-eaten"
Periostitis
Soft tissue mass

imaging (MRI) is preferable for soft tissue masses, and computerized tomography (CT) and/or MRI for bone lesions.

ISOTOPE SCANNING

Technetium, thallium, gallium, and fluorodeoxyglucose positron emission tomography (FDG-PET) are the four major radioisotope scans that may be utilized in the workup of a bone or soft tissue mass. Although thallium and gallium have limited roles, technetium (Tc)-99 radioisotope scans are utilized to assess the degree of osteoblastic activity of a given lesion of bone. In general, Tc-99 scans are quite sensitive, with a few exceptions, for active lesions of bone. Accordingly, Tc-99 scans are excellent screening tools for remote lesions (Figure 1-6). The best indication for a bone scan is suspected multiple bony lesions such as those commonly seen in metastatic carcinomas and lymphomas of bone. Isotope bone scanning is far simpler to perform, is less expensive, and requires less total body irradiation than skeletal surveys. It is common

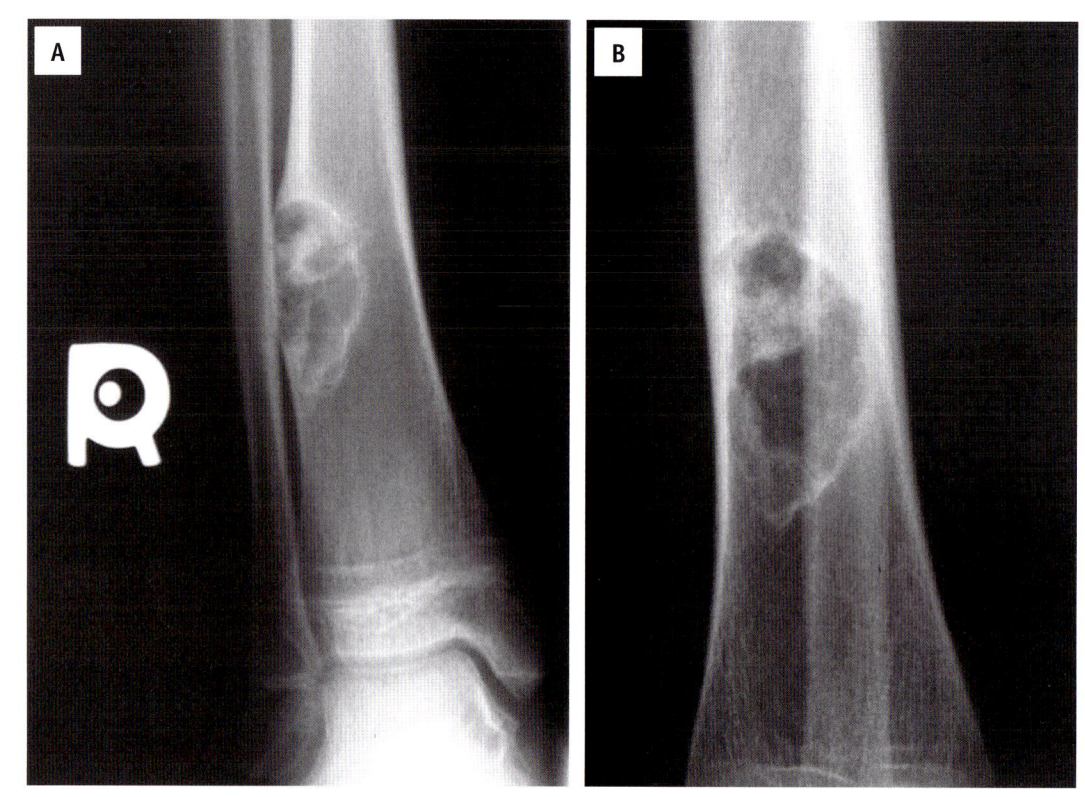

FIGURE 1-4

A, Anteroposterior and **(B)** lateral radiograph of the distal tibia and fibula reveals a well-circumscribed, metaphyseal, eccentric, cortically based, radiolucent lesion that is diagnostic of a nonossifying fibroma of bone.

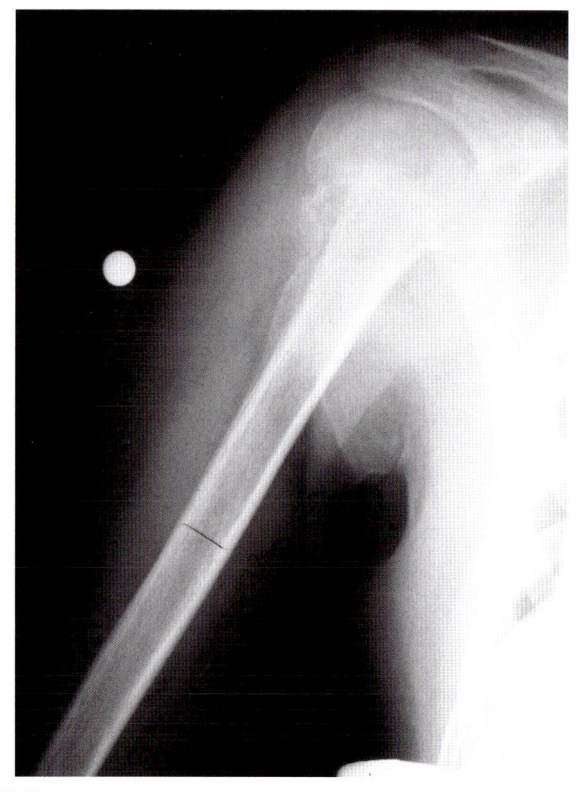

FIGURE 1-5

Anteroposterior radiograph of the proximal humerus demonstrates an infiltrative or permeative process with significant periosteal reaction. On biopsy, this tumor was an osteosarcoma.

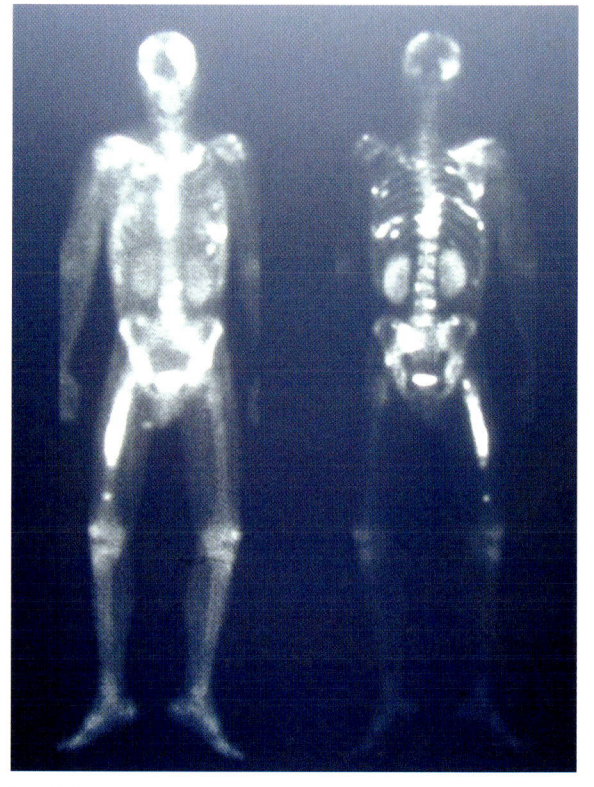

FIGURE 1-6

Technetium bone scan demonstrating widespread metastatic carcinoma to bone.

CHAPTER 1 Approach to the Diagnosis of Bone and Soft Tissue Tumors

practice to use serial isotope scans to manage patients with suspected metastatic disease and at the same time evaluate the effectiveness of their systemic therapy programs.

Isotope scanning is also used in the staging process of a primary sarcoma such as an osteosarcoma to make sure that the patient does not have an asymptomatic remote skeletal lesion. Tc-99 scans are also useful in distinguishing blastic lesions of bone. Given that the study reflects metabolic activity, an enostosis (bone island) would not demonstrate significant increased activity as compared with a blastic prostate metastasis. Inflammatory disease and trauma will also show increased activity. It is important to note, however, that multiple myelomas and metastatic squamous cell carcinoma may not demonstrate technetium uptake (i.e., false-negative results). Skeletal surveys are preferable to screen for additional sites of involvement in such cases.

FDG-PET has proved to be an effective modality in diagnosing and staging many types of cancers, yet its use in soft tissue and bone tumors is less well established. FDG-PET may aid in determining benignity from malignancy, facilitate biopsies to determine the most representative tissue within heterogenous masses, and detect local and distant recurrences in sarcomas. Response to therapy, prognostication, or both are also potential applications for FDG-PET imaging.

COMPUTED TOMOGRAPHY

CT remains a standard imaging procedure for use in well-selected clinical situations. Perhaps the best indication for CT is for smaller lesions that involve cortical structures of bone or spine (Figure 1-7). In such cases, CT is superior to MRI, because the resolution of cortical bone using MRI is inferior. CT scan of the lung is the modality of choice for evaluating the patient with a sarcoma for possible lung metastases. Abdominal CT scan is invaluable in surveying for a primary tumor in patients who have bone metastases. For tumors involving the pelvis and sacrum, CT can help to elucidate the extent of bone involvement, although MRI is helpful in this area as well (Figure 1-8).

MAGNETIC RESONANCE IMAGING

MRI has its greatest application in the evaluation of noncalcific soft tissue lesions. The two most commonly used MRI variations are the T1- and T2-weighted spin-echo imaging techniques (Figure 1-9). Unlike CT scanning, MRI allows for excellent imaging in the longitudinal planes, as well as the axial plane. MRI can also demonstrate the normal anatomy of soft structures, including nerves and vessels, and this nearly eliminates the need for arteriography and myelograms. The use of

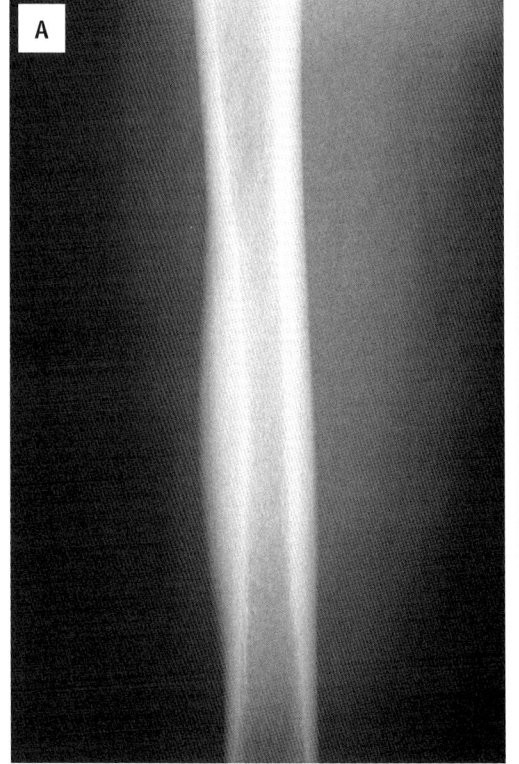

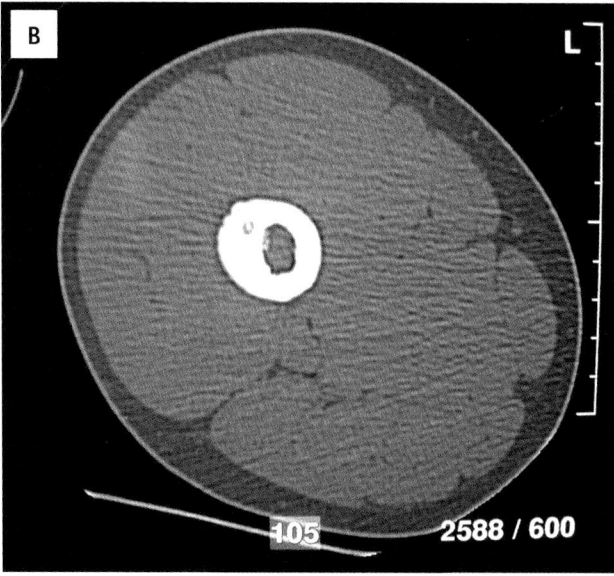

FIGURE 1-7

A, Anteroposterior radiograph of the femoral diaphysis demonstrates nonspecific cortical thinning. **B,** Computed tomographic scan through the area reveals a nidus establishing the diagnosis of osteoid osteoma.

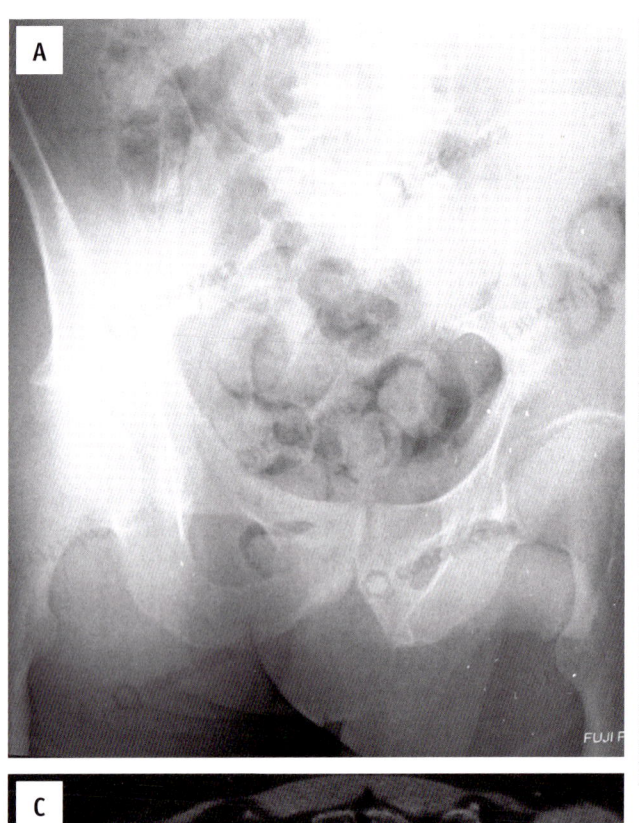

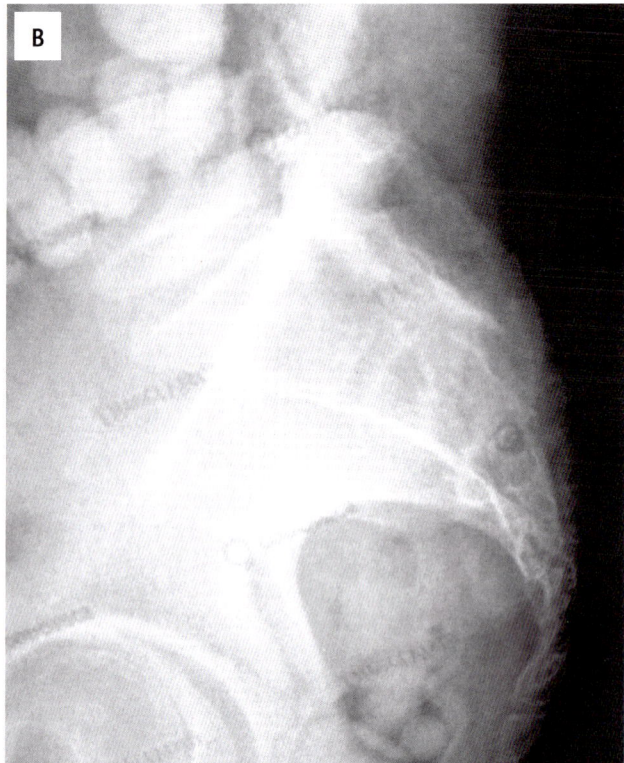

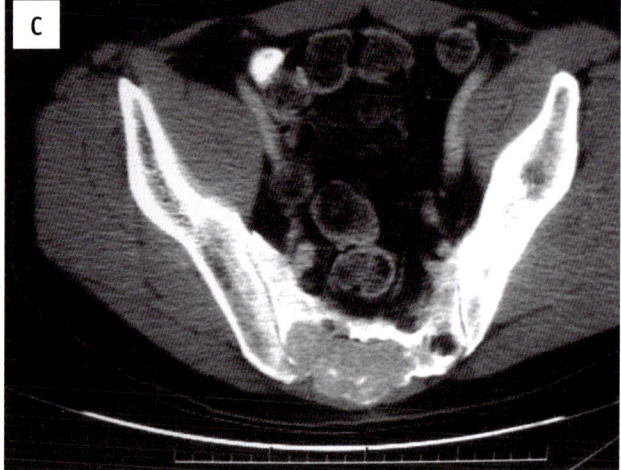

FIGURE 1-8

A, Anteroposterior and **(B)** lateral radiographs of the sacrum show an ill-defined lesion. **C**, Computed tomographic scan demonstrates the extent of the lesion.

the contrast agent gadolinium enables assessment of the vascularity of the neoplasm and aids in the determining of necrosis. MRI has helped to advance extremity-sparing surgery by allowing the surgeon to better anticipate his or her intraoperative surgical findings, thereby facilitating surgical resection.

LABORATORY STUDIES

BIOPSY

The biopsy should usually be the final staging procedure. Although the biopsy can distort the imaging studies, such as MRI, pathologic evaluation and interpretation may require information provided by the prior workup. Complications relating to the biopsy are not infrequent. Accordingly, careful preoperative planning is imperative. The imaging studies will aid the surgeon in selecting the best site for a tissue diagnosis. In most cases, the best diagnostic tissue will be found at the periphery of the tumor, where it interfaces with normal tissue. For example, in the case of a malignant bone tumor, soft tissue invasion usually exists outside the bone, and this area can be sampled without violating cortical bone, and thus without causing a fracture at the biopsy site. If a medullary specimen is needed, a small round or oval hole should be cut to decrease the

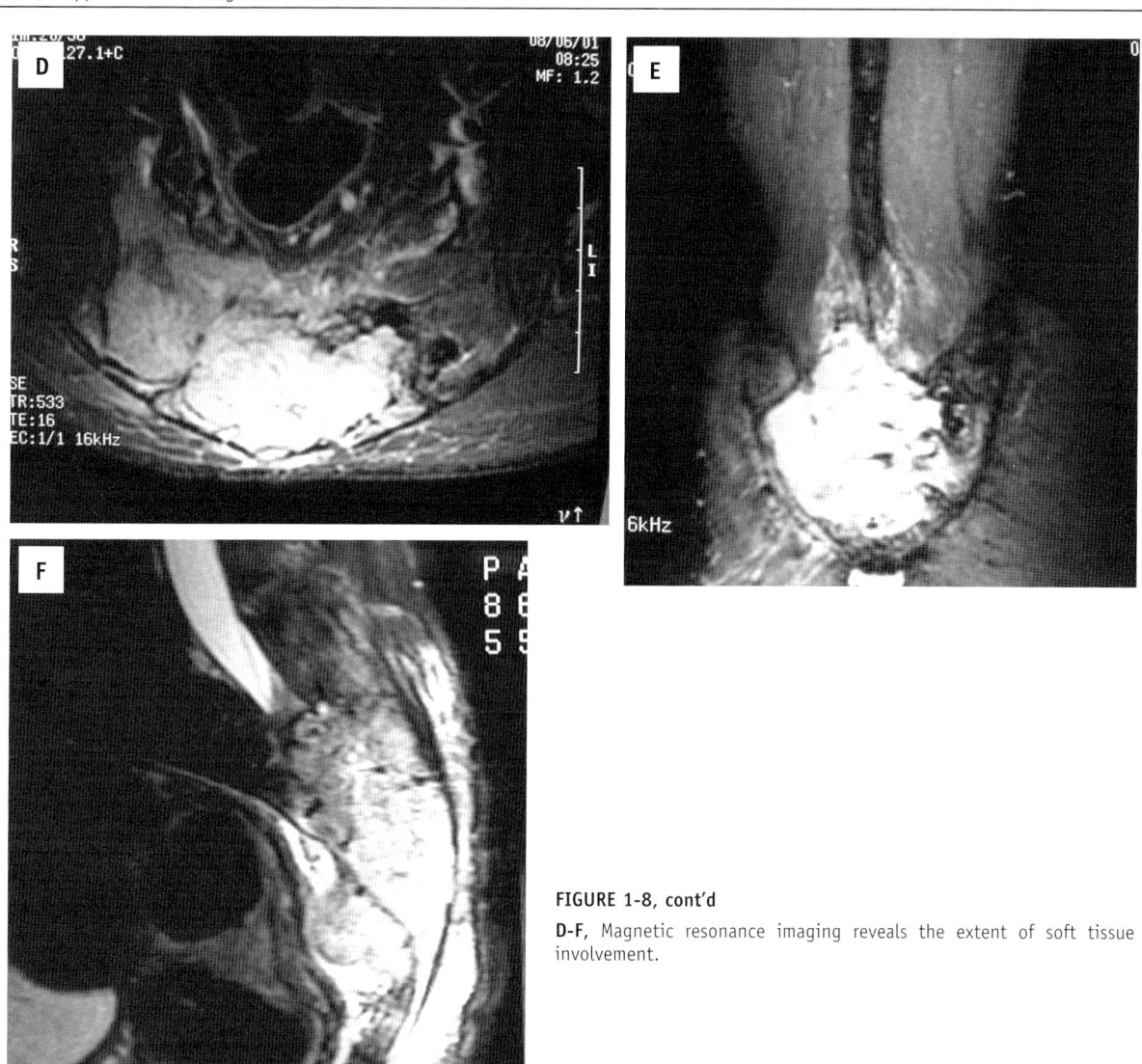

CHAPTER 1   Approach to the Diagnosis of Bone and Soft Tissue Tumors   11

FIGURE 1-8, cont'd
D-F, Magnetic resonance imaging reveals the extent of soft tissue involvement.

chance of fracture. If the medullary specimen is malignant, the cortical hole should be plugged with bone wax or bone cement to reduce soft tissue contamination after the procedure.

Obtaining adequate specimen is critical. Frozen section allows determination of whether appropriate tissue has been obtained. A few experienced tumor centers may make a definitive diagnosis based on a frozen section, allowing the surgeon to proceed with definitive operative treatment of the tumor. However, freezing artifact can cause overinterpretation of the material; therefore, an aggressive resection should always be deferred until the permanent analysis is complete. Additional studies beyond conventional light microscopy, such as immunocytochemistries and cytogenetics, may also be necessary to establish the diagnosis. Furthermore, experimental protocols are in place at some institutions using complementary DNA microarrays, comparative genomic hybridization, fluorescent in situ hybridization, and proteomics necessitating supplemental tissue. Vigilant communication among pathologists, surgeons, and research investigators is critical.

The placement of the biopsy site is a major consideration whether the chosen technique is percutaneous or open. If the surgeon or other interventionalist is inexperienced and not familiar with surgical oncologic

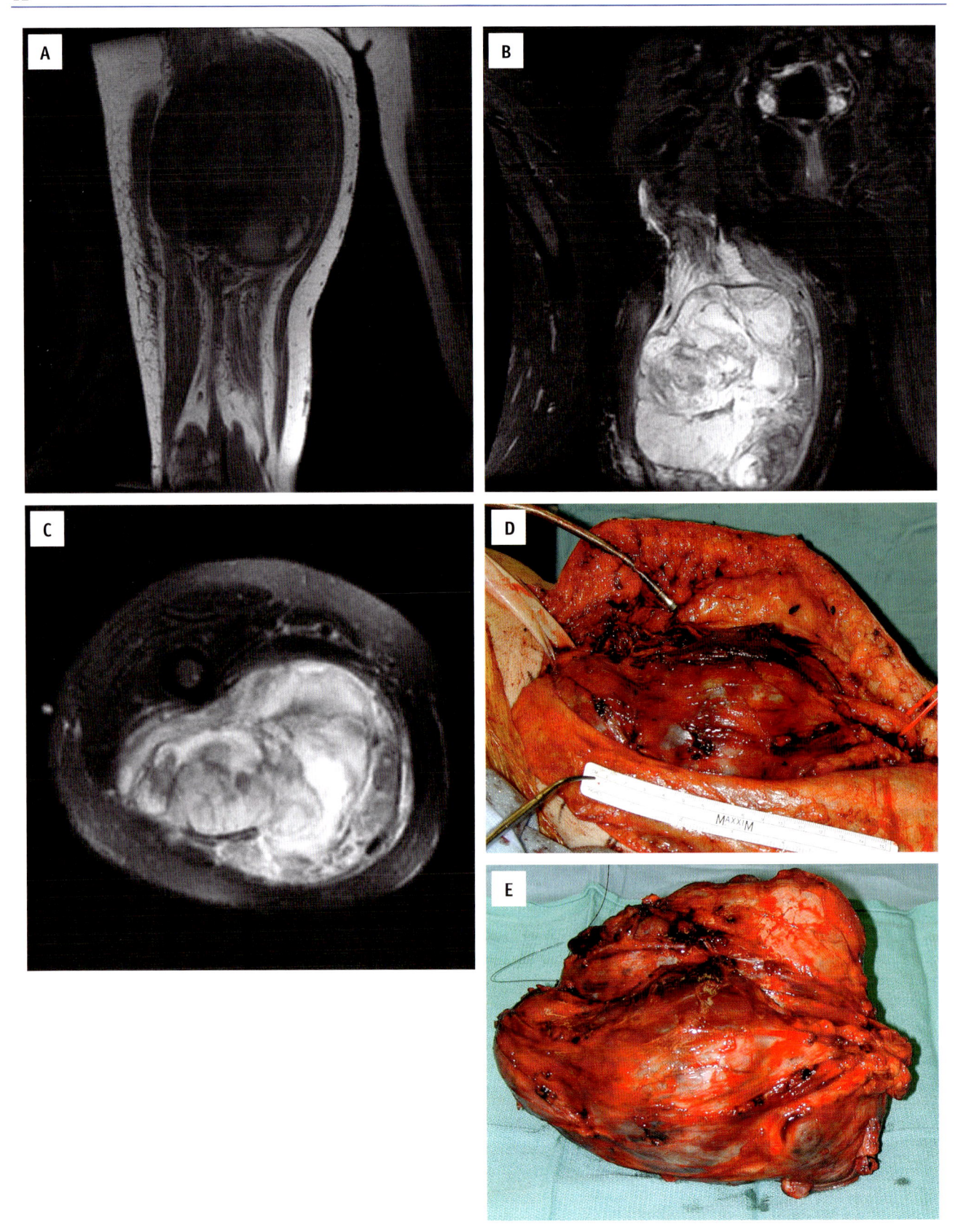

FIGURE 1-9
A, T1-weighted coronal, **(B)** T2-weighted coronal, and **(C)** T2-weighted transverse magnetic resonance images of a malignant peripheral nerve sheath tumor. **D**, Intraoperative photograph. **E**, Resected specimen.

principles, a serious contamination of a vital structure such as the popliteal artery or sciatic nerve may occur. Such an error may necessitate an amputation instead of a limb-sparing procedure. To avoid this problem in the case of a suspected malignant condition, the surgeon who performs the biopsy should be the same surgeon who will perform the definitive operative procedure.

Transverse incisions should be avoided, because removing the entire biopsy site with the widely resected subadjacent tumor mass is difficult. Adequate hemostasis is mandatory to avoid formation of a contaminating hematoma. A drain may be helpful but frequently unnecessary. If a drain is used, it must be placed in line with the incision.

Needle biopsies, either core or fine needle, can be used by experienced tumor centers, especially for lesions that are easily diagnosed, such as metastatic carcinomas or round cell tumors. Because the subtype of sarcoma is proving to be important, architecture of the tumor is generally needed. This requires a core biopsy rather than a fine needle aspirate. Core biopsies also allow the surgeon or interventionalist to sample various areas of the tumor to avoid sampling error in a heterogeneous tumor. In the case of a deep pelvic lesion or a spinal lesion, a CT-guided needle biopsy is ideal because it avoids excessive multicompartmental contamination.

In general, excisional biopsies are discouraged unless the lesion is particularly small (< 2-3 cm) or in an area where a cuff of healthy, uninvolved tissue of at least 1 cm can be removed as well. This would hopefully avoid a second procedure to remove the entire biopsy site if the lesion is found to be malignant.

CULTURES

Infections can mimic neoplasms and visa versa. Ewing sarcoma is all too frequently misdiagnosed as osteomyelitis. It is always a good habit to obtain adequate specimen for bacterial culture (anaerobic and aerobic), as well as fungal and acid-fast bacillus cultures, if clinical suspicion warrants. Different laboratories process these cultures in various ways; therefore, the surgeon or person obtaining the biopsy must check with the microbiology laboratory, before biopsy, to assure adequate handling.

GRADING OF SOFT TISSUE AND BONE SARCOMAS

A number of different grading systems have been proposed over the years for soft tissue and bone sarcomas, utilizing 2 tiered, 3 tiered, and 4 tiered stratification schemes. For soft tissue sarcomas, the most widely used and clinically validated grading systems are those of the National Cancer Institute (NCI system) and French Federation of Cancer Centers (FNCLCC system), both of which are 3 tiered systems (Grade 1, Grade 2, Grade 3). At the present time, the FNCLCC grading system is considered by most soft tissue pathologists to offer the best combination of ease of use, interobserver agreement, and predictive power, and is thus the recommended grading system of the World Health Organization and the College of American Pathologists. For these reasons, we too recommend use of the FNCLCC grading system for soft tissue sarcomas. There is no universally accepted grading system for bone tumors. We have therefore chosen to use the consensus system detailed in the 2009 College of American Pathologists Protocol for the Examination of Specimens from Patients with Tumors of Bone.

GRADING OF SOFT TISSUE TUMORS

The FNCLCC grade is based on 3 parameters: differentiation, mitotic activity, and necrosis. Each of these parameters receives a score: differentiation (1 to 3), mitotic activity (1 to 3), and necrosis (0 to 2). The scores are summed to produce a grade.

Grade 1: 2 or 3
Grade 2: 4 or 5
Grade 3: 6 to 8

DIFFERENTIATION

Tumor differentiation is scored as follows (see Table 1-3).

Score 1: Sarcomas closely resembling normal, adult mesenchymal tissue
Score 2: Sarcomas of certain histologic type
Score 3: Synovial sarcomas, embryonal sarcomas, undifferentiated sarcomas, and sarcomas of doubtful tumor type

Tumor differentiation is the most problematic aspect of the FNCLCC system. Its use is subjective and does not include every subtype of sarcoma. Nevertheless, it is an integral part of the system, and an attempt should be made to assign a differentiation score (Table 1-3).

MITOSIS COUNT

The count is made in the most mitotically active area in 10 successive high-power fields (HPFs) (use the X40 objective).

Score 1: 0 to 9 mitoses per 10 HPFs
Score 2: 10 to 19 mitoses per 10 HPFs
Score 3: 20 or more mitoses per 10 HPFs.

TABLE 1-3
Tumor Differentiation Score According to Histologic Type in the Updated Version of the French Federation of Cancer Centers Sarcoma Group System

Tumor Differentiation

Histologic Type	Score
Well differentiated liposarcoma	1
Myxoid liposarcoma	2
Round cell liposarcoma	3
Pleomorphic liposarcoma	3
Dedifferentiated liposarcoma	3
Fibrosarcoma	2
Myxofibrosarcoma (myxoid malignant fibrous histiocytoma [MFH])	2
Typical storiform MFH (sarcoma, NOS)	3
MFH, pleomorphic type (patternless pleomorphic sarcoma)	3
Giant cell and inflammatory MFH (pleomorphic sarcoma, NOS with giant cells or inflammatory cells)	3
Well differentiated leiomyosarcoma	1
Conventional leiomyosarcoma	2
Poorly differentiated / pleomorphic / epithelioid leiomyosarcoma	3
Biphasic / monophasic synovial sarcoma	3
Poorly differentiated synovial sarcoma	3
Pleomorphic rhabdomyosarcoma	3
Mesenchymal chondrosarcoma	3
Extraskeletal osteosarcoma	3
Ewing sarcoma / PNET	3
Malignant rhabdoid tumor	3
Undifferentiated sarcoma	3

From the CAP Soft Tissue Tumor Protocol with permission (in press).

Tumor Necrosis

Determined on histologic sections.

Score 0: No tumor necrosis
Score 1: Less than or equal to 50% tumor necrosis
Score 2: More than 50% tumor necrosis

Modification of the FNCLCC System for Staging

The proposed 7th Edition of American Joint Committee on Cancer (AJCC) staging system for soft tissue tumors recommends the FNCLCC 3-grade system but effectively collapses into high grade and low grade. This means that FNCLCC grade 2 tumors are considered "high grade" for the purposes of stage grouping.

Grading of Bone Tumors

Bone tumor grading has traditionally been based on a combination of histologic diagnosis and the Broders grading system, which assesses cellularity and degree of anaplasia. The 7th edition of the AJCC Cancer Staging Manual recommends a 4 grade system, with grades 1 and 2 considered "low-grade" and grade 3 and 4 "high-grade". The 2009 CAP Bone Tumor Protocol recommends a pragmatic approach, based principally on histologic classification. Under this system, central low-grade osteosarcoma and parosteal osteosarcoma are considered Grade 1 sarcomas, with periosteal osteosarcoma considered Grade 2, and all other osteosarcomas considered Grade 3. Other Grade 3 bone sarcomas include malignant giant cell tumor, Ewing sarcoma/PNET, angiosarcoma, and dedifferentiated chondrosarcoma.

Chondrosarcomas are graded based on cellularity, cytologic atypia, and mitotic activity. Grade 1 chondrosarcoma is similar histologically to enchondroma, but shows radiographic or histologic evidence of aggressive growth (i.e., permeation). Grade 2 chondrosarcomas show greater cellularity, cytologic atypia, hyperchromasia and nuclear enlargement; or display prominent myxoid change. Grade 3 chondrosarcomas display notable hypercellularity and nuclear pleomorphism and have easily identifiable mitotic figures.

Chordomas are not graded, but are considered low-grade sarcomas. Dedifferentiated chordomas are categorically high-grade sarcomas. Adamantinomas are considered low-grade sarcomas. Sarcomas of types that occur in both bone and soft tissue (e.g., mesenchymal chondrosarcoma, leiomyosarcoma, undifferentiated pleomorphic sarcoma (so-called "malignant fibrous histiocytoma")) are graded according to the FNCLCC system, as described above.

Bone Tumor Grades (Summary)

Grade 1 (Low Grade)
   Low-grade central osteosarcoma
   Parosteal osteosarcoma
   Adamantinoma
Grade 2
   Periosteal osteosarcoma
Grade 3 (High Grade)
   Malignant giant cell tumor
   Ewing sarcoma / PNET
   Dedifferentiated chondrosarcoma

Conventional osteosarcoma
Telangiectactic osteosarcoma
Small cell osteosarcoma
Secondary osteosarcoma
High-grade surface osteosarcoma
Variable Grade
Conventional chondrosarcoma of bone (grades 1 to 3)
Soft-tissue type sarcomas (e.g., leiomyosarcoma)
Ungraded
Chordoma, conventional
Chordoma, dedifferentiated (high grade)

STAGING SYSTEMS

Staging refers to an assessment of the grade of the tumor and the extent to which the disease has spread. Several staging systems are used, but all have the purpose of helping the physician plan a logical treatment program and establish a prognosis for the patient. The two major systems are discussed here.

AMERICAN JOINT COMMITTEE OF CANCER

The American Joint Committee of Cancer (AJCC) system of staging is used by most surgical oncologists when dealing with soft tissue and bone sarcomas (Table 1-4). It has a four-point scale for classifying tumors as grade 1, 2, 3, or 4 on the basis of their histologic appearance. A grade 1 or 2 tumor in the AJCC system is equivalent to a stage I tumor in the Enneking system; grade 3 or 4 is equivalent to Enneking stage II.

SYSTEM OF THE AMERICAN MUSCULOSKELETAL TUMOR SOCIETY (ENNEKING SYSTEM)

The Enneking system addresses the unique problems related to sarcomas of the extremities and applies to tumors of the bone, as well as those of soft tissue. Although utilized by orthopedic oncologists, this system is slowly giving way to the uniformity of the AJCC system. The Enneking system has a three-point scale for classifying tumors as stage I, II, or III on the basis of their histologic and biologic appearance and their likelihood of metastasizing to regional lymph nodes or distant sites such as the lung. Stage I refers to low-grade sarcomas with less than 25% chance of metastasis. Stage II refers to high-grade sarcomas with more than 25% chance of metastasis. Stage III is for either low- or high-grade tumors that have metastasized to a distant site such as a lymph node, lung, or other distant organ system.

The Enneking system further classifies tumors on the basis of whether they are intracompartmental (type A) or extracompartmental (type B) in nature. Type A tumors are constrained by anatomic boundaries such as muscle fascial planes and stand a better chance for local control of tumor growth with surgical removal than do type B tumors. A lesion contained in a single muscle belly or a bone lesion that has not broken out into the surrounding soft tissue would be classified as a type A tumor. A lesion in the popliteal space, axilla, pelvis, or midportion of the hand or foot would be classified as a type B tumor. Although compartmentalization of a tumor is an important concept, studies have shown that the size of the tumor rather than whether it is contained within a compartment is more prognostic. Larger tumors, greater than 5 cm, have a worse prognosis.

TABLE 1-4

American Joint Committee on Cancer Staging System for Soft Tissue and Bone Sarcomas

Soft Tissue Sarcoma Staging

I: T1a,1b,2a,2b N0 M0 G1-2/4 G1/3
II: T1a,1b,2a,2b N0 M0 G3-4/4 G2-3/3
III: T2b N0 M0 G3-4/4 G2-3/3
IV: Any T N1 M0, any G
Any T N0 M1, any G
T $\leq$ 5 cm: T1a = superficial; T1b = deep
T > 5 cm: T2a = superficial; T2b = deep

Bone Sarcoma Staging

IA: G1-2 T1 N0 M0
IB: G1-2 T2 N0 M0
IIA: G3-4 T1 N0 M0
IIB: G3-4 T2 N0 M0
III: any G T3 N0 M0
IVA: any G, T N0 M1a
IVB: any G, T N1 any M
Any G, T, N M1b
T1: $\leq$8 cm
T2: >8 cm
T3: discontiguous (skip)
M1: distant metastases
M1a: lung
M1b: other

A low-grade fibrosarcoma located inside the fascial plane of the biceps muscle and having no evidence of metastasis would be classified as a stage IA tumor. A typical malignant osteosarcoma of the distal femur with breakthrough into the surrounding muscle as determined by MRI would be classified as a stage IIB lesion. If CT scanning showed metastatic involvement of the lung, the osteosarcoma would then be classified as a stage IIIB lesion.

SUGGESTED READINGS

Overview

1. Moley JF, Eberlein TJ: Soft-tissue sarcomas. Surg Clin North Am 2000;80(2):687-708.
2. Zahm SH, Fraumeni JF Jr: The epidemiology of soft tissue sarcoma. Semin Oncol 1997;24:504-514.

Evaluation of Tumors

1. Anderson GS, Brinkmann F, Soulen MC, et al: FDG positron emission tomography in the surveillance of hepatic tumors treated with radiofrequency ablation. Clin Nucl Med 2003;28:192-197.
2. Anderson J, Gordon T, McManus A, et al: Detection of the PAX3-FKHR fusion gene in paediatric rhabdomyosarcoma: A reproducible predictor of outcome? Br J Cancer 2001;85:831-835.
3. Antonescu CR, Elahi A, Healey JH, et al: Monoclonality of multifocal myxoid liposarcoma: Confirmation by analysis of TLS-CHOP or EWS-CHOP rearrangements. Clin Cancer Res 2000;6:2788-2793.
4. Bredella MA, Caputo GR, Steinbach LS: Value of FDG positron emission tomography in conjunction with MR imaging for evaluating therapy response in patients with musculoskeletal sarcomas. AJR Am J Roentgenol 2002;179:1145-1150.
5. Brenner W, Bohuslavizki KH, Eary JF: PET imaging of osteosarcoma. J Nucl Med 2003;44:930-942.
6. Durbin M, Randall RL, James M, et al: Ewing's sarcoma masquerading as osteomyelitis. Clin Orthop 1998;357:176-185.
7. Eary JF, O'Sullivan F, Powitan Y, et al: Sarcoma tumor FDG uptake measured by PET and patient outcome: A retrospective analysis. Eur J Nucl Med Mol Imaging 2002;29:1149-1154.
8. Franzius C, Schober O: Assessment of therapy response by FDG PET in pediatric patients. Q J Nucl Med 2003;47:41-45.
9. Hain SF, O'Doherty MJ, Bingham J, et al: Can FDG PET be used to successfully direct preoperative biopsy of soft tissue tumours? Nucl Med Commun 2003;24:1139-1143.
10. Johnson GR, Zhuang H, Khan J, et al: Roles of positron emission tomography with fluorine-18-deoxyglucose in the detection of local recurrent and distant metastatic sarcoma. Clin Nucl Med 2003;28:815-820.
11. Mankin HJ, Mankin CJ, Simon MA: The hazards of the biopsy, revisited. J Bone Joint Surg Am 1996;78:656-663.
12. Miettinen M, Lasota J: Gastrointestinal stromal tumors—definition, clinical, histological, immunohistochemical, and molecular genetic features and differential diagnosis. Virchows Arch 2001;438:1-12.
13. Randall RL, Mann JA, Johnston JO: Orthopedic soft-tissue tumors. Prim Care 1996;23:241-261.
14. Randall RL, Wade M, Albritton K, et al: Retrieval yield of total and messenger RNA. in mesenchymal tissue ex vivo. Clin Orthop 2003;415:59-63.
15. Skrzynski MC, Biermann JS, Montag A, et al: Diagnostic accuracy and charge savings of outpatient care needle biopsy compared with open biopsy of musculoskeletal tumors. J Bone Joint Surg Am 1996;78:644-649.

Grading of Soft Tissue and Bone Sarcomas

1. Fletcher CDM, Unni KK, Mertens F, et al: Pathology and genetics of tumours of soft tissue and bone. Lyon: IARC Press, 2000.

Staging Systems

1. Bertario L, Russo A, Sala P: Genotype and phenotype factors as determinants of desmoid tumors in patients with familial adenomatous polyposis. Int J Cancer 2001;95:102-107.
2. Cormier JN, Patel SR, Herzog CE, et al: Concurrent ifosfamide-based chemotherapy and irradiation. Analysis of treatment-related toxicity in 43 patients with sarcoma. Cancer 2001;92:1550-1555.
3. dos Santos NR, de Bruijn DR, van Kessel AG: Molecular mechanisms underlying human synovial sarcoma development. Genes Chromosomes Cancer 2001;30:1-14.
4. Enneking WF: A system of staging musculoskeletal neoplasms. Clin Orthop 1985;204:9-24.
5. Flemming DJ, Murphey MD, Carmichael BB, Bernard SA: Primary tumors of the spine. Semin Musculoskelet Radiol 2000;4:299-320.
6. Gallazzi MB, Arborio G, Garbagna PG, et al: Percutaneous radio-frequency ablation of osteoid osteoma: Technique and preliminary results. Radiol Med 2001;102:329-334.
7. Gibbs J, Huang PP, Lee RJ, et al: Malignant fibrous histiocytoma: An institutional review. Cancer Invest 2001;19:23-27.
8. Greene FL, Page DL, Fleming ID, et al: AJCC Cancer Staging Manual, 6th ed. New York, Springer, 2002.
9. Hayes-Jordan AA, Spunt SL, Poquette CA, et al: Nonrhabdomyosarcoma soft tissue sarcomas in children: Is age at diagnosis an important variable? J Pediatr Surg 2000;35:948-953.
10. Kilpatrick SE, Geisinger KR, King TS, et al: Clinicopathologic analysis of HER-2/neu immunoexpression among various histologic subtypes and grades of osteosarcoma. Mod Pathol 2001;14:1277-1283.
11. Ladanyi M: Fusions of the SYT and SSX genes in synovial sarcoma. Oncogene 2001;20:5755-5762.
12. Maitra A, Roberts H, Weinberg AG, Geradts J: Aberrant expression of tumor suppressor proteins in the Ewing family of tumors. Arch Pathol Lab Med 2001;125:1207-1212.
13. Mandahl N: etal: Cytogenetic aberrations and their prognostic impact in chondrosarcoma. Genes Chromosomes Cancer 2002;33:188-200.
14. Meis-Kindblom JM, Sjögren H, Kindblom LG, et al: Cytogenetic and molecular genetic analyses of liposarcoma and its soft tissue simulators: Recognition of new variants and differential diagnosis. Virchows Arch 2001;439:141-151.
15. Nishio J, Iwasaki H, Ohjimi Y, et al: Supernumerary ring chromosomes in dermatofibrosarcoma protuberans may contain sequences from 8q11.2-qter and 17q21-qter: A combined cytogenetic and comparative genomic hybridization study. Cancer Genet Cytogenet 2001;129:102-106.
16. Oberlin O, Deley MC, Bui BN, et al: Study of the French Society of Paediatric Oncology (EW88 study). Br J Cancer 2001;85:1646-1654.
17. Ogose A, Hotta T, Kawashima H, et al: Elevation of serum alkaline phosphatase in clear cell chondrosarcoma of bone. Anticancer Res 2001;21:649-655.
18. Oliveira AM, Nascimento AG: Grading in soft tissue tumors: Principles and problems. Skeletal Radiol 2001;30:543-559.
19. Orvieto E, Furlanetto A, Laurino L, Del Tos AP: Myxoid and round cell liposarcoma: A spectrum of myxoid adipocytic neoplasia. Semin Diagn Pathol 2001;18:267-273.
20. Park YK, Park HR, Chi SG, et al: Overexpression of p53 and absent genetic mutation in clear cell chondrosarcoma. Int J Oncol 2001;19:353-357.
21. Scully SP, Ghert MA, Zurakowski D, et al: Pathologic fracture in osteosarcoma: Prognostic importance and treatment implications. J Bone Joint Surg Am 2002;84-A:49-57.
22. Shields CJ, Winter DC, Kirwan WO, Redmond HP: Desmoid tumours. Eur J Surg Oncol 2001;27:701-706.
23. Simon MA, Finn HA: Diagnostic strategy for bone & soft tissue tumors. J Bone Joint Surg Am 1993;75:622-631.
24. Sluga M, Windhager R, Lang S, et al: The role of surgery and resection margins in the treatment of Ewing's sarcoma. Clin Orthop 2001;(392):394-399.
25. Smith SE, Kransdorf MJ: Primary musculoskeletal tumors of fibrous origin. Semin Musculoskelet Radiol 2000;4:73-88.
26. Sørensen SA, Mulvihill JJ, Nielsen A: Long-term follow-up of von Recklinghausen neurofibromatosis: Survival and malignant neoplasms. N Engl J Med 1986;314:1010-1015.
27. Spillane AJ: A'Hern R, Judson IR: Synovial sarcoma: A clinicopathologic, staging, and prognostic assessment. J Clin Oncol 2000;18:3794-3803.

28. Tallini G, Dorfman H, Brys P, et al: Correlation between clinicopathological features and karyotype in 100 cartilaginous and chordoid tumours. A report from the Chromosomes and Morphology (CHAMP) Collaborative Study Group. J Pathol 2002;196:194–203.
29. Vikkula M, Boon LM, Mulliken JB: Molecular genetics of vascular malformations. Matrix Biol 2001;20:327–335.
30. Weisstein JS, Majeska RJ, Klein MJ, Einhorn TA: Detection of c-fos expression in benign and malignant musculoskeletal lesions. J Orthop Res 2001;19:339–345.
31. Zhou H, et al: Her-2/neu staining in osteosarcoma: Association with increased risk of metastasis. Sarcoma 2001;5(S1):9.

2

Adjuvant Techniques – Immunohistochemistry, Cytogenetics, and Molecular Genetics

Andrew L. Folpe · Enrique de Alava

IMMUNOHISTOCHEMISTRY
- Overview
- Immunohistochemistry in the Differential Diagnosis of Small, Blue, Round Cell Tumors
- Monomorphic Spindle Cell Neoplasms
- Poorly Differentiated Epithelioid Tumors
- Pleomorphic Spindle Cell Tumors

MOLECULAR PATHOLOGY
- Overview
- Methods of Detection of Specific Genetic Events in Soft Tissue and Bone Tumors

IMMUNOHISTOCHEMISTRY

OVERVIEW

This section covers selected applications of immunohistochemistry (IHC) in the diagnosis of soft tissue and bone neoplasms. This section emphasizes applications of IHC to common differential diagnoses in soft tissue and bone pathology, including: (1) small, blue, round cell tumors; (2) monomorphic spindle cell tumors; (3) epithelioid tumors; and (4) pleomorphic spindle cell tumors. It is not possible in this brief section to provide a detailed discussion of each antigen, and the reader is referred to larger, more comprehensive textbooks of soft tissue and bone pathology. Table 2-1 summarizes the most widely used IHC markers for sarcoma diagnosis. Table 2-2 provides an overview of markers expressed by specific common tumor types.

It cannot be overemphasized that IHC is an *adjunctive* diagnostic technique to traditional morphologic methods in soft tissue and bone pathology, as in any other area of surgical pathology. It is critical to recognize that the diagnosis of many soft tissue tumors does not require IHC (e.g., adipocytic tumors), and that no markers or combinations of markers will distinguish benign from malignant tumors (e.g., the distinction of nodular fasciitis from leiomyosarcoma). Furthermore, specific markers do not exist for certain mesenchymal cell types and their tumors. Lastly, it is important to acknowledge that a subset of soft tissue tumors defy classification, even with exhaustive IHC, electron microscopy (EM), and genetic study.

IMMUNOHISTOCHEMISTRY IN THE DIFFERENTIAL DIAGNOSIS OF SMALL, BLUE, ROUND CELL TUMORS

This differential diagnosis includes both sarcomas and nonsarcomas. Nonsarcomatous neoplasms that might be legitimately included in this differential diagnosis include lymphoma, melanoma, and in an older patient, small cell carcinoma. Sarcomas that should be included in the differential diagnosis include Ewing sarcoma/primitive neuroectodermal tumor (ES/PNET), rhabdomyosarcoma (RMS), poorly differentiated synovial sarcoma (PDSS), and desmoplastic round cell tumor. Table 2-3 presents a screening panel of antibodies and the expected results for these tumors. The results of this panel dictate what additional studies are needed to confirm a specific diagnosis.

Additional IHC Workup Depending on Suspected Diagnosis

1. *Small-cell carcinoma:* Confirm with antibodies to chromogranin A or synaptophysin.
2. *Melanoma:* Confirm with antibodies to melanosome-specific proteins (gp100, Melan-A, tyrosinase, microphthalmia transcription factor). A small number of melanomas may be S-100 protein-negative, and occasional melanomas express cytokeratin or desmin. Small-cell melanomas of the sinonasal tract are frequently S-100 protein–negative/HMB45-positive (Figure 2-1).
3. *Lymphoma:* Lymphoblastic lymphoma may be CD45-negative and CD99/FLI1–positive, which can easily result in a misdiagnosis as ES/PNET. Terminal deoxynucleotide transferase may be critical in arriving

TABLE 2-1
Commonly Used Immunohistochemistry Markers in Sarcoma Diagnosis

Antigen	Diagnoses
Cytokeratins	Carcinomas, epithelioid sarcoma, synovial sarcoma, some angiosarcomas and leiomyosarcomas, mesothelioma, extrarenal rhabdoid tumor, myoepithelial tumors
Vimentin	Sarcomas, melanoma, some carcinomas and lymphomas
Desmin	Benign and malignant smooth and skeletal muscle tumors
Glial fibrillary acidic protein	Gliomas, some schwannomas, myoepithelial tumors
Neurofilaments	Neuroblastic tumors
Pan-muscle actin	Benign and malignant smooth and skeletal muscle tumors, myofibroblastic tumors and pseudotumors
Smooth muscle actin	Benign and malignant smooth muscle tumors, myofibroblastic tumors and pseudotumors, myoepithelial tumors
Caldesmon	Benign and malignant smooth muscle tumors
Myogenic nuclear regulatory proteins (myogenin, MyoD1)	Rhabdomyosarcoma
S-100 protein	Melanoma, benign and malignant peripheral nerve sheath tumors, cartilaginous tumors, normal adipose tissue, Langerhans cells, myoepithelial tumors
Epithelial membrane antigen	Carcinomas, epithelioid sarcoma, synovial sarcoma, perineurioma, meningioma, anaplastic large-cell lymphoma
CD31	Benign and malignant vascular tumors
Von Willebrand factor (factor VIII–related protein)	Benign and malignant vascular tumors
CD34	Benign and malignant vascular tumors, solitary fibrous tumor, hemangiopericytoma, epithelioid sarcoma, dermatofibrosarcoma protuberans
CD99 (MIC2 gene product)	Ewing sarcoma/primitive neuroectodermal tumor, some rhabdomyosarcomas, some synovial sarcomas, lymphoblastic lymphoma
CD45 (leukocyte common antigen)	Non-Hodgkin's lymphoma
Terminal deoxynucleotide transferase (TdT)	Lymphoblastic lymphoma
CD30 (Ki-1)	Anaplastic large-cell lymphoma, embryonal carcinoma
CD68 and CD163	Macrophages, fibrohistiocytic tumors, granular cell tumors, various sarcomas, melanomas, carcinomas
Melanosome-specific antigens (HMB-45, Melan-A, tyrosinase, microphthalmia transcription factor)	Melanoma, PEComa, clear-cell sarcoma, melanotic schwannoma
Claudin-1	Perineurioma
Mdm2 and CDK4	Well-differentiated liposarcoma
Glut-1	Perineurioma, infantile hemangioma
INI1	Expression lost in extrarenal rhabdoid tumor and epithelioid sarcoma
TLE1	Synovial sarcoma
TFE3	Alveolar soft part sarcoma
WT1 (carboxy-terminus)	Desmoplastic small round cell tumor
Protein kinase C-θ	Gastrointestinal stromal tumor
Brachyury	Chordoma
Osteocalcin	Osteogenic sarcoma

TABLE 2-2
Markers Useful in the Diagnosis of Selected Tumor Types

Tumor Type	Useful Marker(s)
Angiosarcoma	CD31, CD34, FLI1, von Willebrand factor
Leiomyosarcoma	Muscle (smooth) actins, desmin, caldesmon
Rhabdomyosarcoma	MyoD1, myogenin; muscle (sarcomeric) actins; desmin
Desmoplastic small round cell tumor	Cytokeratins, vimentin, desmin, carboxyl-terminal WT1
Chordoma	Cytokeratins, S100 protein, brachyury
Ewing sarcoma/Primitive neuroectodermal tumor	CD99 (p30/32-MIC2), FLI-1
Synovial sarcoma	Cytokeratin, EMA, TLE1
Epithelioid sarcoma	Cytokeratin, CD34, INI1 (loss of expression)
Malignant peripheral nerve sheath tumor	S-100, CD57, nerve growth factor receptor, EMA, claudin-1, Glut-1
Liposarcoma	mdm2, CDK4
Chondrosarcoma	S-100 protein
Osteogenic sarcoma	Osteocalcin
Kaposi sarcoma	CD31, CD34, VEGFR3, LANA
Myoepithelial tumors	Cytokeratins, smooth muscle actin, S100 protein, glial fibrillary acidic protein
Myofibroblastic lesions (e.g., nodular fasciitis)	Smooth muscle actins
Gastrointestinal stromal tumor	CD117a (c-kit), CD34, protein kinase θ
Hemangiopericytoma, solitary fibrous tumor	CD34
Glomus tumors	Smooth muscle actins, type IV collagen
Angiomatoid (malignant) fibrous histiocytoma	Desmin, EMA, CD68
Alveolar soft part sarcoma	TFE3
Perivascular epithelioid cell neoplasms	Smooth muscle actins, melanocytic markers

EMA, epithelial membrane antigen; LANA, latency associated nuclear antigen.

TABLE 2-3
Screening Panel for Small, Blue, Round Cell Tumors

Antibody To	SCCA	Melanoma	Lymphoma	PNET	RMS	PDSS	DRCT
Pan-cytokeratin	Positive	Variable	Negative	Variable	Rare	Positive	Positive
S-100 protein	Negative	Positive	Negative	Variable	Rare	Variable	Negative
CD45	Negative	Negative	Positive	Negative	Negative	Negative	Negative
TdT	Negative	Negative	Positive	Negative	Negative	Negative	Negative
Desmin	Negative	Variable	Negative	Rare	Positive	Negative	Positive
CD99	Negative	Negative	Variable	Positive	Variable	Positive	Rare

DRCT, desmoplastic round cell tumor; PDSS, poorly differentiated synovial sarcoma; PNET, primitive neuroectodermal tumor; RMS, rhabdomyosarcoma; SCCA, small cell carcinoma; TdT, terminal deoxynucleotide transferase.

FIGURE 2-1

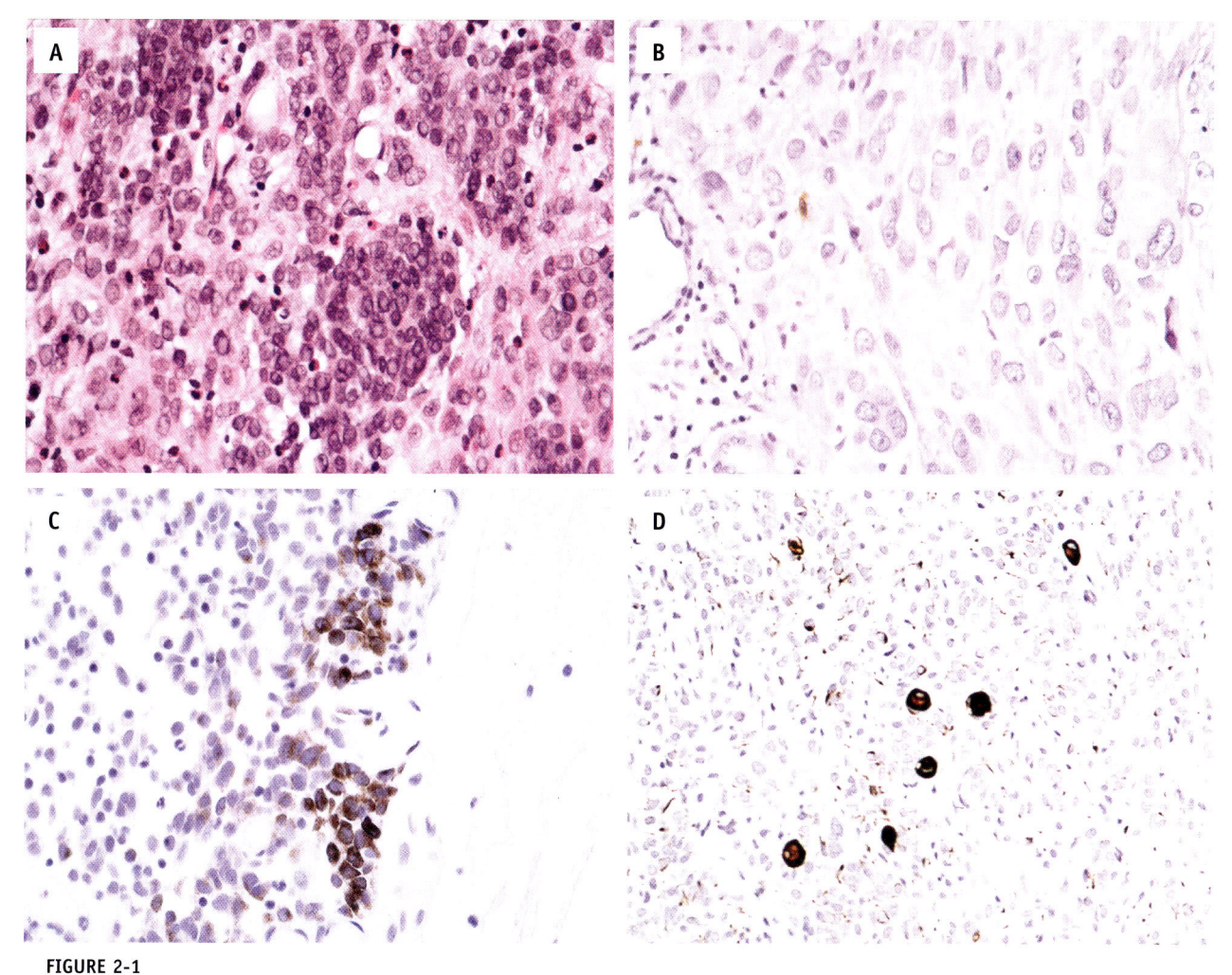

A, Small-cell malignant melanoma illustrating a number of potential pitfalls in the immunodiagnosis of melanoma. This particular case was negative for S-100 protein **(B)** (note positive internal control: Langerhans cell), only focally positive for HMB45 **(C)**, and showed anomalous expression of desmin **(D)**. Anomalous intermediate filament expression is seen in 10% to 15% of melanomas.

at the correct diagnosis. In adults and children, anaplastic large-cell lymphomas, including the small-cell variant, may also be CD45-negative. CD30 is useful here (Figure 2-2).
4. *ES/PNET*: ES/PNETs are unique among small, blue, round cell tumors in that they do not usually express CD56. This finding may be useful in cases with equivocal CD99 expression or anomalous cytokeratin/desmin expression. Demonstration of FLI1 protein expression may also be helpful (Figure 2-3).
5. *RMS*: Confirm with myogenin or MyoD1 (Figure 2-4).
6. *PDSS*: Cytokeratin expression may be patchy or absent in some cases. Epithelial membrane antigen (EMA) and high-molecular-weight cytokeratins may be positive in such cases. Uniform, strong, nuclear expression of TLE1 protein is specific for PDSS.
7. *Desmoplastic small round cell tumor (DSRCT)*: Carboxyl-terminal WT1 antibodies can assist in confirmation (Figure 2-5).

MONOMORPHIC SPINDLE CELL NEOPLASMS

The differential diagnosis of monomorphic spindle cell tumors often includes such entities as fibrosarcoma (usually arising in dermatofibrosarcoma protuberans [DFSP]), monophasic synovial sarcoma, malignant peripheral nerve sheath tumor (MPNST), and solitary fibrous tumor. Particularly in the abdomen, this differential diagnosis may also include a gastrointestinal stromal tumor (GIST), true smooth muscle tumors, and cellular schwannoma. Table 2-4 presents a screening immunohistochemical panel and the expected result for each tumor.

Additional IHC Workup Depending on Suspected Diagnosis
1. *Synovial sarcoma*: Cytokeratin and EMA expression may be focal in synovial sarcomas. Expression

FIGURE 2-2

A, Lymphoblastic lymphoma showing diffuse membranous expression of CD99. **B**, Such cases may easily be confused with Ewing sarcoma, particularly because they are invariably also positive for FLI1 protein. **C**, Demonstration of terminal deoxynucleotide transferase expression is invaluable in this differential diagnosis.

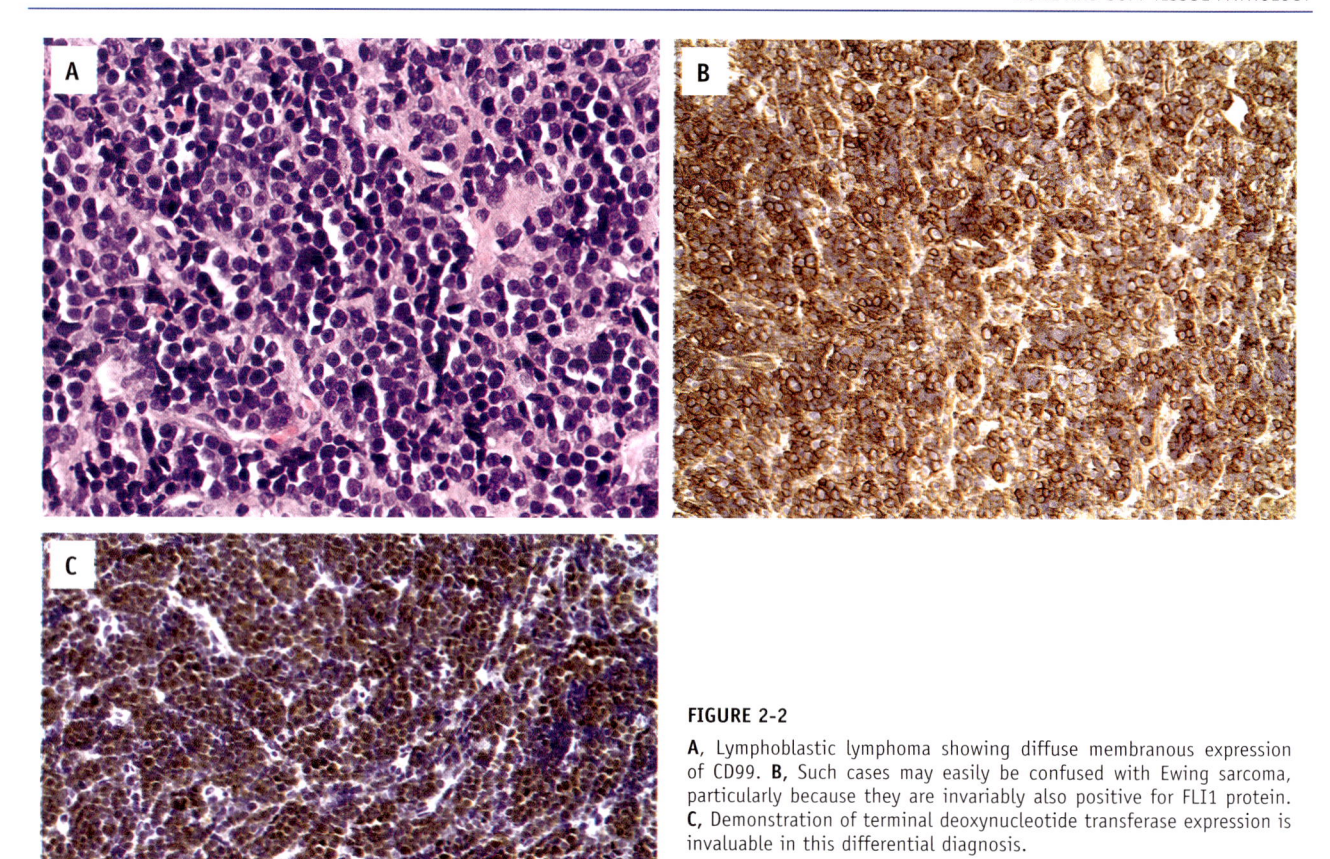

of CD34 is exceptionally rare in synovial sarcoma. TLE1 expression may be helpful (Figure 2-6).
2. *MPNST and cellular schwannoma:* S-100 protein expression is often weak and focal in MPNST but is diffuse and strong in cellular schwannoma. EMA, claudin-1, and Glut-1 expression may be seen in MPNST with perineurial differentiation (Figure 2-7).
3. *Fibrosarcoma* (arising in DFSP): CD34 expression may be seen only in the DFSP component and lost in the fibrosarcoma component. Smooth muscle actin (SMA) expression, indicative of myofibroblastic differentiation, may be present (Figure 2-8).
4. *Solitary fibrous tumor:* Malignant solitary fibrous tumor may show anomalous cytokeratin expression.
5. *GIST:* Expression of protein kinase C-θ may be valuable in cases with weak or absent CD117 expression. GIST may be variably positive for both SMA and S-100 protein but are typically desmin-negative (Figure 2-9).

POORLY DIFFERENTIATED EPITHELIOID TUMORS

The differential diagnosis of poorly differentiated epithelioid tumors includes carcinoma, melanoma, lymphoma (including anaplastic large-cell lymphoma), and epithelioid soft tissue tumors such as epithelioid sarcoma, myoepithelioma, and angiosarcoma. A screening panel for this differential diagnosis is presented in Table 2-5. This initial screening panel can make a specific diagnosis of melanoma, lymphoma, or anaplastic large-cell lymphoma, but generally it is not able to discriminate carcinoma from epithelioid sarcoma or epithelioid angiosarcoma (EAS). In the axial skeleton, this differential diagnosis should also include chordoma. These tumors can be reliably distinguished with the additional panel of antibodies listed in Table 2-5.
Additional IHC Workup Depending on Suspected Diagnosis

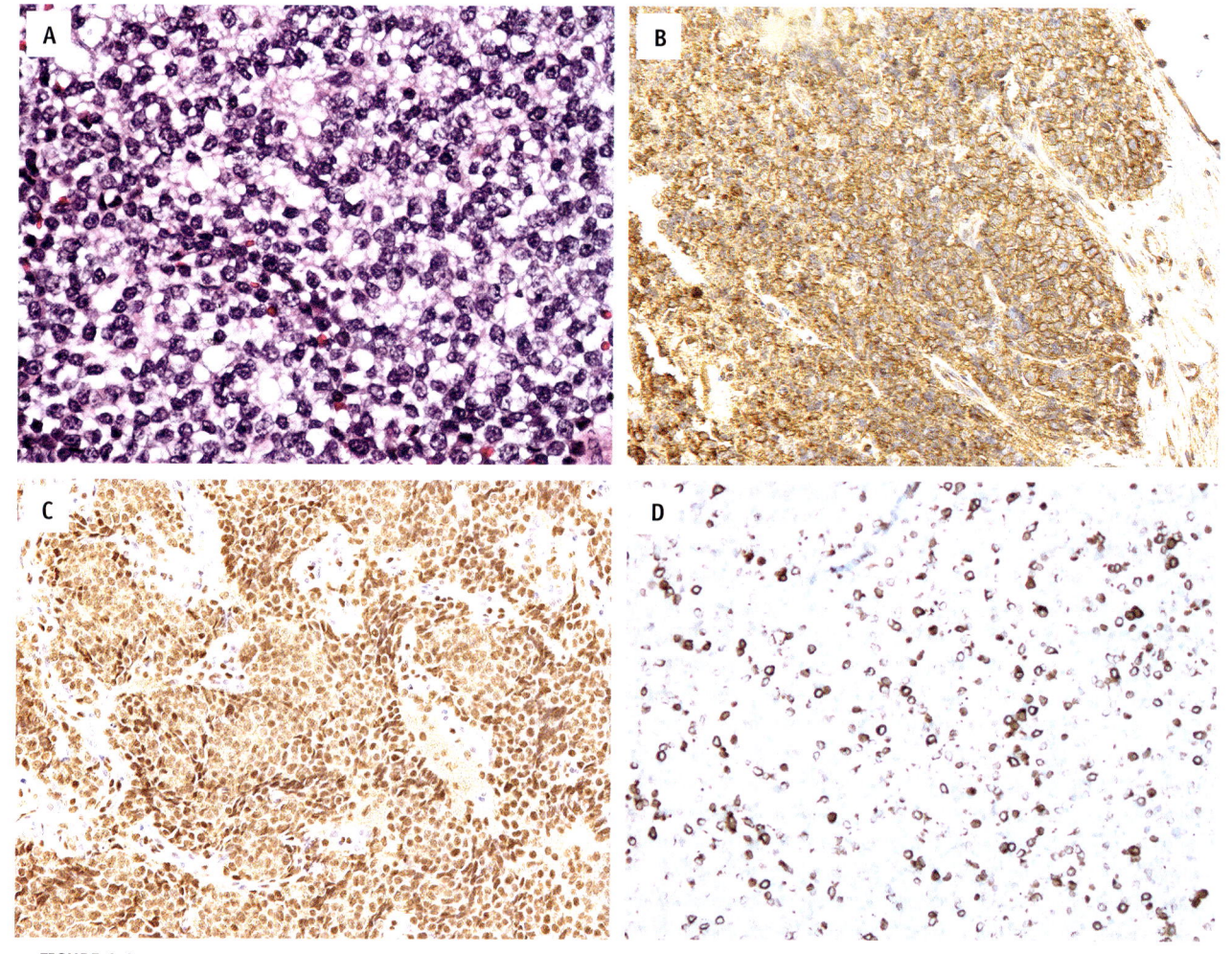

FIGURE 2-3

A, Ewing sarcoma/primitive neuroectodermal tumor showing typical strong membranous expression of CD99 **(B)** and nuclear expression of FLI1 protein **(C). D,** Anomalous cytokeratin expression may be seen in up to 25% of Ewing sarcoma tumors.

1. *Carcinoma:* INI1 expression is retained in carcinomas, unlike more than 90% of epithelioid sarcomas. Lineage-specific markers (e.g., TTF-1, CDX-2, estrogen receptor/progesterone recepter) are also of great value, depending on the clinical scenario.
2. *Melanoma and epithelioid malignant peripheral nerve sheath tumor:* Both are typically diffusely S-100 protein–positive. E-MPNST does not express melanocytic markers such as HMB45 or Melan-A.
3. *Lymphoma:* Anaplastic lymphoma kinase 1 (ALK-1) protein is expressed by many anaplastic large cell lymphoma (ALCL).
4. *Chordoma:* Brachyury is a sensitive and specific marker of chordomas and should be included in the workup of epithelioid tumors in the axial skeleton (Figure 2-10).
5. *Myoepithelioma:* Coexpression of cytokeratin, S-100 protein, SMA, and glial fibrillary acidic protein is diagnostic of myoepithelioma, although any individual marker may be negative in a given tumor.
6. *Epithelioid sarcoma:* Coexpression of CD34 is seen in 50% of epithelioid sarcomas but not in carcinomas. INI-1 expression is lost in more than 90% of epitheloid sarcomas (Figure 2-11).
7. *EAS:* Expression of FLI1 protein may be helpful in the distinction of EAS from carcinoma and epithelioid sarcoma. Unlike many carcinomas and epithelioid sarcoma, EAS does not express high-molecular-weight cytokeratins (Figure 2-12).

PLEOMORPHIC SPINDLE CELL TUMORS

It is critical to realize that histologic findings *trump* IHC for many pleomorphic malignant neoplasms in soft tissue and bone. For example, the finding of pleomorphic lipoblasts, osteoid, or low-grade chondrosarcoma establishes the diagnoses of pleomorphic liposarcoma, osteosarcoma, or dedifferentiated chondrosarcoma, respectively, regardless of the immunophenotype of the pleomorphic tumor cells. In addition, it can be argued that the most clinically relevant use of IHC in the differential diagnosis of a pleomorphic

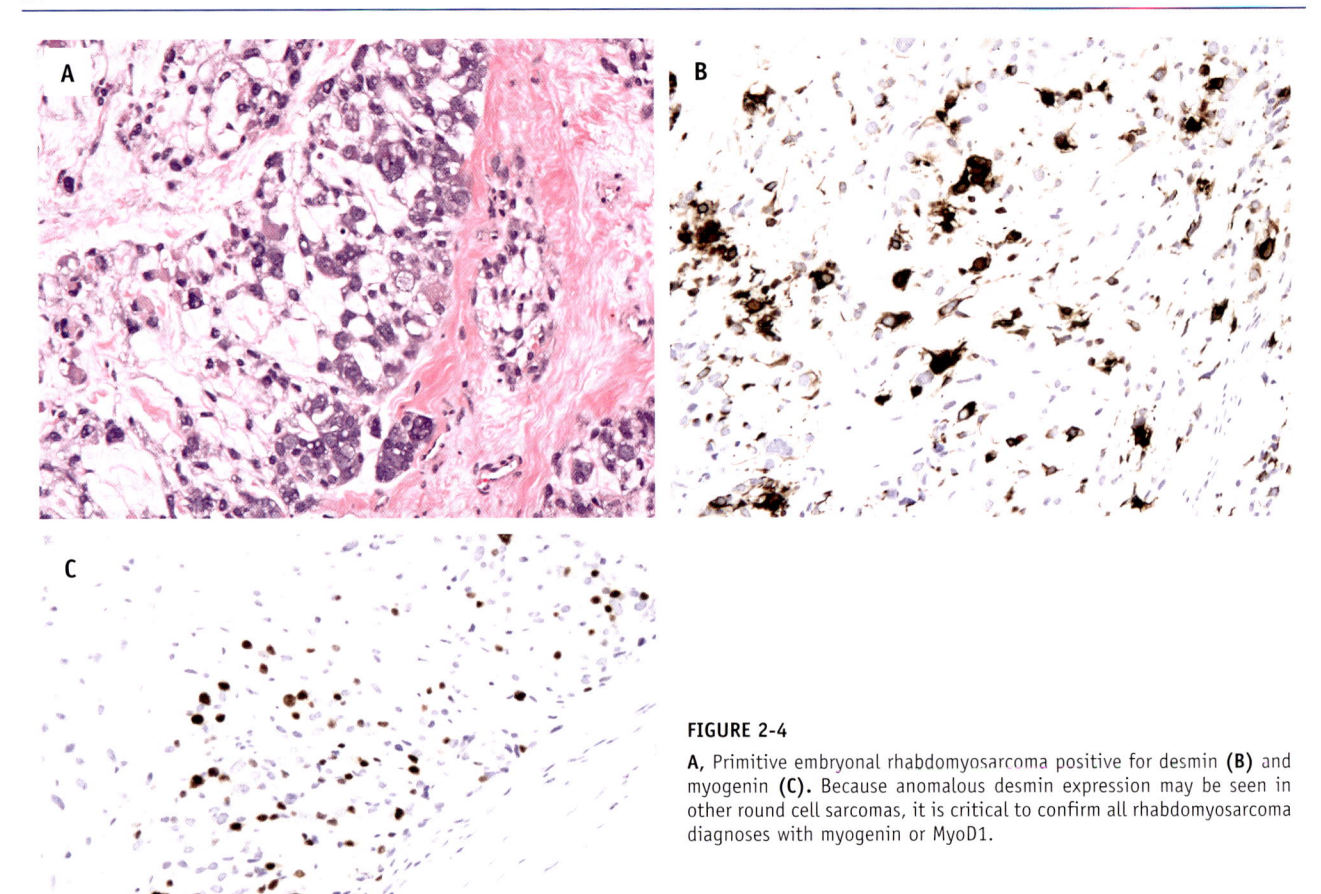

FIGURE 2-4
A, Primitive embryonal rhabdomyosarcoma positive for desmin **(B)** and myogenin **(C)**. Because anomalous desmin expression may be seen in other round cell sarcomas, it is critical to confirm all rhabdomyosarcoma diagnoses with myogenin or MyoD1.

spindle cell tumor in soft tissue or bone is to exclude the possibility of a nonmesenchymal neoplasm, such as metastatic carcinoma or melanoma. There is, however, increasing evidence that the prognosis for pleomorphic sarcomas showing myogenous differentiation is worse than that of other pleomorphic sarcomas; therefore, an attempt should be made to identify such tumors with careful histologic examination and ancillary IHC for muscle markers. Table 2-6 presents an IHC panel for the evaluation of pleomorphic spindle cell tumors.

Additional IHC Workup Depending on Suspected Diagnosis

1. *Carcinoma:* markers of specific primary sites (e.g., TTF-1, CDX-2, ER/PR, prostatic-specific antigen)
2. *Melanoma:* melanocytic markers (e.g., HMB45, Melan-A)
3. *ALCL:* ALK-1 protein
4. *Leiomyosarcoma:* caldesmon, absence of myogenin/MyoD1 (Figure 2-13A,B)
5. *RMS:* myogenin/MyoD1
6. *Undifferentiated pleomorphic sarcoma:* limited SMA expression, indicative of myofibroblastic differentiation, may occasionally be seen; rare cases show focal anomalous cytokeratin expression; occasional cases may show focal desmin expression in the absence of SMA, caldesmon, or myogenin/MyoD1 expression and are probably best not considered as showing evidence of myogenous differentiation; the presence or absence of expression of putative *histiocytic* markers such as CD68 or CD163 is not helpful, because these are highly nonspecific markers (see Figure 2-13C,D)

MOLECULAR PATHOLOGY

OVERVIEW

The cause of sarcomas is not well understood. Some environmental risk factors have been associated with certain types of sarcoma including vinyl chloride, which is associated with hepatic angiosarcoma, and ionizing radiation, which is associated with a variety of sarcomas. Although four familial cancer syndromes have been

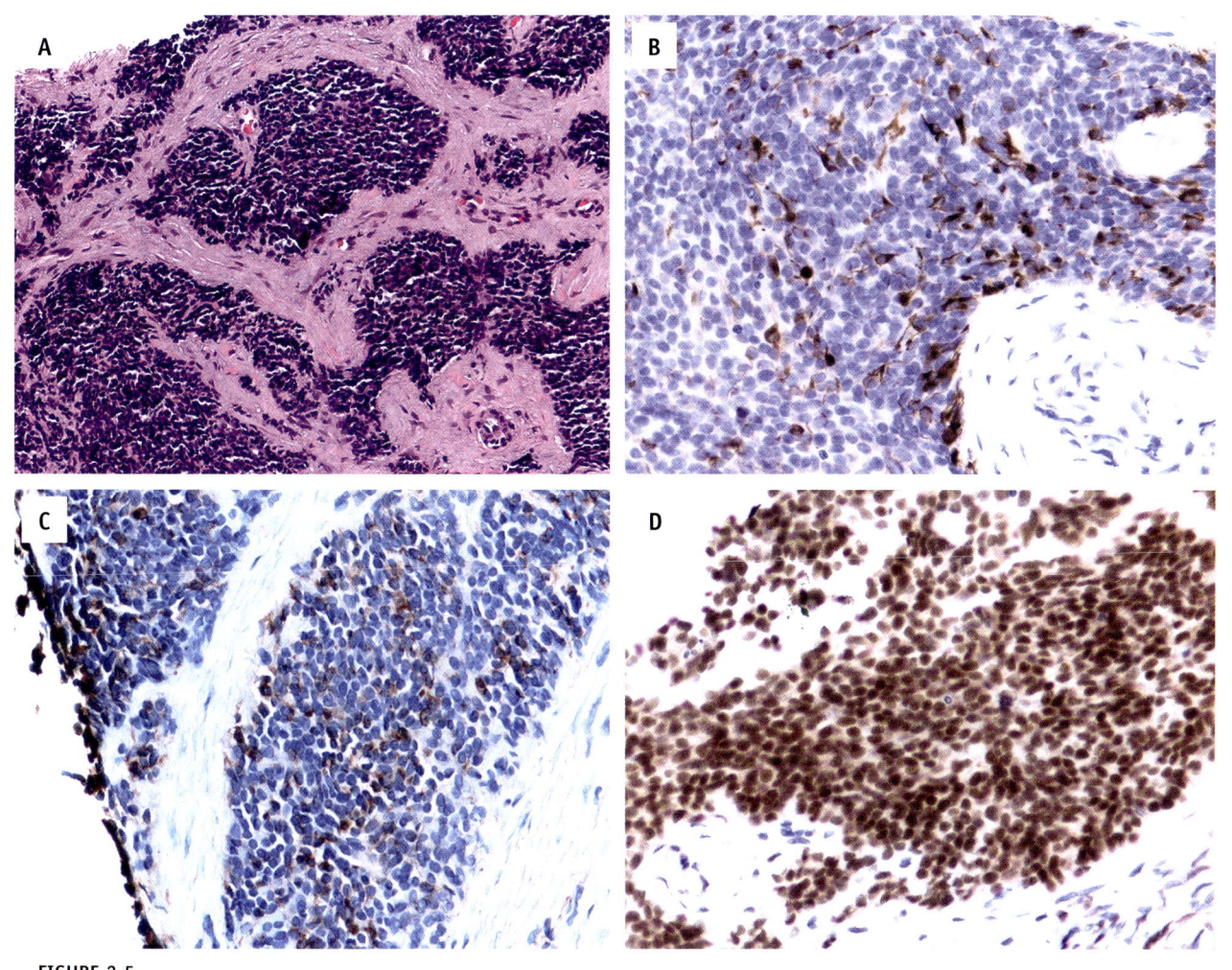

FIGURE 2-5

A, Desmoplastic small round cell tumor showing characteristic coexpression of desmin **(B)** and cytokeratin **(C).** Nuclear positivity using a carboxyl-terminal antibody to WT1 protein **(D)** confirms the presence of the diagnostic EWS-WT1 fusion protein seen in this tumor.

TABLE 2-4
Screening Panel for Monomorphic Spindle Cell Tumors

Antigen	SS	MPNST	FS/DFSP	SMT	SFT	GIST	Cellular Schwannoma
Pan-cytokeratin	Positive	Negative	Negative	Rare	Rare	Negative	Negative
S-100 protein	Variable	Positive	Negative	Rare	Negative	Variable	Positive
CD34	Negative	Variable	Variable	Rare	Positive	Variable	Negative
Smooth muscle actin	Negative	Negative	Variable	Positive	Negative	Variable	Negative
CD117 (c-kit)	Negative	Negative	Negative	Negative	Negative	Positive	Negative

FS/DFSP, fibrosarcoma (arising in dermatofibrosarcoma protuberans); GIST, gastrointestinal stromal tumor; MPNST, malignant peripheral nerve sheath tumor; SFT, solitary fibrous tumor; SMT, true smooth muscle tumor; SS, synovial sarcoma.

FIGURE 2-6

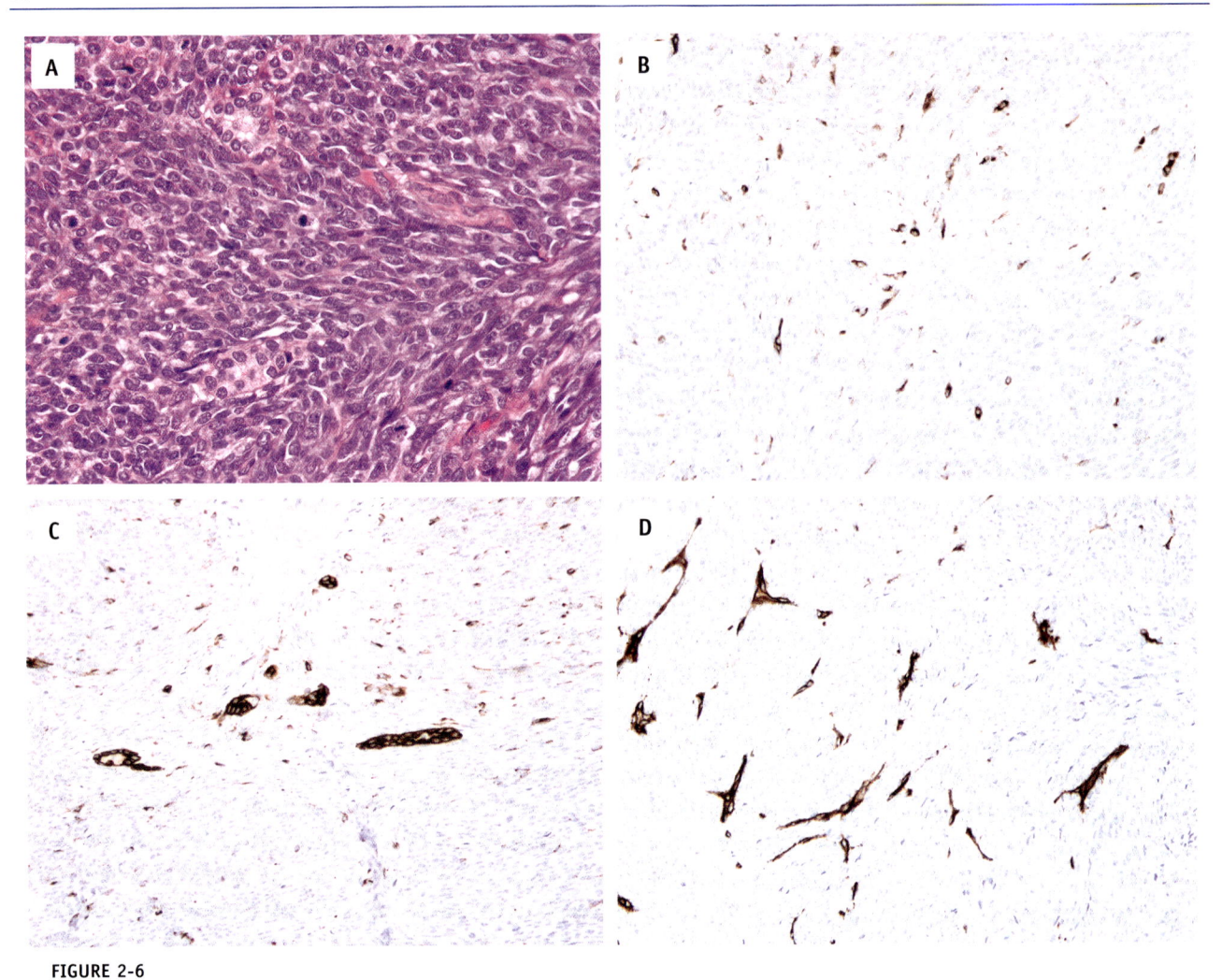

A, Synovial sarcoma showing two small *occult* glands. Immunostains for low-molecular-weight cytokeratins **(B)** and epithelial membrane antigen **(C)** show scattered positive cells, as are typically seen in synovial sarcoma. **D**, The absence of CD34 expression is helpful in distinguishing monophasic synovial sarcomas from malignant solitary fibrous tumors and malignant peripheral nerve sheath tumors.

associated with sarcomas, the majority of them appear to occur through acquired mutations. Detection of such mutations, in its clinicopathologic context, is the main purpose of molecular pathology, whose usefulness in the diagnosis and treatment of sarcomas is covered in this section. Table 2-7 lists selected cytogenetic and molecular genetic alterations, the detection of which may be of value in the diagnosis of soft tissue and bone tumors.

Generally speaking, sarcomas can be divided into two groups depending on the complexity of their molecular alterations. The first group of sarcomas, more frequently found in children and adolescents, shows relatively simple karyotypes, generally with balanced translocations. From a molecular standpoint, these are characterized either by the formation of fusion genes derived from such translocations or by point mutations, which are presumed to be important in the pathogenesis of these tumors.

The second group of sarcomas, typically found in older adults, is characterized by a complex karyotype and the lack of fusion genes. Examples of these tumor types include osteogenic sarcoma, leiomyosarcoma, and undifferentiated pleomorphic sarcoma (so-called malignant fibrous histiocytoma). These tumors are characterized by chromosomal and genomic instability, with increasing karyotypic abnormality and histologic pleomorphism over time.

Mutations in tumor suppressor genes, such as *p53* or *RB*, may be found in both groups of sarcoma and are likely related to tumor progression. These markers have prognostic rather than diagnostic significance.

METHODS OF DETECTION OF SPECIFIC GENETIC EVENTS IN SOFT TISSUE AND BONE TUMORS

REVERSE TRANSCRIPTASE–POLYMERASE CHAIN REACTION

Reverse transcriptase–polymerase chain reaction (RT-PCR) is believed by some authors to represent the method of choice to detect chromosomal translocations

CHAPTER 2 Adjuvant Techniques

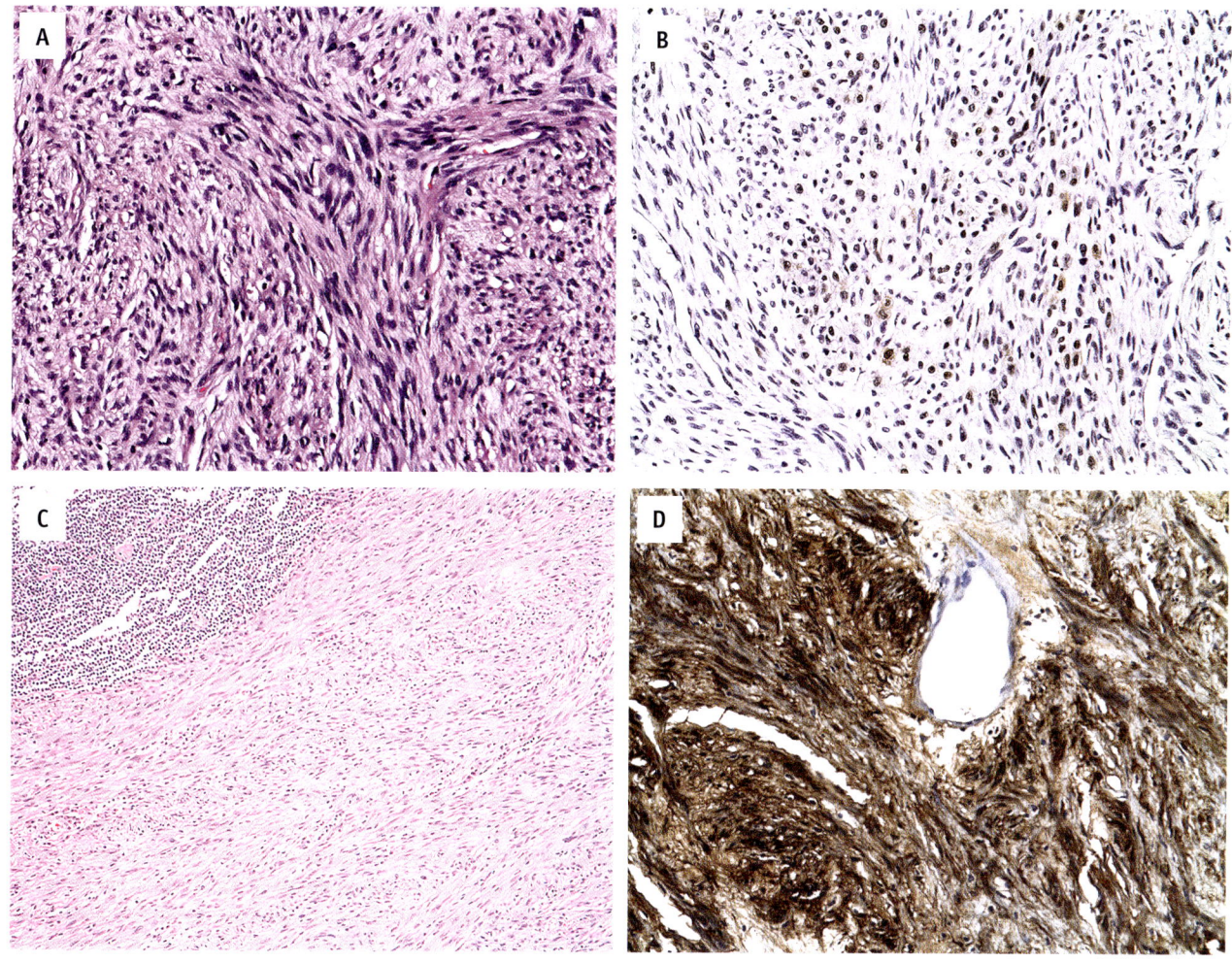

FIGURE 2-7
A, Malignant peripheral nerve sheath tumor showing only weak and patchy expression of S-100 protein **(B)**. This is in contrast with cellular schwannoma **(C)**, which typically shows uniform, intense S-100 protein expression **(D)**.

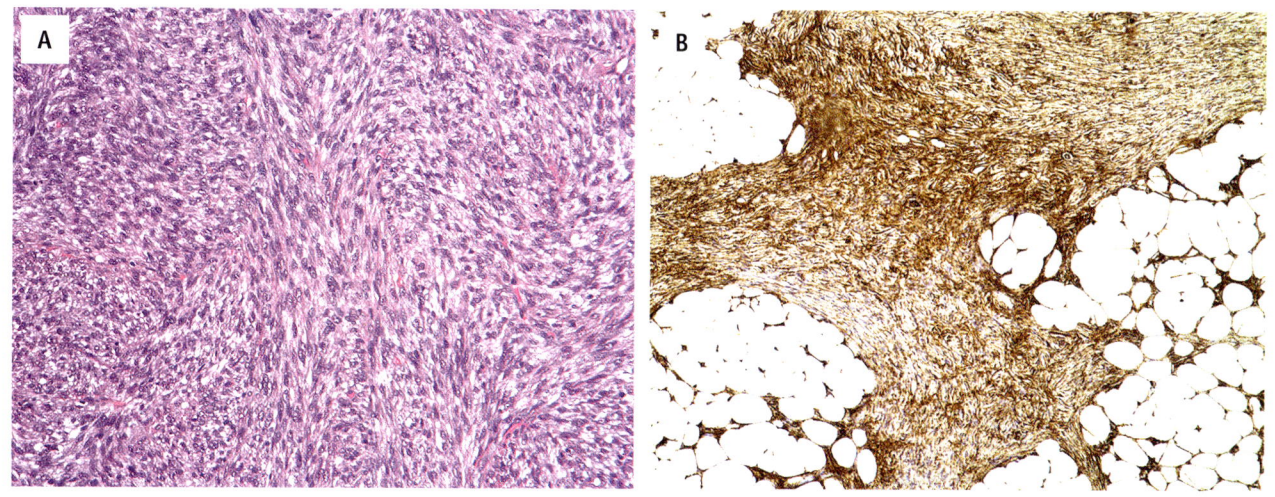

FIGURE 2-8
A, Fibrosarcomatous dermatofibrosarcoma showing intense CD34 expression in better differentiated areas. **B**, The fibrosarcomatous component may show diminished or even absent CD34 expression.

FIGURE 2-9

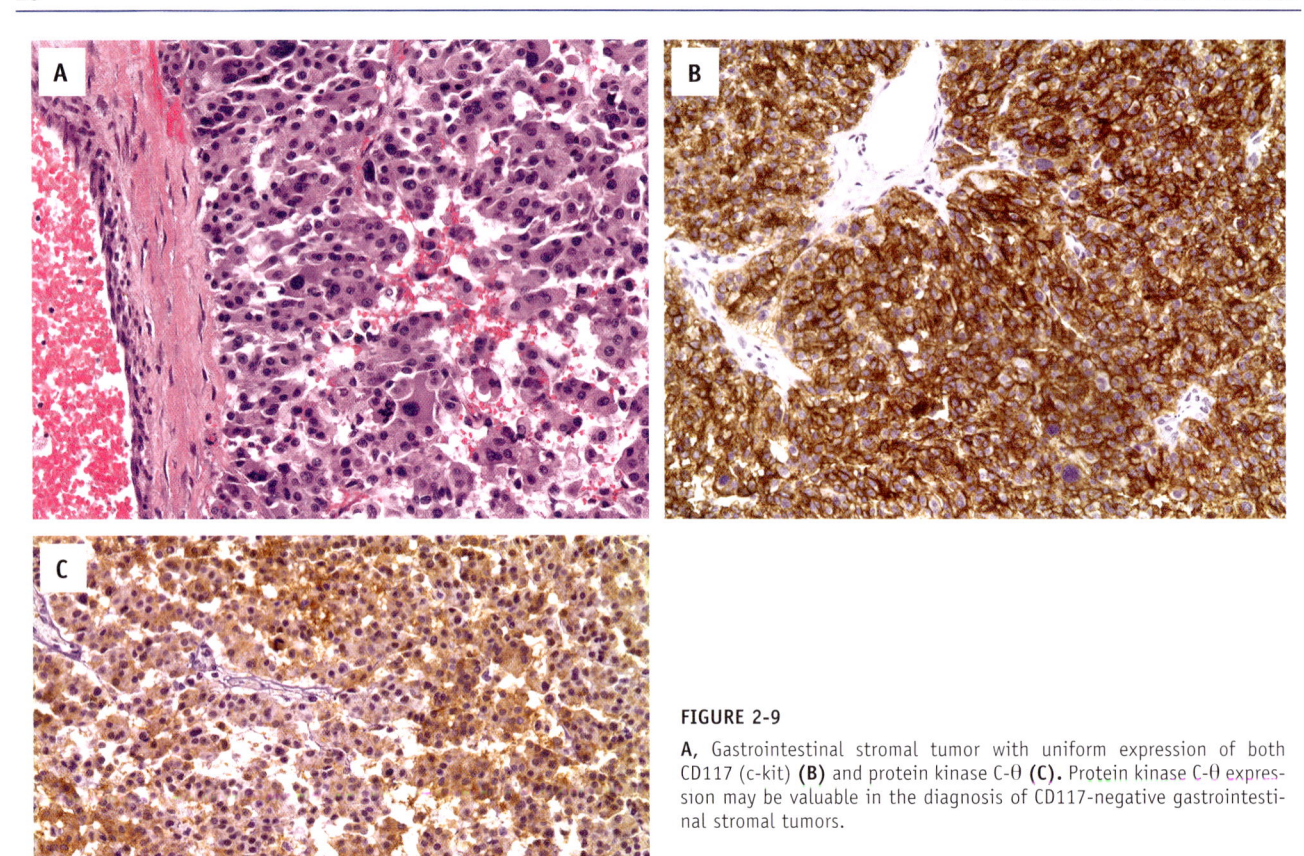

A, Gastrointestinal stromal tumor with uniform expression of both CD117 (c-kit) **(B)** and protein kinase C-θ **(C).** Protein kinase C-θ expression may be valuable in the diagnosis of CD117-negative gastrointestinal stromal tumors.

in clinical specimens. This technique has two steps (Figure 2-14). In the first step, complementary DNA (cDNA) is synthesized from RNA using the RT enzyme. In a second step, the cDNA is amplified by means of conventional PCR, using exonic primers for characteristic sequences that flank the translocation breakpoints. The amplified products are separated by agarose gel electrophoresis. Optionally, the DNA content from the agarose gel can be transferred to a nylon membrane and incubated with DNA probes complementary to the expected sequence (Southern blot). This increases the sensibility and the specificity. Appropriate negative and positive controls must be used (with water and without RT). Translocation breakpoints are usually within certain intronic sequences; nevertheless, they are not site specific. As a result, the fusion structure generated at the genomic DNA level is less predictable than the one generated at the RNA level, where a constant number of exons from each gene is present. For that reason, RNA is the preferred starting material for the detection of translocations in sarcomas. Although RT-PCR is now routinely performed in formalin-fixed, paraffin-embedded materials, the best source of good-quality RNA is fresh-frozen material, which should ideally be saved on suspected sarcoma cases. Cytologic material, typically obtained by fine-needle aspiration (FNA), is an excellent source of RNA of high quality for cytogenetic and molecular studies.

FLUORESCENT IN SITU HYBRIDIZATION

The term *hybridization* refers to the process of joining two complementary sequences of DNA or RNA. The probes are labeled with fluorescent molecules, allowing the detection of the sequence of interest. The probes used in the study of mesenchymal tumors hybridize to specific parts of the genome, such as the centromeric region of a given chromosome, or to a particular sequence of interest. This technique allows detection of fusions, when gene-specific probes are used for each of the genes involved in the fusion (Figure 2-15), or alternatively, detection of gene rearrangements of one particular gene (i.e., *EWS*) using probes flanking the breakpoints of the translocation, in what are called *breakapart probes*. The

TABLE 2-5
Screening Panel for Epithelioid Neoplasms

Antigen	CA	Melanoma/E-MPNST	Lymphoma	Chordoma	Myoepithelioma	Epithelioid sarcoma	EAS
Cytokeratin	Positive	Variable in melanoma, negative in E-MPNST	Negative	Positive	Negative	Positive	Variable
S-100 protein	Negative	Positive	Negative	Positive	Negative	Negative	Negative
CD45	Negative	Negative	Positive in conventional B- and T-cell lymphomas, negative in most ALCL	Negative	Negative	Negative	Negative
CD30	Negative	Negative	Negative in most conventional B and T cell lymphomas, positive in ALCL	Negative	Positive	Negative	Negative
CD31	Negative	Negative	Negative	Negative	Negative	Negative	Positive

ALCL, anaplastic large cell lymphoma; CA, carcinoma; EAS, epithelioid angiosarcoma; E-MPNST, epithelioid malignant peripheral nerve sheath tumor.

advantage of fluorescent in situ hybridization (FISH) is that reliable results can be obtained when the amount of available tissue is scarce or when there is only paraffin-embedded material, or when only cytologic material (FNA or touch preps) is available. Nonetheless, the drawback of the technique is that a fluorescence microscope is required, which makes integration of this technique a difficult task for a small laboratory of pathology.

The competitive in situ hybridization technique, in which immunofluorescence is substituted by a chromogenic molecule (similar to those used in IHC), has already been used in diagnostic routine for the detection of gene amplifications, having a performance similar to that of FISH, and in the near future could be used to detect chromosomal translocations in sarcomas if appropriated chromogens are developed.

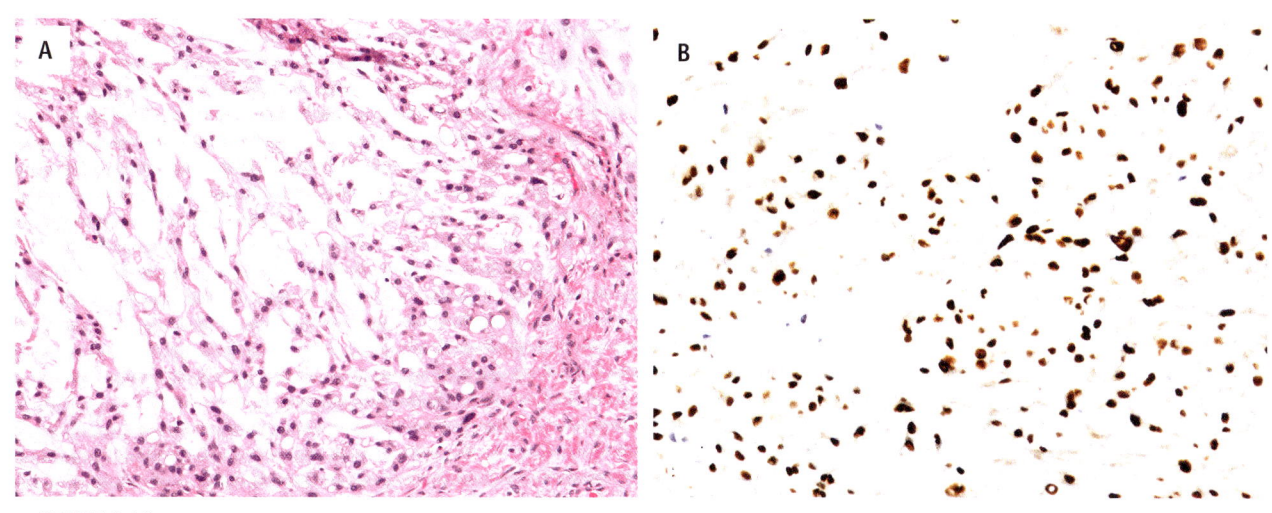

FIGURE 2-10
A, Chordoma showing strong nuclear expression of brachyury **(B)**, a specific marker of notochord-derived tumors. (**B**, *Courtesy of Dr. G. Petur Nielsen, Department of Pathology, Massachusetts General Hospital, Boston, MA.*)

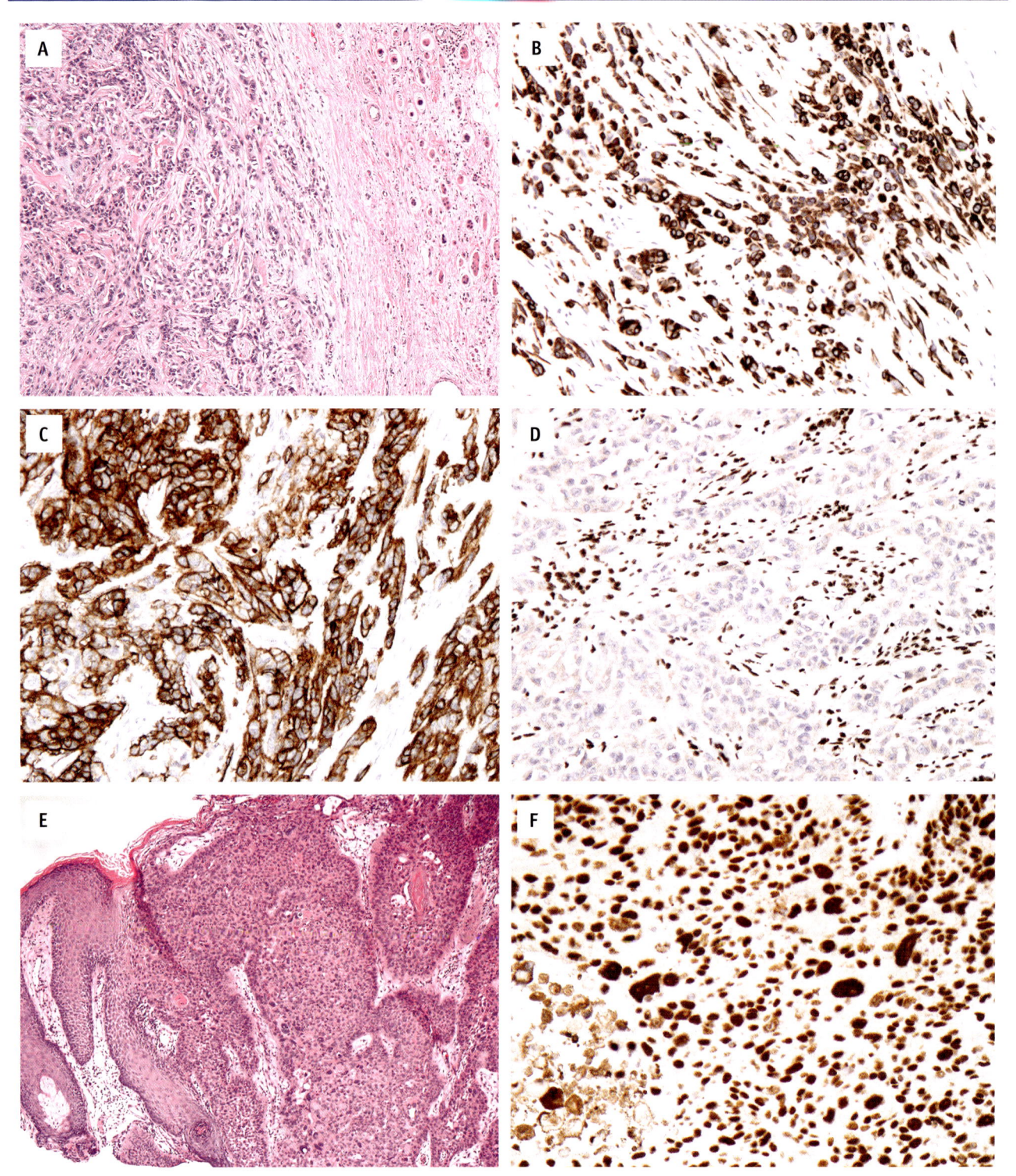

FIGURE 2-11

A, Epithelioid sarcoma showing strong expression of cytokeratins **(B)**, CD34 **(C)**, and loss of INI-1 protein expression **(D).** Normal lymphocytes serve as a positive internal control for INI-1 expression. In contrast, carcinomas, such as this squamous cell carcinoma **(E)**, essentially always show retention of INI-1 expression **(F).**

CHAPTER 2 Adjuvant Techniques

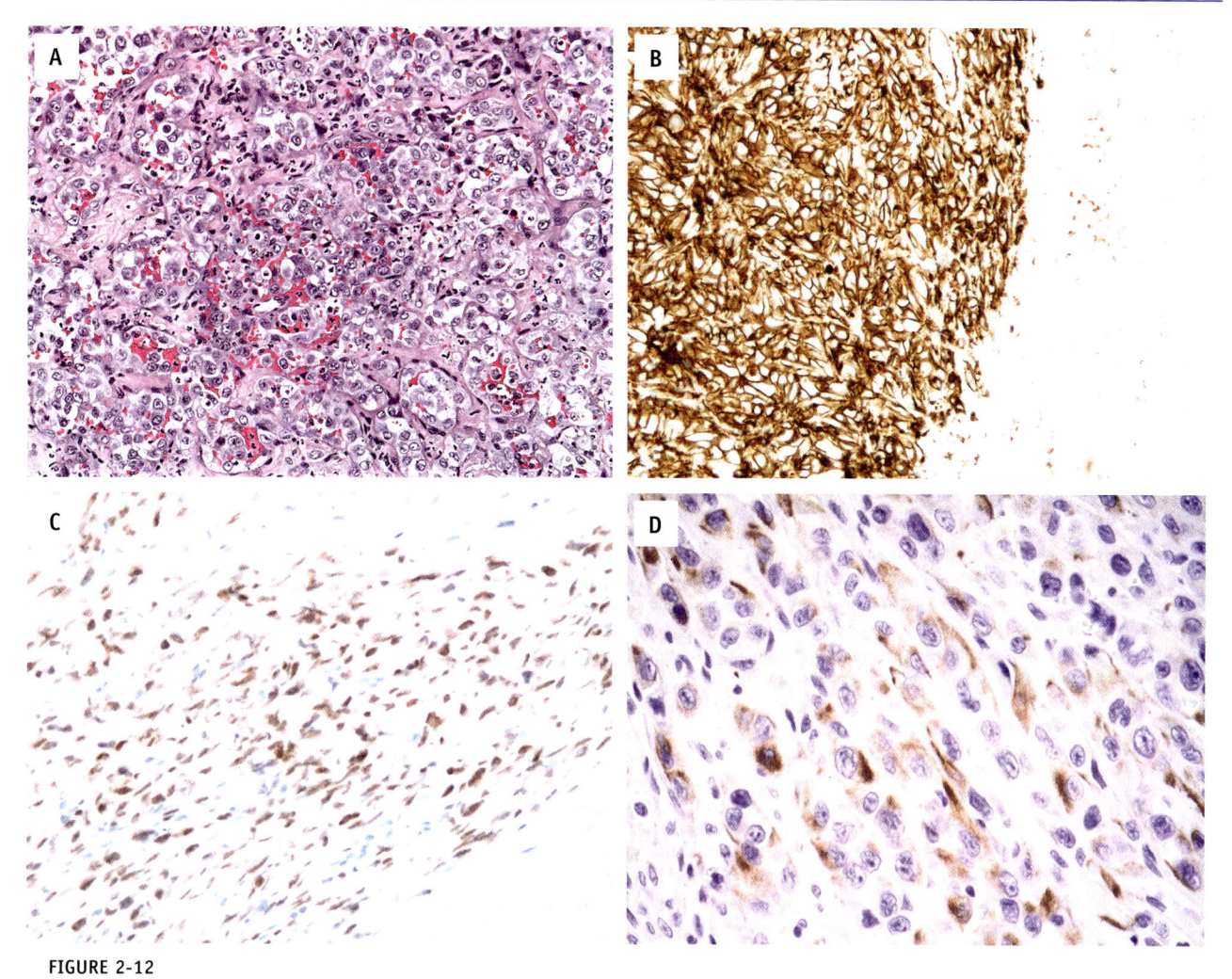

FIGURE 2-12
A, Epithelioid angiosarcoma diffusely positive for CD31 **(B)** and FLI1 protein **(C)**. Cytokeratin expression may be seen in up to 50% of epithelioid angiosarcomas **(D)**, potentially resulting in confusion with other epithelioid tumors, such as epithelioid sarcoma and carcinoma.

TABLE 2-6
Immunohistochemistry Panel for the Evaluation of Pleomorphic Spindle Cell Neoplasms

Antigen	CA	Melanoma	ALCL	LMS	RMS	UDPS (MFH)
Cytokeratin	Positive	Variable	Negative	Variable	Negative	Negative
S-100 protein	Negative	Positive	Negative	Negative	Negative	Negative
CD30	Negative	Negative	Positive	Variable	Negative	Negative
Smooth muscle actin	Negative	Negative	Negative	Positive	Negative	Variable
Desmin	Negative	Variable	Negative	Variable	Positive	Negative

ALCL, anaplastic large cell lymphoma; CA, carcinoma; LMS, leiomyosarcoma; RMS, rhabdomyosarcoma; UDPS (MFH), undifferentiated pleomorphic sarcoma (malignant fibrous histiocytoma).

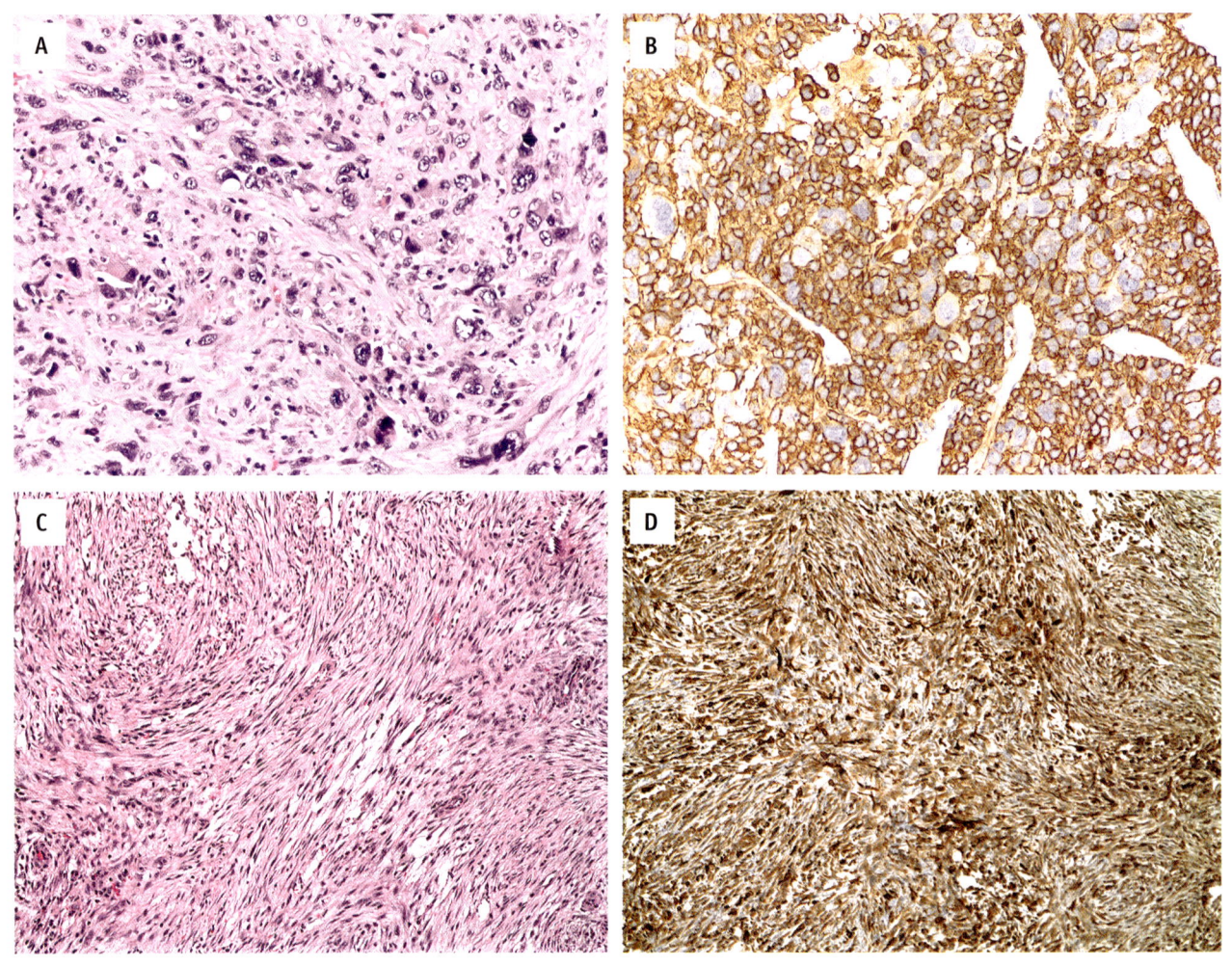

FIGURE 2-13

A, Poorly differentiated leiomyosarcoma showing uniform expression of smooth muscle actin **(B)**. Identification of myogenous differentiation may be of prognostic value in pleomorphic sarcomas. It is important to remember that so-called fibrohistiocytic markers, such as CD68, have no value in the diagnosis of pleomorphic sarcomas. This is illustrated by this case of nodular fasciitis **(C)**, which was submitted in consultation with a suggested diagnosis of *malignant fibrous histiocytoma*, partially on the basis of this strongly positive CD68 immunostain **(D)**.

ACQUIRED ALTERATIONS

SOMATICALLY ACQUIRED

Five different types of mutations can be detected in sarcomas:

Deletion: loss of a segment (arm, gene, or few base pairs) of genetic material from a chromosome

Amplification: production of many copies from a gene whose structure is otherwise normal

Translocation: exchange of genetic material between two nonhomologous chromosomes; balanced translocation, in which there is no net loss or gain of chromosomal material, is the most frequent type of translocation

Inversion: chromosomal rearrangement in which a segment of genetic material is broken away from the chromosome, inverted from end to end, and reinserted into the chromosome at the same breakage site

Point mutation: a mutation resulting from single nucleotide base change

FAMILIAL SYNDROMES

Four well-characterized familial cancer syndromes are associated with sarcomas.
- Patients with *germline mutations* of *RB* have a much higher frequency of osteosarcoma than general population.
- Patients with *Li–Fraumeni syndrome*, with germline mutations of the *p53* gene, have an increased incidence of a variety of sarcomas, typically before the age of 40.
- Another type of sarcoma, *MPNST*, frequently occurs in the setting of neurofibromatosis type 1, which is associated with germline loss of *NF1* gene.
- Finally, a *GIST familial syndrome* has been described in a family whose patients bear germline mutations in *c-kit* gene.

CHAPTER 2 Adjuvant Techniques

TABLE 2-7
Selected Cytogenetic and Molecular Genetic Alterations in Soft Tissue and Bone Sarcomas

Tumor Type	Cytogenetic Features	Molecular Features	Prevalence Rate
ES/PNET	t(11;22)(q24;q12)	EWS-FLI1	95%
	t(21;22)(q22;q12)	EWS-ERG	5%
	t(7;22)(p22;q12)	EWS-ETV1	<1%
	t(2;22)(q33;q12)	EWS-E1AF	<1%
	t(1;22)(q42;q12)	EWS-?	<1%
	t(2;22)(q33;q12)	EWS-FEV	<1%
	t(17;22)(q12;q12)	EWS-ETV4	<1%
DSRCT	t(11;22)(p13;q12)	EWS-WT1	100%
Myxoid-round cell liposarcoma	t(12;16)(q13;p11)	TLS-CHOP	95%
	t(12;22)(q13;q12)	EWS-CHOP	5%
Extraskeletal myxoid liposarcoma	t(9;22)(q22;q12)	EWS-CHN(TEC)	75%
	t(9;17)(q22;q11)	hTAFII68-CHN(TEC)	?
Clear cell sarcoma	t(12;22)(q13;q21)	EWS-ATF1	91%
	t(2;22)(q34;q12)	EWS-CREB1	?
Synovial sarcoma	t(X;18)(p11.23;q11)	SS18-SSX1	65%
	t(X;18)(p11.21;q11)	SS18-SSX2	35%
	t(X;18)(p11;q11)	SS18- SSX4	<1%
	t(X;20)(p11;q13.3)	SS18L1-SSX1	<1%
Gastrointestinal stromal tumor	Various	KIT mutations	95%
Extrarenal rhabdoid tumor/proximal type epithelioid sarcoma	22q deletion	INI inactivation	>90%
Alveolar rhabdomyosarcoma	t(2;13)(q35;q14)	PAX3-FKHR	75%
	t(1;13)(p36;q14)	PAX7-FKHR	10%
Dermatofibrosarcoma protuberans/ giant cell fibroblastoma	t(17;22)(q22;q13)	COL1A1-PDGFB	>90%
Infantile fibrosarcoma	t(12;15)(p13;q25)	ETV6-NTRK3	
Alveolar soft part sarcoma	der(17)t(X;17)(p11;q25)	TFE3-ASPL	
Inflammatory myofibroblastic tumor	t(1;2)(q21;p23)	TPM3/TPM4-ALK	
	t(2;17)(p23;q23)	CLTC2-ALK	
Low-grade fibromyxoid sarcoma	t(7;16)(q34; p11)	FUS/CREB3L2	>95%
		FUS/CREB3L1	1%
Angiomatoid (malignant) fibrous histiocytoma	t(12;16)(16p11; 12q13)	FUS-ATF1	10%
	t(12;22)(q13;q12)	EWSR1-ATF1	40%
	t(2;22)(q34;q12)	EWSR1-CREB1	>50%
Well-differentiated and dedifferentiated liposarcoma	12q13-15 amplification	CDK4 and MDM2	
Aneurysmal bone cyst	t(16;17)	CDH11-USP6	

DSRCT, desmoplastic small round cell tumor; ES/PNET, Ewing sarcoma primitive neuroectodermal tumor.

Mutations with Diagnostic Significance

Translocations

Many types of sarcomas are characterized by specific chromosomal translocations (see Table 2-7). Indeed, major advances have been accomplished in the understanding of its pathogenesis. The fusion genes generated from these chromosomal translocations are probably an initial and necessary event in tumor type formation in various sarcomas. These translocations disrupt certain genes and juxtapose portions of them, creating fusion genes with new structure and function because of the reassortment of functional domains habitually found in separated molecules. These chimeric fusion proteins are often transcription factors—that is, proteins that bind to regulatory regions of certain genes and help to control their expression. In many cases, they are involved in certain key functions for the cell, such as cellular proliferation or survival. As a result of these translocations, fusion genes represent almost always aberrant transcription factors. The two most notable exceptions are

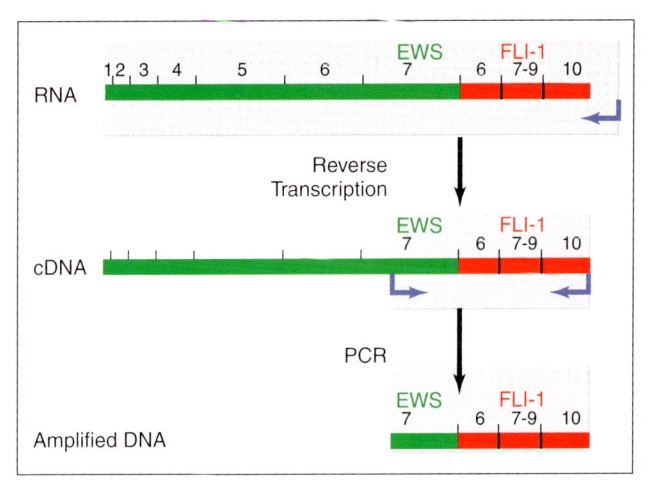

FIGURE 2-14

Reverse transcriptase–polymerase chain reaction (RT-PCR). This technique has two steps. In the first one (top half), RNA is reverse transcribed to complementary DNA (cDNA), whereas in the second one, a specific segment of cDNA, containing the junction of the fused genes, is amplified. The example corresponds to the EWS-FLI1 fusion, characteristic of Ewing tumors, but can be applied to all translocation-bearing sarcomas.

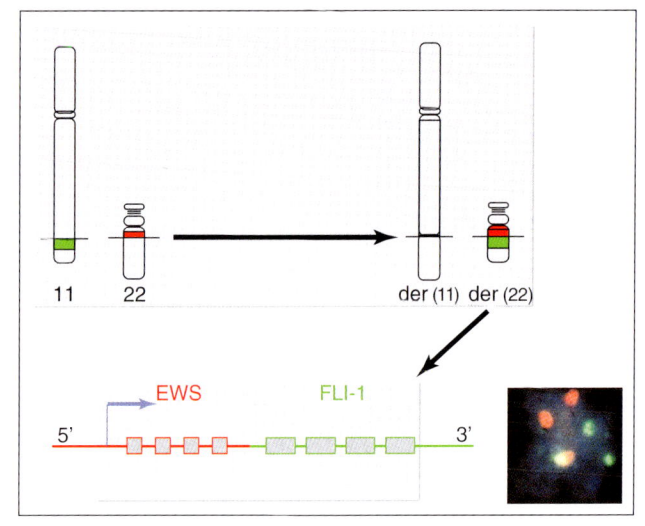

FIGURE 2-15

Fluorescent in situ hybridization (FISH). FISH can be used to identify translocations on cytologic or tissue simples through the use of probes labeled with fluorescent dyes. In this particular example of a fusion-detecting FISH, *EWS* gene in chromosome 22 is represented in red and FLI1 in green. The top shows how the translocation rearranges both genes, and the bottom represents the fusion gene itself. (inset) Corresponds to a FISH experiment of a Ewing tumor and shows a triploid cell in which two red and two green signals, corresponding to the nonrearranged alleles, are seen together with a fusion signal, with a yellowish red color.

the *COL1A1-PDGFB* of dermatofibrosarcoma protuberans, which is a growth factor, and the *ETV6-NTRK3* of congenital fibrosarcoma, which corresponds to a protein with tyrosine kinase activity. Because fusion genes and their products are considered tumor specific and observed in practically all the cases of many types of sarcomas, their characterization is important not only to improve the understanding of the oncogenic process from a pathogenetic standpoint, but also to identify new diagnostic and therapeutic possibilities.

Specific Translocations and Their Tumor Types

Synovial sarcoma has a characteristic chromosomal translocation, t(X;18), that results in the fusion of *SS18* (SYT) gene at chromosome 18 to *SSX* genes, which has two different copies, *SSX1* and *SSX2*, located in two subregions of chromosome Xp11 (23 and 21, respectively); some rarer fusions also exist (Figure 2-16). The fusion encodes an aberrant nuclear transcription factor that alters chromatin remodeling, probably inducing changes in the gene expression patterns. Transcripts may be detected in almost all synovial sarcomas by means of RT-PCR. Synovial sarcoma provides a clear example of the correlation that can exist between the fusion transcript type, prognosis, and tumoral phenotype. *SYT-SSX1* fusions are associated with biphasic synovial sarcoma in both epithelioid and spindle-cell elements, whereas the monophasic variant contains, in most cases, *SYT-SSX2* fusions. It has been suggested that patients with *SYT-SSX2* have a relatively lower risk for relapse, whereas those with *SYT-SSX1* variant have a greater proliferative rate and worse prognosis, although this remains controversial.

About 85% of patients with Ewing tumor (including PNET) have *EWS-FLI1* fusions; *EWS-ERG* fusions are present in 10% of cases, whereas 3% corresponds to fusions between *EWS* and other members of the *ETS* family of transcription factors. These are characteristic for this type of neoplasia, because PCR studies from other small round cell tumors, which enter into its differential diagnosis, such as neuroblastomas, RMSs, adamantinomas, or giant cell tumor of bone, lack these particular gene fusions. In addition to the prognostic factors habitually used in clinical practice (stage, primary tumor site, tumor volume, age, and treatment response), recent studies have evaluated the contribution of molecular heterogeneity to the prognosis in Ewing tumor. This neoplasm presents at least 18 structural possibilities of fusion genes.

Two possible sources of variability exist (Figure 2-17): on the one hand, the fusion partner of *EWS* (FLI1, ERG, ETV1, E1A, or FEV), and on the other, the location of breakpoints within the genes involved. It has been established that for localized Ewing tumor, patients who express the most common chimeric transcript (fusion of *EWS* exon 7 to FLI1 exon 6) have better prognosis than those with other fusion transcript types.

In the DSRCT, the *EWS* gene is fused to *WT1* gene. *WT1* gene was initially described as an altered tumor suppressor gene in Wilms tumor; as a matter of fact, *EWS-WT1* is the first example of a constant rearrangement of a tumor suppressor gene. *EWS-WT1* chimeric transcript has been found in 97% of studied cases, which makes this a useful diagnostic marker. It also suggests that the chimeric protein is important for tumor development.

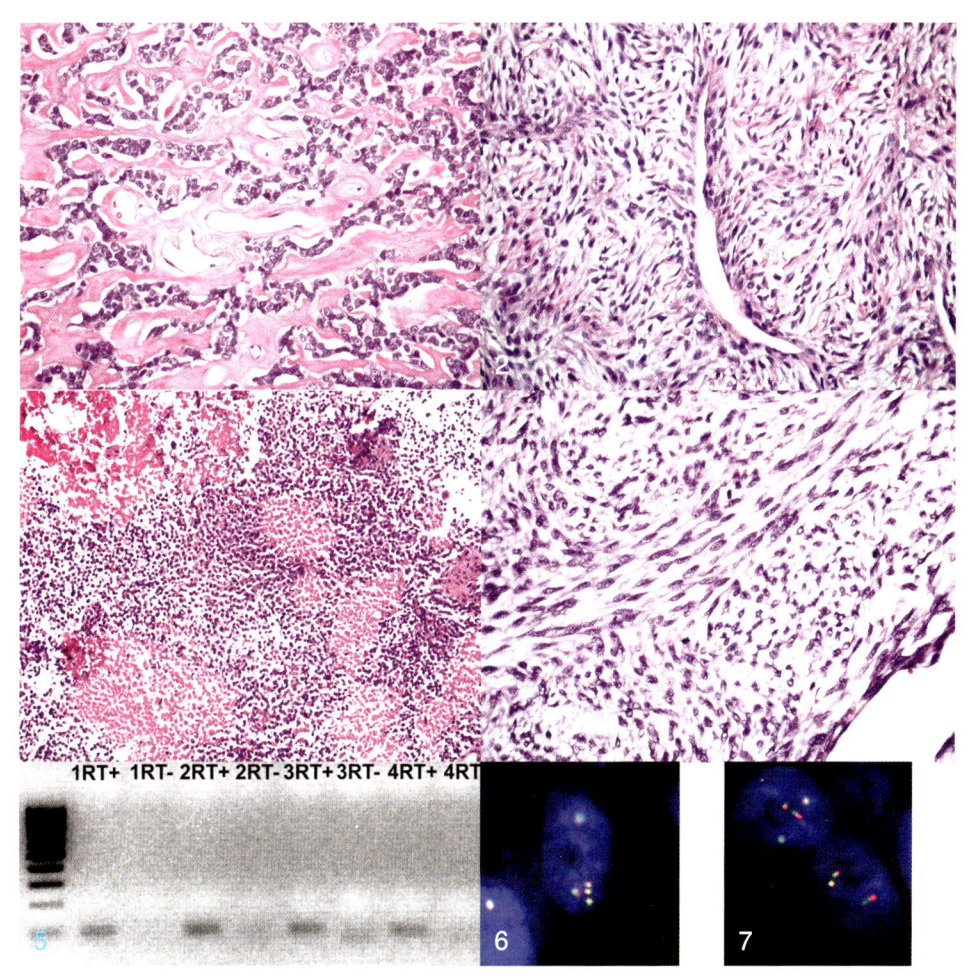

FIGURE 2-16

Detection of translocations is particularly useful in the routine diagnostic workup when sarcomas appear in uncommon clinicopathologic settings. The plate shows four examples of synovial sarcoma. *Image 1* corresponds to a poorly differentiated synovial sarcoma in the ankle of a 5-year-old boy; differential diagnosis included a soft tissue myoepithelioma and Ewing tumor. *Image 2* (7-year-old girl) had a striking hemangiopericytomatous pattern, and an infantile hemangiopericytoma was in the differential. *Image 3* affected the soft tissues of the leg of a 24-year-old woman and corresponded to a largely necrotic small round cell tumor; Ewing tumor was in the differential. *Image 4* is a synovial sarcoma growing in the mandible bone of a 66-year-old man. *Image 5* shows reverse transcriptase–polymerase chain reaction (RT-PCR) study for *SYT-SSX2* fusions, showing in all of them amplification of a 110-base pair segment; RT-negative controls were used in each case. *Image 6* is a fluorescent in situ hybridization (FISH) study of image 1 with breakapart probes for *EWS* gene showing that the *EWS* gene is not rearranged in this particular sample. *Image 7* shows similar results for image 3.

As in many other sarcomas, it is a matter of an aberrant transcription factor, which modulates the expression of genes that coincide, at least partially, with *WT1* gene targets. One of them is platelet-derived growth factor-α (PDGFA), a fibroblastic growth factor that probably contributes to the characteristic desmoplastic stroma of this neoplasia. BAIAP3 is another transcription factor; it regulates the process of exocytosis and, therefore, that of growth factor secretion.

EWS joins to *ATF1* and less commonly to *CREB1* in *clear cell sarcoma of soft parts* (malignant melanoma of soft tissue). As in Ewing tumor, *EWS* joins to the DNA-binding domain of a transcription factor. In contrast with wild-type *ATF1*, *EWS-ATF1* fusion functions as a transcriptional activator, probably deregulating genes habitually controlled by *ATF1*.

EWS-CHN fusion, generated from a t(9;22), is observed in *extraskeletal myxoid chondrosarcoma* and not chondrosarcomas of bone, including those with myxoid change. *CHN* encodes a nuclear receptor with a DNA-binding domain. The fusion protein contains the N-terminal *EWS* domain joined to in-frame *CHN*, which generates a nuclear receptor that is more active than native. This receptor acts on cell proliferation control modulating its response to diverse growth factors. Less frequent variants of this fusion also exist.

An *EWS* analogous gene, *TLS/FUS*, is present in the 90% of cases of *myxoid/round cell liposarcoma (TLS/FUS-CHOP)*. *CHOP* is, again, a transcription factor. In *TLS-CHOP* fusion, the DNA-binding domain of *CHOP* replaces the RNA-binding domain of *TLS*. Myxoid and round cell liposarcoma relation is confirmed by the detection of *TLS-CHOP* in tumors composed, in part or completely, of round cells. Approximately 5% of cases show *EWS-CHOP* fusions, where *EWS* has an analogous role to *TLS/FUS*. Therefore, the RNA-binding proteins *TLS* and *EWS* seem to be functionally similar, whereas the component that contributes the DNA-binding domain, *CHOP*, is tumor specific.

Alveolar RMS is associated with recurring chromosomal translocations, including t(2;13), and less commonly t(1;13), which result in the fusion of *PAX3* and *PAX7* genes, respectively, to the *FKHR* gene located at 13q14 (forkhead in RMS; currently called also *FOXO1A*). *PAX* genes are transcription factors involved in embryonic development, which are necessary for the genesis of certain organs. In particular, *PAX3* and *PAX7* are expressed in the neural tube, being key as much for its adequate formation as for the myoblast migration to the upper and lower extremities. *PAX3* can suppress myoblast differentiation, which may contribute to its undifferentiated phenotype. Fusion gene amplifications have been detected in some tumors with *PAX7-FKHR* fusions, which indicate that translocation and amplification might be not only sequential but also complementary mechanisms in the genesis of this neoplasm. In the case of the *PAX3-FKHR* fusion, *PAX* overexpression of transcriptional origin, not associated to gene amplification, is detected. These differences in *PAX3* and *PAX7* overexpression mechanism are analogous to those observed on the clinical level. *PAX7-FKHR* tumors tend to arise in younger patients, usually associated to better survival and lower metastasis rates compared with those who have *PAX3-FKHR* fusions, despite having a similar morphology.

Dermatofibrosarcoma protuberans and *giant cell fibroblastoma* have a translocation, t(17;22), that results in the fusion of *COL1A1*, a gene of collagen, and *PDGFB*, a gene that encodes a growth factor protein. Because of the genomic structure of the fusion, this results in *PDGFB* being placed under *COL1A1* promoter control, which eliminates the elements that repress the transcription of *PDGFB*. *PDGFB-COL1A1* acts, probably, as an autocrine growth factor.

In *congenital (infantile) fibrosarcoma*, the translocation t(12;15) joins *ETV6* (TEL) gene to *NTRK3* (neurotrophin-3 receptor; TRKC). Curiously, this fusion can also be observed in mesoblastic nephroma, acute myeloblastic leukemia, and breast secretory carcinoma, a rare variant of invasive ductal carcinoma of the breast. *ETV6-NTRK3* is a chimeric tyrosine kinase that can contribute to oncogenesis deregulating signal transduction pathways generated by *NTRK3*.

Translocations not only occur in malignant tumors but also in lesions thought to be pseudoneoplastic, such as *aneurysmal bone cyst*, in which a t(16;17) (usually) generates gene fusions *CDH11-USP6*. It should be noted that sarcomas are not the only nonhematologic tumors bearing translocations. Good examples in the carcinoma group include secretory breast carcinoma, most childhood renal carcinomas, papillary and follicular carcinoma of the thyroid, mucoepidermoid carcinoma (some), and midline poorly differentiated carcinoma.

Understanding the molecular mechanisms implied in the genesis of the different sarcomas may have important consequences in the therapeutic management of the patients with such neoplasms. This is due, in part, to the potential role that these genetic alterations have as targets for therapeutic intervention. As mentioned earlier, some chimeric proteins have tyrosine kinase activity; some of them would be able to respond to imatinib (Gleevec)

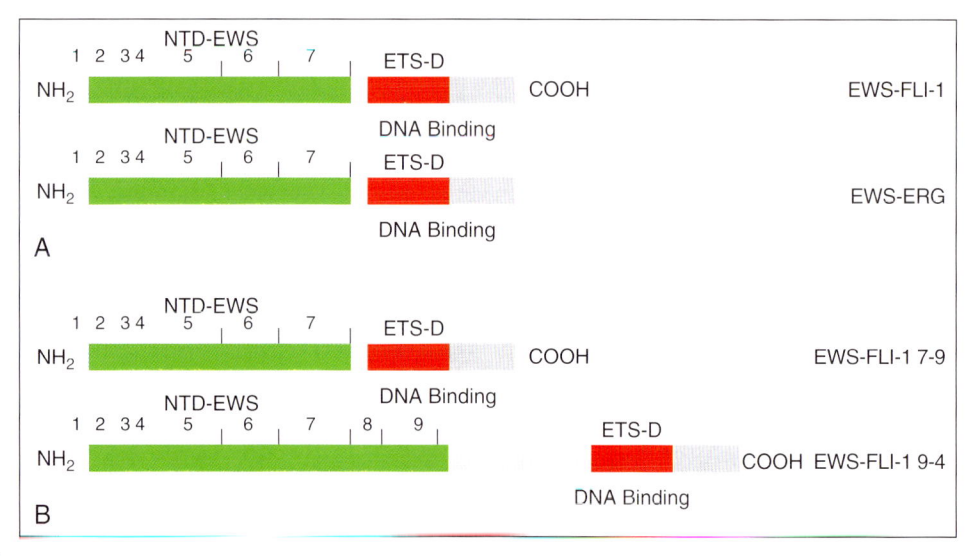

FIGURE 2-17

Structural of the chimeric proteins and their variability. The structure of chimeric proteins that are found in Ewing tumor is an example of that observed in the majority of the chimeric proteins of sarcomas. EWS-FLI1 or EWS-ERG chimeric proteins contain the N-terminal EWS domain (green), joined to the C-terminal domain of FLI1 or ERG *(diagonal stripes)*. The last one has the DNA-binding ETS domain (red in FLI1, green in ERG). Small numbers represent the exons that participate in the fusion. Fusion gene variability in Ewing tumor. **A,** It depends, first, on the fusion partner of EWS. **B,** Second, for a specific fusion type (represented here as EWS-FLI1), several possibilities exist depending on the number of exons that participate in the fusion. The top half of this section shows the shortest fusion (EWS ex.7-FLI1 ex.9), whereas the bottom shows longest one (EWS ex.9-FLI1 ex.4). Gene fusion structure in Ewing tumor is correlated to prognosis.

(dermatofibrosarcoma protuberans, DSRCT), whereas other chimeric proteins will be targets of new drugs.

Point Mutations

Aside from the translocations, mutations (such as gain-of-function mutations of *c-kit* in the GIST, or the loss of function mutations of *hSNF5/INI1* in extrarenal rhabdoid tumors and epithelioid sarcomas) are genetic alterations also found in sarcomas.

Practical Significance of Mutation Detection in Sarcomas

C-*kit* mutations in GIST serve as an excellent practical model of the impact of mutation detection on patient care and outcome in sarcomas. (This subject is also covered in greater depth in Chapter 8.) Constitutive activation of KIT oncoprotein is observed in many GISTs. However, the activation of such protein is ligand independent, because KIT protein in GIST has suffered various structural changes that permit its activation through *autophosphorylation* and *oligomerization*, even in absence of ligand. Nevertheless, evidence has been reported of a small number of GISTs where other mechanisms of activation exist as, for example, *PDGFR* mutations, and there are also GISTs in which detection of *c-kit* mutations does not occur, for example, in patients with neurofibromatosis type 1. In absence of ligand, normal KIT protein is a monomer in which certain domains, fundamentally juxtamembrane domain (exon 11), inhibit kinase activity. The activation occurs when stem cell factor interacts with KIT causing its autophosphorylation. This eliminates KIT basal inhibitory structural conformation, which causes a phosphorylation of KIT and of its substrates, triggering at least two important signaling pathways, namely, mitogen-activated protein kinase and AKT, which regulate, in turn, cell survival and proliferation (Figure 2-18). KIT

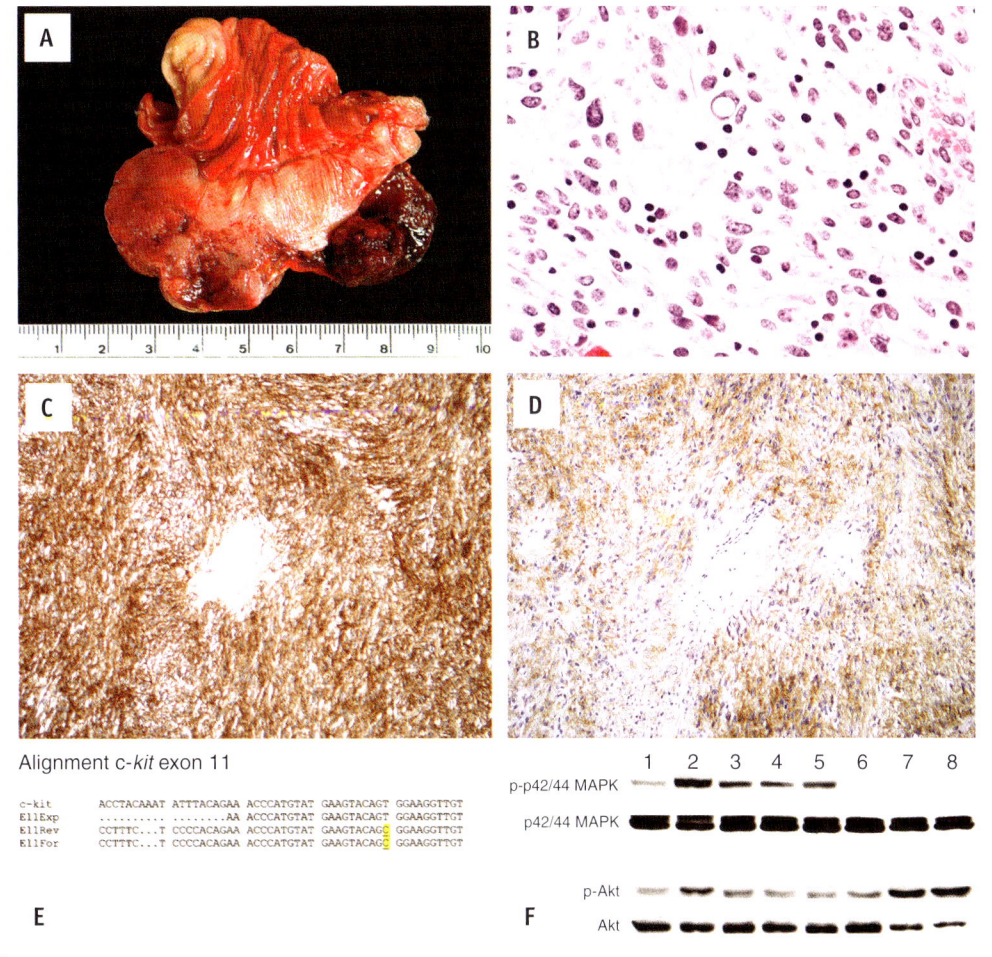

FIGURE 2-18

Molecular pathology of a small-bowel gastrointestinal stromal tumor (GIST) of a 68-year-old woman. **A,** Gross picture showing a fleshy mass invading the wall of the intestine. **B,** The tumor had a high mitotic count and a focally epithelioid appearance. **C,** Tumor cells were immunoreactive with anti-KIT antibody. **D,** Immunoreactivity using a specific antibody to detect phosphorylated (active) KIT (Tyr 703), showing weaker but consistent immunoreactivity. **E,** The tumor had a point mutation in c-*kit* exon 11 (codon 557, T substituted for C). **F,** Western blot analysis showing that the tumor (lane 1) and other GISTs showed activation of mitogen-activated protein kinase (MAPT) and AKT signaling pathways, pointing out other possible therapeutical targets. (**A,** *Courtesy of Dr. Pablo Gonzalvo, Jarrio-Asturias, Spain.*)

TABLE 2-8
Fusion Proteins That Carry Tyrosine Kinase Activity

Tumor	Protein	Response to Imatinib
Dermatofibrosarcoma protuberans	COL1A1-PDGFB*	Yes
Desmoplastic small round cell tumor	EWS-WT1*	Potentially
Infantile fibrosarcoma	ETV6-NTRK3	No
Myofibroblastic inflammatory tumor	TMP3/TPM4/ CLTC2-ALK	No

*Through platelet-derived growth factor (PDGF) receptor signaling.

gain-of-function mutations, as are observed in GIST, can be divided into two large groups: those that affect kinase domains and enzymatic activity, and those that affect regulatory sequences (e.g., juxtamembrane domain) but not enzymatic activity. This difference is important because the use of certain therapeutic molecules to inhibit KIT, such as imatinib (Gleevec), depends on the location of its mutations. Imatinib acts through its binding to kinase or enzymatic domains. Thus, when GISTs have c-*kit* mutations that affect kinase or enzymatic domains, imatinib will not be efficacious because of the absence of an intact kinase domain. In fact, disease-free survival in patients with GIST treated with imatinib is lower if mutations are present in exon 17 of KIT (which encodes for one of the tyrosine kinase domains) rather than if they are present in the juxtamembrane domain (Table 2-8).

SUGGESTED READINGS

Immunohistochemistry

1. Azumi N, Battifora H: The distribution of vimentin and keratin in epithelial and nonepithelial neoplasms. A comprehensive immunohistochemical study on formalin- and alcohol-fixed tumors. Am J Clin Pathol 1987;88:286–296.
2. Bacchi CE, Bonetti F, Pea M, et al: HMB-45. A review. Appl Immunohistochem 1996;73–85.
3. Barnoud R, Sabourin JC, Pasquier D, et al: Immunohistochemical expression of WT1 by desmoplastic small round cell tumor: A comparative study with other small round cell tumors. Am J Surg Pathol 2000;24:830–836.
4. Blay P, Astudillo A, Buesa JM, et al: Protein kinase C theta is highly expressed in gastrointestinal stromal tumors but not in other mesenchymal neoplasias. Clin Cancer Res 2004;10;(12 pt 1):4089–4095.
5. Brown DC, Theaker JM, Banks PM, et al: Cytokeratin expression in smooth muscle and smooth muscle tumours. Histopathology 1987;11:477–486.
6. Busam KJ, Jungbluth AA: Melan-A, a new melanocytic differentiation marker. Adv Anat Pathol 1999;6:12–18.
7. Cassidy M, Loftus B, Whelan A, et al: KP-1: Not a specific marker. Staining of 137 sarcomas, 48 lymphomas, 28 carcinomas, 7 malignant melanomas and 8 cystosarcoma phyllodes. Virchows Arch 1994;424:635–640.
8. Collini P, Sampietro G, Bertulli R, et al: Cytokeratin immunoreactivity in 41 cases of ES/PNET confirmed by molecular diagnostic studies. Am J Surg Pathol 2001;25:273–274.
9. Dei Tos AP, Wadden C, Calonje E, et al: Immunohistochemical demonstration of glycoprotein p30/32(MIC2) (CD99) in synovial sarcoma: A potential cause of diagnostic confusion. Applied Immunohistochemistry 1995;3:168–173.
10. Fanburg-Smith JC, Miettinen M: Angiomatoid "malignant" fibrous histiocytoma: A clinicopathologic study of 158 cases and further exploration of the myoid phenotype. Hum Pathol 1999;30: 1336–1343.
11. Fletcher CD, Berman JJ, Corless C, et al: Diagnosis of gastrointestinal stromal tumors: A consensus approach. Hum Pathol 2002;33: 459–465.
12. Folpe AL: MyoD1 and myogenin expression in human neoplasia: A review and update. Adv Anat Pathol 2002;9:198–203.
13. Folpe AL, Chand EM, Goldblum JR, et al: Expression of Fli-1, a nuclear transcription factor, distinguishes vascular neoplasms from potential mimics. Am J Surg Pathol 2001;25:1061–1066.
14. Folpe AL, Goldblum JR, Rubin BP, et al: Morphologic and immunophenotypic diversity in Ewing family tumors: A study of 66 genetically confirmed cases. Am J Surg Pathol 2005;29:1025–1033.
15. Folpe AL, Schmidt RA, Chapman D, et al: Poorly differentiated synovial sarcoma: Immunohistochemical distinction from primitive neuroectodermal tumors and high-grade malignant peripheral nerve sheath tumors. Am J Surg Pathol 1998;22:673–682.
16. Furlong MA, Mentzel T, Fanburg-Smith JC: Pleomorphic rhabdomyosarcoma in adults: A clinicopathologic study of 38 cases with emphasis on morphologic variants and recent skeletal muscle-specific markers. Mod Pathol 2001;14:595–603.
17. Gerald WL, Miller HK, Battifora H, et al: Intra-abdominal desmoplastic small round-cell tumor. Report of 19 cases of a distinctive type of high-grade polyphenotypic malignancy affecting young individuals. Am J Surg Pathol 1991;15:499–513.
18. Gown AM, Vogel AM, Hoak D, et al: Monoclonal antibodies specific for melanocytic tumors distinguish subpopulations of melanocytes. Am J Pathol 1986;123:195–203.
19. Gray MH, Rosenberg AE, Dickersin GR, et al: Cytokeratin expression in epithelioid vascular neoplasms. Hum Pathol 1990;21:212–217.
20. Gu M, Antonescu CR, Guiter G, et al: Cytokeratin immunoreactivity in Ewing's sarcoma: Prevalence in 50 cases confirmed by molecular diagnostic studies. Am J Surg Pathol 2000;24:410–416.
21. Guillou L, Wadden C, Kraus MD, et al: S-100 protein reactivity in synovial sarcomas: A potentially frequent diagnostic pitfall. Immunohistochemistry 1996;4:167–175.
22. Hill DA, Pfeifer JD, Marley EF, et al: WT1 staining reliably differentiates desmoplastic small round cell tumor from Ewing sarcoma/primitive neuroectodermal tumor. An immunohistochemical and molecular diagnostic study. Am J Clin Pathol 2000;114:345–353.
23. Hoot AC, Russo P, Judkins AR, et al: Immunohistochemical analysis of hSNF5/INI1 distinguishes renal and extra-renal malignant rhabdoid tumors from other pediatric soft tissue tumors. Am J Surg Pathol 2004;28:1485–1491.
24. Hornick JL, Fletcher CD: Immunohistochemical staining for KIT (CD117) in soft tissue sarcomas is very limited in distribution. Am J Clin Pathol 2002;117:188–193.
25. Kahn HJ, Marks A, Thom H, et al: Role of antibody to S100 protein in diagnostic pathology. Am J Clin Pathol 1983;79:341–347.
26. Meis-Kindblom JM, Kindblom LG: Angiosarcoma of soft tissue: A study of 80 cases. Am J Surg Pathol 1998;22:683–697.
27. Miettinen M: Immunoreactivity for cytokeratin and epithelial membrane antigen in leiomyosarcoma. Arch Pathol Lab Med 1988;112:637–640.
28. Miettinen M: Keratin subsets in spindle cell sarcomas. Keratins are widespread but synovial sarcoma contains a distinctive keratin polypeptide pattern and desmoplakins. Am J Pathol 1991;138:505–513.
29. Miettinen M, Fanburg-Smith JC, Virolainen M, et al: Epithelioid sarcoma: An immunohistochemical analysis of 112 classical and variant cases and a discussion of the differential diagnosis. Hum Pathol 1999;30:934–942.
30. Motegi A, Sakurai S, Nakayama H, et al: PKC theta, a novel immunohistochemical marker for gastrointestinal stromal tumors (GIST), especially useful for identifying KIT-negative tumors. Pathol Int 2005;55:106–112.

31. Ordonez NG: Desmoplastic small round cell tumor: II: An ultrastructural and immunohistochemical study with emphasis on new immunohistochemical markers. Am J Surg Pathol 1998;22:1314–1327.
32. Parham DM, Dias P, Kelly DR, et al: Desmin positivity in primitive neuroectodermal tumors of childhood. Am J Surg Pathol 1992;16:483–492.
33. Parham DM, Webber B, Holt H, et al: Immunohistochemical study of childhood rhabdomyosarcomas and related neoplasms. Results of an Intergroup Rhabdomyosarcoma study project. Cancer 1991;67:3072–3080.
34. Perry A, Fuller CE, Judkins AR, et al: INI1 expression is retained in composite rhabdoid tumors, including rhabdoid meningiomas. Mod Pathol 2005;18:951–958.
35. Rangdaeng S, Truong LD: Comparative immunohistochemical staining for desmin and muscle-specific actin. A study of 576 cases. Am J Clin Pathol 1991;96:32–45.
36. Rossi S, Orvieto E, Furlanetto A, et al: Utility of the immunohistochemical detection of FLI-1 expression in round cell and vascular neoplasm using a monoclonal antibody. Mod Pathol 2004;17:547–552.
37. Sebire NJ, Gibson S, Rampling D, et al: Immunohistochemical findings in embryonal small round cell tumors with molecular diagnostic confirmation. Appl Immunohistochem Mol Morphol 2005;13:1–5.
38. Stevenson A, Chatten J, Bertoni F, et al: CD99 (p30/32MIC2) Neuroectodermal/Ewing's sarcoma antigen as an immunohistochemical marker. Review of more than 600 tumors and the literature experience. Appl Immunohistochem 1994;2:231–240.
39. Truong LD, Rangdaeng S, Cagle P, et al: The diagnostic utility of desmin. A study of 584 cases and review of the literature. Am J Clin Pathol 1990;93:305–314.
40. van de Rijn M, Rouse R: CD34: A review. Appl Immunohistochem 1994;2:71–80.
41. Wang NP, Marx J, McNutt MA, et al: Expression of myogenic regulatory proteins (myogenin and MyoD1) in small blue round cell tumors of childhood. Am J Pathol 1995;147:1799–1810.
42. Weiss SW, Langloss JM, Enzinger FM: Value of S-100 protein in the diagnosis of soft tissue tumors with particular reference to benign and malignant Schwann cell tumors. Lab Invest 1983;49:299–308.
43. Weiss SW, Nickoloff BJ: CD-34 is expressed by a distinctive cell population in peripheral nerve, nerve sheath tumors, and related lesions. Am J Surg Pathol 1993;17:1039–1045.
44. Westra WH, Gerald WL, Rosai J: Solitary fibrous tumor. Consistent CD34 immunoreactivity and occurrence in the orbit. Am J Surg Pathol 1994;18:992–998.
45. White W, Shiu MH, Rosenblum MK, et al: Cellular schwannoma. A clinicopathologic study of 57 patients and 58 tumors. Cancer 1990;66:1266–1275.
46. Zarbo RJ, Gown AM, Nagle RB, et al: Anomalous cytokeratin expression in malignant melanoma: One- and two-dimensional western blot analysis and immunohistochemical survey of 100 melanomas. Mod Pathol 1990;3:494–501.

Molecular Pathology

1. Antonescu CR, Tschernyavsky SJ, Woodruff JM, et al: Molecular diagnosis of clear cell sarcoma: Detection of EWS-ATF1 and MITF-M transcripts and histopathological and ultrastructural analysis of 12 cases. J Mol Diagn 2002;4:44–52.
2. Antonescu CR, Viale A, Sarran L, et al: Gene expression in gastrointestinal stromal tumors is distinguished by KIT genotype and anatomic site. Clin Cancer Res 2004;10:3282–3290.
3. Bennicelli JL, Barr FG: Chromosomal translocations and sarcomas. Curr Opin Oncol 2002;14:412–419.
4. Blay P, Astudillo A, Buesa JM, et al: Protein kinase C theta is highly expressed in gastrointestinal stromal tumors but not in other mesenchymal neoplasias. Clin Cancer Res 2004;10:4089–4095.
5. Cook JR, Dehner LP, Collins MH, et al: Anaplastic lymphoma kinase (ALK) expression in the inflammatory myofibroblastic tumor: A comparative immunohistochemical study. Am J Surg Pathol 2001;25:1364–1371.
6. de Alava E: Transcripts, transcripts, everywhere. Adv Anat Pathol 2001;8:264–272.
7. de Alava E, Gerald WL: Molecular biology of the Ewing's sarcoma/primitive neuroectodermal tumor family. J Clin Oncol 2000;18:204–213.
8. de Alava E, Kawai A, Healey JH, et al: EWS-FLI1 fusion transcript structure is an independent determinant of prognosis in Ewing's sarcoma. J Clin Oncol 1998;16:1248–1255.
9. Guillou L, Coindre J, Gallagher G, et al: Detection of the synovial sarcoma translocation t(X;18) (SYT;SSX) in paraffin-embedded tissues using reverse transcriptase-polymerase chain reaction: A reliable and powerful diagnostic tool for pathologists. A molecular analysis of 221 mesenchymal tumors fixed in different fixatives. Hum Pathol 2001;32:105–112.
10. Heinrich MC, Corless CL, Duensing A, et al: PDGFRA activating mutations in gastrointestinal stromal tumors. Science 2003;299:708–710.
11. Heinrich MC, Rubin BP, Longley BJ, et al: Biology and genetic aspects of gastrointestinal stromal tumors: KIT activation and cytogenetic alterations. Hum Pathol 2002;33:484–495.
12. Kawai A, Woodruff J, Healey JH, et al: SYT-SSX gene fusion as a determinant of morphology and prognosis in synovial sarcoma. N Engl J Med 1998;338:153–160.
13. Kumar S, Pack S, Kumar D, et al: Detection of EWS-FLI-1 fusion in Ewing's sarcoma/peripheral primitive neuroectodermal tumor by fluorescence in situ hybridization using formalin-fixed paraffin-embedded tissue. Hum Pathol 1999;30:324–330.
14. Ladanyi M, Bridge JA: Contribution of molecular genetic data to the classification of sarcomas. Hum Pathol 2000;31:532–538.
15. Ladanyi M, Chan WC, Triche TJ, et al: Expression profiling of human tumors: The end of surgical pathology?. J Mol Diagn 2001;3:92–97.
16. Nielsen TO, West RB, Linn SC, et al: Molecular characterisation of soft tissue tumours: A gene expression study. Lancet 2002;359:1301–1307.
17. Oliveira AM, Hsi BL, Weremowicz S, et al: USP6 (Tre2) fusion oncogenes in aneurysmal bone cyst. Cancer Res 2004;64:1920–1923.
18. Schleiermacher G, Peter M, Oberlin O, et al: Increased risk of systemic relapses associated with bone marrow micrometastasis and circulating tumor cells in localized Ewing tumor. J Clin Oncol 2003;21:85–91.
19. Segal NH, Pavlidis P, Noble WS, et al: Classification of clear-cell sarcoma as a subtype of melanoma by genomic profiling. J Clin Oncol 2003;21:1775–1781.
20. Singer S, Rubin BP, Lux ML, et al: Prognostic value of KIT mutation type, mitotic activity, and histologic subtype in gastrointestinal stromal tumors. J Clin Oncol 2002;20:3898–3905.
21. Sorensen PH, Lynch JC, Qualman SJ, et al: PAX3-FKHR and PAX7-FKHR gene fusions are prognostic indicators in alveolar rhabdomyosarcoma: A report from the children's oncology group. J Clin Oncol 2002;20:2672–2679.
22. Tognon C, Knezevich SR, Huntsman D, et al: Expression of the ETV6-NTRK3 gene fusion as a primary event in human secretory breast carcinoma. Cancer Cell 2002;2:367–376.
23. Tuveson DA, Fletcher JA: Signal transduction pathways in sarcoma as targets for therapeutic intervention. Curr Opin Oncol 2001;13:249–255.
24. van de Rijn M, Rubin BP: Gene expression studies on soft tissue tumors. Am J Pathol 2002;161:1531–1534.
25. West RB, Corless CL, Chen X, et al: The novel marker, DOG1, is expressed ubiquitously in gastrointestinal stromal tumors irrespective of KIT or PDGFRA mutation status. Am J Pathol 2004;165:107–113.

Section II

Soft Tissue Pathology

3 Fibroblastic and Fibrohistiocytic Tumors
Louis Guillou · Andrew L. Folpe

4 Adipocytic Tumors
Angelo Paolo Dei Tos

5 Smooth Muscle Tumors
Andrea T. Deyrup

6 Skeletal Muscle Tumors
Raf Sciot

7 Tumor of Perivascular Cells
Andrew L. Folpe · Louis Guillou

8 Gastrointestinal Stromal Tumor
Brian P. Rubin

9 Vascular Tumors of Soft Tissue
Andrew L. Folpe

10 Nerve Sheath and Neuroectodermal Tumors
Julie C. Fanburg-Smith

11 Osteocartilaginous Tumors
John X. O'Connell

12 Tumors of Synovial Tissue
G. Petur Nielsen · John X. O'Connell

13 Tumors of Miscellaneous Type or Uncertain Lineage
Andrew L. Folpe

3 Fibroblastic and Fibrohistiocytic Tumors

Louis Guillou · Andrew L. Folpe

FIBROBLASTIC/MYOFIBROBLASTIC TUMORS
- Introduction
- Nodular Fasciitis and Variants (Ossifying Fasciitis, Cranial Fasciitis, Intravascular Fasciitis, Proliferative Fasciitis, Proliferative Myositis, Ischemic Fasciitis)
- Fibroma of Tendon Sheath
- Elastofibroma
- Fibrous Hamartoma of Infancy
- Calcifying Aponeurotic Fibroma
- Superficial Fibromatoses
- Deep (Desmoid-Type) Fibromatoses
- Inflammatory Myofibroblastic Tumor/Inflammatory Fibrosarcoma
- Myxoinflammatory Fibroblastic Sarcoma (Inflammatory Myxohyaline Tumor of Distal Extremities with Reed–Sternberg or Virocyte-like Cells, Acral Myxoinflammatory Fibroblastic Sarcoma)
- Adult Fibrosarcoma and Variants (Low-Grade Fibromyxoid Sarcoma/Hyalinizing Spindle Cell Tumor with Giant Rosettes, Sclerosing Epithelioid Fibrosarcoma, Myxofibrosarcoma)
- Infantile Fibrosarcoma

FIBROHISTIOCYTIC TUMORS
- Introduction
- Benign Fibrous Histiocytomas and Variants
- Juvenile Xanthogranuloma and Reticulohistiocytoma
- Xanthoma
- Atypical Fibroxanthoma
- Dermatofibrosarcoma Protuberans (Including Bednar Tumor and Giant Cell Fibroblastoma)
- Angiomatoid (Malignant) Fibrous Histiocytoma
- Plexiform Fibrohistiocytic Tumor
- Soft Tissue Giant Cell Tumor (of Low Malignant Potential)
- Undifferentiated Pleomorphic Sarcoma (So-Called Pleomorphic Malignant Fibrous Histiocytoma, Including Giant-Cell and Inflammatory Variants)

FIBROBLASTIC/MYOFIBROBLASTIC TUMORS

INTRODUCTION

The group of fibroblastic/myofibroblastic tumors encompasses those tumors that are essentially composed of fibroblasts and myofibroblasts (Box 3-1).

NODULAR FASCIITIS AND VARIANTS (Ossifying Fasciitis, Cranial Fasciitis, Intravascular Fasciitis, Proliferative Fasciitis, Proliferative Myositis, Ischemic Fasciitis)

Nodular fasciitis is a common, self-limiting, pseudosarcomatous reactive process that is mainly composed of fibroblasts and myofibroblasts. The morphologic variants of nodular fasciitis are discussed briefly below.

CLINICAL FEATURES

Nodular fasciitis is a common, solitary, subcutaneous lesion that occurs mostly in young and middle-aged adults (20 to 50 years of age), with no sex predilection. Patients describe a small (< 2 to 3 cm), sometimes painful mass that develops rapidly (often < 1 month). It can be seen anywhere in the body but is most common in the upper extremities (50% of cases), especially in the subcutaneous tissue of the forearm. It is infrequent in hands and feet, and rare in more unusual locations (e.g., vulva, lymph node capsule, parotid gland, dermis). A previous history of trauma is given in 10% to 20% of cases.

Box 3-1: MAIN HISTOLOGIC TUMOR TYPES AND SUBTYPES IN THE FIBROBLASTIC/MYOFIBROBLASTIC TUMOR CATEGORY

Nodular fasciitis
Proliferative fasciitis
Proliferative myositis
Ischemic fasciitis (atypical decubital fibroplasia)
Myositis ossificans/fibroosseous pseudotumor of digits
Elastofibroma
Fibrous hamartoma of infancy
Myofibroma/myofibromatosis
Fibromatosis colli*
Juvenile hyaline fibromatosis*
Inclusion body (digital) fibromatosis*
Fibroma of tendon sheath
Desmoplastic fibroblastoma (collagenous fibroma)*
Mammary-type fibroblastoma*
Calcifying aponeurotic fibroma
Angiomyofibroblastoma*
Cellular angiofibroma*
Nasopharyngeal angiofibroma*
Nuchal-type fibroma*
Gardner fibroma*
Calcifying fibrous pseudotumor*
Giant cell angiofibroma
Pleomorphic fibroma of skin*
Superficial fibromatosis
Deep-desmoid–type fibromatosis
Lipofibromatosis*
Solitary fibrous tumor of soft tissues
Inflammatory myofibroblastic tumor, inflammatory fibrosarcoma
Low-grade myofibroblastic sarcoma*
Myxoinflammatory fibroblastic sarcoma (inflammatory myxohyaline tumor)
Infantile fibrosarcoma
Adult fibrosarcoma
Myxofibrosarcoma
Low-grade fibromyxoid sarcoma (and hyalinizing spindle cell tumor with giant rosettes)
Sclerosing epithelioid fibrosarcoma

*These entities will not be considered in this chapter because of their rarity.

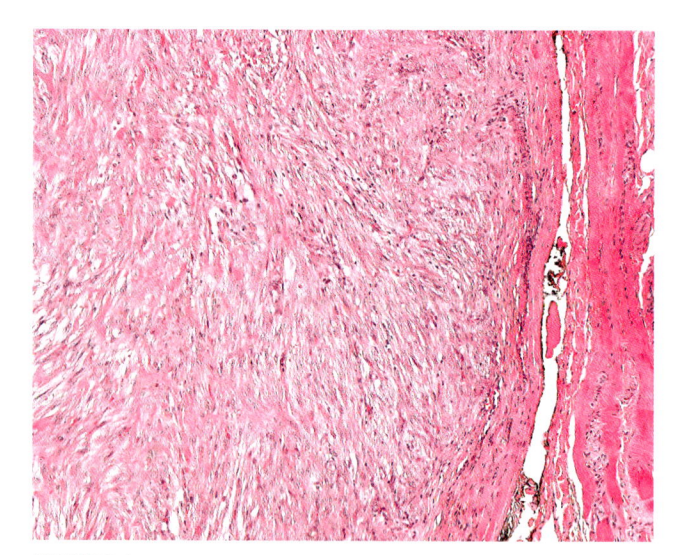

FIGURE 3-1
Nodular fasciitis presenting as a 3.5-cm, well-circumscribed, nonencapsulated intramuscular nodule in the left thigh of a 13-year-old boy.

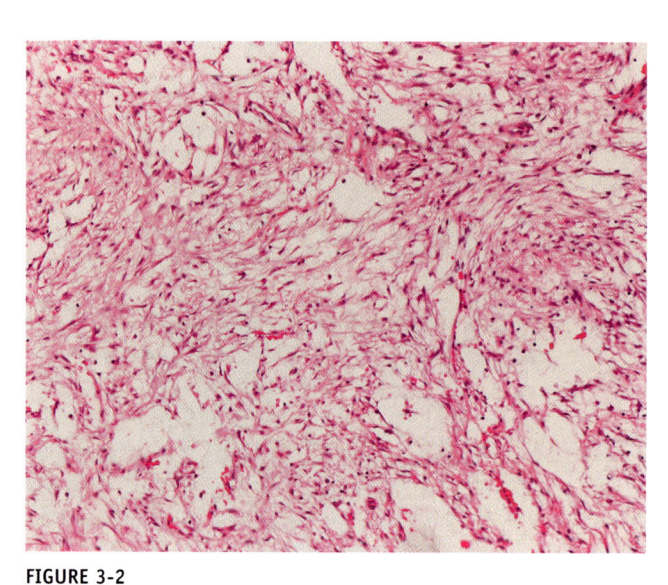

FIGURE 3-2
Nodular fasciitis.
Loosely textured fascicles of nonatypical myofibroblasts with microcysts containing histiocytes.

PATHOLOGIC FEATURES

GROSS FINDINGS

Nodular fasciitis presents as a solitary, well-circumscribed but nonencapsulated, nodule usually less than 3 cm in diameter (Figure 3-1). This nodule is often found within the fibrous septa of the deep subcutis, although deep soft tissues can be involved; in this location (intramuscular), it tends to be larger than its subcutaneous counterpart. On section, recently developed lesions have a myxoid appearance, whereas old lesions are more fibrous and firmer.

MICROSCOPIC FINDINGS

The morphology of nodular fasciitis varies according to the age of the lesion. Early lesions are usually variably cellular, consisting of fibroblasts and myofibroblasts arranged in short, irregular fascicles, set in a loosely textured myxoid matrix (feathery pattern) (Figure 3-2). The cells are plump, with abundant eosinophilic, somewhat fibrillary cytoplasm, resembling cell cultures or granulation tissue. Nuclei are often vesicular and contain a single prominent nucleolus (Figure 3-3). Mitoses can be numerous but almost never abnormal. The lesion tends to extend along the fibrous septa from which it arises, and is often surrounded and infiltrated by numerous inflammatory elements (lymphoid aggregates, plasma cells). It may also contain numerous, centripetally oriented capillaries. Cystic change, interstitial hemorrhage, and minute collections of intralesional histiocytes are quite frequent. Long-standing lesions are less cellular and more fibrotic, containing areas of marked hyaline fibrosis

CHAPTER 3 Fibroblastic and Fibrohistiocytic Tumors

NODULAR FASCIITIS—FACT SHEET

Definition
- A pseudosarcomatous, self-limiting, reactive process composed of fibroblasts and myofibroblasts

Incidence and Location
- Common, mostly subcutaneous, soft tissue lesion
- Upper extremities, trunk, head, and neck most frequently affected

Morbidity and Mortality
- Benign, self-limiting process

Sex, Race, and Age Distribution
- More common in young adults
- No race or sex predilection

Clinical Features
- Rapidly growing (1 to 2 months), sometimes painful nodule

Radiologic Features
- Calcifications in a soft tissue mass may be possible

Prognosis and Treatment
- Benign process
- Local recurrences < 2%
- Simple excision is curative

NODULAR FASCIITIS—PATHOLOGIC FEATURES

Gross Findings
- 2- to 3-cm, solitary, well-circumscribed nodule
- Myxoid appearance of early/active lesions; old lesions are more fibrous

Microscopic Findings
- Variably cellular, fascicular proliferation of fibroblasts and myofibroblasts
- Usually grows along fibrous septa of hypodermis
- Myxoid (early lesions) to collagenized (long-standing lesions) extracellular matrix
- Mitoses often numerous, especially in young lesions; abnormal mitoses absent
- Inflammation prominent around the lesion
- Osteoclast-like multinucleated giant cells in 10% of cases

Genetics
- Usually diploid

Immunohistochemical Findings
- Myofibroblasts: diffusely positive for smooth muscle actin, muscle-specific actin (clone HHF35), and calponin; focally positive for desmin; mostly negative for h-caldesmon and S=100 protein

Differential Diagnosis
- Nodular fasciitis, cellular phase with myxoid changes: myxoma, myxofibrosarcoma, malignant peripheral nerve sheath tumor (MPNST), myxoid dermatofibrosarcoma
- Nodular fasciitis, cellular phase without myxoid changes: fibrous histiocytoma, cellular schwannoma, fibrosarcoma, leiomyosarcoma, spindle cell carcinoma, spindle cell melanoma
- Nodular fasciitis, fibrotic phase: fibroma, desmoplastic fibroblastoma, neurofibroma
- Nodular fasciitis with ganglion-like cells: rhabdomyosarcoma, pleomorphic sarcomas, ganglioneuroblastoma
- Ossifying nodular fasciitis: osteosarcoma
- Ischemic fasciitis: myxofibrosarcoma, epithelioid sarcoma

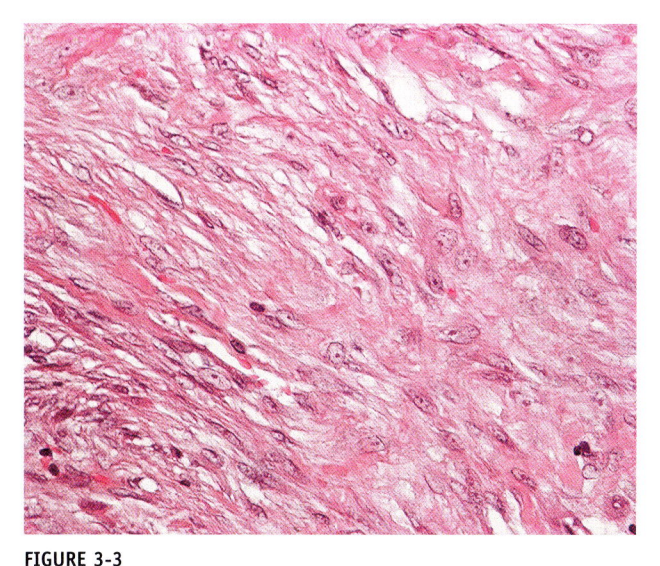

and, sometimes, cystic change. About 10% of nodular fasciitis contains osteoclast-like multinucleated giant cells. By definition, bone metaplasia is a prominent feature of ossifying fasciitis and parosteal fasciitis but may also be observed in cranial or conventional (nodular) fasciitis.

VARIANTS OF NODULAR FASCIITIS

Ossifying fasciitis (also called *fasciitis ossificans*) is simply a variant of fasciitis that contains foci of metaplastic bone. *Cranial fasciitis* develops from the galea aponeurotica, occurring mostly in male infants during the first year of life. It may erode and even penetrate the underlying bone, and is visible on plain radiographs as a lytic lesion of the calvarium. *Intravascular fasciitis* is a rare variant of fasciitis that grows into and obstructs medium-size veins and, less often, arteries. It may have a multinodular growth pattern inside the same vessel. It is mostly observed in the subcutaneous tissue of the upper limbs or in the head and neck.

Proliferative fasciitis and *proliferative myositis* are similar to nodular fasciitis but contain ganglion-like myofibroblastic cells. Proliferative fasciitis is usually seen in the subcutaneous tissue of the upper limbs of middle-aged adults (40 to 60 years), whereas proliferative myositis mainly affects the muscles of the trunk and shoulder girdle. The key feature of these two lesions is the presence,

FIGURE 3-3
Nodular fasciitis.
Myofibroblast nuclei are vesicular and contain a single central nucleolus.

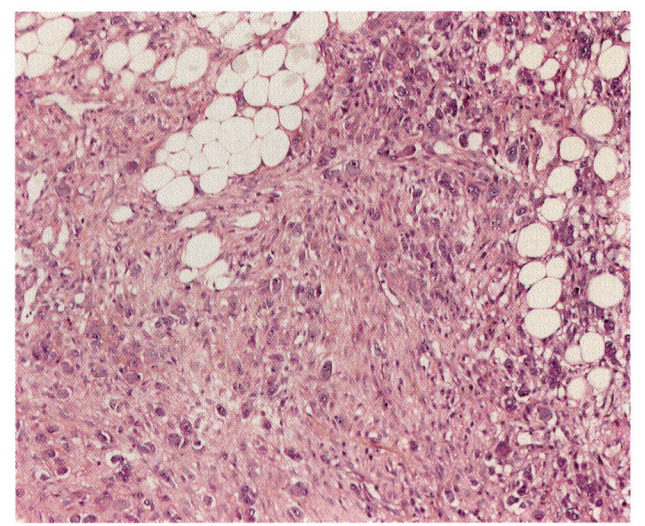

FIGURE 3-4
Proliferative fasciitis.
Ganglion-like giant cells are readily visible, set in a collagenous matrix.

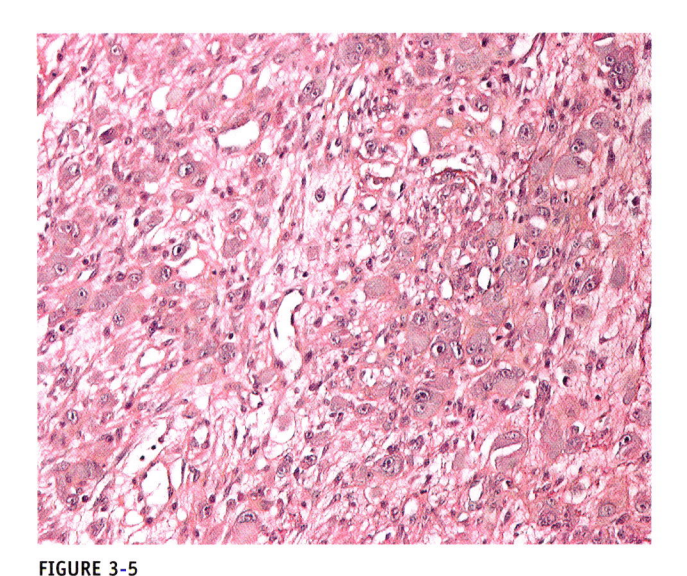

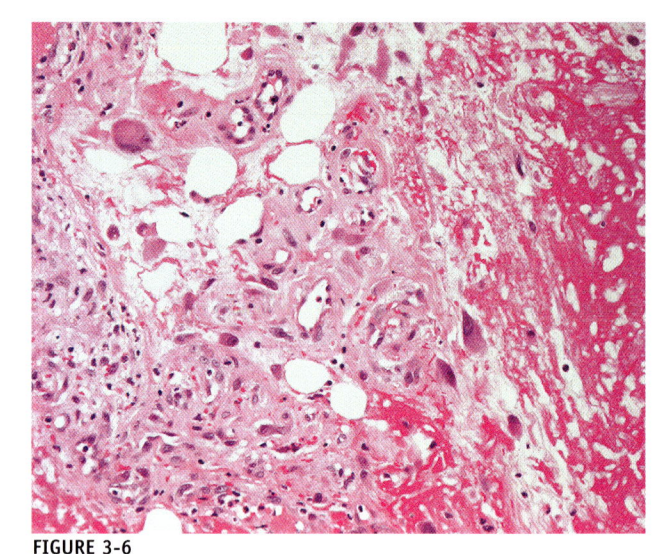

FIGURE 3-6
Ischemic fasciitis.
Fibrin deposition is visible in addition to other features of nodular/proliferative fasciitis, including ganglion-like cells.

FIGURE 3-5
Proliferative fasciitis.
Uninucleated or binucleated ganglion-like cells with abundant basophilic cytoplasm, vesicular nuclei, and prominent central nucleoli.

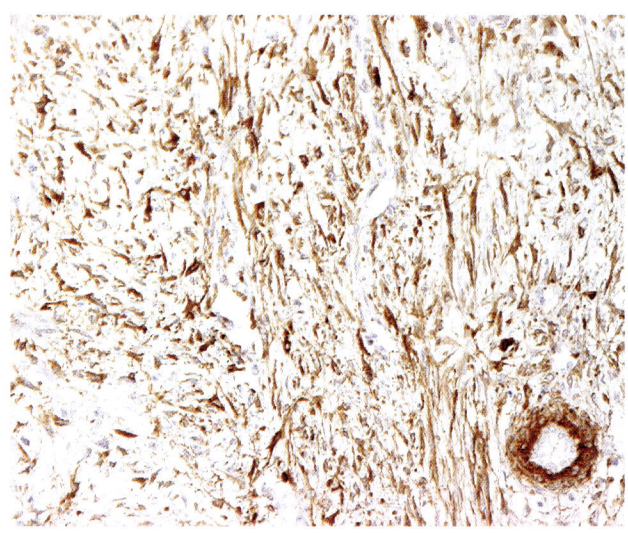

FIGURE 3-7
Nodular fasciitis.
Myofibroblasts are strongly and diffusely positive for smooth muscle actin.

in addition to the other features of nodular fasciitis, of ganglion-like myofibroblasts, having abundant basophilic cytoplasm and one or two, often eccentric, vesicular nuclei with prominent nucleoli (Figures 3-4 and 3-5). They tend to form small clusters. In children, proliferative fasciitis may be cellular and mitotically active, consisting almost exclusively of ganglion-like cells, and may thus mimic rhabdomyosarcoma or epithelioid sarcoma. In proliferative myositis, areas of fibroblastic tissue containing ganglion-like cells alternate with foci of atrophic skeletal muscle to give a typical *checkerboard* pattern. *Ischemic fasciitis* (also called *atypical decubital fibroplasia*) may be considered a variant of proliferative fasciitis. This lesion usually involves the soft tissues overlying bony prominences such as the shoulder, the chest wall, and the sacrococcygeal and greater trochanter regions. It occurs mainly in elderly (70 to 90 years) and physically debilitated or immobilized patients, and may present as a large (< 10 cm) mass. Histologically, it characteristically contains a central zone of fibrinoid necrosis, surrounded by areas resembling proliferative and nodular fasciitis (Figure 3-6).

ANCILLARY STUDIES

IMMUNOHISTOCHEMISTRY

Myofibroblasts in nodular fasciitis are usually strongly, diffusely positive for smooth muscle actin (Figure 3-7), muscle-specific actin (clone HHF35), and calponin, and focally for desmin. H-caldesmon and S-100 protein are usually not expressed. Occasional reactivity for epithelial markers (cytokeratins, epithelial membrane antigen (EMA), or both) is observed in visceral lesions. The ganglion-like cells in proliferative fasciitis and myositis are often negative for muscle markers and express vimentin only.

GENETICS

Assessment of DNA ploidy in nodular fasciitis and related lesions has revealed a diploid pattern in most cases.

DIFFERENTIAL DIAGNOSIS

Because nodular fasciitis is so highly proliferative, it is commonly mistaken for a sarcoma. Predominantly, myxoid lesions are likely to be confused with myxofibrosarcoma (myxoid malignant fibrous histiocytoma), highly cellular lesions may resemble conventional undifferentiated pleomorphic sarcoma (malignant fibrous histiocytoma), and lesions containing ganglion-like cells or rhabdomyoblast-like cells can mimic embryonal or pleomorphic rhabdomyosarcoma and other pleomorphic sarcomas. Importantly, nodular fasciitis tends to be small and superficial, whereas most sarcomas are large and deeply situated. Important clues to the diagnosis of nodular fascitis include the short, randomly arranged fascicles, the absence of a well-developed thick-walled vasculature, the absence of nuclear pleomorphism or hyperchromatism, and the presence of microcystic change. Intravascular forms of nodular fasciitis commonly contain osteoclast-like giant cells and may resemble giant cell tumors of soft parts; the absence of associated metaplastic bone and the predominantly intravascular growth pattern are useful clues that favor a diagnosis of intravascular fasciitis. Long-standing, predominantly fibrous or hyalinized lesions may mimic various benign fibroblastic lesions, such as fibroma of tendon sheath or desmoplastic fibroma (collagenous fibroma), or even chondroid tumors, such as extraskeletal myxoid chondrosarcoma. Attention to areas of typical nodular fasciitis should allow for the resolution of this differential diagnosis in most cases without great difficulty.

PROGNOSIS AND TREATMENT

Nodular fasciitis is a benign, self-limiting, reactive process. Simple excision is the treatment of choice. Local recurrences are exceptional (less than 2% of cases).

FIBROMA OF TENDON SHEATH

Fibroma of tendon sheath is a benign fibroblastic proliferation of the tendon sheath. It may represent a site-specific variant of nodular fasciitis.

CLINICAL FEATURES

Fibroma of tendon sheath typically presents as a relatively small (< 3 cm), long-standing, firm mass of the distal extremities, particularly the hands. Most patients are between 20 and 50 years of age.

PATHOLOGIC FEATURES

GROSS FINDINGS

Fibroma of tendon sheath presents as a firm, fibrous mass with a vaguely lobular appearance, reminiscent of giant cell tumor of tendon sheath. Pigmentation is absent, however.

MICROSCOPIC FINDINGS

The lesion is well-circumscribed and vaguely lobular, and is composed of bland fibroblastic cells embedded in a collagenized background. Small areas of more cellular spindle cell proliferation may be present, essentially identical to nodular fasciitis. Elongated, cleft-like spaces lined by flattened cells are typically present (Figure 3-8).

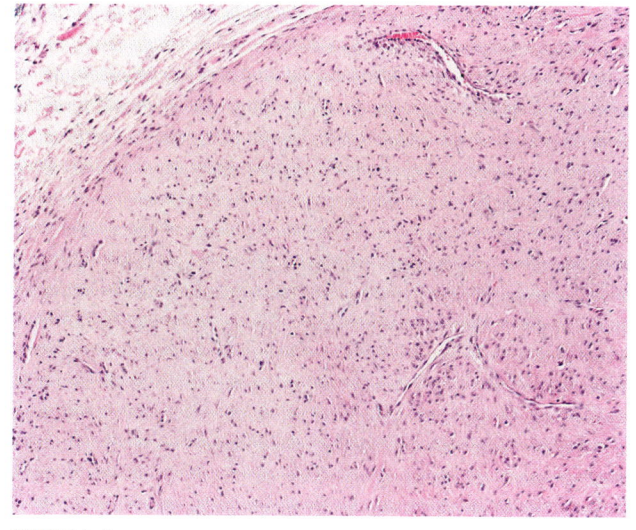

FIGURE 3-8

Fibroma of tendon sheath, consisting of well-circumscribed nodule of bland myofibroblastic cells, with characteristic crescentic vascular spaces.

FIBROMA OF TENDON SHEATH—FACT SHEET
Definition
▸▸ A fibrous lesion observed in a tendon sheath
Incidence and Location
▸▸ Infrequent
▸▸ Mostly hands (tendon sheaths)
Morbidity and Mortality
▸▸ Benign
▸▸ Recurrence in up to 20% to 25% of cases
Sex, Race, and Age Distribution
▸▸ Primarily adult men (20 to 50 years of age)
Clinical Features
▸▸ Well-circumscribed, painless nodule
▸▸ Sometimes finger triggering/pain
Prognosis and Treatment
▸▸ Benign
▸▸ May recur (up to 20% to 25% of cases)
▸▸ Do not metastasize
▸▸ Excision/reexcision usually curative

FIBROMA OF TENDON SHEATH—PATHOLOGIC FEATURES
Gross Findings
▸▸ Small (0.5 to 2 cm), well-circumscribed nodule
Microscopic Findings
▸▸ Multilobulated architecture
▸▸ Hypocellular, fibrous appearance but variations in cellularity possible
▸▸ Contains thin-walled curvilinear vessels or stromal clefts
Immunohistochemical Findings
▸▸ Reactivity for vimentin
▸▸ Focal reactivity for smooth muscle actin possible
▸▸ Negativity for desmin, CD34, keratins, and S-100 protein
Differential Diagnosis
▸▸ Nodular fasciitis
▸▸ Fibrous histiocytoma
▸▸ Superficial fibromatosis
▸▸ Localized giant cell tumor of tendon sheath with few giant cells

Rare cases may show degenerative cytologic atypia (pleomorphic fibroma of tendon sheath). Microcystic change, as seen in nodular fasciitis, is typically absent; when present, the distinction from nodular fasciitis may be difficult if not arbitrary.

ANCILLARY STUDIES

IMMUNOHISTOCHEMISTRY

Fibroma of tendon sheath is a predominantly myofibroblastic lesion and shows an immunophenotype identical to nodular fasciitis, with expression of muscle actins and vimentin but usually not desmin.

GENETIC FINDINGS

Fibromas of tendon sheath have been reported to contain translocations involving the long arm of chromosome 2, including t(2;11)(q31-32;q12).

DIFFERENTIAL DIAGNOSIS

Fibroma of tendon sheath tends to lack the short, randomly arranged cellular fascicles and the microcystic change seen in classic examples of nodular fasciitis. It does, however, closely resemble more hyalinized examples of fasciitis, and may, in fact, represent a site-specific variant. Benign fibrous histiocytomas lack a lobular growth pattern, show peripheral collagen trapping, and often contain *secondary elements,* such as siderophages, multinucleated giant cells, and foamy macrophages. Giant cell tumors of tendon sheath are composed principally of rounded histiocyte-like cells, admixed with larger eosinophilic cells, siderophages, foamy macrophages, and osteoclast-like giant cells. Superficial fibromatoses are infiltrative, cellular tumors that typically arise from the palmar or plantar soft tissues, rather than the tendon sheath.

PROGNOSIS AND TREATMENT

Fibroma of tendon sheath is entirely benign and requires only simple excision.

ELASTOFIBROMA

CLINICAL FEATURES

Elastofibroma is a fibroclastic soft tissue pseudotumor of elderly persons (60 to 70 years) that develops in the connective tissues between the lower scapula and the chest wall. Repetitive trauma is thought to be causative, with many patients reporting a history of intensive manual work. Elastofibroma is more frequent in women than in men, and can be bilateral. It presents as a slow-growing, generally painless soft tissue mass.

CHAPTER 3 Fibroblastic and Fibrohistiocytic Tumors

ELASTOFIBROMA—FACT SHEET

Definition
▸ A fibroelastic soft tissue pseudotumor containing large, round or ragged, elastic fiber fragments

Location
▸ Connective tissue between lower scapula and chest wall

Morbidity and Mortality
▸ Benign process
▸ Repetitive trauma as causative factor

Sex, Race, and Age Distribution
▸ More frequent in women
▸ Elderly patients (60 to 70 years)

Clinical Features
▸ Slow-growing, generally painless soft tissue mass

Radiologic Features
▸ Poorly circumscribed fibrofatty mass

Prognosis and Treatment
▸ Benign, nonrecurring lesion
▸ Simple excision curative

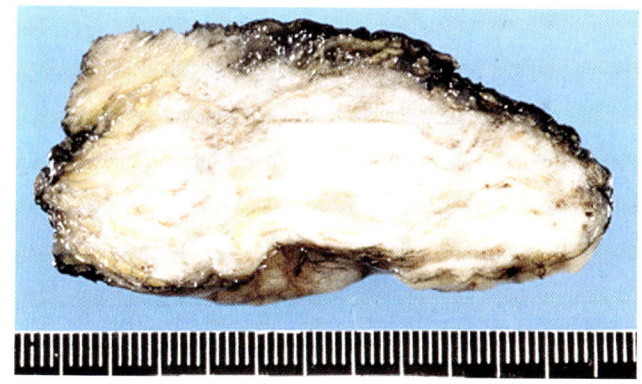

ELASTOFIBROMA—PATHOLOGIC FEATURES

Gross Findings
▸ Median size: 6 to 8 cm
▸ Cut section: whitish fibrous areas interspersed with mature adipose tissue

Microscopic Findings
▸ Mixture of eosinophilic, bead-like, or jagged elastic fiber fragments, fibrous tissue, and mature adipose tissue

Differential Diagnosis
▸ Fibroma
▸ Desmoplastic fibroblastoma

FIGURE 3-9
Elastofibroma.
Characteristic intimate admixture of fibrous and adipocytic areas.

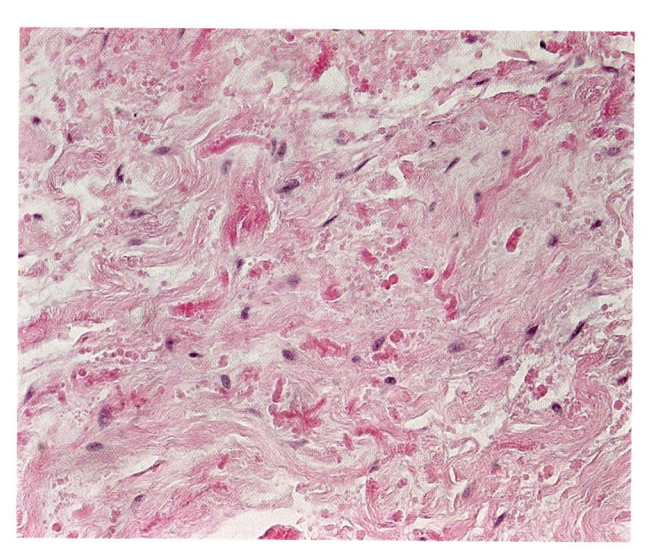

FIGURE 3-10
Elastofibroma.
Fibroadipocytic tissue containing numerous large, fragmented elastic fibers.

PATHOLOGIC FEATURES

GROSS FINDINGS

Elastofibromas measure 5 to 10 cm in maximal diameter. On sectioning, the lesion is composed of mature adipose tissue intermixed with whitish firm fibrous tissue (Figure 3-9).

MICROSCOPIC FINDINGS

The cardinal feature is the presence of numerous large, eosinophilic, fragmented elastic fibers, forming round or jagged beads in aggregates or cords, scattered throughout a hypocellular myxocollagenous stroma admixed with some mature adipose tissue (Figure 3-10). Myxoid and even cystic change can be observed in the nonfatty component. This nonencapsulated lesion may infiltrate adjacent tissues (skeletal muscle, periosteum, or both).

ANCILLARY STUDIES

Elastin stains may help in identifying the fragmented elastic fibers (Figure 3-11).

DIFFERENTIAL DIAGNOSIS

Fibroma and desmoplastic fibroblastoma may be confused with elastofibroma, although neither of them contains the fragmented elastic fibers that are diagnostic of the lesion. Location beneath the lower scapula is also highly suggestive of elastofibroma.

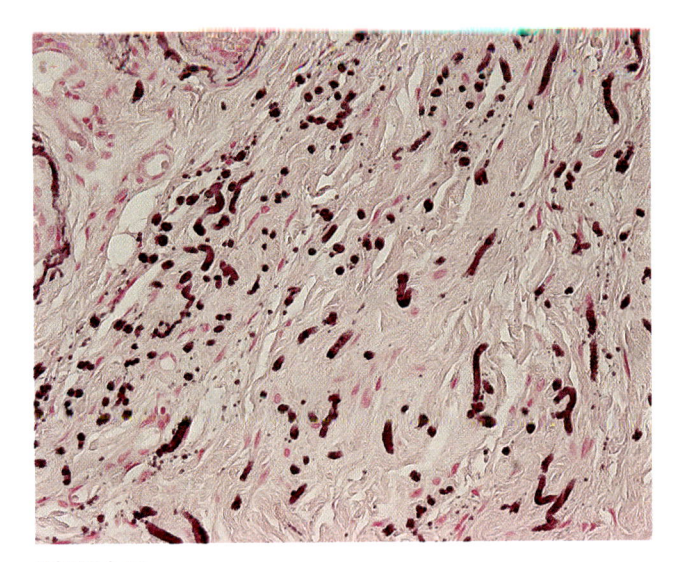

FIGURE 3-11
Elastofibroma.
Abnormal elastic fibers are easily identified using elastin stains.

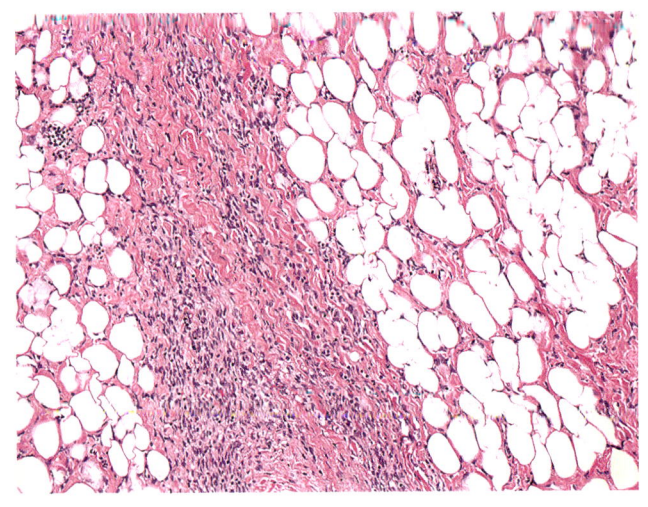

FIGURE 3-13
Hyalinized area within fibrous hamartoma of infancy.

PROGNOSIS AND TREATMENT

Elastofibroma is a benign, nonrecurring lesion. Simple excision is curative.

FIBROUS HAMARTOMA OF INFANCY

CLINICAL FEATURES

Fibrous hamartoma of infancy most often occurs during the first 2 years of life, when it presents as a small, superficial, rapidly growing mass. The lesion is two to three times more common in male than in female infants. The axilla and upper trunk are the most common affected sites, but fibrous hamartoma of infancy has been rarely reported in a wide variety of other soft tissue locations. Almost all tumors are solitary; familial cases have not been reported.

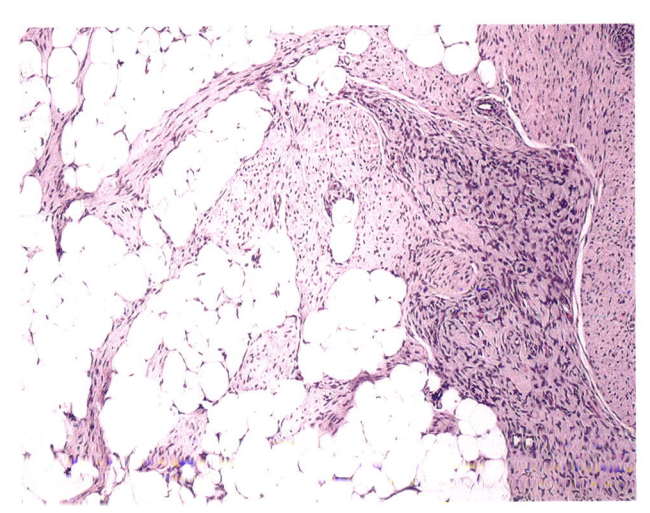

PATHOLOGIC FEATURES

GROSS FINDINGS

Fibrous hamartoma of infancy appears as a poorly circumscribed, variably fatty-appearing, firm mass of relatively small size (usually < 5 cm).

MICROSCOPIC FINDINGS

Microscopically, fibrous hamartoma of infancy shows a triphasic, organoid appearance, with an admixture of well-differentiated fibroblastic fascicles, resembling fibromatosis, mature adipose tissue, and myxoid zones of primitive-appearing mesenchymal cells having a round to stellate shape (Figure 3-12). Hyalinized zones with cracking artifact, reminiscent of giant cell fibroblastoma, may be present (Figure 3-13). Mitotic activity and necrosis are absent.

ANCILLARY STUDIES

IMMUNOHISTOCHEMISTRY

Fibrous hamartomas of infancy commonly express CD34. Occasional cases may show limited expression of smooth muscle actin or desmin, or both, in the fibroblastic component.

FIGURE 3-12
Fibrous hamartoma of infancy, showing a characteristic *triphasic pattern*, with mature fat, bland fibroblastic fascicles, and nodules of primitive mesenchymal cells.

> **FIBROUS HAMARTOMA OF INFANCY—FACT SHEET**
>
> **Definition**
> ▸▸ A benign, likely neoplastic tumor of infancy showing a distinctive triphasic appearance
>
> **Location**
> ▸▸ Most commonly involves axilla and upper chest wall but may involve other soft tissue sites
>
> **Morbidity and Mortality**
> ▸▸ Benign process
> ▸▸ Sex, race, and age distribution
> ▸▸ Most common in male infants
>
> **Clinical Features**
> ▸▸ Rapidly growing, poorly circumscribed, superficially located mass
>
> **Prognosis and Treatment**
> ▸▸ Benign with limited potential for local recurrence
> ▸▸ Complete excision curative

> **FIBROUS HAMARTOMA OF INFANCY—PATHOLOGIC FEATURES**
>
> **Gross Findings**
> ▸▸ Median size: 3 to 5 cm
> ▸▸ Poorly circumscribed, variably fatty, fibrous appearing
>
> **Microscopic Findings**
> ▸▸ Triphasic appearance, with mature fibroblastic zones, mature fat, and myxoid, primitive mesenchyme
>
> **Differential Diagnosis**
> ▸▸ Giant cell fibroblastoma
> ▸▸ Myofibroma/myofibromatosis
> ▸▸ Lipofibromatosis
> ▸▸ CAF

Genetic Findings

Few genetic studies of fibrous hamartoma have been reported without consistent results.

Differential Diagnosis

The hyalinized zones of fibrous hamartoma of infancy may be confused with giant cell fibroblastoma, especially in CD34-positive examples. Careful attention to the triphasic growth pattern of fibrous hamartoma and the absence of small areas resembling dermatofibrosarcoma protuberans (DFSP) should allow this distinction. Lipofibromatosis (infantile fibromatosis) contains both fibroblastic and adipocytic areas, but lacks the primitive mesenchyme seen in fibrous hamartoma. Calcifying aponeurotic fibroma (CAF) occurs in more distal locations and shows distinctive calcifications surrounded by palisaded, epithelioid cells. Myofibroma/myofibromatosis shows a zonated growth pattern, with a peripheral myoid zone and more central *hemangiopericytoma(HPC)-like* zones, often with necrosis.

Prognosis and Treatment

Fibrous hamartomas may recur locally but are cured with complete excision. They are benign lesions that lack metastatic capacity. Despite their name, they most likely represent benign neoplasms rather than hamartomas.

CALCIFYING APONEUROTIC FIBROMA

Clinical Features

CAF typically presents as a slowly growing, painless mass of the hands or feet. Some cases may have a long preclinical duration. Most cases occur in patients between 8 and 14 years of life, although rare cases may involve younger children and older adults. Rare cases present in proximal soft tissue locations, such as the thigh.

Pathologic Features

Gross Findings

CAFs appear as small (< 3 cm), firm, variably circumscribed lesions that merge with the surrounding tendons, skeletal muscle, and adipose tissue. On cut section, they typically have a gritty, partially calcified, fibrous appearance.

Microscopic Findings

CAFs are characterized by an infiltrative proliferation of relatively mature-appearing fibroblastic cells, which surround small foci of calcification and chondroid-like matrix (Figure 3-14). Immediately adjacent to the calcified and chondroid zones, the fibroblastic cells assume a more epithelioid appearance, radiating away from the calcified areas in linear arrays and nuclear palisades (Figure 3-15). Osteoclastic giant cells, occasionally numerous, may be present, and ossification may rarely be seen. Mitoses are infrequent, and pleomorphism and necrosis are not seen. Extraordinarily rare cases of CAF have been reported to progress to sarcoma.

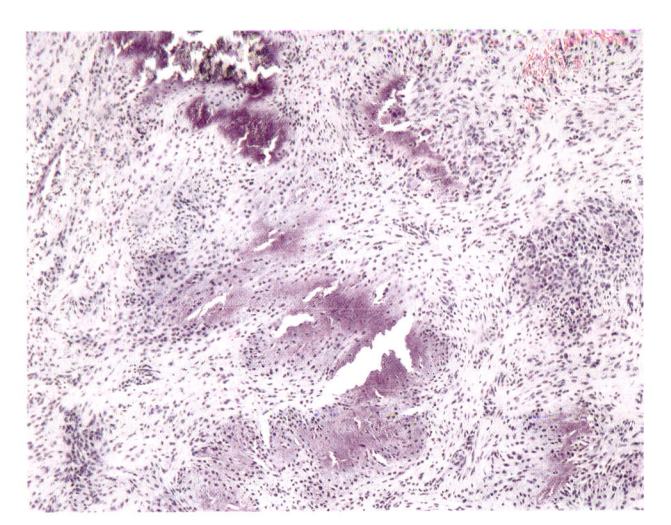

FIGURE 3-14
Calcifying aponeurotic fibroma, consisting of an infiltrative proliferation of bland fibroblastic cells, with abrupt cartilaginous differentiation.

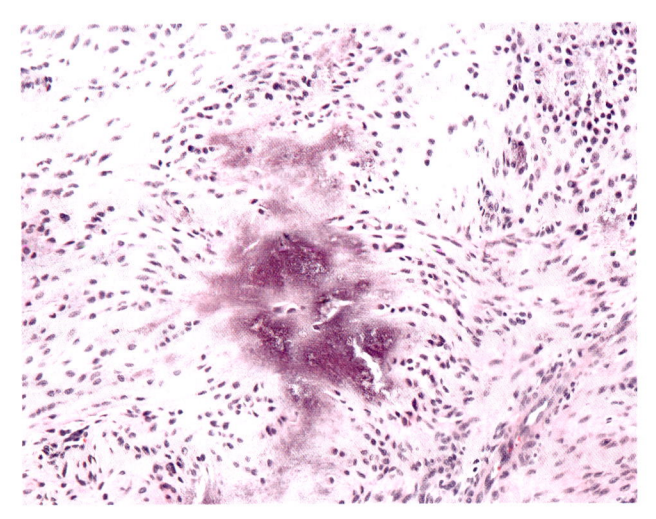

FIGURE 3-15
A radial orientation of epithelioid cells surrounding zones of calcification and cartilaginous differentiation is typical of calcifying aponeurotic fibroma.

CALCIFYING APONEUROTIC FIBROMA—FACT SHEET

Definition
- A benign, locally recurring fibroblastic tumor of the distal extremities of childhood, characterized by distinctive calcifications

Location
- Hands and feet

Morbidity and Mortality
- Significant potential for local recurrence. Extremely rare cases with progression to fully malignant sarcoma.

Sex, Race, and Age Distribution
- Most common in children 8 to 14 years old but may occur in younger children and older adults.

Clinical Features
- Slowly growing, painless mass of hands and feet

Prognosis and Treatment
- Frequently recurs locally; requires wide excision

CALCIFYING APONEUROTIC FIBROMA—PATHOLOGIC FEATURES

Gross Findings
- Median size: 3 cm
- Variably circumscribed, fibrous with gritty areas

Microscopic Findings
- Infiltrative fascicles of mature fibroblasts with distinctive zones of calcification and cartilage formation; chondroid zones are often surrounded by palisaded, epithelioid fibroblastic cells; osteoclastic giant cells in some

Differential Diagnosis
- Lipofibromatosis
- Synovial sarcoma
- Calcified chondroma of soft parts
- Palmar/plantar fibromatosis

ANCILLARY STUDIES

IMMUNOHISTOCHEMISTRY

CAFs typically express only vimentin.

GENETIC FINDINGS

No consistent genetic findings have been reported.

DIFFERENTIAL DIAGNOSIS

Like CAF, lipofibromatosis (juvenile fibromatosis) usually occurs in the distal extremities of children. However, it lacks the calcification and cartilage formation seen in CAF, and contains mature adipose tissue. Monophasic synovial sarcomas may contain calcifications but are composed of clearly malignant-appearing, hyperchromatic, spindled cells arranged in fascicles, with alternating zones of hyper and hypocellularity. Immunostains for cytokeratins and epithelial membrane antigen (EMA), and molecular analysis for the t(X;18) may be helpful in selected cases. Calcified chondromas of soft parts usually occur in older patients and lack the fibroblastic areas that usually make up the majority of CAFs. Palmar and plantar fibromatoses are more cellular and lack calcifications.

CHAPTER 3 Fibroblastic and Fibrohistiocytic Tumors

PROGNOSIS AND TREATMENT

CAFs commonly recur locally and require wide excision. As noted earlier, extremely rare cases have been reported to progress to sarcoma, with metastases.

SUPERFICIAL FIBROMATOSES

CLINICAL FEATURES

Superficial *palmar fibromatosis* (Dupuytren disease or contracture) is the most common type of fibromatosis. The condition affects mainly adult patients, with a strong predilection for male individuals and an increasing incidence with advancing age; almost 20% of the general population is affected by the age of 65. For unknown reasons, palmar fibromatosis occurs most commonly in Northern Europeans and is rare in the black population. Patients present with slowly growing, small subcutaneous nodules, plaques, or cord-like indurations involving the dermis or underlying fascia of the palm. These nodules may lead to contractures that usually predominate on the ulnar side of the palm, affecting the fourth and fifth fingers. Dupuytren disease may be bilateral (50% of cases), and the soles of feet (Ledderhose disease) may be affected simultaneously or metachronously. An association exists between Dupuytren disease and trauma, alcoholism, diabetes, epilepsy, and chronic lung disease. Coexistence with other superficial fibromatoses (penile fibromatosis, knuckle pads) has also been described, but not with deep fibromatoses. *Plantar lesions* are more common in children and adolescents, occurring within the plantar aponeurosis, usually in non–weight-bearing areas. They usually present as solitary or multiple firm nodules that hurt after long standing or walking. Plantar contractures are rare.

PATHOLOGIC FEATURES

GROSS FINDINGS

The lesion consists of single or multiple nodules 0.5 to 2 cm in diameter, attached to a thickened aponeurosis. On cut section, these nodules are firm and grayish.

MICROSCOPIC FINDINGS

On light microscopic examination, the nodule presents as a monotonous, variably collagenized, fascicular proliferation of uniform, nonatypical fibroblasts (Figure 3-16). Some mitotic figures may be visible,

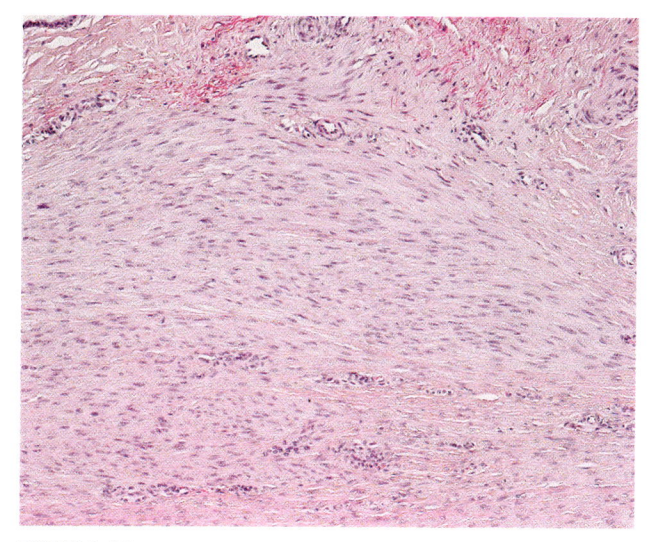

FIGURE 3-16
Superficial fibromatosis, showing a cellular, monotonous fascicular proliferation of nonatypical fibroblasts and myofibroblasts.

SUPERFICIAL FIBROMATOSES—FACT SHEET

Definition
- Benign, recurring but nonmetastasizing, infiltrative, fibroblastic proliferations arising in the palmar or plantar soft tissues

Incidence and Location
- Relatively frequent
- Palmar and plantar locations

Morbidity and Mortality
- Benign, recurring lesion
- Dupuytren disease may be bilateral (50% of cases)
- Superficial fibromatoses may coexist in different locations in the same patient
- Possible association between superficial fibromatoses and trauma, alcoholism, or other diseases (diabetes, epilepsy, chronic lung disease, among others)
- No association with deep fibromatoses

Sex, Race, and Age Distribution
- Middle- to advanced-aged adults
- Predominates in male individuals (three to four times more frequent than in female individuals)
- More common in Northern Europeans
- Plantar lesions more common in children and adolescents

Clinical Features
- Slow-growing small nodules or plaques, or cord-like indurations of the palm
- Contractures

Radiologic Features
- Ill-defined mass

Prognosis and Treatment
- Benign, recurring lesion; no metastases
- Dermofasciectomy followed by skin grafting recommended to prevent recurrences

> **SUPERFICIAL FIBROMATOSES—PATHOLOGIC FEATURES**
>
> **Gross Findings**
> - Single or multiple nodules
> - Size: 0.5 to 2 cm
>
> **Microscopic Findings**
> - Monotonous, fascicular lesion composed of nonatypical fibroblasts in a collagenous background
> - Mitotic figures visible
> - Extracellular collagen abundant in long-standing lesions
> - Hypercellularity frequent in plantar fibromatosis
>
> **Genetics**
> - Trisomy 7 and 8, and loss of Y in Dupuytren disease
> - Trisomy 8 and 14 in Ledderhose disease
>
> **Immunohistochemical Findings**
> - Positivity for vimentin
> - Focal expression of smooth muscle actin
> - Negativity for CD34, keratins, EMA, and S-100 protein
>
> **Differential Diagnosis**
> - Synovial sarcoma
> - MPNST
> - Fibrosarcoma
> - Desmoid-type fibromatosis

especially in early (cellular) lesions. The lesion originates from, and blends into, the palmar or plantar aponeurosis and extends into the overlying subcutaneous fat. Lesions of long duration are less cellular and more collagenized. Some may contain cartilaginous or osseous metaplastic foci. Plantar lesions are often quite hypercellular and may be confused with a spindle cell sarcoma.

ANCILLARY STUDIES

IMMUNOHISTOCHEMISTRY

Immunohistochemically, the spindle cells stain variably for smooth muscle actin and, less frequently, for desmin, in accordance with their myofibroblastic differentiation. Aberrant nuclear expression of beta-catenin protein may be seen.

GENETICS

Chromosomal abnormalities have been described in Dupuytren disease, including trisomy 7 and 8, and loss of the Y chromosome. Familial cases have also been reported. Although beta-catenin protein expression may be present, gene mutations are absent.

DIFFERENTIAL DIAGNOSIS

Diagnosing superficial fibromatoses in their conventional form is usually not a problem for pathologists. However, some cellular forms, especially of plantar fibromatosis, may be confused with sarcomas, especially fibrosarcoma, synovial sarcoma, or MPNST. Clinical presentation (large size and deep situation for sarcomas), immunohistochemical profile (positivity for epithelial markers in synovial sarcoma, focal reactivity for S-100 protein in MPNST), and the presence of specific chromosomal abnormalities [e.g., t(X;18) (p11;q11) for synovial sarcoma] are of great help in making the distinction. Desmoid-type fibromatoses, which may occur in the distal extremities, typically are less cellular than superficial fibromatoses and are composed of longer fascicles of bland fibroblastic cells arrayed about a thin-walled, dilated vasculature. Beta-catenin gene mutations are seen in more than 90% of desmoid-type fibromatoses.

PROGNOSIS AND TREATMENT

Superficial fibromatoses have a strong tendency for local recurrence. Fasciectomy/aponeurectomy followed by skin grafting is the recommended treatment whenever possible to prevent these recurrences.

DEEP (DESMOID-TYPE) FIBROMATOSES

CLINICAL FEATURES

Deep fibromatoses (desmoid tumors) all share the same morphology but differ in their presentation according to the site of development. Classically, deep fibromatoses are divided into abdominal, extra-abdominal, and intra-abdominal forms.

Abdominal desmoid tumors, which develop from the musculoaponeurotic structures of the abdominal wall, tend to occur in young women during pregnancy or during the first year after childbirth, suggesting some hormonal role in their pathogenesis. *Extra-abdominal desmoid tumors* are mostly observed in muscles and aponeuroses of limb girdles (notably shoulder and pelvic regions), chest wall, back, proximal limbs (thigh), and head and neck of young to middle-aged adults. Fibromatoses of the head and neck are more frequent in children, and these tumors tend to be more cellular and locally aggressive. Desmoids are rarely observed in the hands and feet. Abdominal and extra-abdominal desmoids usually present as painless, slow-growing, deep-seated, firm, and

DEEP (DESMOID-TYPE) FIBROMATOSES—FACT SHEET

Definition
- A benign, infiltrative, fibroblastic/myofibroblastic neoplasm that tends to recur but does not metastasize

Incidence and Location
- One of the most frequent soft tissue lesions: three to four cases per million population per year
- Abdominal desmoids: abdominal wall
- Extra-abdominal desmoids: shoulder, pelvic girdle, thoracic wall, back, thigh, head and neck region
- Intra-abdominal desmoids: mesentery, pelvis, retroperitoneum

Morbidity and Mortality
- Local recurrences frequent, depending on the extent of surgery
- Does not metastasize
- May occur in the context of Gardner syndrome

Sex, Race, and Age Distribution
- Abdominal desmoids: adult women (30 to 40 years)
- Extra-abdominal desmoids
  - Adults (15 to 60 years): equal distribution among male and female individuals
  - Children: more frequent in girls than boys, head and neck region

Clinical Features
- Slow-growing, painless, deep-seated mass
- Large size (5 to 10 cm)
- Compression symptoms frequent
- Abdominal fibromatosis that occur during or shortly after pregnancy
- Intra-abdominal desmoid tumors may be associated with Gardner syndrome

Radiologic Features
- Deep-seated homogeneous masses with infiltrative borders
- Erosion of underlying bone possible
- Myxoid changes sometimes observed

Prognosis and Treatment
- Recurring but nonmetastasizing lesions
- Rarely cause death
- Treatment
  - Wide excision plus adjuvant irradiation for symptomatic tumors
  - Simple follow-up and/or low-dose chemotherapy for asymptomatic tumors

DEEP (DESMOID-TYPE) FIBROMATOSES—PATHOLOGIC FEATURES

Gross Findings
- Tumors of large size (5 to 10 cm on average)
- Fascicular/trabecular appearance on cut section

Microscopic Findings
- Fascicular architecture (storiform growth pattern possible)
- Nonatypical, mitotically active, spindle-shaped cells
- Abundant collagenous extracellular matrix
- Well-formed, often gaping muscular vessels
- Infiltrative borders
- Keloidal collagen sometimes present (mesenteric fibromatosis)
- Myxoid changes occasional

Genetics
- Trisomy 8, 20, or both (30% of cases)
- Inactivation (mutations, deletions) of the APC gene in familial cases (Gardner syndrome)
- Mutations in the beta-catenin gene in sporadic desmoid tumors
- Retinoblastoma (Rb) and p53 gene alterations rarely observed

Immunohistochemical Findings
- Diffuse positivity for smooth muscle actin
- Varying expression of desmin and beta-catenin (nuclear expression for beta-catenin)
- Negativity for CD34, S-100 protein, keratins, EMA, and CD117

Differential Diagnosis
- Nodular fasciitis and other reactive myofibroblastic lesions
- Scar tissue
- Idiopathic fibroinflammatory processes (retractile mesenteritis, Ormond disease)
- Desmoplastic fibroblastoma
- Neurofibroma
- Fibrosarcoma
- Low-grade fibromyxoid sarcoma
- Low-grade MPNST
- Monophasic synovial sarcoma (for cellular lesions)

---

poorly circumscribed masses. Some tumors come to medical attention because of neurologic compression symptoms or limitation of motion. In 5% of cases, the disease is multicentric, with subsequent lesions often developing near the initial site. Rarely, extra-abdominal and abdominal desmoids may coexist in the same patient.

Intra-abdominal desmoid tumors develop in the mesentery, pelvis, and/or retroperitoneum of young to middle-aged adults (20 to 35 years). These tumors remain asymptomatic for a long time until they reach a large size (often ≥ 10 cm in maximal diameter). Pelvic fibromatoses that develop mainly in the iliac fossa are often misdiagnosed as ovarian neoplasms. These lesions may encroach on the urinary bladder, vagina, or rectum, or may compress large vessels resulting in a wide range of presenting symptoms, for example, pain, gastrointestinal bleeding, or obstructive symptoms; retroperitoneal tumors are also often large and asymptomatic unless they compress adjacent structures such as ureters, causing hydronephrosis. Trauma is a potential cause of development: more than half of patients had prior abdominal surgery. Mesenteric fibromatosis, the commonest form of intra-abdominal fibromatoses, may be sporadic or associated with Gardner syndrome.

PATHOLOGIC FEATURES

GROSS FINDINGS

Most desmoid tumors are solitary, firm, grossly circumscribed masses with infiltrative borders. They measure between 5 and 10 cm in greatest dimension.

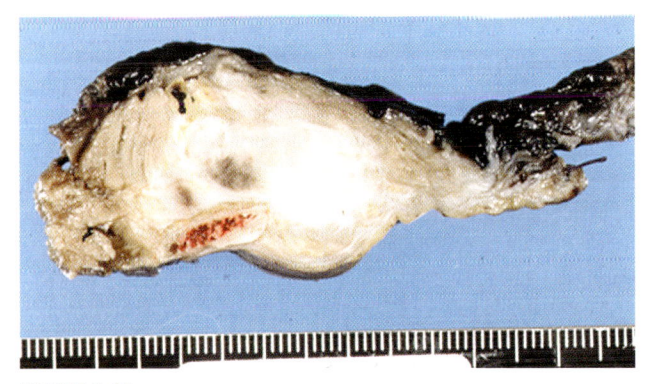

FIGURE 3-17
Gross photograph of a recurrent desmoid tumor of the chest wall in a 71-year-old man. The tumor is an ill-defined, intramuscular, fascicular, whitish mass with infiltrative borders, abutting on a rib.

Sectioning reveals a fascicular, whitish surface resembling leiomyoma or scar tissue (Figure 3-17). Myxoid or cystic change, or both, is occasionally present and may be prominent, especially in intra-abdominal tumors (Figure 3-18). Necrosis is absent.

MICROSCOPIC FINDINGS

Histologically, desmoids are poorly demarcated, uniform, monotonous, fascicular proliferations of spindle shaped fibroblasts and myofibroblasts (Figure 3-19). A storiform growth pattern may be present focally. The spindle-to-stellate tumor cells have a slightly fibrillary cytoplasm with ill-defined borders and bland nuclei with one to three small nucleoli (Figure 3-20). The amount of extracellular matrix observed between the cells varies from one lesion to another, but individual nuclei do not appear to touch each other or overlap. Some lesions can be cellular, mimicking fibrosarcoma, whereas others are markedly collagenized, sometimes

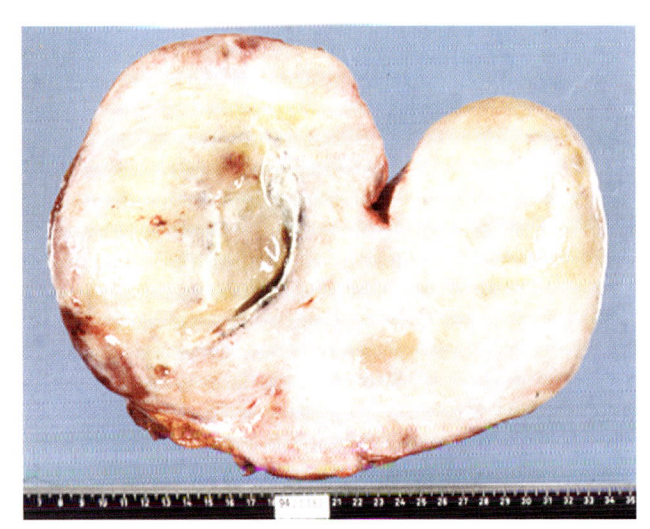

FIGURE 3-19
Intra-abdominal desmoid tumor.
Monotonous fascicular proliferation of bland myofibroblasts with a relatively well-developed, collagenous extracellular matrix.

with a peculiar, keloid-like collagen, especially in mesenteric fibromatosis (Figure 3-21). Well-formed, sometimes gaping vessels with distinctive muscular walls and/or some degree of perivascular hyalinization are also characteristically observed in desmoids. Mitoses may be present in cellular lesions; atypical mitoses and cellular pleomorphism are absent. Characteristically, desmoid tumors have infiltrative borders, encroaching on the surrounding skeletal muscle. As a result, atrophic or regenerative skeletal muscle fibers entrapped by the lesion are commonly observed toward the edges (Figure 3-22), together with lymphoid aggregates. Areas of myxoid change resulting in a fasciitis-like morphology are quite common in early lesions, whereas calcifications, chondroid metaplastic

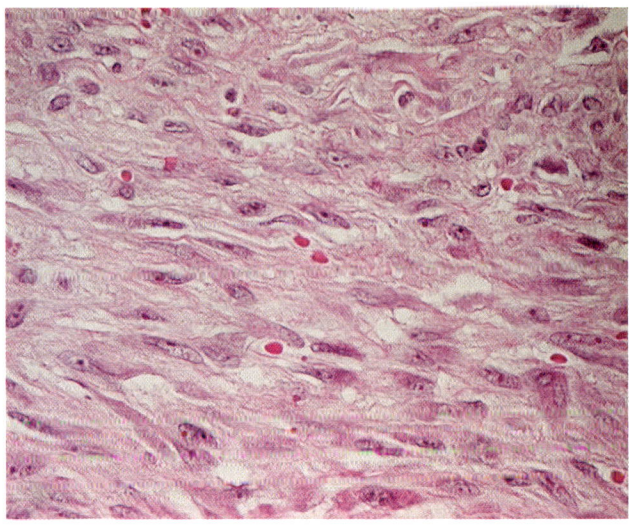

FIGURE 3-18
Sporadic desmoid tumor of the mesentery in a 46-year-old woman. The lesion measured 27 cm and was well-circumscribed with a fascicular appearance. Focal myxoid and cystic changes are visible.

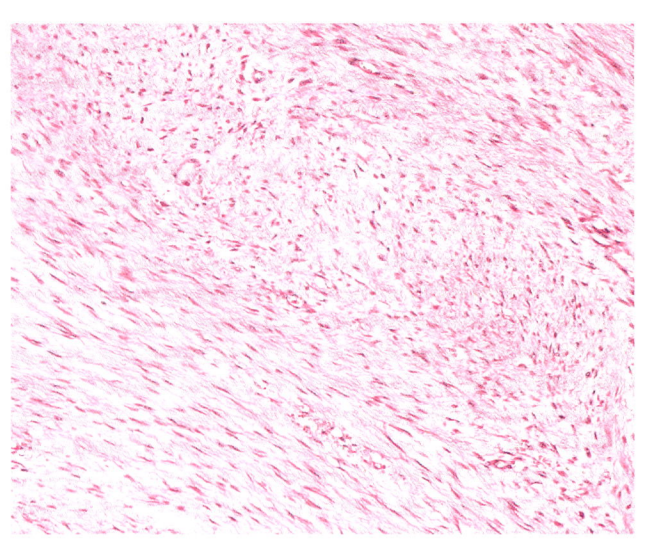

FIGURE 3-20
Intra-abdominal desmoid tumor.
Proliferating myofibroblasts with bland, vesicular nuclei containing one or two small nucleoli.

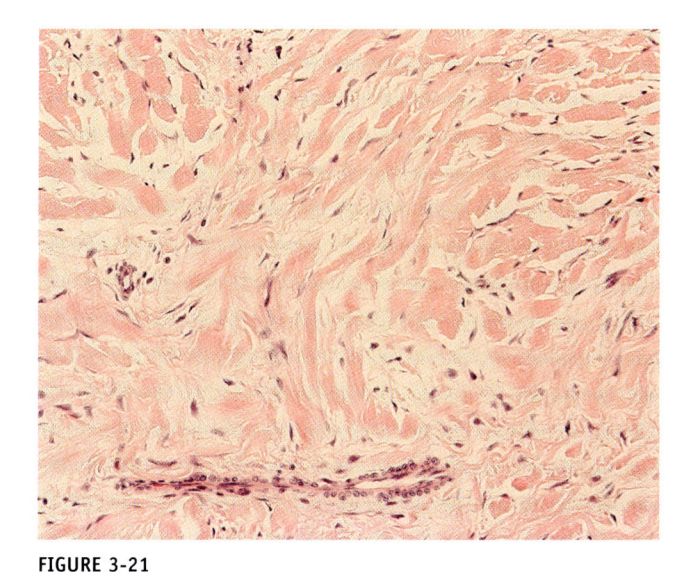

CHAPTER 3 Fibroblastic and Fibrohistiocytic Tumors

FIGURE 3-21
Intra-abdominal desmoid tumor.
The lesion is markedly collagenized, with bands of keloid-like collagen. The vessels in desmoid tumors are typically thin walled and dilated, and often show perivascular edema.

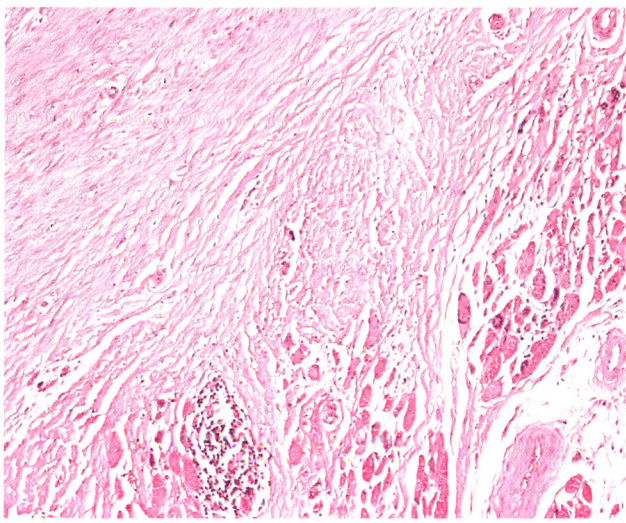

FIGURE 3-23
Desmoid tumor.
Strong positivity for smooth muscle actin in a myofibroblastic *tram-track* pattern.

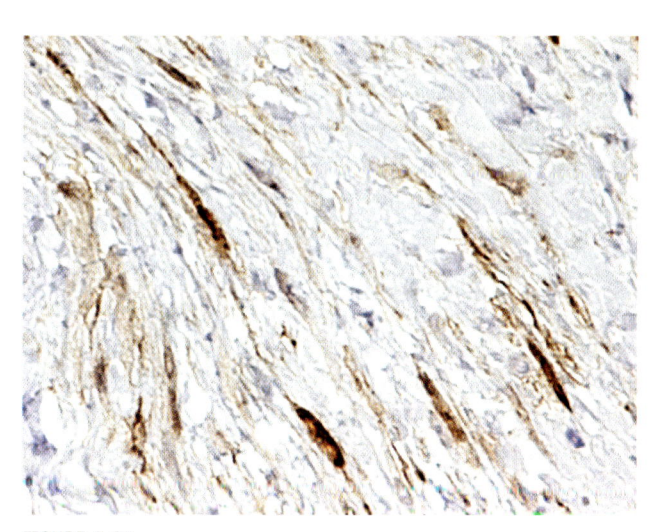

FIGURE 3-22
Desmoid tumor.
Infiltrative borders encroaching on the surrounding skeletal muscle.

FIGURE 3-24
Desmoid tumor.
Aberrant nuclear accumulation of beta-catenin detected by immunohistochemistry.

foci, and/or osteoid metaplastic foci are occasionally observed in long-standing neoplasms.

ANCILLARY STUDIES

IMMUNOHISTOCHEMISTRY

Desmoids are consistently positive, at least focally, for smooth muscle actin (Figure 3-23). Focal expression of desmin is also common. CD34, keratins, EMA, CD117, and S-100 protein are not usually expressed. Beta-catenin is variably expressed in the cytoplasm and/or nucleus of tumor cells, but only nuclear staining is considered specific (Figure 3-24).

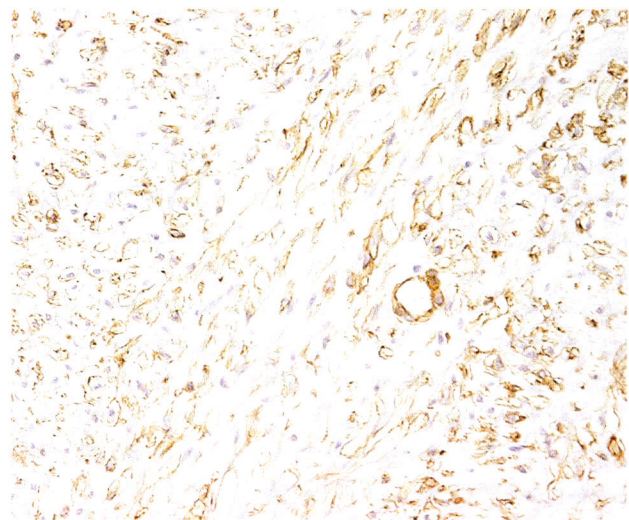

GENETICS

About one third of desmoid-type fibromatoses have trisomy of chromosomes 8 or 20, or both. Patients with Gardner syndrome often show point mutations or allelic deletions of the APC tumor suppressor gene on chromosome arm 5q, leading to gene inactivation. The presence of an abnormal APC protein prevents normal binding to the beta-catenin protein and degradation of the latter, which thus accumulates in the cytoplasm or nucleus, or both, of the cells and is detectable by immunohistochemistry. In sporadic desmoid tumors, the APC gene is intact, but mutations are observed in the beta-catenin gene. This results in the production of an abnormal stabilized beta-catenin protein, which accumulates in the cytoplasm, nucleus, or both.

DIFFERENTIAL DIAGNOSIS

Desmoid tumors showing prominent myxoid change may be confused with nodular fasciitis or any reactive myofibroblastic proliferation. The distinction can be made by the large size of the lesion, deep location, and monotonous histologic appearance with low mitotic activity. Highly collagenized lesions should be differentiated from scar tissue. Sometimes, this distinction is almost impossible, notably in those patients with previous operations at the same site for the same condition. Desmoplastic fibroblastoma, which is usually less cellular than desmoid tumor and lacks a fascicular growth pattern, and neurofibroma, which consists of bland S-100 protein–positive spindled cells with wavy nuclei admixed with bundles of eosinophilic collagen also enter in the differential diagnosis. Cellular variants of desmoid tumor may be confused with malignant lesions. However, desmoids lack the cellular atypia, numerous and atypical mitoses, and tumor necrosis typical of fibrosarcoma or monophasic synovial sarcoma. Low-grade fibromyxoid sarcoma and low-grade MPNST should also be distinguished from desmoid tumors. Desmoid tumors are more fascicular and show neither the whorled or swirling pattern nor the alternating presence of fibrous and myxoid areas that typify low-grade fibromyxoid sarcomas. Desmoid tumors may show myxoid changes particularly when intra-abdominal, but the cells have plump vesicular nuclei and are consistently and more diffusely positive for smooth muscle actin. In addition, nuclear atypia, curvilinear/plexiform vessels resembling those of a myxofibrosarcoma, and giant rosettes are not features of desmoid tumors. Low-grade MPNSTs are less fascicular than desmoid tumors, showing cellular and myxoid areas with spindle cells that are positive for S-100 protein, at least focally. In the mesentery and retroperitoneum, desmoid tumors should also be differentiated from rare idiopathic fibrosclerosing inflammatory processes such as retractile mesenteritis and Ormond disease. The latter are heterogeneous in their histologic appearance, showing a varying admixture of cellular fibroblastic areas, fibrous (poorly cellular) zones, inflammatory areas containing numerous plasma cells and lymphocytes, and foci of liponecrosis with or without lymphocytic venulitis.

PROGNOSIS AND TREATMENT

Desmoid tumors do not metastasize, but they have a strong tendency for local recurrence and may ultimately invade structures such as large vessels, large nerves, or viscera. They rarely cause death—the 5-year survival rate is more than 90%. Complete surgical excision with tumor-free margins is the treatment of choice, but this may result in significant morbidity. The recurrence rate is less than 50% for widely resected tumors. Adjuvant irradiation is recommended, especially for those patients with marginal excisions. Antiestrogen agents (tamoxifen), chemotherapy, or both have been administered with variable success. The current trend in the treatment of desmoid tumors is to refrain from operating on all but those patients with highly symptomatic tumors; the others are followed up and/or are given low doses of methotrexate or doxorubicin (Adriamycin) to stabilize the lesion.

INFLAMMATORY MYOFIBROBLASTIC TUMOR/INFLAMMATORY FIBROSARCOMA

CLINICAL FEATURES

Inflammatory myofibroblastic tumor (IMT) (previously called *inflammatory pseudotumor* or *plasma cell granuloma*) is primarily a tumor of children and young adults (median age, 9 years), with a slight female predilection. The lungs, omentum, mesentery, and soft tissues are predominantly affected, although it may be found virtually anywhere in the body. Forty percent to 45% of extrapulmonary IMTs occur in the omentum and mesentery. Lesions in these two sites mostly affect children and adolescents, whereas pulmonary lesions predominate in adults. Symptoms depend on the site of the lesion: Patients with pulmonary IMT may describe dyspnea, chest pain, or both; abdominal tumors may cause discomfort or gastrointestinal tract obstruction. A significant proportion of IMTs (up to 30%) are associated with systemic symptoms (e.g., weight loss, fever, or night sweats) and/or laboratory abnormalities (e.g., anemia, thrombocytosis, hyperglobulinemia, or increased erythrocyte sedimentation rate) that disappear when the tumor is removed but may reappear if it recurs.

PATHOLOGIC FEATURES

GROSS FINDINGS

IMT is a circumscribed, solitary nodular mass of variable size, 1 to 17 cm (mean diameter, 6 cm). Multiple nodules are seen in about one-third of cases. On section, it has a myxoid or fleshy appearance. Hemorrhagic changes, tumor necrosis, and/or calcifications may be observed. In hollow organs (e.g., urinary bladder), IMT often presents as bloody, infiltrative polyps, measuring between 2 and 10 cm (median, 3 to 5 cm).

MICROSCOPIC FINDINGS

Three basic histologic patterns can be recognized. In the first pattern, plump myofibroblasts are loosely dispersed in an abundant edematous/myxoid extracellular matrix, together with numerous dilated vessels (granulation tissue–like capillaries), extravasated erythrocytes, lymphocytes, plasma cells, and eosinophils (Figures 3-25 and 3-26). Mitoses can be numerous but not atypical. The second growth pattern consists of a denser, storiform or fascicular spindle cell proliferation, with a prominent inflammatory infiltrate consisting predominantly of lymphocytes and plasma cells (Figure 3-27). Lymphoid follicles with germinal centers may be seen. Ganglion cell–like myofibroblasts with vesicular nuclei, prominent nucleoli, and abundant eosinophilic/amphophilic cytoplasm are frequently seen in these two patterns. In the third pattern, the lesion is less cellular and more collagenized, resembling a scar or desmoid fibromatosis with marked inflammation. Calcifications and/or foci of bone metaplasia may be observed. Malignant IMT (inflammatory fibrosarcoma) is characterized by clusters of polygonal, ganglion-like, or epithelioid atypical cells with vesicular nuclei and prominent nucleoli and numerous, often atypical mitoses.

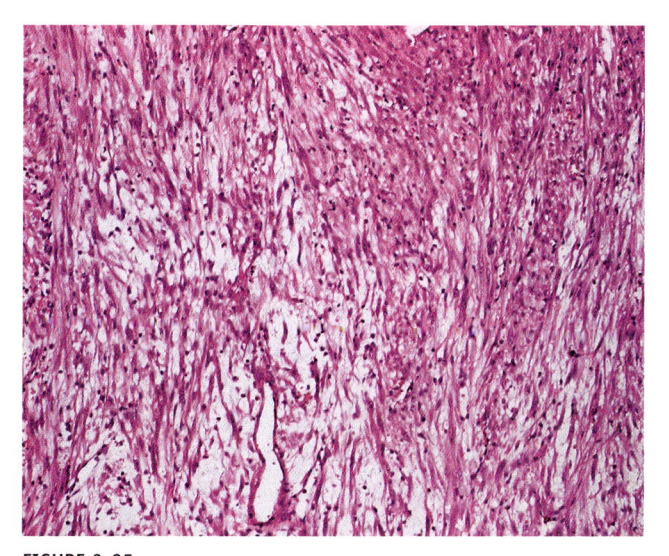

ANCILLARY STUDIES

IMMUNOHISTOCHEMISTRY

Myofibroblasts in IMT are usually focally to diffusely positive for smooth muscle actin (Figure 3-28), calponin, and desmin. They can also show some reactivity for cytokeratins (about 30% of cases), especially in lesions of the genitourinary tract (70% to 90% of the cases). Alkaline (ALK) reactivity is detectable in myofibroblast cytoplasm in about 50% of cases (Figure 3-29). The cells are negative for myogenin, h-caldesmon, S-100 protein, and CD117.

GENETICS

As opposed to adults older than 40 years, IMT in children and young adults often contains clonal rearrangements of the 2p23 region, resulting in ALK receptor tyrosine kinase gene activation and overexpression of the ALK kinase domain. ALK protein activation is restricted to the myofibroblastic component of IMT, in which it may be detected by immunohistochemistry.

FIGURE 3-25
Inflammatory myofibroblastic tumor.
Plump myofibroblasts dispersed in an abundant edematous/myxoid extracellular matrix, containing numerous lymphocytes and plasma cells.

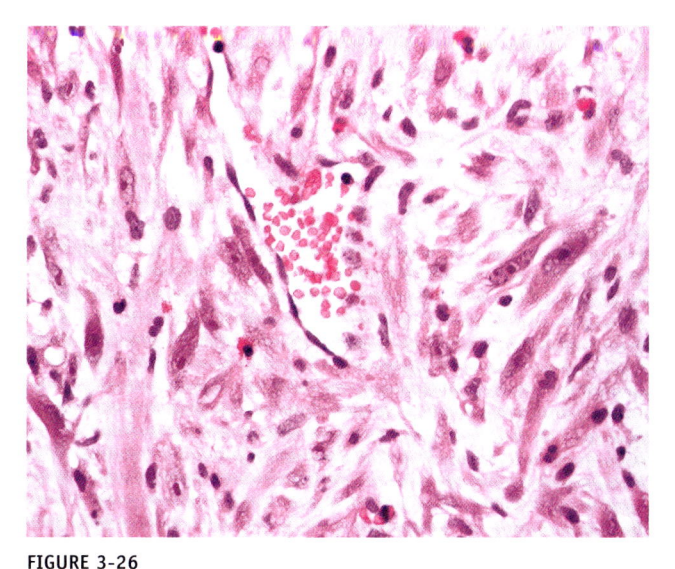

FIGURE 3-26
Inflammatory myofibroblastic tumor.
Ganglion-like myofibroblasts with abundant, basophilic, and fibrillary cytoplasm, and prominent nucleoli.

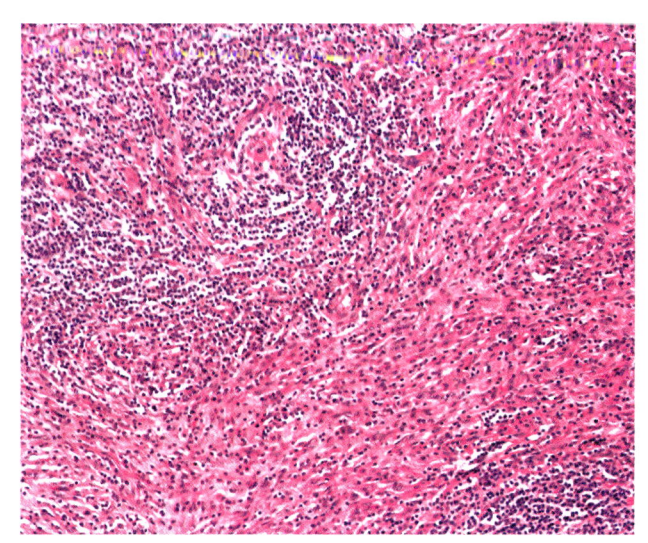

FIGURE 3-27
Inflammatory myofibroblastic tumor.
Admixture of myofibroblasts, lymphocytes, and plasma cells. Lymphoid follicles with germinal centers are visible.

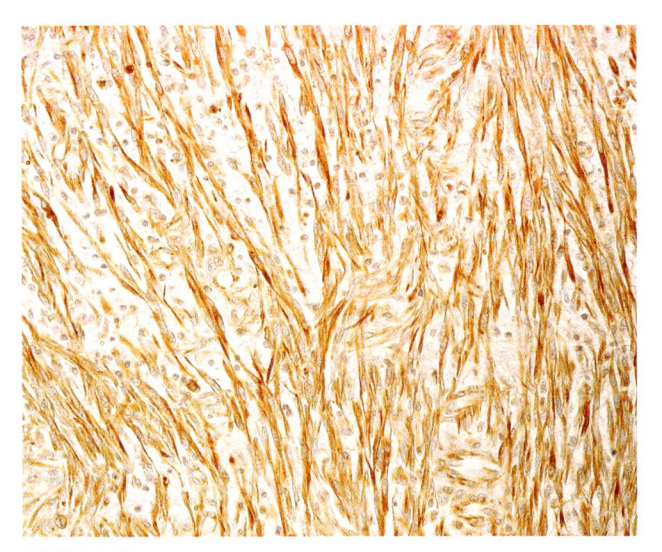

FIGURE 3-28
Inflammatory myofibroblastic tumor.
Strong positivity for smooth muscle actin.

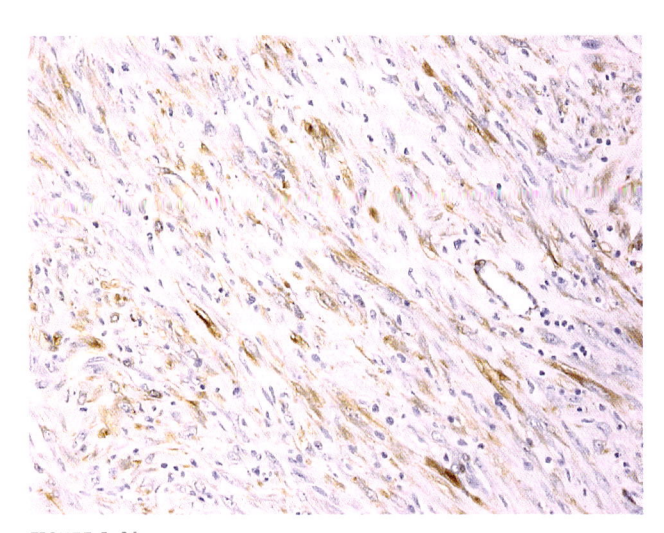

FIGURE 3-29
Inflammatory myofibroblastic tumor.
Cytoplasmic expression of ALK1 in tumor cells.

INFLAMMATORY MYOFIBROBLASTIC TUMOR/INFLAMMATORY FIBROSARCOMA—FACT SHEET

Definition
- A distinctive lesion composed of myofibroblasts, lymphocytes, plasma cells, and eosinophils

Incidence and Location
- Rare
- Predominate in lungs, soft tissues, and abdominal viscera (mesentery, omentum, genitourinary tract)

Morbidity and Mortality
- Mostly benign behavior; rare cases metastasize

Sex, Race, and Age Distribution
- Children and young adults; pulmonary form more common in middle age
- Slight female predominance

Clinical Features
- Pulmonary IMT: chest pain and dyspnea
- Abdominal IMT: pain, discomfort, gastrointestinal obstruction
- Mass, fever, and/or weight loss frequent
- Anomalous laboratory findings (anemia, hyperglobulinemia, increased erythrocyte sedimentation rate) occasional

Radiologic Features
- Heterogeneous lobulated solid mass
- Calcifications may be present

Prognosis and Treatment
- 30% to 40% recurrence rate for extrapulmonary and extravesical IMT (5% to 10% for pulmonary lesions; 25% for lesions from urinary bladder)
- Metastasis in less than 5% of cases
- Treatment: wide excision whenever possible
- Regression under anti-inflammatory agents (corticoids) possible

---

DIFFERENTIAL DIAGNOSIS

The differential diagnosis depends on the histologic appearance of the lesion. When the tumor is predominantly myxoid and mitotically active, it resembles a reactive pseudosarcomatous lesion such as granulation tissue, nodular fasciitis, or proliferative fasciitis (if ganglion-like cells are numerous). When IMTs are markedly cellular, smooth muscle neoplasms, fibrous histiocytoma, inflammatory cell–rich gastrointestinal stromal tumors, and dendritic cell neoplasms must be considered. In the liver and spleen, most lesions resembling IMT actually correspond to dendritic cell tumors. Immunoreactivity for CD21 and CD35, signs of Epstein–Barr virus infection in follicular dendritic cell tumors, and S-100 and CD1a positivity in interdigitating dendritic cell tumors are useful features in this setting. Benign myofibroblastic spindle-cell lesions associated with infections, especially with mycobacterial infections, should also be distinguished from IMT. Special stains (methenamine silver and Ziehl stains) should always be performed, especially if the patient is immunodeficient or treated with corticosteroids. When IMTs are relatively sclerotic and less cellular, desmoid-type fibromatosis, scarring, and calcifying fibrous pseudotumor are potential mimics. Some overlap exists between calcifying fibrous pseudotumor and IMT, and it is possible that the former is no more than a late fibrosing stage of the latter. In the retroperitoneum, mesentery, and mediastinum, sclerosing IMT should be distinguished from well-differentiated sclerosing/inflammatory liposarcoma, sclerosing lymphoma, sclerosing carcinoma, Hodgkin's lymphoma, and all fibrosclerosing inflammatory processes that occur in disimmune/autoimmune diseases.

CHAPTER 3 Fibroblastic and Fibrohistiocytic Tumors

INFLAMMATORY MYOFIBROBLASTIC TUMOR/INFLAMMATORY FIBROSARCOMA—PATHOLOGIC FEATURES

Gross Findings
- Circumscribed multinodular mass
- Whitish to myxoid
- Mean diameter: 6 cm (range, 1 to 17 cm)

Microscopic Findings
- Three patterns:
  1. Fairly dispersed spindled fibroblasts/myofibroblasts; some ganglion-like myofibroblasts
  Prominent inflammation (lymphocytes, plasma cells, eosinophils)
  Edematous/myxoid background with numerous vessels
  2. Dense, fascicular myofibroblastic proliferation
  Prominent inflammatory infiltrate/plasma cell aggregates/lymphoid nodules
  Variably myxoid to collagenized background
  Ganglion-like myofibroblasts
  3. Moderate to hypocellular myofibroblastic proliferation
  Well-developed collagenized extracellular matrix
- Malignant IMT (inflammatory fibrosarcoma) characterized by:
  - Atypical, polygonal, ganglion-like/epithelioid cells with vesicular nuclei and prominent nucleoli
  - Numerous/atypical mitoses

Genetics
- Clonal rearrangements of the 2p23 region
- ALK gene activation frequent in IMT of children and young adults, rare in adults older than 40 years
- ALK gene activation frequent in IMT of urinary bladder

Immunohistochemical Findings
- Focal or diffuse reactivity for smooth muscle actin, calponin, and desmin
- Cytokeratin reactivity in about 30% of cases (especially in lesions from urinary bladder)
- Cytoplasmic ALK reactivity in about 50% of cases (70% to 90% in tumors from urinary bladder)
- Negativity for myogenin, h-caldesmon, S-100 protein, and CD117

Differential Diagnosis
- Granulation tissue/reactive processes
- Nodular fasciitis
- Fibrous histiocytoma
- GIST
- Spindle cell carcinoma
- Dendritic cell neoplasms
- Desmoid-type fibromatosis
- Well-differentiated sclerosing/inflammatory liposarcoma
- Sclerosing lymphoma/Hodgkin's disease
- Autoimmune-associated fibrosing processes (Ormond disease, sclerosing mediastinitis)

Malignant forms of IMT/inflammatory fibrosarcoma should be differentiated from malignant fibrous histiocytoma, inflammatory leiomyosarcoma, rhabdomyosarcoma, and spindle cell carcinoma. Clinical presentation (children), tumor site (intra-abdominal lesion), and immunohistochemical profile (positivity for ALK) help in making the distinction.

PROGNOSIS AND TREATMENT

Extrapulmonary IMT has an overall recurrence rate of 30% to 40%. The recurrence rate is significantly lower in pulmonary lesions (5%) and in lesions from the urinary bladder (25%). A minority (<5%) produce metastasis.

Wide excision is the treatment of choice. Tumor regression has been described with anti-inflammatory (corticosteroid) treatment.

MYXOINFLAMMATORY FIBROBLASTIC SARCOMA (Inflammatory Myxohyaline Tumor of Distal Extremities with Reed–Sternberg or Virocyte-like Cells, Acral Myxoinflammatory Fibroblastic Sarcoma)

CLINICAL FEATURES

Myxoinflammatory fibroblastic sarcoma (MIFS) is a rare, recently described soft tissue of low-grade malignancy that most often occurs in acral locations. MIFS typically affects middle-aged adults, with a peak incidence in the fourth to fifth decades of life. Approximately two-thirds of cases involve the upper extremity and one-third the lower, although rare cases have been reported in more proximal locations, including the trunk. Patients typically have a slow-growing, infiltrative, occasionally painful mass.

PATHOLOGIC FEATURES

GROSS FINDINGS

MIFSs typically appear as multinodular, poorly circumscribed, friable masses of white-tan tissue. Most cases are relatively small (3 to 4 cm).

MICROSCOPIC FINDINGS

MIFSs show a distinctive admixture of hyalinized, inflammatory, and myxoid areas (Figure 3-30). The inflammatory areas may predominate, creating the low-power appearance of an inflammatory or infectious process. Neutrophils, eosinophils, lymphocytes, and histiocytes may be present, in variable numbers. Within the hyalinized and myxoid zones are found aggregates of bizarre-appearing tumor cells, often with giant macronucleoli, reminiscent of cytomegalovirus-infected cells or Reed–Sternberg cells (Figure 3-31). Pseudolipoblast-like fibroblastic cells are usually easily identified within the myxoid areas (Figure 3-32). Mitotic figures may be present but are typically sparse. Small foci of necrosis are occasionally seen.

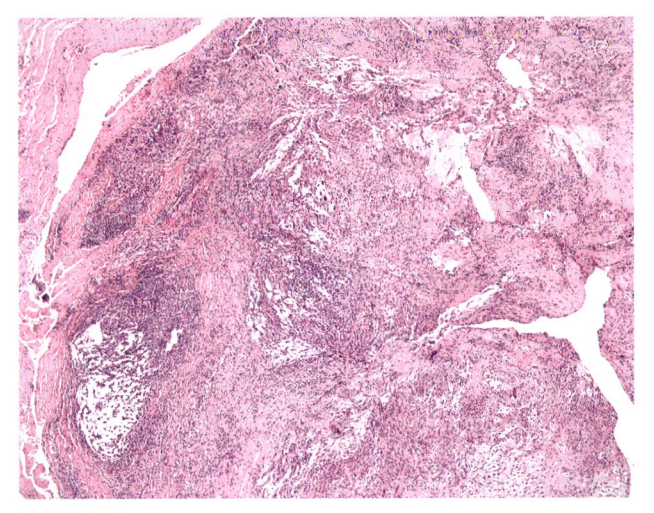

FIGURE 3-30
Myxoinflammatory fibroblastic sarcoma, showing a characteristic admixture of hyalinized, myxoid, and inflammatory areas.

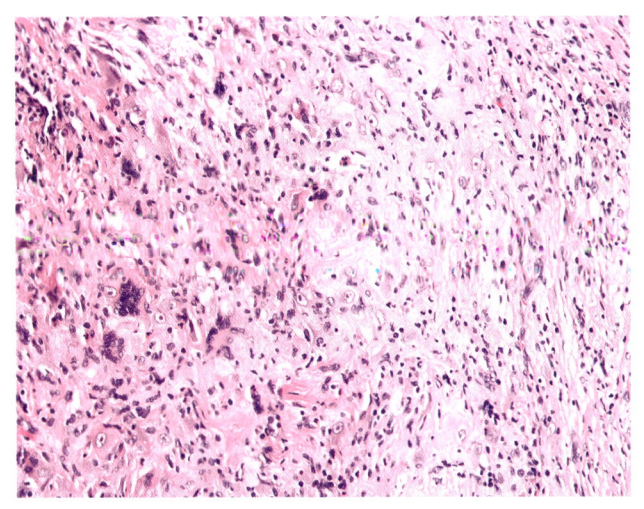

FIGURE 3-31
Inflammatory cells and bizarre-appearing tumor cells with prominent macronucleoli in myxoinflammatory fibroblastic sarcoma.

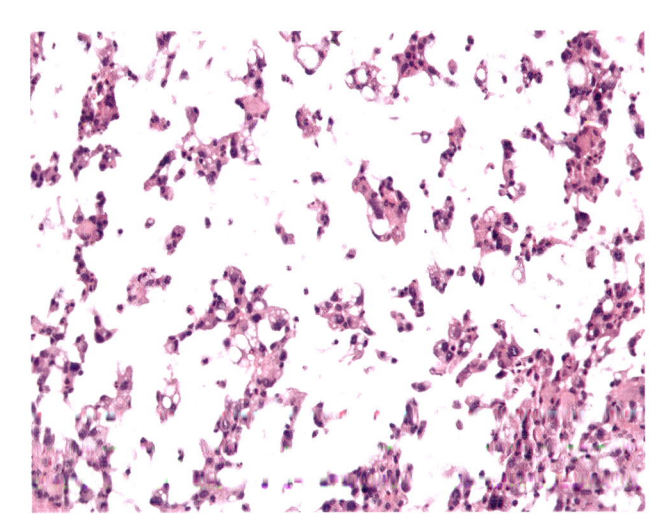

FIGURE 3-32
Myxoid area in myxoinflammatory fibroblastic sarcoma, with pseudolipoblasts.

MYXOINFLAMMATORY FIBROBLASTIC SARCOMA—FACT SHEET

Definition
▸▸ A distinctive low-grade sarcoma of the distal extremities, characterized by an admixture of hyalinized, myxoid, and inflammatory areas

Location
▸▸ Acral sites; two-thirds upper extremities, one-third lower extremities; rare cases in proximal locations including trunk

Morbidity and Mortality
▸▸ Significant potential for aggressive, destructive local recurrence; rare cases with lymph node and lung metastases

Sex, Race, and Age Distribution
▸▸ Middle-aged adults; no sex predilection

Clinical Features
▸▸ Slow-growing, occasionally painful mass of distal extremities

Prognosis and Treatment
▸▸ Frequent local recurrence, occasionally necessitating amputation; requires wide excision; selected cases may require adjuvant radiotherapy

---

MYXOINFLAMMATORY FIBROBLASTIC SARCOMA—PATHOLOGIC FEATURES

Gross Findings
▸▸ Median size: 3 cm
▸▸ Poorly circumscribed, friable, fibrous to myxoid appearing

Microscopic Findings
▸▸ Hyalinized and myxoid areas that contain bizarre tumor cells with giant macronucleoli; pseudolipoblasts in myxoid areas; mixed acute and chronic inflammatory cell infiltrate; low mitotic rate with infrequent necrosis

Differential Diagnosis
▸▸ Myxofibrosarcoma
▸▸ Infection/inflammatory process
▸▸ Giant cell tumor of tendon sheath
▸▸ Hodgkin's lymphoma

A well-developed, arborizing, thick-walled vasculature, as seen in myxofibrosarcoma, is not seen.

Ancillary Studies

Immunohistochemistry

The neoplastic cells of MIFS routinely express vimentin and are positive for CD34 in roughly 25% of cases. Occasional cases may be cytokeratin and smooth muscle actin positive.

Genetic Findings

No consistent genetic findings have been reported.

Differential Diagnosis

Inflammatory and infectious lesions lack the clearly malignant cells seen in MIFS, as well as the distinctive admixture of hyalinized and myoid zones. Soft tissue Hodgkin's lymphoma is extremely rare, and the cells of MIFS lack CD30 and CD15 expression, seen in Reed–Sternberg cells. Myxofibrosarcoma (myxoid malignant fibrous histiocytoma) is typically larger and more proximally located, occurs in older adults, and shows a well-developed arborizing vasculature, which is absent in MIFS. Giant cell tumors of tendon sheath lack the prominent cytologic atypia and the acute inflammatory cells seen in MIFSs. IMTs usually occur in much younger patients, contain fascicles of relatively bland myofibroblasts, and seldom occur in distal locations.

Prognosis and Treatment

MIFS is considered a low-grade sarcoma, with significant potential for aggressive local recurrence, sometimes necessitating amputation, and limited potential for lymph node and distant metastases. Exceptional cases of MIFS show histologic progression to high-grade sarcoma; the significance of this finding is uncertain, but likely reflects a significantly more aggressive lesion. MIFS require wide excision, with consideration of adjuvant radiotherapy in selected cases.

ADULT FIBROSARCOMA AND VARIANTS
(Low-Grade Fibromyxoid Sarcoma/Hyalinizing Spindle Cell Tumor with Giant Rosettes, Sclerosing Epithelioid Fibrosarcoma, Myxofibrosarcoma)

Clinical Features

Conventional fibrosarcoma is a relatively rare neoplasm of adult patients (30 to 60 years) that occurs slightly more frequently in men. Most patients describe a deep-seated, often slow-growing, large solitary mass. A significant proportion of cases occur at the site of former injury, in burn scars, or in previously irradiated fields (postradiation fibrosarcoma). The lower extremities are predominantly affected (thigh), followed by the trunk.

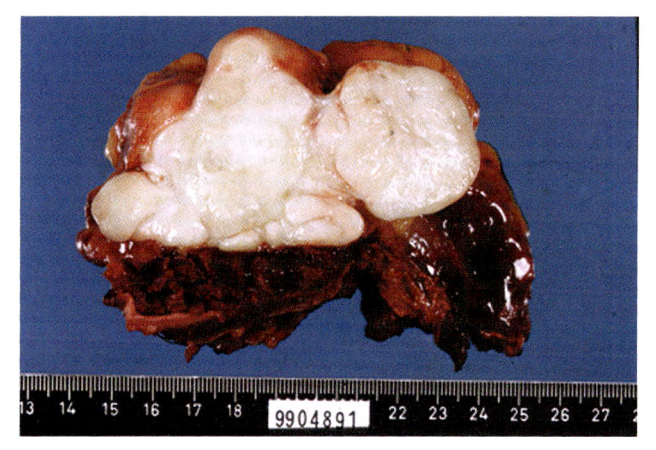

FIGURE 3-33
Gross photograph of a low-grade fibromyxoid sarcoma, showing a lobulated, glistening, leiomyoma-like, whitish mass.

Low-grade fibromyxoid sarcoma is an unusual variant of fibrosarcoma that was not recognized as a malignant neoplasm until 1987. It usually presents as a long-standing, painless mass that occurs preferentially in the deep soft tissues of the limbs (thigh), limb girdles (shoulder), and trunk of young adults (median age, 35 years), with a slight predilection for male individuals.

Sclerosing epithelioid fibrosarcoma is an uncommon, distinctive, often painful variant of fibrosarcoma that occurs in adults (median age, 43 years) with equal sex distribution. The tumor develops predominantly in the limbs (especially lower limbs) and limb girdles, and is deep seated in most cases.

Myxofibrosarcoma, previously called *myxoid malignant fibrous histiocytoma*, is a relatively common sarcoma of older patients (50 to 70 years), mostly found in the deep dermis and subcutaneous fat of limbs and limb girdles. About one third of the cases are deep seated, developing in fascia and skeletal muscle. This is a slow-growing, often painless tumor that affects men and women equally.

Pathologic Features

Gross Findings

Conventional fibrosarcomas are large, well-circumscribed, solitary masses, measuring 3 to 8 cm. On section, the tumor is whitish, fleshy, and may contain foci of necrosis or hemorrhage, or both. *Low-grade fibromyxoid sarcomas* are also well-demarcated, sometimes lobulated. Cut section shows a fibrous or fibromyxoid, whitish, glistening mass, bearing some resemblance to a uterine leiomyoma (Figure 3-33). *Sclerosing epithelioid fibrosarcoma* is a well-circumscribed, lobulated tumor that may have calcifications, cystic change, or myxoid change on sectioning. As with low-grade fibromyxoid sarcoma, necrosis is uncommon. *Myxofibrosarcoma* is typically located in the subcutaneous fat, growing along fibrous septa and forming more or less gelatinous nodules (Figure 3-34). Large tumors are often deep-seated, and partially necrotic and/or hemorrhagic.

MICROSCOPIC FINDINGS

Conventional fibrosarcoma is composed of monotonous, uniform fibroblast-like spindle cells that have little cytoplasm and grow in long fascicles separated by regular collagen fibers, giving the classic *herringbone* growth pattern (Figure 3-35). Tumor cell bundles may also intersect at right angles. Mitoses are readily visible. Focal cartilage or bone metaplasia, or both, can occasionally be seen; giant or multinucleated cells are generally absent. Extracellular collagen deposition is usually more pronounced in postradiation fibrosarcoma, as bundles of thick, hyalinized collagen separating the tumor cells. Poorly differentiated cases are more cellular and pleomorphic, with more numerous mitotic figures, less collagen, and some necrosis.

In its classic form, *low-grade fibromyxoid sarcoma* consists of spindle-shaped tumor cells forming sweeping fascicles or whorls, in a collagenous and myxoid background (Figures 3-36 and 3-37). The cells have pale eosinophilic cytoplasm and deceptively bland, ovoid, or tapered nuclei with one or two small nucleoli and occasional nuclear inclusions (Figure 3-38). Mitotic figures are rare, and there is no necrosis. The stroma is focally collagenous; in the myxoid areas, curvilinear or plexiform vessels resembling those of a myxoid liposarcoma are readily visible. Although grossly well-circumscribed, the tumor often infiltrates the surrounding tissues on microscopic examination. Some tumors may contain clusters of large rosettes, consisting of cores of hyalinized collagen surrounded by rounded, epithelioid-looking tumor cells. When they are numerous, the lesion has been described as *hyalinizing spindle cell*

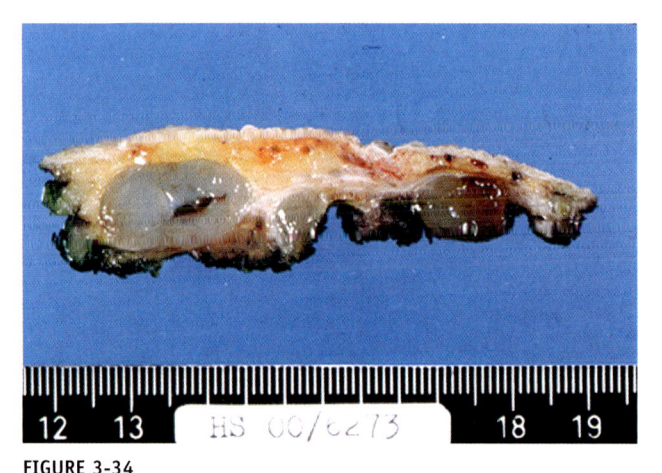

FIGURE 3-34
Gross photograph of a myxofibrosarcoma.
Several myxoid nodules are visible in the subcutaneous fat.

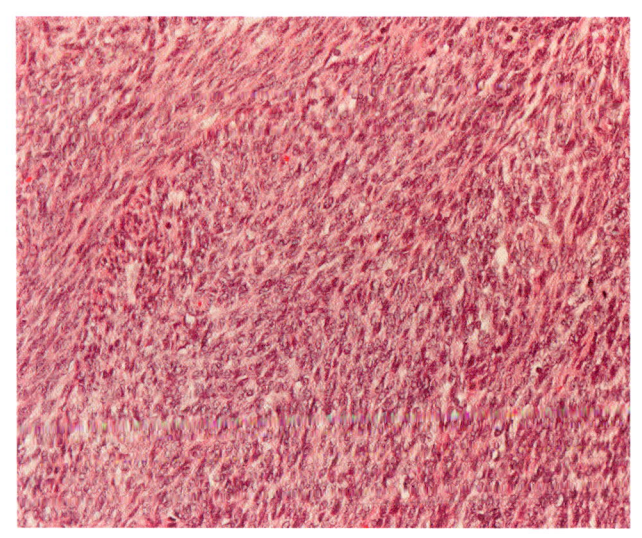

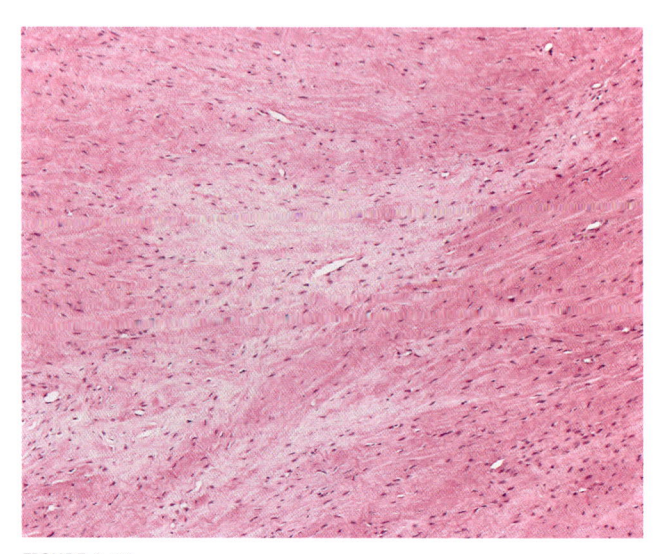

FIGURE 3-36
Low-grade fibromyxoid sarcoma.
Hypocellular mass with alternating collagenous and myxoid areas.

FIGURE 3-35
Conventional adult fibrosarcoma.
Monotonous spindle cells in a *herringbone* pattern.

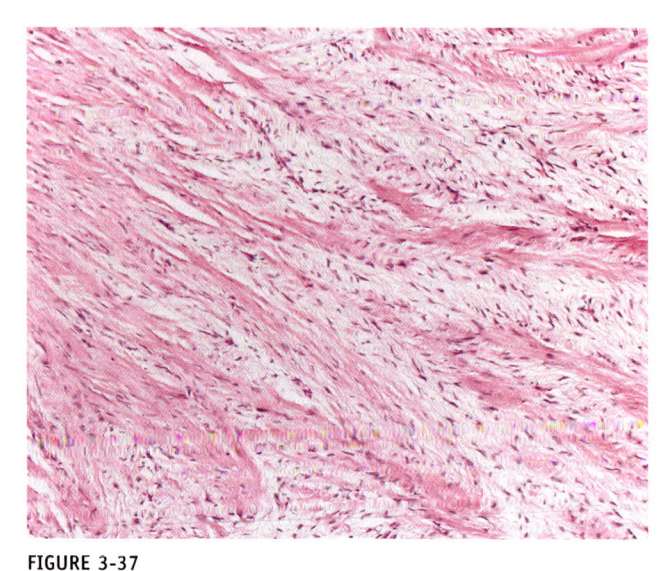

FIGURE 3-37
Low-grade fibromyxoid sarcoma.
Fascicular arrangement of tumor cells, with alternating collagenous and myxoid areas.

tumor with giant rosettes (Figure 3-39). Fifteen to 20% of low-grade fibromyxoid sarcomas contain intermediate- or high-grade, densely cellular areas resembling conventional fibrosarcoma. Recurrent tumors also tend to be more cellular and mitotically active, at least focally.

Sclerosing epithelioid fibrosarcoma consists of peculiar, epithelioid or clear tumor cells, arranged in strands, nests, or acini and embedded in a densely hyalinized collagenous matrix (Figure 3-40). Nuclei are often round and relatively bland, and mitotic activity is minimal. Sclerotic hypocellular areas coexist with more cellular zones resembling conventional fibrosarcoma. Myxoid change, foci of cartilage, and/or bone metaplasia and calcified foci are frequently observed. The tumor often infiltrates the surrounding tissues and may even infiltrate the periosteum or the underlying bone, or both.

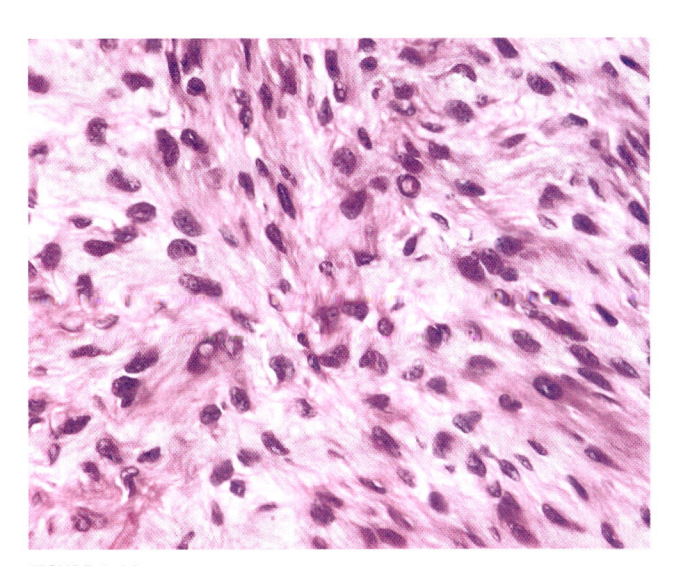

Myxofibrosarcoma is a nodular, variably myxoid lesion. Unfortunately, no consensus exists on the extent of the myxoid areas required for the diagnosis of myxofibrosarcoma: whereas some authors require at least 50%, 10% is enough for others. Low-, intermediate-, and high-grade tumors have been described, depending on the respective proportions of myxoid and nonmyxoid components. Low-grade myxofibrosarcomas are predominantly myxoid; the tumor is hypocellular and contains distinctive curvilinear vessels (Figure 3-41). Tumor cells, which have enlarged hyperchromatic nuclei, tend to aggregate around vessels. Vacuolated cells containing acid mucin and resembling lipoblasts are also found. Mitotic figures are rare. In high-grade lesions, the malignant fibrous histiocytoma-like component predominates but myxoid foci are still recognizable (Figure 3-42). Nuclear pleomorphism is

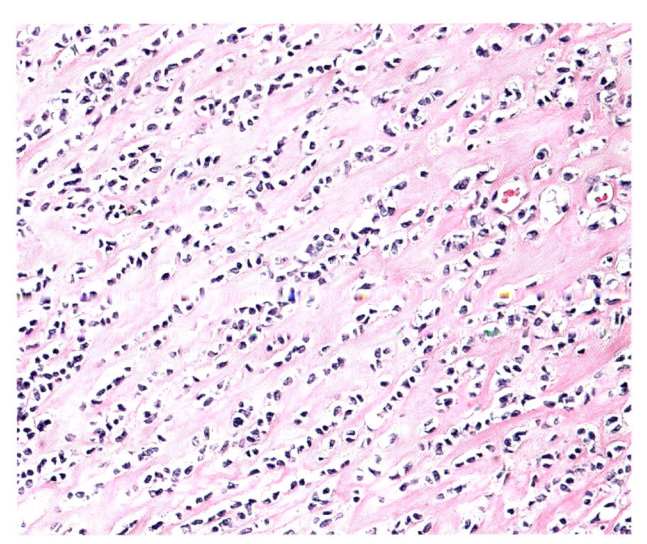

FIGURE 3-38
Low-grade fibromyxoid sarcoma.
Pseudonuclear inclusions are evident in this cellular zone.

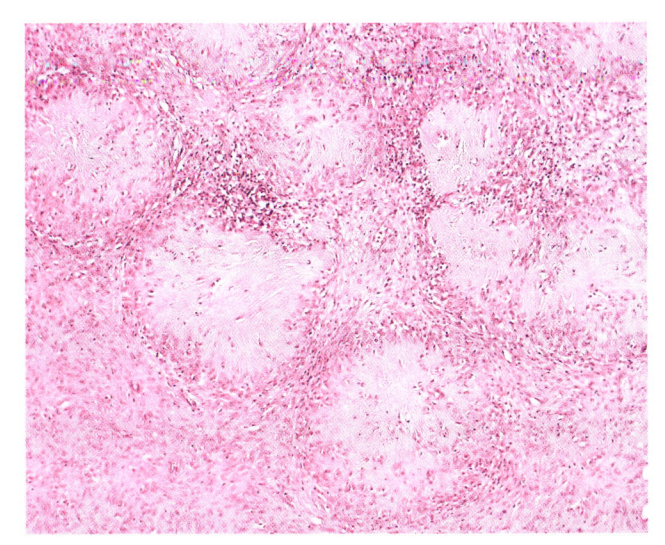

FIGURE 3-40
Sclerosing epithelioid fibrosarcoma.
Cords of epithelioid-to-clear cells embedded in a densely hyalinized collagenous matrix.

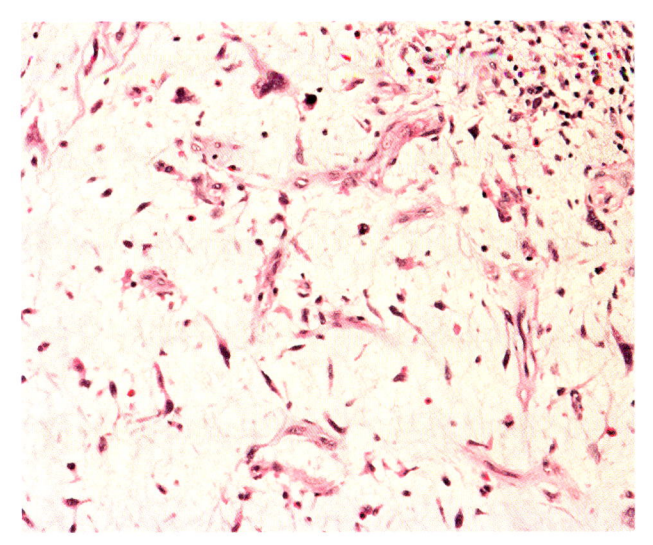

FIGURE 3-39
Hyalinizing spindle cell tumor with giant rosettes, a rosette-rich variant of low-grade fibromyxoid sarcoma. Giant rosettes consist of cores of hyalinized collagen surrounded by rounded, epithelioid tumor cells.

FIGURE 3-41
Low-grade myxofibrosarcoma.
Curvilinear vessels and tumor cells with enlarged hyperchromatic nuclei are evident in this myxoid nodule.

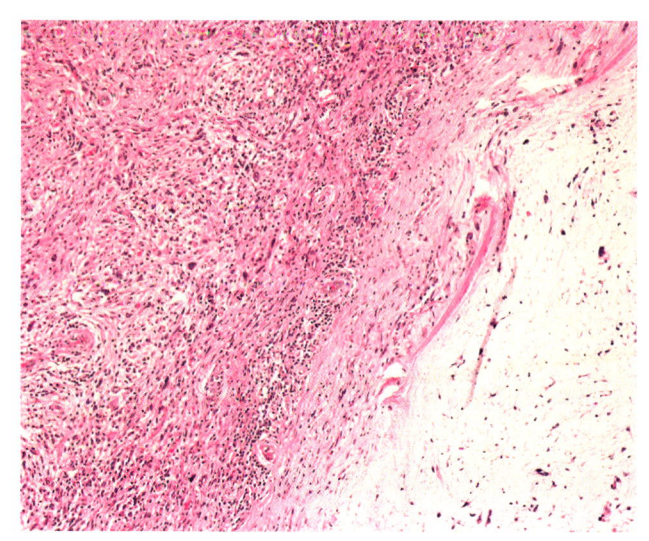

FIGURE 3-42
High-grade myxofibrosarcoma.
High-grade areas adjacent to low-grade/myxoid foci.

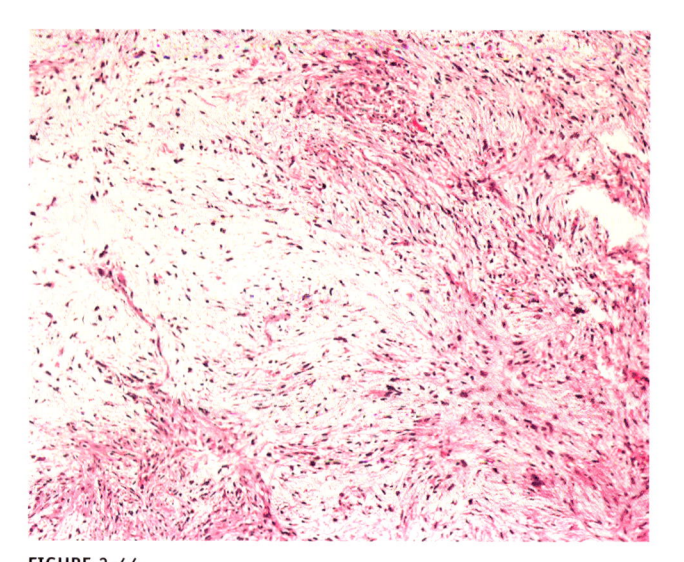

FIGURE 3-44
Intermediate-grade myxofibrosarcoma showing cellularity and cellular atypia intermediate between high- and low-grade forms.

evident, multinucleated giant cells and necrosis are common, and mitotic figures, including abnormal mitoses, are readily visible (Figure 3-43). Cellularity and cellular atypia in intermediate-grade myxofibrosarcomas are between low- and high-grade forms (Figure 3-44). Subcutaneous cases of myxofibrosarcoma can grow quite a way along subcutaneous fibrous septa from the main lesion.

ANCILLARY STUDIES

IMMUNOHISTOCHEMISTRY

In *conventional fibrosarcoma,* tumor cells express vimentin only. Focal reactivity for smooth muscle actin is also possible. S-100 and epithelial markers are not expressed. *Low-grade fibromyxoid sarcoma* cells may also focally express smooth muscle actin and, more rarely, CD34 or desmin. They are generally negative for S-100 protein and EMA. Unlike the other variants, cells in *sclerosing epithelioid fibrosarcoma* may express various antigens, including bcl-2 (90% of cases), p53 protein, S-100 protein, EMA (50% of cases), and cytokeratins (10% of cases). CD34, CD45, desmin, smooth muscle actin, and HMB45 are generally not expressed. In *myxofibrosarcoma,* the cells stain diffusely for vimentin and occasionally for smooth muscle actin. They are negative for S-100 protein, CD34, and CD68.

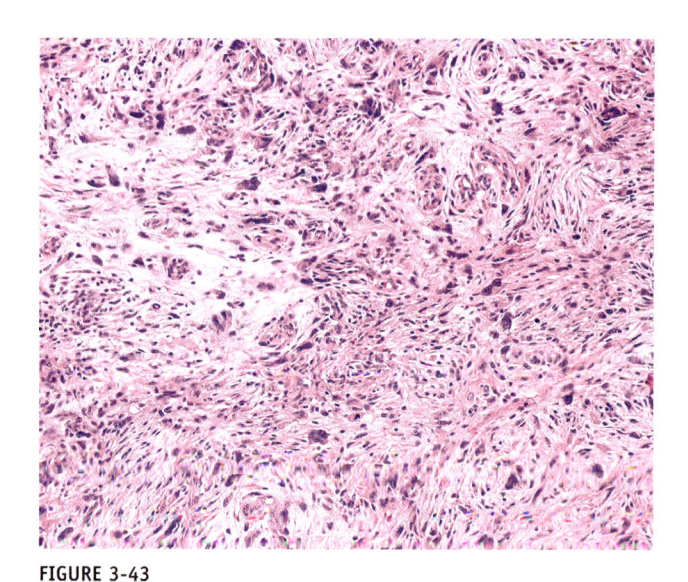

GENETICS

Recurrent and specific chromosomal abnormalities have not yet been observed in fibrosarcoma and its variants, with the exception of low-grade fibromyxoid sarcoma. A significant proportion of low-grade fibromyxoid sarcomas bear a t(7;16) (q33;p11) reciprocal translocation or contain supernumerary ring chromosomes composed of material from chromosomes 7 and 16. Chimeric FUS/CREB3L2 fusion transcripts can be detected in this tumor type, using reverse transcription–polymerase chain reaction (RT-PCR) or fluorescence in situ hybridization (FISH).

DIFFERENTIAL DIAGNOSIS

Conventional fibrosarcoma is a diagnosis of exclusion, meaning that monophasic synovial sarcoma and MPNST, two important mimics, must be ruled out. As opposed to fibrosarcoma, tumor cells in monophasic synovial sarcoma express epithelial markers (EMA, cytokeratins, or both)

FIGURE 3-43
High-grade myxofibrosarcoma.
Nuclear pleomorphism, giant tumor cells, and mitotic figures, including abnormal mitoses, are common features in high-grade zones.

and bear the t(X;18)(p11;q11) (SYT-SSX) translocation. Unlike fibrosarcoma, MPNSTs are positive for S-100 protein in 50% to 60% of cases, and often also for CD34. In the subcutis, any fibrosarcoma-like tumor should prompt a search for a DFSP with fibrosarcomatous transformation. CD34 positivity is important in this context, and the periphery of the tumor and the deep dermis should be carefully examined for areas of more conventional dermatofibrosarcoma. Spindle cell melanoma and carcinoma can be ruled out by their reactivity for S-100 protein and melan-A, and keratins and EMA, respectively. Conventional fibrosarcoma must also be differentiated from benign lesions such as nodular fasciitis in its active phase and the deep variant of fibrous histiocytoma. As opposed to fibrosarcoma, nodular fasciitis is a small, subcutaneous tumor composed of bland myofibroblasts and some inflammatory cells in a variably myxoid matrix. Fibrous histiocytoma is generally small, and displays a storiform and/or an HPC-like rather than a fascicular growth pattern; there are also various inflammatory elements present, including xanthoma cells. Hypocellular and/or markedly collagenous variants of fibrosarcoma may be confused with desmoid tumor or fibroma but will always be more cellular and more mitotically active.

Classic *low-grade fibromyxoid sarcoma* may resemble benign lesions such as fibroma, neurofibroma, perineurioma, and desmoid tumor. However, neurofibroma and perineurioma are positive for S-100 protein and EMA, respectively. Deep fibromatoses (desmoid tumors) are more uniform, lack myxoid nodules, have a more fascicular growth pattern, and are usually reactive for smooth muscle actin and often focally for desmin. Among malignant tumors, low-grade MPNST (focal S-100 positivity), the myxoid variant of dermatofibrosarcoma (CD34 positivity), and the low-grade variant of myxofibrosarcoma (subcutaneous location, greater degree of nuclear pleomorphism) are most likely to be confused with low-grade fibromyxoid sarcoma. When giant rosettes are present, leiomyoma, neuroblastoma-like schwannoma, and metastatic low-grade endometrial stromal sarcoma must also be considered but can easily be excluded on immunohistochemical grounds.

The differential diagnosis of *sclerosing epithelioid fibrosarcoma* is wide. This tumor should be differentiated primarily from signet-ring-cell carcinoma (especially infiltrating lobular carcinoma), sclerosing lymphoma, epithelioid synovial sarcoma, clear cell sarcoma, MPNST, paraganglioma, and extraskeletal osteosarcoma. In this context, previous medical history, clinical presentation, immunohistochemical features, and molecular data should all be taken into consideration.

Low-grade myxofibrosarcoma may be confused with myxoma and nodular fasciitis, as well as with low-grade fibromyxoid sarcoma and myxoid liposarcoma, because of the presence of plexiform vessels and vacuolated cells. However, myxoma, nodular fasciitis, and low-grade fibromyxoid sarcoma all occur in young to middle-aged adults, and lack cellular atypia and hyperchromatic nuclei. *High-grade myxofibrosarcoma* may be confused with any pleomorphic sarcomas, as well as with the recently described inflammatory myxohyaline tumor (also called *myxoinflammatory fibroblastic sarcoma*).

PROGNOSIS AND TREATMENT

The local recurrence rate of *conventional fibrosarcoma* is 20% to 45% at 5 years. As for any sarcoma, wide excision with tumor-free margins followed by adjuvant radiation therapy is the gold standard for therapy; for patients thus treated, the recurrence rate is between 10% and 20%. The metastatic rate is 20% to 30% at 5 years, depending on tumor grade. Metastases are mainly to lungs but also to bone; lymph node metastases are rare. Patients with high-grade tumors may benefit from adjuvant chemotherapy. Overall, the 5-year survival rate

---

ADULT FIBROSARCOMA AND VARIANTS—FACT SHEET

Definition
- *Conventional fibrosarcoma*: a malignant tumor composed of fibroblasts arranged in a herringbone pattern, with varying amounts of collagen in the background
- *Low-grade fibromyxoid sarcoma*: a rare sarcoma consisting of an admixture of myxoid and collagenized zones, with whorls of deceptively bland spindle cells and prominent curved vessels
- *Sclerosing epithelioid fibrosarcoma*: a distinctive variant of fibrosarcoma, in which strands or nests of epithelioid tumor cells are embedded in a densely collagenous matrix
- *Myxofibrosarcoma*: a fibroblastic lesion with a variably myxoid stroma, nuclear pleomorphism, and a distinctive vascular pattern

Incidence and Location
- *Conventional fibrosarcoma*: rare; lower extremities (thigh), trunk
- *Low-grade fibromyxoid sarcoma*: rare; deep soft tissues of limbs (thigh), limb girdles, trunk
- *Sclerosing epithelioid fibrosarcoma*: rare; deep soft tissues of limbs and limb girdles
- *Myxofibrosarcoma*: one of the most common sarcomas of elderly patients
  - Limbs and limb girdles; two-thirds in lower dermis or subcutis, one-third in deep soft tissues

Morbidity and Mortality
- *Conventional fibrosarcoma*: overall 5-year survival rate: 40% to 60%
  - Metastases occurring in lungs and bone (vertebra)
- *Low-grade fibromyxoid sarcoma*: 5-year overall survival: more than 95% if initial tumor is adequately treated
  - Late metastases common, mostly to lungs
- *Sclerosing epithelioid fibrosarcoma*: local recurrence rate: 50%
  - Metastatic rate: 40% to 80%, to lungs, pleura, and bone
  - Overall 5-year survival rate: 70%
- *Myxofibrosarcoma*: recurrences in up to 50% to 60%, regardless of grade
  - Metastases in 20% to 35%, only in intermediate- and high-grade lesions (lungs, bone, lymph nodes)

(Continued)

ADULT FIBROSARCOMA AND VARIANTS—FACT SHEET—con't

Sex, Race, and Age Distribution
- *Conventional fibrosarcoma:* younger adults (30 to 60 years), slightly more frequent in men
- *Low-grade fibromyxoid sarcoma:* young adults (median age, 35 years), slightly more frequent in men
- *Myxofibrosarcoma:* older adults (50 to 70 years), no sex predilection
- *Sclerosing epithelioid fibrosarcoma:* adults (median age, 43 years), no sex predilection

Clinical Features
- *Conventional fibrosarcoma:* Large, deep-seated, slow-growing, solitary mass
  - May occur at site of prior injury, burn, or radiotherapy (postirradiation fibrosarcoma)
- *Low-grade fibromyxoid sarcoma:* Deep, painless mass that may have been present for a long time
- *Sclerosing epithelioid fibrosarcoma:* deep-seated, sometimes painful mass
- *Myxofibrosarcoma:* slow-growing, painless mass
  - Two-thirds in lower dermis or subcutis, one-third deep to fascia

Radiologic Features
- *Conventional fibrosarcoma:* if in contact with bone, may be visible periosteal reaction
- *Low-grade fibromyxoid sarcoma:* cystic change may be visible
- *Sclerosing epithelioid fibrosarcoma:* may be focally calcified
- *Myxofibrosarcoma:* necrosis and hemorrhage may be visible

Prognosis and Treatment
- *Conventional fibrosarcoma:* 5-year overall local recurrence rate: 20% to 45% (10% to 20% for adequately resected tumors)
  - 5-year metastatic rate: 20% to 30%
  - Adverse prognostic factors: high histologic grade, high cellularity, high mitotic activity (> 20/10 hpf), tumor size larger than 5 cm, tumor necrosis, deep location
  - Treatment: wide excision with tumor-free margins plus adjuvant radiation therapy; adjuvant chemotherapy recommended for high-grade tumors
- *Low-grade fibromyxoid sarcoma*
  - For adequately resected primaries:
  Local recurrence rate: 10%
  Metastatic rate: 5% to 10%
  - Adverse prognostic factors: marginal resection and, possibly, high-grade areas
  - Treatment: wide excision with tumor-free margins; adjuvant radiation therapy recommended
- *Sclerosing epithelioid fibrosarcoma*
  - Adverse prognostic factors: proximal location, large tumor size, male sex
- *Myxofibrosarcoma:* overall recurrence rate of 50%, unrelated to histologic grade
  - Overall metastatic rate of 20% to 35%, grade-dependent (only in high-grade lesions)
  - Low-grade lesions may give higher-grade recurrences
  - Mortality higher in deep-seated and high-grade lesions, and if local recurrence occurs within 12 months of initial therapy

ADULT FIBROSARCOMA VARIANTS—PATHOLOGIC FEATURES

Gross Findings
- *Conventional fibrosarcoma:* well-defined solitary masses, 3 to 8 cm
  - Whitish and fleshy on section; may contain necrotic or hemorrhagic foci
- *Low-grade fibromyxoid sarcoma:* well-defined, sometimes lobulated; homogeneous tan appearance
- *Sclerosing epithelioid fibrosarcoma:* well-circumscribed, lobulated, median size of 7 to 10 cm
  - Firm and whitish, sometimes with calcifications or cystic/myxoid change
- *Myxofibrosarcoma:*
  - Subcutaneous lesions: multiple glistening gray-white nodules
  - Deep lesions: solitary poorly defined mass, may have necrosis or hemorrhage

Microscopic Findings
- *Conventional fibrosarcoma:* monotonous, uniform, bipolar spindle cells with scant cytoplasm and tapered nuclei
  - Long, sweeping bundles in a herringbone pattern
  - Collagenous stroma may be abundant (postradiation sarcoma) or minimal (high-grade lesions)
  - Mitotic activity moderate
  - Little or no pleomorphism, giant or multinucleated cells
  - Necrosis: mostly in high-grade lesions
- *Low-grade fibromyxoid sarcoma:* admixture of collagenous and myxoid zones, with abrupt transition from one to the other
  - Bland spindle cells with oval nuclei and pale eosinophilic cytoplasm
  - Sweeping fascicles or whorls
  - Curvilinear or plexiform vessels, especially visible in myxoid areas
  - Mitotic activity low; no necrosis
- *Sclerosing epithelioid fibrosarcoma:* strands or nests of epithelioid or clear cells with uniform, round, or oval nuclei
  - Mitotic activity low
  - Dense collagenous background
  - May be more cellular areas resembling conventional fibrosarcoma
  - HPC-like vascular pattern
- *Myxofibrosarcoma:* Cells with enlarged, hyperchromatic, often pleomorphic nuclei
  - Variably myxoid background
  - May be lipoblast-like cells
  - Mitotic activity low
  - Curvilinear, thin-walled blood vessels

Genetics
- *Conventional fibrosarcoma:* no specific findings yet described
- *Low-grade fibromyxoid sarcoma:* t(7;16) reciprocal translocation, or ring chromosomes with material from 7 and 16
- *Sclerosing epithelioid fibrosarcoma:* no specific findings yet described
- *Myxofibrosarcoma:* no specific findings yet described

Immunohistochemical Findings
- *Conventional fibrosarcoma, myxofibrosarcoma, and low-grade fibromyxoid sarcoma*
  - Constant positivity for vimentin
  - Focal positivity for smooth muscle actin possible
  - S-100 protein, EMA, keratins negative

---

is 40% to 60%, regardless of grade. Adverse prognostic factors include high histologic grade, high cellularity with minimal collagen deposition, high mitotic activity (> 20/10 hpf), large tumor size (> 5 cm), tumor necrosis, and deep location.

(Continued)

ADULT FIBROSARCOMA VARIANTS—PATHOLOGIC FEATURES—con't

» *Sclerosing epithelioid fibrosarcoma*
  » Constantly vimentin positive
  » bcl-2 positive in 90% of cases
  » p53, S-100 protein, EMA, keratins may be positive in a minority of cases

Differential Diagnosis

» *Conventional fibrosarcoma*
  » Monophasic fibrous synovial sarcoma
  » MPNST
  » DFSP with fibrosarcomatous transformation (if located in the subcutis)
  » Nodular fasciitis and fibrous histiocytoma
  » Fibromatosis
  » *Low-grade fibromyxoid sarcoma*
  » *Classic low-grade fibromyxoid sarcoma:*
  Fibroma
  Neurofibroma
  Perineurioma
  Deep fibromatosis (desmoid tumor)
  MPNST
  Myxofibrosarcoma
  Myxoid variant of dermatofibrosarcoma
  Spindle cell liposarcoma
  » *Low-grade fibromyxoid sarcoma with giant rosettes:*
  Soft tissue leiomyoma
  Neuroblastoma-like schwannoma
  Metastatic low-grade endometrial stromal sarcoma with smooth muscle differentiation
» *Sclerosing epithelioid fibrosarcoma*
  » Carcinoma (signet ring cell carcinoma)
  » Melanoma
  » Synovial sarcoma
  » MPNST
  » Extraskeletal chondrosarcoma and osteosarcoma
  » Dedifferentiated liposarcoma
» *Myxofibrosarcoma*
  » Low-grade:
  Nodular fasciitis
  Myxoma/cellular myxoma/juxta-articular myxoma
  Myxoid liposarcoma
  » High-grade:
  Inflammatory myxohyaline tumor/myxoinflamatory fibroblastic sarcoma
  Pleomorphic liposarcoma
  Dedifferentiated liposarcoma
  High-grade MPNST
  Metastatic carcinoma and melanoma

For *low-grade fibromyxoid sarcomas* adequately resected *ab initio*, the local recurrence rate is close to 10% and the metastatic rate is close to 15%. Metastases are mainly to lungs and pleura, also to bone, and can occur late in the course of the disease (15 to 25 years after initial excision). The presence of small high-grade areas in an otherwise low-grade lesion is not currently believed to be prognostically significant. Wide excision with tumor-free margins is the optimal surgical treatment. Adjuvant radiation therapy is recommended by some authors.

About 50% of patients with *sclerosing epithelioid fibrosarcoma* have local recurrences. Metastases develop in 40% to 80% of patients, mainly in the lungs but also in pleura, bone, and soft tissues. Five-year survival is around 70%. Proximal location, large tumor size, and male sex are important adverse prognostic factors.

The clinical behavior of *myxofibrosarcoma* depends on its histologic grade and on the extent of resection. Local recurrences occur in about 50% of cases, often because of inadequate initial excisions. It is not unusual for recurrences to show signs of upgrading with an increase in cellularity, pleomorphism, and mitotic activity, and conversely, a reduction of the myxoid component. Metastases to lungs and bone are mostly observed in high-grade, deep-seated tumors (20% to 35%); they are rare in low-grade lesions. The overall 5-year survival rate is 60% to 70%.

INFANTILE FIBROSARCOMA

CLINICAL FEATURES

Infantile fibrosarcoma (also called *congenital fibrosarcoma*) is an unusual tumor of infants and young children. It presents as a large, painless, solitary, rapidly growing mass of distal extremities (foot, ankle, lower leg, forearm, wrist, hand) involving the superficial and deep soft tissues. The trunk and the head and neck region may more rarely be involved. The overlying skin is often reddened or ulcerated. The tumor is present at birth in 30% to 40% of cases.

PATHOLOGIC FEATURES

GROSS FINDINGS

Infantile fibrosarcoma is a poorly circumscribed and lobulated neoplasm measuring 5 to 15 cm in diameter. Cut section reveals a fleshy, grayish aspect. Necrotic, hemorrhagic, and/or myxoid areas can be observed.

MICROSCOPIC FINDINGS

At low power, infantile fibrosarcoma is a densely cellular neoplasm composed of intersecting bundles of monotonous spindle cells (Figure 3-45). Nuclear pleomorphism is not a feature, and collagen deposition is often minimal. The mitotic activity is usually brisk and the tumor contains numerous interstitial lymphocytes. Dilated and/or branching, HPC-like vessels are often seen (Figure 3-46). Dystrophic calcification, areas of hemorrhage or necrosis, and foci of extramedullary hematopoiesis may be visible.

INFANTILE FIBROSARCOMA—FACT SHEET

Definition
- A tumor of infants, which resembles classic adult fibrosarcoma histologically and which predominantly involves the distal extremities

Incidence and Location
- 12% of soft tissue malignancies in infants
- 36% to 80% of cases are congenital or occur in the first year of life
- Rare after 2 years of age
- Distal extremities (60% of cases); trunk, head, and neck region

Morbidity and Mortality
- Local recurrence in 5% to 50% of cases
- Metastases in less than 10% of cases
- Mortality rate: 4% to 25%

Sex, Race, and Age Distribution
- Slight male predominance

Clinical Features
- Congenital in 30% to 40% of cases
- Large, painless, rapidly enlarging mass
- Overlying skin reddened or ulcerated

Prognosis and Treatment
- Local recurrences in 5% to 50% of cases
- Metastases in less than 10% of cases
- Treatment: complete surgical excision with or without adjuvant chemotherapy

INFANTILE FIBROSARCOMA—PATHOLOGIC FEATURES

Gross Findings
- Poorly circumscribed, lobular mass
- Size: 5 to 15 cm

Microscopic Findings
- Densely cellular
- Intersecting fascicles of spindle cells; nuclear pleomorphism usually absent
- Numerous mitoses
- Numerous interstitial lymphocytes
- Hemangiopericytoma-like vascular pattern often apparent
- Infiltration of surrounding tissues

Genetics
- t(12;15)(p13;q26) reciprocal translocation involving *NTRK3* and *ETV6* genes
- Trisomy of chromosomes 8, 11, 17, and 20

Immunohistochemical Findings
- Positivity for vimentin
- Variable reactivity with smooth muscle actin
- Occasional reactivity with desmin, CD34, S-100 protein, or keratins
- EMA negative

Differential Diagnosis
- Conventional (adult-type) fibrosarcoma
- Synovial sarcoma (monophasic variant)
- MPNST
- Infantile hemangiopericytoma and myofibromatosis
- Spindle cell rhabdomyosarcoma
- Infantile fibromatosis (cellular variant)

Although grossly well delineated, this neoplasm commonly infiltrates the surrounding soft tissues on microscopic examination. Rarely, recurring infantile fibrosarcoma may be more pleomorphic. Areas resembling infantile myofibromatosis or infantile hemangiopericytoma are observed in so-called composite tumors.

ANCILLARY STUDIES

IMMUNOHISTOCHEMISTRY

Spindle cells in infantile fibrosarcoma express vimentin and smooth muscle actin in 30% of cases. Occasional reactivity for desmin, CD34, S-100 protein, or keratins may be seen. EMA is not expressed.

GENETICS

Most infantile fibrosarcomas bear a reciprocal t(12;15)(p13;q26) translocation. The two genes involved are the *NTRK3* gene (a receptor tyrosine kinase gene) on chromosome 15q, and the *ETV6* (TEL) gene on chromosome 12p. A similar genetic profile is observed in cellular congenital mesoblastic nephroma. The ETV6/NTRK3 fusion protein is oncogenic, and is detectable in frozen and paraffin-embedded tissue using RT-PCR or in situ hybridization. Trisomy of chromosomes 11, 20, 17, and 8 are also characteristically observed in infantile fibrosarcoma.

DIFFERENTIAL DIAGNOSIS

Conventional (adult-type) fibrosarcoma, monophasic synovial sarcoma, MPNST, infantile myofibromatosis, infantile fibromatosis (cellular variant)/infantile hemangiopericytoma, malignant hemangiopericytoma, and spindle cell rhabdomyosarcoma are the main differential diagnoses to be considered. Age at presentation and the presence of interstitial lymphocytes within the tumor distinguish infantile fibrosarcoma from the adult form. Synovial sarcomas are almost always positive for cytokeratins, EMA, or both. MPNSTs are rare in infants and are often attached to large nerves. Infantile myofibromatosis, infantile hemangiopericytoma, and cellular

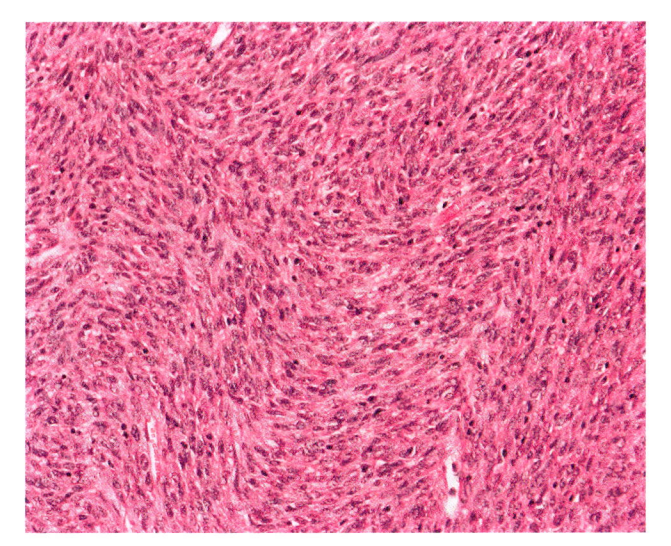

FIGURE 3-45
Infantile fibrosarcoma.
Intersecting fascicles of monotonous spindle cells, resembling conventional (adult-type) fibrosarcoma, with rare interspersed lymphocytes.

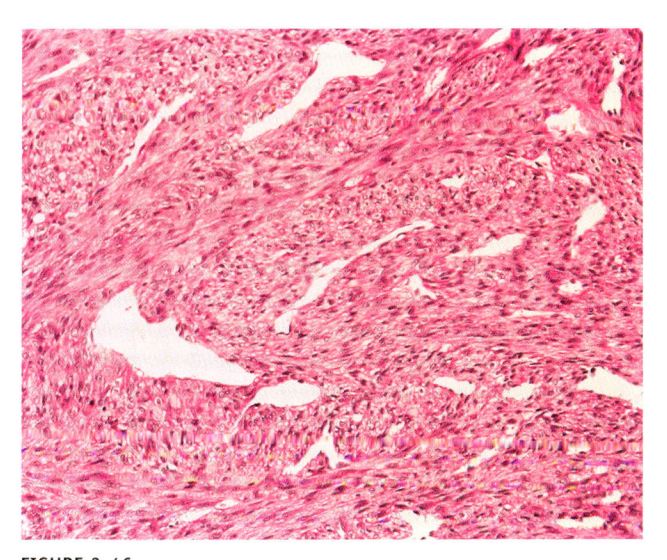

FIGURE 3-46
Infantile fibrosarcoma.
Spindle cell proliferation with branching, hemangiopericytoma-like vessels.

infantile fibromatosis may be morphologically indistinguishable from infantile fibrosarcoma. The two former entities are related, benign neoplasms, whereas infantile fibromatosis is a recurring but nonmetastasizing lesion; in all three, the tumor cells are positive, at least focally, for smooth muscle actin and variably positive for desmin. Cytogenetics and molecular biology are crucial for distinguishing between these entities. Spindle cell rhabdomyosarcoma usually occurs in the paratesticular and head and neck regions in children. The tumor cells, which have a fibrillary elongated cytoplasm, are positive for desmin and myogenin, and show ultrastructural features of skeletal muscle differentiation.

PROGNOSIS AND TREATMENT

Although large, and histologically worrisome, infantile fibrosarcoma carries a good prognosis. It can recur (5% to 50% of cases depending on the extent of the surgical excision) but metastasizes rarely (< 10% of cases). The mortality rate ranges from 4% to 25%; the 5-year survival rate is 75% to 84%. Rare cases of spontaneous regression have been described. Complete surgical excision, if possible, is the treatment of choice. Amputation may be required for huge unresectable tumors. Adjuvant/neoadjuvant chemotherapy or adjuvant radiotherapy has also been proved effective in selected cases.

FIBROHISTIOCYTIC TUMORS

INTRODUCTION

The group of fibrohistiocytic tumors encompasses those tumors that are composed, partly or exclusively, of fibroblasts, myofibroblasts, and tumor cells (including multinucleated giant cells) showing some evidence of phagocytic activity. In keeping with the recent World Health Organization (WHO) classification of tumors of soft tissue and bone, pleomorphic malignant fibrous histiocytoma, which was previously regarded as the most common adult soft tissue sarcoma, is now considered an undifferentiated pleomorphic sarcoma NOS. The so-called myxoid variant of malignant fibrous histiocytoma (currently called *myxofibrosarcoma*) remains a discrete entity. By contrast, giant cell and inflammatory subtypes of malignant fibrous histiocytoma, which share

---

MAIN HISTOLOGIC TUMOR TYPES AND SUBTYPES IN THE FIBROHISTIOCYTIC TUMOR CATEGORY

Benign fibrous histiocytomas
Dermal benign fibrous histiocytomas
Subcutaneous and deep benign fibrous histiocytomas
Juvenile xanthogranuloma, reticulohistiocytoma
Xanthoma
Atypical fibroxanthoma
Giant cell tumor of tendon sheath, localized type (nodular tenosynovitis)
Giant cell tumor of tendon sheath, diffuse type (pigmented villonodular synovitis)
DFSP
Giant cell fibroblastoma
Plexiform fibrohistiocytic tumor
Angiomatoid fibrous histiocytoma
Giant cell tumor of soft tissue (of low malignant potential)
Undifferentiated high-grade sarcoma (so-called *malignant fibrous histiocytoma*)

some morphologic features with other unrelated tumors, are no longer considered distinct entities.

BENIGN FIBROUS HISTIOCYTOMAS AND VARIANTS

CLINICAL FEATURES

Benign fibrous histiocytoma is a common lesion of the dermis and subcutis. Dermal lesions are also called *dermatofibromas*. Benign fibrous histiocytoma can be seen in every part of the body but is more frequently encountered in extremities of young to middle-aged adults (20 to 40 years). It has a female predominance. The lesions may be solitary or multiple. Several variants have been described, of which the cellular, aneurysmal, and atypical forms have potential for local recurrence (25% of cases).

PATHOLOGIC FEATURES

GROSS FINDINGS

Conventional fibrous histiocytoma presents as an indurated, well-delineated plaque or nodule, measuring usually less than 1 cm in maximal diameter. Aneurysmal benign fibrous histiocytomas may occasionally be large (>5 cm).

MICROSCOPIC FINDINGS

Fibrous histiocytoma consists of a circumscribed, variably cellular monomorphic population of spindle cells arranged in fascicles and storiform patterns, which may be intermixed with multinucleated giant cells (Touton giant cells), foamy macrophages, siderophages, and interstitial fibrosis (Figures 3-47 and 3-48). Thickened collagen bundles are classically observed at the periphery, surrounded by lesional cells (Figure 3-49). The overlying epidermis is often hyperplastic. Cellular fibrous histiocytomas are highly cellular lesions, showing a storiform (Figure 3-50) or fascicular growth pattern, with little collagen deposition. They may resemble leiomyosarcomas in the marked eosinophilic appearance of tumor cells arranged in a predominantly fascicular growth pattern. They tend to be larger (up to 2.5 cm) than common dermatofibroma, often extending into subcutis (30% of cases). Mitoses are numerous (often ≥ 3/10 hpf), and foci of necrosis (10%) or vascular invasion, or both, may be observed. Intralesional aneurysmal changes are characteristic of the aneurysmal variant of fibrous histiocytoma (Figure 3-51). Vascular spaces are often bordered directly by multinucleated cells, siderophages, or both. The pseudovascular lumina are frequently occupied by foamy siderophages or Touton giant cells containing lipid and hemosiderin (Figure 3-52). The atypical (pseudosarcomatous) fibrous histiocytoma variant contains numerous pleomorphic (monster) cells with enlarged hyperchromatic nuclei, resulting in a pseudosarcomatous appearance (Figure 3-53). Mitoses are sometimes numerous in this variant, and atypical mitoses are occasionally seen, especially in pleomorphic areas. Fibrous histiocytomas of the subcutis and/or deep soft tissue are more uniform in appearance, showing a storiform growth pattern and a peculiar hemangiopericytoma-like vascularization formed by branching vessels. They are often

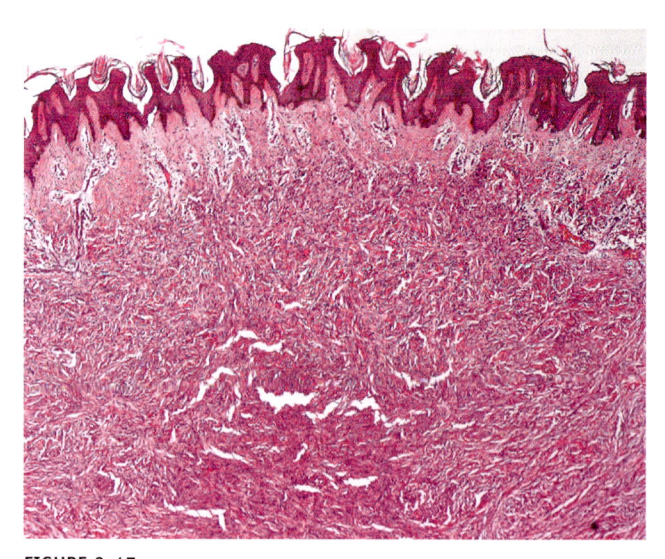

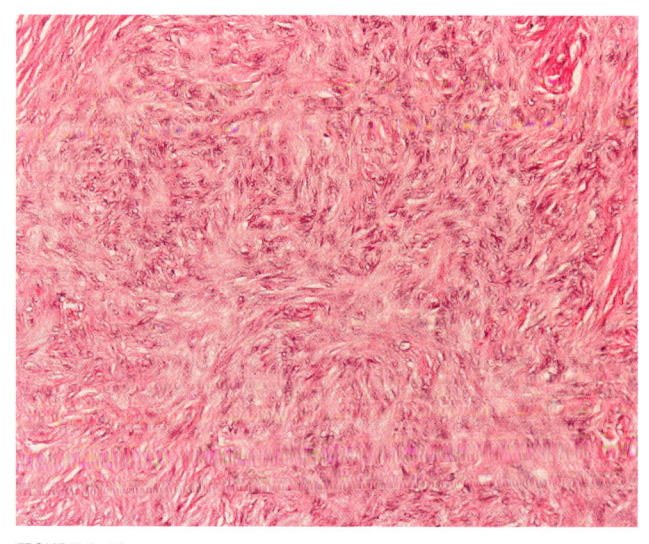

FIGURE 3-47
Benign fibrous histiocytoma.
A circumscribed but noncapsulated fibrohistiocytic dermal proliferation. The overlying epidermis is hyperplastic.

FIGURE 3-48
Benign fibrous histiocytoma.
Storiform arrangement of tumor cells.

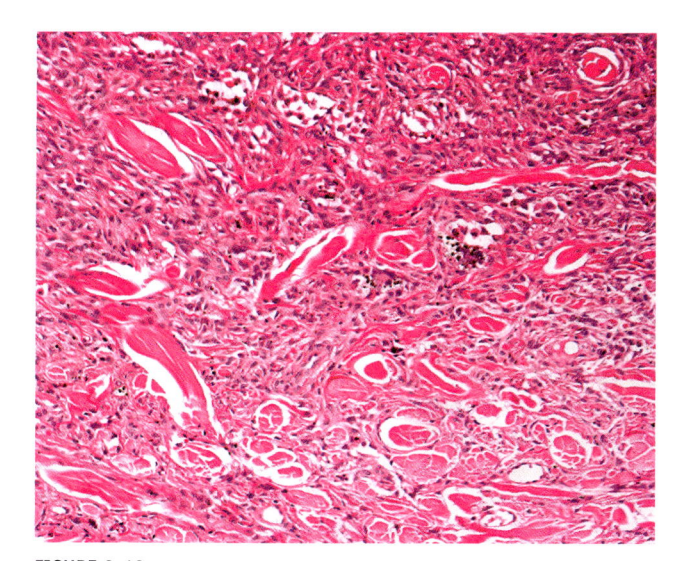

FIGURE 3-49
Benign fibrous histiocytoma.
Thickened collagen bundles are classically observed at the interface between the lesion and the surrounding dermis.

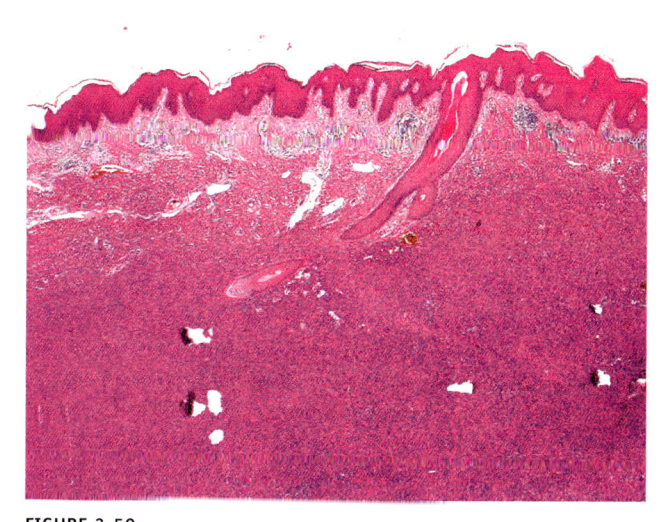

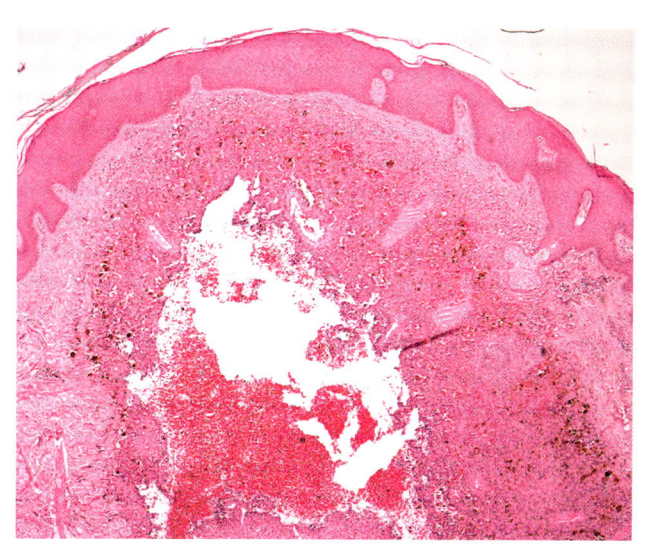

FIGURE 3-51
Aneurysmal benign fibrous histiocytoma.
A low-power view showing central aneurysmal change.

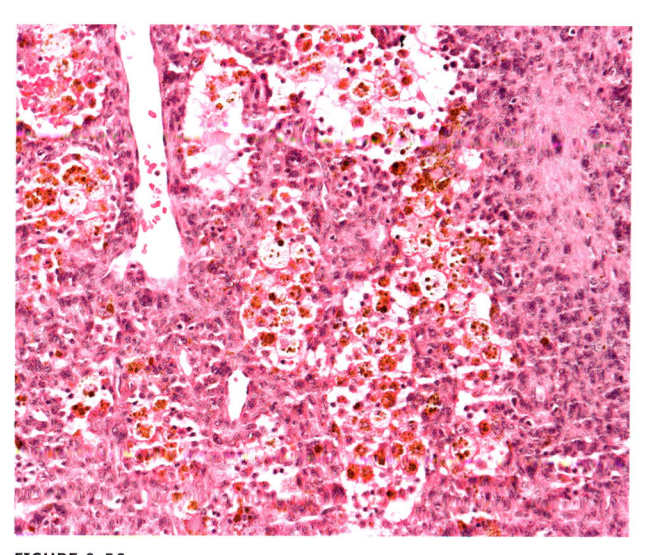

FIGURE 3-50
Cellular benign fibrous histiocytoma.
A fascicular proliferation of bland, lightly eosinophilic spindled cells growing in short fascicles.

FIGURE 3-52
Aneurysmal benign fibrous histiocytoma.
Hemosiderin deposits, and vascular spaces occupied by hemosiderophages and foamy histiocytes are readily visible at high-power magnification.

well demarcated and can be encapsulated. Local recurrences are observed in up to 30% of cases. Several other more unusual fibrous histiocytoma variants have been described, including epithelioid fibrous histiocytoma, clear cell dermatofibroma, granular cell dermatofibroma, and lipidized *(ankle-type)* fibrous histiocytoma.

ANCILLARY STUDIES

IMMUNOHISTOCHEMISTRY

Immunohistochemically, the spindle cells are usually negative for CD34 and positive for factor XIIIa and KiM1p, as opposed to the cells in DFSP. The histiocytic cells, including multinucleated giant cells, express CD68 (clone KP1, PGM1, or both). Deep fibrous histiocytomas often contain a subpopulation of CD34-positive cells.

GENETICS

The true nature, neoplastic or reactive, of benign fibrous histiocytoma has long been disputed. Clonal cytogenetic changes may be seen in up to 38% of cases, favoring a neoplastic process. Karyotypic abnormalities are more frequent in the cellular variant and are different from those in DFSP.

BENIGN FIBROUS HISTIOCYTOMAS—FACT SHEET

Definition
- A benign fibrohistiocytic proliferation of dermis or superficial subcutis, or both

Incidence and Location
- Most common soft tissue tumor of skin
- Mostly in extremities; may be multiple (one-third of cases)

Morbidity and Mortality
- Benign, usually nonrecurring (< 5%)
- Cellular, aneurysmal, and atypical variants recur in up to 25% of cases

Sex, Race, and Age Distribution
- Early to middle-aged adults, no race predilection
- Tend to be more frequent in female individuals

Clinical Features
- Elevated or flat, well-delineated, painless, often indurated, red to brown skin lesion

Prognosis and Treatment
- Complete excision is curative

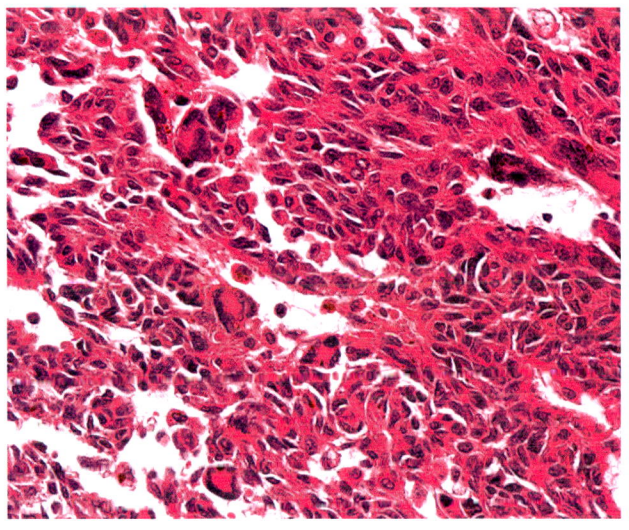

BENIGN FIBROUS HISTIOCYTOMAS—PATHOLOGIC FEATURES

Gross Findings
- Small (≤ 2 cm) plaque-like or nodular well-circumscribed lesion

Microscopic Findings
- Dermal lesion, may extend into subcutis
- Storiform growth pattern
- Foamy macrophages, Touton giant cells, and siderophages common
- Areas of increased cellularity, cellular atypia, and mitotic figures occasional
- Thickened collagen bundles at the periphery of the lesion
- Accompanying epidermal hyperplasia
- *Variants:* growth patterns predominantly fascicular and hemangiopericytoma-like in cellular and deep fibrous histiocytomas, respectively; numerous pleomorphic, *monster* cells in atypical (pseudosarcomatous) fibrous histiocytoma. prominent epithelioid cytomorphology in epithelioid fibrous histiocytoma

Genetics
- Clonal proliferations with karyotypic aberrations

Immunohistochemical Findings
- Tumor cell positivity for CD68 and factor XIIIa; negative for CD34
- Occasional positivity for smooth muscle actin; desmin usually negative

Differential Diagnosis
- DFSP (conventional and cellular fibrous histiocytoma)
- Leiomyosarcoma (cellular fibrous histiocytoma)
- Malignant fibrous histiocytoma (aneurysmal and atypical fibrous histiocytoma)
- Spitz nevus and melanoma (epithelioid fibrous histiocytoma)

FIGURE 3-53
Atypical benign fibrous histiocytoma.
Cellular atypia, pleomorphic hyperchromatic nuclei, and mitoses, including abnormal mitoses, characterize this variant of benign fibrous histiocytoma. The majority of this lesion showed more typical features of benign fibrous histiocytoma.

DIFFERENTIAL DIAGNOSIS

The cellular, aneurysmal, and atypical variants of fibrous histiocytoma are the most likely to be confused with a malignant lesion, especially leiomyosarcoma, DFSP, and malignant fibrous histiocytoma. Leiomyosarcoma may develop in the dermis or subcutis. It is generally more fascicular and contains fewer inflammatory elements than fibrous histiocytomas. In addition, leiomyosarcoma is usually diffusely positive for smooth muscle actin and h-caldesmon, and focally positive for desmin, which is not the case for cellular fibrous histiocytoma. DFSP is a noninflammatory, diffusely infiltrating process developing in deep dermis, often extending into subcutis. It shows a more monotonous storiform appearance than fibrous histiocytoma, and lacks giant and xanthomatous cells. Unlike fibrous histiocytoma, DFSP is positive for CD34 and generally contains only a limited number of factor XIIIa–positive cells. Deep fibrous histiocytomas showing a prominent hemangiopericytomatous pattern should be distinguished from solitary fibrous tumor. Malignant fibrous histiocytomas usually present as large (> 3 cm), pleomorphic to myxoid subcutaneous lesions with cellular atypia and numerous, often atypical, mitoses. Epithelioid fibrous histiocytoma should be differentiated from reticulohistiocytoma, Spitz nevus, and melanoma.

Prognosis and Treatment

Fibrous histiocytomas are benign lesions. Recurrences are rare (<5% of cases), often after incomplete local excisions. Cellular, aneurysmal, and atypical variants of fibrous histiocytoma are prone to recur more frequently (up to 25% of cases). Reexcision is usually curative. Rare occurrence of metastases have been reported with cellular, aneurysmal, and atypical variants of fibrous histiocytomas, often after multiple recurrences.

JUVENILE XANTHOGRANULOMA AND RETICULOHISTIOCYTOMA

Clinical Features

Juvenile xanthogranuloma is a non-X (non-Langerhans cell) form of histiocytosis that occurs predominantly (but not exclusively) in infancy and childhood. It presents as single or multiple skin nodules, sometimes accompanied by synchronous or metachronous lesions in deep soft tissues and/or viscera (lung, epicardium, eye, oral cavity, testis). About half of the lesions develop on the head and neck, followed by the trunk and extremities; 15% to 30% occur in individuals older than 20 years. No associations have been made with serum lipid abnormalities.

Solitary reticulohistiocytoma is a benign skin lesion that overlaps with the adult variant of juvenile xanthogranuloma. It occurs especially in men, at any body site but with a predilection for the head and neck, as a solitary small painless nodule. Solitary reticulohistiocytoma should be separate from the rare multicentric reticulohistiocytosis, a systemic disease occurring predominantly in female individuals, characterized by multiple skin lesions variably associated with systemic symptoms (arthritis, pyrexia, weight loss), with systemic disease (Sjögren syndrome, systemic lupus erythematosus), and occasionally with visceral malignancies.

Pathologic Features

Gross Findings

Juvenile xanthogranulomas usually measure 1.5 cm or less in maximal diameter. They are usually solitary in children older than 2 years and in adults. Reticulohistiocytoma likewise presents as a solitary small (≤ 1.5 cm) lesion.

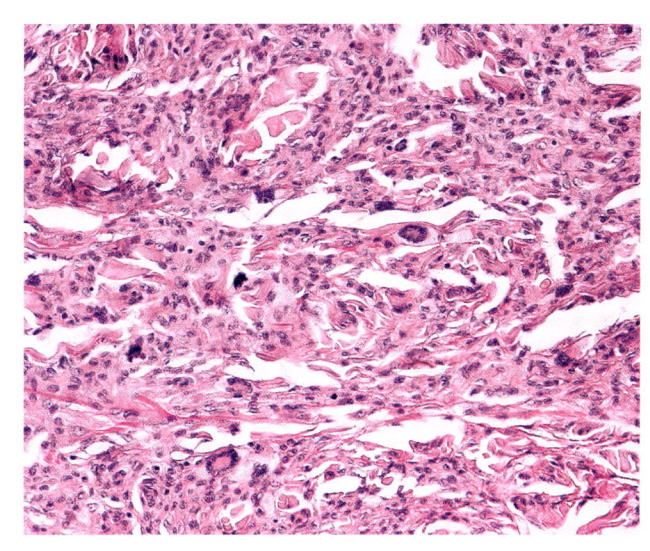

FIGURE 3-54
Juvenile xanthogranuloma.
Dermal/subcutaneous accumulation of nonatypical histiocytes and Touton-type multinucleated giant cells.

Microscopic Findings

Cutaneous lesions consist of dermal/subcutaneous accumulations of nonatypical histiocytes, eosinophils, and Touton multinucleated giant cells in varying proportions. The overlying epidermis is not hyperplastic. The morphologic aspect varies according to the amount of lipid present in the cytoplasm of the histiocytes. Early lesions are predominantly composed of nonlipidized histiocytes and rarely contain Touton giant cells (Figure 3-54), whereas older lesions usually contain numerous xanthomatous histiocytes, Touton giant cells, eosinophils, and some degree of interstitial fibrosis, sometimes resulting in a reticulohistiocytoma-like appearance. Mitoses are scarce. Fibrosis often predominates in long-standing lesions, and these are often difficult to separate from conventional fibrous histiocytomas. In contrast with the cutaneous lesions of juvenile xanthogranuloma, deep lesions are often misleading because of a less specific appearance. They are quite cellular, more monomorphous, less lipidized, and contain few, if any, Touton giant cells.

Reticulohistiocytoma is composed of sheets of histiocytes with abundant eosinophilic cytoplasm (Figures 3-55 and 3-56). Multinucleated giant cells are commonly observed, as well as lymphocyte aggregates. Although rare, mitotic figures can occasionally be seen.

Ancillary Studies

Immunohistochemistry

The histiocytic tumor cells in both entities stain positively for CD68 (clones KP1 and PGM1) and also for CD31. Juvenile xanthogranuloma may be strongly

JUVENILE XANTHOGRANULOMA AND RETICULOHISTIOCYTOMA—FACT SHEET

Definition
▸▸ A benign (fibro)histiocytic proliferation of dermis or superficial subcutis, or both

Incidence and Location
▸▸ Infrequent
▸▸ Head and neck are most common regions

Morbidity and Mortality
▸▸ Benign, nonrecurring lesions; juvenile xanthogranuloma may regress with time

Sex, Race, and Age Distribution
▸▸ Juvenile xanthogranuloma most common in infancy and childhood with no sex predilection; 15% to 30% observed in adults
▸▸ Solitary reticulohistiocytoma most common in adult men

Clinical Features
▸▸ Small nodular skin lesions, solitary for reticulohistiocytoma, may be multiple for juvenile xanthogranuloma
▸▸ Juvenile xanthogranuloma may develop in deep soft tissues, parenchymal organs, or both

Prognosis and Treatment
▸▸ Simple excision is curative
▸▸ Juvenile xanthogranuloma may regress spontaneously with time

FIGURE 3-55
Reticulohistiocytoma.
Dermal accumulation of enlarged, somewhat glassy appearing histiocytes.

positive for factor XIIIa. They are always negative for CD1a and often negative for S-100 protein.

DIFFERENTIAL DIAGNOSIS

Langerhans cell histiocytosis (previously called *histiocytosis X*) involving the skin is the main differential diagnosis of juvenile xanthogranuloma. As opposed to juvenile xanthogranuloma, cells in the former condition are more spindly, with coffee-bean nuclei; they are positive for S-100 protein and CD1a. Touton cells are not a feature of Langerhans cell histiocytosis. Granular cell tumor (in the case of nonlipidized lesions), storage diseases, and benign fibrous histiocytoma are also differential diagnoses to consider. Reticulohistiocytomas characterized by marked cellular pleomorphism should also be distinguished from malignancies such as melanoma, carcinoma, or pleomorphic sarcomas (malignant fibrous histiocytoma).

JUVENILE XANTHOGRANULOMA AND RETICULOHISTIOCYTOMA—PATHOLOGIC FEATURES

Gross Findings
▸▸ Usually small (≤ 1.5-cm) nodular lesions
▸▸ Juvenile xanthogranuloma may be multiple
▸▸ Numerous lesions in multicentric reticulohistiocytosis

Microscopic Findings
▸▸ Dermal accumulations of histiocytes (with striking eosinophilic cytoplasm in reticulohistiocytoma), Touton giant cells, and eosinophils
▸▸ Variable interstitial fibrosis

Immunohistochemical Findings
▸▸ Histiocytes are positive for CD68; negative for CD1a and, often, S-100 protein
▸▸ Histiocytes are negative for factor XIIIa in multicentric reticulohistiocytosis

Differential Diagnosis
▸▸ Langerhans cell histiocytosis (histiocytosis X)
▸▸ Granular cell tumor (in case of nonlipidized lesions)
▸▸ Lipid storage diseases
▸▸ Benign fibrous histiocytoma
▸▸ Melanoma, carcinoma, and pleomorphic sarcomas for reticulohistiocytomas with marked cellular pleomorphism

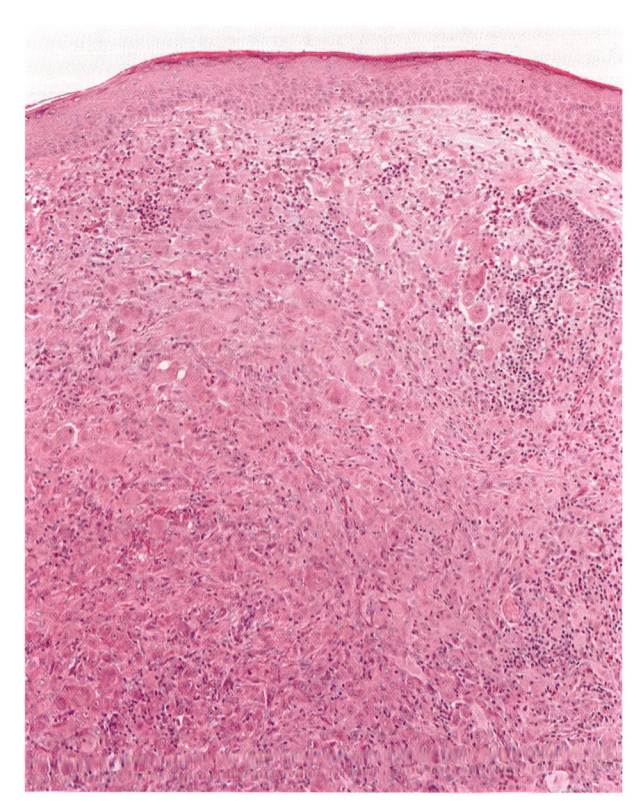

PROGNOSIS AND TREATMENT

Juvenile xanthogranuloma and solitary reticulohistiocytoma are benign, nonrecurring lesions. Skin lesions of juvenile xanthogranuloma often stabilize with time

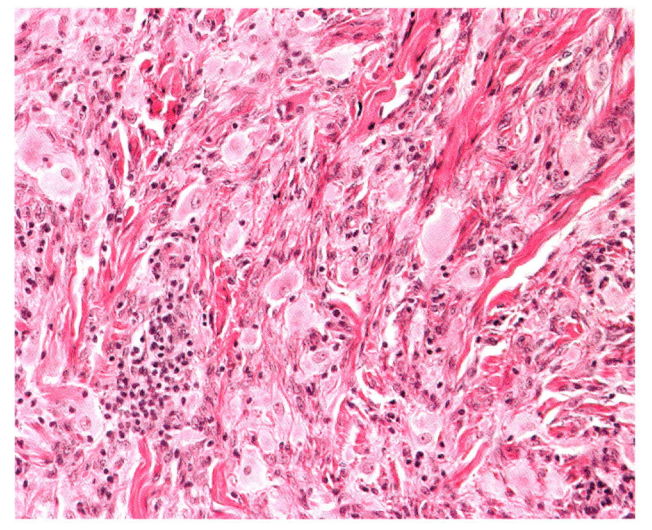

CHAPTER 3 Fibroblastic and Fibrohistiocytic Tumors

FIGURE 3-56
High-power view of reticulohistiocytoma showing histiocytic cells with abundant eosinophilic cytoplasm and vesicular nuclei.

and may even regress. For deep lesions of juvenile xanthogranuloma and for solitary reticulohistiocytoma, simple excision is curative.

XANTHOMA

CLINICAL FEATURES

Xanthoma represents a localized collection of lipid-laden histiocytes. It occurs mostly in the skin and subcutis of patients with alterations in serum lipids such as hyperlipoproteinemias. Several clinical forms of cutaneous xanthomas have been described including eruptive, plane, and tuberous xanthomas. Xanthelasma is xanthomas of the eyelid, mostly observed in normolipemic persons. Xanthomas of deep soft tissues usually develop in tendon, tendon sheath, or synovium. Tendinous xanthomas are usually associated with hypercholesterolemia. They develop predominantly in the finger, wrist, and ankle (Achilles tendon) as painless, slow-growing masses. Tuberous xanthomas, which are most characteristic of familial dysbetalipoproteinemia, present as nodular lesions on elbows, knees, and buttocks. They may resolve with treatment of the underlying hyperlipidemia.

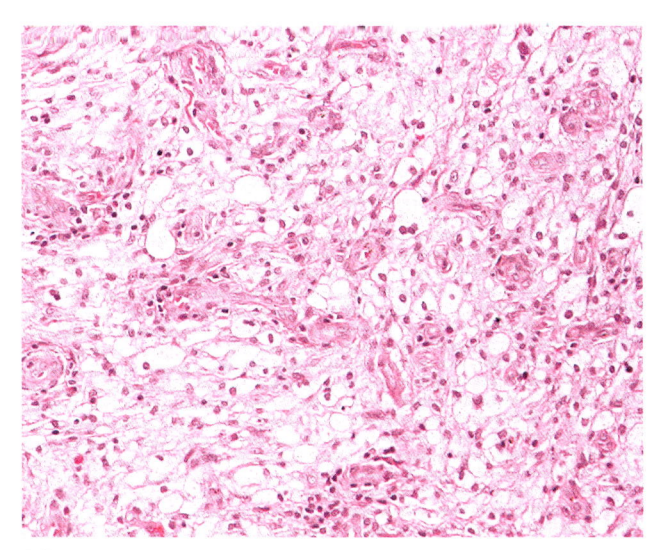

PATHOLOGIC FEATURES

GROSS FINDINGS

Xanthomas present generally as well-circumscribed white or yellow to brown masses.

MICROSCOPIC FINDINGS

Tuberous and tendinous xanthomas show a varying admixture of foamy histiocytes (Figure 3-57), cholesterol clefts, foreign body giant cells, lymphocytes aggregates, and fibrosis. Xanthelasma is composed predominantly of xanthoma cells with little fibrosis.

XANTHOMA—FACT SHEET

Definition
▸▸ Localized collection of lipid-laden histiocytes

Incidence and Location
▸▸ Frequent in patients with hyperlipidemia
▸▸ Mostly in skin and subcutis, less frequent in deep soft tissues (tendons of hand and feet)

Clinical Features
▸▸ Well-circumscribed, often multiple slow-growing masses

Prognosis and Treatment
▸▸ Simple excision of the mass in case of compromised function
▸▸ Treatment of hyperlipidemia

FIGURE 3-57
Xanthoma.
The lesion is composed predominantly of foamy histiocytes.

XANTHOMA—PATHOLOGIC FEATURES

Gross Findings
▸▸ Well-circumscribed white or yellow to brown masses

Microscopic Findings
▸▸ Varying admixture of foamy histiocytes, foreign body giant cells, cholesterol clefts, fibrosis, and lymphocytes

DIFFERENTIAL DIAGNOSIS

Deep-seated tuberous xanthomas may be mistaken clinically for a sarcoma. However, histologic examination and existence of hypercholesterolemia are diagnostic.

PROGNOSIS AND TREATMENT

Removal of the mass is indicated in case of compromised joint function. Alterations in serum lipids should also be corrected. Masses may recur unless hyperlipidemia is corrected.

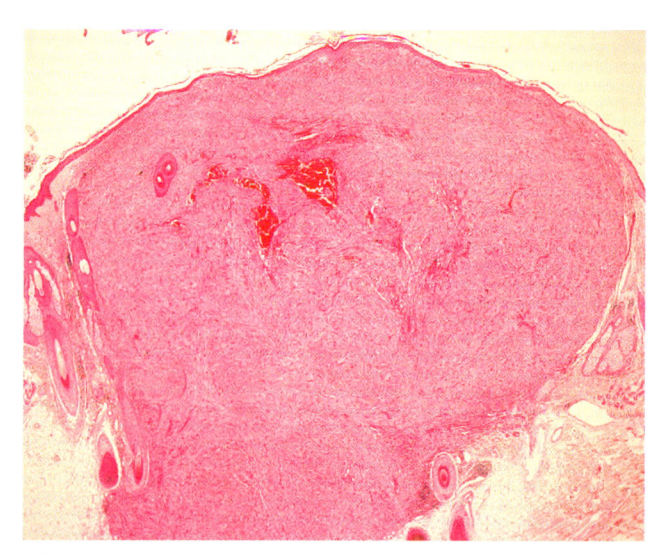

ATYPICAL FIBROXANTHOMA

CLINICAL FEATURES

Atypical fibroxanthoma almost always occurs on sun-exposed skin, mainly on the head and neck, in the elderly. The tumor appears as a solitary small nodule or bleeding ulcer. Radiation (solar, occupational, or therapeutic) is a predisposing factor, as demonstrated by the frequent association between atypical fibroxanthoma and basal cell or squamous cell carcinomas.

PATHOLOGIC FEATURES

GROSS FINDINGS

Atypical fibroxanthomas are solitary and small (< 2 cm) cutaneous nodules or ulcers (Figure 3-58).

MICROSCOPIC FINDINGS

Microscopically, atypical fibroxanthomas are virtually indistinguishable from storiform/pleomorphic malignant fibrous histiocytomas. They consist of well-circumscribed dermal proliferations of plump, spindle-to-pleomorphic cells with enlarged hyperchromatic nuclei set in a variably collagenized extracellular matrix (Figure 3-59). Mononucleated and multinucleated giant tumor cells and mitoses, including atypical mitoses, are common. The overlying epidermis is usually not hyperplastic unless ulcerated. Dilated capillaries, inflammatory changes, and solar elastosis are usually present at the periphery of the lesion. Little or no extension of the lesion into the subcutis occurs. Although most atypical fibroxanthomas are predominantly composed of giant pleomorphic cells, a few of them may essentially be composed of spindle cells, resembling leiomyosarcoma. Tumor necrosis is not a feature of atypical fibroxanthoma.

FIGURE 3-58
Atypical fibroxanthoma.
Low-power view showing a small, well-circumscribed, atypical dermal lesion occurring in association with actinic damage.

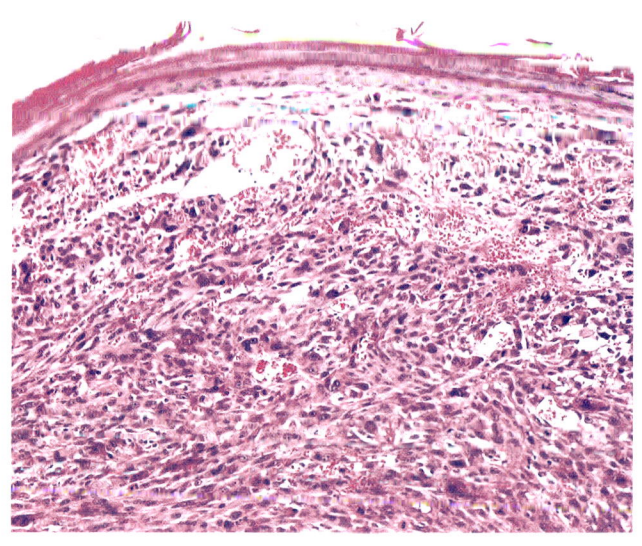

FIGURE 3-59
Atypical fibroxanthoma.
Dermal proliferation of spindle-to-giant pleomorphic cells with hyperchromatic nuclei and mitotic figures, including atypical mitoses.

ANCILLARY STUDIES

IMMUNOHISTOCHEMISTRY

The tumor cells in atypical fibroxanthomas usually express CD68 (clones KP1 and PGM1) and, often focally, smooth muscle actin. They are negative for cytokeratins, desmin, and S-100 protein.

ATYPICAL FIBROXANTHOMA—FACT SHEET

Definition
▸▸ A pleomorphic tumor mostly found on sun-damaged skin (elderly)
▸▸ Incidence and location, sex, race, and age distribution
▸▸ Frequent; no sex predilection
▸▸ Head and neck (elderly)
▸▸ Distal extremities and trunk (young adults)

Morbidity and Mortality
▸▸ Benign clinical course; seldom recur; metastasis exceptional

Clinical Features
▸▸ Small nodule (< 2 cm)
▸▸ Ulcer
▸▸ Sun-exposed skin in most cases

Prognosis and Treatment
▸▸ Simple excision is curative; local recurrences and/or metastases exceptional

ATYPICAL FIBROXANTHOMA—PATHOLOGIC FEATURES

Gross Findings
▸▸ Small dermal nodule (< 2 cm)
▸▸ Ulceration/bleeding frequent

Microscopic Findings
▸▸ Proliferation of spindle to pleomorphic cells
▸▸ Giant tumor cells
▸▸ Numerous mitoses, may be atypical
▸▸ Solar elastosis of adjacent skin
▸▸ Absence of tumor necrosis
▸▸ No extension into subcutis

Immunohistochemical Findings
▸▸ Positivity for CD68 and, frequently, for CD99 (75% of cases)
▸▸ Focal reactivity for smooth muscle actin
▸▸ Negative for desmin, CD34, keratins, and S-100 protein

Differential Diagnosis
▸▸ Spindle cell/sarcomatoid carcinoma
▸▸ Melanoma
▸▸ Malignant fibrous histiocytoma
▸▸ Spindle cell angiosarcoma (scalp)

DIFFERENTIAL DIAGNOSIS

Atypical fibroxanthoma is a diagnosis of exclusion. Before giving a diagnosis of atypical fibroxanthoma, one must be sure that the lesion is not a sarcomatoid carcinoma (positivity for keratins, EMA, or both) or a melanoma (positivity for S-100 protein). Malignant fibrous histiocytoma is usually found in the deep portion of the subcutis and is larger than atypical fibroxanthoma. In general, the term *atypical fibroxanthoma* should be reserved for small (< 1.5 cm), dermal-based lesions that occur in sun-damaged skin, with no more than minimal involvement of the subcutis. The spindle cell variant of atypical fibroxanthoma may be difficult to separate from leiomyosarcoma. The latter, however, shows a prominent fascicular growth pattern and is diffusely positive for smooth muscle actin and focally positive for desmin and/or h-caldesmon. When dealing with a lesion of the scalp, spindle cell angiosarcoma (positivity for CD31, CD34, or both) should enter the differential diagnosis.

PROGNOSIS AND TREATMENT

Simple excision is the treatment of choice. Local recurrence (often with invasion of deep soft tissue) and metastasis are exceptional.

DERMATOFIBROSARCOMA PROTUBERANS (Including Bednar Tumor and Giant Cell Fibroblastoma)

CLINICAL FEATURES

DFSP, Bednar tumor, and giant cell fibroblastoma are considered fibrohistiocytic tumors of intermediate malignancy because they have significant potential for local recurrence but a low risk for metastasis. Most frequently seen on the trunk and proximal extremities of middle-aged adults, DFSP presents clinically as a slow-growing (often for several years) nodular mass or as an ill-defined plaque-like infiltration of the skin. In some cases, cutaneous involvement may be subtle or even absent, and the tumor may present as a subcutaneous mass. Men are more commonly affected than women. DFSP may occur in the pediatric age group, where the lesion may coexist with giant cell fibroblastoma. Giant cell fibroblastoma is considered a juvenile form of DFSP. It usually develops in the dermis and subcutis of infants and children younger than 5 years. Boys are more often affected than girls. Pure giant cell fibroblastoma is exceptional in adults. The lesion presents as a painless nodule or plaque frequently located on proximal extremities and trunk.

PATHOLOGIC FEATURES

GROSS FINDINGS

Advanced stage lesions present as single or multiple nodular growths involving the skin or subcutis, or both, whereas earlier lesions present as plaque-like or

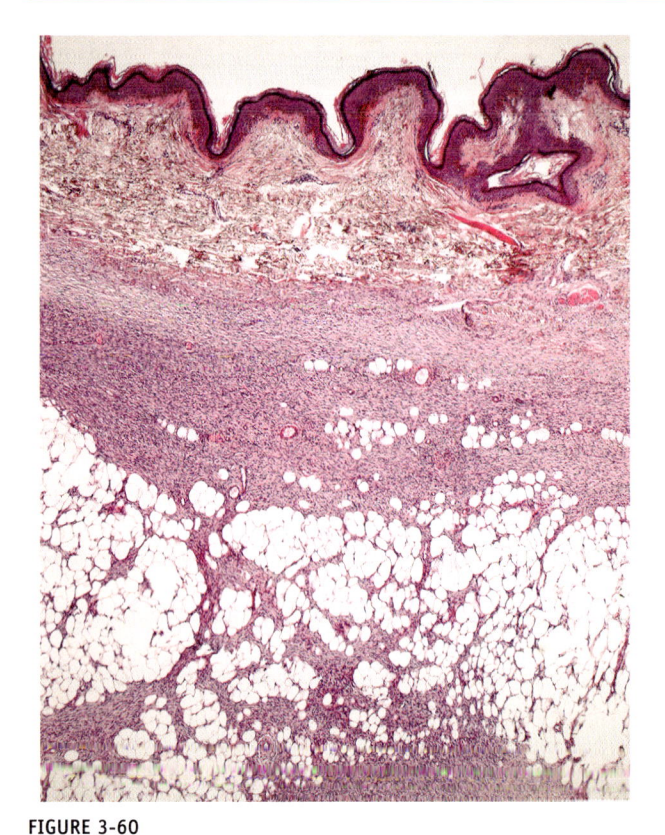

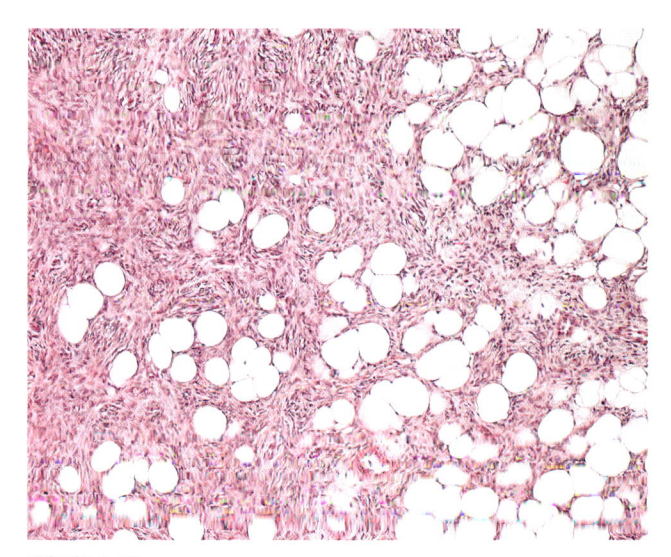

FIGURE 3-60
Dermatofibrosarcoma protuberans.
Infiltration of deep dermis and subcutis by the lesion in a honeycomb pattern. The superficial dermis is spared.

localized skin induration. Multinodular presentation is often seen in local recurrences. The average size of the lesion is approximately 5 cm at the time of surgery. Giant cell fibroblastoma usually presents as a painless myxoid/mucoid nodule between 1 and 8 cm in greatest diameter (median, 3 cm).

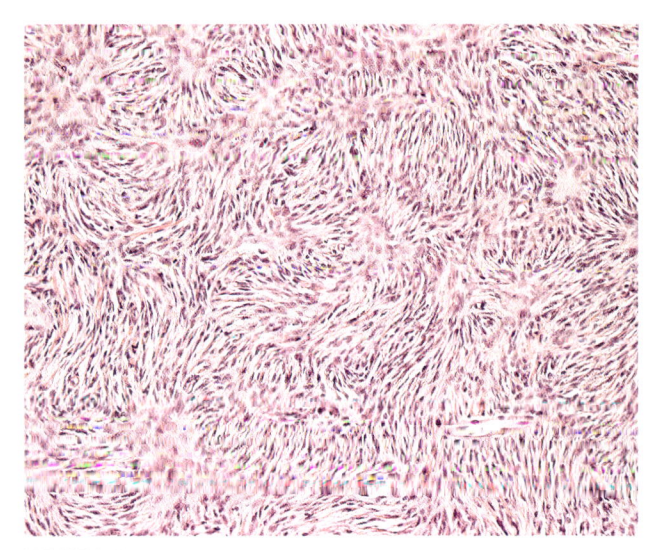

MICROSCOPIC FINDINGS

DFSP is a diffusely infiltrating spindle cell proliferation that develops, in most cases, at the interface between dermis and subcutis (Figure 3-60). In rare cases, it develops almost exclusively in the subcutis with minimal dermal involvement. An uninvolved (grenz) zone of dermis separates the lesion from the overlying epidermis, which is not hyperplastic. The spindle cell proliferation displays a typical monotonous storiform growth pattern (Figure 3-61). Cellular atypia is minimal, and mitoses are scarce. Characteristically, the lesion infiltrates the subcutaneous adipose tissue in a lace-like or honeycomb pattern (Figure 3-62). In the deep regions, the tumor spreads along the connective tissue septa, sparing adnexa. Myxoid change, multinucleated giant cells similar to those observed in giant cell fibroblastoma, and myoid nodules are occasionally observed.

Some dermatofibrosarcomas may contain areas resembling conventional fibrosarcoma, with a hypercellular, fascicular pattern of growth (Figure 3-63). In these areas, nuclear pleomorphism is more pronounced and mitoses more numerous (> 5 mitoses per 10 hpf). Rarely, dermatofibrosarcoma may contain areas resembling storiform/pleomorphic malignant fibrous histiocytoma. High-grade sarcomatous changes in dermatofibrosarcoma may be observed de novo, as well as in recurrences. Bednar tumor corresponds to a pigmented variant of DFSP in which spindled melanin pigment-containing cells are identified.

Giant cell fibroblastomas are proliferations of short spindle cells set in a variably myxoid to collagenous background (Figure 3-64). Pseudovascular spaces (so-called *angiectid spaces*) are commonly found, often

FIGURE 3-61
Dermatofibrosarcoma protuberans.
Typical storiform growth pattern. Cellular atypia is absent.

FIGURE 3-62
Dermatofibrosarcoma protuberans.
Infiltration of subcutaneous fat in a typical lace-like or honeycomb pattern.

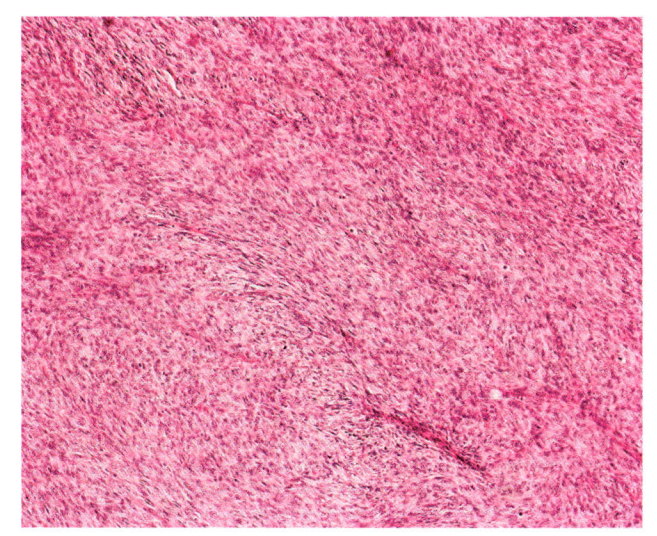

FIGURE 3-63
Fibrosarcomatous change in a dermatofibrosarcoma protuberans.
Cellularity and mitotic activity are significantly increased.

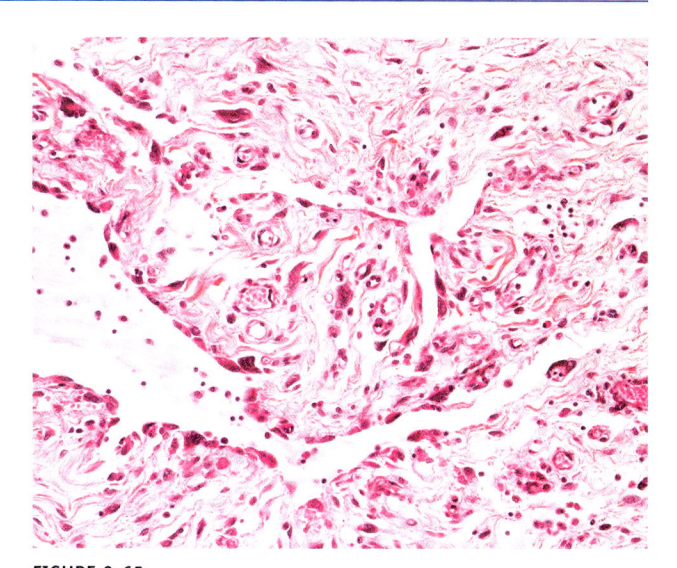

FIGURE 3-65
Giant cell fibroblastoma.
Multinucleated giant cells with smudged chromatin lining pseudovascular (angiectid) spaces.

bordered by multinucleated-appearing giant cells or by hyperchromatic cells with smudged chromatin (Figure 3-65). Hypocellular/collagenous or myxoid areas may alternate with hypercellular areas. Mitotic figures are rare, and no tumor necrosis is present. Areas morphologically indistinguishable from conventional DFSP may also occasionally be observed, resulting in the so-called hybrid lesions. The transition from one pattern to the other may be quite abrupt or gradual, and this can be seen in primary lesions, as well as in subsequent recurrences. A giant cell fibroblastoma may recur with the overall appearance of a conventional dermatofibrosarcoma, and vice versa.

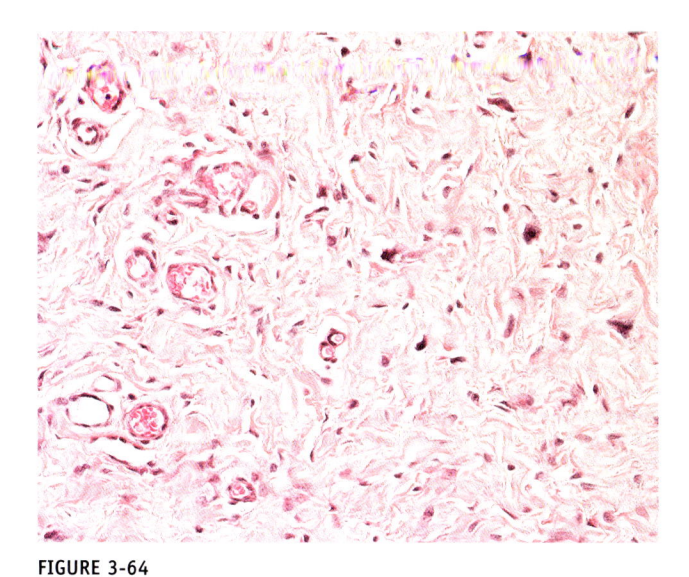

ANCILLARY STUDIES

IMMUNOHISTOCHEMISTRY

The spindle cells in conventional DFSP are characteristically diffusely positive for CD34 (Figure 3-66). Occasional reactivity with S-100 protein and smooth muscle actin may also be observed. Apolipoprotein A1 has also been reported as a sensitive marker of DFSP but has not been widely tested. The spindle cells in Bednar tumor are usually S-100 negative, despite the presence of melanin pigment. Myoid nodules are consistently positive for smooth muscle actin. Desmin, EMA, and cytokeratins are not expressed in DFSP. CD34 reactivity is generally retained in areas of fibrosarcomatous changes with, however, a significant reduction of the staining intensity.

Tumor cells in giant cell fibroblastoma are classically positive for CD34, including the giant cells. CD31, S-100 protein, and epithelial markers are not expressed.

GENETICS

DFSP, Bednar tumor, and giant cell fibroblastoma share similar molecular abnormalities: the presence of supernumerary ring chromosomes consisting of amplified sequences from chromosomes 17 and 22, and/or the presence of t(17;22), a balanced reciprocal translocation that fuses the platelet-derived growth factor β-chain (PDGF-β) gene to the collagen type 1 α1 *(COL1A1)* gene. This fusion protein, which has a PDGF-β–type effect, participates in cell proliferation and sarcoma maintenance through paracrine/autocrine stimulation.

FIGURE 3-64
Giant cell fibroblastoma.
Spindle cells and multinucleated giant cells distributed within a heavily collagenized matrix.

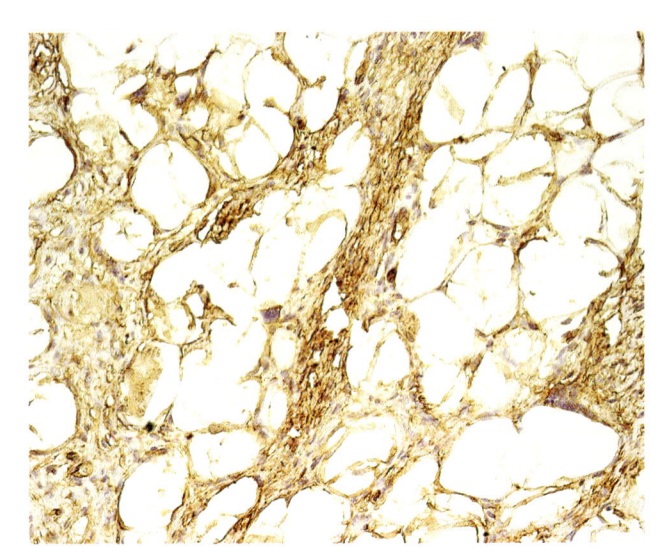

FIGURE 3-66
Dermatofibrosarcoma protuberans.
Spindled tumor cells are diffusely positive for CD34.

Inhibition of PDGF receptor using blocking agents such as imatinib mesylate (Gleevec), a tyrosine kinase inhibitor, shown some efficacy in the treatment of recurrent or metastatic dermatofibrosarcoma. Ring chromosomes are predominantly observed in dermatofibrosarcoma of adult patients, whereas the t(17;22) translocation is mostly seen in dermatofibrosarcoma of children and in giant cell fibroblastoma.

DIFFERENTIAL DIAGNOSIS

Benign fibrous histiocytoma is the most important differential diagnosis. As opposed to DFSP, benign fibrous histiocytoma is smaller, more superficial, less monotonous, less storiform, and more eosinophilic/myoid-looking in its appearance, is often associated with epidermal hyperplasia, and is CD34 negative. In myxoid DFSP, the storiform pattern is less obvious, contrasting with the prominent plexiform vasculature that resembles that of myxoid liposarcoma. CD34 positivity and absence of lipoblasts in dermatofibrosarcoma are key features. It is important to make the distinction between fibrosarcomatous changes in DFSP and conventional fibrosarcoma because the latter is more aggressive and metastasizes more frequently. As opposed to dermatofibrosarcoma with fibrosarcomatous changes, conventional fibrosarcomas are large and deep-seated, CD34 negative tumors. Neurofibroma and low-grade MPNST may also be confused with dermatofibrosarcoma; however, these two tumors are positive for S-100 protein in addition to CD34.

Giant cell fibroblastoma should be differentiated from giant cell angiofibroma, solitary fibrous tumor, myxoid malignant fibrous histiocytoma, fibrous hamartoma of

---

DERMATOFIBROSARCOMA PROTUBERANS—FACT SHEET

Definition
▸▸ A recurring but rarely metastasizing skin tumor of young to middle-aged adults; may also occur in children

Incidence and Location
▸▸ Infrequent
▸▸ Trunk, groin, and proximal extremities commonly affected
▸▸ Exceptional in hands and feet

Morbidity and Mortality
▸▸ Tumor of intermediate malignancy (low-grade sarcoma)
▸▸ Local recurrences common (10% to 50% of cases), metastases rare (< 5% of the cases)

Sex, Race, and Age Distribution
▸▸ More frequent in male individuals
▸▸ Middle-aged adults; rare in children

Clinical Features
▸▸ Nodular or plaque-like painless cutaneous tumor
▸▸ Slow-growing lesion (over several years)

Prognosis and Treatment
▸▸ Wide excision with tumor-free margins is curative
▸▸ Local recurrence in 10% to 50% of cases, after inadequate excision
▸▸ Metastases rare (<5%)
▸▸ High-grade fibrosarcomatous changes seem not to be associated with an increased risk for local recurrence and distant metastases

---

DERMATOFIBROSARCOMA PROTUBERANS—PATHOLOGIC FEATURES

Gross Findings
▸▸ Plaque-like skin lesion
▸▸ Single or multiple nodular skin masses

Microscopic Findings
▸▸ Monotonous spindle cell proliferation
▸▸ Diffuse infiltration of dermis or superficial subcutis, or both
▸▸ Storiform growth pattern
▸▸ Absence of cellular atypia, mitoses rare
▸▸ Infiltration of subcutaneous fat in a honeycomb pattern

Genetics
▸▸ Ring chromosomes
▸▸ t(17;22) (PDGF-β; COL1A1) reciprocal translocation

Immunohistochemical Findings
▸▸ Diffusely positive for CD34
▸▸ Occasional reactivity for smooth muscle actin and S-100 protein
▸▸ Negativity for keratins, EMA, and desmin

Differential Diagnosis
▸▸ Benign fibrous histiocytoma
▸▸ Neurofibroma
▸▸ Fibrosarcoma
▸▸ MPNST
▸▸ Malignant fibrous histiocytoma
▸▸ Myxoid liposarcoma (in case of prominent myxoid changes)

CHAPTER 3 Fibroblastic and Fibrohistiocytic Tumors

GIANT CELL FIBROBLASTOMA—FACT SHEET

Definition
- A juvenile form of DFSP

Incidence and Location
- Rare
- Proximal extremities and trunk mostly affected

Morbidity and Mortality
- May recur; does not metastasize

Sex, Race, and Age Distribution
- More frequent in male individuals
- Tumor of childhood

Clinical Features
- Slow-growing painless nodule

Prognosis and Treatment
- Tends to recur but does not metastasize
- Wide excision is curative

GIANT CELL FIBROBLASTOMA—PATHOLOGIC FEATURES

Gross Findings
- Small skin nodule (average size, 3 cm)

Microscopic Findings
- Spindle to pleomorphic cells
- Variably collagenized matrix
- Multinucleated-appearing giant cells bordering pseudovascular spaces
- Mitoses rare, no necrosis
- May contain areas of conventional DFSP

Genetics
- Most common abnormality: t(17;22) (PDGF-β, COL1A1) translocation
- Less frequent: ring chromosome

Immunohistochemical Findings
- Positivity for CD34
- Negativity for S-100, CD31, and epithelial markers

Differential Diagnosis
- Giant cell angiofibroma
- Solitary fibrous tumor
- Fibrous hamartoma of infancy
- Malignant fibrous histiocytoma
- Myxoid liposarcoma if the lesion shows prominent myxoid changes

---

infancy, and myxoid liposarcoma for those cases showing prominent myxoid changes. Angiectid spaces and CD34 reactivity are features shared by both giant cell fibroblastoma and giant cell angiofibroma. As opposed to the former, giant cell angiofibroma is a well-circumscribed, nonrecurring lesion that is usually found in the orbital region. Areas of conventional DFSP are not found in giant cell angiofibroma or in solitary fibrous tumor. Malignant fibrous histiocytoma is more cellular and composed of more pleomorphic, atypical, and mitotically active tumor cells. Fibrous hamartoma of infancy usually occurs in the axillary region and shows triphasic histology, with fibromatosis-like zones, mature fat, and primitive mesenchyme. Fibrous hamartoma and DFSP/GCFB are both CD34 positive, and immunohistochemistry is not helpful in this distinction. Myxoid liposarcoma is a deep-seated tumor that displays a characteristic delicate plexiform vascular network, which is not as evident in giant cell fibroblastoma with prominent myxoid changes. In addition, the former contains lipoblasts, a feature not observed in giant cell fibroblastoma.

PROGNOSIS AND TREATMENT

Conventional dermatofibrosarcoma recurs locally in 10% to 50% of cases, often after incomplete excisions. Distant metastases are observed in less than 5% of cases, almost all of which most likely contain small areas of fibrosarcoma. Fibrosarcomatous changes were thought to be associated with an increased risk for local and distant recurrences, but a recent study showed that this is not the case if the lesion is adequately excised, that is, widely excised with tumor-free margins. Actually, the risk for local recurrence correlates with the extent of the excision, and a minimum of a 3-cm excision margin is currently recommended for dermatofibrosarcoma. Dermatofibrosarcoma metastasizes to the lungs and, less frequently, to the regional lymph nodes. Radiotherapy has been proposed for unresectable tumors or after margin-positive resections. Imatinib mesylate (Gleevec), a tyrosine kinase inhibitor, may have some potential value in the treatment of recurrent or metastatic dermatofibrosarcoma.

Giant cell fibroblastoma recurs in up to 50% of cases but does not metastasize. As for DFSP, a lower recurrence rate should be expected if lesions are excised with tumor-free margins.

ANGIOMATOID (MALIGNANT) FIBROUS HISTIOCYTOMA

Angiomatoid (malignant) fibrous histiocytoma (AMFH) is a rare mesenchymal tumor of uncertain differentiation, which has recently been shown to be translocation associated. It is traditionally considered a fibrohistiocytic tumor of intermediate malignancy, although it is perhaps better considered a mesenchymal tumor of uncertain differentiation.

CLINICAL FEATURES

AMFH typically occurs in children and young adults. AMFH usually occurs in the subcutis or deep dermis and presents as a solitary mass, most commonly in the extremities. Clinically, they may resemble hematoma, hemangioma, or a benign cyst. These tumors may be associated with a variety of systemic manifestations including fevers, weight loss, anemia, polyclonal gammopathy, and rarely, a Castleman disease–like lymphadenopathy, which resolve after excision of the tumor.

PATHOLOGIC FEATURES

GROSS FINDINGS

AMFH typically appears as a small, hemosiderin stained, subcutaneous mass. Cystic change is commonly present (Figure 3-67).

MICROSCOPIC FINDINGS

Histologically, AMFH is characterized by the presence of a dense, fibrous capsule and a surrounding lymphocytic infiltrate, mimicking metastatic disease involving a lymph node (Figure 3-68). This chronic inflammatory infiltrate is generally most prominent around the periphery of the tumor and may show germinal center formation. The blood-filled cystic spaces for which this tumor is named are present in most, but not all, cases, and are lined by flattened tumor cells rather than true endothelium. The cells of AMFH are histiocytoid to spindled in appearance and are arranged in a variety of growth patterns, including sheets, meningioma-like whorls, and short fascicles (Figure 3-69). AMFHs are most often cytologically bland, although occasional cases may show striking pleomorphism, a finding that does not appear to have clinical significance. The mitotic rate is typically low. Cases without the large cystic spaces show at least some evidence of hemorrhage, such as intracellular hemosiderin or focal hemorrhage. In some cases, this hemorrhage may be extensive and elicit a striking desmoplastic reaction surrounding minute tumor cell nodules, obscuring the underlying neoplasm (Figure 3-70).

ANCILLARY STUDIES

IMMUNOHISTOCHEMISTRY

The cells of AMFH have a unique immunophenotype, with coexpression of desmin, EMA, and CD68 in more than 60% of cases (Figures 3-71 and 3-72). Although rare, AMFH may show muscle actin expression, but they are never myogenin or MyoD1 positive, distinguishing them from rhabdomyosarcomas. AMFH does not express endothelial markers, such as CD31, CD34, or factor VIII–related antigen.

GENETIC FINDINGS

At the genetic level, AMFH is characterized by t(12;22) (FUS-ATF1), t(11;22) (EWS-ATF1), and most recently, t(11;22) (EWS-CREB1) in roughly equal percentages of tumors. These gene fusions may be demonstrated by RT-PCR or FISH, in fixed tissues. Notably, identical EWS-ATF1 and EWS-CREB1 fusions are seen

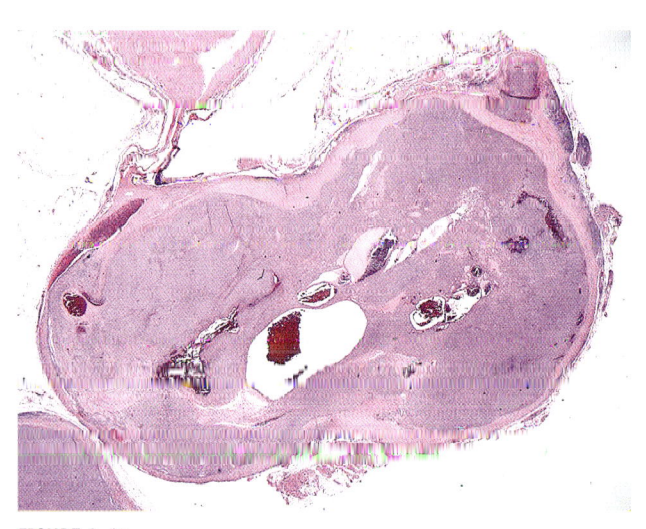

FIGURE 3-67
Low-power view of angiomatoid (malignant) fibrous histiocytoma, showing a fibrous capsule, lymphoid aggregates, and blood-filled spaces.

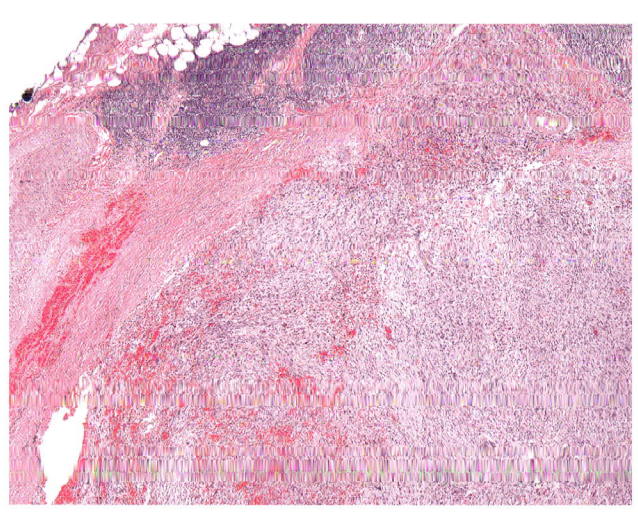

FIGURE 3-68
Peripheral zone in angiomatoid (malignant) fibrous histiocytoma, with a fibrous capsule and a proliferation of histiocytoid spindled cells in fascicular and whorled patterns.

in clear cell sarcomas of soft tissue and the gastrointestinal tract, emphasizing the need to integrate molecular findings with morphology and immunohistochemistry.

PROGNOSIS AND TREATMENT

Wide surgical excision and careful follow-up are recommended for patients with AMFH. Metastases are most common to lymph nodes, and patients may achieve long survival time and cure with resection of metastatic lesions. Lesions of the head and neck have a worse prognosis because of the difficulty in achieving complete resection in these anatomic locations. No evidence has been reported to suggest that adjuvant therapy plays a role in the primary management of this tumor.

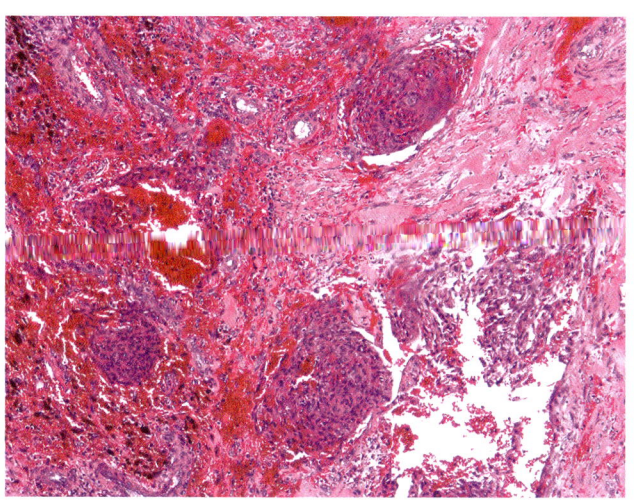

DIFFERENTIAL DIAGNOSIS

The differential diagnosis of AMFH includes dermatofibroma with aneurysmal/hemosiderotic change (aneurysmal benign fibrous histiocytoma), metastatic tumor in a lymph node, various vascular neoplasms, follicular dendritic cell tumor, and rhabdomyosarcoma. Careful examination of aneurysmal dermatofibroma will show characteristic infiltration of spindled cells among preexisting collagen bundles, a storiform growth pattern, and a more polymorphous cell population, with siderophages and foamy macrophages. The characteristic cell of aneurysmal dermatofibroma is also a spindled cell, rather than the distinctly histiocytoid cell of AMFH.

The dense capsule and the surrounding lymphoid infiltrate seen in AMFH may closely simulate a

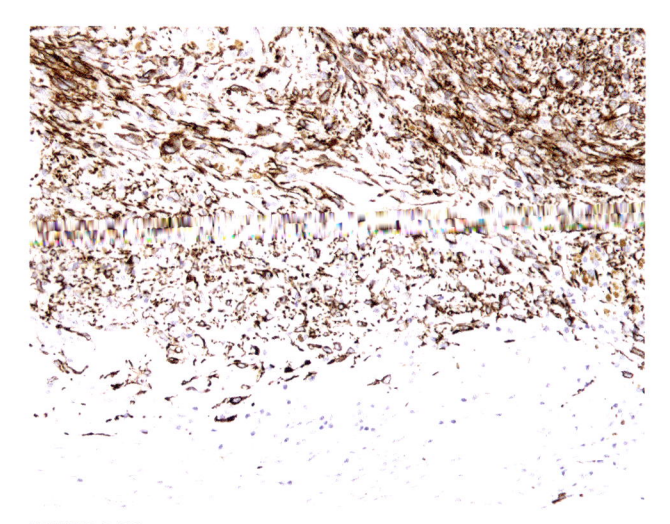

FIGURE 3-69
Some angiomatoid (malignant) fibrous histiocytoma may elicit striking desmoplasia, leaving only small nodules of identifiable tumor in a hemosiderin-laden fibrotic background.

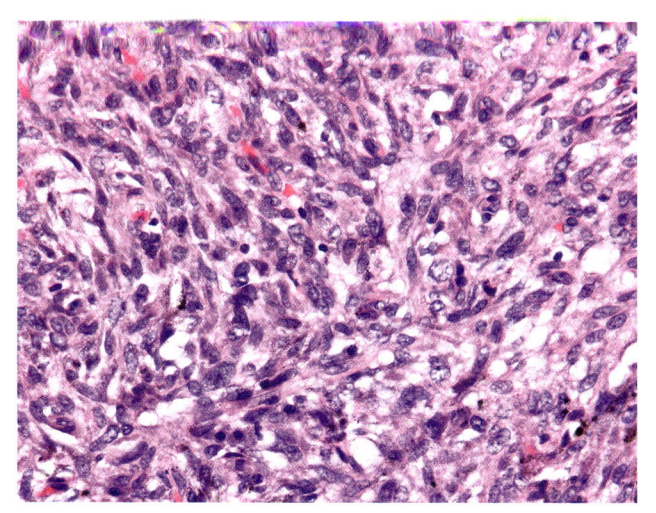

FIGURE 3-71
Anomalous desmin expression in angiomatoid (malignant) fibrous histiocytoma.

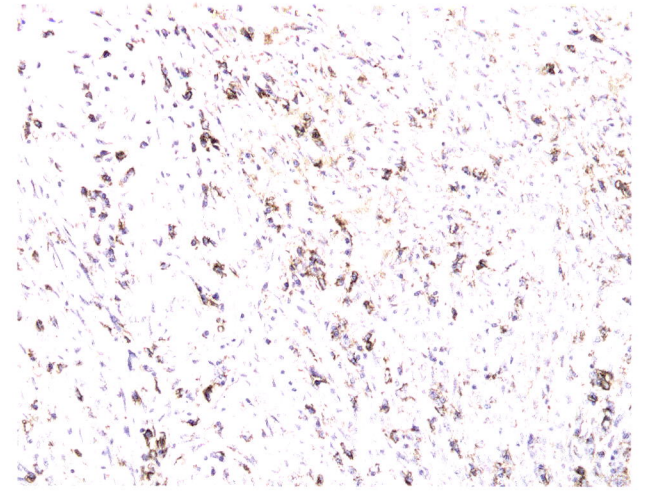

FIGURE 3-70
High-power view of angiomatoid (malignant) fibrous histiocytoma, showing intracytoplasmic hemosiderin.

FIGURE 3-72
Epithelial membrane antigen expression in angiomatoid (malignant) fibrous histiocytoma.

metastatic neoplasm in a lymph node. Careful evaluation discloses the absence of the structures found in normal lymph nodes, such as a subcapsular sinus or afferent lymphatics.

The angiomatoid and cystic features of AMFH may raise the question of a vascular neoplasm, such as an epithelioid hemangioma or even an angiosarcoma. Careful attention to the presence of the characteristic fibrous capsule and chronic inflammatory cell infiltrate, the absence of expression of endothelial markers, and the absence of true vasoformation should allow this distinction without great difficulty.

Follicular dendritic cell tumors may closely resemble AMFH but tend to lack a fibrous pseudocapsule and intracytoplasmic hemosiderin, and contain numerous intermixed small lymphocytes. Follicular dendritic cell tumors express markers such as CD21, CD35, and clusterin, and are negative for desmin and EMA.

Finally, desmin-positive AMFH in children may be confused with rhabdomyosarcomas, likely reflecting the natural tendency for pathologists to *rule out* rhabdomyosarcoma in any unusual pediatric tumor. Unlike rhabdomyosarcomas, which are typically large and deeply seated, AMFHs are small, superficially located masses. Careful histologic evaluation of AMFH reveals cytologically bland, histiocytoid cells, unlike the clearly malignant round cells, strap cells, and eosinophilic giant cells of rhabdomyosarcoma. Importantly, AMFHs do not express myogenin or MyoD1, which are present in nearly all rhabdomyosarcomas.

PLEXIFORM FIBROHISTIOCYTIC TUMOR

CLINICAL FEATURES

Plexiform fibrohistiocytic tumor (PFHT) is an unusual fibrohistiocytic tumor of intermediate malignancy that most commonly presents as a dermal or subcutaneous mass of the extremities in children or young adults. Any anatomic site may be involved, although location in the head is rare.

PATHOLOGIC FEATURES

GROSS FINDINGS

Lesions appear as firm, fixed, small dermal and subcutaneous nodule or nodules. Sectioning reveals small, firm, white nodules.

MICROSCOPIC FINDINGS

PFHT typically grows as a poorly circumscribed, plexiform proliferation of multiple small nodules, each

---

ANGIOMATOID (MALIGNANT) FIBROUS HISTIOCYTOMA—FACT SHEET

Definition
- A recurring but rarely metastasizing superficial soft tissue tumor of children and young adults

Incidence and Location
- Rare
- Most common in extremities
- Head and neck tumors may be difficult to completely resect

Morbidity and Mortality
- Tumor of intermediate malignancy (low-grade sarcoma)
- Local recurrences common (10% to 50% of cases), metastases rare (< 5% of the cases)

Sex, Race, and Age Distribution
- Either sex
- Most common in children

Clinical Features
- Hemorrhagic, cystic, superficial soft tissue mass
- May be associated with systemic symptoms

Prognosis and Treatment
- Wide excision with tumor-free margins is curative in most cases
- Local recurrence in 10% to 50% of cases
- Metastases rare (< 5%), may metastasize to lymph nodes

ANGIOMATOID (MALIGNANT) FIBROUS HISTIOCYTOMA—PATHOLOGIC FEATURES

Gross Findings
- Nodular, cystic, hemorrhagic mass, usually larger than 3 cm

Microscopic Findings
- Fibrous pseudocapsule with lymphoid infiltrate
- Blood-filled, pseudovascular spaces in more than 50% of cases
- Bland histiocytoid to spindled cells arranged in short fascicles, whorls, and sheets
- Intracytoplasmic hemosiderin deposition
- Occasional cases with striking cytologic atypia

Genetics
- t(12;22) (FUS-ATF1), t(11;22) (EWS-ATF1), and t(11;22) (EWS-CREB1) in roughly equal percentages of tumors

Immunohistochemical Findings
- Frequent coexpression of desmin, EMA, and CD68
- Negative for dendritic cell markers, myogenin/MyoD1

Differential Diagnosis
- Aneurysmal benign fibrous histiocytoma
- Lymph node metastasis
- Vascular neoplasms
- Follicular dendritic cell tumor
- Rhabdomyosarcoma

composed of an admixture of rounded mononuclear cells and osteoclast-like giant cells (Figure 3-73). These nodules are often surrounded by short fascicles of fibroblasts and myofibroblasts, which mingle with the round cell nodules (Figure 3-74). Lesions may consist largely or even entirely of either the mononuclear and giant cells or the spindled fibroblastic cells (Figure 3-75). The mononuclear cells typically resemble cytologically bland histiocytes, although rare pleomorphic variants occur. Mitotic activity is typically low.

ANCILLARY STUDIES

IMMUNOHISTOCHEMISTRY

The spindled component often expresses smooth muscle actin in a myofibroblastic *(tram-track)* pattern, and the rounded cells and osteoclasts are usually CD68 positive. CD68 immunostaining may be valuable in bringing out a subtle, multinucleated giant cell population in a predominantly fibroblastic tumor. Desmin, cytokeratins, CD34, and S-100 protein are negative. NKI/C3, a marker frequently expressed by cellular neurothekeoma, is typically negative, assisting in this sometimes difficult differential diagnosis.

GENETIC FINDINGS

No consistent genetic event has been identified in PFHT.

PROGNOSIS AND TREATMENT

PFHTs recur in between 12% and 40% of cases but have a low risk for metastatic disease. Lymph node and pulmonary metastases have been reported in fewer than five patients altogether. These tumors should be treated with wide excision and careful long-term follow-up.

DIFFERENTIAL DIAGNOSIS

The differential diagnosis of PFHT includes soft tissue giant cell tumor, granulomatous inflammation, cellular neurothekeoma, fibromatosis, and fibrous hamartoma of infancy. The nodules of rounded cells and osteoclasts seen in PFHT are indistinguishable from the tumor nodules of soft tissue giant cell tumor, and in cases lacking a prominent spindled component, this distinction may be difficult, if not arbitrary. Features that should suggest PFHT include younger patient age, a plexiform growth pattern with minute nodules (as opposed to the coarser

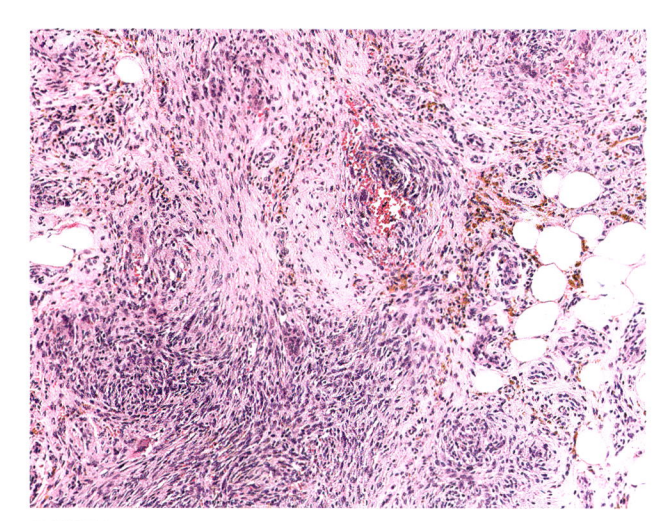

FIGURE 3-73
Plexiform fibrohistiocytic tumor, consisting of a multinodular, plexiform proliferation of nodules of osteoclastic giant cells and mononuclear cells, surrounded by fibroblastic fascicles.

multinodular pattern of soft tissue giant cell tumor), and the absence of metaplastic bone or aneurysmal bone cyst–like areas.

The presence of nodules of histiocyte-like mononuclear cells with admixed giant cells may suggest the possibility of a granulomatous process. However, PFHT contains osteoclast-like, rather than Langerhans-type, giant cells. Central necrosis is not a feature of the histiocytic and giant-cell–rich nodules of PFHT.

Cases of PFHT with relative predominance of the fibroblastic component and only rare or absent mononuclear cell nodules may be confused with fibromatoses. However, fibromatosis typically does not grow in a plexiform fashion, is usually deeply seated rather than cutaneous, and shows longer, sweeping fascicles with characteristic thin-walled dilated blood vessels.

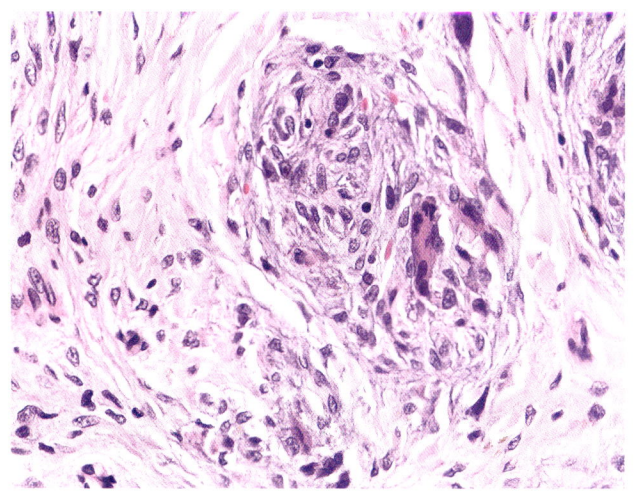

FIGURE 3-74
High-power view of mononuclear cells, osteoclastic giant cells, and surrounding fibroblasts.

PLEXIFORM FIBROHISTIOCYTIC TUMOR—FACT SHEET
Definition ▸▸ A recurring but rarely metastasizing superficial soft tissue tumor of children and young adults
Incidence and Location ▸▸ Rare ▸▸ Any location; rare in head/neck
Morbidity and Mortality ▸▸ Tumor of intermediate malignancy (low-grade sarcoma) ▸▸ Local recurrences common (10% to 50% of cases), metastases rare (<1% of cases)
Sex, Race, and Age Distribution ▸▸ Either sex ▸▸ Most common in children
Clinical Features ▸▸ Multinodular superficial soft tissue mass
Prognosis and Treatment ▸▸ Wide excision with tumor-free margins is recommended ▸▸ Local recurrence in 10% to 50% of cases ▸▸ Metastases extremely rare (<1%); may metastasize to lymph nodes

PLEXIFORM FIBROHISTIOCYTIC TUMOR—PATHOLOGIC FEATURES
Gross Findings ▸▸ Small, superficial, multinodular mass ▸▸ May be fixed to underlying tissues
Microscopic Findings ▸▸ Plexiform growth pattern ▸▸ Minute nodules of rounded histiocyte-like cells, with intermixed osteoclast-like giant cells, surrounded by fibroblastic fascicles ▸▸ May be composed of predominantly round cells or spindled cells ▸▸ Rare cases with striking cytologic atypia
Genetics ▸▸ No consistent abnormality
Immunohistochemical Findings ▸▸ Mononuclear cells and osteoclast-like giant cells express CD68 ▸▸ NKI/C3 negative
Differential Diagnosis ▸▸ Soft tissue giant cell tumor ▸▸ Granulomatous disease ▸▸ Fibromatosis ▸▸ Cellular neurothekeoma

Cellular neurothekeoma grows in a distinctly nodular fashion, with small nests of generally bland epithelioid cells, separated by thin fibrous septae. This multinodular growth pattern may closely mimic examples of PFHT that lack a prominent fibroblastic component. However, unlike PFHT, cellular neurothekeomas lack osteoclast-like giant cells and tend to show more cytologic variation. Expression of NKI/C3 may also help to distinguish cellular neurothekeoma from PFHT.

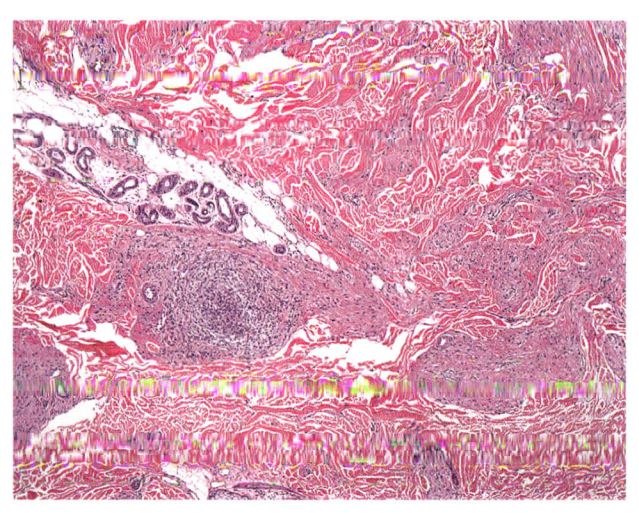

Fibrous hamartomas of infancy may display a somewhat plexiform growth pattern, reminiscent of PFHT. Recognition of the typical triphasic histology of fibrous hamartoma, with fibroblastic fascicles, fat, and most importantly, nodules and whorls of primitive mesenchymal tissue is critical for this distinction. Fibrous hamartoma also typically occurs in much younger patients than does PFHT, and lacks fibrohistiocytic nodules and osteoclast-like giant cells.

SOFT TISSUE GIANT CELL TUMOR (of Low Malignant Potential)

Soft tissue giant cell tumor, also known as *giant cell tumor of low malignant potential*, is the soft tissue counterpart of giant cell tumor of bone. It is considered a fibrohistiocytic tumor of intermediate malignancy by the WHO.

CLINICAL FEATURES

Soft tissue giant cell tumors typically present as multinodular masses in the skin or subcutis of young to middle-aged adults, although occasional cases may present as more deeply seated masses or in children.

FIGURE 3-75
Some plexiform fibrohistiocytic tumors may consist largely of either fibroblastic or mononuclear elements. This example showed only a single nodule of mononuclear cells.

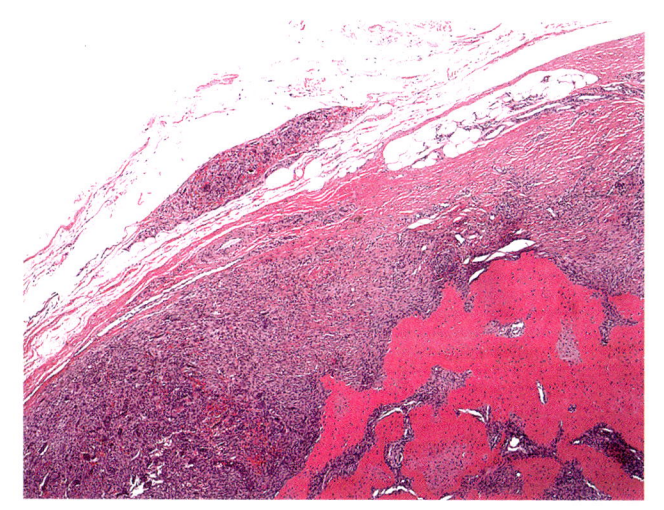

CHAPTER 3 Fibroblastic and Fibrohistiocytic Tumors

FIGURE 3-76
Soft tissue giant cell tumor, showing a multinodular proliferation of osteoclastic giant cells and mononuclear cells, with a shell of woven bone.

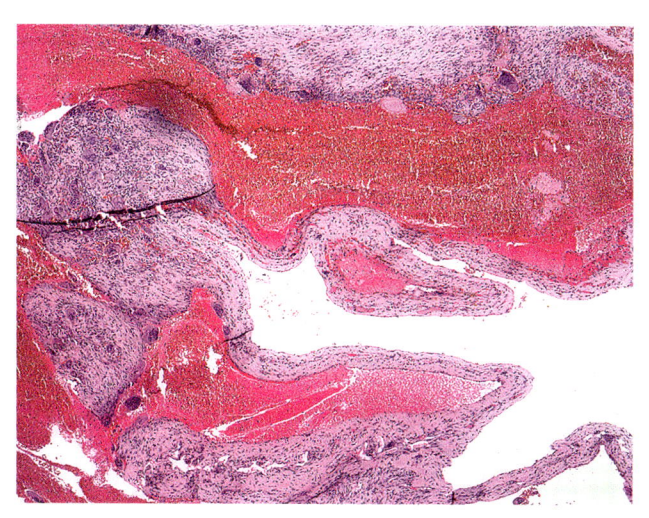

FIGURE 3-78
Aneurysmal bone cyst–like changes in soft tissue giant cell tumor.

PATHOLOGIC FEATURES

GROSS FINDINGS

Soft tissue giant cell tumors appear as thickenings or small nodules in the dermis and subcutis. Foci of hemorrhage may be present. Calcified lesions may have a gritty character.

MICROSCOPIC FINDINGS

The tumors typically show involvement of the deep dermis and subcutis by a multinodular mass, sometimes with a surrounding shell of metaplastic, woven bone (Figure 3-76). The individual tumor nodules are essentially identical to giant cell tumor of bone, with a mixture of osteoclast-like giant cells, bland mononuclear cells, and short fascicles of bland spindled cells (Figure 3-77). Mitotic figures are usually easily identified, but atypical forms are not. Vascular involvement by the tumor is common. Other changes that may be seen on occasion include spindled fibrohistiocytic proliferations of the type seen in giant cell tumors of bone, aneurysmal bone cyst–like changes including metaplastic bone and angiectatic spaces, and rarely cartilage (Figure 3-78). Necrosis, atypical mitotic figures, and severe cytologic atypia are not seen.

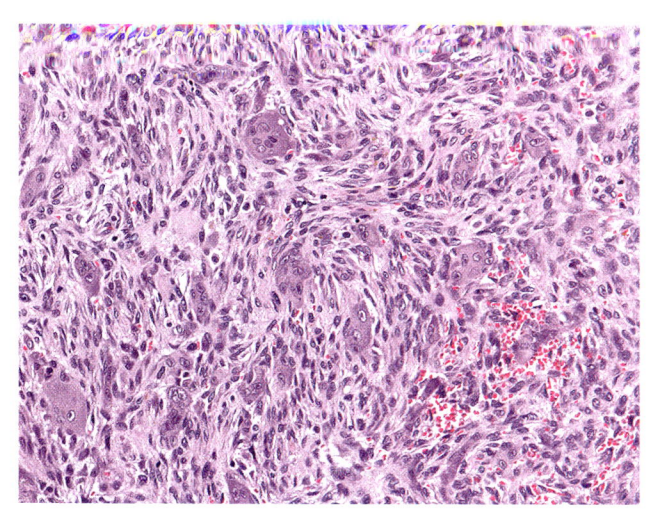

ANCILLARY STUDIES

IMMUNOHISTOCHEMISTRY

The mononuclear cells of soft tissue giant cell tumor are essentially always CD68 positive and have been reported in some series to be positive for smooth muscle actin in more than 75% of cases. Desmin, cytokeratins, CD31, CD34, and S-100 protein are negative.

GENETIC FINDINGS

No consistent genetic abnormality has been identified.

PROGNOSIS AND TREATMENT

Soft tissue giant cell tumors have significant capacity for local recurrence, but only metastasize in extremely rare instances. Metastasizing soft tissue giant cell tumors may be analogized to rare *benign metastasizing* giant cell tumors of bone. The locally recurring potential of

FIGURE 3-77
The histologic features of soft tissue giant cell tumor are essentially identical to those of giant cell tumor of bone.

SOFT TISSUE GIANT CELL TUMOR—FACT SHEET

Definition
- A recurring but rarely metastasizing superficial soft tissue tumor of adults

Incidence and Location
- Rare
- Any location

Morbidity and Mortality
- Tumor of intermediate malignancy (low-grade sarcoma)
- Local recurrences common (10% to 50% of cases), metastases extremely rare (< 1% of the cases)

Sex, Race, and Age Distribution
- Either sex
- Most common in adults

Clinical Features
- Dermal and subcutaneous thickening and nodularity, often with calcification

Prognosis and Treatment
- Wide excision with tumor-free margins is curative in most cases
- Local recurrence in 10% to 50% of cases, after inadequate excision
- Metastases rare (< 1%)

SOFT TISSUE GIANT CELL TUMOR—PATHOLOGIC FEATURES

Microscopic Findings
- Identical to giant cell tumor of bone
- Sheets of osteoclast-like giant cells and bland mononuclear cells
- Mitotic activity common
- Cytologic atypia, necrosis, and atypical mitotic forms are not seen
- Aneurysmal bone cyst-like changes and fibrohistiocytic spindle cell proliferation may be seen
- Extension into small vessels may be present

Genetics
- No recurrent genetic event

Immunohistochemical Findings
- Mononuclear cells and osteoclast-like giant cells express CD68; mononuclear cells may also express smooth muscle actins

Differential Diagnosis
- Osteoclast-rich sarcomas, carcinoma, melanomas, and lymphomas
- Tenosynovial giant cell tumor
- Intravascular nodular fasciitis

these tumors is most likely related to their multinodular growth pattern, and wide excision should be curative in most cases. The behavior of superficially and deeply located soft tissue giant cell tumor appears to be similar.

DIFFERENTIAL DIAGNOSIS

The differential diagnosis of soft tissue giant cell tumor includes both benign and malignant entities. Essentially any malignant neoplasm may contain large numbers of osteoclast-like giant cells on occasion, including various sarcomas, melanoma, carcinomas, and even lymphomas. It cannot be overemphasized that soft tissue giant cell tumor shows little, if any, cytologic atypia, and lacks atypical mitotic figures and necrosis. Any osteoclast-rich lesion showing such features should be carefully examined for potential histologic clues (e.g., gland formation, osteoid production) and immunostained with a panel of markers to include cytokeratins, S-100 protein, smooth muscle actins, desmin, and possibly hematolymphoid markers.

Soft tissue giant cell tumor may also be mistaken for benign tumors, such as tenosynovial giant cell tumors or giant-cell–rich forms of nodular fasciitis. Tenosynovial giant cell tumor differs from soft tissue giant cell tumor by virtue of its usual location near joint spaces or bursae, a generally uninodular rather than multinodular growth pattern, prominent stromal hyalinization, and the generally more mixed population of small synoviocyte-like cells, siderophages, foamy histiocytes, and lymphocytes. Metaplastic bone production is not seen in tenosynovial giant cell tumor. Nodular fasciitis may show considerable numbers of osteoclastic giant cells, both in association with hemorrhage and in intravascular variants (intravascular fasciitis). Recognition of more typical areas of fasciitis, characterized by somewhat randomly arrayed bland myofibroblastic cells, commonly with associated microcystic change, should allow this distinction in most cases. Intravascular fasciitis will also show the majority of the tumor to be within distended blood vessels, in contrast with soft tissue giant cell tumor, in which the bulk of the tumor is situated in the dermis.

UNDIFFERENTIATED PLEOMORPHIC SARCOMA (So-Called Pleomorphic Malignant Fibrous Histiocytoma, Including Giant-Cell and Inflammatory Variants)

The term *pleomorphic malignant fibrous histiocytoma* is reserved for high-grade soft tissue sarcomas that fail to show any specific line of differentiation using currently available ancillary techniques. Ten years ago, malignant fibrous histiocytoma was the most common sarcoma type of adults. Since then, it has been realized that the morphology of malignant fibrous histiocytoma, as defined by Enzinger and colleagues, is a nonspecific one shared by many poorly differentiated neoplasms, including carcinomas, melanomas, and lymphomas. *Undifferentiated pleomorphic sarcoma* is now the preferred term for designating those tumors in which epithelial, melanotic, and lymphoid differentiation have been excluded, and an evident mesenchymal line of differentiation cannot be proved.

Two variants of undifferentiated pleomorphic sarcoma with specific features have been described: the undifferentiated pleomorphic sarcoma with giant cells (so-called giant cell malignant fibrous histiocytoma) and the undifferentiated pleomorphic sarcoma with prominent inflammation (also designated by the term *inflammatory malignant fibrous histiocytoma*). The giant cell variant, mostly observed in deep soft tissue of the limbs or trunk, is best thought of as simply an osteoclastic giant-cell–rich variant of undifferentiated pleomorphic sarcoma. The inflammatory form of undifferentiated pleomorphic sarcoma is often associated with systemic symptoms (fever, weight loss, leukocytosis, eosinophilia) and predominates in the retroperitoneum. It has recently been appreciated that a large majority of so-called *inflammatory malignant fibrous histiocytomas of the retroperitoneum* are, in fact, inflammatory forms of dedifferentiated liposarcoma.

CLINICAL FEATURES

Undifferentiated pleomorphic sarcomas occur most frequently in the limbs (especially lower limbs) of middle to advanced-aged adults, with a male predominance. More than 90% of cases arise in the deep soft tissues and present as large, often necrotic tumors. Rapidly growing tumors may be painful.

PATHOLOGIC FEATURES

GROSS FINDINGS

Undifferentiated pleomorphic sarcomas present as large (5- to 15-cm), well-circumscribed, often pseudoencapsulated, deep-seated masses. Subcutaneous lesions usually measure less than 5 cm in maximal diameter. Cut surface often shows hemorrhagic, myxoid, and/or necrotic changes (Figure 3-79).

MICROSCOPIC FINDINGS

The lesion is composed by an admixture of spindled and pleomorphic cells, set in a collagenous to myxoid extracellular matrix. Cellularity is variable and cellular atypia, nuclear pleomorphism, mitoses, abnormal mitoses, areas of tumor necrosis, histiocyte-like cells, foamy cells, and giant tumor cells with enlarged, polylobulated

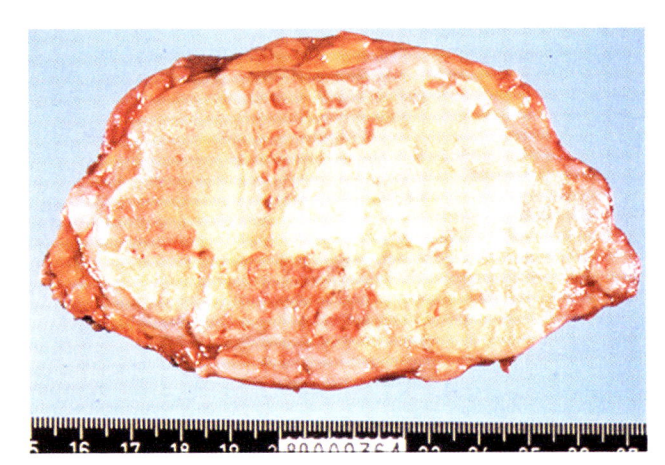

FIGURE 3-79
Gross photograph of undifferentiated high-grade pleomorphic sarcoma (so-called *malignant fibrous histiocytoma*). Areas of necrosis are visible as whitish areas.

nuclei are commonly observed (Figure 3-80). The spindled cells show morphologic features reminiscent of fibroblasts/myofibroblasts. By definition, the neoplastic cells should not show any other line of specific differentiation.

In contrast with the conventional variant, the giant cell variant contains numerous, benign-looking, osteoclast-like multinucleated giant cells (Figure 3-81). In some cases, however, these giant cells may show malignant features. The inflammatory variant is characterized by a reduced number of pleomorphic tumor cells that are often masked by a prominent inflammatory infiltrate composed mainly of histiocytes, xanthoma cells, neutrophils, and eosinophils (Figures 3-82 and 3-83). It is not rare to see phagocytosis of inflammatory cells by tumor cells.

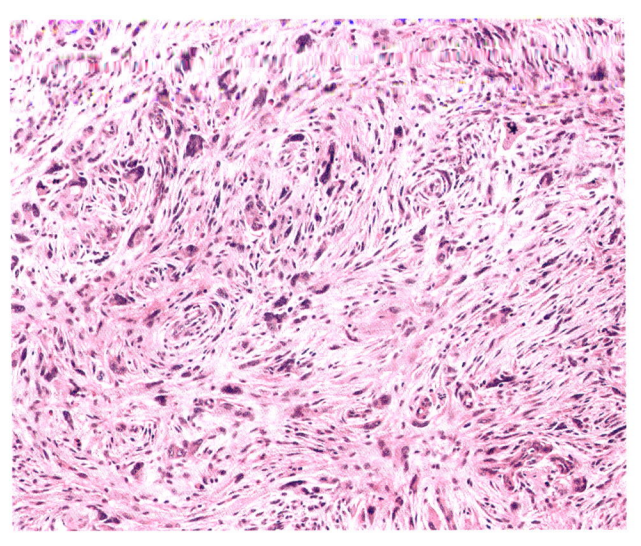

FIGURE 3-80
Undifferentiated high-grade pleomorphic sarcoma.
Numerous spindle and pleomorphic tumor cells are set in a variably collagenized extracellular matrix. An abnormal mitosis is also visible.

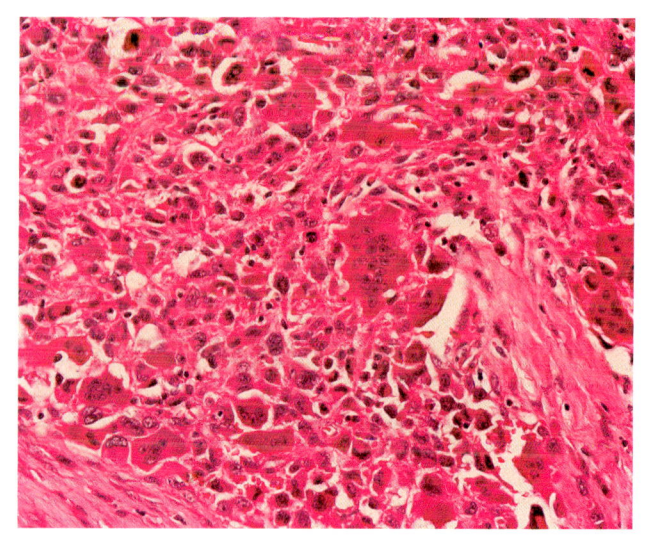

FIGURE 3-81
Undifferentiated high-grade pleomorphic sarcoma with giant cells (giant cell variant of malignant fibrous histiocytoma).
In addition to spindle and pleomorphic cells, the tumor contains numerous benign-looking osteoclast-like giant cells.

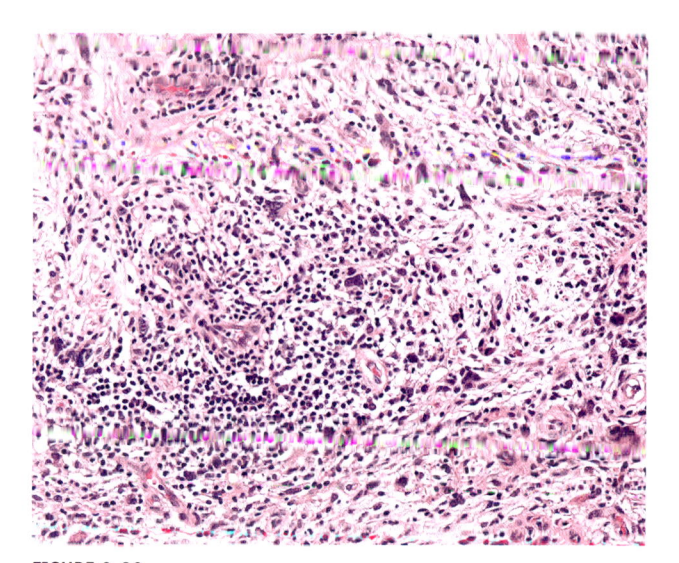

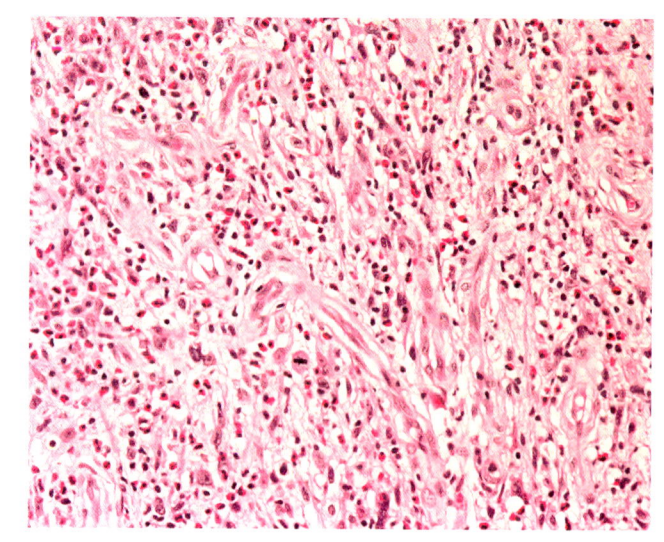

FIGURE 3-83
Undifferentiated high-grade pleomorphic sarcoma with prominent inflammation (inflammatory variant of malignant fibrous histiocytoma).
The inflammatory infiltrate consists predominantly of eosinophils.

FIGURE 3-82
Undifferentiated high-grade pleomorphic sarcoma with prominent inflammation (inflammatory variant of malignant fibrous histiocytoma).
Malignant tumor cells are rare, masked by a prominent lymphoplasmacytic infiltrate.

ANCILLARY STUDIES

IMMUNOHISTOCHEMISTRY

It is common for undifferentiated pleomorphic sarcomas to show some limited foci of smooth muscle actin reactivity, but S-100 protein, desmin, H-caldesmon, and epithelial markers are usually not expressed. If they are, the diagnosis of undifferentiated pleomorphic sarcoma should be questioned and a search for a specific line of differentiation pursued. Histiocytic antigens (e.g., α1-antitrypsin, α1-antichymotrypsin, CD68, lysozyme) are of no utility.

GENETICS

Undifferentiated pleomorphic sarcomas have complex karyotypes. No specific structural or numerical abnormalities have been proved to be useful for identification purposes.

DIFFERENTIAL DIAGNOSIS

Undifferentiated pleomorphic sarcoma is a diagnosis of elimination. Before giving such a diagnosis, all other potential mimics should have been ruled out, including metastatic carcinomas (lung, kidney), melanoma, lymphoma, pleomorphic rhabdomyosarcoma, pleomorphic leiomyosarcoma, pleomorphic liposarcoma, pleomorphic MPNST, liposarcoma with high-grade dedifferentiated areas, and high-grade myxofibrosarcoma. Extensive sampling, careful examination of slides (looking for lipoblasts or rhabdomyoblasts), and ancillary techniques (immunohistochemistry, electron microscopy, genetics) are critical in this context.

The giant-cell–rich variant of undifferentiated pleomorphic sarcoma should be differentiated from other giant cell–rich neoplasms, namely, giant-cell–rich carcinomas (e.g., pancreas, thyroid, breast, kidney), extraskeletal osteosarcomas, giant-cell–rich leiomyosarcomas, giant-cell–rich malignant mesenchymomas, and giant cell tumors of soft tissue. Inflammatory undifferentiated pleomorphic sarcoma should be distinguished from lymphoma, Hodgkin's disease, and any inflammatory processes or neoplasia including inflammatory carcinomas, inflammatory leiomyosarcomas, and IMTs.

UNDIFFERENTIATED PLEOMORPHIC SARCOMA—FACT SHEET

Definition
▸▸ A highly malignant pleomorphic neoplasm lacking any specific line of differentiation

Incidence and Location
▸▸ True incidence difficult to determine
▸▸ Location: lower limbs, trunk

Sex, Race, and Age Distribution
▸▸ Middle- to advanced-aged adults
▸▸ Male predominance

Clinical Features
▸▸ Large, deep-seated mass
▸▸ Prognosis and treatment
▸▸ 5-year survival rate: 30% to 50%
▸▸ Wide excision followed by irradiation is the treatment of choice
▸▸ More indolent clinical course for the inflammatory variant

UNDIFFERENTIATED PLEOMORPHIC SARCOMA—PATHOLOGIC FEATURES

Gross Findings
▸▸ Large (5- to 15-cm), well-circumscribed neoplasm
▸▸ Deep soft tissues

Microscopic Findings
▸▸ Admixture of spindled and pleomorphic cells
▸▸ Giant tumor cells with enlarged or multiple pleomorphic nuclei
▸▸ Collagenous to myxoid extracellular matrix
▸▸ Cellular atypia and nuclear pleomorphism
▸▸ Mitoses, abnormal mitoses
▸▸ Tumor necrosis
▸▸ *Giant cell variant*: numerous osteoclast-like giant cells
▸▸ *Inflammatory variant*: numerous xanthoma cells and neutrophils, few tumor cells

Genetics
▸▸ Complex karyotype; no specific chromosomal abnormalities

Immunohistochemical Findings
▸▸ Limited reactivity for smooth muscle actin
▸▸ Negativity for desmin, h-caldesmon, S-100 protein, and epithelial markers

Differential Diagnosis
▸▸ Metastasis from carcinoma or melanoma
▸▸ Lymphoma
▸▸ Dedifferentiated liposarcoma (retroperitoneum)
▸▸ Other pleomorphic sarcomas (rhabdomyosarcoma, leiomyosarcoma, liposarcoma, MPNST, high-grade myxofibrosarcoma)
▸▸ *Giant cell variant*: other giant-cell–rich neoplasms (extraskeletal osteosarcoma, giant-cell–rich leiomyosarcoma, giant cell tumor of soft tissue)
▸▸ *Inflammatory variant*: lymphoma, IMT, abscess

PROGNOSIS AND TREATMENT

Undifferentiated pleomorphic sarcomas, including the giant-cell–rich variant, are aggressive; 30% to 50% of patients die within 5 years after diagnosis. Again, it is important for therapeutic purposes that mimics are carefully ruled out, such as carcinomas, melanoma, lymphoma, and the potentially less aggressive dedifferentiated (retroperitoneal) liposarcoma. Wide excision followed by irradiation is the treatment of choice. Adjuvant chemotherapy may be considered in selected cases (e.g., young patients).

The inflammatory form of undifferentiated pleomorphic sarcoma, which corresponds to dedifferentiated liposarcomas in most cases, shows a more indolent clinical course.

SUGGESTED READINGS

Nodular Fasciitis

1. Bernstein KE, Lattes R: Nodular (pseudosarcomatous) fasciitis, a nonrecurrent lesion: Clinicopathologic study of 134 cases. Cancer 1982;49:1668-1678.
2. Chung EB, Enzinger FM: Proliferative fasciitis. Cancer 1975;36:1450-1458.
3. Daroca PJ Jr., Pulitzer DR, LoCicero J III: Ossifying fasciitis. Arch Pathol Lab Med 1982;106:682-685.
4. Enzinger FM, Dulcey F: Proliferative myositis. Report of thirty-three cases. Cancer 1967;20:2213-2223.
5. Lauer DH, Enzinger FM: Cranial fasciitis of childhood. Cancer 1980;45:401-406.
6. Meis JM, Enzinger FM: Proliferative fasciitis and myositis of childhood. Am J Surg Pathol 1992;16:364-372.
7. Montgomery EA, Meis JM: Nodular fasciitis. Its morphologic spectrum and immunohistochemical profile. Am J Surg Pathol 1991;15:942-948.
8. Montgomery EA, Meis JM, Mitchell MS, et al: Atypical decubital fibroplasia. A distinctive fibroblastic pseudotumor occurring in debilited patients. Am J Surg Pathol 1992;16:708-715.
9. Perosio PM, Weiss SW: Ischemic fasciitis: A juxta-skeletal fibroblastic proliferation with a predilection for elderly patients. Mod Pathol 1993;6:69-72.
10. Shimizu S, Hashimoto H, Enjoji M: Nodular fasciitis. An analysis of 250 patients. Pathology 1984;16:161-166.

Fibroma of Tendon Sheath

1. Chung EB, Enzinger FM: Fibroma of tendon sheath. Cancer 1979;44:1945-1954.
2. Humphreys S, McKee PH, Fletcher CDM: Fibroma of tendon sheath: A clinicopathologic study. J Cutan Pathol 1986;13:331-338.
3. Pulitzer DR, Martin PC, Reed RJ: Fibroma of tendon sheath. A clinicopathologic study of 32 cases. Am J Surg Pathol 1989;13:472-479.

Elastofibroma

1. Nagamine N, Nohara Y, Ito E: Elastofibroma in Okinawa. A clinicopathologic study of 170 cases. Cancer 1982;50:1794-1805.

Superficial Fibromatoses

1. Burge P, Hoy G, Regan P, et al: Smoking, alcohol and the risk of Dupuytren's contracture. J Bone Joint Surg Br 1997;79:206-210.

2. de Wever I, Dal Cin P, Fletcher CD, et al: Cytogenetic, clinical, and morophologic correlations in 78 cases of fibromatosis. A report from the CHAMP Study Group. CHromosomes And Morphology. Mod Pathol 2000;13:1080–1085.
3. Mikkelsen OA: Dupuytren's disease: Initial symptoms, age of onset and spontaneous course. Hand 1977;9:11–15.

Deep (Desmoid–Type) Fibromatosis

1. de Wever I, Dal Cin P, Fletcher CD, et al: Cytogenetic, clinical, and morphologic correlations in 78 cases of fibromatosis. A report from the CHAMP Study Group. CHromosomes And Morphology. Mod Pathol 2000;13:1080–1085.
2. Gurbuz AK, Giardello FM, Petersen GM, et al: Desmoid tumours in familial adenomatous polyposis. Gut 1994;35:377–381.
3. Kouho H, Aoki T, Hisaoka M, et al: Clinicopathological and interphase cytogenetic analysis of desmoid tumours. Histopathology 1997;31:336–341.
4. Merchant NB, Lewis JJ, Woodruff JM, et al: Extremity and trunk desmoid tumors: A multifactorial analysis of outcome. Cancer 1999;86:2045–2052.
5. Miyaki M, Konishi M, Kikuchi-Yanoshita R, et al: Coexistence of somatic and germ-line mutations of APC gene in desmoid tumors from patients with familial adenomatous polyposis. Cancer Res 1993;53:5079–5082.
6. Miyoshi Y, Iwao K, Nawa G, et al: Frequent mutations in the beta-catenin gene in desmoid tumors from patients without familial adenomatous polyposis. Oncol Res 1998;10:591–594.
7. Reitamo JJ, Hayry P, Nykyri E, et al: The desmoid tumor. I. Incidence, sex, age, and anatomical distribution in the Finnish population. Am J Clin Pathol 1982;77:665–673.

Inflammatory Myofibroblastic Tumor/Inflammatory Fibrosarcoma

1. Chan JKC: Inflammatory pseudotumor: A family of lesions of diverse nature and etiologies. Adv Anat Pathol 1996;3:156–171.
2. Coffin CM, Dehner LP, Meis-Kindblom JM: Inflammatory myofibroblastic tumor, inflammatory fibrosarcoma, and related lesions. An historical review with differential diagnostic considerations. Semin Diagn Pathol 1998;15:102–110.
3. Coffin CM, Humphrey PA, Dehner LP: Extrapulmonary inflammatory myofibroblastic tumor: A clinical and pathological survey. Semin Diagn Pathol 1998;15:85–101.
4. Coffin CM, Patel A, Perkins S, et al: ALK1 and p80 expression and chromosomal rearrangements involving 2p23 in inflammatory myofibroblastic tumor. Mod Pathol 2001;14:569–576.
5. Cook JR, Dehner LP, Collins MH, et al: Anaplastic lymphoma kinase (ALK) expression in the inflammatory myofibroblastic tumor. A comparative immunohistochemical study. Am J Surg Pathol 2001;25:1364–1371.
6. Freeman A, Geddes N, Munson P, et al: Anaplastic lymphoma kinase (ALK 1) staining and molecular analysis in inflammatory myofibroblastic tumours of the bladder: A preliminary clinicopathological study of nine cases and review of the literature. Mod Pathol 2004;17:765–771.
7. Meis-Kindblom JM, Kjellström C, Kindblom LG: Inflammatory fibrosarcoma: Update, reappraisal, and perspective on its place in the spectrum of inflammatory myofibroblastic tumors. Semin Diagn Pathol 1998;15:133–143.
8. Pomplun S, Goldstraw P, Davies SE, et al: Calcifying fibrous pseudotumour arising within an inflammatory pseudotumour: Evidence of progression from one lesion to the other. Histopathology 2000;37:380–382.

Myxoinflammatory Fibroblastic Sarcoma

1. Meis-Kindblom JM, Kindblom LG: Acral myxoinflammatory fibroblastic sarcoma. A low grade tumor of the hands and feet. Am J Surg Pathol 1998;22:911–924.
2. Montgomery EA, Devaney KO, Giordano TJ, et al: Inflammatory myxohyaline tumor of distal extremities with virocyte or Reed-Sternberg-like cells: A distinctive lesion with features simulating inflammatory conditions, Hodgkin's disease, and various sarcomas. Mod Pathol 1998;11:384–391.

Adult Fibrosarcoma and Variants

1. Antonescu CR, Rosenblum MK, Pereira P, et al: Sclerosing epithelioid fibrosarcoma: A study of 16 cases and confirmation of a clinicopathologically distinct tumor. Am J Surg Pathol 2001;25:699–709.
2. Evans HL: Low-grade fibromyxoid sarcoma. A report of 12 cases. Am J Surg Pathol 1993;17:595–600.
3. Folpe AL, Lane KL, Paull G, et al: Low-grade fibromyxoid sarcoma and hyalinizing spindle cell tumor with giant rosettes: A clinicopathologic study of 73 cases supporting their identity and assessing the impact of high-grade areas. Am J Surg Pathol 2000;24:1353–1360.
4. Goodlad JR, Mentzel T, Fletcher CD: Low grade fibromyxoid sarcoma: Clinicopathological analysis of eleven new cases in support of a distinct entity. Histopathology 1995;26:229–237.
5. Guillou L, Benhattar J, Gengler C, et al: Translocation-positive low-grade fibromyxoid sarcoma: Clinicopathologic and molecular analysis of a series expanding the morphologic spectrum and suggesting potential relationship to sclerosing epithelioid fibrosarcoma: A study from the French Sarcoma Group. Am J Surg Pathol 2007;31:1387–1402.
6. Huang HY, Lal P, Qin J, et al: Low-grade myxofibrosarcoma: A clinicopathologic analysis of 49 cases treated at a single institution with simultaneous assessment of the efficacy of 3-tier and 4-tier grading systems. Hum Pathol 2004;35:612–621.
7. Lane KL, Shannon RJ, Weiss SW: Hyalinizing spindle cell tumor with giant rosettes: A distinctive tumor closely resembling low-grade fibromyxoid sarcoma. Am J Surg Pathol 1997;21:1481–1488.
8. Meis-Kindblom JM, Kindblom LG, Enzinger FM: Sclerosing epithelioid fibrosarcoma. A variant of fibrosarcoma simulating carcinoma. Am J Surg Pathol 1995;19:979–993.
9. Mentzel T, Calonje E, Wadden C, et al: Myxofibrosarcoma. Clinicopathologic analysis of 75 cases with emphasis on the low-grade variant. Am J Surg Pathol 1996;20:391–405.
10. Merck C, Angervall L, Kindblom LG, et al: Myxofibrosarcoma. A malignant soft tissue tumor of fibroblastic histiocytic origin. A clinicopathologic and prognostic study of 110 cases using multivariate analysis. Acta Pathol Microbiol Immunol Scand Suppl 1983;282:1–40.
11. Panagopoulos I, Storlazzi CT, Fletcher CD, et al: The chimeric FUS/CREB3l2 gene is specific for low-grade fibromyxoid sarcoma. Genes Chromosomes Cancer 2004;40:218–228.
12. Pritchard DJ, Soule EH, Taylor WF, et al: Fibrosarcoma—a clinicopathologic and statistical study of 199 tumors of the soft tissues of the extremities and trunk. Cancer 1974;33:888–897.
13. Scott SM, Reiman HM, Pritchard DJ, et al: Soft tissue fibrosarcoma. A clinicopathologic study of 132 cases. Cancer 1989;64:925–931.
14. Weiss SW, Enzinger FM: Myxoid variant of malignant fibrous histiocytoma. Cancer 1977;39:1672–1685.
15. Zamecnik M, Michal M: Low-grade fibromyxoid sarcoma: A report of eight cases with histologic, immunohistochemical, and ultrastructural study. Ann Diagn Pathol 2000;4:207–217.

Infantile Fibrosarcoma

1. Bourgeois JM, Knezevich SR, Mathers JA, et al: Molecular detection of the ETV6-NTRK3 gene fusion differentiates congenital fibrosarcoma from other childhood spindle cell tumors. Am J Surg Pathol 2000;24:937–946.
2. Chung EB, Enzinger FM: Infantile fibrosarcoma. Cancer 1976;38:729–739.
3. Coffin CM, Jaszcz W, O'Shea PA, et al: So-called congenital-infantile fibrosarcoma: Does it exist and what is it? Pediatr Pathol 1994;14:133–150.
4. Rubin BP, Chen CJ, Morgan TW, et al: Congenital mesoblastic nephroma t(12;15) is associated with ETV6-NTRK3 gene fusion: Cytogenetic and molecular relationship to congenital (infantile) fibrosarcoma. Am J Pathol 1998;153:1451–1458.
5. Sheng WQ, Hisaoka M, Okamoto S, et al. Congenital-infantile fibrosarcoma. A clinicopathologic study of 10 cases and molecular detection of the ETV6-NTRK3 fusion transcripts using paraffin-embedded tissue. Am J Clin Pathol 2001;115:348–355.

Benign Fibrous Histiocytomas and Variants

1. Calonje E, Fletcher CDM: Aneurysmal benign fibrous histiocytoma: Clinicopathological analysis of 40 cases of a tumour frequently misdiagnosed as a vascular neoplasm. Histopathology 1995;26:323–331.

2. Calonje E, Mentzel T, Fletcher CDM: Cellular benign fibrous histiocytoma. Clinicopathologic analysis of 74 cases of a distinctive variant of cutaneous fibrous histiocytoma with frequent recurrence. Am J Surg Pathol 1994;18:668–676.
3. Fletcher CDM: Benign fibrous histiocytoma of subcutaneous and deep soft tissue: A clinicopathologic analysis of 21 cases. Am J Surg Pathol 1990;14:801–809.
4. Kaddu S, McMenamin ME, Fletcher CD: Atypical fibrous histiocytoma of the skin: Clinicopathologic analysis of 59 cases with evidence of infrequent metastasis. Am J Surg Pathol 2002;26:35–46.
5. Vanni R, Fletcher CDM, Sciot R, et al: Cytogenetic evidence of clonality in cutaneous benign fibrous histiocytomas: A report of the CHAMP Study Group. Histopathology 2000;37:212–217.

Juvenile Xanthogranuloma and Reticulohistiocytoma

1. Nascimento AG: A clinicopathologic and immunohistochemical comparative study of cutaneous and intramuscular forms of juvenile xanthogranuloma. Am J Surg Pathol 1997;21:645–652.
2. Sonoda T, Hashimoto H, Enjoji M: Juvenile xanthogranuloma. Clinicopathologic analysis and immunohistochemical study of 57 cases. Cancer 1985;56:2280–2286.
3. Zelger B, Cerio R, Soyer HP, et al: Reticulohistiocytoma and multicentric reticulohistiocytosis. Histopathologic and immunophenotypic distinct entities. Am J Dermatopathol 1994;16:577–584.

Xanthoma

1. Cruz PD Jr, East C, Bergstresser PR: Dermal, subcutaneous, and tendon xanthomas: Diagnostic markers for specific lipoprotein disorders. J Am Acad Dermatol 1988;19:95–111.

Atypical Fibroxanthoma

1. Calonje E, Wadden C, Wilson-Jones E, et al: Spindle cell non-pleomorphic atypical fibroxanthoma: Analysis of a series and delineation of a distinctive variant. Histopathology 1993;22:247–254.
2. Fretzin DF, Helwig EB: Atypical fibroxanthoma of the skin. A clinicopathologic study of 140 cases. Cancer 1973;31:1541–1552.
3. Leong AS-Y, Milios J: Atypical fibroxanthoma of the skin: A clinicopathological and immunohistochemical study and a discussion of its histogenesis. Histopathology 1987;11:463–475.
4. Longacre TA, Smoller BR, Rouse RV: Atypical fibroxanthoma. Multiple immunohistologic profiles. Am J Surg Pathol 1993;17:1199–1206.
5. Silvis NG, Swanson PE, Manivel JC, et al: Spindle cell and pleomorphic neoplasms of the skin. A clinicopathologic and immunohistochemical study of 30 cases, with emphasis on atypical fibroxanthomas. Am Dermatopathol 1988;10:9–19.

Dermatofibrosarcoma Protuberans (Including Bednar Tumor and Giant Cell Fibroblastoma)

1. Alguacil-Garcia A: Giant cell fibroblastoma recurring as dermatofibrosarcoma protuberans. Am J Surg Pathol 1991;15:798–801.
2. Bowne WB, Antonescu CR, Leung DH, et al: Dermatofibrosarcoma protuberans: A clinicopathologic analysis of patients treated and followed at a single institution. Cancer 2000;88:2711–2720.
3. Dal Cin P, Polito P, Van Eyken P: et al: Anomalies of chromosome 17 and 22 in giant cell fibroblastoma. Cancer Genet Cytogenet 1997;97:165–166.
4. Dupree WB, Langloss JM, Weiss SW: Pigmented dermatofibrosarcoma protuberans (Bednar tumor): A pathologic, ultrastructural, and immunohistochemical study. Am J Surg Pathol 1985;9:630–639.
5. Goldblum JR: Giant cell fibroblastoma: A report of three cases with histologic and immunohistological evidence of a relationship to dermatofibrosarcoma protuberans. Arch Pathol Lab Med 1996;120:1052–1055.
6. Goldblum JR, Reith JD, Weiss SW: Sarcomas arising in dermatofibrosarcoma protuberans: A reappraisal of biologic behavior in eighteen cases treated by wide local excision with extended clinical follow-up. Am J Surg Pathol 2000;24:1125–1130.

7. Mentzel T, Beham A, Katenkamp D, et al: Fibrosarcomatous (high-grade) dermatofibrosarcoma protuberans: Clinicopathologic and immunohistochemical study of a series of 41 cases with emphasis on prognostic significance. Am J Surg Pathol 1998;22:576–587.
8. Minoletti F, Miozzo M, Pedeutour F, et al: Involvement of chromosomes 17 and 22 in dermatofibrosarcoma protuberans. Genes Chromosom Cancer 1995;13:62–65.
9. Pedeutour F, Simon MP, Minoletti F, et al: Translocation, t(17;22)(q22;q13), in dermatofibrosarcoma protuberans: A new tumor-associated chromosome rearrangement. Cytogenet Cell Genet 1996;72:171–174.
10. Rubin BP, Fletcher JA, Fletcher CDM: The histologic, genetic, and biological relationships between dermatofibrosarcoma protuberans and giant cell fibroblastoma: An unexpected story. Adv Anat Pathol 1997;4:336–341.
11. Shmookler BM, Enzinger FM, Weiss SW: Giant cell fibroblastoma. A juvenile form of dermatofibrosarcoma protuberans. Cancer 1989;64:2154–2161.
12. Simon MP, Pedeutour F, Sirvent N, et al: Deregulation of the platelet-derived growth factor B-chain gene via fusion with collagen gene COL1A1 in dermatofibrosarcoma protuberans and giant-cell fibroblastoma. Nat Genet 1997;15:95–98.
13. Terrier-Lacombe MJ, Guillou L, Maire G, et al: Dermatofibrosarcoma protuberans, giant cell fibroblastoma, and hybrid lesions in children: Clinicopathologic comparative analysis of 28 cases with molecular data—a study from the French Federation of Cancer Centers Sarcoma Group. Am J Surg Pathol 2003;27:27–39.
14. Wang J, Hisaoka M, Shimajiri S, et al: Detection of COL1A1-PDGFB fusion transcripts in dermatofibrosarcoma protuberans by reverse transcription-polymerase chain reaction using archival formalin-fixed, paraffin-embedded tissues. Diagn Mol Pathol 1999;8:113–119.

Angiomatoid (Malignant) Fibrous Histiocytoma

1. Antonescu CR, Dal Cin P, Nafa K, et al: EWSR1-CREB1 is the predominant gene fusion in angiomatoid fibrous histiocytoma. Genes Chromosomes Cancer 2007;46:1051–1060.
2. Costa MJ, Weiss SW: Angiomatoid malignant fibrous histiocytoma. A follow-up study of 108 cases with evaluation of possible histologic predictors of outcome. Am J Surg Pathol 1990;14:1126–1132.
3. Enzinger FM: Angiomatoid malignant fibrous histiocytoma: A distinct fibrohistiocytic tumor of children and young adults simulating a vascular neoplasm. Cancer 1979;44:2147–2157.
4. Fanburg-Smith JC, Miettinen M: Angiomatoid malignant fibrous histiocytoma: A clinicopathologic study of 158 cases and further exploration of the myoid phenotype. Hum Pathol 1999;30:1336–1343.
5. Rossi S, Szuhai K, Ijszenga M, et al: EWSR1-CREB1 and EWSR1-ATF1 fusion genes in angiomatoid fibrous histiocytoma. Clin Cancer Res 2007;13:7322–7328.

Plexiform Fibrohistiocytic Tumor

1. Enzinger FM, Zhang RY: Plexiform fibrohistiocytic tumor presenting in children and young adults. An analysis of 65 cases. Am J Surg Pathol 1988;12:818–826.
2. Hollowood K, Holley MP, Fletcher CD: Plexiform fibrohistiocytic tumour: Clinicopathological, immunohistochemical and ultrastructural analysis in favour of a myofibroblastic lesion. Histopathology 1991;19:503–513.
3. Remstein ED, Arndt CA, Nascimento AG: Plexiform fibrohistiocytic tumor: Clinicopathologic analysis of 22 cases. Am J Surg Pathol 1999;23:662–670.

Soft Tissue Giant Cell Tumor

1. Billings SD, Folpe AL: Cutaneous and subcutaneous fibrohistiocytic tumors of intermediate malignancy: An update. Am J Dermatopathol 2004;26:141–155.
2. Folpe AL, Morris RJ, Weiss SW: Soft tissue giant cell tumor of low malignant potential: A proposal for the reclassification of malignant giant cell tumor of soft parts. Mod Pathol 1999;12:894–902.

3. O'Connell JX, Wehrli BM, Nielsen GP, et al: Giant cell tumors of soft tissue: A clinicopathologic study of 18 benign and malignant tumors. Am J Surg Pathol 2000;24:386-395.
4. Oliveira AM, Dei Tos AP, Fletcher CD, et al. Primary giant cell tumor of soft tissues: A study of 22 cases. Am J Surg Pathol 2000;24: 248-256.

Undifferentiated Pleomorphic Sarcoma

1. Coindre JM, Hostein I, Maire G, et al: Inflammatory malignant fibrous histiocytomas and dedifferentiated liposarcomas: Histological review, genomic profile, and MDM2 and CDK4 status favour a single entity. J Pathol 2004;203:822-830.
2. Fletcher CDM: Pleomorphic malignant fibrous histiocytoma: Fact or fiction? A critical reappraisal based on 159 tumors diagnosed as pleomorphic sarcoma. Am J Surg Pathol 1992;16:213-228.
3. Hollowood K, Fletcher CD: Malignant fibrous histiocytoma: Morphologic pattern or pathologic entity? Semin Diagn Pathol 1995;12:210-220.
4. Khalidi HS, Singleton TP, Weiss SW: Inflammatory malignant fibrous histiocytoma: Distinction from Hodgkin's disease and non-Hodgkin's lymphoma by a panel of leukocyte markers. Mod Pathol 1997;10:438-442.
5. Kyriakos M, Kempson RL: Inflammatory malignant fibrous histiocytoma. An aggressive and lethal lesion. Cancer 1976;37:1584-1606.
6. Mentzel T, Calonje E, Fletcher CD. Leiomyosarcoma with prominent osteoclast-like giant cells. Analysis of eight cases closely mimicking the so-called giant cell variant of malignant fibrous histiocytoma. Am J Surg Pathol 1994;18:258-265.
7. Mentzel T, Fletcher CD: Malignant mesenchymomas of soft tissue associated with numerous osteoclast-like giant cells mimicking the so-called giant cell variant of malignant fibrous histiocytoma. Virchows Arch 1994;424:539-545.
8. Weiss SW, Enzinger FM: Malignant fibrous histiocytoma: An analysis of 200 cases. Cancer 1978;41:2250-2266.

4

Adipocytic Tumors

Angelo Paolo Dei Tos

- Lipoma
- Lipomatosis of Nerve
- Angiolipoma
- Spindle Cell and Pleomorphic Lipoma
- Lipoblastoma and Lipoblastomatosis
- Hibernoma
- Myolipoma
- Chondroid Lipoma
- Well-Differentiated Liposarcoma/Atypical Lipomatous Tumors
- Dedifferentiated Liposarcoma
- Myxoid Liposarcoma
- Pleomorphic Liposarcoma

The category of adipocytic tumors includes several entities, all sharing in variable features of lipomatous differentiation. Diagnostic criteria appear to be well established; however, since the late 1990s, several studies have led to significant conceptual changes, in part as a consequence of the interactions between genetics and pathology. Adipocytic tumor represents the commonest group of mesenchymal lesions.

LIPOMA

Lipoma represents a benign, mature adipocytic proliferation. Lipomas are the most common human mesenchymal neoplasm.

CLINICAL FEATURES

Benign lipomas tend to occur in adults with a peak incidence between the fourth and sixth decades of life. A greater incidence in male individuals is observed. A statistically significant association with obesity is reported. Lipomas can arise anywhere both in the superficial and deep soft tissues. Those lesions arising within or in between skeletal muscles are labeled intramuscular and intermuscular lipomas, respectively. Lipomas can also arise in the gastrointestinal tract, most often in the submucosa of the small and large bowels. Lipomas usually present clinically as a painless mass. Approximately 5% of patients present with multiple lesions. Other variants include dermal lipomas and synovial lipoma. Rarely, patients can present with a diffuse overgrowth of adipose tissue known as lipomatosis. Clinically, lipomatosis is subclassified in symmetric, asymmetric, pelvic, and mediastinoabdominal forms.

PATHOLOGIC FEATURES

GROSS FINDINGS

Benign lipomas are usually soft, well-circumscribed masses featuring a yellow cut surface, ranging in size between 1 and 25 cm. However, deep-seated lesions tend to attain a larger size than superficial ones. A thin capsule is usually seen.

MICROSCOPIC FINDINGS

Lipomas are composed of a uniform proliferation of mature adipocytes featuring minimal variation in size and shape (Figure 4-1A). Occasionally, the presence of metaplastic bone or cartilage (so-called *osteolipoma* and *chondrolipoma*), as well as of extramedullary hematopoiesis, can be observed. The presence of fibrous tissue and myxoid change has justified the use of terms such as *fibrolipoma* and *myxolipoma*, respectively. Intramuscular/intermuscular lipomas harbor skeletal muscle fibers showing variable degrees of atrophy (see Figure 4-1B).

ANCILLARY STUDIES

IMMUNOHISTOCHEMISTRY

Benign lipomas are diffusely positive for S 100 protein.

LIPOMA—FACT SHEET

Definition
» A benign, uniform proliferation of mature adipocytes

Incidence and Location
» Trunk and limbs but can occur anywhere in the superficial or deep soft tissues

Sex and Age Distribution
» More frequent in male than female individuals; peak incidence between fourth and fifth decades of life

Clinical Features
» Slow-growing, painless mass

Prognosis and Treatment
» Lipoma is a benign neoplasm; complete surgical removal is curative

LIPOMA—PATHOLOGIC FEATURES

Gross Findings
» Well-circumscribed, capsulated mass with a yellow cut surface

Microscopic findings
» Lobules of uniform mature adipocytes

Fine-Needle Aspiration Biopsy Findings
» Aggregates of mature adipose tissue

Genetics
» Rearrangements of the 12q13-15 region mostly with 3q22; deletion of 13q; rearrangement of 6p21-23

Immunohistochemical Features
» Positive for S-100 protein

Differential Diagnosis
» Uniformity of cell size and shape, and lack of cytologic atypia distinguishes lipoma from atypical lipomatous tumors

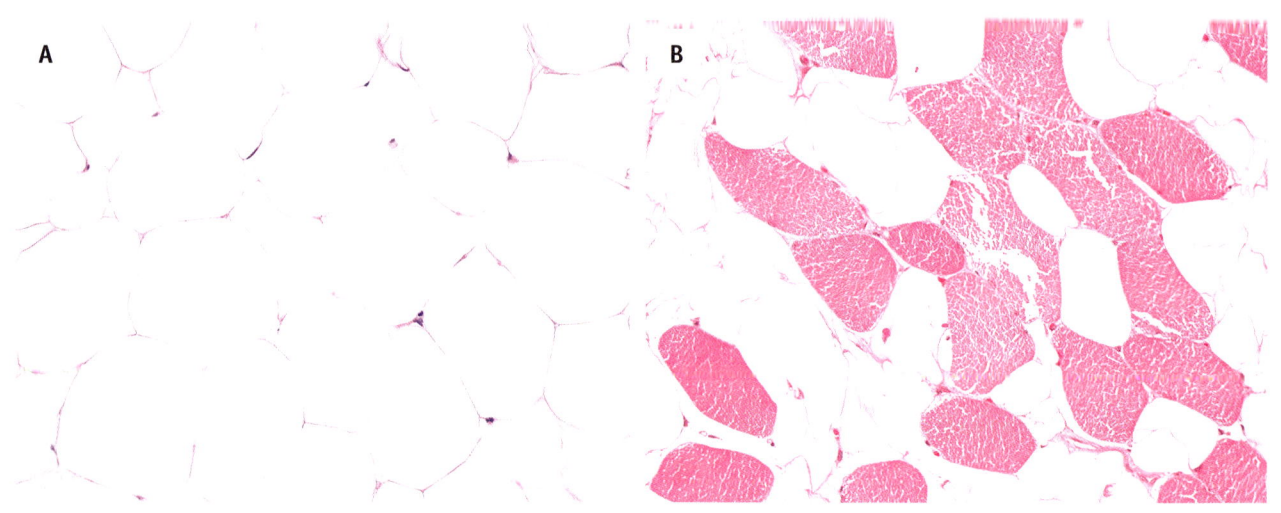

FIGURE 4-1
A, A uniform proliferation of adipocytes is generally observed in benign lipoma. **B,** The presence of mature adipocytes intermingled with normal striated muscle fibers represent the hallmark of intramuscular lipoma.

CYTOGENETICS

Cytogenetics of ordinary benign lipomas appears to be more interesting than their somewhat boring morphology, featuring an abnormal karyotype in about half of cases. Three main categories can be identified: (1) rearrangements of the 12q13-15 region mostly with 3q22; (2) a deletion of 13q; and (3) a rearrangement of 6p21-23. The target gene in 12q13-15 is a member of the high mobility group protein (HMG) gene family *HMGA2*.

DIFFERENTIAL DIAGNOSIS

The diagnosis of benign lipomas is usually straightforward. The absence of cytologic atypia in both adipocytes and stromal cells, as well as the uniform size of fat cells, allows separation from atypical lipomatous tumor/lipoma-like, well-differentiated liposarcoma. Sometimes intramuscular lipoma needs to be distinguished from intramuscular hemangioma that, alongside a complex vascular network, frequently features extensive fatty atrophy of muscle fibers.

PROGNOSIS AND TREATMENT

Lipomas are benign lesions whose complete local excision is curative. By contrast, intramuscular lipomas are characterized by a high incidence of local recurrence that can be avoided only by complete removal of the involved muscle.

LIPOMATOSIS OF NERVE

Lipomatosis of nerve (so-called *fibrolipomatous hamartoma of nerve*) is represented by a fibrolipomatous proliferation of epineurium with consequent enlargement of the affected nerve.

CLINICAL FEATURES

Lipomatosis of nerve most commonly affects the median nerve (followed by ulnar nerve) of patients between the first and the third decades of life. One-third of patients feature macrodactyly. Lesions can present at birth.

HISTOLOGIC FEATURES

GROSS FINDINGS

Grossly, a fusiform enlargement of the affected nerve is seen. The presence of adipose tissue confers a yellow cut surface.

MICROSCOPIC FINDINGS

Mature adipose tissue, associated with a fibrous component, infiltrates the epineurial and perineurial compartments of the affected nerves (Figure 4-2). Perineurial concentric fibrosis is constantly present, whereas microfasciculation is more rarely encountered.

ANCILLARY STUDIES

IMMUNOHISTOCHEMISTRY

Lipomatosis of nerve is a histologic diagnosis in which immunohistochemistry plays only the role of highlighting the various components of nerve fibers.

DIFFERENTIAL DIAGNOSIS

The diagnosis of lipomatosis of nerve is usually straightforward. The occasional presence of microfasciculation may raise the differential diagnosis with intraneural perineurioma.

PROGNOSIS AND TREATMENT

Lipoma of nerve is a benign lesion whose local excision may lead to severe functional damage. Conservative surgical approaches are therefore recommended.

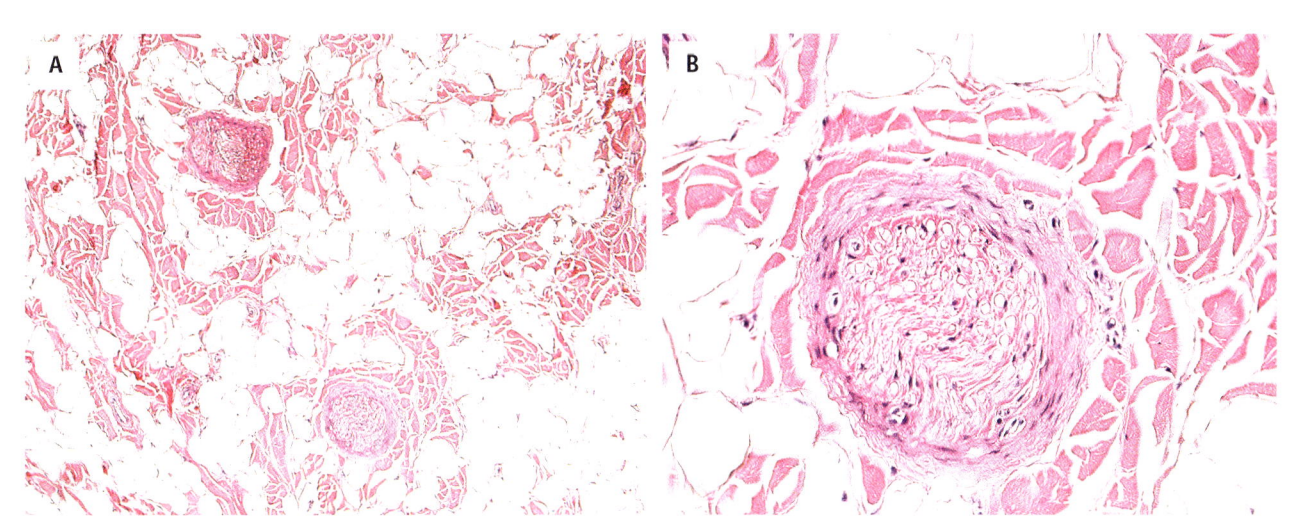

FIGURE 4-2
A-B, Fibrofatty expansion of the epineurial and perineurial compartments of the affected nerves.

LIPOMATOSIS OF NERVE—FACT SHEET

Definition
- Fibrolipomatous proliferation of the epineurium of a nerve

Incidence and Location
- Rare condition mostly occurring in the median nerve

Sex and Age Distribution
- More common in male than female individuals; first to third decades of life

Clinical Features
- Gradual enlargement of the affected part.

Prognosis and Treatment
- Lipomatosis of nerve is a benign condition; attempt of surgical removal may lead to severe functional impairment

LIPOMATOSIS OF NERVE—PATHOLOGIC FEATURES

Gross Findings
- Fusiform enlargement of the affected nerve

Microscopic Findings
- Fibrofatty proliferation located within the epineurial and perineurial compartments of a nerve

Immunohistochemistry
- Epithelial membrane antigen staining of perineurium highlights the compartmentalization of adipocytic proliferation

Differential Diagnosis
- Intraneural perineurioma

ANGIOLIPOMA—FACT SHEET

Definition
- Benign adipocytic lesion featuring a capillary-sized vascular network

Incidence and Location
- Subcutis of forearm, trunk, and upper arm

Sex and Age Distribution
- More common in male than female individuals; late second decade of life

Clinical Features
- Painful, multiple subcutaneous nodules

Prognosis and Treatment
- Benign lesion; local excision curative

ANGIOLIPOMA—PATHOLOGIC FEATURES

Gross Findings
- Encapsulated yellowish to red nodules

Microscopic Findings
- Mature adipocytic proliferation associated with a capillary-sized vascular network that contains fibrin microthrombi

Genetics
- Normal karyotype

Immunohistochemical Features
- Positive for S-100 protein; positive for endothelial markers in the vascular component

Differential Diagnosis
- Cellular angiolipoma may be mistaken for Kaposi sarcoma or angiosarcoma

ANGIOLIPOMA

Angiolipoma represents a benign adipocytic lesion featuring a variable capillary-sized vascular network.

CLINICAL FEATURES

Angiolipoma usually presents as multiple, painful subcutaneous nodules. Peak incidence is between the second and the third decades of life. They most frequently affect the upper limbs (approximately two thirds occur in the forearm), followed by the trunk and the lower limbs.

PATHOLOGIC FEATURES

GROSS FINDINGS

Angiolipomas are well-circumscribed, encapsulated nodular lesions, most often smaller than 2 cm, the cut surface of which varies from yellow to red according to the prevalence of adipocytic or vascular components.

MICROSCOPIC FINDINGS

Angiolipomas are composed of a mature adipocytic proliferation associated with a variable vascular network. In the latter component, a predominantly capillary-sized proliferation is detected (Figure 4-3A). Characteristically, blood vessels contain fibrin microthrombi, representing the diagnostic hallmark of this lesion (see Figure 4-3B). The amount of the capillary proliferation can

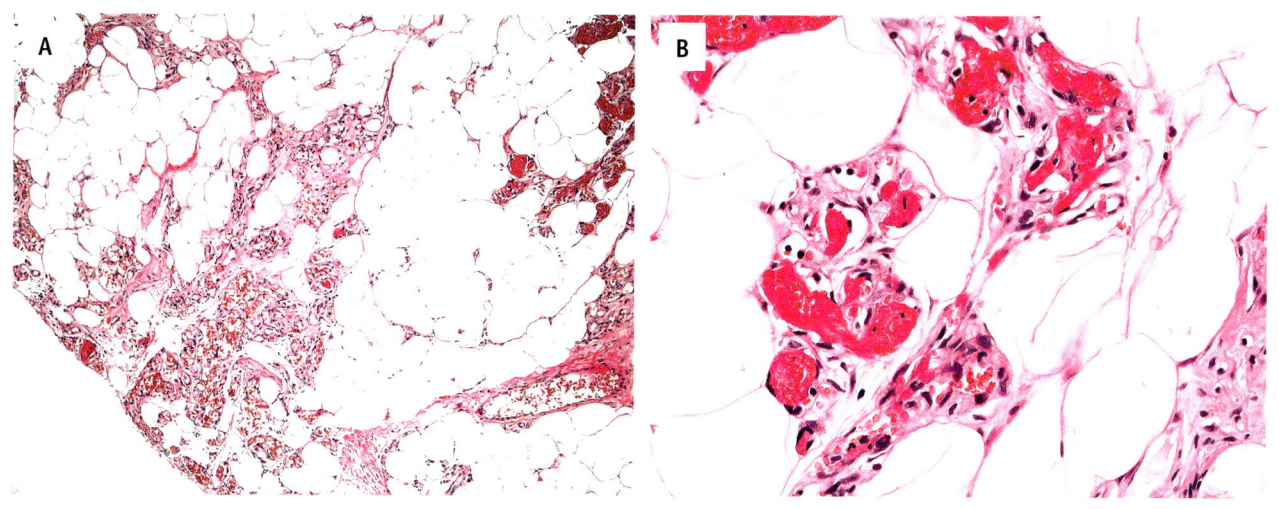

FIGURE 4-3
A, Angiolipomas are composed of a mature adipocytic proliferation associated with a variable vascular component. **B,** Blood vessels contain fibrin microthrombi, representing the diagnostic hallmark of angiolipoma.

vary from minimal to abundant, to the extent that the adipocytic component can be overlooked.

ANCILLARY FEATURES

CYTOGENETICS

Cytogenetically, angiolipomas are almost unique among adipocytic neoplasms because they represent the only entity that lacks any karyotypic aberrations.

DIFFERENTIAL DIAGNOSIS

Most diagnostic problems with angiolipoma are with lesions laying at the extremes of the spectrum. Sometimes the vascular component can be minimal and, therefore, overlooked; sometimes it is predominant to the extent that the lesion is mistaken for a vascular lesion, including angiosarcoma and Kaposi sarcoma.

PROGNOSIS AND TREATMENT

Angiolipomas are benign lesions. Local excision is curative, and local recurrence never occurs.

SPINDLE CELL AND PLEOMORPHIC LIPOMA

Spindle cell and pleomorphic lipoma represents a spectrum of benign adipocytic neoplasm featuring a spindle cell proliferation associated with coarse, eosinophilic collagen fibers. Rarely, multinucleated, hyperchromatic cells may be present.

CLINICAL FEATURES

Spindle cell and pleomorphic lipoma most often arise as a painless subcutaneous mass located in the posterior aspect of the neck or in the upper back. Peak incidence is between the fourth and the fifth decade, and the male-to-female ratio is 10:1.

PATHOLOGIC FEATURES

GROSS FINDINGS

Spindle cell and pleomorphic lipoma is usually less well-circumscribed than ordinary lipomas. The color of cut surface varies from yellow to white-gray depending on the relative amount of adipocytic and spindle cell component. Rarely, a predominantly myxoid appearance is present.

MICROSCOPIC FINDINGS

Microscopically, spindle cell lipoma is composed of a bland spindle cell proliferation admixed with brightly eosinophilic, coarse collagen fibers (Figure 4-4A). Rarely, a myxoid stroma is present that can become prominent (see Figure 4-4B). In these cases, it is possible to detect the formation of angiectoid spaces resulting in a pseudoangiomatous growth pattern. The adipocytic component can predominated or sometimes be focal (see Figure 4-4C). Pleomorphic lipoma represents part of the spectrum of this lesion, wherein bizarre, hyperchromatic, sometimes multinucleated cells are

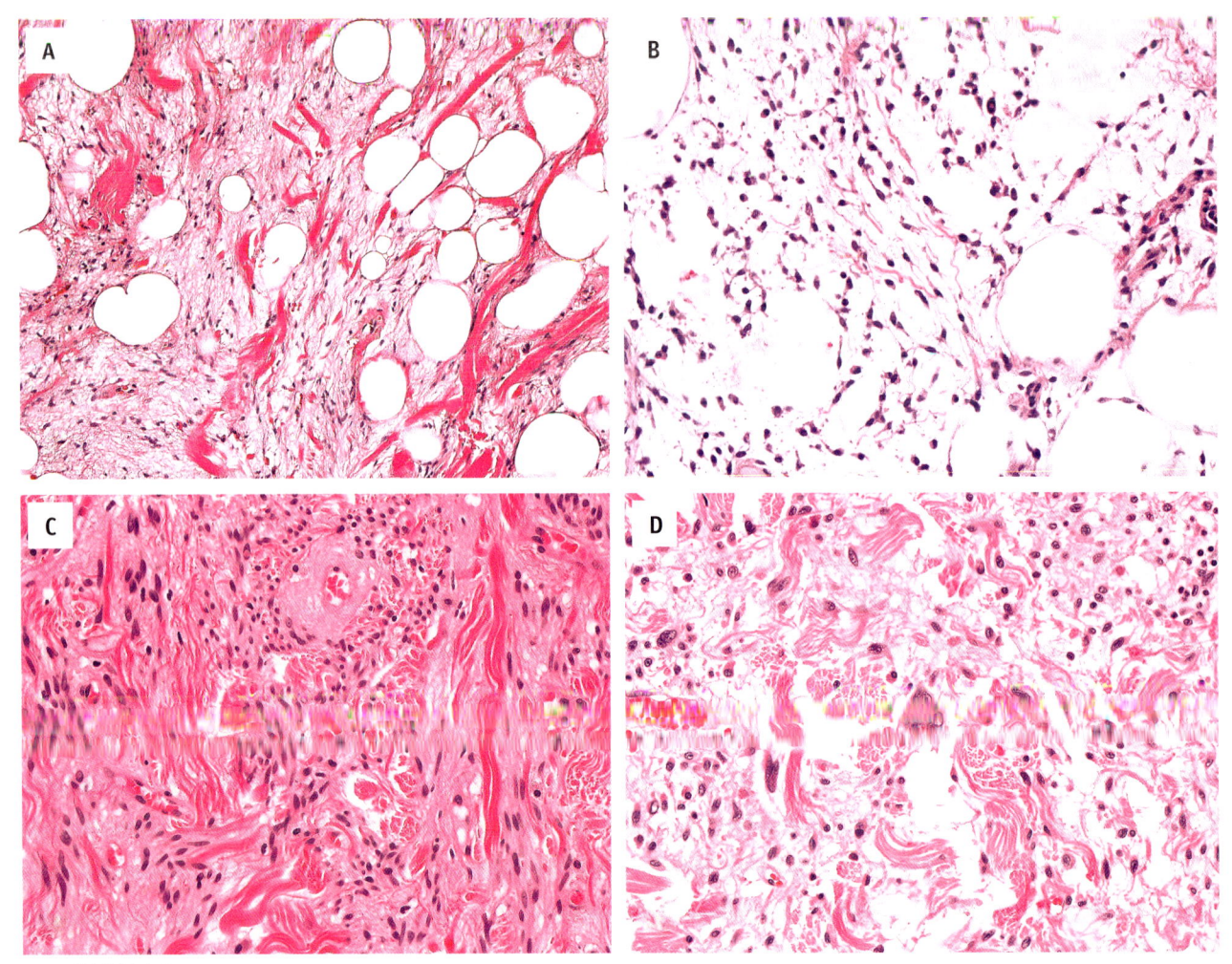

FIGURE 4-4

A, Eosinophilic coarse collagen bundles, bland spindle cells, and mature adipocytes are the main components of spindle cell lipoma. **B,** Myxoid change in spindle cell lipoma may lead to diagnostic confusion with myxoid liposarcoma. **C,** In cellular variants of spindle cell lipoma, the adipocytic component can be minimal. **D,** Floret-like multinucleated giant cell represents a typical feature of spindle cell and pleomorphic lipoma.

SPINDLE CELL AND PLEOMORPHIC LIPOMA—FACT SHEET

Definition
▸▸ A spectrum of benign lesion composed of an admixture of mature adipocytes, spindle cells, and hyperchromatic, multinucleated giant cells

Incidence and Location
▸▸ Posterior neck and upper back

Sex and Age Distribution
▸▸ More frequent in males than female individuals; peak incidence in fourth and fifth decades of life

Clinical Features
▸▸ Asymptomatic, mobile lump in the subcutis of the posterior neck

Prognosis and Treatment
▸▸ Benign lesion; local excision curative

SPINDLE CELL AND PLEOMORPHIC LIPOMA—PATHOLOGIC FEATURES

Gross Findings
▸▸ Oval, yellowish to grayish mass

Microscopic Findings
▸▸ Admixture of mature adipocytes, spindle cells, and ropey collagen bundles; hyperchromatic mononucleated and multinucleated (floret-like) giant cells are present at the pleomorphic end of the spectrum

Genetics
▸▸ Chromosomal aberrations of 13q and 16q

Immunohistochemical Features
▸▸ CD34+

Differential Diagnosis
▸▸ The presence of lipoblasts may lead to a diagnosis of atypical lipomatous tumor

associated with the typical morphology of spindle cell lipoma (see Figure 4-4D). Lipoblasts occasionally may be present.

ANCILLARY FINDINGS

IMMUNOHISTOCHEMISTRY

Spindle cell lipoma is characterized by diffuse positivity for CD34.

CYTOGENETICS

Loss of material from the region 16q13-qter together with 13q deletions is observed, therefore supporting separation from both ordinary lipoma and atypical lipomatous tumor/well-differentiated liposarcoma.

DIFFERENTIAL DIAGNOSIS

Extensive myxoid degeneration may raise the differential diagnosis with myxoid liposarcoma. Spindle cell lipoma lacks the typical plexiform vascular network, and atypia is minimal. Pleomorphic lipoma, because of cytologic atypia, may be confused with pleomorphic sarcomas. However, pleomorphic lipoma is usually less cellular, and in contrast with pleomorphic sarcomas, mitoses are exceptional.

PROGNOSIS AND TREATMENT

Spindle cell and pleomorphic lipoma are entirely benign, and local excision is curative.

LIPOBLASTOMA AND LIPOBLASTOMATOSIS

Lipoblastoma is a rare, benign, adipocytic tumor of infancy composed of immature (fetal) adipose tissue. It may occur as a localized lesion (lipoblastoma) or as a diffuse proliferation (lipoblastomatosis).

CLINICAL FEATURES

Lipoblastoma occurs predominantly in the first 3 years of life and is more common in boys. The most frequently affected anatomic site is the extremities, followed by the mediastinum, the retroperitoneum, the trunk, and the head and neck area. Most frequently, it presents as a well-demarcated nodule confined to the subcutis (lipoblastoma) or infiltrating the underlying muscle (lipoblastomatosis). Maximum size usually does not exceed 5 cm.

PATHOLOGIC FEATURES

GROSS FINDINGS

Grossly, lipoblastomas are well-circumscribed. Cut surface exhibits a lobulated appearance, and color varies from white to yellow. The presence of gelatinous area may vary from focal to predominant.

MICROSCOPIC FINDINGS

Microscopically, lipoblastoma is characterized by a proliferation of adipocytes in varying stages of differentiation, organized in a lobular growth pattern (Figure 4-5A). The number of lipoblasts is variable and depends on the duration of the lesion. Long-standing lipoblastomas may show complete maturation, therefore resembling an ordinary lipoma. The stroma can be myxoid and associated with a plexiform vascular network mimicking myxoid liposarcoma (see Figure 4-5B). In lipoblastomatosis, the lobular architecture is usually much less evident.

ANCILLARY FINDINGS

CYTOGENETICS

Lipoblastoma is characterized by a specific rearrangement involving the 8q11-q13 region. Two fusion genes have been reported to be involved: *HAS2/PLAG1* and *COL1A2/PLAG1*. *PLAG1* maps at 8q12. These fusion genes seem to utilize the so called *promoter-swapping mechanism*.

DIFFERENTIAL DIAGNOSIS

The most important differential diagnosis of lipoblastoma is with myxoid liposarcoma. The young age of the patient, the lobular growth pattern, and the absence of cytologic atypia represent useful clues; however, rare cases exist in which, because of significant morphologic overlap, genetic analysis may be necessary.

PROGNOSIS AND TREATMENT

Lipoblastoma is a benign lesion whose complete excision is curative. Local recurrence is observed in approximately 15% of lipoblastomatosis cases.

LIPOBLASTOMA AND LIPOBLASTOMATOSIS—FACT SHEET

Definition
- Benign adipocytic tumor composed of immature (fetal) adipose tissue.

Incidence and Location
- Extremities, mediastinum, retroperitoneum, trunk, head and neck

Sex and Age Distribution
- More common in boys than girls; first 3 years of life

Clinical Features
- Well-demarcated subcutaneous nodule (lipoblastoma) or lesion infiltrating the underlying muscle (lipoblastomatosis)

Prognosis and Treatment
- Benign lesion; local excision curative; 15% recurrence rate for lipoblastomatosis

LIPOBLASTOMA AND LIPOBLASTOMATOSIS—PATHOLOGIC FEATURES

Gross Findings
- Well-circumscribed, lobular lump

Microscopic Findings
- Proliferation of adipocytes in varying stages of differentiation in lobular organization

Genetics
- Rearrangement of 8q11-q13 region

Immunohistochemical Features
- Positive for S-100 protein

Differential Diagnosis
- Myxoid liposarcoma

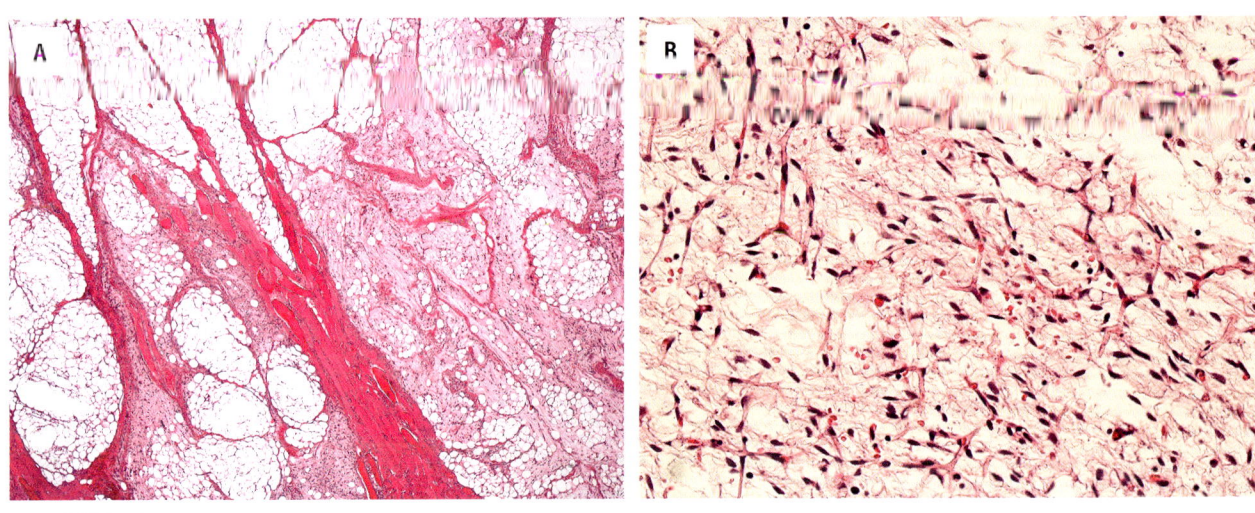

FIGURE 4-5
A, Lobulation is one of the distinctive low-power features of lipoblastoma. **B**, Myxoid background and plexiform vascular network may cause morphologic overlap with myxoid liposarcoma.

HIBERNOMA

Hibernoma is a benign adipocytic tumor characterized by a brown fat cell component variably intermingled with mature white adipose tissue.

CLINICAL FEATURES

Hibernoma tends to occur in the subcutis of young adults (peak incidence is in the third and fourth decades of life). A minority of cases may be deep seated within somatic muscles. The most frequently affected anatomic sites are represented by the thigh followed by the trunk, the upper limbs, and the head and neck area. Rarely, it may occur at a visceral location. Hibernoma most often presents as a painless, slow-growing mass.

PATHOLOGIC FEATURES

GROSS FINDINGS

Grossly, hibernomas tend to be well-circumscribed, ranging between 2 and 20 cm in diameter. Cut surface features a lobular appearance with a color varying from

CHAPTER 4 Adipocytic Tumors

HIBERNOMA—FACT SHEET

Definition
- Benign tumor composed of brown fat cells admixed with mature white adipose tissue

Incidence and Location
- Thigh, trunk, upper limbs, and head and neck

Sex and Age Distribution
- More frequent in male than female individuals; peak incidence in the third and fourth decades of life

Clinical Features
- Painless, slow-growing mass

Prognosis and Treatment
- Benign lesion; complete excision is curative

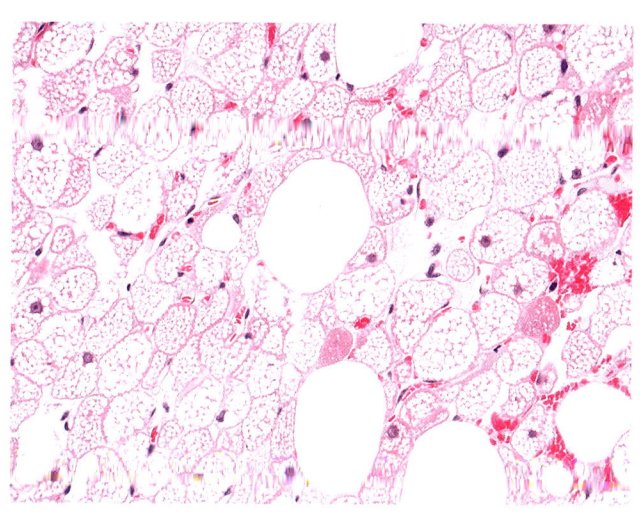

HIBERNOMA—PATHOLOGIC FEATURES

Gross Findings
- Well-circumscribed, often lobulated, with brown to yellow cut surface

Microscopic Findings
- A proliferation of multivacuolated brown adipocytes admixed with a variable amount of white adipose tissue

Genetics
- Rearrangements of the 11q13-21 and 10q22 regions

Immunohistochemical Features
- Positive for S-100 protein

Differential Diagnosis
- Well-differentiated liposarcoma with hibernoma-like features

FIGURE 4-6
The cytoplasm of brown fat cells of hibernoma may vary from pale to intensely eosinophilic.

yellow to brown according to the relative amount of brown and white adipose tissue.

MICROSCOPIC FINDINGS

Microscopically, the majority of hibernomas are composed of a proliferation of multivacuolated brown adipocytes that contain granular cytoplasm and centrally located nuclei (Figure 4-6). The cytoplasm of brown fat cells may vary from pale to intensely eosinophilic. Mitotic activity is usually absent, as is cytologic atypia. In rare cases, myxoid degeneration of the stroma can be present. The brown fat component is most often admixed with a variable amount of ordinary adipose tissue.

ANCILLARY STUDIES

IMMUNOHISTOCHEMISTRY

The diagnosis of hibernoma is relatively straightforward, and immunohistochemistry does not play a major role. As in most adipocytic lesions, S-100 protein is usually positive.

GENETICS

Cytogenetic analysis most often reveals structural rearrangements of the 11q13-21 region and less often of 10q22. At the molecular level, the presence of deletion of the multiple endocrine neoplasia 1 *(MEN1)* gene has been reported.

DIFFERENTIAL DIAGNOSIS

Hibernoma-like features can be observed occasionally in atypical lipomatous tumors and well-differentiated liposarcoma.

PROGNOSIS AND TREATMENT

Hibernomas are benign neoplasm irrespective of morphologic variations, and local excision is curative.

MYOLIPOMA

Myolipoma, also known as lipoleiomyoma, is a benign neoplasm characterized morphologically by coexistence of a mature adipocytic and smooth muscle cell proliferation.

MYOLIPOMA—FACT SHEET

Definition
▸▸ Benign neoplasm composed of mature adipocytes and smooth muscle cells

Incidence and Location
▸▸ Abdomen, retroperitoneum

Sex and Age Distribution
▸▸ More frequent in female than male individuals; peak incidence in the fifth and sixth decades of life

Clinical Features
▸▸ Painless, palpable mass

Prognosis and Treatment
▸▸ Benign lesion; surgical excision curative

MYOLIPOMA—PATHOLOGIC FEATURES

Gross Findings
▸▸ Large encapsulated mass with a yellow-white cut surface

Microscopic Findings
▸▸ Mature adipocytic tissue intermingled with bundles of differentiated smooth muscle fibers

Immunohistochemical Features
▸▸ S-100 protein positive (adipocytes), desmin positive, SMA positive (smooth muscle cells)

Differential Diagnosis
▸▸ Leiomyoma with fatty metaplasia

CLINICAL FEATURES

Myolipoma most frequently arises in the pelvis and in the abdomen, followed by the retroperitoneum of adult patients. Peak incidence is in the fifth and sixth decades of life, and male individuals appear to be affected less frequently than female individuals.

PATHOLOGIC FEATURES

GROSS FINDINGS

Myolipoma is macroscopically most often appears as a large, encapsulated mass, ranging in size between 10 and 20 cm, with a yellow-white cut surface. Necrosis is constantly absent.

MICROSCOPIC FINDINGS

Myolipoma is characterized by a distinctive, biphasic, morphologic picture composed of mature adipocytic tissue intermingled with bundles of differentiated smooth muscle fibers (Figure 4-7). Importantly, cytologic atypia must be absent both in the smooth muscle and in the adipocytic component.

ANCILLARY STUDIES

IMMUNOHISTOCHEMISTRY

The presence of dual adipocytic and smooth muscle differentiation can be easily confirmed immunohistochemically by demonstration of desmin and/or smooth muscle actin immunopositivity.

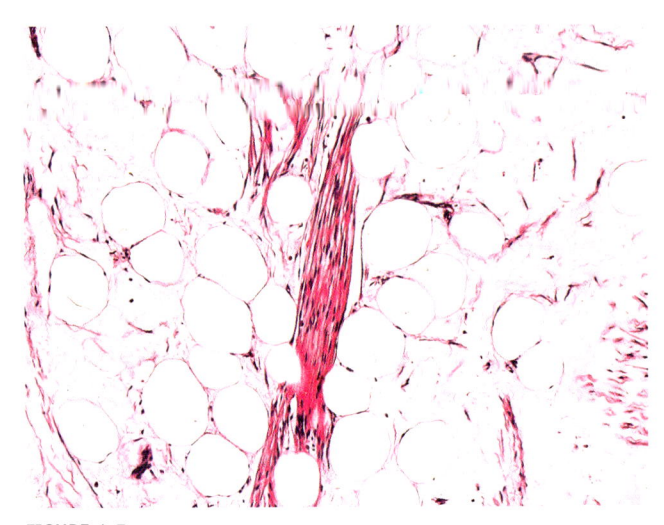

FIGURE 4-7
Myolipoma is composed of mature fat and smooth muscle cells.

DIFFERENTIAL DIAGNOSIS

The most important differential diagnosis of myolipoma is represented by leiomyomas with extensive fatty degeneration, which usually lack the uniformly spaced distribution of adipocytes that is typically observed in myolipoma. Atypical lipomatous tumors may also contain foci of smooth muscle differentiation.

PROGNOSIS AND TREATMENT

Myolipoma is an entirely benign lesion whose complete surgical removal is curative.

CHONDROID LIPOMA

Chondroid lipoma is a rare, benign, fatty tumor, first reported under the name *extraskeletal chondroma with lipoblast-like cells*.

CLINICAL FEATURES

Chondroid lipoma usually presents as a well-defined, deep-seated lesion located in the limbs, trunk, and head and neck region of women.

PATHOLOGIC FEATURES

GROSS FINDINGS

Chondroid lipoma is usually well-circumscribed, capsulated, and sometimes multilobular. Cut surface is yellowish as consequence of the presence of adipose tissue.

MICROSCOPIC FINDINGS

Microscopically, it is composed of an admixture of mature adipocytes, eosinophilic chondroblast-like cells, and vacuolated cells set in myxochondroid background (Figure 4-8A). One of the most striking features is the presence of vacuolated cells that cannot be distinguished

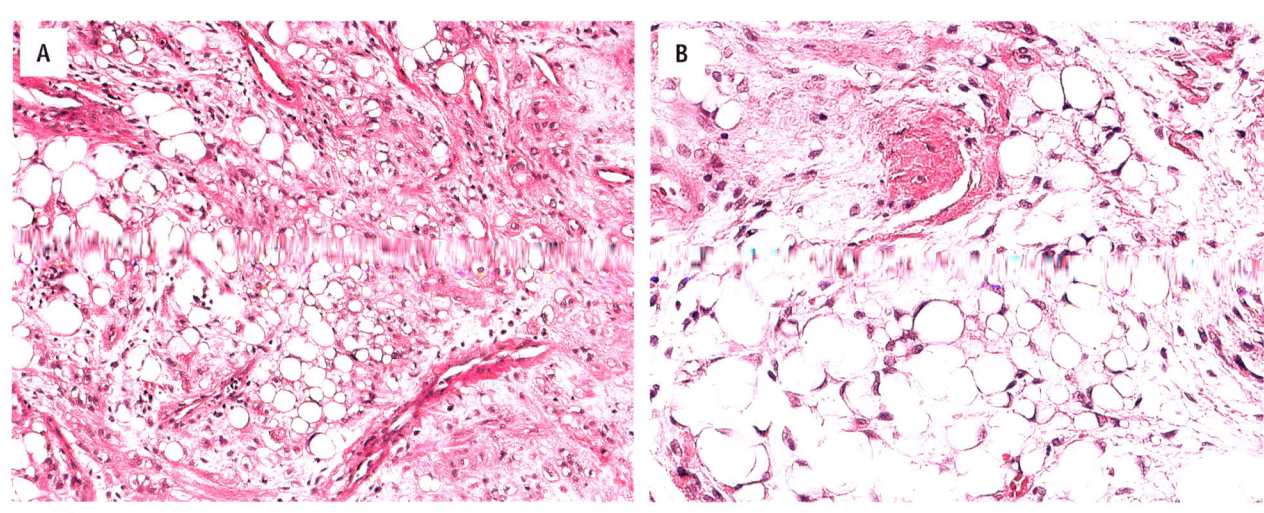

FIGURE 4-8
A-B, Cords and sheets of eosinophilic epithelioid cells associated with lipoblasts are seen in chondroid lipoma.

CHONDROID LIPOMA—FACT SHEET

Definition
» Benign adipocytic tumor composed of lipoblasts and mature fat set in a chondroid matrix

Incidence and Location
» Limbs, trunk, head and neck

Sex and Age Distribution
» More frequent in female than male individuals; peak incidence in the fifth and sixth decades of life

Clinical Features
» Deep-seated, painless mass

Prognosis and Treatment
» Benign lesion; surgical excision curative.

CHONDROID LIPOMA—PATHOLOGIC FEATURES

Gross Findings
» Well-circumscribed, capsulated with a yellowish cut surface

Microscopic Findings
» Admixture of mature adipocytes, chondroblast-like cells, and lipoblasts set in myxochondroid background

Ultrastructural Features
» Immature cells sharing features of embryonal fat and cartilage, lipoblasts, and preadipocytes

Genetics
» 11q13 aberrations

Immunohistochemical Features
» Positive for S-100 protein

Differential Diagnosis
» Myxoid liposarcoma, extraskeletal myxoid chondrosarcoma

from ordinary lipoblasts (see Figure 4-8B). It should be stressed that the use of the term *pseudolipoblast* in this context is misleading because it more properly indicates cells with vacuolated cytoplasm that mimic true lipoblasts.

ANCILLARY STUDIES

ULTRASTRUCTURE

Electron microscopy reveals immature cells that share features of embryonal fat and cartilage, lipoblasts, and preadipocytes.

IMMUNOHISTOCHEMISTRY

Immunohistochemically, S-100 protein decorates most neoplastic cells.

GENETICS

Chondroid lipoma contains complex rearrangements that involve chromosomes 1 and 2. Recently, a t(11;16)(q13;p12-13) translocation has been reported.

DIFFERENTIAL DIAGNOSIS

The differential diagnosis of chondroid lipoma includes myxoid liposarcoma, the recognition of which is greatly helped by the presence of a highly distinctive plexiform capillary-sized vascular network. Extraskeletal myxoid chondrosarcoma presents a more pronounced lobular architecture associated with peripheral accentuation of cellularity. In contrast with common belief, S-100 protein immunopositivity is encountered in not more than 20% of extraskeletal myxoid chondrosarcomas.

PROGNOSIS AND TREATMENT

Chondroid lipoma is an entirely benign lesion. Complete surgical removal is curative.

WELL-DIFFERENTIATED LIPOSARCOMA/ ATYPICAL LIPOMATOUS TUMORS

Well-differentiated liposarcoma represents about 40% to 45% of all liposarcomas. Four subtypes of well-differentiated liposarcoma are recognized by the 2002 World Health Organization (WHO) classification: adipocytic (or lipoma-like), sclerosing, inflammatory, and spindle cell.

CLINICAL FEATURES

Well-differentiated liposarcoma tends to occur equally in the retroperitoneum or the limbs and, more rarely, in the spermatic cord and the mediastinum.

PATHOLOGIC FEATURES

GROSS FINDINGS

Well-differentiated liposarcoma is usually well-circumscribed. Cut surface tends to be uniformly yellow in the lipoma-like variant. The variable presence of fibrous tissue correlates with the presence of white-gray areas.

MICROSCOPIC FINDINGS

Lipoma-like, well-differentiated liposarcoma is composed of mature adipocytes that exhibit marked variation in cell size with at least focal nuclear atypia (Figure 4-9A). Scattered hyperchromatic stromal cells are sometimes encountered (see Figure 4-9B). An important point is represented by the fact that the number of lipoblasts (monovacuolated or multivacuolated cells featuring hyperchromatic, scalloped nucleus) in well-differentiated liposarcoma may vary from many to none. Lipoblasts for a long time have been considered as virtually diagnostic of liposarcoma; however, the presence of lipoblasts does not make (or is required for) a diagnosis of liposarcoma. Moreover, several benign adipocytic lesions (e.g., lipoblastoma, pleomorphic lipoma, chondroid lipoma) may contain lipoblasts.

Sclerosing liposarcoma tends to occur most frequently in the retroperitoneum and in the paratesticular region. Microscopically, the presence of scattered, distinctive, bizarre stromal cells, as well as of rare multivacuolated lipoblasts set in a fibrillary collagenous background, represents the main histologic finding (see Figure 4-9C). Not infrequently, the fibrous component can be overrepresented to the extent that lipogenic areas can be missed.

In rare instances, well-differentiated liposarcoma may exhibit the presence of a dense, chronic inflammatory infiltrate that can obscure the adipocytic nature of the neoplasm (see Figure 4-9D). Polyphenotypic lymphoplasmacytic aggregates are most often detected, but cases exist in which a T-cell population represents the main inflammatory component.

The single new variant of well-differentiated liposarcoma described during the 2000s is represented by spindle cell liposarcoma. Spindle cell liposarcoma occurs in adults and exhibits an anatomic distribution comparable

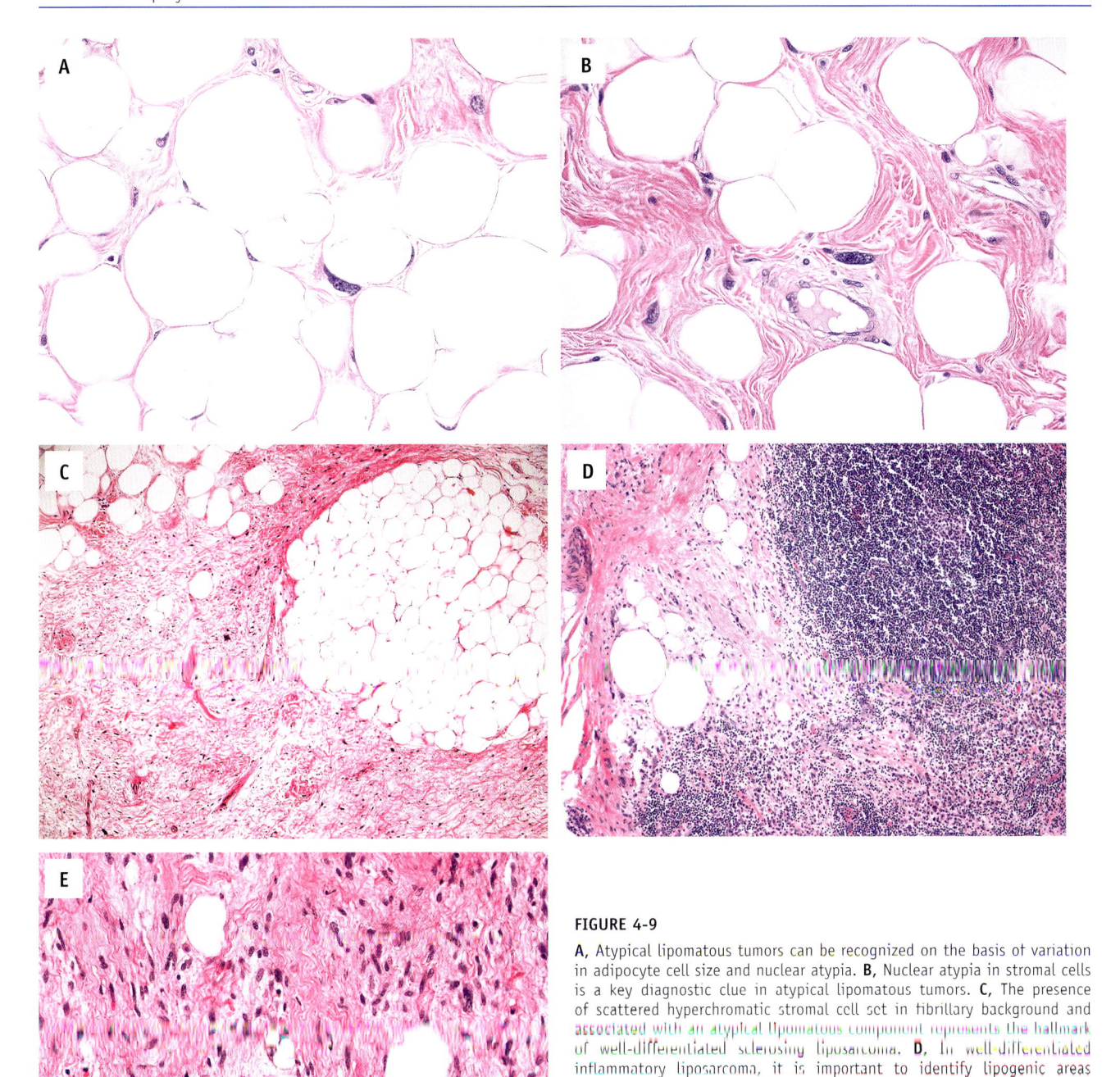

CHAPTER 4 Adipocytic Tumors 109

FIGURE 4-9

A, Atypical lipomatous tumors can be recognized on the basis of variation in adipocyte cell size and nuclear atypia. **B,** Nuclear atypia in stromal cells is a key diagnostic clue in atypical lipomatous tumors. **C,** The presence of scattered hyperchromatic stromal cell set in fibrillary background and associated with an atypical lipomatous component represents the hallmark of well-differentiated sclerosing liposarcoma. **D,** In well-differentiated inflammatory liposarcoma, it is important to identify lipogenic areas that can be obscured by the presence of the inflammatory infiltrate. **E,** The presence of a neural-like spindle cell proliferation set in a fibrous background and associated with an atypical lipomatous component represents the typical morphologic picture of spindle cell liposarcoma. A multivacuolated lipoblast is seen.

with that of the other well-differentiated liposarcoma subtypes; however, a tendency to involve the subcutis was observed in the first series. The main morphologic feature of spindle cell liposarcoma is the presence of a bland spindle cell proliferation reminiscent of a neural neoplasm set in a fibrous and/or myxoid background, and associated with an atypical lipomatous component that usually includes lipoblasts (see Figure 4-9E).

ANCILLARY STUDIES

IMMUNOHISTOCHEMISTRY

Immunohistochemically, most adipocytic tumors express S-100 protein that may play a role in highlighting the presence of lipoblasts. Expression of *MDM2* and *CDk4* may play a diagnostic role.

Genetics

Karyotypic analysis of well-differentiated liposarcoma has shown that this group of mesenchymal neoplasms is characterized by the presence of ring or giant marker chromosomes, or both. Both rings and giant markers contain amplified sequences derived from the 12q13-15 chromosome region, wherein they map several proto-oncogenes such as *MDM2*, *CDK4*, *HMGA2*, *SAS*, *GLI*, *DDTI3*, *OS1*, and *OS9*, all playing important roles in the molecular pathogenesis of human neoplasia. Interestingly, concomitant amplification of *HMGA2*, *MDM2*, and *CDK4*, as well as overexpression of the proteins thereof, has been recently demonstrated in well-differentiated liposarcomas.

Differential Diagnosis

The differential diagnosis of well-differentiated lipoma-like liposarcoma is mainly with benign lipoma. Variation in adipocytic size and presence of cytologic atypia represents the main diagnostic clues. Well-differentiated inflammatory liposarcoma has to be distinguished mainly from nonadipocytic lesions such as inflammatory myofibroblastic tumor and Castleman disease. These lesions should be sampled extensively to avoid diagnostic confusion and to prevent overlooking the adipocytic component. The differential diagnoses of spindle cell liposarcoma include benign and malignant lesions such as spindle cell lipoma, neurofibroma, dermatofibrosarcoma protuberans, malignant peripheral nerve sheath tumors, well-differentiated sclerosing liposarcoma, and low-grade fibromyxoid sarcoma (Evans tumor). In this context, the presence of lipoblasts represents a helpful diagnostic clue.

Prognosis and Treatment

Well-differentiated liposarcoma is characterized by a 30% risk for local recurrence but is incapable of metastasis unless it undergoes dedifferentiation. It was for this reason that, in 1979, Harry Evans suggested the use of alternative terms such as *atypical lipoma* or *atypical lipomatous tumour*. After a long debate, the 2002 WHO Classification of Soft Tissue Tumors reached a consensus on the fact that the terms *atypical lipomatous tumor* and *well-differentiated liposarcoma* are synonyms. The choice of terminology should be based on the principle of avoiding either inadequate or excessive treatment.

Anatomic site represents the most relevant prognostic factor. Overall mortality rate is close to 0% for lesions arising in surgically amenable soft tissues, but increases up to 80% for lesions that occur in the retroperitoneum. Standard treatment for atypical lipomatous tumor is represented by complete surgical removal with negative margins.

WELL-DIFFERENTIATED LIPOSARCOMA/ATYPICAL LIPOMATOUS TUMORS—FACT SHEET

Definition
- Proliferation of mature adipocytes exhibiting marked variation in cell size with at least focal nuclear atypia

Incidence and Location
- Retroperitoneum, limbs, spermatic cord, mediastinum

Sex and Age Distribution
- More frequent in male than female individuals; peak incidence in the sixth decade of life

Clinical Features
- Slow-growing, painless mass

Prognosis and Treatment
- Anatomic site represents the main prognostic factor; complete excision is virtually curative but difficult to achieve in the retroperitoneum

---

WELL-DIFFERENTIATED LIPOSARCOMA/ATYPICAL LIPOMATOUS TUMORS—PATHOLOGIC FEATURES

Gross Findings
- Well-circumscribed mass with a uniformly yellow cut surface (lipoma-like variant); the variable presence of fibrous tissue (all variants) correlates with the presence of white-gray areas

Microscopic Findings
- Mature adipocytic proliferation with variation in shape and size, associated with nuclear atypia in fat or stromal cells, or both
- Additional key features are the presence of hyperchromatic, bizarre stromal cells in the sclerosing subtype, a heavy lymphoplasmacytic infiltrate in the inflammatory subtype, and a predominantly spindle cell proliferation in the spindle cell subtype
- The number of lipoblasts is extremely variable

Genetics
- Ring chromosome and giant marker chromosomes; amplification 12q12-15 region

Immunohistochemical Features
- S-100 positivity in lipogenic areas; nuclear expression of *MDM2* and *CDK4*

Differential Diagnosis
- Lipoma-like, well differentiated liposarcoma is separated from benign lipoma on the basis of adipocyte variation in size and shape and/or cytologic atypia; spindle cell liposarcoma can be mistaken for a neural or fibroblastic/myofibroblastic neoplasm; inflammatory liposarcoma can be confused with lymphoproliferative disorders

DEDIFFERENTIATED LIPOSARCOMA

The term *dedifferentiated liposarcoma* was first used by Harry Evans in 1979 to define the transition from low-grade to high-grade nonlipogenic morphology within a well-differentiated liposarcoma. In the 2002 WHO classification it specified that nonlipogenic areas may not be necessarily high grade. The concept of dedifferentiation had been previously introduced by David Dahlin in the context of the description of tumor progression in chondrosarcoma.

Clinical Features

Dedifferentiated liposarcoma occurs most frequently in the retroperitoneum of adults. Men are more frequently affected than women. Dedifferentiation in well-differentiated liposarcoma occurs more frequently in the primary tumor (90%) than in recurrences (10%).

Pathologic Features

Gross Findings

Multinodular mass with yellow cut surface, containing firm tan-gray areas. Sometimes a distinct firm nodule is seen in the context of adipose tissue.

Microscopic Findings

The transition usually from well-differentiated liposarcoma to high-grade sarcoma tends to be abrupt (Figure 4-10A); however, rare cases exist in which this can be more gradual, and exceptionally low-grade and high-grade areas appear to be intermingled. Morphologically dedifferentiated areas overlap with undifferentiated pleomorphic sarcoma (formerly storiform and pleomorphic variant of malignant fibrous histiocytoma) or less frequently with high-grade myxofibrosarcoma (see Figure 4-10B). Dedifferentiated liposarcoma may exhibit heterologous differentiation in about 5% to 10% of cases, most often myogenic (see Figures 4-10C,D) or osteosarcomatous/chondrosarcomatous, and more rarely angiosarcomatous. Occasionally, dedifferentiated liposarcoma may contain peculiar whorls of spindle cells somewhat reminiscent of neural or meningothelial structures, often associated with metaplastic bone formation (see Figure 4-10E). Ultrastructural features may suggest follicular dendritic cell differentiation; however, this has not been confirmed immunohistochemically. Sometimes dedifferentiated liposarcoma exhibits the presence of fascicles of bland spindle cells with a cellularity intermediate between well-differentiated sclerosing liposarcoma and usual high-grade areas. *Low-grade dedifferentiation* is the term proposed to describe these areas. The grade of dedifferentiated areas does not affect the outcome.

Ancillary Studies

Immunohistochemistry

The presence of heterologous elements can be highlighted by use of appropriate differentiation markers. Overexpression of MDM2 and CDK4 in both

---

DEDIFFERENTIATED LIPOSARCOMA—FACT SHEET

Definition
- A liposarcoma showing transition from well-differentiated liposarcoma to high-grade nonlipogenic sarcoma

Incidence and Location
- Retroperitoneum > limbs

Sex and Age Distribution
- More common in male than female individuals; peak incidence in the sixth decade of life

Prognosis and Treatment
- Metastatic rate less than 20%; overall survival at 5 years: 60% to 70%; surgical excision as wide as possible

---

DEDIFFERENTIATED LIPOSARCOMA—PATHOLOGIC FEATURES

Gross Findings
- Multinodular mass with yellow cut surface, containing firm tan-gray areas

Microscopic Findings
- Transition (either abrupt or gradual) from well-differentiated liposarcoma to high-grade nonlipogenic sarcoma

Genetics
- Ring and giant marker chromosome associated with complex chromosome aberrations

Immunohistochemical Features
- Heterologous differentiation is associated with expression of appropriate differentiation markers

Differential Diagnosis
- Other pleomorphic sarcomas (most often pleomorphic leiomyosarcoma), sarcomatoid carcinoma

lipogenic and nonlipogenic components is consistently observed.

CYTOGENETICS AND MOLECULAR GENETICS

Dedifferentiated liposarcoma usually shows the presence of ring or giant marker chromosomes, or both, as in well-differentiated liposarcoma, although superimposed additional aberrations have been reported. At the molecular level, a significant increase of both overexpression and amplification of *MDM2* in the high-grade areas has been observed, which may account for the tumor progression in this subset of sarcomas. However, at variance with high-grade pleomorphic sarcomas that most often present concomitant *MDM2* amplification and *TP53* mutations (being significantly related to poor clinical outcome) in dedifferentiated liposarcoma, *TP53* is almost always unaffected.

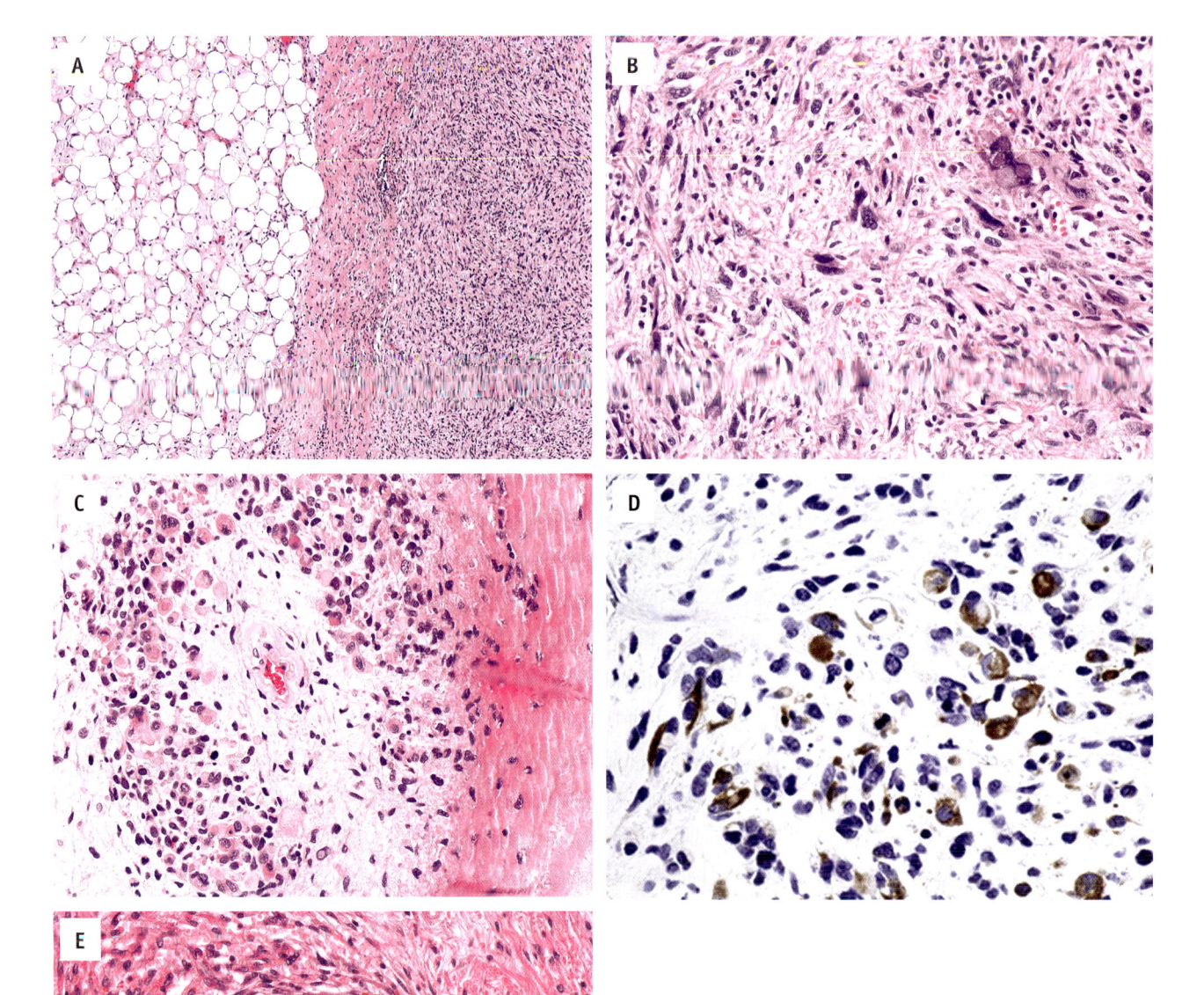

FIGURE 4-10
A, Abrupt transition from low-grade lipogenic areas to high-grade undifferentiated pleomorphic sarcoma is frequently seen in dedifferentiated liposarcoma. **B,** In dedifferentiated liposarcoma, the high-grade nonlipogenic component most often overlaps with "malignant fibrous histiocytoma"–like pleomorphic sarcoma. **C,** Heterologous differentiation represented by rhabdomyoblasts is seen in the example of dedifferentiated liposarcoma. **D,** Desmin immunopositivity is seen in the rhabdomyoblastic component. **E,** A peculiar whorling growth pattern is rarely seen in dedifferentiated liposarcoma. Neoplastic cells have been defined as exhibiting either a meningothelial-like or neural-like morphology.

DIFFERENTIAL DIAGNOSIS

Dedifferentiated liposarcomas need to be kept separate from other pleomorphic sarcomas (most often pleomorphic leiomyosarcoma) that occur in the retroperitoneum, as well as from nonsarcomatous lesions such as sarcomatoid carcinoma.

PROGNOSIS AND TREATMENT

The biologic behavior of dedifferentiated liposarcoma represents one of the most fascinating enigmas of tumor biology: (1) despite high-grade morphology, it tends to be less aggressive than other types of high-grade pleomorphic sarcomas; (2) dedifferentiated liposarcoma can recur as an entirely well-differentiated liposarcoma; and (3) in contrast with well-differentiated liposarcoma, dedifferentiation is associated with a 20% to 25% metastatic rate; however, mortality is more related to uncontrolled local recurrences than to metastatic spread. Standard treatment is represented by wide surgical resection. In the retroperitoneal location, resection should include adjacent viscera.

MYXOID LIPOSARCOMA

Myxoid liposarcoma represents the second larger group of adipocytic malignancies accounting for about 30% to 35% of all liposarcomas. Myxoid liposarcoma forms a morphologic continuum that includes a hypercellular neoplasm composed of oval to round cell neoplastic cells, formerly known as *round cell liposarcoma*.

CLINICAL FEATURES

Clinically, myxoid and round cell liposarcoma occur predominantly in the limbs, whereas the retroperitoneal location is exceptional. Peak incidence is between the third and the fifth decades of life, and both sexes are equally affected. Myxoid liposarcoma tends to recur repeatedly and metastasize to both bone and soft tissue locations including the retroperitoneum.

PATHOLOGIC FEATURES

GROSS FINDINGS

Myxoid liposarcomas are usually well-circumscribed, multinodular, gelatinous lesions. The presence of hypercellular (round cell) areas may confer a fleshy appearance.

MICROSCOPIC FINDINGS

Purely myxoid liposarcoma is composed of a hypocellular bland spindle cell proliferation set in a myxoid background, often featuring mucin pooling. Lipoblasts are most often monovacuolated and tend to cluster around vessels or at the periphery of the lesion. The most distinctive morphologic clue is represented by the presence of a capillary network organized in a plexiform pattern (Figure 4-11A).

Myxoid/round cell liposarcoma is defined by the presence of hypercellular areas, most frequently originating in a perivascular distribution, composed of undifferentiated round cells showing increased nuclear grade, frequent mitotic activity, and nuclear overlapping. Such foci may compose between 5% and 80% of the entire tumor mass (see Figure 4-11B). Pure round cell liposarcoma is a rare neoplasm in which hypercellularity or round cell differentiation accounts for more than 80% of tumor tissue (see Figure 4-11C). Adipocytic differentiation in pure round cell liposarcoma is often hardly appreciable, but the presence of S-100 immunopositivity in the majority of cases may be diagnostically helpful. As Evans suggested, transition to hypercellular/round cell areas is commonly observed in myxoid liposarcoma, therefore providing strong evidence in favor of the concept that myxoid and round cell liposarcoma represents a morphologic continuum of myxoid adipocytic neoplasia. Recently, these morphologic observations have gained the conclusive support of genetic analysis by demonstrating that myxoid and round cell liposarcoma exhibit exactly the same characteristic chromosome translocation.

ANCILLARY STUDIES

IMMUNOHISTOCHEMISTRY

Myxoid liposarcoma usually exhibits S-100 immunopositivity, which tends to be retained also in the hypercellular/round cell areas.

CYTOGENETICS AND MOLECULAR GENETICS

Myxoid liposarcoma is characterized by two main karyotypic aberrations: a t(12;16) that fuses the *DDIT3* gene on 12q13 (a member of the CCAAT/enhancer binding protein family involved in adipocyte differentiation) with the *FUS* (or *TLS*) gene on 16p11, and t(12;22) that fuses *DDIT3* with *EWS* on 22q12. The normal function of the *DDIT3* gene is to promote growth arrest, but as a consequence of the translocation, such an antiproliferative activity is lost. Trisomy 8 has been also observed as

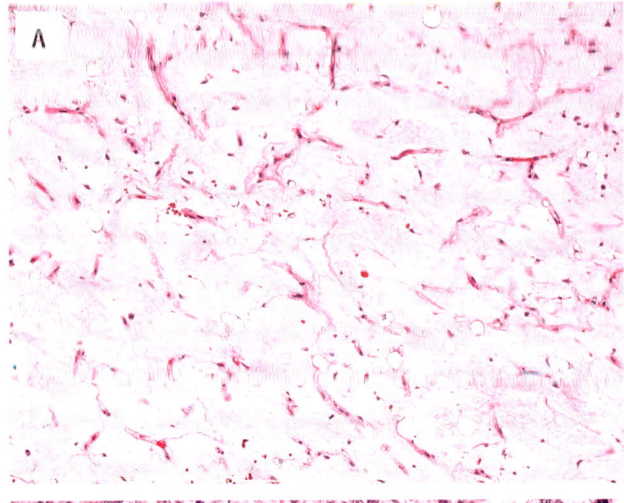

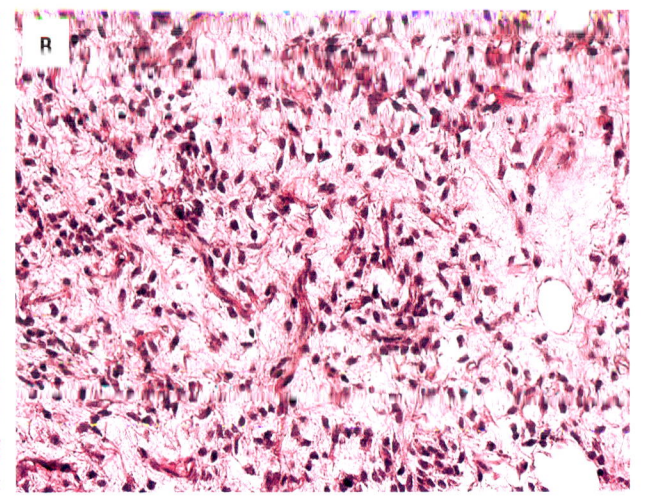

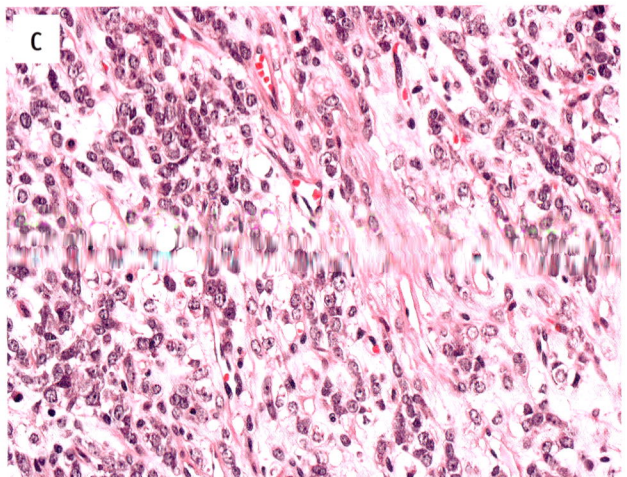

FIGURE 4-11

A, A cytologically bland spindle cell proliferation set in a myxoid background and associated with a distinctive plexiform capillary network represents the histologic hallmark of pure myxoid liposarcoma. **B**, In myxoid and round cell liposarcoma pure myxoid liposarcoma hypercellular foci begin to form around blood vessels. **C**, In high-grade "round cell" liposarcoma, adipocytic differentiation can be minimal.

MYXOID LIPOSARCOMA—FACT SHEET

Definition
- A variably cellular myxoid adipocytic neoplasm composed of spindle and/or round cells, monovacuolated lipoblasts, and associated with a plexiform vascular network

Incidence and Location
- 30% of liposarcomas and 10% of all sarcomas; deep soft tissues of the limbs

Sex and Age Distribution
- Both sexes equally affected; peak incidence in the fourth decade of life

Clinical Features
- Slow growing mass in the limbs; disease can be multifocal

Prognosis and Treatment
- Overall survival: 90% for purely myxoid lesions and 40% for high-grade "round cell" lesions at 5 years; wide surgery can be associated to adjuvant therapy in high-grade tumors

---

MYXOID LIPOSARCOMA—PATHOLOGIC FEATURES

Gross Findings
- Multinodular, well-demarcated, gelatinous mass

Microscopic Findings
- A proliferation of spindle cell and monovacuolated lipoblasts set in a richly vascularized myxoid stroma

Genetics
- (12;16)(q13;p11) fusing *DDIT3* with *TLS*, and t(12;22)(q13;q11) fusing *DDIT3* and *EWS*

Immunohistochemical Features
- Positive for S-100 protein

Differential Diagnosis
- Low-grade myxofibrosarcoma and myxoid chondrosarcoma

a nonrandom secondary change. Molecular analysis of myxoid liposarcoma has shown that *TP53* gene mutations occur in approximately one-third of cases, but these are independent from tumor grade. Overexpression of MDM2 protein represented the only parameter that correlated with tumor progression in this subset of sarcomas.

Differential Diagnosis

Myxoid liposarcoma must be differentiated from low-grade myxofibrosarcoma (a myxoid neoplasm composed of atypical stromal cells and pseudolipoblasts associated with thick-walled, arborizing blood vessels) and myxoid chondrosarcoma (a multinodular myxoid neoplasm showing oval to round cells organized in strands and cords, clustering at the periphery of the nodules).

Prognosis and Treatment

The presence of hypercellularity or round cell differentiation is associated with worsening of prognosis. Different cutoff values, ranging between 5% and 25%, have been set by independent studies. A reliable assessment of the percentage of hypercellular areas is difficult to achieve because it may be hampered by inadequate sampling, as well as by that degree of subjectivity that is an intrinsic part of morphologic evaluation. For the time being, it appears safer to consider any amount of hypercellularity as prognostically relevant and, if this exceeds 25%, to consider the lesion high grade. Standard treatment is represented by wide surgical resection. In high-grade lesions, adjuvant therapy (radiotherapy, chemotherapy, or both) may be indicated. Recently, the use of a marine-derived alkaloid labeled trabectedin (ET743) has proved extremely effective in the treatment of metastatic myxoid liposarcoma.

PLEOMORPHIC LIPOSARCOMA

Pleomorphic liposarcoma represents the rarest form of liposarcoma and represents a high-grade lipogenic pleomorphic sarcoma.

Clinical Features

Clinically, pleomorphic liposarcoma represents an aggressive neoplasm most often occurring in the limbs of older adults (the lower extremity, particularly the thigh, is the most frequent location) with a peak incidence between the fifth and sixth decade of life. It slightly predominates in the male sex. The trunk and the retroperitoneum represent less frequently affected anatomic sites. Rare cases of pleomorphic liposarcomas have been also reported in the skin; however, in these rare cases, clinical outcome appears mostly benign, with complete removal being usually curative.

Pathologic Features

Gross Findings

Pleomorphic liposarcoma exhibits gross features of high-grade sarcomas. Usually these neoplasms are well-circumscribed, fleshy, with variable amount of necrosis.

Microscopic Findings

Pleomorphic liposarcoma is a high-grade pleomorphic sarcoma that shows histologic evidence of adipocytic differentiation and represents the rarest variant of liposarcoma. The main diagnostic clue to define adipocytic differentiation in a pleomorphic sarcoma is the presence of lipoblasts, and it requires a careful histopathologic examination of an optimally sampled neoplasm. Lipoblasts are frequently large and show irregular, hyperchromatic, scalloped nuclei with prominent nucleoli, set in a multivacuolated cytoplasm. Nuclear pseudoinclusions and multinucleation are frequent findings. Most cases tend to fit into three main categories: approximately two-thirds are represented by a high-grade pleomorphic/spindle cell sarcoma with scattered lipoblasts or sheets of lipoblasts (Figure 4-12A), in less than one-third a high-grade pleomorphic sarcoma with epithelioid areas and scattered lipoblasts is seen (see Figure 4-12B), and a minority of cases overlap morphologically with intermediate- to high-grade myxofibrosarcoma except for the presence of lipoblasts (see Figure 4-12C). More rarely, pleomorphic liposarcoma in entirely composed of pleomorphic, multivacuolated lipoblasts (see Figure 4-12D).

Ancillary Studies

Immunohistochemistry

S-100 protein immunoreactivity may help highlight the presence of multivacuolated lipoblasts in those cases in whom adipocytic differentiation tends to be focal and, therefore, easily overlooked.

Genetics

Similar to most pleomorphic high-grade sarcomas, pleomorphic liposarcomas tend to exhibit complex karyotypes.

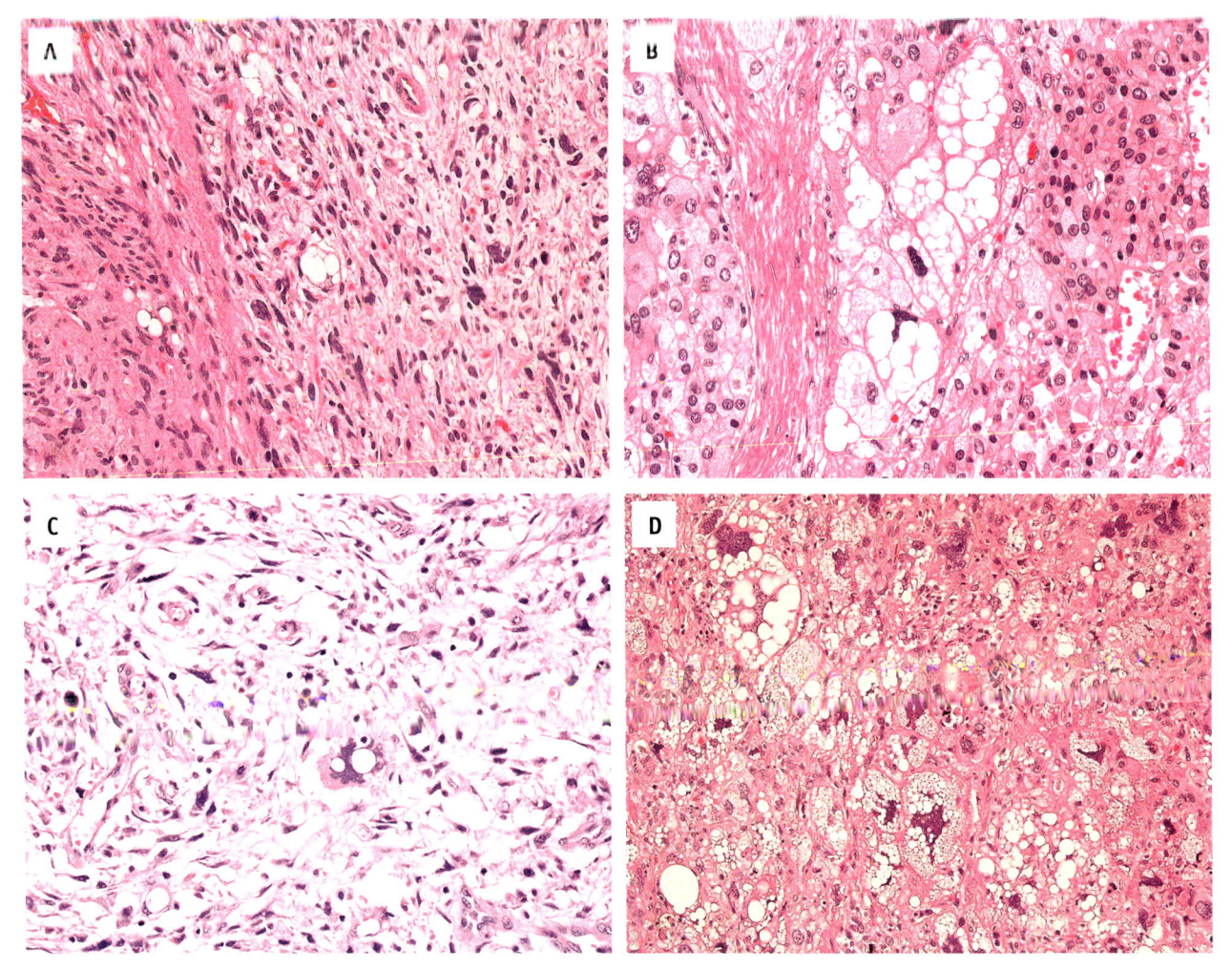

FIGURE 4-12

A, In this example of pleomorphic liposarcoma, a high-grade pleomorphic/spindle cell sarcoma with scattered lipoblasts is shown. **B,** Pleomorphic liposarcoma can feature an epithelioid cell component associated with pleomorphic lipoblasts. **C,** A myxofibrosarcoma-like morphology with lipoblasts is one of the possible presentations of pleomorphic liposarcoma. **D,** Rarely, pleomorphic liposarcoma can be entirely composed of pleomorphic lipoblasts.

PLEOMORPHIC LIPOSARCOMA—FACT SHEET

Definition
- A pleomorphic high-grade sarcoma that contains a variable number of lipoblasts

Incidence and Location
- 5% of liposarcomas and 20% of pleomorphic sarcomas; extremities

Sex and Age Distribution
- Elderly patients; both sexes equally affected

Clinical Features
- Enlarging firm mass

Prognosis and Treatment
- Overall mortality rate is 50%; wide surgery may be associated to adjuvant chemotherapy

PLEOMORPHIC LIPOSARCOMA—PATHOLOGIC FEATURES

Microscopic Findings
- Three main presentations are recognized: a high-grade pleomorphic/spindle cell sarcoma with scattered lipoblasts or sheets of lipoblasts; a pleomorphic sarcoma with epithelioid areas and scattered lipoblasts; a neoplasm mimicking intermediate- to high-grade myxofibrosarcoma except for the presence of lipoblasts

Fine-Needle Aspiration Biopsy Findings
- Collection of pleomorphic lipoblasts

Genetics
- Complex karyotypic aberrations

Immunohistochemical Features
- S-100 protein may highlight the presence of lipoblasts

Differential Diagnosis
- Other pleomorphic sarcomas subtypes

DIFFERENTIAL DIAGNOSIS

The main differential diagnosis of pleomorphic liposarcoma is with other subtypes of high-grade pleomorphic sarcoma and with dedifferentiated liposarcoma. The recognition of even focal adipocytic differentiation in an otherwise pleomorphic sarcoma represents the most important diagnostic clue and permits distinction from other pleomorphic sarcoma subtypes. In dedifferentiated liposarcoma, the high-grade component is usually nonlipogenic and always associated with a well-differentiated liposarcomatous component.

PROGNOSIS AND TREATMENT

Pleomorphic liposarcoma is a high-grade sarcoma associated with poor survival. Metastatic rate is between 30% and 50%, and overall mortality ranges between 40% and 50%. Standard treatment is represented by wide surgical resection associated with adjuvant therapy (radiotherapy, chemotherapy, or both).

SUGGESTED READINGS

Lipoma

1. Nielsen GP, Mandahl N: Lipomas In Fletcher CDM, Maertens F, Unni KK, (eds): Pathology and Genetics. WHO Classification of Soft Tissue Tumors. Lyon, France: IARC Press, 2002, pp 20–22.
2. Petit MR, Mols R, Schoenmakers EFPM, et al: LPP, the preferred fusion partner gene of HMGIC in lipomas, is a novel member of the LIM protein gene family. Genomics 1996;86:118–129.
3. Schoenmakers EFPM, Wanchura S, Mols R, et al: Recurrent rearrangements in the high mobility group protein gene, HMGI-C, in benign mesenchymal tumours. Nat Genet 1995;10:436–444.

Lipomatosis of Nerve

1. Derli E, Roncaroli F, Fibrolipomatous hamartoma of a cranial nerve. Histopathology 1994;24:591–592.
2. Boren WL, Henry RE Jr, Wintch K: MR diagnosis of fibrolipomatous hamartoma of nerve: Association with nerve territory-oriented macrodactyly (macrodystrophia lipomatosa). Skeletal Radiol 1995;24:296–297.
3. Silverman TA, Enzinger FM: Fibrolipomatous hamartoma of nerve. A clinicopathologic analysis of 26 cases. Am J Surg Pathol 1985;9:7–14.

Angiolipoma

1. Dixon AY, McGregor DH, Lee SH: Angiolipomas: An ultrastructural and clinicopathological study. Hum Pathol 1981;112:739–747.
2. Hunt SJ, Santa Cruz DJ, Barr RJ: Cellular angiolipoma. Am J Surg Pathol 1990;14:75–81.
3. Sciot R, Akerman M, Dal Cin P, et al: Cytogenetic analysis of subcutaneous angiolipoma: Further evidence supporting its difference from ordinary pure lipomas: A report from the CHAMP study group. Am J Surg Pathol 1997;21:441–444.

Spindle Cell and Pleomorphic Lipoma

1. Azzopardi JG, Iocco J, Salm R: Pleomorphic lipoma: a tumour simulating liposarcoma. Histopathology 1983;7:511–523.
2. Dal Cin P, Sciot R, Polito P, et al: Lesions of 13q may occur independently of deletion of 16q in spindle cell/pleomorphic lipoma. Histopathology 1997;31:222–225.
3. Enzinger FM, Harvey DA: Spindle cell lipoma. Cancer 1975;36:1852–1859.
4. Fletcher CDM, Martin Bates E: Spindle cell lipoma: A clinicopathologic study with some original observations. Histopathology 1987;11:803–817.
5. Hawley IC, Krausz T, Evans DJ, et al: Spindle cell lipoma: A pseudoangiomatous variant. Histopathology 1994;24:565–569.
6. Shmookler BM, Enzinger FM: Pleomorphic lipoma: A benign tumor simulating liposarcoma. A clinicopathologic analysis of 48 cases. Cancer 1981;47:126–133.
7. Suster S, Fisher C: Immunoreactivity for the human hematopoietic progenitor cell antigen (CD34) in lipomatous tumor. Am J Surg Pathol 1997;22:863–872.

Lipoblastoma and Lipoblastomatosis

1. Chung EB, Enzinger FM: Benign lipoblastomatosis. An analysis of 35 cases. Cancer 1973;32:482–492.
2. Dal Cin P, Sciot R, De Wever I, et al: New discriminative chromosomal marker in adipose tissue tumors. The chromosome 8q11-q13 region in lipoblastoma. Cancer Genet Cytogenet 1994;78:232–235.
3. Hibbard MK, Kozakewich HP, Dal Cin P, et al: PLAG1 fusion gene in lipoblastoma. Cancer Res 2000;60:4869–4872.
4. Mentzel T, Calonje E, Fletcher CDM: Lipoblastoma and lipoblastomatosis: A clinicopathological study of 14 cases. Histopathology 1993;23:527–533.
5. Vellios F, Baez J, Shumacker HB: Lipoblastomatosis: A tumor of fetal fat different from hibernoma. Report of a case with observations on the embryogenesis of human adipose tissue. Am J Pathol 1958;34:1149–1159.

Hibernoma

1. Fletcher CDM, Akerman M, Dal Cin P, et al: Correlation between clinicopathological features and karyotype in lipomatous tumors. Am J Pathol 1996;148:623–630.
2. Furlong MA, Fanburg-Smith JC, Miettinen M: The morphologic spectrum of hibernoma: A clinicopathologic study of 170 cases. Am J Surg Pathol 2001;25:809–881.
3. Gisselson G, Hoglund M, Mertens F, et al: Hibernomas are characterized by homozygous deletions in the multiple endocrine neoplasia type 1 region. Metaphase fluorescence in situ hybridization reveals complex rearrangements not detected by conventional cytogenetics. Am J Pathol 1999;155:61–66.
4. Merkel H: On a pseudolipoma of the breast (peculiar fat tumor). Beitr Pathol Anat 1906;39:152–157.

Myolipoma

1. Evans HL: Smooth muscle in atypical lipomatous tumors. A report of three cases. Am J Surg Pathol 1990;14:714–718.
2. Meis JM, Enzinger FM: Myolipoma of soft tissue. Am J Surg Pathol 1991;15:121–125.

Chondroid Lipoma

1. Chan JKC, Lee KC, Saw D: Exstraskeletal chondroma with lipoblast-like cells. Hum Pathol 1986;17:1285–1287.
2. Meis JM, Enzinger FM: Chondroid lipoma. A unique tumor simulating liposarcoma and myxoid chondrosarcoma. Am J Surg Pathol 1993;17:1103–1112.

Well-Differentiated Liposarcoma/Atypical Lipomatous Tumors

1. Argani P, Facchetti F, Inghirami G, et al: Lymphocyte-rich well-differentiated liposarcoma: Report of nine cases. Am J Surg Pathol 1997;21:884–895.
2. Binh MB, Garau XS, Guillou L, et al: Reproducibility of MDM2 and CDK4 staining in soft tissue tumors. Am J Clin Pathol 2006;125:693–697.
3. Dei Tos AP, Doglioni C, Piccinin S: et al: Coordinated expression and amplification of the MDM2, CDK4 and HMGI-C genes in atypical lipomatous tumours. J Pathol 2000;190:531–536.
4. Dei Tos AP, Mentzel T, Newman PL, et al: Spindle cell liposarcoma: A hitherto unrecognized variant of well-differentiated liposarcoma: Analysis of six cases. Am J Surg Pathol 1994;18:913–921.
5. Dei Tos AP, Pedetour F: Well-differentiated liposarcoma. In Fletcher CDM, Maertens F, Unni KK (eds): Pathology and Genetics. WHO Classification of Soft Tissue Tumors. Lyon, France, IARC Press, 2002, pp 35–37.
6. Enzinger FM, Winslow DJ: Liposarcoma. A study of 103 cases. Virchows Arch Path Anat 1962;335:367–388.
7. Evans HL: Atypical lipomatous tumor, its variants, and its combined forms: A study of 61 cases, with a minimum follow-up of 10 years. Am J Surg Pathol 2007;31:1–14.
8. Evans HL: Liposarcoma and atypical lipomatous tumours: A study of 66 cases followed for a minimum of 10 years. Surg Pathol 1988;1:41–54.
9. Evans HL, Soule EH, Winkelmann RK: Atypical lipoma, atypical intramuscular lipoma, and well differentiated retroperitoneal liposarcoma. A reappraisal of 30 cases formerly classified as well-differentiated liposarcoma. Cancer 1979;43:574–584.
10. Kraus MD, Guillou L, Fletcher CDM: Well-differentiated inflammatory liposarcoma: An uncommon and easily overlooked variant of a common sarcoma. Am J Surg Pathol 1997;21:518–527.
11. Stout AP: Liposarcoma: The malignant tumour of lipoblasts. Ann Surg 1944;119:86–107.

Dedifferentiated Liposarcoma

1. Coindre JM, Hostein I, Maire G, et al: Inflammatory fibrous histiocytoma and dedifferentiated liposarcoma: Histological review, genomic profile, and MDM2 and CDK4 status favour a single entity. J Pathol 2004;203:822–830.
2. Dei Tos AP, Doglioni C, Piccinin S, et al: Molecular abnormalities of the p53 pathway in dedifferentiated liposarcoma. J Pathol 1997;181:8–13.
3. Dei Tos AP, Pedetour F: Dedifferentiated liposarcoma. In Fletcher CDM, Maertens F, Unni KK (eds): Pathology and Genetics. WHO Classification of Soft Tissue Tumors. Lyon, France: IARC Press, 2002, pp 38–39.
4. Elgar F, Goldblum JR: Well-differentiated liposarcoma of the retroperitoneum: A clinicopathologic analysis of 20 cases, with particular attention to the extent of low-grade dedifferentiation. Mod Pathol 1997;10:113–120.
5. Evans HL: Atypical lipomatous tumor, its variants, and its combined forms: A study of 61 cases, with a minimum follow-up of 10 years. Am J Surg Pathol 2007;31:1–14.
6. Evans HL: Liposarcoma: A study of 55 cases with a reassessment of its classification. Am J Surg Pathol 1979;3:507–523.
7. Fletcher CDM, Akerman M, Dal Cin P, et al: Correlation between clinicopathological features and karyotype in lipomatous tumours. Am J Pathol 1996;148:623–630.
8. Henricks WH, Chu YC, Goldblum JR, et al: Dedifferentiated liposarcoma: A clinicopathologic analysis of 155 cases with proposal for an expanded definition of dedifferentiation. Am J Surg Pathol 1997;21:271–281.
9. McCormick D, Mentzel T, Beham A, et al: Dedifferentiated liposarcoma. Clinicopathologic analysis of 32 cases suggesting a better prognostic subgroup among pleomorphic sarcomas. Am J Surg Pathol 1994;18:1213–1223.
10. Mertens F, Fletcher CDM, Dal Cin P, et al: Cytogenetic analysis of 46 pleomorphic soft tissue sarcomas and correlation with morphologic and clinical features: A report of the CHAMP study group. CHromosomes and MorPhology. Genes Chromosomes Cancer 1998;22:16–25.
11. Nascimento AG, Kurtin PJ, Guillou L, et al: Dedifferentiated liposarcoma. A report of nine cases with a peculiar neurallike whorling pattern associated with metaplastic bone formation. Am J Surg Pathol 1998;22:945–955.

Myxoid Liposarcoma

1. Dei Tos AP, Doglioni C, Piccinin S, et al: Molecular aberrations of the G1-S cell cycle checkpoint in myxoid and round cell liposarcoma. Am J Pathol 1997;151:1531–1539.
2. Dei Tos AP, Wadden C, Fletcher CDM: S-100 protein staining in liposarcoma. Its diagnostic utility in the high grade myxoid (round cell) variant. Appl Immunohistochem 1996;4:95–101.
3. Fletcher CDM: Will we ever reliably predict prognosis in a patient with myxoid and round cell liposarcoma? Adv Anat Pathol 1997;2:108–113.
4. Grosso F, Jones RL, Demetri GD, et al: Efficacy of trabectedin (ET-743) in advanced pre-treated myxoid liposarcomas. Lancet Oncol 2007;8(7):595–602.
5. Kilpatrick SE, Doyon J, Choong PFM, et al: The clinicopathologic spectrum of myxoid and round cell liposarcoma. A study of 95 cases. Cancer 1996;77:1450–1458.
6. Knight JC, Renwick PJ, Dal Cin P, et al: Translocation t(12;16) (q13;p11) in myxoid liposarcoma and round cell liposarcoma: Molecular and cytogenetic analysis. Cancer Res 1995;55:24–27.
7. Orvieto E, Furlanetto A, Laurino L, et al: Myxoid and round cell liposarcoma: A spectrum of myxoid adipocytic neoplasia. Semin Diagn Pathol 2001;18:267–273.
8. Smith TA, Easley KA, Goldblum JR: Myxoid/round cell liposarcoma of the extremities. A clinicopathologic study of 29 cases with particular attention to extent of round cell liposarcoma. Am J Surg Pathol 1996;20:171–180.
9. Tallini G, Akerman M, Dal Cin P, et al: Combined morphologic and karyotypic study of 28 myxoid liposarcomas. Implications for a revised morphologic typing. A report from the CHAMP group. Am J Surg Pathol 1996;20:1047–1055.

Pleomorphic Liposarcoma

1. Dei Tos AP: Pleomorphic sarcomas: Where are we now? Histopathology 2006;48:51–62.
2. Gebhard S, Coindre JM, Michels JJ, et al: Pleomorphic liposarcoma: Clinicopathologic, immunohistochemical, and follow-up analysis of 63 cases: A study from the French Federation of Cancer Centers Sarcoma Group. Am J Surg Pathol 2002;26:601–616.
3. Hornick JL, Bosenberg MW, Mentzel T, et al: Pleomorphic liposarcoma: Clinicopathologic analysis of 57 cases. Am J Surg Pathol 2004;28:1257–1267.
4. Oliveira AM, Nascimento AG: Pleomorphic liposarcoma. Semin Diagn Pathol 2001;18:274–285.

5 Smooth Muscle Tumors
Andrea T. Deyrup

LEIOMYOMA
- Pilar Leiomyoma
- Leiomyomas of the External Genitalia
- Leiomyoma of Deep Soft Tissue
- Vascular Leiomyoma (Angioleiomyoma)
- Leiomyoma of the Retroperitoneum

LEIOMYOSARCOMA
- Cutaneous Leiomyosarcoma
- Leiomyosarcomas of Deep Soft Tissue
- Vascular Leiomyosarcoma
- Retroperitoneal Leiomyosarcoma
- Epstein–Barr Virus–Associated Smooth Muscle Tumors

Depending on the site, smooth muscle neoplasms can be common (e.g., in female genital tract) or rare (in somatic soft tissue). Moreover, the incidence of benign (leiomyoma) versus malignant (leiomyosarcoma) smooth muscle tumors (SMTs) and the criteria for differentiating the two are also strongly correlated with location.

Most SMTs arise in association with pre-existing smooth muscle (e.g., pilar, uterine, and vascular SMTs). In addition, SMTs are one of the rare mesenchymal neoplasms that can be associated with an infectious agent: Epstein–Barr virus (EBV) in immunocompromised patients.

LEIOMYOMA

Leiomyomas are categorized according to site of origin as pilar, genital, vascular, or arising in the deep soft tissue or retroperitoneum. They tend to be well circumscribed, though not encapsulated. On cut section, they usually have a firm, whorled surface that ranges from white to gray. Microscopically, they are composed of well-differentiated smooth muscle cells that are characterized by a spindled shape, brightly eosinophilic cytoplasm, and blunt-ended, cigar-shaped nuclei (Figure 5-1). Cytoplasmic vacuolation and a perinuclear clear zone may be seen. Benign SMTs express a wide range of antigens including desmin, smooth muscle actin, muscle specific actin, calponin, h-caldesmon, and smooth muscle myosin heavy chain. All of these may be expressed or only a subset. In addition, focal expression of cytokeratin and S-100 protein are occasionally noted. In differentiating smooth muscle cells from myofibroblasts, h-caldesmon can be useful because it is not usually expressed by the latter.

The most important entity to be considered in the differential diagnosis of a benign SMT is a malignant SMT, namely, a leiomyosarcoma. In nongynecologic sites, criteria are quite strict and allow only minimal cytologic atypia, no coagulative necrosis, and a mitotic index of no more than 1 per 50 high power fields (hpf).

In most cases, simple excision is adequate therapy. Although these tumors may recur, they do not metastasize.

PILAR LEIOMYOMA

CLINICAL FEATURES

Pilar leiomyoma is a relatively rare tumor that arises from the arrector pili smooth muscles in the subcutis. They affect primarily adolescents and young adults, though they can be seen in any age group. Typically, they present either as clusters of cutaneous red to brown papules or, more rarely, as a single nodule, and they are frequently painful. The most common site is the extremities; truncal lesions, when they occur, are often multiple. A familial association has been reported, and these patients have an increased incidence of uterine leiomyomas and renal cell carcinoma.

PATHOLOGIC FEATURES

GROSS FINDINGS

Pilar leiomyomas are poorly circumscribed tumors, located in the subcutis, and are generally less than 2 cm in maximum dimension.

MICROSCOPIC FINDINGS

Unlike the orderly, intersecting arrangement of tumor cells seen in most tumors of well-differentiated smooth muscle, pilar leiomyomas have a more disorganized architecture, similar to the normal arrangement of arrector pili smooth muscle cells (Figure 5-2). The tumor cells are brightly eosinophilic with blunt-ended, somewhat vesicular nuclei. Focal nuclear atypia of the degenerative type may be seen, but mitoses are absent. Abundant collagen separates individual tumor cells and bundles of cells, and at the periphery, an infiltrative pattern may be appreciated.

DIFFERENTIAL DIAGNOSIS

The primary consideration in the differential diagnosis for pilar leiomyoma is benign fibrous histiocytoma (BFH). The latter is composed of slender spindled cells that are commonly admixed with secondary elements including giant cells and xanthoma cells, and usually express factor XIIIa.

PROGNOSIS AND TREATMENT

Solitary nodules are adequately treated by simple excision; however, in cases with multiple tumors, surgical excision may not be feasible. In the latter setting, tumors gradually progress with enlargement of existing lesions and development of new tumors. Pain may contribute significantly to morbidity in these patients.

LEIOMYOMAS OF THE EXTERNAL GENITALIA

CLINICAL FEATURES

Leiomyomas of the external genitalia occur in adults, are usually painless, and arise in the dartoic muscles of the scrotum and the muscles of the deep dermis of the vulva. The most common clinical presentation in female individuals is a mass in the labia majora that may be clinically interpreted as a Bartholin cyst. Scrotal tumors are most common in white men between the fourth and sixth decades of life. They can attain a significant size and are often clinically diagnosed as cysts.

PATHOLOGIC FEATURES

GROSS FINDINGS

Genital leiomyomas are usually solitary nodules. Vulvar tumors are generally better circumscribed than tumors arising in the scrotum. On cut section, they display a characteristic white, whorled appearance, and calcifications may be present.

MICROSCOPIC FINDINGS

Histologically, vulvar leiomyomas are composed primarily of bland spindled cells, although epithelioid morphology can be seen. Myxoid stroma and hyalinization are also common. Vulvar leiomyomas are probably composed of hormonally responsive smooth muscle, and as in gynecologic SMTs, the criteria for malignancy are somewhat less stringent; if only one of the following criteria is met, the tumor is considered a leiomyoma: moderate-to-severe cytologic atypia, size greater than or equal to 5 cm, infiltrative margins, and greater than or equal to 5 mitotic figures per 10 hpf. SMTs in this location with

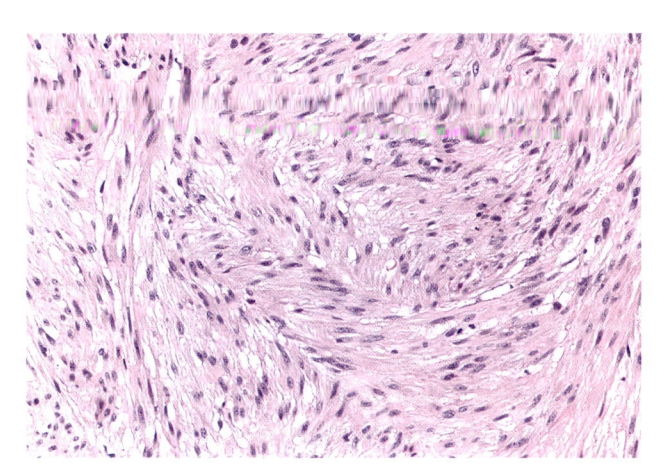

FIGURE 5-1
Leiomyoma composed of fascicles of bland spindled cells with blunt-ended nuclei and cytoplasmic vacuolation.

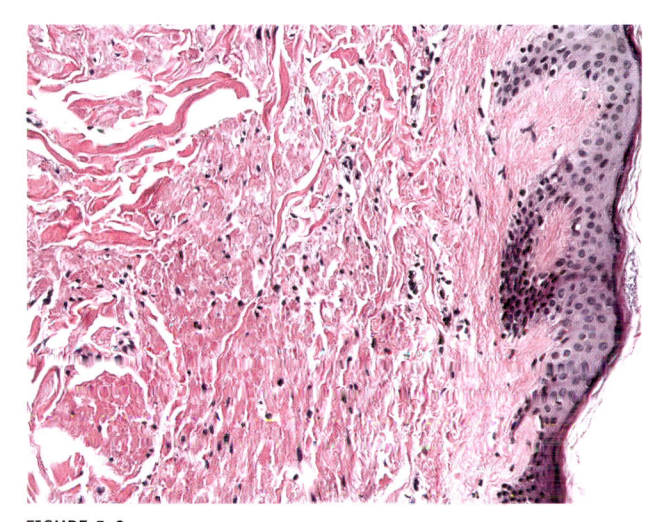

FIGURE 5-2
Pilar leiomyoma.

two of these features are considered benign but termed atypical leiomyomas, and if three criteria are met, the lesion is considered a leiomyosarcoma.

Scrotal leiomyomas are generally well circumscribed, although they may be focally infiltrative (Figure 5-3). They may display degenerative-type cytologic atypia that, in the absence of hypercellularity and mitotic activity, is not worrisome. Lymphoid aggregates are sometimes associated with these tumors.

IMMUNOHISTOCHEMISTRY

In addition to muscle-specific antigens, vulvar leiomyomas usually express estrogen and progesterone receptors. This is not seen in scrotal tumors.

DIFFERENTIAL DIAGNOSIS

Smooth muscle hyperplasia in the scrotum can mimic an SMT. However, unlike leiomyomas in this site, these lesions are less compact and display a more orderly architecture. In the vulva, cellular angiofibroma, a well-circumscribed tumor that is composed of bland spindled cells admixed with wispy collagen and fat, may be considered in the differential diagnosis; however, these tumors are negative for muscle-specific antigens and tend to be more reminiscent histologically of spindle cell lipomas than SMTs.

PROGNOSIS AND TREATMENT

Complete excision is curative.

LEIOMYOMA OF DEEP SOFT TISSUE

CLINICAL FEATURES

Leiomyomas of deep soft tissue are extremely rare, because most SMTs in this clinical setting are malignant. These tumors most commonly present as a single nodule located in the extremities and predominantly affect young or middle-aged adults.

PATHOLOGIC FEATURES

GROSS FINDINGS

Leiomyomas of deep soft tissue are well-circumscribed, fusiform-to-spherical, white-to-gray tumors that can grow to a substantial size: tumors larger than 30 cm have been reported. If significant myxoid areas are present, the tumor may appear focally gelatinous.

MICROSCOPIC FINDINGS

Histologically, leiomyomas are composed of intersecting fascicles of well-differentiated smooth muscle cells that are characterized by a spindled shape, eosinophilic cytoplasm, and blunt-ended, cigar-shaped nuclei. Myxoid change and hyalinization are commonly seen, as are calcifications (Figures 5-4 and 5-5). Necrosis, brisk mitotic activity (greater than 1 per 50 hpf), and significant cytologic atypia are not seen. The presence of any of these findings suggests a diagnosis of leiomyosarcoma.

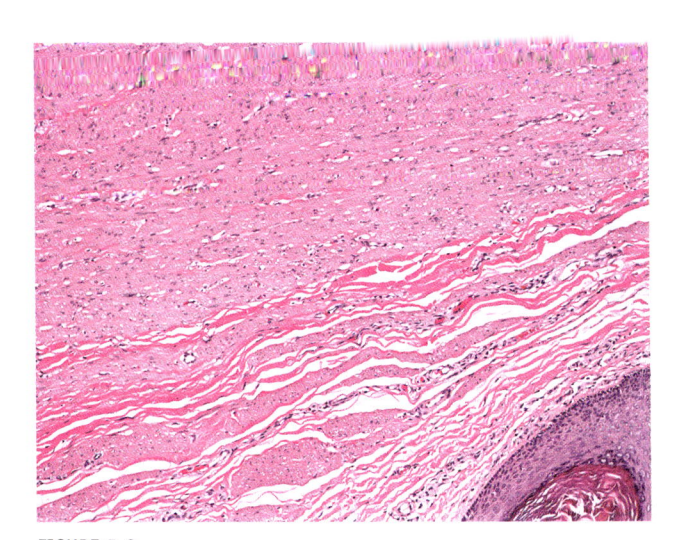

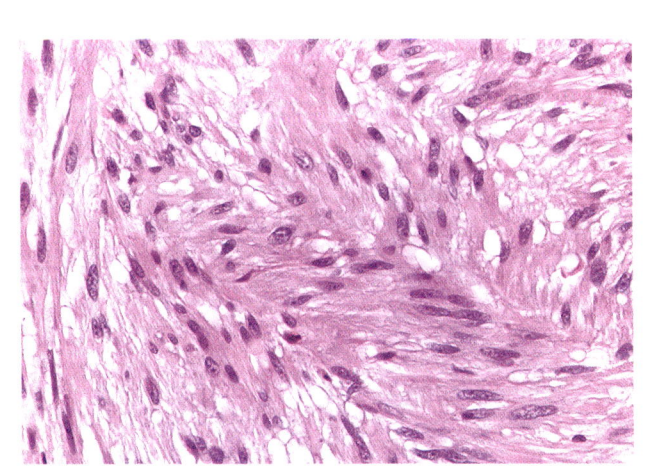

FIGURE 5-3
Scrotal leiomyoma with peripheral infiltration.

FIGURE 5-4
Leiomyoma of deep soft tissue displaying bland nuclear features and cytoplasmic vacuolation.

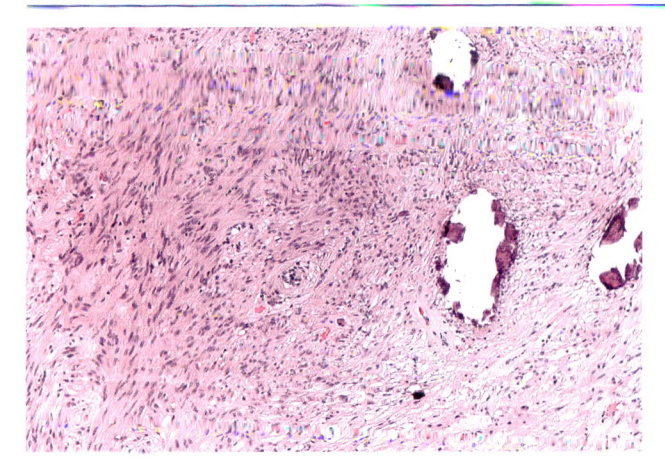

FIGURE 5-5
Calcifications in leiomyoma of deep soft tissue.

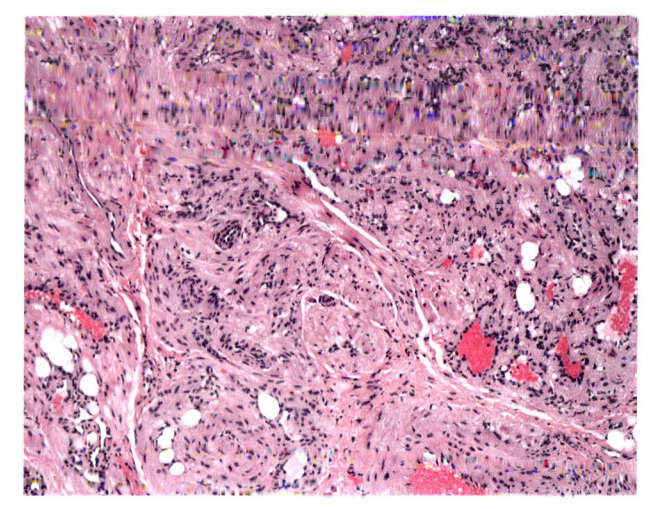

FIGURE 5-6
Vascular leiomyoma showing merging of smooth muscle cells with vessel wall.

IMMUNOHISTOCHEMISTRY

Smooth muscle actin, desmin, and h-caldesmon are at least focally expressed in leiomyomas of deep soft tissue.

DIFFERENTIAL DIAGNOSIS

Leiomyomas with nuclear palisading can suggest a diagnosis of schwannoma; the latter lesion, however, is usually encapsulated and is always S-100 protein positive.

VASCULAR LEIOMYOMA (ANGIOLEIOMYOMA)

CLINICAL FEATURES

Vascular leiomyomas occur in a wide age range, with an increased incidence in patients between the fourth and sixth decades of life. Most cases present as solitary nodules that are superficially located in the subcutis or, rarely, the deep dermis. The extremities, particularly the lower leg, are the most common site. Pain is a common symptom. The solid subtype of vascular leiomyoma has a marked female predominance, is usually located on the extremities, and is often painful. In contradistinction, the venous subtype shows a slight predilection for male individuals, is often located on the head, and is rarely painful.

PATHOLOGIC FEATURES

GROSS FINDINGS

Vascular leiomyomas are well-circumscribed, white-to-gray nodules, generally less than 2 cm in maximum dimension. Calcifications can sometimes be appreciated macroscopically.

MICROSCOPIC FINDINGS

Three histologic subtypes of vascular leiomyoma have been identified: solid, venous, and cavernous. All subtypes are composed of proliferating, well-differentiated smooth muscle cells and vessels. Calcification, myxoid change, and hyalinization are common findings, but degenerative atypia is rarely seen. Criteria for "symplastic" leiomyoma (leiomyoma with degenerative nuclear atypia) of somatic soft tissue have not been elaborated, and any nuclear atypia should raise suspicion for malignancy. The solid subtype is the most common and is characterized by intersecting fascicles of bland spindled cells with a well-developed, thin-walled vasculature. In contrast, the vessels in venous vascular leiomyomas are thick walled, and the constituent smooth muscle cells merge with surrounding muscle bundles (Figure 5-6). Cavernous vascular leiomyoma displays a similar merging of vessel wall and smooth muscle; however, the vessels in this tumor are thin walled and dilated, as the name implies.

IMMUNOHISTOCHEMISTRY

In addition to diffuse smooth muscle actin and desmin expression, rare cytokeratin-positive cells can be seen.

DIFFERENTIAL DIAGNOSIS

The combination of proliferating smooth muscle cells and vessels has a distinctive appearance, and the differential diagnosis is limited, although glomus tumors should be considered. Glomus cells are actually considered to be variants of smooth muscle cells; consequently, immunohistochemistry is not particularly useful. In glomangiomyomas, glomus cells blend with smooth muscle cells in a manner similar to the merging of vessel smooth muscle and proliferating smooth muscle in vascular leiomyomas. In glomangiopericytomas, spindled glomus cells can mimic proliferating smooth muscle. However, in both glomangiomyomas and glomangiopericytomas, distinctive round cells with regular, distinct nuclei are present, at least focally.

PROGNOSIS AND TREATMENT

Vascular leiomyomas are benign and are adequately treated by complete excision. Local recurrence is rare.

LEIOMYOMA OF THE RETROPERITONEUM

CLINICAL FEATURES

Like leiomyomas of the vulva, leiomyomas of the retroperitoneum are believed to originate in hormone-sensitive smooth muscle. They occur almost exclusively in women, usually in the perimenopausal period. Because of their location, they may reach a significant size by the time of diagnosis.

PATHOLOGIC FEATURES

GROSS FINDINGS

Retroperitoneal leiomyomas tend to be large, well-circumscribed, lobulated masses that are similar in appearance to uterine leiomyomas—that is, firm, whorled, white-to-yellow cut surface. Like uterine leiomyomas, cystic degeneration and hemorrhage may be apparent.

MICROSCOPIC FINDINGS

A fibrous pseudocapsule is often present in leiomyomas of the retroperitoneum. The tumors are composed of well-differentiated smooth muscle cells arranged in a cord-like or reticular pattern, similar to that seen in uterine leiomyomas (Figure 5-7). Cytologic atypia is minimal and mitotic activity is very low. Hyaline necrosis may be present, but coagulative necrosis is not. Fatty metaplasia and epithelioid change may be seen, identical to uterine leiomyomas.

IMMUNOHISTOCHEMISTRY

Unlike leiomyomas in other sites, retroperitoneal leiomyomas commonly express estrogen and progesterone receptors, in addition to smooth muscle-specific antigens.

DIFFERENTIAL DIAGNOSIS

The primary consideration in the differential diagnosis of retroperitoneal leiomyomas is SMT of uncertain malignant potential and leiomyosarcoma. Although the criteria for

---

LEIOMYOMA—FACT SHEET

Definition
- Benign mesenchymal tumor with smooth muscle differentiation that is classified according to location as pilar, genital, vascular, deep soft tissue, and retroperitoneal

Incidence and Location
- Pilar: uncommon; extremities > trunk, hair-bearing skin
- Genital: uncommon; scrotum, vulva
- Deep soft tissue: rare; extremities
- Vascular: rare; extremities, particularly lower leg
- Retroperitoneal: slightly more common; retroperitoneum

Morbidity and Mortality
- Pilar: when multiple, there can be significant morbidity secondary to pain
- Genital: none
- Deep soft tissue: none
- Vascular: may be painful
- Retroperitoneal: none

Sex and Age Distribution
- Pilar leiomyoma: equal sex distribution; adolescents/young adults
- Genital leiomyoma: more common in female than male individuals; adults
- Deep leiomyoma: equal sex distribution; young adults to middle-aged adults
- Vascular leiomyomas: solid type, more common in female than male individuals; venous type, more common in male than female individuals; middle-aged to older adults
- Retroperitoneal: much more frequent in female than male individuals; perimenopausal

Clinical Features
- Pilar: single or multiple; often painful
- Genital: single can attain significant size; painless
- Deep: enlarging mass
- Vascular: single; often painful
- Retroperitoneal: pain; mass effect

Prognosis and Treatment
- Complete surgical excision is the appropriate treatment

LEIOMYOMA—PATHOLOGIC FEATURES

Gross Findings
▸▸ Circumscribed to infiltrative pilar, with a rubbery texture, whorled surface and white-to-gray coloring; hemorrhage, cystic change, myxoid stroma, and calcifications may be apparent

Microscopic Findings
▸▸ Pilar: thickened, haphazardly arranged bundles of well-differentiated smooth muscle cells; infiltrative to well circumscribed
▸▸ Genital, deep soft tissue, vascular, retroperitoneal: well-circumscribed to focally infiltrative bundles of well-differentiated smooth muscle cells
▸▸ All types: no significant (moderate-to-severe) cytologic atypia, significant mitotic activity (less than 1 mitosis per 50 hpf) in all except vulvar leiomyomas, which may have up to 3 mitoses per 50 hpf, or coagulative tumor necrosis

Immunohistochemical Features
▸▸ Expression of desmin, smooth muscle actin, muscle-specific actin, calponin, h-caldesmon, and smooth muscle myosin heavy chain

Differential Diagnosis
▸▸ Pilar: BFH
▸▸ Genital: hyperplastic scrotal smooth muscle, cellular angiofibroma
▸▸ Deep soft tissue: schwannoma, leiomyosarcoma
▸▸ Vascular: glomangiomyoma/glomangiopericytoma
▸▸ Retroperitoneal: cellular schwannoma, leiomyosarcoma, GIST

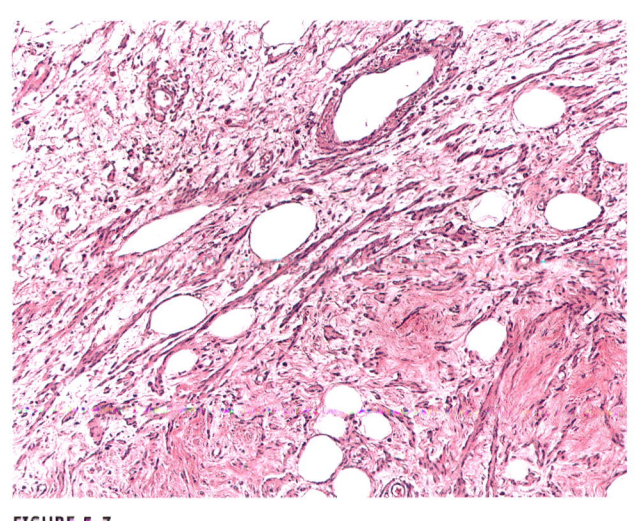

FIGURE 5-7
Cord-like pattern in leiomyoma of the retroperitoneum.

malignancy in uterine SMTs are well established, the significance of increased cellularity, mitotic activity, and cytologic atypia are less clear in retroperitoneal leiomyomas. Generally speaking, SMTs that display greater than 3 mitotic figures per 50 hpf or have coagulative tumor necrosis should not be considered to be benign. It is important to emphasize that mitotic activity may be seen in retroperitoneal leiomyomas in women but is far more worrisome in somatic locations or in men. Rare retroperitoneal leiomyomas may show striking cytologic atypia in the absence of other worrisome features, akin to "symplastic" leiomyomas of the uterus.

Extragastrointestinal stromal tumor (eGIST) and cellular schwannoma are two other entities to be considered. eGIST is typically more cellular than leiomyoma, may have epithelioid areas, and is usually CD117 positive, often CD34 positive, focally SMA positive, and rarely desmin positive. Cellular schwannoma also consists of spindled cells but has additional histologic findings such as foamy macrophages and hyalinized blood vessels. Furthermore, these tumors are strongly and diffusely positive for S-100 protein.

PROGNOSIS AND TREATMENT

Simple excision is curative.

LEIOMYOSARCOMA

Leiomyosarcomas of soft tissue are rare tumors that account for only about 10% of soft tissue sarcomas. They can be divided into four groups, depending on site of origin: cutaneous, deep soft tissue, vascular, and retroperitoneal. Leiomyosarcomas are diagnosed primarily in middle-aged and older adults and predominate in the retroperitoneum. They also occur in the extremities and are often associated with large blood vessels. Microscopically, they range from well to poorly differentiated, the former composed of spindled cells similar to those seen in leiomyomas but with mild cytologic atypia and increased mitotic activity or necrosis, and the latter including tumors that can be difficult to identify as showing smooth muscle differentiation. Epithelioid morphology, myxoid change, and a prominent inflammatory infiltrate can be seen. Leiomyosarcomas display immunohistologic evidence of smooth muscle differentiation including actins, desmin, calponin, and h-caldesmon. However, it should be noted that actin expression can be somewhat nonspecific and can also be seen in sarcomas of myofibroblasts. Aside from wholly cutaneous leiomyosarcomas that are amenable to curative surgical excision, leiomyosarcomas have a poor prognosis and aggressive clinical course.

CUTANEOUS LEIOMYOSARCOMA

CLINICAL FEATURES

Cutaneous leiomyosarcomas arise from the arrector pili and dartoic muscles. They occur over a wide age range, with increased incidence in middle age. Conflicting evidence exists whether it predominates in the male or female sex. These tumors are most common on the extremities, particularly on the extensor surface. Usually, they present as solitary nodules that may cause ulceration or discoloration of the overlying epidermis. Grouped nodules have also been described; however, these lesions must be distinguished from metastatic leiomyosarcoma. They are small: usually less than 2 cm and rarely as large as 5 cm.

Pathologic Features

Gross Findings

Cutaneous leiomyosarcomas arise in the subcutis and may be well to poorly circumscribed. They may be lobular or pedunculated. The cut surface varies in color from white to tan to gray and may have a whorled appearance.

Microscopic Findings

Most cutaneous leiomyosarcomas are well to moderately differentiated, although they may display significant cytologic atypia and brisk mitotic activity (Figure 5-8). They can be either well-circumscribed or diffusely infiltrative (Figure 5-9). Epithelioid morphology is rarely seen.

Immunohistochemistry

Smooth muscle actin is usually diffusely expressed, although desmin may be seen only focally. Occasionally cytokeratin expression is seen.

Differential Diagnosis

Nodular fasciitis, cellular BFH, and cellular myofibromas should be considered in the differential diagnosis of cutaneous leiomyosarcoma. The brisk mitotic activity and hypercellularity seen in nodular fasciitis can mimic a sarcomatous process; however, areas of microcystic breakdown, extravasated red blood cells, and thin-walled blood vessels combined with the clinical history of a rapidly growing lesion in a younger patient aid in diagnosis. Cellular BFH shares several histologic features with cutaneous leiomyosarcoma, including a fascicular architecture, eosinophilic spindled cells, and increased mitotic activity. The lesional cells, however, generally have a more tapered nucleus and are associated with giant cells, foam cells, and inflammatory cells. Moreover, the overlying epidermis is usually hyperplastic. Factor XIIIa, which can be used to distinguish BFHs from pilar leiomyomas, is not helpful here because cellular BFHs rarely express this marker. In addition, cellular BFH may be focally actin positive, though only rarely desmin positive.

Cellular myofibromas also have brisk mitotic activity. Unlike cutaneous leiomyosarcomas, however, they have a biphasic pattern composed of myoid nodules with associated hypercellular spindled areas. They generally affect younger patients and may be multifocal.

Epithelioid cutaneous leiomyosarcoma should be distinguished from malignant melanoma and epithelioid sarcoma. Malignant melanoma is usually positive for S-100 protein and other melanocytic markers, may have a junctional component, and is often associated with a lymphocytic infiltrate. Epithelioid sarcoma occurs primarily on the extremities of young patients, is positive for cytokeratins, and often displays necrosis with peripheral palisading.

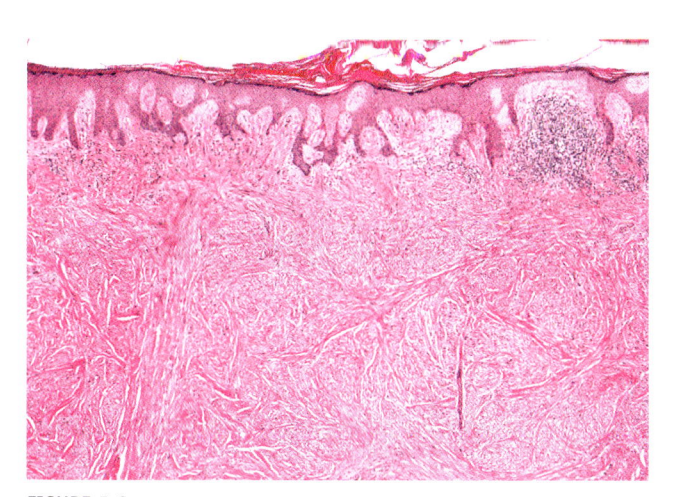

FIGURE 5-8
Pilar leiomyosarcoma displaying fascicular architecture and cytologic atypia.

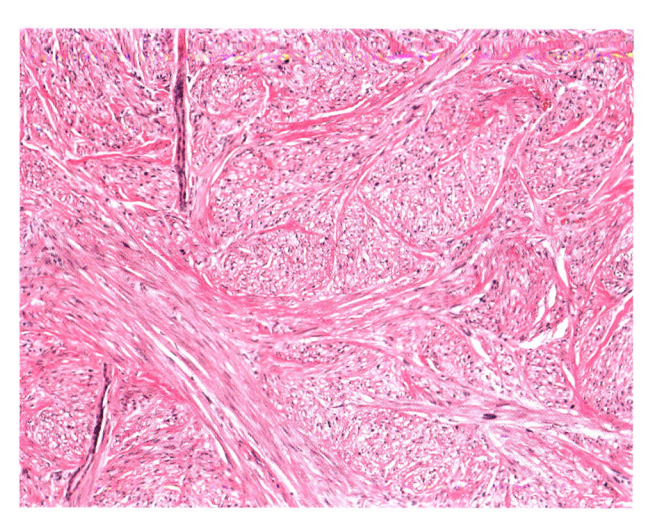

FIGURE 5-9
Diffusely infiltrative pilar leiomyosarcoma.

PROGNOSIS AND TREATMENT

Like most superficially located malignancies, cutaneous leiomyosarcomas have an excellent prognosis. Although they may recur if simply enucleated, metastasis is rare. Wide local excision with negative surgical margins is considered appropriate treatment.

LEIOMYOSARCOMAS OF DEEP SOFT TISSUE

CLINICAL FEATURES

Leiomyosarcoma of somatic soft tissue primarily affects middle-aged and older patients of both sexes. They usually arise in the lower extremities and present as an enlarging mass that is generally somewhat smaller, on the range of 5 cm, than leiomyosarcomas of the retroperitoneum.

PATHOLOGIC FEATURES

GROSS FINDINGS

Macroscopically, these tumors often appear circumscribed and may have a multinodular appearance. They have a fleshy, variegated surface, ranging from white to tan with areas of hemorrhage, necrosis, and cystic change.

MICROSCOPIC FINDINGS

Careful histologic examination often reveals an associated vessel; unlike vascular leiomyosarcomas *(vide infra)*, the vessels are of small caliber and may be obliterated by the expanding tumor. Generally speaking, most leiomyosarcomas of deep soft tissue are moderately differentiated and are composed of atypical spindled cells arranged, sometimes focally, in intersecting fascicles (Figure 5-10).

LEIOMYOSARCOMA—FACT SHEET

Definition
- Malignant mesenchymal tumor with smooth muscle differentiation that can be categorized as cutaneous, vascular, or arising in deep soft tissue or the retroperitoneum

Incidence and Location
- Cutaneous: rare; extremities
- Deep soft tissue: rare; lower extremities
- Vascular: extremely rare; IVC
- Retroperitoneal: most common; retroperitoneum
- EBV-SMT: rare; primarily lung and liver, but any location possible

Morbidity and Mortality
- Cutaneous, low
- Deep soft tissue, high
- Vascular, high
- Retroperitoneal, high
- EBV-SMT, generally related to underlying disease

Sex and Age Distribution
- Cutaneous: more frequent in male than female sex; younger adults
- Deep soft tissue: equal distribution among sexes; middle-aged adults
- Vascular: more frequent in female than male sex; adults
- Retroperitoneal: more frequent in female than male sex; adults
- EBV-SMT: equal distribution among sexes; all ages

Clinical Features
- Cutaneous, deep soft tissue, retroperitoneal: slow-growing mass
- Vascular: evidence of vascular obstruction, including edema
- EBV-SMT: growing mass or incidental finding related to surveillance

Prognosis and Treatment
- Cutaneous: complete surgical excision
- Deep soft tissue, vascular, retroperitoneal: surgical excision and adjuvant therapy
- EBV-SMT: surgical excision, questionable value of reduced immunosuppression/adjuvant therapy

---

LEIOMYOSARCOMA—PATHOLOGIC FEATURES

Gross Findings
- Fleshy red to tan, poorly circumscribed tumor that may have areas of necrosis, myxoid degeneration, or cystic change

Microscopic Findings
- Cutaneous: well-differentiated smooth muscle cells with brisk mitotic activity
- Deep soft tissue: well to moderately differentiated smooth muscle cells with brisk mitotic activity, a fascicular architecture, and often associated with a vessel wall
- Vascular: moderately to poorly differentiated smooth muscle cells with brisk mitotic activity/necrosis
- Retroperitoneal: moderately to poorly differentiated smooth muscle cells that may show areas of anaplasia or necrosis
- Cutaneous, deep soft tissue, vascular, and retroperitoneal: nuclear atypia visible on scanning magnification (4×), necrosis and/or mitotic activity greater than 1 per 50 hpf
- EBV-SMT: dual cell population of well-differentiated spindled cells and small, primitive round cells; prominent lymphocytic infiltrate; necrosis uncommon

Immunohistochemical Features
- Expression of desmin, smooth muscle actin, muscle-specific actin, calponin, h-caldesmon, and smooth muscle myosin heavy chain
- EBV RNA in EBV-SMT

Differential Diagnosis
- Cutaneous: cellular BFH
- Deep soft tissue, vascular (extremity): monophasic synovial sarcoma, fibrosarcoma, MPNST
- Retroperitoneal, IVC: eGIST, cellular schwannoma, dedifferentiated liposarcoma
- EBV-SMT: benign nerve sheath tumor, lymphoproliferative disorder

Mitotic activity can be brisk, but a mitotic index as low as 1 per 10 hpf can be seen in leiomyosarcomas of deep soft tissue. Occasionally, anaplasia similar to that seen in malignant fibrous histiocytomas can be seen.

DIFFERENTIAL DIAGNOSIS

In well to moderately differentiated tumors, fibrosarcoma, malignant peripheral nerve sheath tumor (MPNST), and monophasic synovial sarcoma should be considered in the differential diagnosis. Unlike the blunt-ended nuclei of smooth muscle cells, the tumor cells of fibrosarcomas tend to be tapered, whereas those of MPNSTs have a wavy or buckled appearance. Monophasic synovial sarcoma generally displays a greater degree of cellular overlap, and the long fascicles of cells do not usually intersect; molecular studies demonstrating the t(X:18) can confirm the diagnosis.

In poorly differentiated tumors, malignant fibrous histiocytoma and pleomorphic rhabdomyosarcoma should be considered; the myofibroblastic rather than smooth muscle immunophenotype, the greater degree of interstitial collagen, and the absence of fascicular architecture can help in identifying the former, whereas myogenin and MyoD1 are specific for skeletal muscle differentiation.

PROGNOSIS AND TREATMENT

Leiomyosarcomas of deep soft tissue are aggressive tumors that metastasize in approximately 40% of cases, usually to the liver and lung. Five-year survival is approximately 65%. Prognosis is influenced by tumor size, patient age, presence of necrosis, and vascular invasion. The degree of differentiation offers only limited information, because even well-differentiated tumors may behave aggressively.

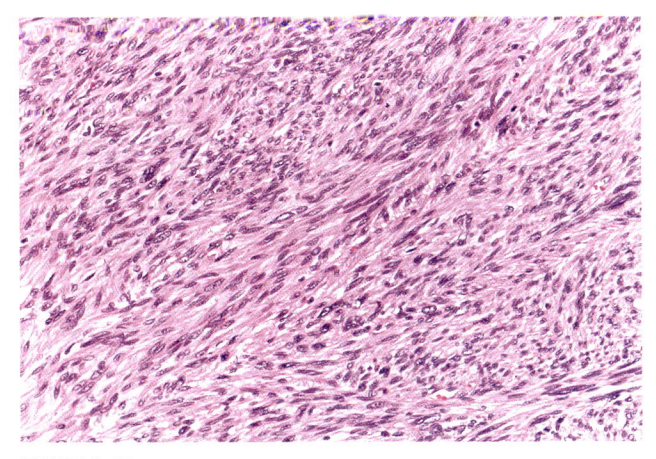

FIGURE 5-10
Fascicular architecture in leiomyosarcoma of deep soft tissue.

VASCULAR LEIOMYOSARCOMA

CLINICAL FEATURES

The term *vascular* leiomyosarcoma is reserved for those tumors arising in large-caliber vessels such as the inferior vena cava (IVC) and large veins of the lower extremity. Distribution in the female sex predominates in tumors arising in the IVC, and there is an increased incidence in the sixth decade of life. Leiomyosarcomas arising in vessels other than the IVC are equally distributed between the male and female sexes. Tumors that originate in the upper portion of the IVC can block the hepatic veins, resulting in Budd–Chiari syndrome, whereas those that arise in the midportion of the IVC can obstruct the renal veins, causing renal dysfunction. Tumors of the lower IVC and large veins of the lower extremity can cause significant lower leg edema.

PATHOLOGIC FEATURES

GROSS FINDINGS

In cases that involve large vessels such as the IVC, a portion of the vascular wall may be seen grossly. These tumors tend to be lobulated, fleshy masses with a mottled white-to-tan appearance.

MICROSCOPIC FINDINGS

Vascular leiomyosarcomas can range from well to poorly differentiated (Figure 5-11). Cytoplasmic and perinuclear vacuolation are common. Cellularity is generally quite high, and necrosis is frequently seen. Focal

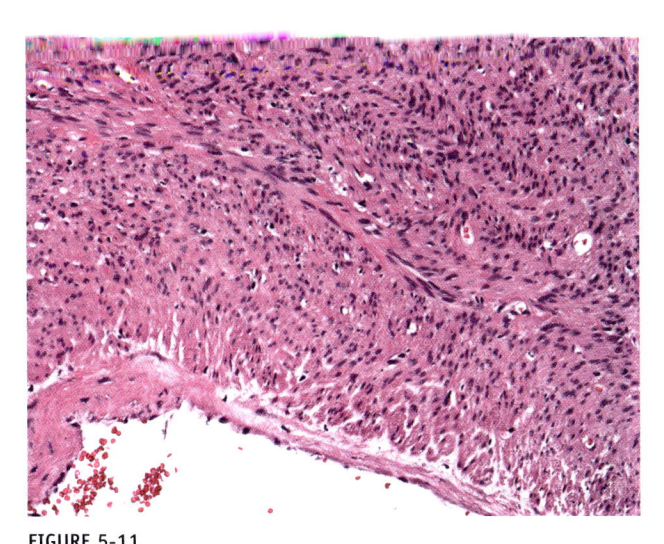

FIGURE 5-11
Leiomyosarcoma arising from a blood vessel.

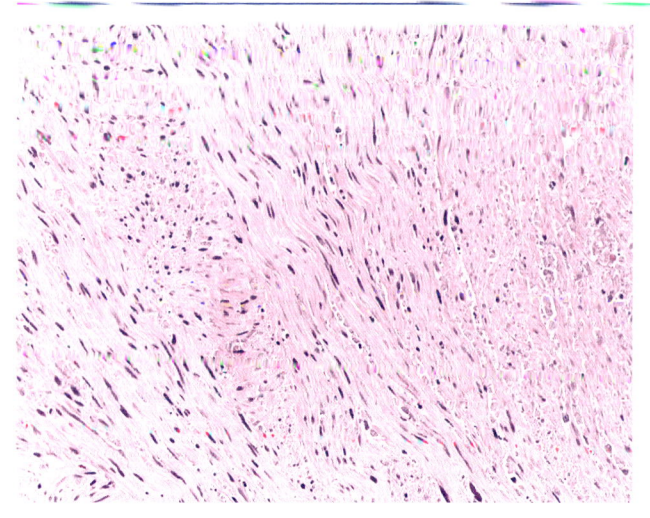

FIGURE 5-12
Focus of necrosis in retroperitoneal leiomyosarcoma.

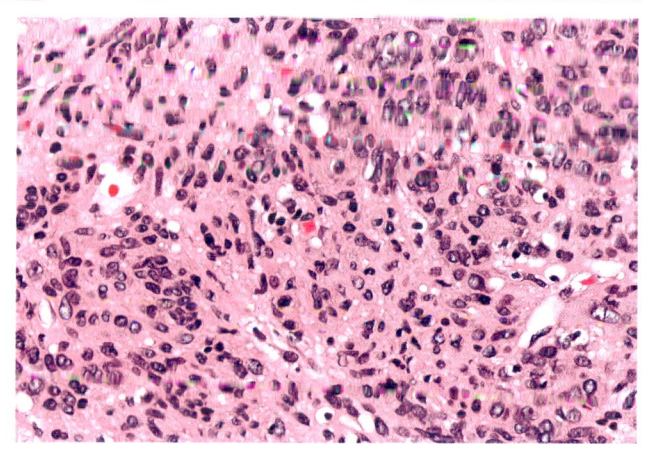

FIGURE 5-13
Epithelioid morphology in retroperitoneal leiomyosarcoma.

areas of myxoid change may be present, but extensive myxoid stroma is distinctly uncommon.

PROGNOSIS AND TREATMENT

Leiomyosarcomas of the large vessels have a poor prognosis, regardless of the degree of differentiation, which may relate to early hematogenous spread related to the site of involvement. In addition, many tumors are unresectable because of their intimate association with critical vascular structures. Metastases can be seen to lung, liver, and brain.

RETROPERITONEAL LEIOMYOSARCOMA

CLINICAL FEATURES

The retroperitoneum and pelvis are the most common sites for leiomyosarcomas. They occur predominantly in women in the fifth to seventh decades of life. Pain may be the presenting symptom. Because of their location, retroperitoneal leiomyosarcomas can reach a significant size before diagnosis, and complete surgical resection can be difficult.

PATHOLOGIC FEATURES

GROSS FINDINGS

Retroperitoneal leiomyosarcomas range in appearance from leiomyomatous (firm, white-to-tan, whorled cut surface) to a fleshy mass that displays areas of hemorrhage, cystic change, or necrosis. Large tumors may involve adjacent organs.

MICROSCOPIC FINDINGS

The histologic appearance of vascular leiomyosarcoma is similar to other leiomyosarcomas: eosinophilic spindled cells arranged in intersecting fascicles and displaying a variable degree of cytologic atypia, mitotic activity, and necrosis (Figure 5-12). Cytoplasmic vacuolation is common, and areas of hyalinization or hypocellularity may be present. Epithelioid morphology and frank anaplasia may be seen (Figure 5-13).

IMMUNOHISTOCHEMISTRY

Retroperitoneal leiomyosarcomas express actin, desmin, and h-caldesmon to a varying degree. Rarely, focal expression of cytokeratin, epithelial membrane antigen, S-100 protein, or CD34 exists.

DIFFERENTIAL DIAGNOSIS

Cellular schwannoma and eGIST should both be considered in the differential diagnosis of retroperitoneal leiomyosarcoma. Immunohistochemistry is helpful in distinguishing these entities, particularly on needle biopsy. eGIST is usually CD117 positive, often CD34 positive, focally SMA positive, and rarely desmin positive. In contrast, cellular schwannoma is strongly and diffusely positive for S-100 protein.

Dedifferentiated liposarcoma, which can have a fascicular appearance and immunohistochemical evidence of myoid differentiation, should also be considered. An associated well-differentiated liposarcomatous component facilitates diagnosis.

PROGNOSIS AND TREATMENT

Retroperitoneal leiomyosarcomas have an extremely high mortality rate, related, at least in part, to the difficulty in achieving clear surgical margins and the large

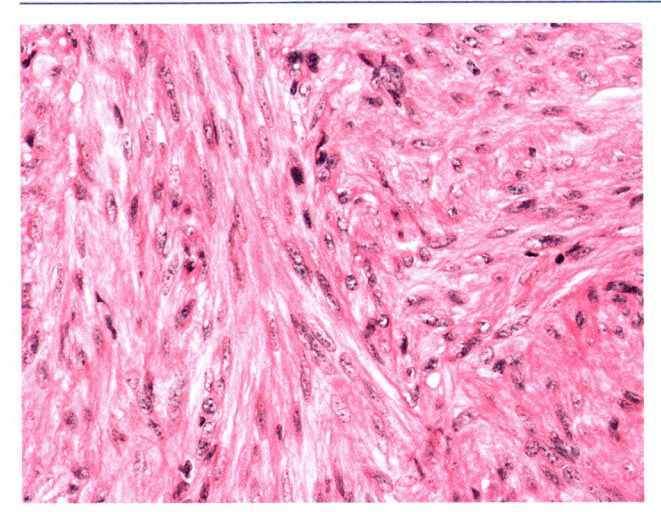

FIGURE 5-14
Epstein–Barr virus–associated smooth muscle tumor showing well-differentiated smooth muscle cells.

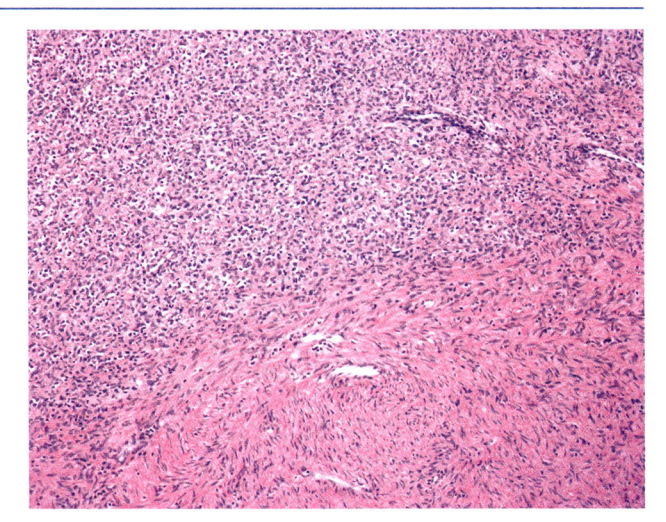

FIGURE 5-15
Round cell population in Epstein–Barr virus–associated smooth muscle tumor.

size attained by these tumors. The lungs and liver are the primary sites for metastasis.

EPSTEIN–BARR VIRUS–ASSOCIATED SMOOTH MUSCLE TUMORS

CLINICAL FEATURES

Epstein–Barr virus–associated smooth muscle tumors (EBV-SMTs) occur in immunocompromised patients of all ages such as those who have acquired immunodeficiency syndrome (AIDS) or who are immunosuppressed subsequent to organ transplantation. Both sexes are affected. These tumors generally arise at least 3 years after transplantation but may be the presenting symptom in AIDS. They can arise in any site, including unusual sites such as endocrine glands and the central nervous system, but occur most commonly in the lungs and liver. They are often multifocal.

PATHOLOGIC FEATURES

GROSS FINDINGS

EBV-SMT can have circumscribed or infiltrative borders and usually appear white to tan with a whorled surface on cross section.

MICROSCOPIC FINDINGS

Cytologic atypia is usually minimal and resembles that of a well-differentiated leiomyosarcoma (Figure 5-14). A dual cell population is often present, which is composed of well-differentiated smooth muscle cells and small, round, primitive smooth muscle cells (Figure 5-15). A lymphocytic infiltrate is common. Necrosis and myxoid change are rare. Mitotic activity is generally low, though it can be significant in some cases.

IMMUNOHISTOCHEMISTRY

These tumors are diffusely positive for actins and usually express desmin only focally. In situ hybridization for early EBV RNA helps confirm the diagnosis.

DIFFERENTIAL DIAGNOSIS

In EBV-SMT with prominent round cell morphology, a lymphoproliferative disorder may be suspected. Expression of actins and absence of lymphocytic markers can discriminate between these two entities. In predominantly spindled tumors, the bland histology may suggest a schwannoma or well-differentiated nerve sheath tumor, neither of which will show the strong actin expression seen in EBV-SMT.

PROGNOSIS AND TREATMENT

EBV-SMT displays neither the completely benign behavior of a leiomyoma nor the frank aggressiveness of a leiomyosarcoma. Patients are more likely to die of their underlying disease or of complications secondary to immunosuppression than of EBV-SMT. Although these tumors are often multifocal, this finding is related to multiple infection events and not metastasis. Surgical excision, when possible, is often curative; however, because of multiple infection events, tumors may arise elsewhere. Radiofrequency ablation has also been attempted. Neither reducing immunosuppression nor adding chemotherapeutic agents has shown convincing efficacy.

SUGGESTED READINGS

1. Bellezza G, Sidoni A, Cavaliere A, et al: Primary cutaneous leiomyosarcoma: A clinicopathological and immunohistochemical study of 7 cases. Int J Surg Pathol 2004;12:39–44.
2. Evans HL, Shipley J: Leiomyosarcoma. Pathology and Genetics. Tumors of Soft Tissue and Bone. Lyon, France: IARC Press, 2002, pp 131–134.
3. Farshid G, Pradhan M, Goldblum J, et al: Leiomyosarcoma of somatic soft tissues: A tumor of vascular origin with multivariate analysis of outcome in 42 cases. Am J Surg Pathol 2002;26:14–24.
4. Fields JP, Helwig EB: Leiomyosarcoma of the skin and subcutaneous tissue. Cancer 1981;47:156–169.
5. Fletcher CDM: Smooth muscle tumors. Diagnostic Histopathology of Tumors. London, Harcourt Publishers Ltd, 2000, pp 1509–1513.
6. Hachisuga T, Hashimoto H, Enjoji M: Angioleiomyoma: A clinicopathologic reappraisal of 562 cases. Cancer 1984;54:126–130.
7. Hasegawa T, Seki K, Yang P, et al: Mechanism of pain and cytoskeletal properties in angioleiomyomas: An immunohistochemical study. Pathol Int 1994;44:66–72.
8. Hashimoto H, Quade B: Leiomyoma of deep soft tissue. Pathology and Genetics. Tumors of Soft Tissue and Bone. Lyon, France, IARC Press, 2002, p 130.
9. Holst VA, Junkins-Hopkins JM, Elenitsas R: Cutaneous smooth muscle neoplasms: Clinical features, histologic findings, and treatment options. J Am Acad Dermatol 2002;46:477–494.
10. Lee ES, Locker J, Nalesnik M, et al: The association of Epstein-Barr virus with smooth-muscle tumors occurring after organ transplantation. N Engl J Med 1995;332:19–25.
11. McClain KL, Leach CT, Jenson HB, et al: Association of Epstein-Barr virus with leiomyosarcomas in children with AIDS. N Engl J Med 1995;332:12–18.
12. Newman PL, Fletcher CD: Smooth muscle tumours of the external genitalia: Clinicopathological analysis of a series. Histopathology 1991;18:523–539.
13. Nielsen GP, Rosenberg AE, Koerner FC, et al: Smooth-muscle tumors of the vulva. A clinicopathological study of 25 cases and review of the literature. Am J Surg Pathol 1996;20:779–793.
14. Raj S, Calonje E, Kraus M, et al: Cutaneous pilar leiomyoma: Clinicopathologic analysis of 53 lesions in 45 patients. Am J Dermatopathol 1997;19:2–9.
15. Weiss SW, Goldblum JR: Benign tumors of smooth muscle. Soft Tissue Tumors. St. Louis, Mosby, 2001, pp 695–704.
16. Weiss SW, Goldblum JR: Leiomyosarcoma. Soft Tissue Tumors. St. Louis, Mosby, 2001, pp 727–746.
17. Weiss SW: Smooth muscle tumors of soft tissue. Adv Anat Pathol 2002;9:351–359.
18. Yokoyama R, Hashimoto H, Daimaru Y, et al: Superficial leiomyomas. A clinicopathologic study of 34 cases. Acta Pathol Japonica 1987;37:1415–1422.

6 Skeletal Muscle Tumors
Raf Sciot

RHABDOMYOMA
- Adult Rhabdomyoma
- Fetal Rhabdomyoma
- Genital Rhabdomyoma
- Embryonal Rhabdomyosarcoma
- Alveolar Rhabdomyosarcoma
- Pleomorphic Rhabdomyosarcoma
- Adult Sclerosing Rhabdomyosarcoma

Mesenchymal tumors that show skeletal muscle differentiation are generally rare, and as opposed to other soft tissue tumors, the benign variants (rhabdomyoma) are much rarer than their malignant counterpart (rhabdomyosarcoma). Nevertheless, rhabdomyosarcomas are an important category because they represent the largest subgroup of sarcomas in children. In addition, thanks to more reliable use of immunohistochemistry, it has become clear that rhabdomyosarcomas are not so rare in adulthood as thought earlier. Accurate subclassification of rhabdomyosarcomas is mandatory in view of prognostic implications. The embryonal and alveolar subtypes are the most frequent rhabdomyosarcomas of childhood, and the pleomorphic type is almost exclusively present in adults. Cytogenetic and molecular genetic analysis has become a powerful tool in the differential diagnosis between embryonal and alveolar rhabdomyosarcoma (mainly the solid variant), as well as with other small, blue round cell tumors. Recently, another type of rhabdomyosarcoma has been described, designated by the term *adult sclerosing rhabdomyosarcoma*.

RHABDOMYOMA

Rhabdomyomas are rare mesenchymal tumors that are classified into the cardiac and extracardiac types. Depending on the degree of differentiation, extracardiac rhabdomyoma is further divided into the fetal and adult type. Genital rhabdomyoma is a differentiated rhabdomyoma of the genital tract. The main problem with rhabdomyomas is that, because of their rarity, they can be difficult to differentiate from rhabdomyosarcomas and other more aggressive tumors.

ADULT RHABDOMYOMA

CLINICAL FEATURES

Adult rhabdomyoma is mainly found in adults, the median age being 60 years, with a 3:1 male sex predominance. The mucosal surface of the oral cavity, larynx and pharynx, and the soft tissues of the neck are most frequently involved. Signs and symptoms relate to these locations (obstruction, mass). On occasion, adult rhabdomyoma is multinodular or even multicentric.

PATHOLOGIC FEATURES

GROSS FINDINGS

Rhabdomyomas are well-delineated, nodular masses that range from 1.5 to about 8 cm.

MICROSCOPIC FINDINGS

On histology, adult rhabdomyoma is an unencapsulated, well-circumscribed lesion composed of nodules of closely packed large polygonal cells. The cells are typically characterized by an abundant, eosinophilic, granular-to-vacuolated cytoplasm (Figure 6-1). Cytoplasmic cross-striations or rod-like inclusions are seen focally. The nucleus is vesicular and centrally or peripherally located. Cell borders are well defined, and the intercellular stroma is usually scant. A PAS stain usually reveals abundant cytoplasmic glycogen, and a Masson trichrome or PTAH stain may reveal the cytoplasmic striations/inclusions to a better advantage. Mitotic figures are generally not present.

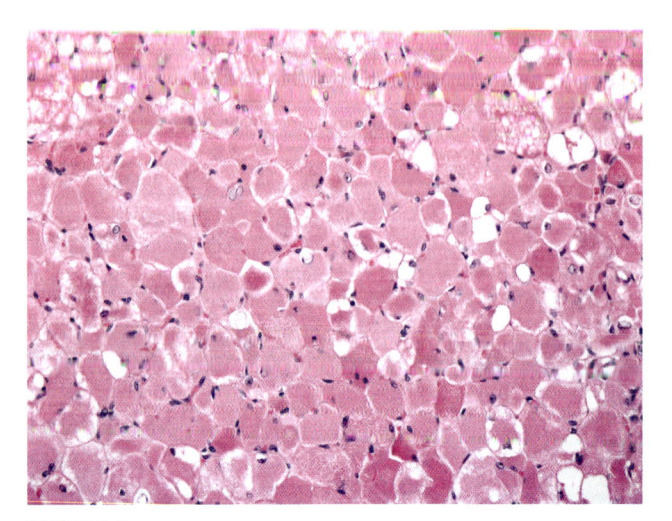

FIGURE 6-1
Adult rhabdomyoma.
Tumor consists of polygonal tumor cells with abundant eosinophilic-to-granular cytoplasm.

ANCILLARY STUDIES

IMMUNOHISTOCHEMISTRY

Cytoplasmic positivity for muscle-specific actin, desmin, and myoglobin is always present. Occasionally, tumor cells may express α smooth muscle actin or S-100 protein.

DIFFERENTIAL DIAGNOSIS

Because of the copious cytoplasm of the tumor cells, adult rhabdomyoma may resemble other tumors with this feature, such as granular cell tumor, crystal-storing histiocytosis, and alveolar soft part sarcoma. Granular cell tumor does not express muscle markers and should be strongly S-100 protein and CD68 positive. Crystal-storing histiocytosis is, in fact, a pure histiocytic proliferation, and thus stains for CD68. Alveolar soft part sarcoma shows a typical alveolar growth pattern, with characteristic PAS-diastase–positive crystalline cytoplasmic inclusions that have pathognomonic ultrastructural features. Expression of desmin and other myogenic markers is described in this sarcoma.

PROGNOSIS AND TREATMENT

Complete surgical excision is the treatment of choice. After incomplete resection, often late, recurrence may occur. No malignant transformation is documented.

FETAL RHABDOMYOMA

CLINICAL FEATURES

Fetal rhabdomyoma is predominantly a tumor of childhood. The median age is 4 years, but presentations in adult life (up to 58 years) are well documented. A slight male sex predominance exists (2.4:1). More than 90% of fetal rhabdomyomas occur in the soft tissues or mucosa of the head and neck. Associations with the nevoid basal cell carcinoma syndrome have been described.

PATHOLOGIC FEATURES

GROSS FINDINGS

Fetal rhabdomyomas are well-delineated solitary masses of 1 to 13 cm, the cut surface of which is more glistening than the adult counterpart.

MICROSCOPIC FINDINGS

These lesions are well delineated but not encapsulated. Depending on the cellularity, the degree of myxoid matrix and the degree of differentiation, one can discriminate between a classic immature fetal rhabdomyoma and an intermediate fetal rhabdomyoma. The first is myxoid, and contains bland spindle cells and fetal myotubes. The latter shows more differentiation and cellularity with bundles of spindled rhabdomyoblasts, and strap-like or ganglion-like rhabdomyoblasts (Figure 6-2). In fact, this intermediate rhabdomyoma, also referred to as juvenile or cellular rhabdomyoma, shows a degree of differentiation in between that of classic fetal rhabdomyoma and adult rhabdomyoma. Fetal rhabdomyoma should not show obvious nuclear atypia, necrosis, or more than an occasional mitotic figure.

ANCILLARY STUDIES

IMMUNOHISTOCHEMISTRY

Skeletal muscle differentiation, with desmin, myoglobin, and muscle-specific actin expression, is always seen. Occasionally, tumor cells may express α smooth muscle actin or S-100 protein.

DIFFERENTIAL DIAGNOSIS

It can be difficult to differentiate fetal rhabdomyoma from embryonal rhabdomyosarcoma. Both are basically variably spindly and myxoid lesions.

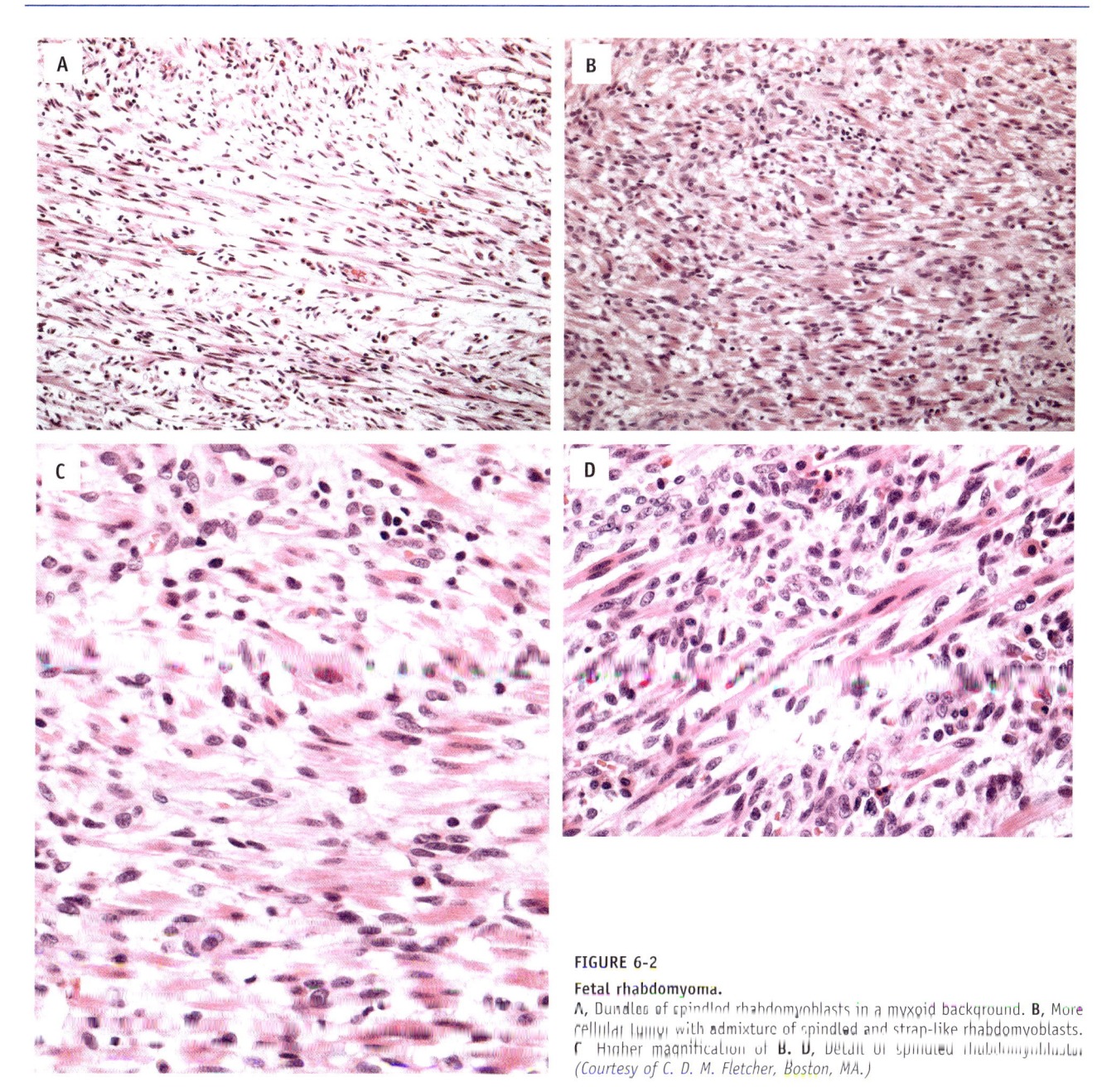

FIGURE 6-2
Fetal rhabdomyoma.
A, Bundles of spindled rhabdomyoblasts in a myxoid background. B, More cellular tumor with admixture of spindled and strap-like rhabdomyoblasts. C, Higher magnification of B. D, Detail of spindled rhabdomyoblasts. *(Courtesy of C. D. M. Fletcher, Boston, MA.)*

Lack of prominent nuclear atypia is the most important criterion separating fetal rhabdomyoma from rhabdomyosarcoma.

PROGNOSIS AND TREATMENT

Complete excision is curative. No malignant behavior is documented.

GENITAL RHABDOMYOMA

CLINICAL FEATURES

Most cases of genital rhabdomyoma present as polypoid lesions of the cervix or vagina of middle-aged women (age range, 30 to 48 years). Rarely, the paratesticular region or epididymis is involved.

PATHOLOGIC FEATURES

GROSS FINDINGS

Genital rhabdomyoma resembles a benign vaginal polyp and is covered by normal smooth mucosa.

MICROSCOPIC FINDINGS

Genital rhabdomyoma shows an advanced degree of skeletal muscle differentiation, with haphazardly arranged round or strap-like rhabdomyoblasts with copious eosinophilic cytoplasm and cross striations. Thus, they resemble the "intermediate" fetal rhabdomyomas of the head and neck. However, in genital rhabdomyoma, the stroma is more fibrous and contains more dilated vessels. In addition, this lesion lacks the more variable cellular morphology and architecture of "intermediate" fetal rhabdomyoma (Figure 6-3).

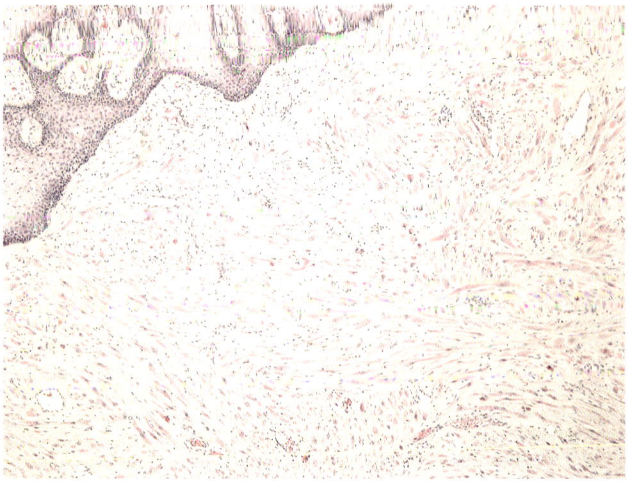

FIGURE 6-3
Low-power view of genital rhabdomyoma.
The epithelium of the vaginal wall is seen at the left upper corner. Tumor consists of eosinophilic rhabdomyoblasts in a fibrous and vascular stroma. *(Courtesy of P. Hogendoorn, Leiden, the Netherlands.)*

ANCILLARY STUDIES

The immunohistochemical features of genital rhabdomyoma are identical to that of the other rhabdomyomas.

RHABDOMYOMA—FACT SHEET

Definition
- Benign mesenchymal tumor with skeletal muscle differentiation divided into the adult, fetal, and genital types, according to degree of differentiation and location. Cardiac rhabdomyomas are not considered here.

Incidence and Location
- Rare
- Adult and fetal rhabdomyoma predominantly involve the head and neck region; genital rhabdomyoma involves the vagina

Morbidity and Mortality
- None

Sex, Race, and Age Distribution
- Adult rhabdomyoma: median age, 60 years (age range, 33 to 80 years); 3:1 male sex predominance
- Fetal rhabdomyoma: median age, 4 years (age range, 3 days to 58 years); 2.4:1 male sex predominance
- Genital rhabdomyoma: median age, 42 years; (age range, 30 to 48 years); presents almost exclusively in female individuals

Clinical Features
- Soft tissue or mucosal mass; symptoms depend on the site of involvement

Prognosis and Treatment
- Total surgical excision is the treatment of choice; no aggressive behavior has been documented

---

RHABDOMYOMA—PATHOLOGIC FEATURES

Gross Findings
- Well-circumscribed mass, the fetal type being more glistening on cut surface, the genital type having a typical polypoid aspect

Microscopic Findings
- Adult type: lobules of closely packed large polygonal cells with abundant eosinophilic granular/vacuolated cytoplasm and vesicular nuclei; cross striations are focally present
- Fetal type: abundant myxoid stroma with primitive spindled cells and myotubules in the classic immature form, more cellular with fascicles of spindled rhabdomyoblasts, and interlacing strap-like or ganglion-like rhabdomyoblasts in the intermediate form
- Genital type: haphazard arrangement of large rhabdomyoblasts embedded in a fibrous stroma with dilated vessels
- No nuclear atypia, significant mitotic activity, or necrosis in any type

Immunohistochemical Features
- Expression of desmin, muscle-specific actin and myoglobin is always present

Differential Diagnosis
- Adult type: granular cell tumor, crystal-storing histiocytosis, alveolar soft part sarcoma
- Fetal type: embryonal rhabdomyosarcoma
- Genital type: vaginal stromal polyp, embryonal rhabdomyosarcoma

DIFFERENTIAL DIAGNOSIS

Because the vagina is a well-known site for embryonal rhabdomyosarcoma, this tumor should be excluded. The lack of any atypia favors a genital rhabdomyoma. A classic vaginal polyp does not show rhabdomyoblastic features.

PROGNOSIS AND TREATMENT

Local, complete excision is adequate treatment of genital rhabdomyoma, and no malignant behavior is documented.

EMBRYONAL RHABDOMYOSARCOMA

CLINICAL FEATURES

Embryonal rhabdomyosarcoma recapitulates the phenotypic and biological features of embryonic skeletal muscle. Embryonal rhabdomyosarcoma is divided into the conventional, botryoid, spindle cell, and anaplastic variant. It is the most frequent sarcoma of childhood, occurring in 3 per 1 million children in the United States younger than 15 years, and it represents 70% to 75% of all rhabdomyosarcomas. Children between 5 and 15 years of age are typically affected (45%), whereas up to 35% occur before the age of 5. Adult cases are rare but well documented. A slight male-to-female predominance (1.2:1) exists. The majority (70%) of U.S. embryonal rhabdomyosarcomas occur in non-Hispanic whites. Incidence figures in Europe mirror those of the United States; eastern and southern Asia have somewhat lower figures. A minority (<9%) of embryonal rhabdomyosarcomas arise in the skeletal musculature of the extremities. The head and neck region is the predominant site of involvement (±47%), with the orbit, eyelid, oropharynx, parotid gland, auditory canal, middle ear, pterygoid fossa, nose, paranasal sinuses, tongue, and cheek being typical sites. The genitourinary system is involved in ±28% of cases, with the urinary bladder, prostate, and paratesticular soft tissues as typical examples. Involvement of visceral organs, retroperitoneum, pelvis, and perineum is rare. The spindle cell variant typically occurs in scrotal soft tissues and head and neck; the botryoid variant occurs in the wall of hollow organs or beneath a mucosal lining. The symptoms generally relate to mass effects and obstruction.

PATHOLOGIC FEATURES

GROSS FINDINGS

Embryonal rhabdomyosarcomas present as poorly circumscribed, fleshy masses of 1 to 32 cm (Figure 6-4). The spindle cell variant is more firm and fibrous, whereas the botryoid variant typically has a grape-like polypoid and more gelatinous appearance.

MICROSCOPIC FINDINGS

Both at the cellular level and the architectural level, the *conventional* variant of embryonal rhabdomyosarcoma recapitulates embryonic skeletal muscle tissue. The most primitive cells are spindled to stellate-like cells with an ovoid nucleus and little amphophilic cytoplasm (Figure 6-5). They hardly show recognizable skeletal muscle differentiation. As these cells mature, they get more cytoplasm,

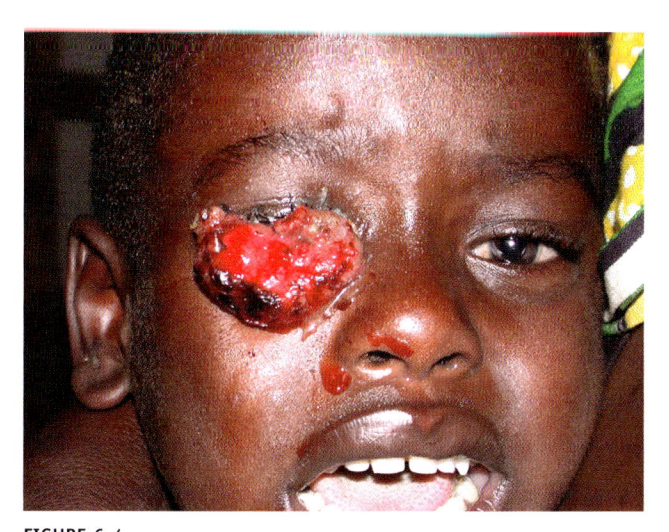

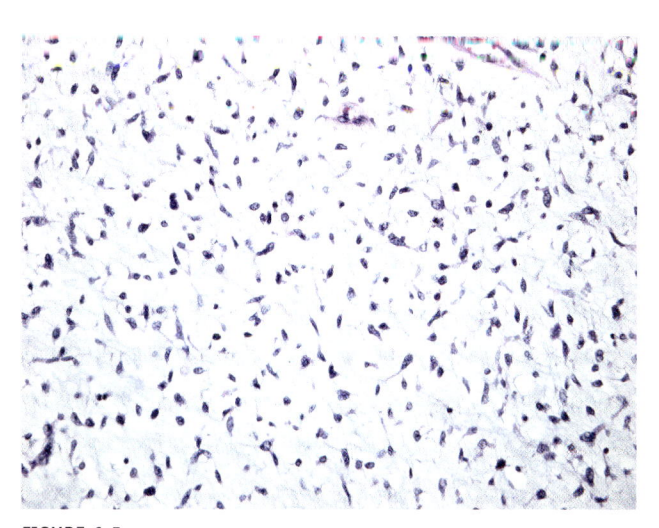

FIGURE 6-4
Young child with protruding and ulcerated orbital embryonal rhabdomyosarcoma.

FIGURE 6-5
Conventional variant of embryonal rhabdomyosarcoma, showing primitive spindled-to-stellate cells in a myxoid background.

which is characteristically intensely eosinophilic and, on occasion, fibrillar (Figure 6-6). The rounded nucleus is often pushed aside. For these rhabdomyoblasts, descriptive terms such as *tadpole*, *strap*, or *spider* cell are used. Cells with (on hematoxylin and eosin stain) recognizable cross-striations are present in only about a third of embryonal rhabdomyosarcomas. They represent the well-differentiated end of the spectrum. The relative proportion between the less or well-differentiated cells is variable from case to case. The tumor cell nuclei vary from spindled to rounded, and most often they contain dense smooth chromatin, the nucleolus being invisible or small and inconspicuous. Few, if any, mitotic figures are found in embryonal rhabdomyosarcomas composed of predominantly well-differentiated cells, whereas up to 30 mitoses per 10 high-power fields are not uncommon in lesions with less differentiated cells. It is striking that tumors removed from patients who have had preoperative chemotherapy or radiation therapy often show prominent differentiation (Figure 6-7). Architecturally, the cells may be tightly packed with little intercellular substance, or can be scattered in an abundant myxoid matrix (Figures 6-5 and 6-8). Most often, the cells are arranged in nondescript sheets. The amount of loose and dense cellularity varies from case to case, as well as within a given tumor. Most of the differentiated or differentiating cells are set within a collagenous matrix, whereas the undifferentiated cells tend to be in a myxoid matrix.

The *botryoid* variant is characterized by a more or less linear arrangement of tightly packed, undifferentiated, spindled to rounded cells with little cytoplasm lying in a parallel band beneath the epithelium. This feature is described as "cambium layer" (Figure 6-9). Beneath the cambium layer, the tumor has the same outlook as conventional embryonal rhabdomyosarcoma. Tumors composed of more than 50% of whorls or fascicles of spindle cells, akin to leiomyosarcoma, constitute the *spindle cell* variant of embryonal rhabdomyosarcoma. The cells have

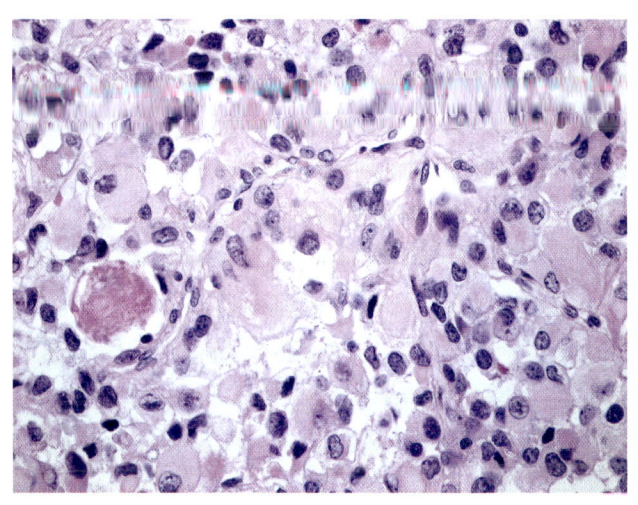

FIGURE 6-6
Typical rhabdomyoblasts with eccentric eosinophilic cytoplasm.

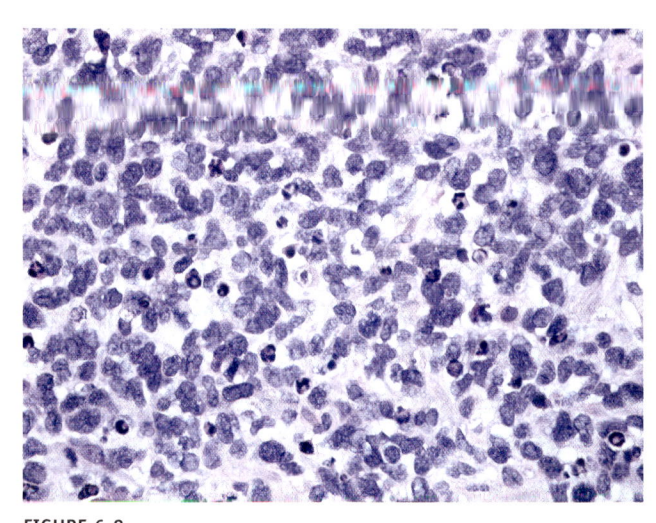

FIGURE 6-8
Highly cellular conventional embryonal rhabdomyosarcoma.

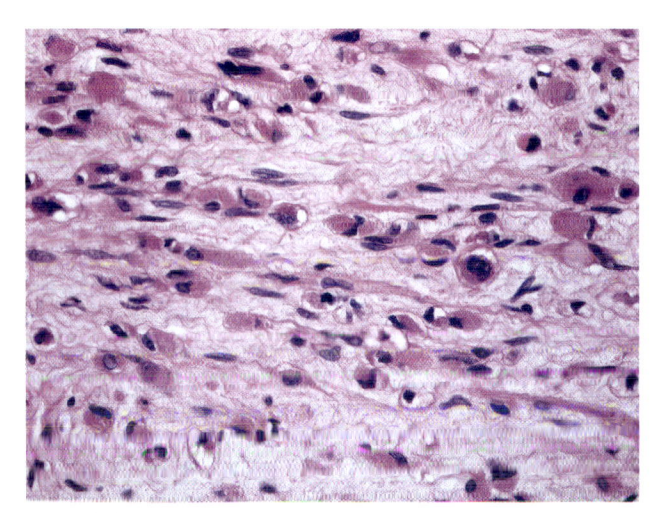

FIGURE 6-7
Embryonal rhabdomyosarcoma after chemotherapy; note the prominence of rhabdomyoblasts.

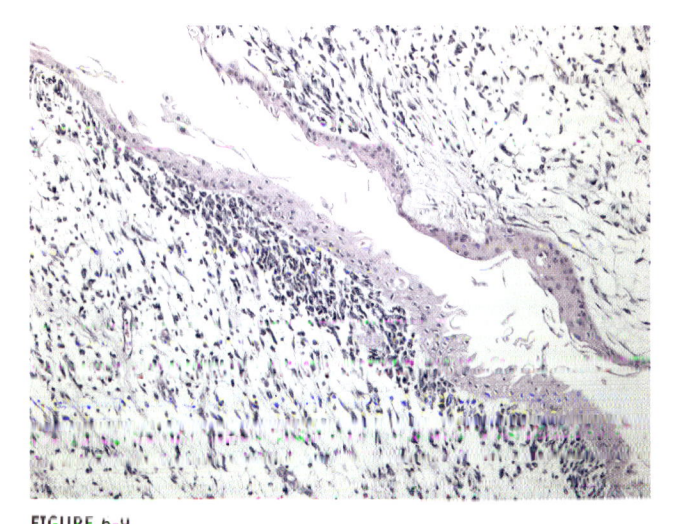

FIGURE 6-9
Botryoid variant of embryonal rhabdomyosarcoma, with "cambium layer" of tightly packed tumor cells beneath the epithelium.

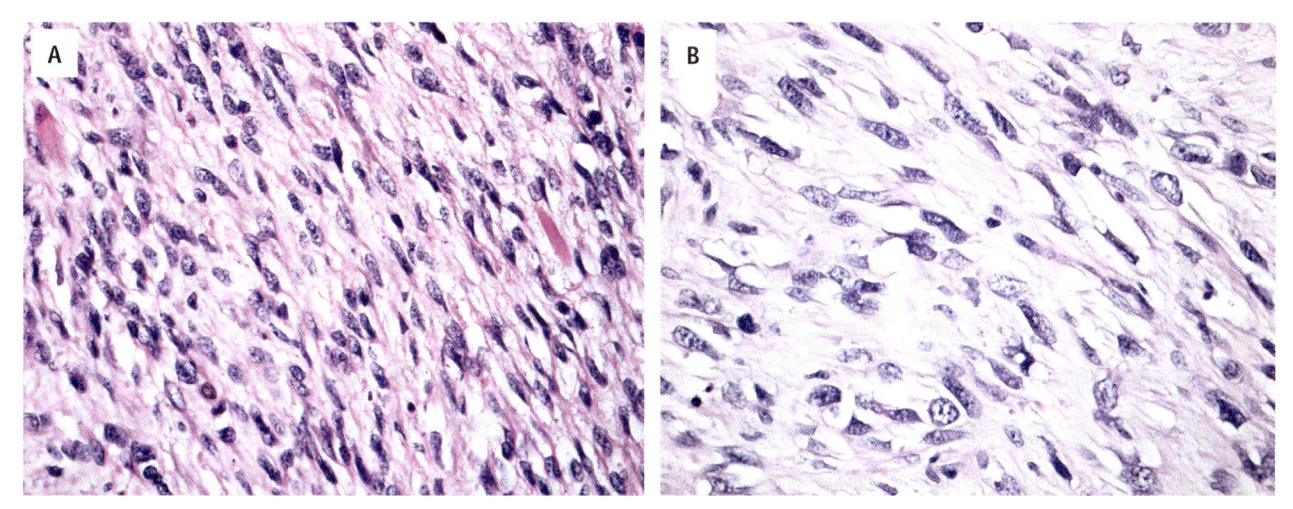

FIGURE 6-10
A, Spindle cell variant of embryonal rhabdomyosarcoma is characterized by fascicles of eosinophilic spindle cells **(B)**, some of which can show prominent paranuclear vacuolisation, as seen in leiomyosarcoma.

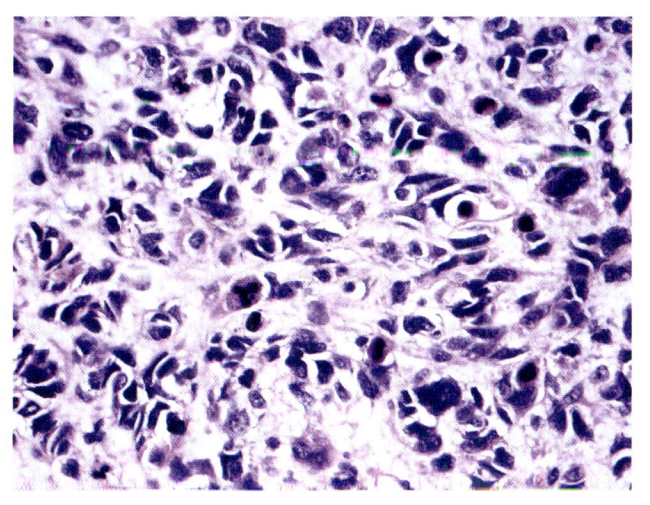

FIGURE 6-11
In the anaplastic variant of embryonal rhabdomyosarcoma, the tumor cells have enlarged hyperchromatic and atypical nuclei. Note the presence of a tripolar mitotic figure.

an eosinophilic fibrillar cytoplasm, cigar-shaped, blunt-ended nuclei, and may also be arranged in a storiform pattern (Figure 6-10). The *anaplastic* variant of embryonal rhabdomyosarcoma is characterized by enlarged, atypical cells with hyperchromatic nuclei that are three times larger than the nuclei of surrounding cells. Atypical mitotic figures are commonly present (Figure 6-11). Generally, the anaplasia must be multifocal or diffuse before the tumor should be denominated as anaplastic.

ANCILLARY STUDIES

IMMUNOHISTOCHEMISTRY

Immunohistochemistry plays a pivotal role in the diagnosis of embryonal rhabdomyosarcoma, to the extent that all embryonal rhabdomyosarcomas, whatever the type, should stain for desmin or for more specific markers such as myogenin or MyoD1 (Figures 6-12 and 6-13). The latter antibodies are currently used as a standard approach for the diagnosis. Desmin expression is usually mirrored by muscle-specific actin immunoreactivity and is present in more than 90% of embryonal rhabdomyosarcomas, except in the anaplastic variant. The proportion of desmin-positive cells may vary considerably from case to case, depending on the number of differentiating/differentiated cells. Because undifferentiated cells do not express desmin, the number of positive cells may be as few as 5%. In the anaplastic variant, desmin expression is present in only about 60% of cases. Myogenin and MyoD1 are myogenic regulatory proteins that are expressed early in skeletal muscle differentiation, before the expression of desmin and actin. Myogenin is expressed in more than 90% of rhabdomyosarcomas. It should be noted that only nuclear staining is specific. In addition, regenerating skeletal muscle fibers may display myogenin expression. Occasional aberrant staining of embryonal rhabdomyosarcomas with cytokeratin, S-100 protein, CD99, and neurofilament has been described.

GENETICS

A consistent diagnostic cytogenetic abnormality for embryonal rhabdomyosarcoma has not been described. Structural and numeric changes are quite frequent, including extra copies of chromosomes 2, 8, and 13. Allelic loss in chromosomal region 11p15 has also been described.

DIFFERENTIAL DIAGNOSIS

Because embryonal rhabdomyosarcoma is a small, blue round cell tumor, a number of entities always enter the differential diagnosis. Ewing sarcoma/primitive

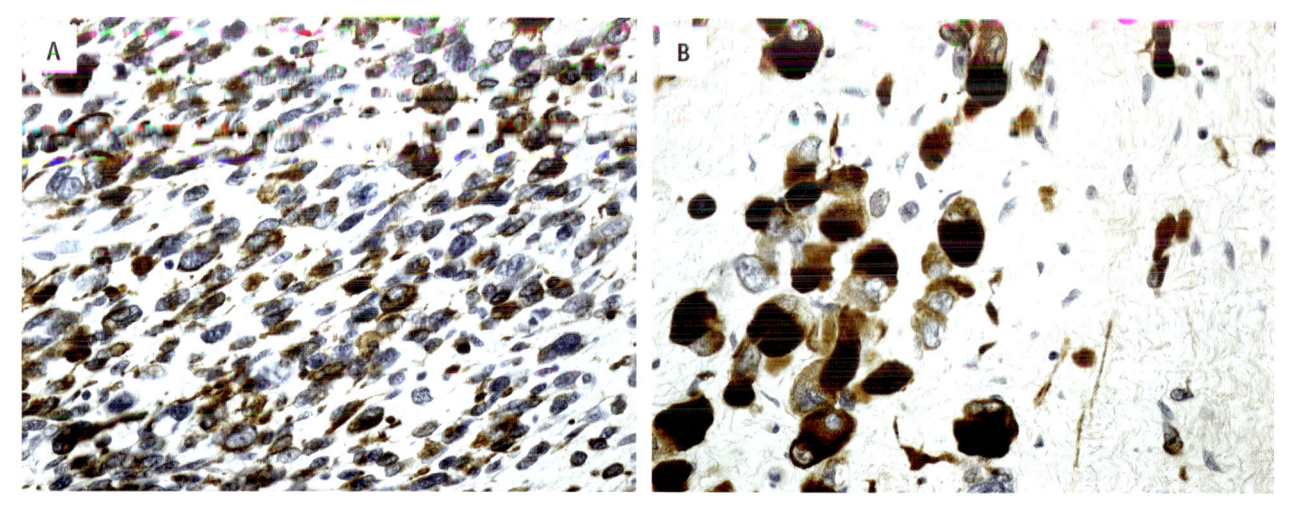

FIGURE 6-12
A, Embryonal rhabdomyosarcoma stained for desmin, revealing cytoplasmic immunoreactivity. **B,** At high power, cross-striation can be seen in some rhabdomyoblasts.

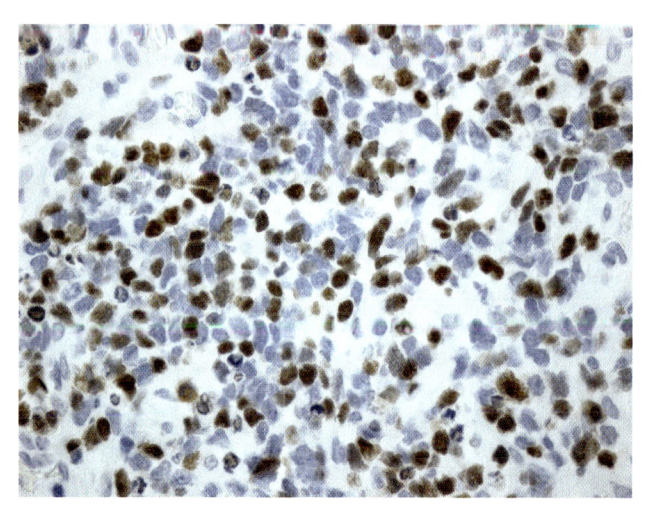

FIGURE 6-13
Myogenin expression in embryonal rhabdomyosarcoma, depicting a typical nuclear staining pattern.

neuroectodermal tumor (PNET) is generally a more uniformly round cell proliferation, without clear-cut spindle cells and cells with eccentric eosinophilic cytoplasm. In addition, a classic Ewing sarcoma/PNET should always express CD99 and is desmin/myogenin/MyoD1 negative. Furthermore, this sarcoma has a characteristic t(11;22)(q12;q24). Neuroblastoma is characterized by hyperchromatic nuclei with granular chromatin and shows a fine, fibrillar stroma. Pseudorosettes may be present and chromogranin/synaptophysin/neurofilament expression can usually be documented, whereas myogenic markers are absent. Nephroblastoma may show skeletal muscle differentiation but also has blastema and epithelial differentiation. Desmoplastic, small, round cell tumor often contains

EMBRYONAL RHABDOMYOSARCOMA—FACT SHEET

Definition
- A primitive soft tissue sarcoma, showing a variable degree of embryonic skeletal muscle differentiation

Incidence and Location
- The most frequent sarcoma of childhood and the most frequent type of rhabdomyosarcoma, occurring in 3 per 1 million children younger than 15 years
- The head and neck region and genitourinary system are most frequently involved; the botryoid variant typically occurs in the wall of hollow organs

Morbidity and Mortality
- Disease-free survival rate of about 70%, depending on stage, histologic type, and location

Sex, Race, and Age Distribution
- Children younger than 10 years are typically affected with a slight male sex predominance
- Incidence figures in Europe mirror those of the United States; eastern and southern Asia have somewhat lower figures; in the United States, non-Hispanic whites are mainly affected

Clinical Features
- Variable and aspecific, depending on site of involvement, and ranging from painful/less mass, obstruction, or bleeding

Prognosis and Treatment
- The botryoid and paratesticular spindle cell variants have a good prognosis (> 90% overall survival rate), the conventional and nonparatesticular spindle cell variants an intermediate prognosis (± 70%), and the anaplastic variant a poor prognosis (±45%)
- Head and neck, genitourinary, and orbital lesions have a better overall prognosis
- Treatment consists of chemotherapy, radiotherapy, and surgery

> **EMBRYONAL RHABDOMYOSARCOMA—PATHOLOGIC FEATURES**
>
> **Gross Findings**
> - Poorly circumscribed masses
> - Spindle cell variant: firm and fibrous
> - Botryoid variant: grape-like polypoid
>
> **Microscopic Findings**
> - Conventional variant: nondescript sheets of cells with a variable density and ranging from undifferentiated spindly/stellate cells to classic rhabdomyoblasts with round nuclei and often eccentric eosinophilic cytoplasm; the intercellular matrix may be sparse or abundant and myxoid
> - Botryoid variant: a cambium layer of tightly packed undifferentiated cells underlining the mucosal surface and overlining a conventional rhabdomyosarcoma-looking part
> - Spindle cell variant: more than 50% fascicles/whorls of leiomyosarcoma-like spindle cells
> - Anaplastic variant: diffuse or multifocal presence of atypical nuclei and mitoses
>
> **Genetics**
> - No consistent and diagnostic changes are present
> - Numeric/structural changes and allelic loss of 11p15 have been described
>
> **Immunohistochemical Features**
> - Staining for desmin, or myogenin/MyoD1 should be present
>
> **Differential Diagnosis**
> - Small, blue round cell tumors (PNET/Ewing sarcoma; neuroblastoma/nephroblastoma; desmoplastic, small, round cell tumor; small-cell synovial sarcoma; lymphoma; rhabdoid tumor; rhabdomyoma; alveolar rhabdomyosarcoma)
> - The spindle cell variant should be differentiated from leiomyosarcoma, myofibroma(tosis), and infantile fibromatosis

desmin-positive cells but has a desmoplastic stroma, strong expression of epithelial markers, and a typical t(11;22)(p13;q12). Small-cell synovial sarcoma should express epithelial markers and no myogenic markers, and is characterized by a t(X;18)(p11.2;q11.2). A non-Hodgkin's lymphoma can be documented by CD45 and B- or T-cell markers. Malignant rhabdoid tumor also shows an eccentric cytoplasm, but the nuclei are more vesicular with prominent nuclei, and the rhabdoid cells should be cytokeratin positive. The differential diagnosis with a rhabdomyoma and the solid variant of alveolar rhabdomyosarcoma is discussed in the respective chapters. The spindle cell variant of embryonal rhabdomyosarcoma should be differentiated from myofibroma(tosis), infantile fibromatosis, and leiomyosarcoma. The latter is unusual in the pediatric age group and does not express myogenin/MyoD1. Myofibroma(tosis) and infantile fibromatosis do not have nuclear atypia, and the first often features a pericytic vascular pattern.

PROGNOSIS AND TREATMENT

Since the introduction of current chemotherapy, modern radiotherapy, and improved surgical procedures, disease-free survival has improved from 20 % to about 70 %. Three factors influence the prognosis: histologic subtype, site, and stage (Intergroup Rhabdomyosarcoma Study clinical group). The botryoid and spindle cell variants have a superior outcome, certainly the paratesticular spindle cell rhabdomyosarcomas. Rhabdomyosarcomas with diffuse anaplasia have a worse outcome. Regarding primary site, head and neck, genitourinary, and orbital lesions have a better overall prognosis. The lungs, lymph nodes, liver, and brain are the most common metastatic sites.

ALVEOLAR RHABDOMYOSARCOMA

CLINICAL FEATURES

Alveolar rhabdomyosarcoma is a high-grade round cell sarcoma characterized by alveolar and solid growth patterns, and shows a variable skeletal muscle differentiation. It mainly affects children and young adults (age range, 2 to 25 years). This aggressive neoplasm is fortunately rare and accounts for only 20 % to 25 % of all rhabdomyosarcomas. Because of the bad prognosis, it is of utmost importance to distinguish alveolar rhabdomyosarcoma from embryonal rhabdomyosarcoma. Moreover, any rhabdomyosarcoma with an alveolar pattern, no matter how focal, behaves like an alveolar rhabdomyosarcoma. These tumors mainly occur in the skeletal muscle of the extremities; additional sites of involvement are head and neck, trunk, and pelvis. No sex, race, or geographic predilection exists. A rapidly growing, painless mass is a frequent sign, with secondary compression/obstruction, depending on the location. Alveolar rhabdomyosarcomas tend to be high-stage lesions at presentation.

PATHOLOGIC FEATURES

GROSS FINDINGS

Alveolar rhabdomyosarcomas are fleshy tumors with a variable amount of hemorrhagic or fibrous tissue, ranging in size from 2 to 8 cm.

MICROSCOPIC FINDINGS

All alveolar rhabdomyosarcomas show round cell features, reminiscent of lymphoma, but with variable rhabdomyoblastic differentiation. The *conventional* type of alveolar rhabdomyosarcoma is characterized by fibrovascular septa that separate the tumor into nests. In the center of these discrete nests, the cells are discohesive, whereas the cells at the edge are attached to each other and to the septa, simulating the alveolar pattern of the lung (Figure 6-14). The tumor cells are relatively large, the largest ones (15 to 30 μm) often showing rhabdomyoblastic differentiation with eccentric eosinophilic cytoplasm, with or without cross striations. The majority of the cells is less differentiated, with a round nucleus and little cytoplasm. Multinucleated giant ("wreath") cells are often present as well and are of help in the (differential) diagnosis (Figure 6-15). In the diagnostically more challenging *solid* variant of alveolar rhabdomyosarcoma, the fibrovascular septa are hardly found, and no discohesive growth pattern is present (Figure 6-16). The tumor cells show the same morphology as in the conventional variant. Occasionally, clear cell changes, anaplastic features, or rhabdoid features may be seen in alveolar rhabdomyosarcoma.

ANCILLARY STUDIES

IMMUNOHISTOCHEMISTRY

As in the embryonal type, expression of desmin and myogenin/MyoD1 is present in most alveolar rhabdomyosarcomas, whatever the type (Figure 6-17). This is particularly helpful in the solid variant. It is of interest that alveolar rhabdomyosarcoma generally stains more diffusely positive for myogenin than does embryonal rhabdomyosarcoma (Figure 6-18). Occasional expression of other, less relevant markers is similar as in the embryonal type.

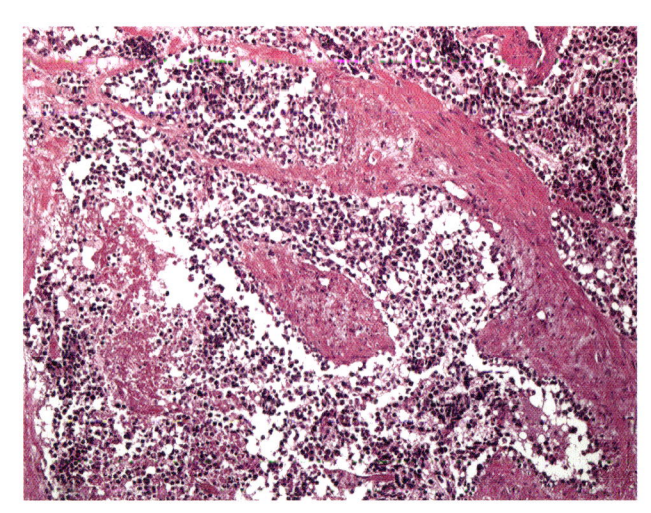

FINE NEEDLE ASPIRATION BIOPSY

In addition to individually dispersed cells, loosely cohesive cell nests are usually present. Often, a striking uniformity of the rounded cells is evident. Rhabdomyoblastic differentiation may be seen.

GENETICS

As described in Chapter 2, alveolar rhabdomyosarcoma exhibits a characteristic t(2;13)(q35;q14) or t(1;13)(p36;q14) as variant translocation.

DIFFERENTIAL DIAGNOSIS

Because alveolar rhabdomyosarcoma is a small, blue round cell sarcoma, the same entities as mentioned in the Embryonal Rhabdomyosarcoma section (see earlier)

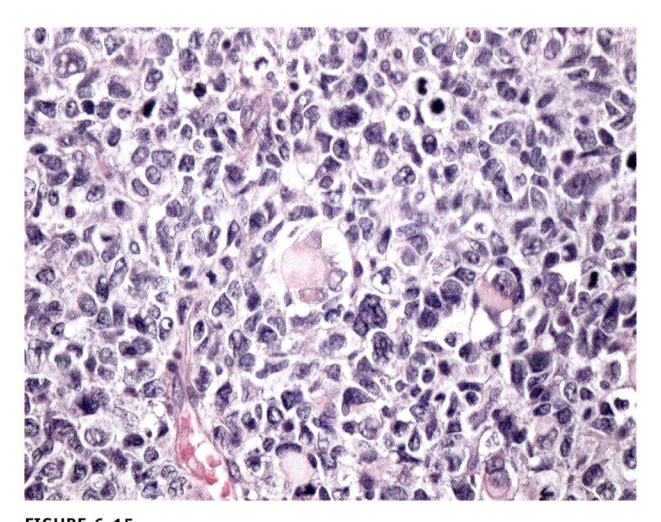

FIGURE 6-15
Wreath cell is the solid variant of alveolar rhabdomyosarcoma.

FIGURE 6-14
Low-power view of the conventional type of alveolar rhabdomyosarcoma with fibrovascular septa to which tumor cells are attached. In the center of the cell nests, the tumor cells are discohesive.

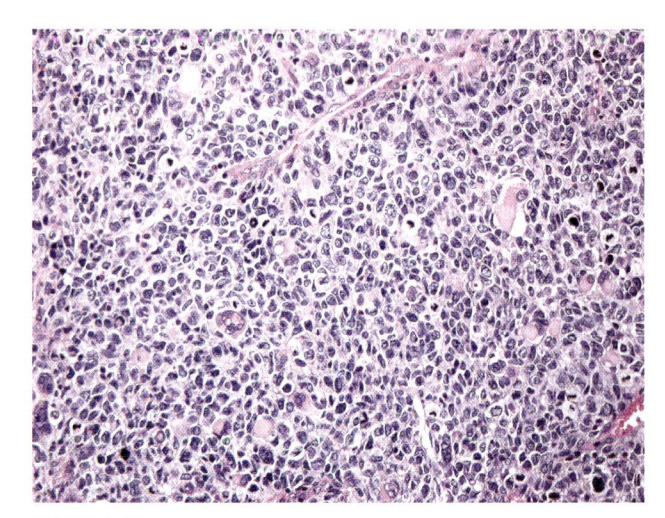

FIGURE 6-16
Solid variant of alveolar rhabdomyosarcoma. Some rhabdomyoblasts are present.

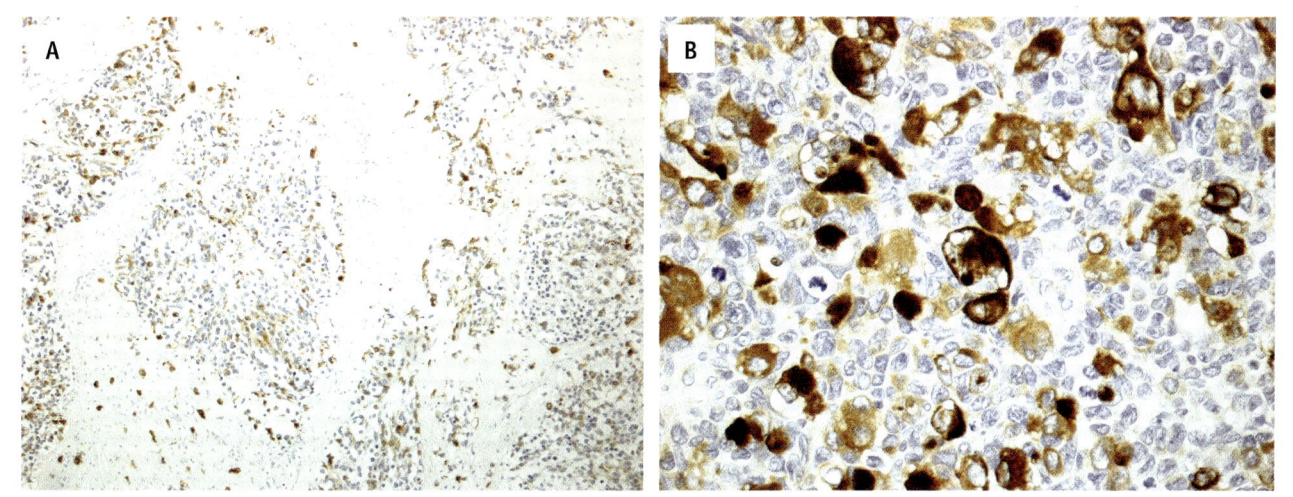

FIGURE 6-17
A, Desmin staining in the conventional and **(B)** solid variant of alveolar rhabdomyosarcoma.

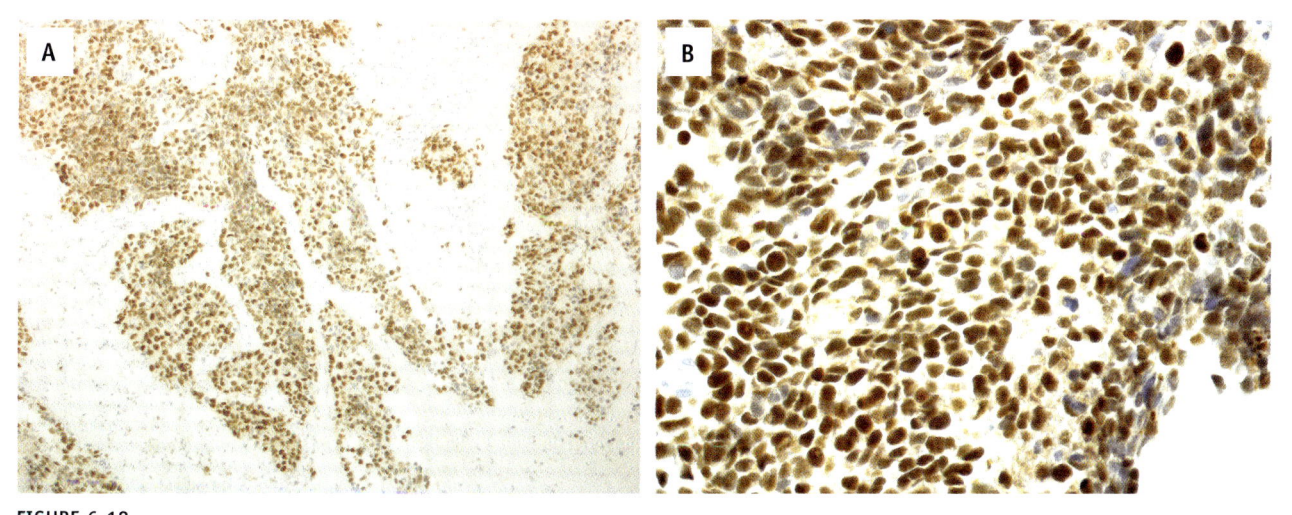

FIGURE 6-18
Myogenin expression in alveolar rhabdomyosarcoma. Note the strong and diffuse immunoreactivity. **A**, Low-power view. **B**, High-power view.

enter the differential diagnosis. This mainly holds true for the solid variant, because the conventional type usually represents a straightforward diagnosis on hematoxylin and eosin sections. Nevertheless, an alveolar growth pattern can also be seen in poorly differentiated carcinomas and, more specifically, in the alveolar soft part sarcoma. Cytokeratin expression and absence of muscle markers obviously disclose a carcinoma. Alveolar soft part sarcoma may be more difficult to rule out because of the same alveolar growth pattern, and because it can be desmin and/or MyoD1 positive. A PAS-diastase stain will, however, show the characteristic crystalline cytoplasmic inclusions of alveolar soft part sarcoma. In addition, alveolar soft part sarcoma does not contain multinucleated giant cells. In view of the prognostic difference, the solid variant of alveolar rhabdomyosarcoma should be differentiated from embryonal rhabdomyosarcoma. In alveolar rhabdomyosarcoma, the nuclei generally are larger and more uniform, and the cells are more consistently rounder. In addition, multinucleated giant cells are not a characteristic feature of embryonal rhabdomyosarcoma, and myogenin expression is more diffuse in the alveolar type.

Prognosis and Treatment

Alveolar rhabdomyosarcoma does not respond well to chemotherapy, and the overall survival rate for all stages is less than 50%. The stage of the disease obviously affects the outcome as in embryonal rhabdomyosarcoma, but stage for stage, the prognosis is much worse in alveolar rhabdomyosarcoma. Metastases are twice as common as in embryonal rhabdomyosarcoma, with a similar distribution. PAX7/FKHR-positive tumors may behave less aggressively than PAX3/FKHR-positive ones.

ALVEOLAR RHABDOMYOSARCOMA—FACT SHEET

Definition
- A high grade round cell sarcoma with an alveolar or solid growth pattern with variable rhabdomyoblastic differentiation

Incidence and Location
- Rare (20% to 25% of all childhood rhabdomyosarcomas)
- Deep soft tissues of the extremities most frequently involved

Morbidity and Mortality
- Overall 5-year survival rate < 50%
- Mixed embryonal/alveolar rhabdomyosarcoma always behaves like the alveolar type

Sex, Race, and Age Distribution
- Children and young adults between 2 and 25 years of age are mainly affected
- No sex or race predominance

Clinical Features
- Rapidly growing mass, with secondary signs/symptoms depending on the location

Prognosis and Treatment
- No efficient therapy is available
- Prognosis dependent on stage but always more aggressive than embryonal rhabdomyosarcoma

ALVEOLAR RHABDOMYOSARCOMA—PATHOLOGIC FEATURES

Gross Findings
- Fleshy mass with variable fibrous/hemorrhagic areas

Microscopic Findings
- Uniform, small, blue round cell neoplasm, with variable rhabdomyoblastic differentiation
- Conventional type: fibrovascular septa delineating discrete nests, the cells in the center of which show a discohesive pattern, whereas the cells at the edge are cohesively attached
- Solid type: fibrovascular septa are only focally present
- Multinucleated giant cells often present

Genetics
- t(2;13)(q35;q14) or t(1;13)(p36;q14) as variant translocation
- Juxtaposition of the PAX3 (chromosome 2) or PAX7 (chromosome 1) with the FKHR on chromosome 13

Immunohistochemical Features
- Staining for desmin should be present or myogenin/MyoD1 should be present
- Myogenin expression more diffuse than in embryonal type of rhabdomyosarcoma

Differential Diagnosis
- Similar as small, blue round cell sarcomas mentioned in embryonal rhabdomyosarcoma section
- Solid type represents the major differential diagnostic problem and should be differentiated from embryonal rhabdomyosarcoma
- Alveolar type should be differentiated from alveolar soft part sarcoma and from undifferentiated carcinoma

PLEOMORPHIC RHABDOMYOSARCOMA

CLINICAL FEATURES

Pleomorphic rhabdomyosarcoma is a high-grade sarcoma consisting of bizarre spindled, rounded, and polygonal cells, some of which display skeletal muscle differentiation, as evidenced by immunohistochemistry or electron microscopy, or both. Pleomorphic rhabdomyosarcoma mainly occurs in predominantly male adults. The deep soft tissue of the lower extremities is typically involved, and the tumor usually presents as a rapidly growing, painful swelling.

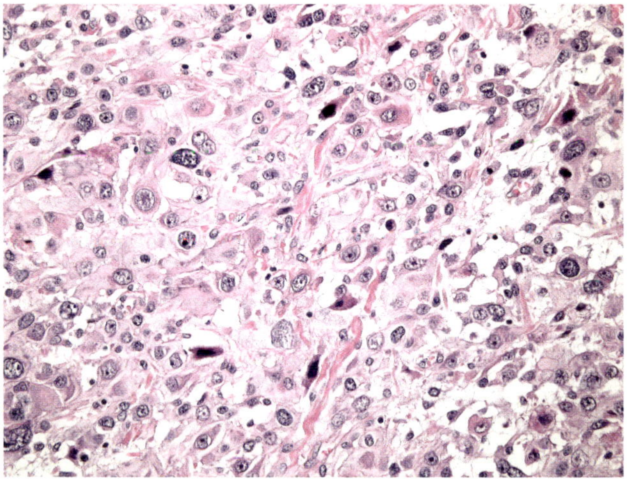

PATHOLOGIC FEATURES

GROSS FINDINGS

Pleomorphic rhabdomyosarcomas are often large tumors (10 to 30 cm), seemingly well circumscribed, and commonly display areas of necrosis and hemorrhage.

FIGURE 6-19
Pleomorphic rhabdomyosarcoma showing bizarre pleomorphic tumor cells with eosinophilic cytoplasm.

MICROSCOPIC FINDINGS

At first glance, pleomorphic rhabdomyosarcoma resembles any type of pleomorphic sarcoma. The tumor cells range from spindly to bizarre, large polygonal to rounded undifferentiated cells. Also, the nuclei display an impressive pleomorphism, with a vesicular to atypical and hyperchromatic aspect. Multinuclear cells are not rare. The cells often have a copious eosinophilic cytoplasm, but convincing cross striations are rare (Figure 6-19). Mitotic figures are often frequent, including atypical mitoses. The architecture varies from a fascicular to storiform to patternless pattern. Areas of necrosis complete the picture.

ANCILLARY STUDIES

IMMUNOHISTOCHEMISTRY

At least some cells must express desmin and myogenin/MyoD1 (Figure 6-20). The expression of the latter markers in pleomorphic rhabdomyosarcoma is usually more limited than in other rhabdomyosarcomas.

GENETICS

Only nonconsistent, highly complex karyotypes have been described.

DIFFERENTIAL DIAGNOSIS

Any type of pleomorphic sarcoma enters the differential diagnosis for pleomorphic rhabdomyosarcoma, and the reader is referred to Chapter 3 on pleomorphic malignant fibrous histiocytoma. In this regard, the finding of myogenin or MyoD1 expression by immunohistochemistry, is crucial. It is of note that other sarcomas may display heterologous rhabdomyosarcomatous differentiation, a Triton tumor and a dedifferentiated

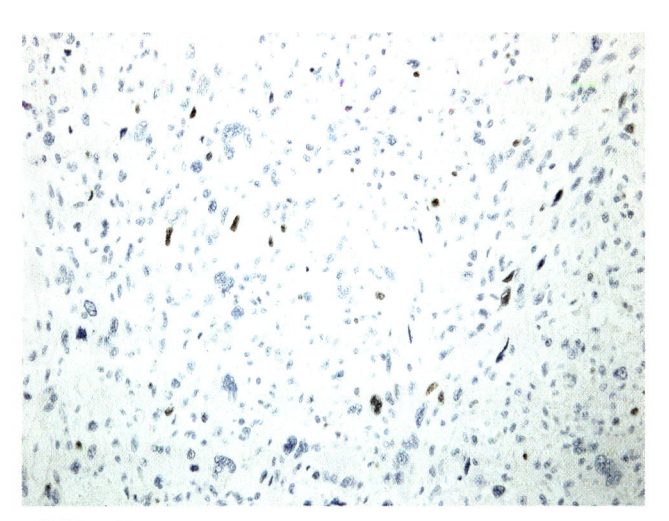

FIGURE 6-20
Scattered myogenin expression in pleomorphic rhabdomyosarcoma.

PLEOMORPHIC RHABDOMYOSARCOMA—FACT SHEET

Definition
▸▸ High-grade pleomorphic sarcoma that displays (often focal) skeletal muscle differentiation by electron microscopy or immunohistochemistry, or both

Incidence and Location
▸▸ Relatively rare tumor with a predilection for the deep soft tissues of the lower extremities

Sex and Age Distribution
▸▸ Usually affects adult men

Clinical Features
▸▸ Rapidly growing, painful mass

Prognosis and Treatment
▸▸ Poor prognosis; most patients die within a year of presentation

---

PLEOMORPHIC RHABDOMYOSARCOMA—PATHOLOGIC FEATURES

Gross Findings
▸▸ Large tumors, often with evidence of necrosis and hemorrhage

Microscopic Findings
▸▸ Spindly to bizarre polygonal atypical cells, arranged in sheets, storiform or patternless patterns
▸▸ Vesicular to atypical hyperchromatic nuclei
▸▸ Necrosis and (atypical) mitoses frequent
▸▸ Cytoplasm can be eosinophilic and copious, but cross-striations are usually absent

Ultrastructural Features
▸▸ Rudimentary sarcomere formation indicates skeletal muscle differentiation

Immunohistochemical Features
▸▸ At least focal presence of desmin and/or myogenin/MyoD1 is essential and diagnostic

Differential Diagnosis
▸▸ Any pleomorphic sarcoma and sarcomas with heterologous rhabdomyoblastic differentiation (dedifferentiated liposarcoma, malignant Triton tumor)

---

liposarcoma being classic examples. Careful sampling, clinical information, and immunohistochemistry may solve the problem. The presence of neurofibromatosis type I or a peripheral nerve location indicates is an malignant peripheral nerve sheath tumor with rhabdomyoblastic differentiation, and a dedifferentiated liposarcoma stains for MDM2.

PROGNOSIS AND TREATMENT

Because of the rarity and flux diagnostic criteria of pleomorphic sarcoma in the past, only few studies are present, and no reliable prognostic factors have been established. Nevertheless, the prognosis of pleomorphic rhabdomyosarcoma is poor, and most patients die of disseminated disease within 1 year of presentation. The lung is the most common site of metastases.

ADULT SCLEROSING RHABDOMYOSARCOMA

Recently, seven cases of an unusual rhabdomyosarcoma have been described, under the names *sclerosing pseudovascular rhabdomyosarcoma in adults* and *sclerosing rhabdomyosarcoma in adults*. These tumors arose in the extremities, orbit, nasopharynx, jaw, and sacrum of patients from 18 to 56 years old. On histology, they showed an abundant hyaline matrix, resembling primitive osteoid or chondroid, and dividing the rounded tumor cells into nests, lobules, or single files (Figure 6-21). An alveolar to pseudovascular pattern was focally present. Cells with rhabdomyoblastic differentiation were rarely present. Desmin expression is present, albeit with an unusual dot-like pattern. Myogenin expression is often less obvious than MyoD1 expression (Figure 6-22). These tumors seem to have the capacity to behave in an aggressive fashion. They should be differentiated from osteosarcoma, chondrosarcoma, sclerosing epithelioid fibrosarcoma, and angiosarcoma, with appropriate immunohistochemical stains being discriminative. It is not clear yet whether these rhabdomyosarcomas are an unusual presentation of embryonal rhabdomyosarcoma or whether they represent a separate entity. They do not show the genetic changes of alveolar rhabdomyosarcoma.

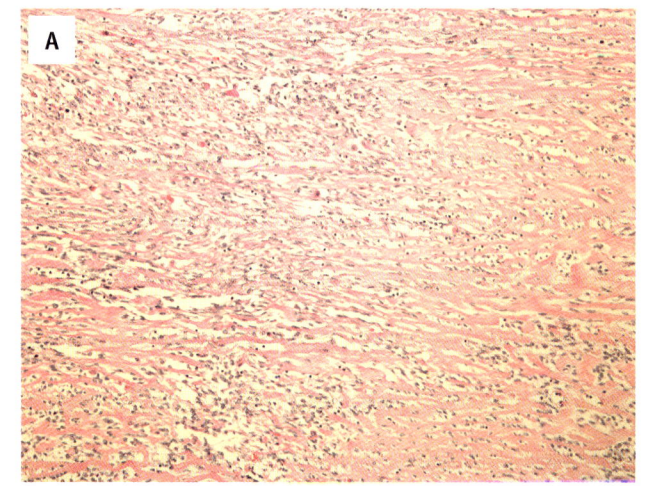

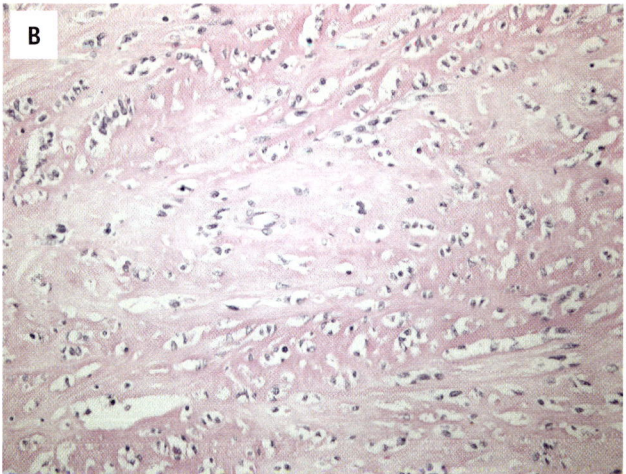

FIGURE 6-21
Adult sclerosing rhabdomyosarcoma.
A-B, Low-power view shows the hyaline-to-chondroid aspect of the matrix. **C,** At high power, some rhabdomyoblasts are present.

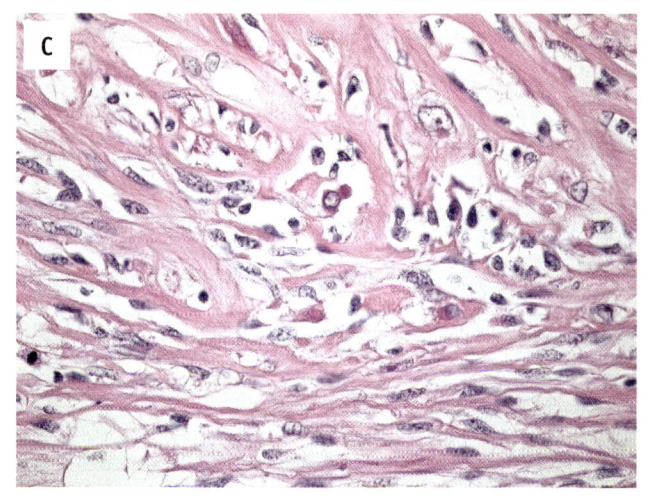

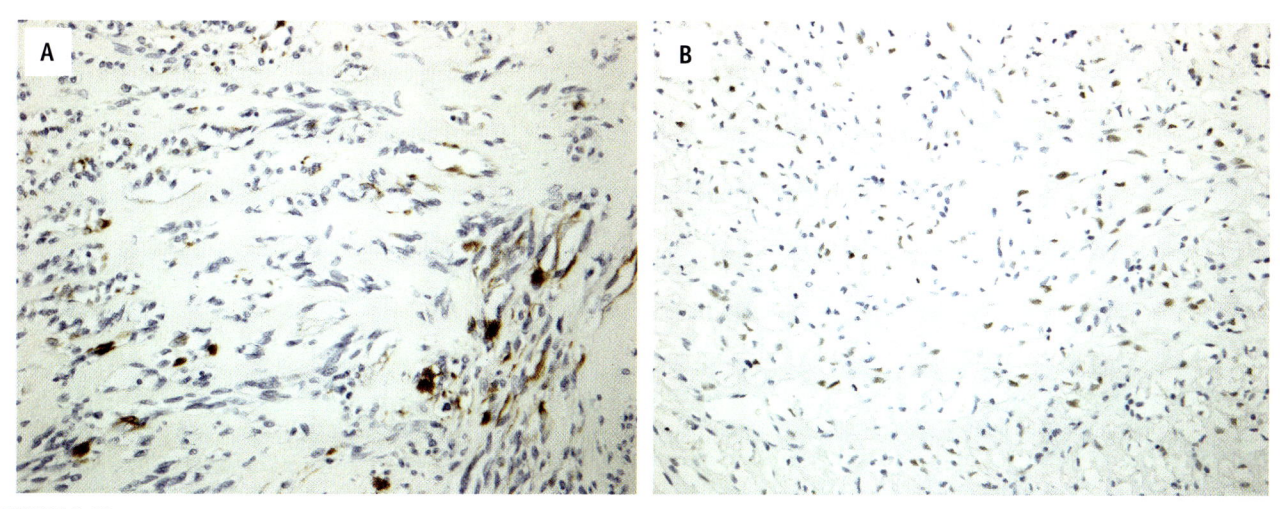

FIGURE 6-22
Adult sclerosing rhabdomyosarcoma **(A)** with desmin and **(B)** myogenin expression.

SUGGESTED READINGS

Rhabdomyoma

1. Kapadia SB, Barr FG: Rhabdomyoma. Pathology & Genetics. Tumours of Soft Tissue & Bone. Lyon, France, IARC Press, 2002, pp 142–145.
2. Kempson RL, Fletcher CDM, Evans HL, et al: Skeletal muscle tumors. Atlas of Tumor Pathology. Tumors of the Soft Tissues. Washington, DC, Armed Forces Institute of Pathology, 2002, pp 257–306.
3. Weiss SW, Goldblum JR: Rhabdomyoma. Soft Tissue Tumors. St. Louis, MO, Mosby, 2001, pp 769–784.

Embryonal Rhabdomyosarcoma

1. Coindre JM: Immunohistochemistry in the diagnosis of soft tissue tumors. Histopathology 2003;43:1–16.
2. Folpe AL: MyoD1 and Myogenin expression in human neoplasia: A review and update. Adv Anat Pathol 2002;9:198–203.
3. Kempson RL, Fletcher CDM, Evans HL, et al: Skeletal muscle tumors. Atlas of Tumor Pathology. Tumors of the Soft Tissues. Washington, DC, Armed Forces Institute of Pathology, 2002, pp 257–306.
4. Maurer HM, Beltangady M, Gehan FA, et al: The Intergroup Rhabdomyosarcoma Study. I. A final report. Cancer 1988;61:209–220.
5. Maurer HM, Gehan EA, Bellangady M, et al: The Intergroup Rhabdomyosarcoma Study. II. Cancer 1993;71:1904–1922.
6. Parham DM, Barr FG: Embryonal rhabdomyosarcoma. Pathology & Genetics. Tumours of Soft Tissue & Bone. Lyon, France, IARC Press, 2002, pp 146–149.
7. Weiss SW, Goldblum JR: Rhabdomyoma. Soft Tissue Tumors. St. Louis, MO, Mosby, 2001, pp 785–837.

Alveolar Rhabdomyosarcoma

1. Kempson RL, Fletcher CDM, Evans HL, et al: Skeletal muscle tumors. Atlas of Tumor Pathology. Tumors of the Soft Tissues. Washington, DC, Armed Forces Institute of Pathology, 2002, pp 257–306.
2. Parham DM, Barr FG: Alveolar rhabdomyosarcoma. Pathology & Genetics. Tumours of Soft Tissue & Bone. Lyon, France, IARC Press, 2002, pp 150–152.
3. Sebire NJ, Malone M: Myogenin and MyoD1 expression in paediatric rhabdomyosarcomas. J Clin Pathol 2003;56:412–416.
4. Sorensen PHB, Lynch JC, Qualman SJ, et al: PAX3-FKHR and PAX-7FKHR gene fusions are prognostic indicators in alveolar rhabdomyosarcoma: A report from the children's oncology group. J Clin Oncol 2002;11:2672–2679.
5. Weiss SW, Goldblum JR: Rhabdomyoma. Soft Tissue Tumors. St. Louis, MO, Mosby, 2001, pp 785–837.

Pleomorphic Rhabdomyosarcoma

1. Furlong MA, Fanburg-Smith JC: Pleomorphic rhabdomyosarcoma in children: Four cases in the pediatric age group. Ann Diagn Pathol 2001;5:199–206.
2. Furlong MA, Mentzel T, Fanburg-Smith JC: Pleomorphic rhabdomyosarcoma in adults: A clinicopathological study of 38 cases with emphasis on morphologic variants and recent skeletal muscle-specific markers. Mod Pathol 2001;14:595–603.
3. Kempson RL, Fletcher CDM, Evans HL, et al: Skeletal muscle tumors. Atlas of Tumor Pathology. Tumors of the Soft Tissues. Washington, DC, Armed Forces Institute of Pathology, 2002, pp 257–306.
4. Montgomery E, Barr FG: Pleomorphic rhabdomyosarcoma. Pathology & Genetics. Tumours of Soft Tissue & Bone. Lyon, France, IARC Press, 2002, pp 150–152.
5. Weiss SW, Goldblum JR: Rhabdomyoma. Soft Tissue Tumors. St. Louis, MO, Mosby, 2001, pp 785–837.

Adult Sclerosing Rhabdomyosarcoma

1. Folpe AL, McKenny JK, Bridge JA, et al: Sclerosing rhabdomyosarcoma in adults. Report of four cases of a hyalinising, matrix-rich variant of rhabdomyosarcoma that may be confused with osteosarcoma, chondrosarcoma, or angiosarcoma. Am J Surg Pathol 2002;26:1175–1183.
2. Mentzel T, Katenkamp D: Sclerosing pseudovascular rhabdomyosarcoma in adults: Clinocopathlogical and immunohistochemical analysis of three cases. Virchows Arch 2000;436:305–311.

7 Tumor of Perivascular Cells
Andrew L. Folpe • Louis Guillou

- Hemangiopericytoma, Solitary Fibrous Tumor of Soft Tissues, and Related Lesions (Giant Cell Angiofibroma, Lipomatous Hemangiopericytoma)
- Myopericytoma Family of Tumors (Infantile Myofibromatosis, Solitary Myofibroma in Infants and Adults, Infantile Hemangiopericytoma, Myopericytoma, Glomangiopericytoma)
- Glomus Tumors (Solid Glomus Tumor, Glomangioma, Glomangiomyoma, Symplastic Glomus Tumor, Glomus Tumor of Uncertain Malignant Potential, Malignant Glomus Tumor/Glomangiosarcoma)
- Atypical and Malignant Glomus Tumors

HEMANGIOPERICYTOMA, SOLITARY FIBROUS TUMOR OF SOFT TISSUES, AND RELATED LESIONS (Giant Cell Angiofibroma, Lipomatous Hemangiopericytoma)

Hemangiopericytoma (HPC) is currently considered by the World Health Organization to be closely related, if not identical, to solitary fibrous tumor (SFT) of soft tissue, with classic HPC representing the cellular phase of this single entity. Although the precise line of differentiation shown by HPC/SFT is still unclear, it seems certain that HPC is not showing differentiation along the lines of true microvascular contractile pericytes. Nevertheless, for historical reasons, both HPC and SFT are discussed in this chapter.

CLINICAL FEATURES

HPCs and SFTs are ubiquitous neoplasms that can be found anywhere in the body. Common locations for classic HPC include the abdomen and retroperitoneum, whereas classic SFT most often arises from the mesothelial surfaces of the thoracic and abdominal cavities. However, HPCs/SFTs may arise in essentially any soft tissue or visceral location, including the meninges, orbit, kidney, lungs, and salivary glands, among others. They are usually observed in middle-aged adults (average age, 50 years) but may be seen in children. Male individuals are affected as frequently as female individuals. Most lesions present as well-circumscribed, slow-growing, painless masses. Large tumors may result in compression symptoms and/or may be associated with paraneoplastic syndromes such as hypoglycemia (caused by the production of an insulin-like growth factor by the tumor cells). Malignant tumors are often locally infiltrative.

PATHOLOGIC FEATURES

GROSS FINDINGS

HPCs/SFTs are well-delineated, solitary, lobulated masses that measure 5 to 8 cm on average. Cut section reveals a multinodular, white-to-gray, firm lesion (Figure 7-1). HPCs/SFTs with adipocytic differentiation (lipomatous HPC and SFT) are often larger and may have a fatty appearance.

MICROSCOPIC FINDINGS

Most HPCs/SFTs are well-circumscribed but nonencapsulated or only partially encapsulated lesions. Classic HPC shows a uniform, well-developed, *staghorn*

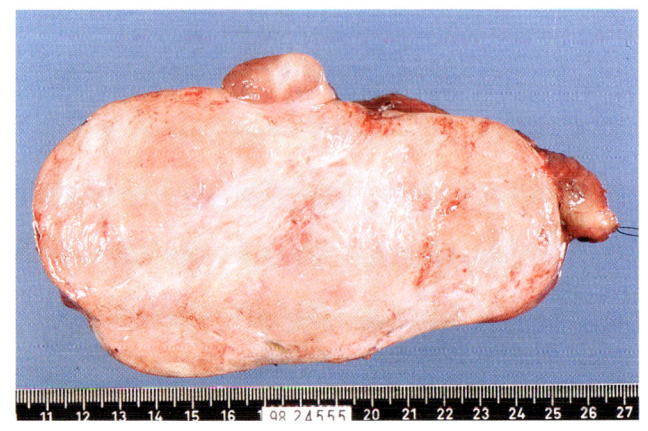

FIGURE 7-1

Gross photograph of a solitary fibrous tumor of soft tissue, showing a large, fibrous-appearing mass.

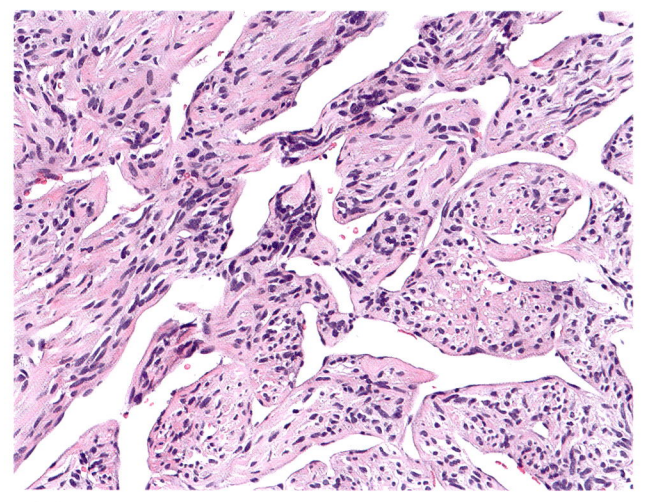

FIGURE 7-2
Cellular zone in solitary fibrous tumor *(hemangiopericytoma)* with a prominent branching, hyalinized vasculature, surrounded by bland ovoid-to-spindled cells.

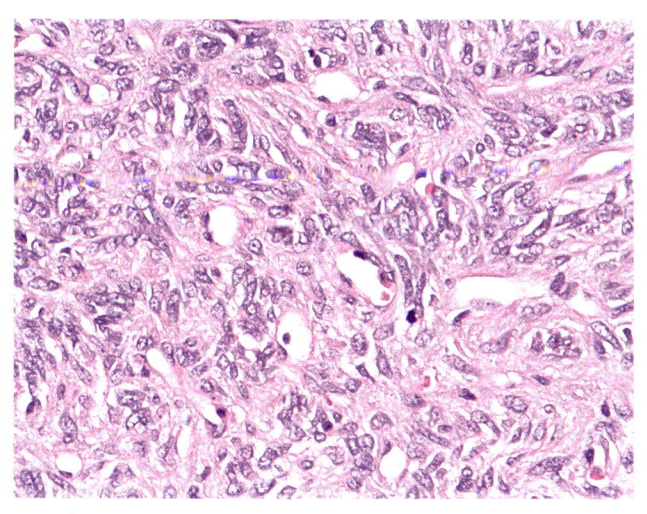

FIGURE 7-3
The more cellular zones of solitary fibrous tumor/hemangiopericytoma typically consist of a moderately cellular proliferation of short spindled cells, arranged in a *patternless* pattern.

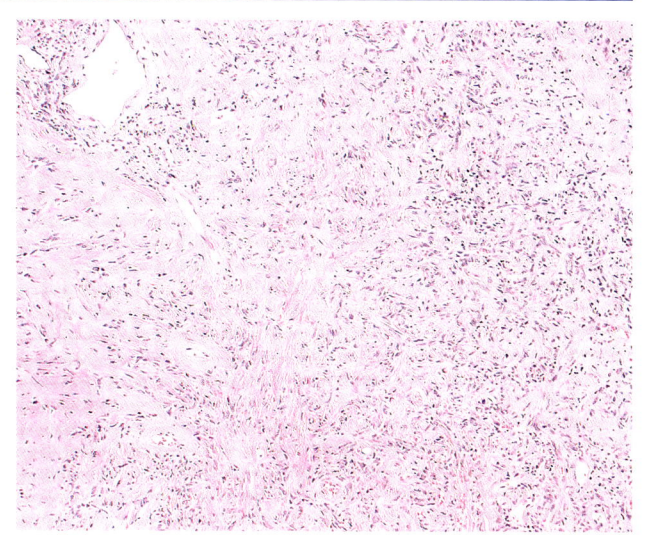

FIGURE 7-4
Classic solitary fibrous tumor of soft tissues showing alternating hypocellular/collagenized and hypercellular zones, with thick-walled vessels.

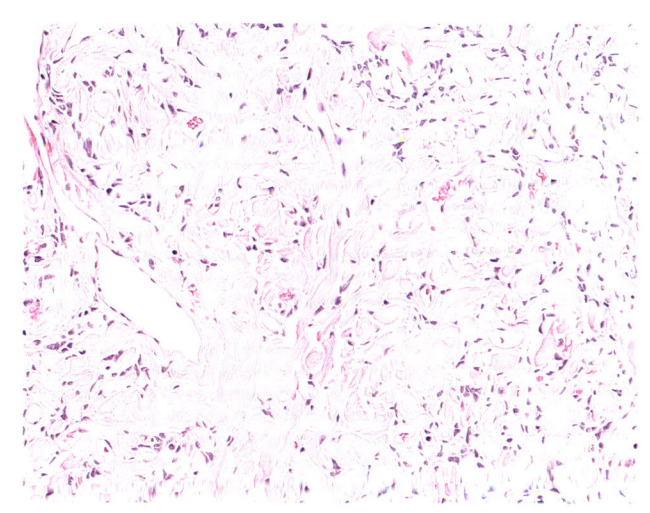

FIGURE 7-5
Solitary fibrous tumor of soft tissue with hyalinized collagen, cracking artifact, and *patternless* growth.

vasculature with perivascular hyalinization, around which are arrayed bland spindled to ovoid cells (Figures 7-2 and 7-3). Classic SFT typically shows small areas identical to classic HPC, but additionally shows broad areas of collagenization, with cracking artifact, as well as fascicular areas, and a *patternless* proliferation of bland, fibroblastic spindled cells (Figures 7-4 and 7-5). Lesions that show hybrid features of classic HPC and SFT are, however, the rule rather than the exception, and there is an increasing trend to regard the classic HPC pattern as simply the cellular phase of SFT. Except in malignant cases, mitoses are scarce, usually between 1 and 3 per 10 high-power fields (hpf). Occasional HPC/SFT may contain pseudovascular spaces lined by multinucleated giant cells (so-called *giant cell angiofibroma*) (Figure 7-6) or may contain abundant mature fat (lipomatous SFT or HPC) (Figure 7-7).

Malignant HPCs/SFTs are hypercellular lesions that usually display infiltrative borders, nuclear pleomorphism, hyperchromasia, areas of tumor necrosis, and/or increased mitotic activity (> 4 mitoses/10 hpf), including atypical mitoses (Figure 7-8).

Ancillary Studies

Immunohistochemistry

Tumors cells in HPC/SFT are characteristically positive for CD34 (90% to 95% of cases) and CD99 (70% of cases) (Figure 7-9). Reactivity for epithelial membrane antigen, bcl2, and smooth muscle actin is observed in about one-third of cases. Occasional focal reactivity for S-100 protein has been described. Nuclear beta-catenin

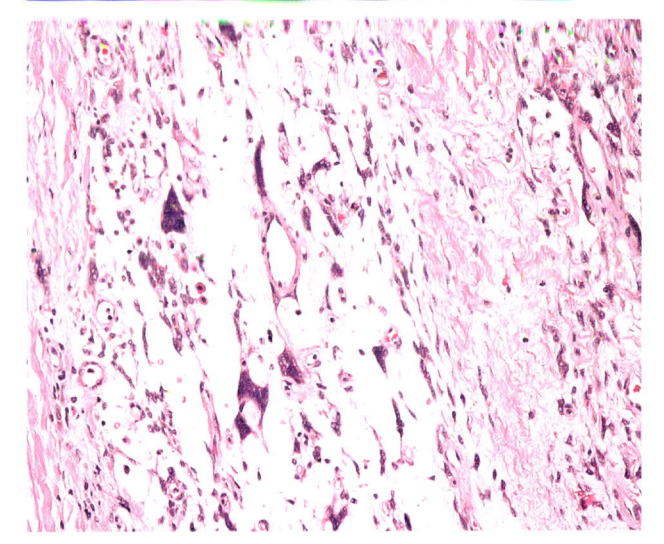

FIGURE 7-6
Solitary fibrous tumor with multinucleated tumor giant cells (so-called giant cell angiofibroma).

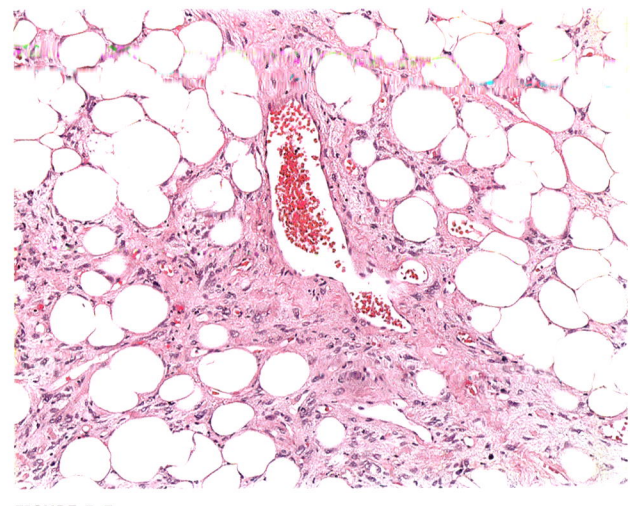

FIGURE 7-7
Lipomatous hemangiopericytoma/solitary fibrous tumor with mature fat.

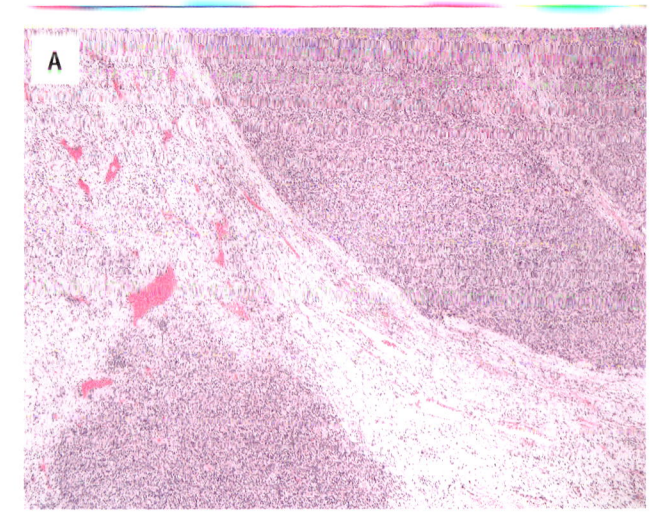

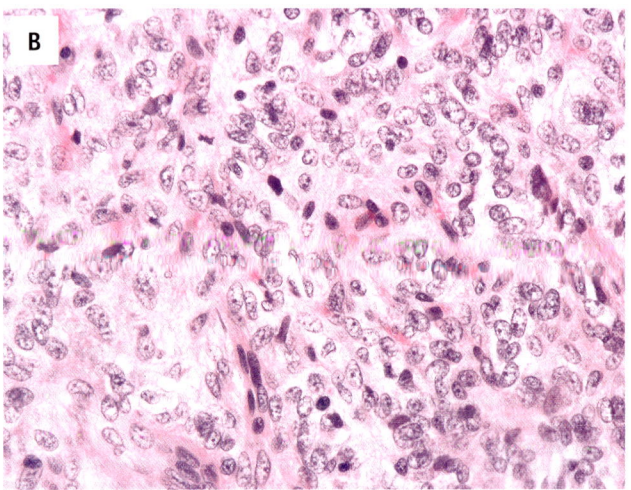

FIGURE 7-8
A, Low-power view of a malignant solitary fibrous tumor of soft tissue showing a clear transition from typical solitary fibrous tumor to much more cellular nodules. **B,** Higher-power examination of the cellular nodules shows mitotically active, malignant-appearing, round-to-spindled cells.

expression may be seen. Immunohistochemistry is usually negative for cytokeratins, desmin, and CD117.

Genetic Studies

No consistent genetic event has been described in SFT or HPC.

Differential Diagnosis

The differential diagnosis of HPC/SFT is wide and depends mainly on the location of the lesion. Classic SFT of the pleura and peritoneum may be confused with desmoplastic mesothelioma, particularly in small biopsies. Attention to the typical vascular pattern of SFT, the absence of cytological atypia, and CD34 and cytokeratin immunostains should allow relatively easy resolution of this differential diagnosis. When situated in the subcutis, HPC/SFT should be differentiated from deep fibrous histiocytoma. The latter shows a more prominent and uniform storiform growth pattern, often contains siderophages and foamy macrophages, and is negative for CD34. In deep soft tissues, cellular and malignant HPC/SFT may resemble synovial sarcoma, malignant peripheral nerve sheath tumor, or low-grade fibromyxoid sarcoma. Synovial sarcoma is almost always negative for CD34 and bears the t(X;18) SYT-SSX translocation, which is not found in SFT. Malignant peripheral nerve sheath tumors are often less circumscribed, less positive for CD34, and usually develop in contact with nerves. Low-grade fibromyxoid sarcoma is more uniform and less cellular in its appearance; it is usually less well circumscribed and does not show the HPC-like vasculature so typical of SFT. In addition, low-grade

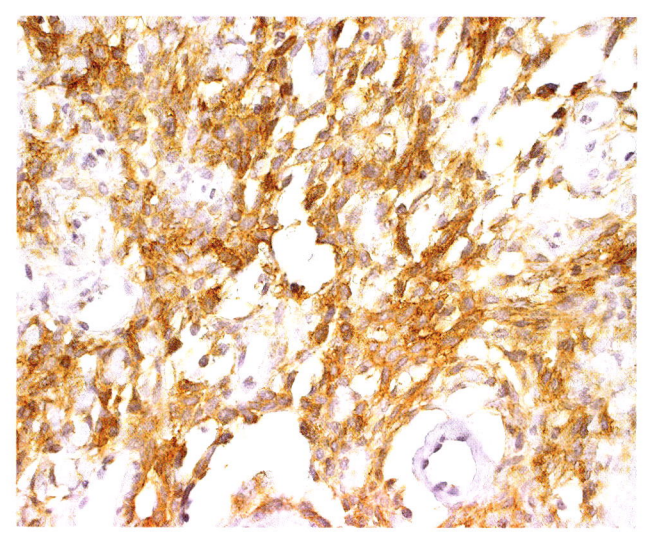

FIGURE 7-9
Solitary fibrous tumor, positive for CD34.

fibromyxoid sarcoma is never diffusely positive for CD34. Intra-abdominal HPC/SFT must be distinguished from gastrointestinal stromal tumors, a lesion that seldom shows a staghorn vascular pattern, and that expresses, in most instances, CD117 (c-kit) in addition to CD34. It is also important to remember that essentially any neoplasm may show an *HPC-like* vascular pattern, in particular, mesenchymal chondrosarcoma, endometrial stromal tumor, thymoma, and various smooth muscle tumors. Clinical history, careful sampling and histologic evaluation, and judicious application of immunostains are the keys to correctly recognizing these various HPC mimics.

Giant cell angiofibroma, which contains numerous giant cells or angiectoid spaces, or both, may be confused with giant cell fibroblastoma. Both lesions are reactive for CD34 but occur in different clinical settings and locations (giant cell fibroblastoma is a juvenile form of dermatofibrosarcoma protuberans, which occurs predominantly in proximal extremities and trunk. Lipomatous HPC should not be confused with a well-differentiated liposarcoma (including the spindle cell variant) or a dedifferentiated liposarcoma, especially if situated in the retroperitoneum. The former does not contain lipoblasts, lacks enlarged hyperchromatic cells, and is negative for

---

HEMANGIOPERICYTOMA, SOLITARY FIBROUS TUMOR OF SOFT TISSUES, AND RELATED LESIONS—FACT SHEET

Definition
- Usually benign tumor showing uncertain line of differentiation (not true microvascular pericytes)

Incidence and Location
- Rare
- Classic HPC most common in retroperitoneum and abdomen
- Classic SFT most common in thoracic cavity and abdomen
- Both may be seen in any soft tissue location
- Orbit is common location for giant-cell–rich SFT (giant cell angiofibroma)

Morbidity and Mortality
- Benign tumors may cause symptoms related to compression of local structures
- Malignant tumors grow in a locally aggressive fashion and may metastasize in 15% to 20% of cases, with death from disease

Sex, Race, and Age Distribution
- No sex predilection
- Adults

Clinical Features
- Large, nonspecific soft tissue mass
- Tumor-induced hypoglycemia in some cases

Prognosis and Treatment
- Most tumors are histologically and clinically benign, and are adequately treated with histologically complete resection
- Occasional histologically benign tumors metastasize (uncertain malignant potential)
- Histologically malignant examples metastasize in 15% to 20% of cases; require wide excision and consideration of adjuvant radiotherapy, chemotherapy, or both

---

HEMANGIOPERICYTOMA, SOLITARY FIBROUS TUMOR OF SOFT TISSUES, AND RELATED LESIONS—PATHOLOGIC FEATURES

Gross Findings
- Large soft tissue mass of deep soft tissue, mesothelial-lined surfaces, or superficial soft tissue

Microscopic Findings
- Hyalinized, branching, *staghorn* blood vessels
- Bland ovoid-to-spindled cells arranged in a *patternless* pattern
- Broad zones of collagen with cracking artifact and spindled fibroblastic zones in classic SFT
- Multinucleated giant cells (giant cell angiofibroma) and mature fat (lipomatous HPC/SFT) in some
- Malignant examples show high-nuclear-grade mitotic activity > 4/10 hpf, necrosis, hemorrhage, infiltrative growth

Immunohistochemical Findings
- Express CD34, CD99, bcl-2
- May show nuclear beta-catenin expression
- Occasionally show cytokeratin expression, more often in malignant tumors

Differential Diagnosis
- Synovial sarcoma
- Malignant peripheral nerve sheath tumor
- Low-grade fibromyxoid sarcoma
- Desmoplastic mesothelioma
- Well-differentiated liposarcoma (lipomatous HPC/SFT)
- Giant cell fibroblastoma (giant cell containing HPC/SFT)

mdm2, cdk4, or both, as opposed to well-differentiated and dedifferentiated liposarcomas.

PROGNOSIS AND TREATMENT

The prognosis of HPC/SFT is unpredictable. Most HPCs/SFTs of soft tissues behave in a benign fashion. Conversely, those located in the mediastinum, abdomen, pelvis, and/or retroperitoneum tend to be locally aggressive and may metastasize. About 10% to 15% of HPCs/SFTs metastasize, sometimes years after removal of the primary tumor, mostly to the lungs, but liver and bone can also be affected. No strict correlation exists between morphology and behavior, although lesions with small size (< 5 cm), low mitotic activity (< 4 mitoses per 10 hpf), low cellularity, and that lack cellular atypia, nuclear pleomorphism, tumor necrosis, and/or infiltrative borders seldom recur after removal. Wide surgical excision with clear margins is the treatment of choice. To date, lesions described as *giant cell angiofibroma* and *lipomatous HPC* have all behaved in an entirely benign fashion.

MYOPERICYTOMA FAMILY OF TUMORS
(Infantile Myofibromatosis, Solitary Myofibroma in infants and Adults, Infantile Hemangiopericytoma, Myopericytoma, Glomangiopericytoma)

Myopericytoma is a unifying term for a group of histologically overlapping lesions, which span a spectrum from infantile HPC (most likely representing the cellular phase of myofibroma in young children), to adult myofibroma and infantile myofibromatosis, to somewhat more glomoid-appearing lesions, termed *myopericytoma* and *glomangiopericytoma*.

CLINICAL FEATURES

Myofibromas principally occur as subcutaneous lesions, often on the head and neck. Lesions may be either solitary (in adults and children) or multiple (infantile myofibromatosis). Myofibromas are approximately twice as common in male as in female individuals. Myopericytomas present as painless masses, most often of the distal extremities, although any location may be involved. Myopericytomas and glomangiopericytomas occur most often in adults, without a sex predilection. Rare intravascular myopericytomas have been reported. Infantile HPCs occur in the first year of life and most often involve the subcutis and oral cavity.

PATHOLOGIC FEATURES

GROSS FINDINGS

Myofibromas, infantile HPCs, and myopericytomas appear grossly as nonspecific soft tissue masses. Central necrosis and calcification may be apparent in myofibroma and infantile HPC. In patients with infantile myofibromatosis, multiple lesions are present in skin, as well as bone, viscera, and deep soft tissues.

MICROSCOPIC FINDINGS

Myofibromas are distinctly zonated lesions, with peripheral hyalinized, distinctly myoid-appearing areas surrounding a core of smaller, pericyte-like cells (Figures 7-10 and 7-11). The peripheral zone may have a basophilic, vaguely chondroid appearance in some cases. The center of the nodule may show necrosis and calcification. The central zone of myofibroma (corresponding

---

MYOPERICYTOMA FAMILY OF TUMORS—FACT SHEET

Definition
- Usually benign tumors of true microvascular pericytes, related to glomus tumors

Incidence and Location
- Uncommon; myofibroma/myofibromatosis is the most common, particularly in children
- Any cutaneous, soft tissue, bone, or visceral location

Morbidity and Mortality
- Solitary myofibromas and almost all myopericytomas are benign
- Multicentric myofibromatosis with visceral involvement results in death in 75% of affected infants

Sex, Race, and Age Distribution
- Myofibromas in children are twice as common in male as female individuals
- Adult myofibromas and myopericytomas occur at any age, without a sex predilection

Clinical Features
- Multicentric myofibromatosis: multiple small lesions in skin, soft tissue, bone, viscera
- Solitary myofibroma and myopericytoma: small, solitary lesion usually in the skin

Prognosis and Treatment
- Excellent prognosis for solitary myofibroma and myopericytoma; cured with simple excision
- Solitary myofibromas in children may spontaneously regress
- Extremely rare malignant myopericytomas may show aggressive local growth
- Multicentric myofibromas in infants with visceral involvement cause death from respiratory or gastrointestinal causes in 75% of cases; low-dose chemotherapy may be of benefit

MYOPERICYTOMA FAMILY OF TUMORS—PATHOLOGIC FEATURES

Gross Findings
- Nonspecific soft tissue and skin masses
- Central necrosis and calcification may be apparent

Microscopic Findings
- Myofibroma: peripheral hyalinized, myoid-appearing spindled zone, central zone of primitive-appearing round to short spindled cells with hemangiopericytomatous vasculature, calcification, and necrosis
- Adult myofibromas may show inverted or disorganized zonation
- Infantile HPC corresponds to the central zone of myofibroma, with only minimal spindling
- Myopericytoma: myoid-appearing, short, spindled cells arranged around small blood vessels, hemangiopericytomatous vascular pattern, glomus-like areas (glomangiopericytoma)

Immunohistochemical Findings
- Positive for smooth muscle actins; negative for desmin and CD34; central zone of myofibroma is less often actin positive

Differential Diagnosis
- Infantile fibrosarcoma (highly cellular myofibroma in children/infantile HPC)
- Glomus tumor
- SFT/HPC
- Angioleiomyoma

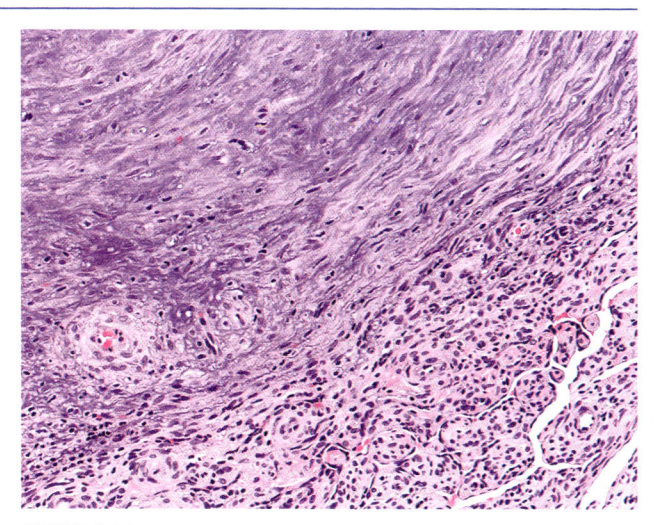

FIGURE 7-10

Adult myofibroma, showing a *reversed* pattern of zonation, with a central myoid area and a peripheral zone composed of rounder cells with a hemangiopericytomatous vascular pattern.

to infantile HPC) may be highly cellular, mitotically active and show necrosis, features that may suggest a sarcoma if one does not identify the better differentiated myoid zones. An HPC-like vascular pattern is frequently present in the central zone. Myofibromas in adults often show a "reversed" pattern of zonation, with a central rather than peripheral myoid zone, or may show a disorganized admixture of myoid and primitive-appearing areas. All myofibromas may show extension into small blood vessels at the periphery of the lesion. Myopericytoma and glomangiopericytoma are best thought of as lesions that have hybrid features somewhere between myofibroma and glomus tumor. These lesions are typically composed of distinctly myoid-appearing, short, eosinophilic, spindled cells, which are arranged around an HPC-like vasculature. *Myoid balls,* reminiscent of the myoid zones in myofibroma, are often present, as are distinctive areas of concentric perivascular growth (Figures 7-12 and 7-13). In some cases, the cells are more glomoid (corresponding to *glomangiopericytoma*), and the histologic features of these cases overlap significantly with glomangiomyoma.

A small number of myopericytomas have been reported to show histologic features of malignancy, including cytological atypia, high mitotic activity, and aggressive invasion of surrounding tissues. The histologic features of such lesions overlap to a significant degree with those of malignant glomus tumors.

ANCILLARY STUDIES

IMMUNOHISTOCHEMISTRY

The peripheral zone of myofibromas and all of the lesional cells of myopericytoma/glomangiopericytoma are strongly smooth muscle actin positive, and typically negative for desmin and CD34. The central zone of myofibroma and infantile HPCs are less often actin positive. CD34 is negative in these areas as well.

GENETICS

No consistent genetic abnormality has been identified.

DIFFERENTIAL DIAGNOSIS

Highly cellular myofibromas and infantile HPCs may be mistaken for other primitive sarcomas, in particular, infantile fibrosarcoma. Although infantile fibrosarcoma may show an HPC-like vascular pattern, it is composed of more spindled, cytologically atypical cells, often with numerous interspersed lymphocytes. Genetic study for the *ETV-NTRK6* fusion gene may be helpful in excluding infantile fibrosarcoma in selected cases. In general, careful inspection of highly cellular myofibromas and infantile HPCs will reveal small peripheral zones of bland, myoid-appearing cells, a reassuring feature. Myopericytomas may closely resemble angioleiomyomas,

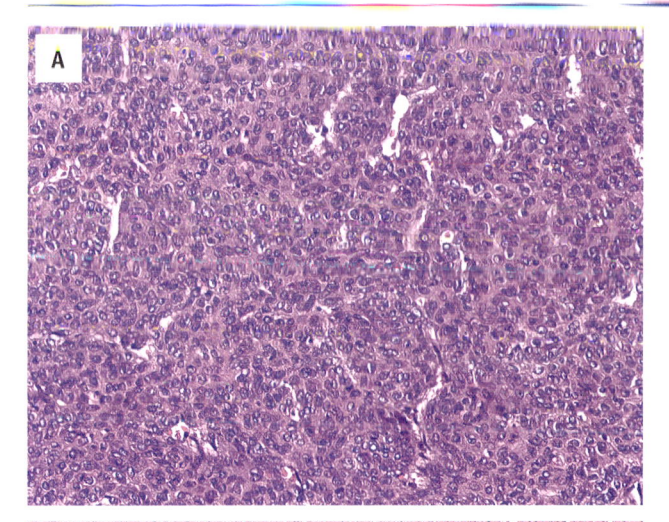

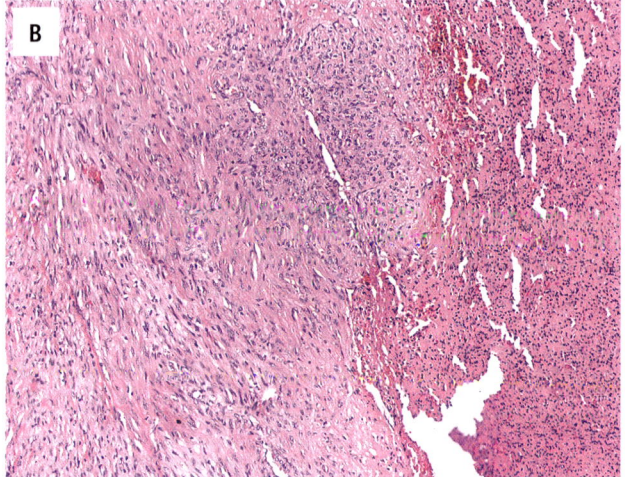

FIGURE 7-11
A, Central zone in infantile myofibroma showing primitive-appearing cells arranged around a branching vasculature. So-called infantile hemangiopericytomas most likely represent myofibromas with predominance of these areas. **B,** Other areas in this tumor showed fascicles of myoid-appearing spindled cells and necrosis, characteristic features of myofibroma.

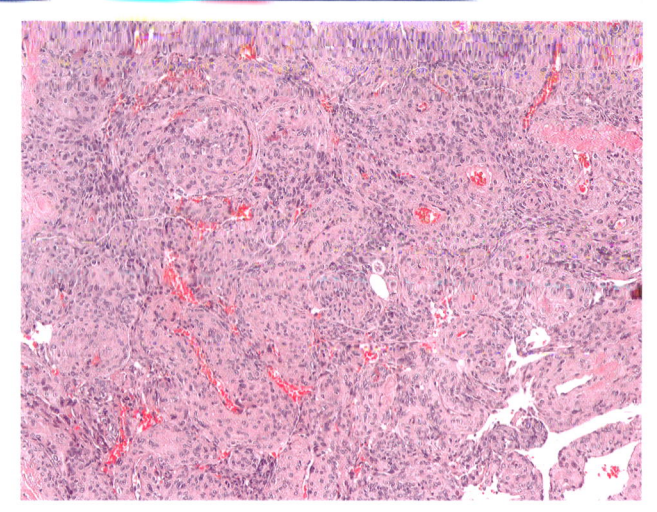

FIGURE 7-12
Myopericytoma showing a cellular proliferation of myoid-appearing spindled cells around many small vessels.

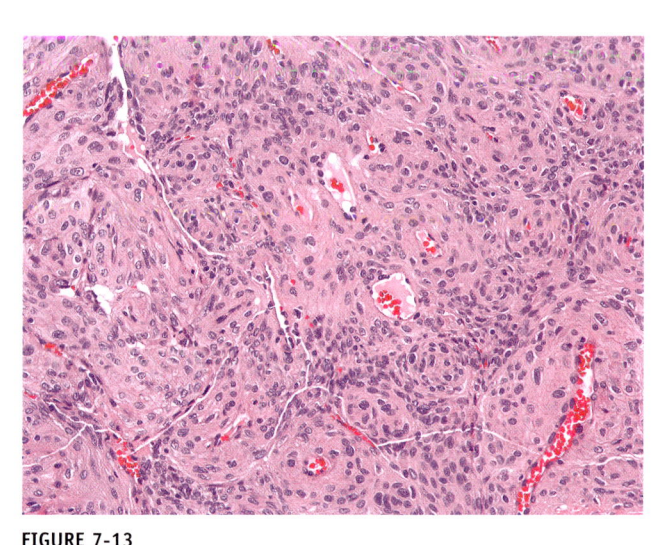

FIGURE 7-13
Concentric perivascular growth in myopericytoma.

although they tend to lack the distinctive thick-walled blood vessel seen in the latter lesion and are composed, in part, of smaller, more glomoid-appearing cells. The distinction between these two benign lesions may, at times, be arbitrary. Similarly, the distinction between myopericytomas with only small areas of spindled growth and glomus tumors that show smooth muscle differentiation (glomangiomyoma) may be difficult, if not impossible.

Prognosis and Treatment

Solitary myofibromas and multiple myofibromas confined to soft tissue and bone have an excellent prognosis, with many lesions regressing spontaneously and others requiring little more than simple excision. Infants with multiple visceral myofibromas have a much more guarded prognosis, with death from respiratory or gastrointestinal causes in up to 75% of affected patients. Low-dose chemotherapy has shown some value in the treatment of infants with multiple visceral myofibromas. Solitary (adult) myofibromas are entirely benign and require only simple excision. Most myopericytomas and glomangiopericytomas are histologically and clinically benign, and are treated with simple excision. Rare malignant myopericytomas have behaved as low grade sarcomas, and require more extensive surgery, possibly with adjuvant radiotherapy.

GLOMUS TUMORS (Solid Glomus Tumor, Glomangioma, Glomangiomyoma, Symplastic Glomus Tumor, Glomus Tumor of Uncertain Malignant Potential, Malignant Glomus Tumor/Glomangiosarcoma)

CLINICAL FEATURES

Glomus tumors typically occur in young adults but may occur at any age. No sex predilection is seen, except in subungual lesions, which are far more common in women. Glomus tumors almost always occur in the skin or superficial soft tissues of the distal extremities, although rare cases occur in deep soft tissue or viscera. Superficially located glomus tumors often present with paroxysms of pain radiating away from the lesion; these symptoms are often exacerbated by changes in temperature, in particular, exposure to cold. Deeply seated glomus tumors typically have no associated symptoms. Glomuvenous malformations (glomangiomas) usually occur in children as nonpainful masses of the distal extremities.

PATHOLOGIC FEATURES

GROSS FINDINGS

Glomus tumors usually present as small (< 1 cm) red-blue nodules in the skin and superficial soft tissues. Subungual glomus tumors may appear as areas of discoloration of the nail bed. Visceral glomus tumors appear as a nonspecific soft tissue mass.

MICROSCOPIC FINDINGS

Typical glomus tumors are subcategorized as *solid glomus tumor*, *glomuvenous malformation (glomangioma)*, and *glomangiomyoma*, depending on the relative prominence of glomus cells, vascular structures, and smooth muscle. Glomus cells are small, uniform, rounded cells with a centrally placed, round nucleus and amphophilic to lightly eosinophilic cytoplasm (Figure 7-14). Each cell is surrounded by basal lamina, seen best on PAS or toluidine blue histochemical stains. Solid glomus tumors are the most common variant, comprising approximately 75% of cases. They are composed of nests of glomus cells surrounding capillary-sized vessels. The stroma may show hyalinization or myxoid change (Figure 7-15). Small cuffs of glomus cells are often seen around small vessels located outside of the main mass. Glomuvenous malformations, previously termed *glomangiomas*, are characterized by a somewhat poorly circumscribed proliferation of cavernous hemangioma-like vascular

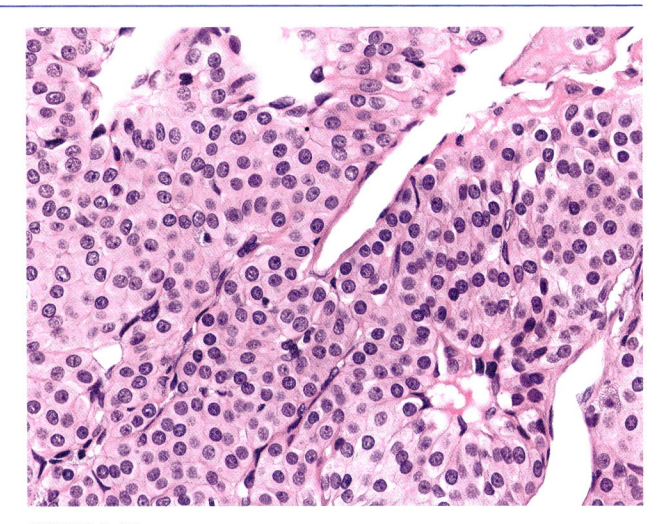

FIGURE 7-14
Typical glomus cells with well-defined cell borders and round, regular nuclei with indistinct nucleoli.

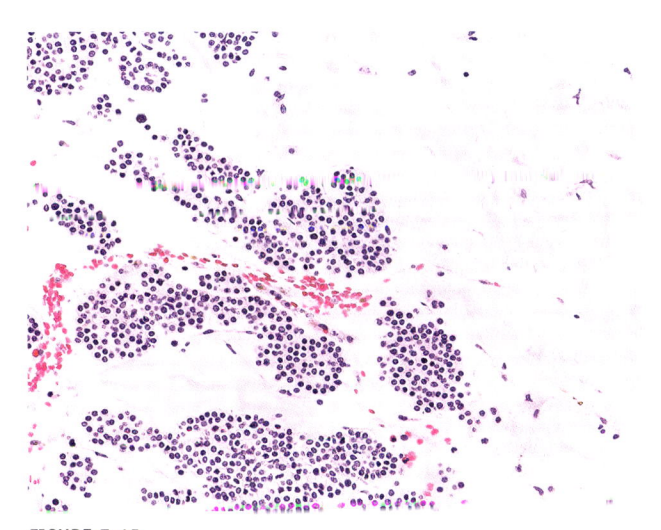

FIGURE 7-15
Hyalinization in a glomus tumor.

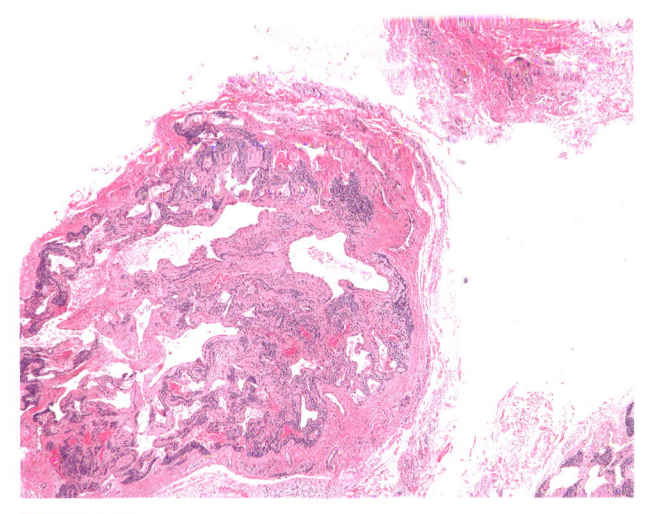

FIGURE 7-16
Glomuvenous malformation (glomangioma), consisting of a well-circumscribed, cavernous hemangioma-like nodule, with perivascular glomus cell proliferation.

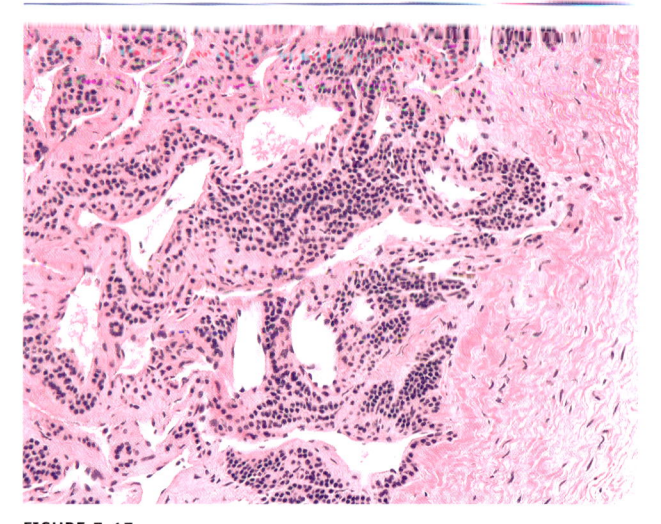

FIGURE 7-17
Higher-power view (compared with Figure 7-16) of glomus cell clustered about thick-walled vessels in glomuvenous malformation.

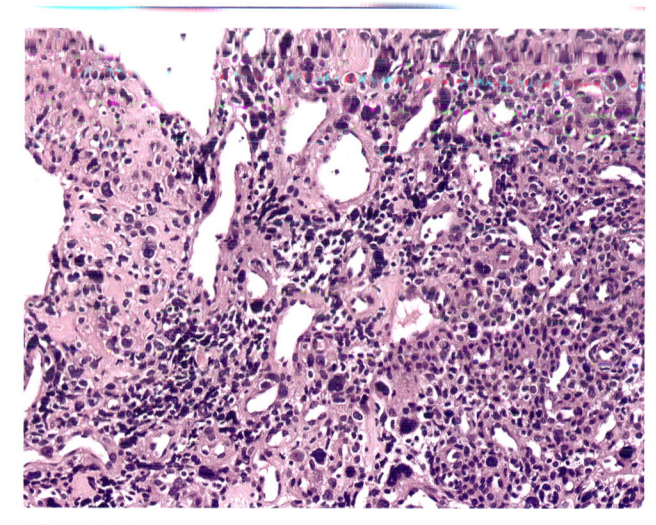

FIGURE 7-19
Symplastic glomus tumor, showing bizarre-appearing giant cells with hyperchromatic nuclei, in a background of typical glomus tumor.

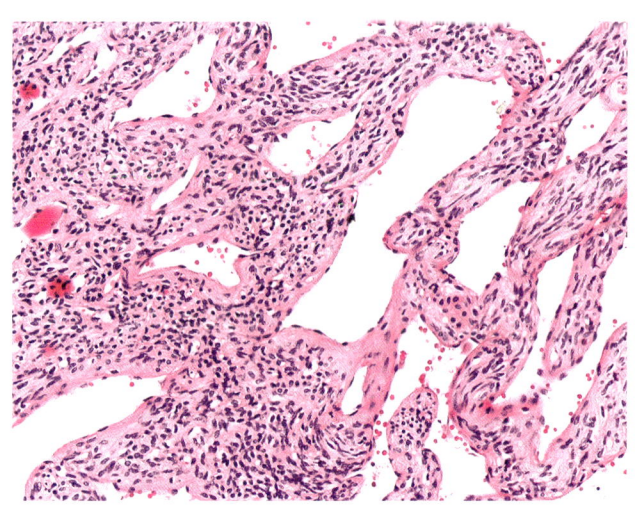

FIGURE 7-18
Glomus tumor with smooth muscle differentiation (glomangiomyoma).

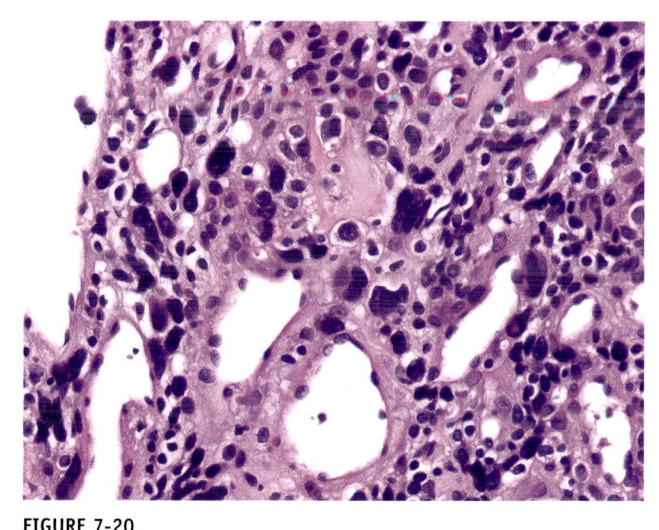

FIGURE 7-20
Hyperchromatic giant cells in *symplastic* glomus tumor.

channels surrounded by small clusters of glomus cells (Figures 7-16 and 7-17). Glomangiomyomas are characterized by a transition from typical glomus cells to elongated cells resembling mature smooth muscle (Figure 7-18).

Rare glomus tumors show striking nuclear atypia in the absence of any other worrisome feature *(symplastic glomus tumor)* (Figures 7-19 and 7-20). The marked nuclear atypia that characterizes these tumors is believed to be a degenerative phenomenon. All cases reported to date have behaved in a benign fashion. Although a single mitotic figure may occasionally be identified in a symplastic glomus tumor, the overall rate should be extremely low (< 1/50 hpf).

ATYPICAL AND MALIGNANT GLOMUS TUMORS

Table 7-1 presents a classification scheme for atypical glomus tumors. Histologically or clinically malignant glomus tumors, or both, are exceedingly rare. Two types of malignant glomus tumors exist. In the first type, a component of preexisting benign glomus tumor is present, often at the periphery of a larger nodule of cytologically atypical, mitotically active, spindle cell sarcoma, which resembles leiomyosarcoma or fibrosarcoma (Figures 7-21 and 7-22). The second type of malignant glomus tumor most often lacks a clear-cut benign component; in this variant, the malignant component retains an overall architectural similarity to benign glomus tumor and

CHAPTER 7 Tumor of Perivascular Cells

TABLE 7-1
Classification of Atypical Glomus Tumors

Category	Criteria
Malignant glomus tumor	High nuclear grade plus mitotic activity *or* Atypical mitotic figures
Symplastic glomus tumor	Marked nuclear atypia alone
Glomus tumor of uncertain malignant potential	Tumors not fulfilling criteria for malignancy but having at least one atypical feature other than pleomorphism (e.g., large size and deep location, without atypia or mitotic activity)

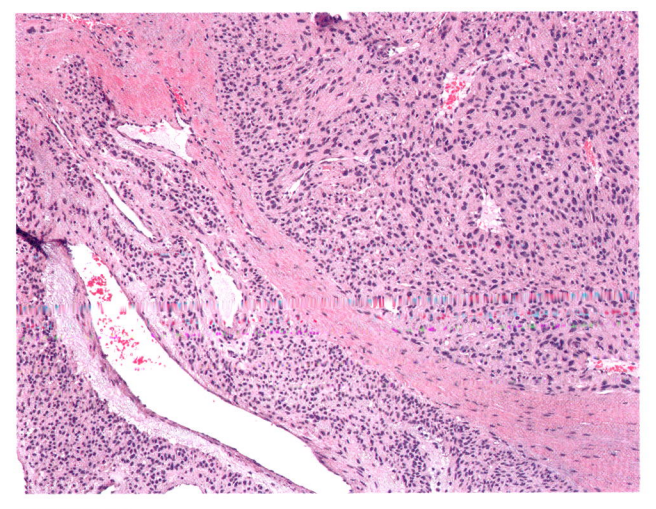

FIGURE 7-21
Malignant glomus tumor showing a clear transition from typical glomus tumor (bottom left) and leiomyosarcoma-like malignant glomus tumor (upper right).

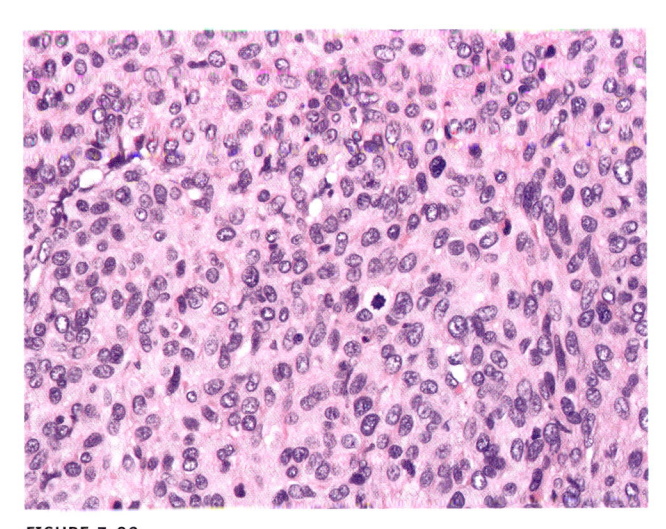

FIGURE 7-22
Malignant-appearing, mitotically active, round to spindled cells in malignant glomus tumor.

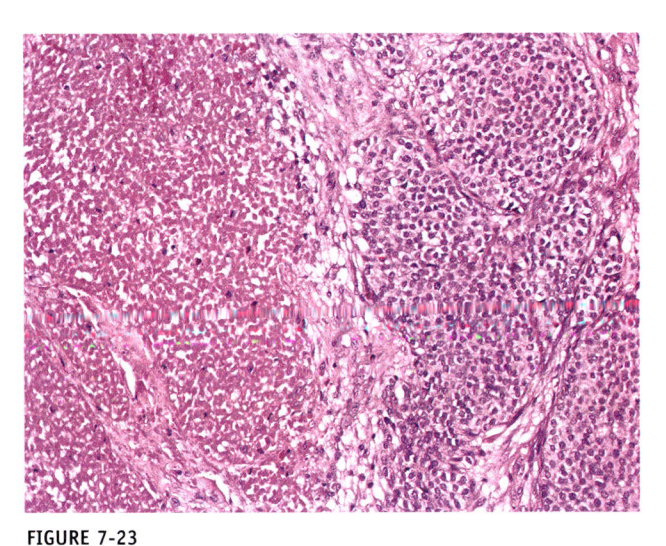

FIGURE 7-23
Round cell pattern and necrosis in a malignant glomus tumor.

consists of sheets of highly malignant-appearing round cells, which by immunohistochemistry express smooth muscle actin and pericellular type IV collagen, but not desmin, cytokeratins, or S-100 protein (Figure 7-23). Glomus tumors that do not fulfill criteria for malignancy, but have at least one atypical feature other than nuclear pleomorphism, should be diagnosed as *glomus tumors of uncertain malignant potential.*

ANCILLARY STUDIES

IMMUNOHISTOCHEMISTRY

Glomus tumors of all types typically express smooth muscle actin and have abundant pericellular type IV collagen production. Desmin and CD34 are usually negative.

GENETICS

Multiple inherited glomuvenous malformations are caused by mutations in the glomulin gene located on chromosome 1p21-22. Glomulin is a normal component

GLOMUS TUMORS—FACT SHEET

Definition
- Mesenchymal tumors that differentiate along the lines of glomus cells, modified smooth muscle cells with a thermoregulatory function

Incidence and Location
- Uncommon
- Most common in skin; extremely rare tumors in deep soft tissue and viscera

Morbidity and Mortality
- Overwhelming majority of glomus tumors are benign
- Extremely rare histologically malignant examples behave as high-grade sarcomas with aggressive local recurrence and distant metastases

Sex, Race, and Age Distribution
- Subungual glomus tumors are far more common in women
- Other glomus tumors usually occur in young adults, without sex predilection
- Glomuvenous malformations (glomangiomas) occur in children

Clinical Features
- Cutaneous and subungual tumors frequently present with pain and cold sensitivity
- Deeply seated and visceral glomus tumors are usually asymptomatic
- Cutaneous and subungual tumors appear as small red-blue nodules or discoloration under the nail bed

Prognosis and Treatment
- Benign glomus tumors and glomuvenous malformations are benign and require only excision
- Rare malignant glomus tumors may metastasize in up to 40% of cases and should be treated as high-grade sarcomas, akin to leiomyosarcomas
- Rare large and deep/visceral glomus tumors have uncertain malignant potential and should be completely resected and the patients followed closely for lung metastases

GLOMUS TUMORS—PATHOLOGIC FEATURES

Gross Findings
- Red-blue cutaneous nodule
- Deeply seated tumors appear as nonspecific masses

Microscopic Findings
- Uniform round cells with well-defined cell borders and centrally placed, round nuclei
- Accentuated perivascular cellularity
- Variably prominent vascular pattern, often HPC-like
- Cells may occasionally spindle and resemble smooth muscle (glomangiomyoma)
- May be hyalinized or myxoid
- Glomuvenous malformations (glomangiomas) have a low-power architecture reminiscent of cavernous hemangioma, surrounded by clusters of glomus cells
- "Symplastic" glomus tumors show striking degenerative cytologic atypia in the absence of other worrisome features (e.g., large size, mitotic activity, necrosis)
- Malignant glomus tumors show high-nuclear-grade and mitotic activity with atypical forms, often with spindling (leiomyosarcoma-like)

Immunohistochemical Findings
- Positive for smooth muscle actin and pericellular collagen type IV
- Negative for desmin and CD34

Differential Diagnosis
- Myopericytic tumors
- HPC/SFT
- Other round cell sarcomas and spindle cell sarcomas (malignant glomus tumors)

---

of vascular smooth muscle during embryogenesis. The genetic events underlying sporadic glomus tumors are not known.

DIFFERENTIAL DIAGNOSIS

The distinction of glomus tumors from tumors in the myopericytoma family of tumors is discussed earlier. It is likely that myopericytic and glomus tumors form a morphologic spectrum, and the distinction of these tumors may, at times, be arbitrary. SFTs/HPCs are typically larger and more deeply situated, consist of ovoid to spindled, rather than round cells, and are CD34 positive and smooth muscle actin negative. Malignant glomus tumors may be confused with spindle cell sarcomas, such as leiomyosarcoma, when they exhibit spindled growth, or with round cell sarcomas, when they consist entirely of malignant glomus cells with round cell morphology. Identification of areas of more typical glomus tumor and demonstration of the typical glomus cell immunophenotype are the keys to these differential diagnoses.

PROGNOSIS AND TREATMENT

Histologically benign glomus tumors and glomus tumor variants are benign neoplasms that require only simple excision. Symplastic glomus tumors also require only simple excision. Glomus tumors of uncertain malignant potential should be resected with histologically negative margins and the patients followed closely for evidence of lung metastases. Histologically malignant glomus tumors are highly aggressive with metastases in approximately 40% of cases, resulting in the death of the patient. These should most likely be managed as one would a conventional leiomyosarcoma of equivalent stage and grade.

SUGGESTED READINGS

Hemangiopericytoma, Solitary Fibrous Tumor of Soft Tissues, and Related Lesions

1. Angervall L, Kindblom LG, Nielsen JM, et al: Hemangiopericytoma: A clinicopathologic, angiographic and microangiographic study. Cancer 1978;42:2412-2427.
2. Dei Tos AP, Seregard S, Calonje E, et al: Giant cell angiofibroma. A distinctive orbital tumor in adults. Am J Surg Pathol 1995;19:1286-1293.
3. England DM, Hochholzer L, McCarthy MJ: Localized benign and malignant fibrous tumors of the pleura. A clinicopathologic review of 223 cases. Am J Surg Pathol 1989;13:640-658.
4. Enzinger FM, Smith BH: Hemangiopericytoma. An analysis of 106 cases. Hum Pathol 1976;7:61-82.
5. Espat NJ, Lewis JJ, Leung D, et al: Conventional hemangiopericytoma: Modern analysis of outcome. Cancer 2002;95:1746-1751.
6. Folpe AL, Devaney K, Weiss SW: Lipomatous hemangiopericytoma: A rare variant of hemangiopericytoma that may be confused with liposarcoma. Am J Surg Pathol 1999;23:1201-1207.
7. Gold JS, Antonescu CR, Hajdu J, et al: Clinicopathologic correlates of solitary fibrous tumors. Cancer 2002;94:1057-1068.
8. Guillou L, Gebhard S, Coindre JM: Orbital and extraorbital giant cell angiofibroma: A giant cell-rich variant of solitary fibrous tumor? Clinicopathologic and immunohistochemical analysis of a series in favor of a unifying concept. Am J Surg Pathol 2000;24:971-979.
9. Moran CA, Suster S, Koss MN: The spectrum of histologic growth patterns in benign and malignant fibrous tumors of the pleura. Semin Diagn Pathol 1992;9:169-180.
10. Nappi O, Ritter JH, Pettinato G, et al: Hemangiopericytoma: Histopathological pattern or clinicopathologic entity? Semin Diagn Pathol 1995;12:221-232.
11. Nielsen GP, O'Connell JX, Dickersin GR, et al: Solitary fibrous tumor of soft tissue: A report of 15 cases, including 5 malignant examples with light microscopic, immunohistochemical, and ultrastructural data. Mod Pathol 1997;10:1028-1037.
12. Suster S, Nascimento AG, Miettinen M, et al: Solitary fibrous tumors of soft tissue. A clinicopathologic and immunohistochemical study of 12 cases. Am J Surg Pathol 1995;19:1257-1266.
13. Vallat-Decouvelaere AV, Dry SM, Fletcher CD: Atypical and malignant solitary fibrous tumors in extrathoracic locations: Evidence of their comparability to intra-thoracic tumors. Am J Surg Pathol 1998;22:1501-1511.

Myopericytoma Family of Tumors

1. Dray MS, McCarthy SW, Palmer AA, et al: Myopericytoma: A unifying term for a spectrum of tumours that show overlapping features with myofibroma. A review of 14 cases. J Clin Pathol 2006;59:67-73.
2. Granter SR, Badizadegan K, Fletcher CD: Myofibromatosis in adults, glomangiopericytoma, and myopericytoma: a spectrum of tumors showing perivascular myoid differentiation. Am J Surg Pathol 1998;22:513-525.
3. Matsuyama A, Hisaoka M, Hashimoto H: Angioleiomyoma: A clinicopathologic and immunohistochemical reappraisal with special reference to the correlation with myopericytoma. Hum Pathol 2007;38:645-651.
4. McMenamin ME, Calonje E: Intravascular myopericytoma. J Cutan Pathol 2002;29:557-561.
5. McMenamin ME, Fletcher CD: Malignant myopericytoma: Expanding the spectrum of tumours with myopericytic differentiation. Histopathology 2002;41:450-460.
6. Mentzel T, Dei Tos AP, Sapi Z, et al: Myopericytoma of skin and soft tissues: Clinicopathologic and immunohistochemical study of 54 cases. Am J Surg Pathol 2006;30:104-113.

Glomus Tumors

1. Boon LM, Mulliken JB, Enjolras O, et al: Glomuvenous malformation (glomangioma) and venous malformation: Distinct clinicopathologic and genetic entities. Arch Dermatol 2004;140:971-976.
2. Brouillard P, Ghassibe M, Penington A, et al: Four common glomulin mutations cause two thirds of glomuvenous malformations (familial glomangiomas): Evidence for a founder effect. J Med Genet 2005;42:e13.
3. Folpe AL, Fanburg-Smith JC, Miettinen M, et al: Atypical and malignant glomus tumors: Analysis of 52 cases, with a proposal for the reclassification of glomus tumors. Am J Surg Pathol 2001;25:1-12.
4. Gaertner EM, Steinberg DM, Huber M, et al: Pulmonary and mediastinal glomus tumors—report of five cases including a pulmonary glomangiosarcoma: A clinicopathologic study with literature review. Am J Surg Pathol 2000;24:1105-1114.
5. Gould EW, Manivel JC, Albores-Saavedra J, et al: Locally infiltrative glomus tumors and glomangiosarcomas. A clinical, ultrastructural, and immunohistochemical study. Cancer 1990;65:310-318.
6. Henning JS, Kovich OI, Schaffer JV: Glomuvenous malformations. Dermatol Online J 2007;13:17.
7. Hiruta N, Kameda N, Tokudome T, et al: Malignant glomus tumor: A case report and review of the literature. Am J Surg Pathol 1997;21:1096-1103.
8. Mayr-Kanhauser S, Behmel A, Aberer W: Multiple glomus tumors of the skin with male-to-male transmission over four generations. J Invest Dermatol 2001;116:475-476.
9. Nuovo M, Grimes M, Knowles D: Glomus tumors: A clinicopathologic and immunohistochemical analysis of forty cases. Surg Pathol 1990;3:31-45.
10. Van Geertruyden J, Lorea P, Goldschmidt D, et al: Glomus tumours of the hand. A retrospective study of 51 cases. J Hand Surg [Br] 1996;21:257-260.
11. Velasco A, Palomar-Asenjo V, Ganan L, et al: Mutation analysis of the SDHD gene in four kindreds with familial paraganglioma: Description of one novel germline mutation. Diagn Mol Pathol 2005;14:109-114.
12. Watanabe K, Sugino T, Saito A, et al: Glomangiosarcoma of the hip: report of a highly aggressive tumour with widespread distant metastases. Br J Dermatol 1998;139:1097-1101.
13. Wetherington RW, Lyle WG, Sangueza OP: Malignant glomus tumor of the thumb: A case report. J Hand Surg [Am] 1997;22:1098-1102.

8

Gastrointestinal Stromal Tumor

Brian P. Rubin

Gastrointestinal stromal tumor (GIST) is the most common mesenchymal tumor of the gastrointestinal tract. Tremendous progress has been made in understanding the molecular pathogenesis of GIST. This has resulted in an improved ability to diagnose and prognosticate GIST, as well as the development of two effective targeted therapies, imatinib mesylate and sunitinib maleate. This chapter highlights these recent developments.

CLINICAL FEATURES

GISTs tend to arise predominantly in middle-aged to older adults with a median age of 58 years. They are slightly more common in men. Approximately 60% arise in the stomach, and 30% arise in the small bowel; the other 10% arise in the esophagus, colon, rectum, gallbladder, appendix, omentum, mesentery, retroperitoneum, and pelvis. Those GISTs that arise in the omentum, mesentery, retroperitoneum, and pelvis are collectively known as extragastrointestinal stromal tumors. Presenting symptoms include anemia or fatigue, or both, caused by ulceration and bleeding, abdominal pain, early satiety or fullness, or abdominal distension. Occasionally, GISTs are discovered incidentally during or after surgery for other reasons such as esophagogastrectomy for esophageal carcinoma. A small subset of GISTs occurs in pediatric patients, predominantly in the setting of Carney's triad (gastric GIST, extra-adrenal paraganglioma, and pulmonary chondroma). Patients with type I neurofibromatosis also have an increased risk for the development of GIST.

RADIOLOGIC FEATURES

Computed tomography (CT) and magnetic resonance imaging (MRI) identify GISTs, and allow preoperative determination of size and involvement of other structures. These modalities are also useful in identifying metastatic lesions. Positron emission tomographic scans have been of particular interest in GISTs because they have been used to monitor response to therapy with imatinib mesylate (see p. 163). Finally, endoscopic ultrasound is being used increasingly to identify GISTs, because this technique is able to localize the lesion within the wall of the gastrointestinal tract. All of these imaging techniques allow localization of lesions for core needle biopsy or fine-needle aspiration (FNA).

PATHOLOGIC FEATURES

GROSS FINDINGS

GISTs arise most commonly from the gastrointestinal wall and are unilobular or multilobular with smooth, circumscribed borders (Figure 8-1). They can protrude inward, leading to ulceration of the mucosa, or outward, resulting in predominantly serosal-based lesions. Occasionally, GISTs can be pedunculated. Some tumors protrude in both directions, resulting in a characteristic dumbbell configuration. The cut surface is fleshy and often cystic. Necrosis, hemorrhage, or both are common.

MICROSCOPIC FINDINGS

GISTs are composed of either epithelioid or spindle-shaped cells. Many cases have combined epithelioid and spindle cell cytomorphologies. Epithelioid GISTs can exhibit either a sheet-like or nested growth pattern (Figure 8-2), whereas spindle cell GISTs tend to adopt a fascicular arrangement of the neoplastic cells (Figure 8-3). Cytologically, GISTs have round-to-elongated nuclei with fine chromatin, inconspicuous nucleoli, and abundant fibrillary cytoplasm (Figure 8-4). Cardinal diagnostic features of GIST include lack of cytologic pleomorphism and low mitotic rate. These features are so consistent that the presence of pleomorphism or a high mitotic rate, or both, should lead to a re-evaluation of the diagnosis of GIST. GISTs frequently exhibit paranuclear vacuoles; sometimes these can be prominent (Figure 8-5). Spindle cell GISTs can show prominent nuclear palisading that mimics schwannoma (Figure 8-6). A small subset of GISTs has acellular collagen bundles known as *skeinoid* fibers that are positive by PAS staining (Figure 8-7), and occasional cases have scattered lymphocytes admixed with the lesional cells. GISTs can exhibit a variety of

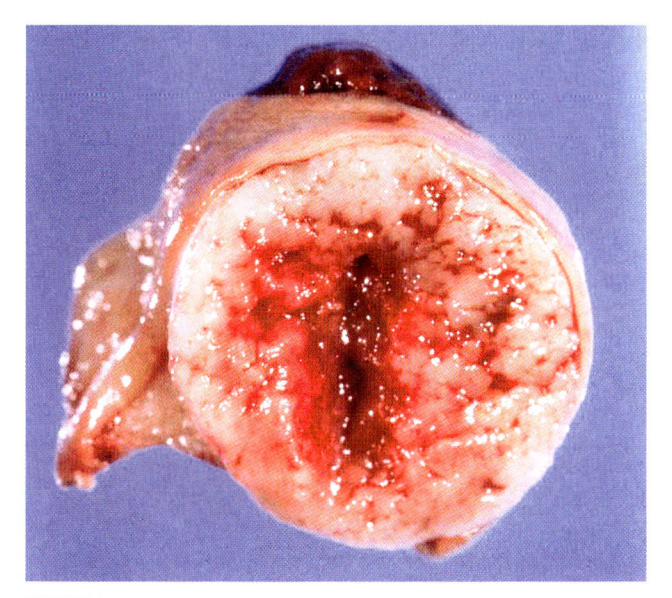

FIGURE 8-1
Gross appearance of gastrointestinal stromal tumor (GIST).
Gross specimen showing a well-circumscribed nodule with a fleshy appearance and central hemorrhage and cyst formation. Note the overlying ulcerated mucosa at the top.

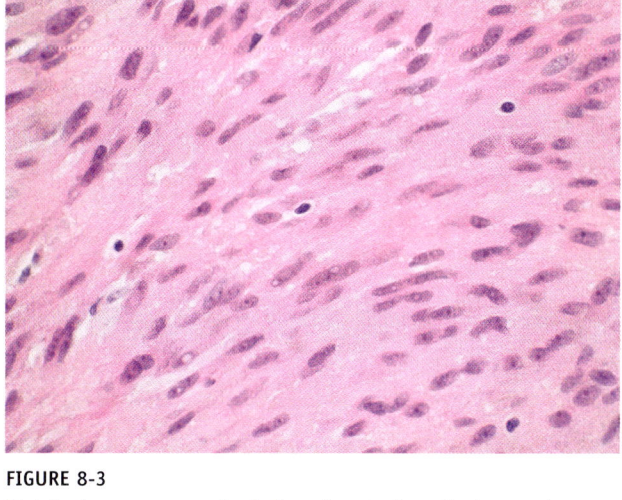

FIGURE 8-3
Histologic appearance of spindle cell gastrointestinal stromal tumor (GIST).
A relatively hypocellular example of a spindle cell GIST with spindle-shaped cells arranged in fascicles. The constituent cells are monomorphic and lack mitotic activity.

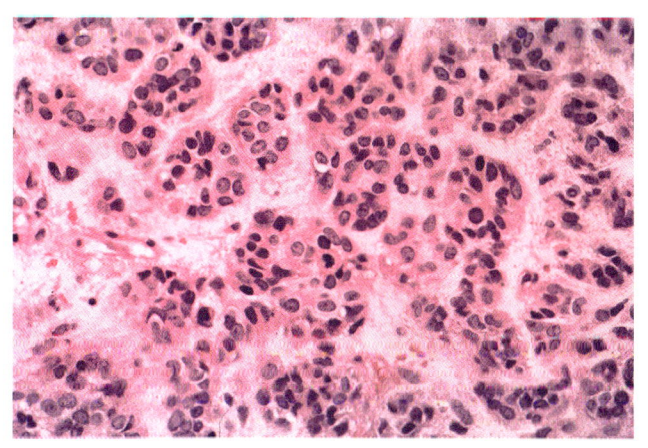

FIGURE 8-2
Histologic appearance of epithelioid gastrointestinal stromal tumor (GIST).
Epithelioid GIST with a nested architectural pattern. Other epithelioid gastrointestinal stromal tumors exhibit a sheet-like growth pattern.

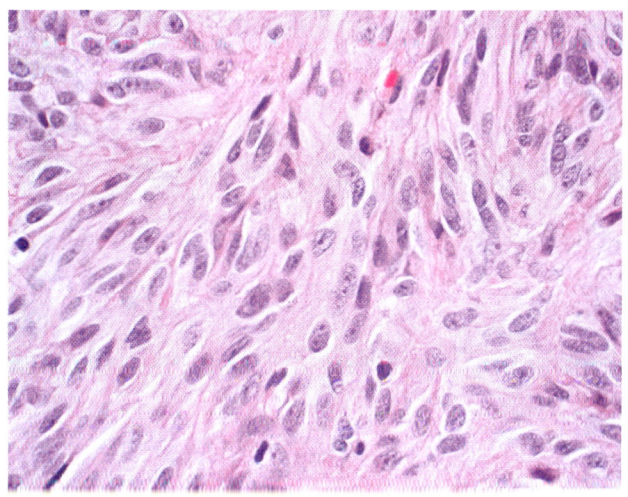

FIGURE 8-4
Gastrointestinal stromal tumor (GIST): Fibrillary cytoplasm.
Note the fibrillary cytoplasm in this cellular spindle cell GIST. The cells have fine chromatin and inconspicuous nucleoli.

vascular patterns ranging from inconspicuous to those lesions with prominent staghorn (hemangiopericytomatous) vessels. The stroma is usually hyalinized but can be edematous and rarely myxoid.

ANCILLARY STUDIES

ULTRASTRUCTURAL FEATURES

Currently, ultrastructural analysis does not play an important role in the diagnosis of GIST. Ultrastructural analysis reveals a variety of features including a relative lack of differentiation to those lesions with incomplete smooth muscle differentiation or neuraxonal differentiation. Importantly, GISTs lack the bundles of actin filaments that are characteristic of true smooth muscle tumors. Although a subset of GISTs previously known as gastrointestinal autonomic tumors (GANTs) were originally defined by ultrastructural analysis as possessing neuraxonal differentiation as defined by bulbous synapse-like structures and interdigitating processes, it is now believed that GANT is part of the spectrum of GIST, and there is no need to subclassify GANTs because they do not possess any meaningful clinicopathologic differences from GISTs.

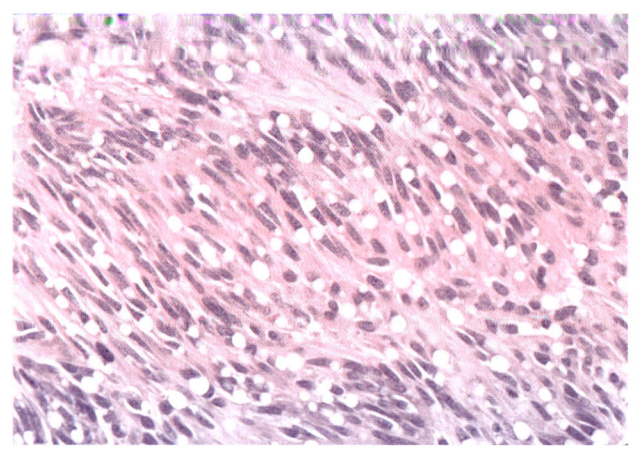

FIGURE 8-5
Gastrointestinal stromal tumor (GIST) with vacuolated cytoplasm.
It is not unusual to find GISTs with striking cytoplasmic vacuolization. This feature was previously thought to be more characteristic of smooth muscle tumors.

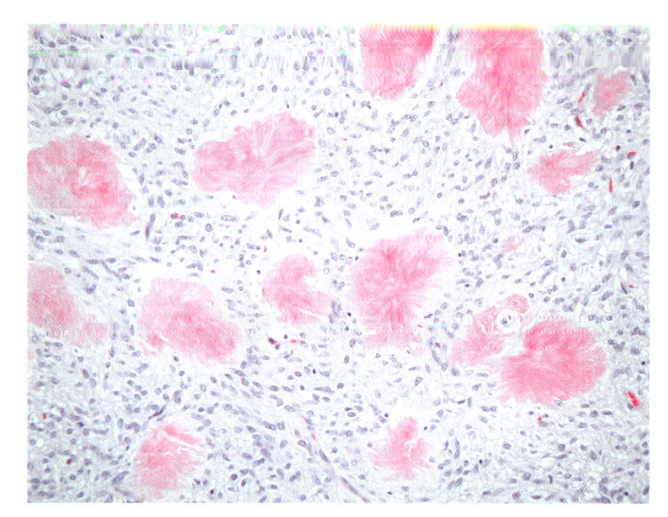

FIGURE 8-7
***Skeinoid* fibers in gastrointestinal stromal tumor (GIST).**
Some GISTs contain acellular collagen bundles known as *skeinoid* fibers, which are particularly prominent in this unusual example.

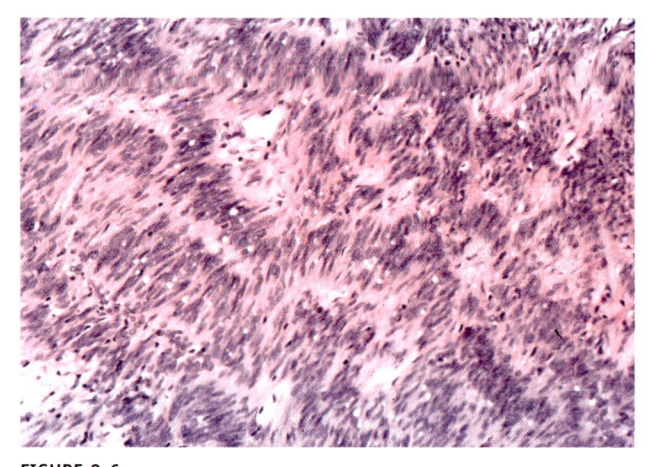

FIGURE 8-6
Gastrointestinal stromal tumor (GIST) with prominent palisading.
Many GISTs exhibit extensive palisading and can mimic schwannoma. Immunohistochemistry for S-100 protein is useful in distinguishing GIST from schwannoma because it fails to exhibit immunoreactivity for S-100 protein.

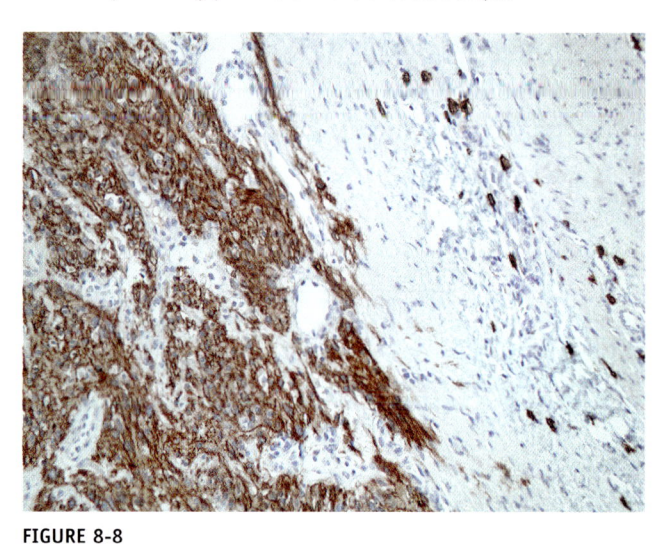

FIGURE 8-8
KIT(CD117) staining in gastrointestinal stromal tumor (GIST).
KIT (CD117) is positive in approximately 95% of GISTs. Most GISTs are diffusely and strongly positive for KIT. Note the isolated mast cells on the right side of the figure. These serve as an excellent internal immunohistochemical control because mast cells are usually found adjacent to most GISTs and are invariably positive for KIT.

IMMUNOHISTOCHEMISTRY

GISTs are positive for KIT (CD117) (95%) (Figure 8-8), CD34 (75%), and smooth muscle actin (40%). They are virtually always negative for S-100 protein and desmin. KIT staining is usually diffuse, strong, and cytoplasmic or membranous but can also exhibit a paranuclear globular staining pattern. Approximately 5% of GISTs is negative for KIT. The majority of these are epithelioid gastric GISTs with *PDGFRA* mutations. These cases should be referred to an expert consultant pathologist for verification.

CYTOGENETICS

GISTs have a characteristic cytogenetic profile that most commonly contains loss of chromosomes 14 and 22 and loss of material from the short arm of chromosome 1 (Figure 8-9). Loss of material from the short arm of chromosomes 9 and 11 is seen less often and is associated with clinically aggressive GISTs.

DNA SEQUENCING

Approximately 80% to 90% of GISTs contain activating *KIT* or *PDGFRA* mutations. DNA sequencing can be used to verify the diagnosis in difficult cases such as KIT immunohistochemistry-negative GIST. Currently, mutational analysis for *KIT* and *PDGFRA* is strongly encouraged if imatinib therapy is initiated for unresectable or metastatic disease. Mutational analysis can be considered for patients with primary disease, particularly those with high-risk tumors.

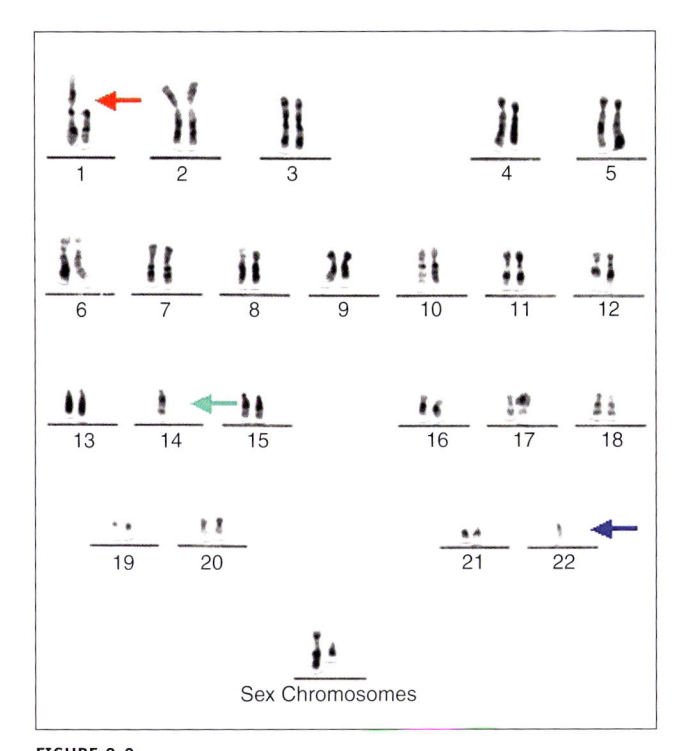

CHAPTER 8 Gastrointestinal Stromal Tumor

FIGURE 8-9
Cytogenetic profile of gastrointestinal stromal tumor (GIST).
Loss of material from the short arm of chromosome 1 *(red arrow)* and monosomy for chromosomes 14 *(green arrow)* and 22 *(blue arrow)* are the most common cytogenetic findings in GIST. Loss of material from the short arm of chromosomes 9 and 11 is less common and is associated with aggressive clinical behavior.

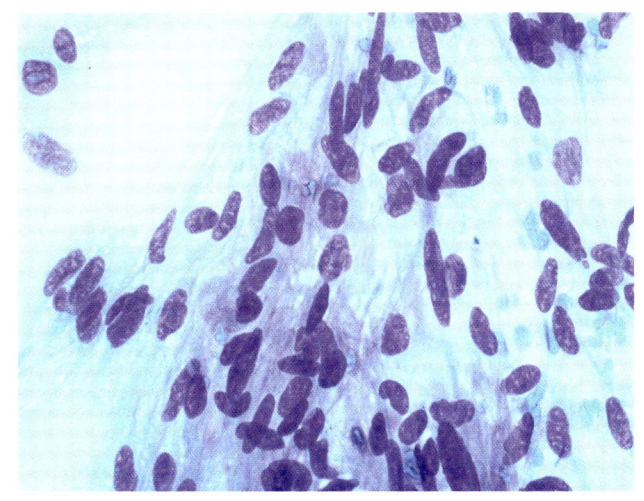

FIGURE 8-10
Cytology of gastrointestinal stromal tumor (GIST).
Fine-needle aspiration (FNA) smear. This smear from an FNA of a gastric lesion consists of a hypercellular proliferation of monomorphic spindle cells with fibrillary cytoplasm and a relative paucity of mitotic figures.

FINE-NEEDLE ASPIRATION BIOPSY

FNA is being used increasingly in the diagnosis of GIST. Cytologic preparations of GIST are cellular and reveal monomorphic epithelioid or spindle cell proliferations with fibrillary cytoplasm and without nuclear pleomorphism or prominent mitotic activity (Figure 8-10).

DIFFERENTIAL DIAGNOSIS

The differential diagnosis of GIST includes true smooth muscle tumors, schwannoma, desmoid fibromatosis, carcinoma, melanoma, and other spindle cell sarcomas, which rarely occur in the gastrointestinal tract, such as synovial sarcoma. True smooth muscle tumors (leiomyoma and leiomyosarcoma), have brightly eosinophilic cytoplasm and most often exhibit spindle cell morphology but can rarely have epithelioid cytomorphology. Leiomyomas tend to arise from the muscularis mucosae, whereas leiomyosarcomas arise from the muscularis propria. In contrast with GIST, leiomyosarcomas exhibit significant cytologic pleomorphism and mitotic activity, and are positive for actin and desmin and negative for KIT by immunohistochemistry. Gastrointestinal schwannomas are most common in the stomach, arise from the bowel wall, and are well-circumscribed. They are usually surrounded by dense aggregates of lymphocytes, and are diffusely and strongly positive for S-100 protein and negative for KIT. Desmoid fibromatosis can involve the bowel wall and is composed of long and broad fascicles of monomorphous, benign appearing spindle cells with palely eosinophilic cytoplasm and oval nuclei with fine chromatin and inconspicuous nucleoli. They have an infiltrative growth pattern and are negative for KIT by immunohistochemistry, although they exhibit variable (usually focal) immunoreactivity for smooth muscle actin, desmin, and S-100 protein. Carcinomas of the gastrointestinal tract can mimic spindle cell or epithelioid GIST. However, they are usually more pleomorphic and mitotically active than GIST, and are positive for cytokeratins and usually negative for KIT. Melanoma frequently metastasizes to the gastrointestinal tract, especially the small bowel, and can have a variety of histologic appearances. Immunohistochemical studies are useful in distinguishing melanoma from GIST because melanomas are positive for S-100 protein, MelanA, HMB-45, and tyrosinase. However, melanomas can exhibit immunoreactivity for KIT, although it is usually less extensive than GIST. Other primary and metastatic sarcomas are rare in the gastrointestinal tract and are usually negative for KIT.

PROGNOSIS AND TREATMENT

Most GISTs exhibit benign clinical behavior. However, approximately half of lesions have the ability to recur locally and metastasize distantly. GISTs have a tendency for intra-abdominal spread and metastasize almost exclusively to the liver. Lymph node metastasis is extremely rare, as is spread outside of the abdominal cavity. The most common site of metastasis outside of the abdomen

TABLE 8-1
Approach for Defining Risk for Aggressive Behavior in Gastrointestinal Stromal Tumors: Risk Stratification of Primary Gastrointestinal Stromal Tumor by Mitotic Index, Size, and Site

Mitotic Index	Size	Risk for Progressive Disease*(%)			
		Gastric	Duodenum	Jejunum/Ileum	Rectum
≤5/50 high-power fields	≤2 cm	None (0%)	None (0%)	None (0%)	None (0%)
	>2 ≤ 5 cm	Very low (1.9%)	Low (8.3%)	Low (4.3%)	Low (8.5%)
	>5 ≤ 10 cm	Low (3.6%)	Insufficient data	Moderate (24%)	Insufficient data
	>10 cm	Moderate (10%)	High (34%)	High (52%)	High (57%)
>5/50 high-power fields	≤2 cm	None to small number of cases	Insufficient data	High to small number of cases	High (54%)
	>2 ≤ 5 cm	Moderate (16%)	High (50%)	High (73%)	High (52%)
	>5 ≤ 10 cm	High (55%)	Insufficient data	High (85%)	Insufficient data
	>10 cm	High (86%)	High (86%)	High (90%)	High (71%)

Data are based on long-term follow-up of 1055 gastric, 629 small intestinal, 144 duodenal, and 111 rectal gastrointestinal stromal tumors.
*Defined as metastasis or tumor-related death.
Adapted from Miettinen M, Lasota J: Gastrointestinal stromal tumors: Pathology and prognosis at different sites. Semin Diagn Pathol 2006;23:70–83, by permission.

is the lungs. Many prognostic factors have been studied in GIST, but anatomic location, mitotic rate, and size are most predictive of behavior. Instead of dividing GISTs into benign and malignant categories, a strategy of risk stratification based on anatomic location, size, and mitotic activity is recommended (Table 8-1).

It has been realized that approximately 95 % of GISTs possess activating mutations within the KIT tyrosine kinase growth factor receptor. In addition, platelet-derived tyrosine kinase growth factor α receptor (PDGFR α) harbors activating mutations in a small percentage of GISTs that lack KIT activation. KIT and PDGFRα activation results in ligand-independent constitutive activation, which is central to promoting oncogenesis. This is important because it is possible to target these oncogenic pathways with imatinib mesylate, a small-molecule ATP analogue, which inhibits both KIT and PDGFRα. This therapy has been shown to be useful in the treatment of the majority of GISTs (Figure 8-11). Variability exists in the exons that are mutated in KIT and PDGFRα, and response to imatinib is dependent on the site of the mutation. Fortunately, the largest number of mutations occurs in exon 11 of KIT, and tumors harboring these mutations respond well to imatinib. For those lesions that do not respond to imatinib or for those that become resistant to imatinib after an initial response, sunitinib maleate has been approved by the U.S. Food and Drug Administration. Sunitinib is also a small-molecule ATP that binds to and inhibits KIT.

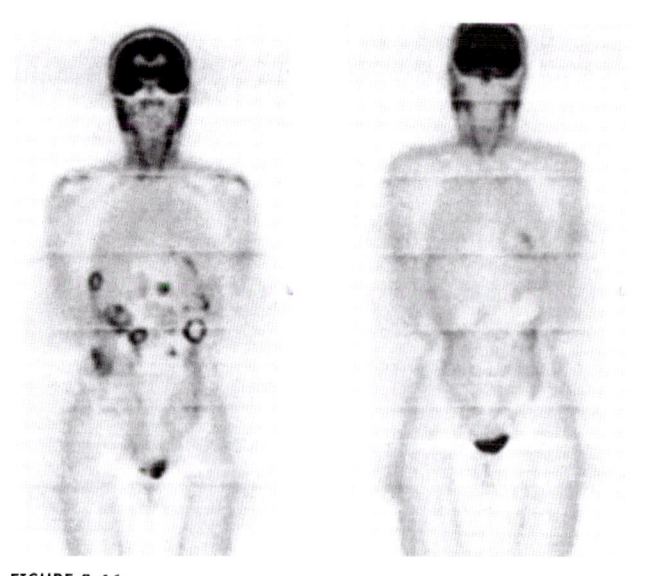

FIGURE 8-11

Treatment of gastrointestinal stromal tumor (GIST) by imatinib mesylate (Gleevec).
Sequential positron emission tomography (PET) scans with fluorodeoxyglucose in a patient with disseminated GIST. Numerous metastases in the liver and upper abdomen are metabolically active before administration of imatinib **(A)**, whereas the lesions have lost metabolic activity 5 weeks after administration of imatinib **(B)**.
(From Joensuu H, Roberts PJ, Sarlomo-Rikala M, et al: Effect of the tyrosine kinase inhibitor STI571 in a patient with a metastatic gastrointestinal stromal tumor. N Engl J Med 2001;344:1052–1056, by permission.)

GASTROINTESTINAL STROMAL TUMOR—FACT SHEET

Definition
▸▸ Most common mesenchymal neoplasm that arises primarily in the gastrointestinal tract

Incidence and Location
▸▸ Annual incidence of approximately 6000 new cases in the United States each year
▸▸ Gastrointestinal GISTs arise in the stomach (60%), small bowel (30%), esophagus, colon, rectum, gallbladder, and appendix (10%)
▸▸ Extragastrointestinal GISTs are rare and arise in the omentum, mesentery, retroperitoneum, and pelvis

Morbidity and Mortality
▸▸ Range of clinical behavior from benign/low-grade to fully malignant lesions
▸▸ Malignant lesions can cause death because of liver metastasis or intra-abdominal dissemination

Sex, Race, and Age Distribution
▸▸ Slightly more common in men
▸▸ Tend to arise in adults, with median age of 58 years
▸▸ Can arise in children and young adults, especially in the setting of Carney's triad

Clinical Features
▸▸ Presenting symptoms include anemia or fatigue, or both, caused by ulceration/bleeding, abdominal pain, early satiety, abdominal distension
▸▸ Incidental lesions are identified in resection specimens that are resected for other reasons, such as gastrectomy for gastric carcinoma
▸▸ Most pediatric cases are associated with Carney's triad (gastric GIST, extra-adrenal paraganglioma, and pulmonary chondroma)

Radiologic and Endoscopic Features
▸▸ Seen on CT and MRI
▸▸ Endoscopic ultrasound useful

Prognosis and Treatment
▸▸ Prognosis is related to risk for aggressive behavior
▸▸ Surgery is the treatment of choice for localized lesions
▸▸ Imatinib mesylate (Gleevec) is useful in the treatment of unresectable GISTs

GASTROINTESTINAL STROMAL TUMOR—PATHOLOGIC FEATURES

Gross Findings
▸▸ Commonly arise from wall of the gastrointestinal tract
▸▸ Unilobular or multilobular with smooth, circumscribed borders
▸▸ Ulceration common
▸▸ Serosal-based pedunculated lesions occur
▸▸ Cut surface is fleshy, often cystic
▸▸ Necrosis, hemorrhage, or both are common

Microscopic Findings
▸▸ Spindle cell lesions arranged in fascicles
▸▸ Epithelioid lesions arranged in nests or sheets
▸▸ Many cases have combined epithelioid and spindle cell cytomorphology
▸▸ Cells have nuclei with fine chromatin and abundant fibrillary cytoplasm
▸▸ Relatively few mitotic figures
▸▸ Pleomorphism rare
▸▸ Some lesions have extensive paranuclear vacuolization, prominent nuclear palisading, or *skeinoid* fibers

Ultrastructural Features
▸▸ Relative lack of differentiation; "incomplete" smooth muscle or neuroaxonal differentiation

Immunohistochemical Features
▸▸ 95% of cases diffusely and strongly positive for KIT (CD117) in membranous, cytoplasmic, or globular pattern
▸▸ Positive for CD34 (75%), smooth muscle actin (40%)
▸▸ Negative for desmin and S-100 protein

Cytogenetics
▸▸ Loss of chromosomes 14 and 22, and loss of material from short arm of chromosome 1 most common
▸▸ Also see loss of material from short arm of chromosomes 9 and 11

Fine-Needle Aspiration Biopsy Findings
▸▸ Cellular monomorphic epithelioid and spindle cell proliferations
▸▸ Fibrillary cytoplasm without nuclear pleomorphism or prominent mitotic activity

Differential Diagnosis
▸▸ True smooth muscle tumors: leiomyoma and leiomyosarcoma
▸▸ Schwannoma
▸▸ Desmoid fibromatosis
▸▸ Melanoma
▸▸ Carcinoma

SUGGESTED READING

1. Demetri GD, Benjamin RS, Blanke CD, et al: NCCN task force report: management of patients with gastrointestinal stromal tumor (GIST) – update of the NCCN clinical practice guidelines. J Natl Compr Canc Netw 2007; 5 Suppl 2:S1–S29.
2. Heinrich MC, Corless CL, Demetri GD, et al: Kinase mutations and imatinib response in patients with metastatic gastrointestinal stromal tumor. J Clin Oncol 2003;21:4342–4349.
3. Heinrich MC, Corless CL, Duensing A, et al: PDGFRA activating mutations in gastrointestinal stromal tumors. Science 2003;299:708–710.
4. Hirota S, Isozaki K, Moriyama Y, et al: Gain-of-function mutations of c-kit in human gastrointestinal stromal tumors. Science 1998;23:577–580.
5. Medeiros F, Corless CL, Duensing A, et al: KIT-negative gastrointestinal stromal tumors: proof of concept and therapeutic implications. Am J Surg Pathol 2004;28:889–894.
6. Miettinen M, Lasota J: Gastrointestinal stromal tumors: pathology and prognosis at different sites. Semin Diagn Pathol 2006; 23:70–83.
7. Rubin BP: Gastrointestinal stromal tumours: an update. Histopathology 2006;48:83–96.
8. Rubin BP, Heinrich MC, Corless CL: Gastrointestinal stromal tumour. Lancet 2007;369:1731–1741, 2007.

# 9 Vascular Tumors of Soft Tissue

Andrew L. Folpe

- **REACTIVE VASCULAR PROLIFERATIONS**
  - Papillary Endothelial Hyperplasia
  - Pyogenic Granuloma (Lobular Capillary Hemangioma)
  - Bacillary Angiomatosis
  - Glomeruloid Hemangioma
- **BENIGN VASCULAR TUMORS**
  - Capillary Hemangioma
  - Cavernous Hemangioma
  - Spindle Cell Hemangioma
  - Deeply Located Hemangiomas Including Angiomatosis
  - Epithelioid Hemangioma (Angiolymphoid Hyperplasia with Eosinophilia)
- **VASCULAR TUMORS OF INTERMEDIATE (BORDERLINE) MALIGNANCY: HEMANGIOENDOTHELIOMAS**
  - Kaposiform Hemangioendothelioma
  - Dabska-Type (Papillary Intralymphatic Angioendothelioma) and Retiform Hemangioendotheliomas
  - Epithelioid Hemangioendothelioma
- **FULLY MALIGNANT VASCULAR TUMORS**
  - Angiosarcoma
  - Kaposi Sarcoma

REACTIVE VASCULAR PROLIFERATIONS

PAPILLARY ENDOTHELIAL HYPERPLASIA

CLINICAL FEATURES

Papillary endothelial hyperplasia (PEH) may occur in any location, but most commonly presents in the superficial soft tissues of the extremities, head, and neck. The thumb is a particularly common location for this process. A history of trauma is occasionally present. PEH may also be superimposed on a preexisting benign vascular lesion, such as an intramuscular hemangioma.

PATHOLOGIC FEATURES

GROSS FINDINGS

PEH typically presents as a small, firm, red-to-blue mass in the superficial soft tissues. Most cases are intravascular, and the lesion may be surrounded by the remnants of a vessel wall or by a fibrous pseudocapsule.

MICROSCOPIC FINDINGS

PEH usually begins within a thrombosed blood vessel, and abundant thrombotic material is usually present (Figure 9-1). On occasion, the process may extend beyond the vessel wall, and thrombotic material and proliferating endothelial cells may be seen in the adjacent soft tissues. Early lesions show ingrowth of endothelial cells into the thrombus, with the formation of pseudopapilla. These papillae are lined by plump, normochromatic endothelial cells, which grow in a single, nonstratified layer (Figure 9-2). Mitotic activity may rarely be focally present. In more fully developed lesions, the endothelial proliferation may create the appearance of interanastomosing vascular channels, simulating angiosarcoma. The bland appearance of the endothelial cells, the overall circumscription of the lesion, and

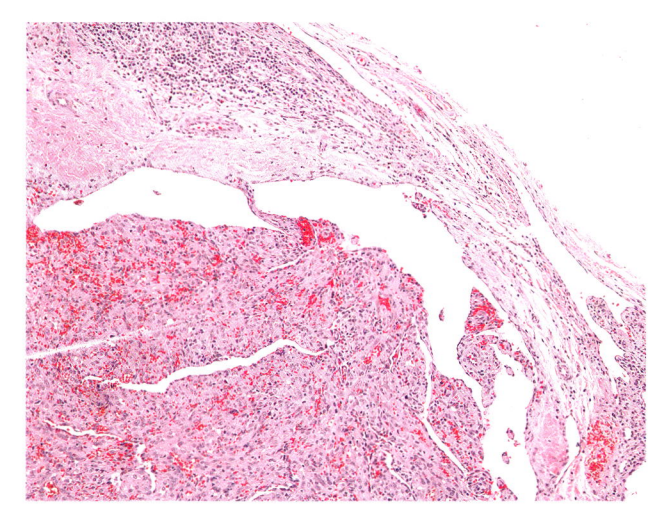

FIGURE 9-1
Intravascular papillary endothelial hyperplasia showing a cellular proliferation of benign endothelial cells within an organizing thrombus.

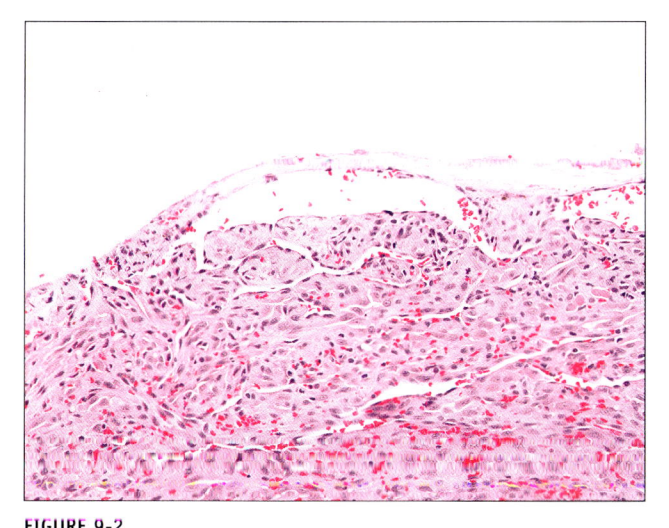

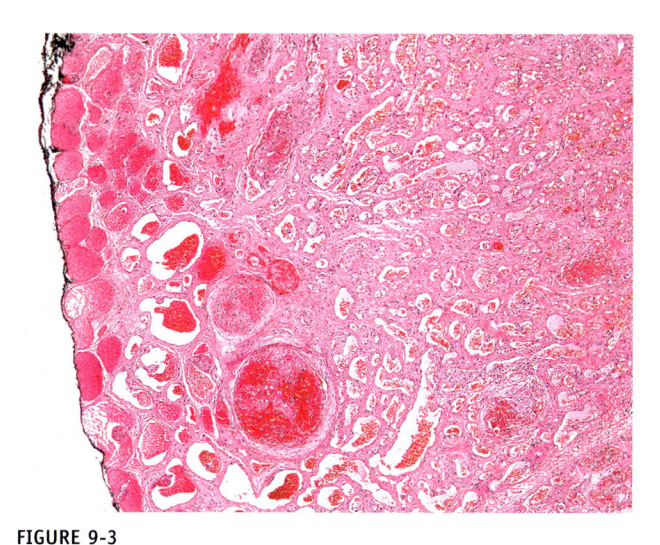

FIGURE 9-3
Capillary hemangioma with superimposed thrombosis and papillary endothelial hyperplasia. Papillary endothelial hyperplasia may occur as a secondary change in any type of vascular tumor.

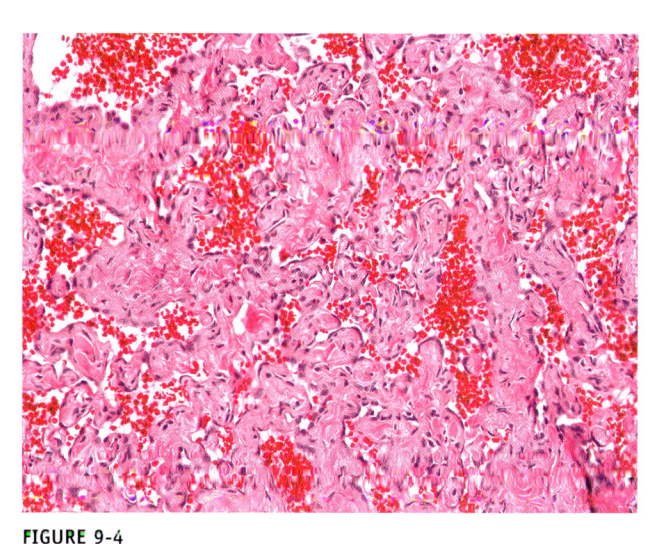

FIGURE 9-2
High-power view of papillary endothelial hyperplasia. Note the bland cytologic features of the endothelial cells and the absence of endothelial cell stratification.

FIGURE 9-4
Organized papillary endothelial hyperplasia within a hemangioma, creating a sinusoidal pattern.

recognition of the typical features of PEH are the keys to avoiding this serious misdiagnosis. PEH may also occur within other vascular tumors, such as hemangiomas (Figures 9-3 and 9-4).

ANCILLARY STUDIES

IMMUNOHISTOCHEMISTRY

The cells of PEH are differentiated endothelial cells, which express markers such as CD31, CD34, FLI1 protein, and von Willebrand factor (vWF, factor VIII–related protein). Immunohistochemistry is seldom necessary in arriving at this diagnosis.

DIFFERENTIAL DIAGNOSIS

As noted earlier, the most important differential diagnostic consideration is angiosarcoma. Most angiosarcomas will present as larger masses, with clear-cut nuclear atypism, frequent mitotic figures, and necrosis. Unlike PEH, which shows overall low-power circumscription, angiosarcomas are diffusely infiltrating lesions. Many cases of PEH arise within blood vessels, a distinctly unusual feature in angiosarcoma. It is important to remember that PEH may engraft itself on essentially any vascular tumor, as well as onto areas of hemorrhage and thrombosis within other types of tumors. Thus, one should always hunt carefully for any evidence of a preexisting neoplasm, particularly in deep locations.

PROGNOSIS AND TREATMENT

PEH is a reactive lesion that requires only simple excision.

PYOGENIC GRANULOMA (Lobular Capillary Hemangioma)

CLINICAL FEATURES

Pyogenic granulomas typically occur on the mucosal surfaces, particularly the mouth, and the skin. Lesions may occasionally be multiple and arise after trauma in roughly one-third of cases. The tumors often have an initial period of rapid growth, followed by stabilization and occasionally regression. Identical mucosal lesions may arise spontaneously during pregnancy (granuloma gravidarum). Rarely, this process may occur within a small vein, so-called *intravascular pyogenic granuloma*.

PATHOLOGIC FEATURES

GROSS FINDINGS

Pyogenic granulomas are typically small, polypoid lesions, which are often ulcerated and friable.

MICROSCOPIC FINDINGS

At low-power magnification, pyogenic granulomas are exophytic, polypoid masses that often are surrounded by an epidermal collarette (Figure 9-5). The

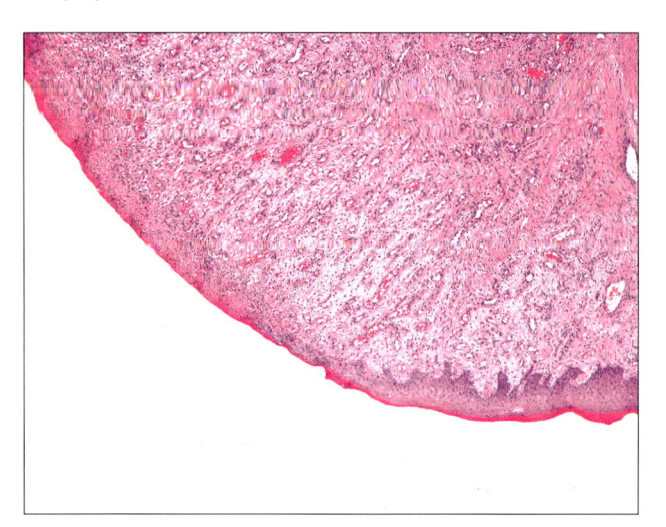

FIGURE 9-5
Ulceration and polypoid growth pattern in pyogenic granuloma.

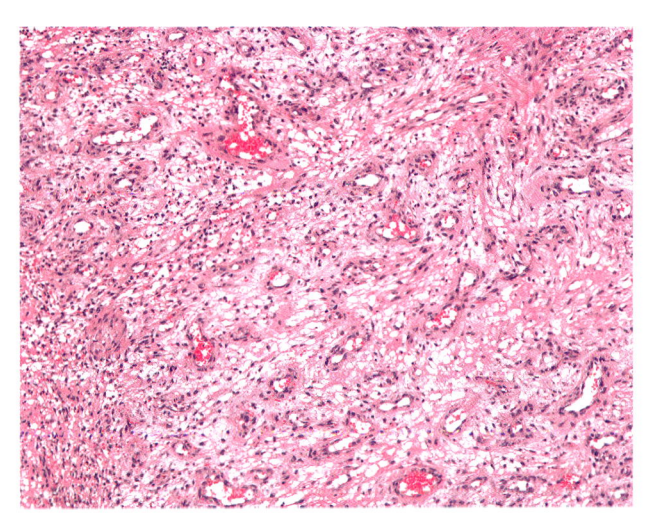

FIGURE 9-6
Pyogenic granuloma, with a lobular proliferation of well-formed capillaries lined by plump endothelial cells, with numerous stromal neutrophils.

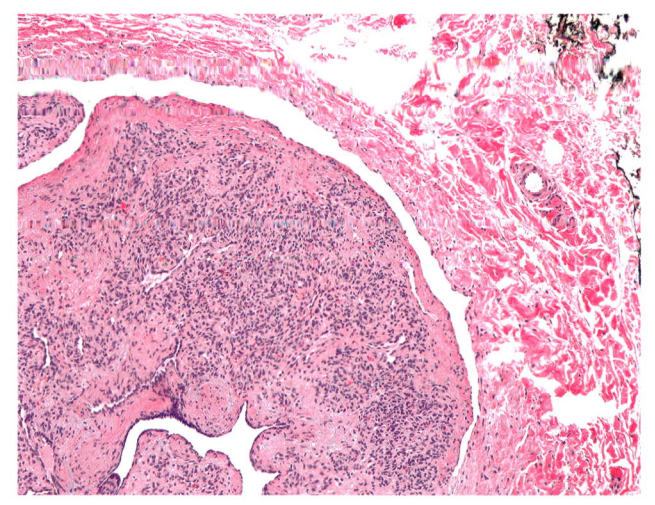

FIGURE 9-7
Intravascular pyogenic granuloma (intravascular lobular capillary hemangioma).

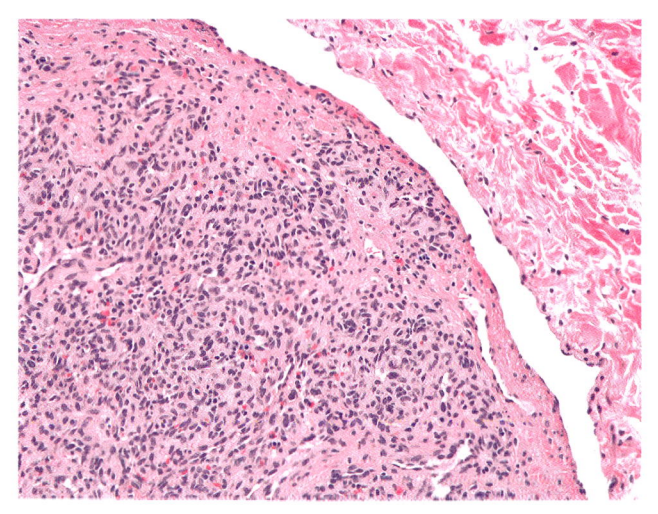

FIGURE 9-8
As in their more common extravascular counterparts, intravascular pyogenic granulomas show a lobular growth pattern of well-formed capillaries.

lesions are well circumscribed and distinctly lobular, with central larger vessels and peripheral aggregates of well-formed capillaries. A mixed acute and chronic inflammatory cell infiltrate is almost always present, similar to that seen in granulation tissue (Figure 9-6). Mitotic activity is often brisk. Necrosis may be seen in association with surface ulceration. Lesions identical to pyogenic granuloma/lobular capillary hemangioma may also occasionally be seen in intravascular locations (intravascular pyogenic granuloma) (Figures 9-7 and 9-8).

ANCILLARY STUDIES

IMMUNOHISTOCHEMISTRY

The cells of pyogenic granuloma express endothelial markers such as CD31, CD34, FLI1 protein, and vWF.

DIFFERENTIAL DIAGNOSIS

The sometimes high cellularity and brisk mitotic activity of pyogenic granuloma occasionally create concern for an angiosarcoma. The most important features distinguishing these two entities are the circumscription and lobular growth pattern seen in pyogenic granuloma and absent in angiosarcoma. Kaposi sarcoma (KS) may, on occasion, show superficial zones with a vaguely lobular growth pattern, suggestive of pyogenic granuloma. However, examination of deeper portions of the biopsy will invariably reveal infiltrative growth, with formation of slit-like vascular spaces by hyperchromatic, vaguely myoid-appearing spindled cells. In difficult cases, immunohistochemistry for human herpes virus type 8 (HHV-8) latency-associated nuclear antigen (LANA) protein (present in KS, absent in pyogenic granuloma) may be helpful. It is also important to recognize that areas reminiscent of pyogenic granuloma may be seen at the surface of almost any ulcerated lesion, including oral squamous cell carcinomas, for example, and one should carefully examine the entire specimen, including the deepest portions, before definitely making this diagnosis.

PROGNOSIS AND TREATMENT

Pyogenic granulomas are usually cured with simple excision. These lesions may recur locally in 10% to 15% of cases, particularly when incompletely excised, and occasionally recur as multiple satellite lesions.

BACILLARY ANGIOMATOSIS

CLINICAL FEATURES

Bacillary angiomatosis is a reactive vascular proliferation caused by infection with the bacteria Bartonella henselae and Bartonella quintana. It occurs almost exclusively in immunocompromised patients, typically men with human immunodeficiency virus (HIV) infection, and usually presents as multiple, elevated, pink skin or mucosal lesions. This process may also involve visceral organs, such as the liver, where it produces peliosis.

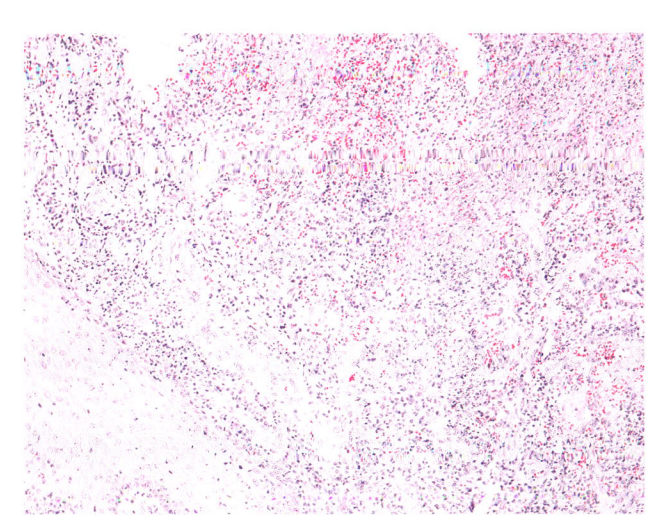

FIGURE 9-9
Bacillary angiomatosis, presenting as an ulcerated dermal nodule composed of blood vessels lined by epithelioid endothelial cells in association with marked acute inflammation.

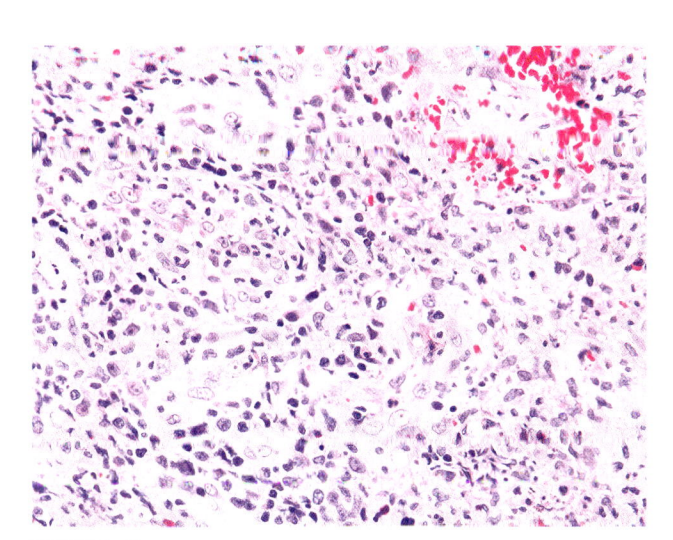

FIGURE 9-10
High-power view of bacillary angiomatosis, showing epithelioid endothelial cells, neutrophils, and eosinophilic debris.

PATHOLOGIC FEATURES

MICROSCOPIC FINDINGS

Bacillary angiomatosis usually shows a vaguely lobular growth pattern, with capillary-sized vessels lined by epithelioid endothelial cells with clear cytoplasm (Figure 9-9). Numerous stromal neutrophils are seen, as are amorphous, eosinophilic aggregates that contain fibrin and bacilli (Figure 9-10). The bacilli may be identified with a Warthin–Starry stain. In the liver, peliosis hepatis is seen, with surrounding aggregates of fibrin and bacilli.

ANCILLARY STUDIES

The cells of bacillary angiomatosis have a typical endothelial immunophenotype.

REACTIVE VASCULAR PROLIFERATIONS—FACT SHEET

Definition
- Reactive proliferations of endothelial cells, sometimes with known infectious or paraneoplastic causative agents

Incidence and Location
- Rare
- Typically cutaneous or mucosal

Morbidity and Mortality
- Pyogenic granulomas are entirely benign
- Bacillary angiomatosis responds to antibiotics and treatment of underlying immunosuppression
- Glomeruloid hemangioma is seen with POEMS syndrome, which has a 5-year survival rate of only 60%

Sex, Race, and Age Distribution
- None for pyogenic granuloma
- Bacillary angiomatosis is more common in HIV-positive men but may be seen in any immunosuppressed patient
- Glomeruloid hemangioma occurs in older patients of either sex

Clinical Features
- Pyogenic granuloma presents as an ulcerated, polypoid mass
- Bacillary angiomatosis presents as multiple, elevated, pink skin or mucosal lesions
- Glomeruloid hemangioma presents as small, red-to-violaceous cutaneous papules, usually on the trunk and proximal extremities

Prognosis and Treatment
- Excellent prognosis for pyogenic granulomas with simple excision
- Bacillary angiomatosis has excellent prognosis with antibiotic therapy, particularly if underlying immunosuppression can be corrected
- Glomeruloid hemangioma is treated with simple excision; treatment of underlying cause of POEMS syndrome may be more difficult

---

DIFFERENTIAL DIAGNOSIS

Occasionally, the vaguely lobular growth pattern and the clear endothelial cells may be relatively inapparent, and bacillary angiomatosis may closely resemble ordinary granulation tissue. Clinical correlation may be valuable here. Careful inspection should reveal the characteristic clear endothelial cells and eosinophilic debris seen in bacillary angiomatosis. The clinical setting of bacillary angiomatosis also often raises the possibility of KS, a lesion that shows as its hallmark spindled cells forming slit-like vascular spaces, rather than lobules of clear, epithelioid cells.

PROGNOSIS AND TREATMENT

Therapy of bacillary angiomatosis is aimed at eradicating the underlying infectious causative agent, most often with erythromycin.

GLOMERULOID HEMANGIOMA

CLINICAL FEATURES

Glomeruloid hemangioma is an extremely rare reactive vascular proliferation seen in patients with POEMS syndrome (polyneuropathy, organomegaly, endocrinopathy, M-protein, skin lesions). Such lesions are seen in roughly 25% to 45% of patients with this syndrome. Although patients with POEMS syndrome may present with other benign vascular tumors (e.g., microvenular hemangioma, cherry hemangioma), glomeruloid hemangiomas appear to be specific to this syndrome.

PATHOLOGIC FEATURES

GROSS FINDINGS

Glomeruloid hemangiomas present as small, red-to-violaceous cutaneous papules, usually on the trunk and proximal extremities.

MICROSCOPIC FINDINGS

Glomeruloid hemangiomas are dermal lesions, consisting of collections of ectatic small vessels containing intraluminal nests of proliferating capillaries, resembling glomeruli. A distinctive feature is the presence of large, vacuolated endothelial cells that contain

> **REACTIVE VASCULAR PROLIFERATIONS—PATHOLOGIC FEATURES**
>
> **Gross Findings**
> - Polypoid mucosal tumor or erythematous skin lesion
>
> **Microscopic Findings**
> - Lobular proliferation of mitotically active, bland endothelial cells in association with ulceration and neutrophilic infiltrate in pyogenic granuloma
> - Vaguely lobular growth pattern, capillary-sized vessels lined by epithelioid endothelial cells with clear cytoplasm, numerous stromal neutrophils and amorphous, eosinophilic aggregates that contain fibrin and bacilli in bacillary angiomatosis
> - Ectatic small vessels that contain intraluminal nests of proliferating capillaries, resembling glomeruli, with large, vacuolated endothelial cells that contain eosinophilic proteinaceous material in glomeruloid hemangioma
>
> **Immunohistochemical Findings**
> - Expression of CD31, CD34, FLI-1 protein, and vWF
>
> **Differential Diagnosis**
> - Pyogenic granuloma: angiosarcoma, KS, reactive vascular proliferations overlying other pathology
> - Bacillary angiomatosis: granulation tissue, KS
> - Glomeruloid hemangioma: Dabska tumor, PEH

eosinophilic proteinaceous material (polytypic immunoglobulin).

ANCILLARY STUDIES

IMMUNOHISTOCHEMISTRY

Glomeruloid hemangiomas express markers of normal endothelium, such as CD31, CD34, and vWF.

DIFFERENTIAL DIAGNOSIS

The differential diagnosis of glomeruloid hemangioma is principally with other vascular tumors that contain intraluminal papillations. PEH contains thrombotic material, shows fibrous stalks lined by plump endothelial cells, and lacks vacuolated cells with eosinophilic inclusions. Papillary intralymphatic angioendothelioma (Dabska tumor, malignant endovascular papillary angioendothelioma) almost always occurs in young children and shows dilated, lymphatic-like spaces, surrounding fibrosis, and hyalinized papillae lined by hyperchromatic, "hobnailed" endothelial cells. Intravascular pyogenic granuloma occurs within larger vessels and shows a distinctly lobular growth pattern.

PROGNOSIS AND TREATMENT

Glomeruloid hemangioma is a reactive lesion that requires only simple excision. Patients with POEMS syndrome have a poor prognosis, with a 5-year survival rate of approximately 60%.

BENIGN VASCULAR TUMORS

CAPILLARY HEMANGIOMA

CLINICAL FEATURES

Capillary hemangiomas are the most common subtype of hemangiomas; they are also the most common subtype of soft tissue tumor in infants and children. Many capillary hemangiomas present either at birth or immediately thereafter and show an initial period of rapid growth, followed by stabilization and eventual involution. In approximately 15% to 20% of infantile cases, multiple hemangiomas are seen. Rare familial capillary hemangioma syndromes have been reported, in association with mutations in chromosome 5. The skin and oral mucosa are by far the most common locations for capillary hemangiomas, although they may occur in essentially any location, including the viscera. In infants, extremely large capillary hemangiomas of the head and neck may be seen as part of the PHACES syndrome (*p*osterior fossa abnormalities, *h*emangiomas of the cervicofacial region, *a*rterial, *c*ardiac, and ocular abnormalities, *s*ternal clefting). Also, in infants, lumbosacral hemangiomas have been associated with occult spinal malformations and other anomalies.

PATHOLOGIC FEATURES

GROSS FINDINGS

Great variation exists in the gross appearance of capillary hemangiomas, depending on their size and depth. Small, superficial hemangiomas may appear as red macules, whereas larger, deeper hemangiomas may appear as firm, blue–violet, tumorous masses.

MICROSCOPIC FINDINGS

All capillary hemangiomas grow as multinodular, well-circumscribed, distinctly lobular proliferations of well-formed capillaries, lined by bland endothelial cells (Figures 9-11 and 9-12). In very young children, these lesions may be highly cellular and solid appearing, with

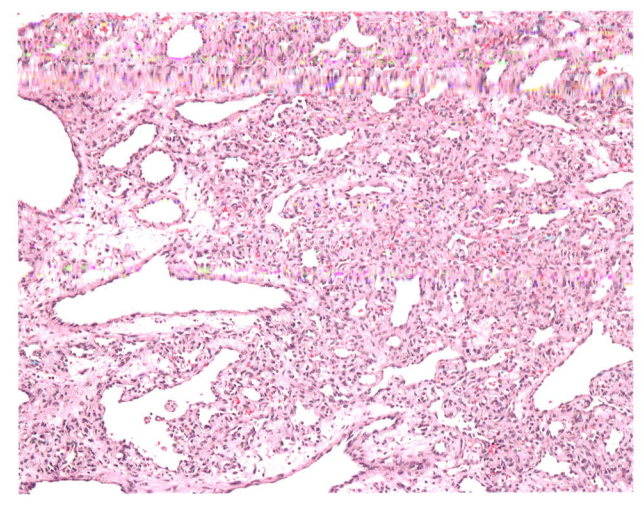

FIGURE 9-11
Typical capillary hemangioma, with a pronounced lobular pattern and numerous small capillaries.

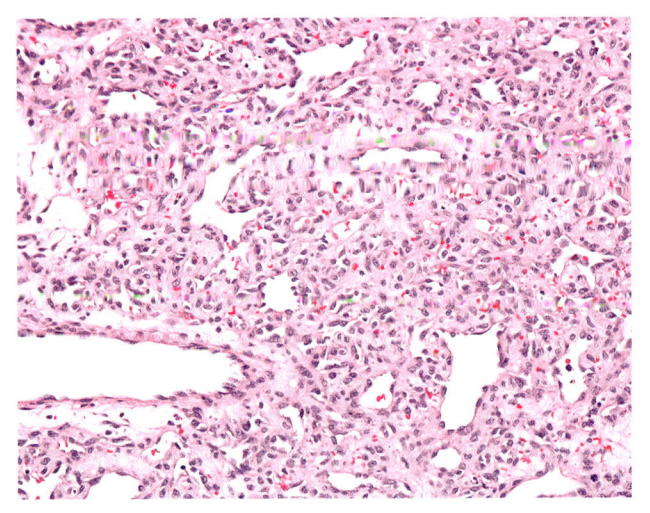

FIGURE 9-12
Small, well-formed capillaries lined by bland endothelial cells in capillary hemangioma.

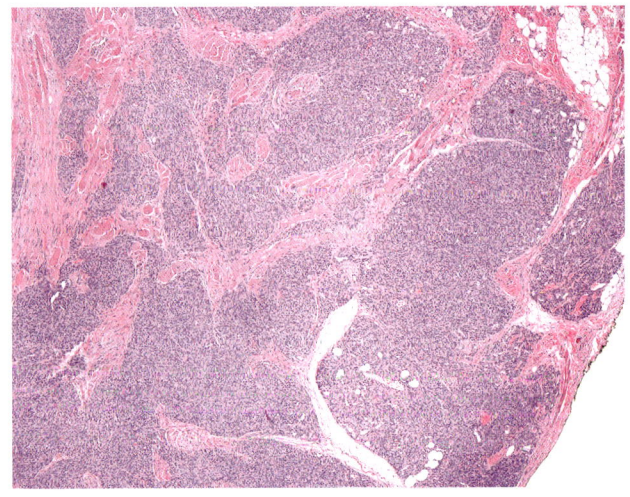

FIGURE 9-13
Cellular capillary hemangioma in a child. The cellularity of these lesions may suggest a round cell sarcoma, particularly in thick sections. Low-power identification of the typical lobular growth pattern is helpful in this situation.

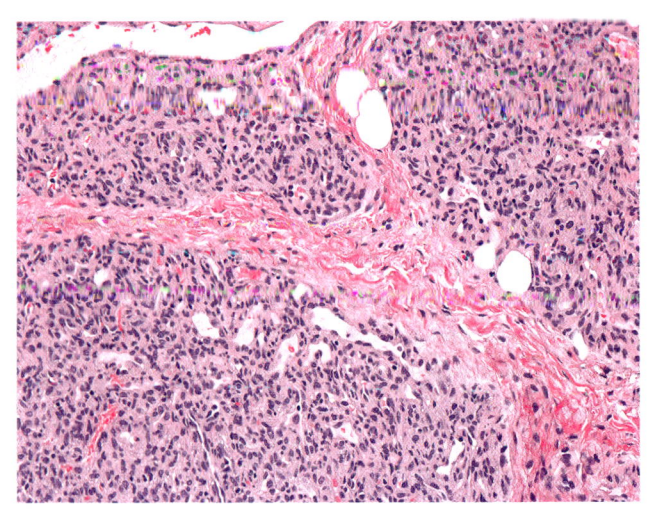

FIGURE 9-14
Although the cellularity of some capillary hemangiomas in children may obscure the lobular growth pattern, careful inspection of well-prepared sections will always show this feature, at least focally.

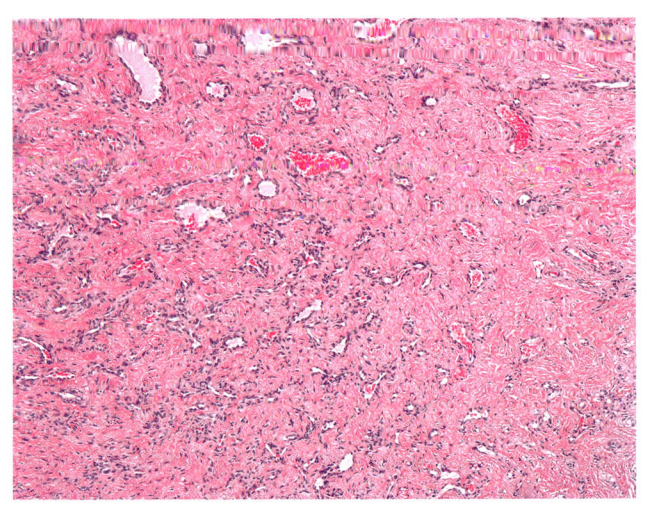

FIGURE 9-15
Atrophic capillary hemangioma in an adult, showing stromal fibrosis and a lobular growth pattern.

only subtle lumen formation, caused by protrusion of the plump endothelial cells into the lumens and the large numbers of pericytic cells *(juvenile hemangioma)* (Figures 9-13 and 9-14). Mitotic figures may be present. Such lesions may be confused with a variety of pediatric round cell malignancies. In older patients (and older tumors), lumen formation is typically much more obvious, because the endothelial cells flatten out and the individual vessels are surrounded by increasing amounts of fibrous connective tissue (Figures 9-15 and 9-16). Old lesions may be largely fibrotic, with only scattered, thin-walled vessels arranged in a vaguely lobular pattern.

CHAPTER 9 Vascular Tumors of Soft Tissue

CAPILLARY HEMANGIOMA—FACT SHEET

Definition
- Benign, regressing tumor of endothelial cells

Incidence and Location
- Most common soft tissue tumor of childhood
- Most common in the skin; may involve any location

Morbidity and Mortality
- Benign, frequently regress spontaneously
- Large capillary hemangiomas may be cosmetically deforming
- Some are associated with various syndromes and congenital malformations

Sex, Race, and Age Distribution
- No race or sex predilection
- Infants and young children

Clinical Features
- Small, superficial hemangiomas appear as red macules
- Larger, deeper hemangiomas appear as firm, blue–violet, tumorous masses

Prognosis and Treatment
- Many spontaneously regress
- Interferon therapy effective for large tumors in potentially dangerous locations
- Antiangiogenic therapy may also be effective for some

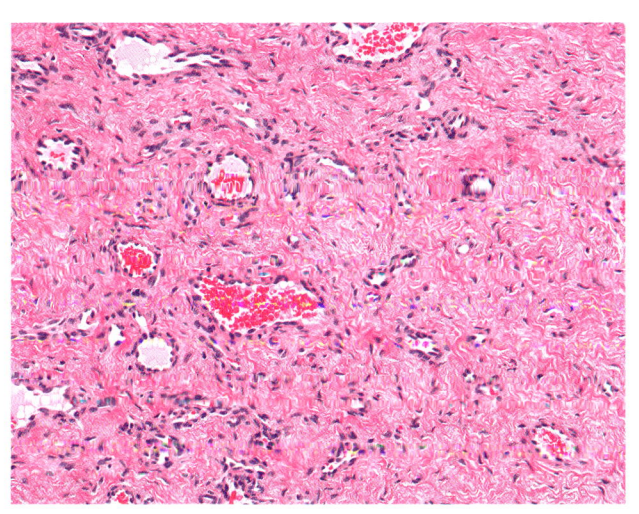

CAPILLARY HEMANGIOMA—PATHOLOGIC FEATURES

Gross Findings
- Polypoid mucosal tumor or erythematous skin lesion

Microscopic Findings
- Multinodular, well-circumscribed, distinctly lobular proliferations of well-formed capillaries, lined by bland endothelial cells
- May be highly cellular, mitotically active, and solid appearing in young children
- Old lesions may be largely fibrotic, with only scattered, thin-walled vessels arranged in a vaguely lobular pattern

Immunohistochemical Findings
- Express CD31, CD34, FLI-1 protein, and vWF
- GLUT-1 positive

Differential Diagnosis
- KHE
- Pediatric round cell tumors

FIGURE 9-16
In older adults, capillary hemangiomas may have a vaguely infiltrative appearance, because of an increase in stromal collagen and flattening of the blood vessels.

Ancillary Studies

Immunohistochemistry

Capillary hemangiomas, particularly cellular juvenile variants, typically contain both endothelial cells (CD31, CD34, vWF positive) and pericytic cells (smooth muscle actin positive). The glucose transporter protein GLUT1 is expressed in all juvenile capillary hemangiomas but not in other vascular malformations or neoplasms; this finding may suggest differentiation along the lines of placental capillary endothelium, rather than normal adult capillary endothelium.

Differential Diagnosis

Highly cellular juvenile capillary hemangiomas may be mistaken for a pediatric round cell malignant neoplasm, such as Ewing sarcoma or rhabdomyosarcoma. This is particularly true if one is evaluating overly thick sections. Careful evaluation of properly prepared sections from even the most cellular juvenile hemangioma will reveal subtle lumen formation, often seen best at the periphery of the tumor. In addition, juvenile hemangiomas are well-circumscribed, unlike malignant round cell tumors, which are infiltrative. Immunohistochemical demonstration of endothelial marker expression may be helpful, especially in cellular cases. Large capillary hemangiomas may also be confused with kaposiform hemangioendothelioma (KHE) and vice versa. KHEs are usually larger than capillary hemangiomas and have infiltrative margins. Although KHEs do show vaguely lobular zones composed of well-formed capillaries, they also contain areas composed of spindled cells that form slit-like vascular spaces, glomeruloid structures that contain fibrin microthrombi and fibrotic stroma, features not seen in capillary hemangioma. KHEs do not express GLUT1 protein, unlike cellular capillary hemangiomas.

Prognosis and Treatment

Treatment of capillary hemangiomas is based on the age of the patient, and the location and size of the tumors. Many tumors in children will spontaneously involute, and these can simply be followed clinically. Larger tumors or those that affect vital structures have been successfully treated with glucocorticosteroids or interferon-α, or both. A role for antiangiogenesis agents in the treatment of unresectable tumors has also been proposed.

CAVERNOUS HEMANGIOMA

Clinical Features

Cavernous hemangiomas also usually occur in young children but are far less frequent than are capillary hemangiomas. Cavernous hemangiomas tend to be larger than capillary hemangiomas and more frequently involve deep structures, with the liver being a particularly common site of visceral involvement. They tend to be less well-circumscribed. Unlike capillary hemangiomas, cavernous hemangiomas do not regress. Cavernous hemangiomas may be associated with consumptive coagulopathy (Kasabach–Merritt syndrome). The association of cavernous hemangiomas of the skin and gastrointestinal tract has been referred to as the *blue rubber bleb nevus syndrome*.

Pathologic Features

Gross Findings

Cavernous hemangiomas may appear as irregular reddish lesions when they involve the skin, or may appear blue or even nonpigmented when they present in deeper soft tissues. On cut section, a *sponge-like* appearance is common.

Microscopic Findings

Cavernous hemangiomas consist of large, dilated, blood-filled spaces, often with fibrotic walls (Figure 9-17). The tumors may be vaguely lobular or consist of elaborately interanastomosing vascular spaces, resembling a sponge. Thrombosis and calcification are common findings, and osseous metaplasia may occasionally be seen. The lining endothelium is usually flattened (Figure 9-18). On occasion, thrombosis and recanalization may produce a sinusoidal pattern (so-called sinusoidal hemangioma).

Ancillary Studies

The cells of cavernous hemangioma have a typical endothelial immunophenotype.

CAVERNOUS HEMANGIOMA—FACT SHEET

Definition
- Benign, nonregressing tumor of endothelial cells

Incidence and Location
- Less common than capillary hemangioma
- More frequently involve deep structures, particularly the liver

Morbidity and Mortality
- Benign, do not regress spontaneously
- May be associated with consumptive coagulopathy (Kasabach–Merritt syndrome)

Sex, Race, and Age Distribution
- No race or sex predilection
- Infants and young children
- Liver lesions are common in adults

Clinical Features
- Cutaneous tumors are irregular and reddish
- May appear blue or even nonpigmented when they present in deeper soft tissues

Prognosis and Treatment
- Nonregressing
- Do not respond to interferons or antiangiogenic therapy
- Require surgical treatment

CAVERNOUS HEMANGIOMA—PATHOLOGIC FEATURES

Gross Findings
- Sponge-like appearance, bloody

Microscopic Findings
- Large, dilated, blood-filled spaces with flattened endothelial lining, often with fibrotic walls
- May be vaguely lobular or consist of elaborately interanastomosing vascular spaces, resembling a sponge
- Thrombosis and calcification commonly seen
- Thrombosis and recanalization may produce a sinusoidal pattern

Immunohistochemical Findings
- Express CD31, CD34, FLI-1 protein, and vWF
- GLUT-1 negative

Differential Diagnosis
- Angiosarcoma
- SCH
- Capillary hemangioma

CHAPTER 9 Vascular Tumors of Soft Tissue

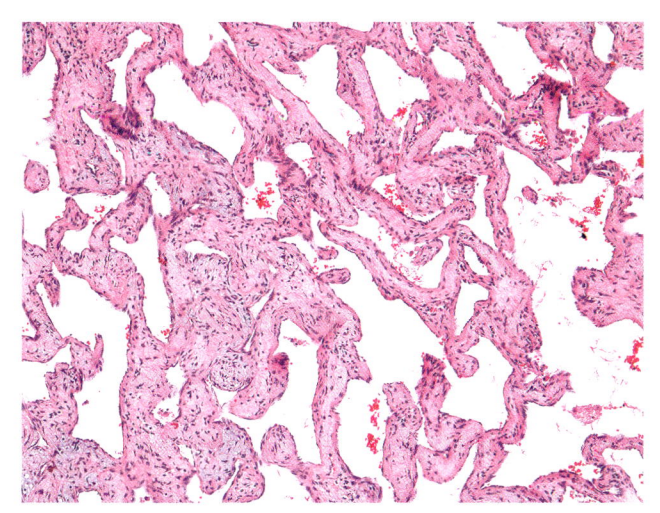

FIGURE 9-17
Cavernous hemangioma showing a characteristic "sieve-like" growth pattern.

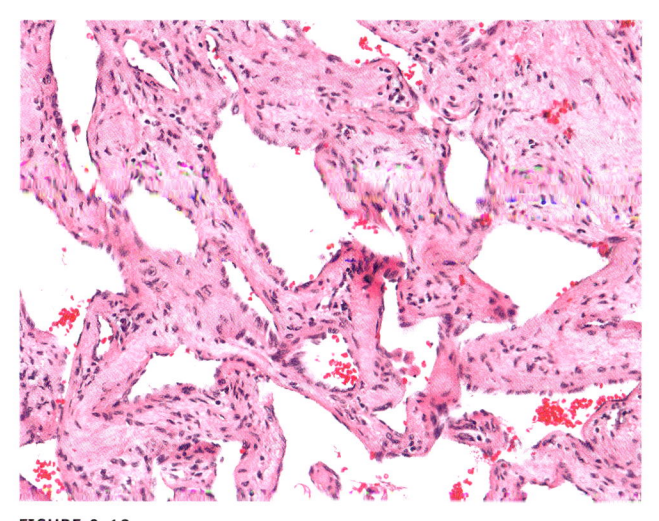

FIGURE 9-18
Vascular channels with fibrous walls, lined by flattened endothelial cells in cavernous hemangioma.

DIFFERENTIAL DIAGNOSIS

Thrombosis, recanalization, and PEH may occur within a preexisting cavernous hemangioma and may impart the appearance of elaborately interanastomosing vascular channels, worrisome for angiosarcoma. Low-power examination, however, reveals these lesions to be well circumscribed at the periphery, unlike the diffusely infiltrating growth seen in angiosarcoma. Angiosarcomas will also show nuclear atypia, mitotic activity, and frequently necrosis. Spindle cell hemangioma (SCH; spindle cell hemangioendothelioma) typically displays areas identical to cavernous hemangioma, admixed with spindled zones reminiscent of KS, and distinctive vacuolated endothelial cells. Recognition of this characteristic admixture of patterns, as well as its frequent association with a damaged-appearing blood vessel, is the key to the recognition of SCH.

PROGNOSIS AND TREATMENT

Cavernous hemangiomas do not regress and may cause local tissue destruction because of compressive effects. They require surgical removal and do not respond to medical therapy. Preoperative embolization may allow the resection of large lesions that involve locations such as the liver.

SPINDLE CELL HEMANGIOMA

SCH was originally described as *spindle cell hemangioendothelioma* and was believed to represent an unusual form of low-grade angiosarcoma. Subsequent studies have convincingly shown it to be a benign and possibly reactive lesion, and it has been reclassified by the World Health Organization as *spindle cell hemangioma (SCH)*.

CLINICAL FEATURES

SCHs typically occur in the dermis or subcutis of the distal extremities in young adults. Rare cases have been reported in deep soft tissue. In a significant subset of patients, the lesions are reported to have been present for many years, without symptoms. Approximately 5% of SCHs occur in patients with Maffucci syndrome (multiple enchondromas and vascular tumors), and one should always raise this possibility in a patient with a new diagnosis of SCH.

PATHOLOGIC FEATURES

GROSS FINDINGS

SCH typically presents as a slow-growing, violaceous, small, solitary, subcutaneous, small mass in the distal extremities.

MICROSCOPIC FINDINGS

SCHs typically grow in a well-circumscribed fashion and frequently are, at least in part, intravascular (Figure 9-19). Organizing thrombi, calcifications, and phleboliths are frequently present. A characteristic feature is the presence of two distinct zones; one characterized by thin-walled, dilated vessels, reminiscent of cavernous hemangioma, and the second by a proliferation of normochromatic, eosinophilic spindle cells, creating *slit-like* vascular spaces. Within these spindled areas, vacuolated, epithelioid cells are identified, a useful diagnostic feature of SCH (Figure 9-20). Mitotic figures are rare, and necrosis is absent. A chronic inflammatory cell infiltrate is absent, helping to distinguish SCH from KS.

Ancillary Studies

Immunohistochemistry

SCH contains a mixture of spindled and epithelioid endothelial cells, which almost always express typical vascular markers such as CD31 and CD34, and smooth muscle/pericytic cells, which variably express smooth muscle actin and desmin. The HHV-8 LANA protein is not present.

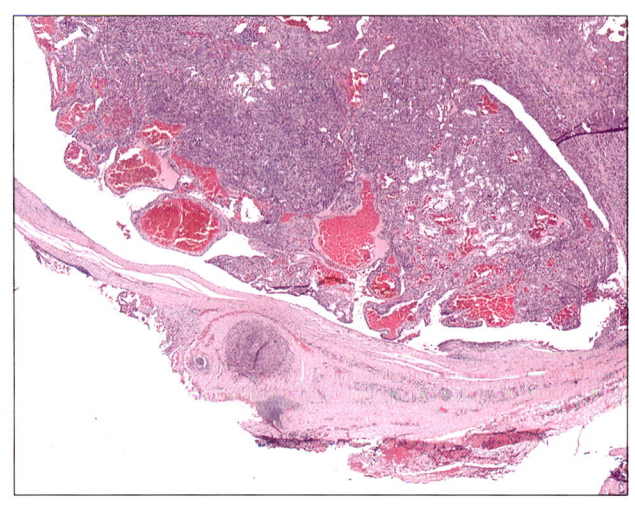

FIGURE 9-19
Spindle cell hemangioma occurring, in part, within a blood vessel. At low power, these lesions typically show a mixture of areas resembling cavernous hemangioma and Kaposi sarcoma.

SPINDLE CELL HEMANGIOMA—FACT SHEET

Definition
- Benign or possibly reactive endothelial tumor, frequently associated with Maffucci syndrome

Incidence and Location
- Rare
- Dermis or subcutis, rarely deep

Morbidity and Mortality
- Benign
- May propagate along damaged vessel with proximal local recurrences

Sex, Race, and Age Distribution
- No sex or race predilection
- Young adults

Clinical Features
- Violaceous nodule in skin or subcutis
- 5% of cases are associated with Maffucci syndrome (hemangiomas and enchondromas)

Prognosis and Treatment
- Benign
- May recur locally through propagation along vessel
- Surgical excision

Differential Diagnosis

SCH is most often mistaken for KS. Although KS may on rare occasions grow in a nodular fashion, it lacks the superb circumscription of SCH, does not show intravascular extension, and invariably shows infiltration of the spindled cells into the surrounding stroma. In addition, KS lacks the admixture of spindled and vacuolated endothelial cells characteristic of SCH, and typically shows an associated chronic inflammatory cell infiltrate. The cells of KS also display a greater degree of nuclear

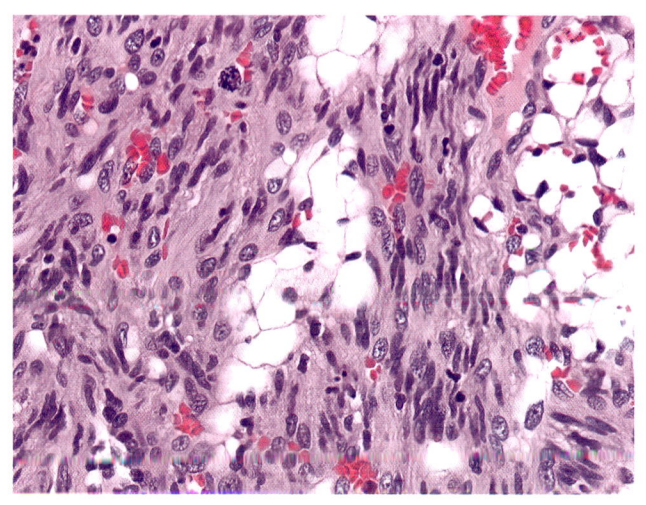

FIGURE 9-20
Diagnostic features of spindle cell hemangioma include an admixture of bland spindled cells (principally pericytes) and vacuolated endothelial cells.

SPINDLE CELL HEMANGIOMA—PATHOLOGIC FEATURES

Gross Findings
- Small, circumscribed
- May be calcified

Microscopic Findings
- Organizing thrombi, calcifications, and phleboliths
- Thin-walled, dilated vessels, reminiscent of cavernous hemangioma
- Normochromatic, eosinophilic spindle cells, creating "slit-like" vascular spaces
- Vacuolated, epithelioid endothelial cells
- Rare mitoses and absent necrosis
- Absent chronic inflammatory cell infiltrate

Immunohistochemical Findings
- Vacuolated endothelial cells express CD31, CD34, FLI-1 protein, and vWF
- Spindled cells are smooth muscle actin (SMA) positive pericytes

Differential Diagnosis
- Angiosarcoma
- KS
- KHE

enlargement and hyperchromasia, contrasting with the bland spindled cells of SCH, and frequently contain intracytoplasmic hyaline globules.

Occasional angiosarcomas show predominantly spindled features and can be confused with SCH. Again, careful attention to the absence of circumscription and the presence of diffusely infiltrating growth should point one toward the correct diagnosis. Most spindled angiosarcomas show focal areas of typical angiosarcoma, characterized by more epithelioid cells forming primitive vascular channels. Angiosarcomas also show significant nuclear atypia, frequent mitoses, and will often have foci of necrosis, all features typically absent in SCH.

In a child, the differential diagnosis of SCH may also include KHE. KHE is characterized by a distinctly lobular proliferation of spindled endothelial cells, surrounded by a fibrous stroma. Dilated blood vessels and lymphatics are often noted in association with the tumors. Features that allow the distinction of SCH from cutaneous KHE include circumscription of the lesion, intravascular growth, the presence of vacuolated epithelioid endothelial cells, and the absence of lobular growth or fibrosis.

PROGNOSIS AND TREATMENT

SCHs are benign tumors, without capacity for metastasis. A significant percentage of patients may have multiple lesions and *local recurrences*. The latter is most likely related to propagation of the process along adjacent, possibly abnormal blood vessels.

DEEPLY LOCATED HEMANGIOMAS INCLUDING ANGIOMATOSIS

CLINICAL FEATURES

Deeply situated hemangiomas, principally intramuscular hemangiomas, account for less than 1% of all vascular tumors. Clinically, deep hemangiomas often present as large, nonspecific masses, which may be confused with a variety of sarcomas. Commonly, deep hemangiomas contain a large component of benign fat and may be mistaken clinically and radiographically for fatty tumors. Deep hemangiomas may occur in any location, including synovium *(synovial hemangioma)* and nerve *(intraneural hemangioma)*. For a lesion to be classified as *angiomatosis*, it must either show extensive involvement of multiple tissues planes, such as skin, subcutis, muscle, and bone, or it must involve more than one muscle in a contiguous fashion.

PATHOLOGIC FEATURES

GROSS FINDINGS

Great diversity exists in the gross appearance of deep hemangiomas, depending on the relative predominance of fat, capillary hemangioma-like, and cavernous hemangioma-like areas.

MICROSCOPIC FINDINGS

Deep hemangiomas may show principally features of capillary hemangioma or cavernous hemangioma, and frequently show an admixture of both areas, as well as larger, malformed vessels resembling both arteries and veins (Figures 9-21 to 9-23). Although

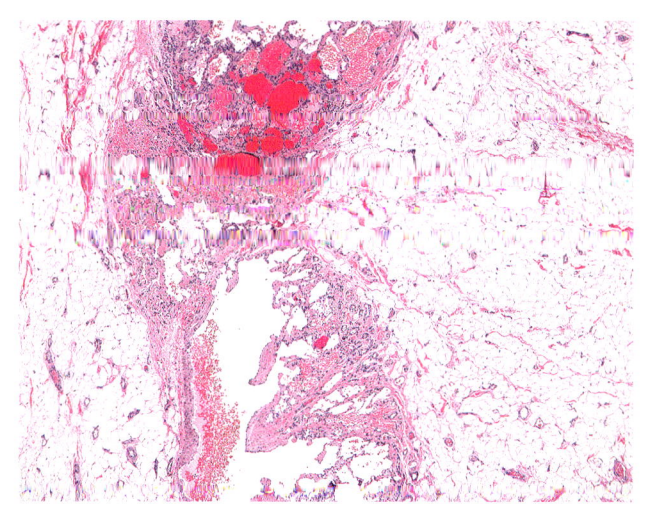

FIGURE 9-21
Intramuscular hemangioma (vascular malformation), with abundant mature adipose tissue, and numerous abnormal vascular channels, resembling arteries, veins, and cavernous hemangioma.

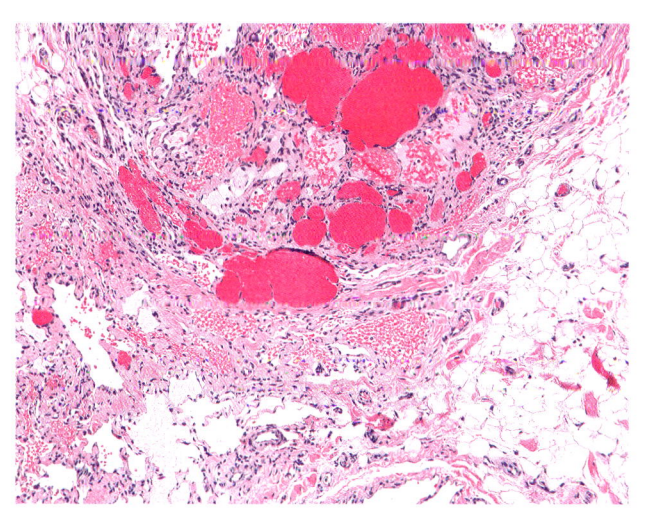

FIGURE 9-22
Abnormal aggregates of vascular channels of different types in intramuscular hemangioma.

DEEPLY LOCATED HEMANGIOMAS INCLUDING ANGIOMATOSIS—FACT SHEET

Definition
- Deeply situated, often progressive, benign vascular tumor
- Angiomatosis must involve multiple tissue planes or involve multiple muscles

Incidence and Location
- <1% of hemangiomas
- Any soft tissue location

Morbidity and Mortality
- May be extensive, locally invasive, and difficult to completely resect

Sex, Race, and Age Distribution
- None

Clinical Features
- Large, nonspecific soft tissue mass
- Large fatty component, often thought of as lipoma

Prognosis and Treatment
- Benign
- Frequent local recurrences
- Treated surgically

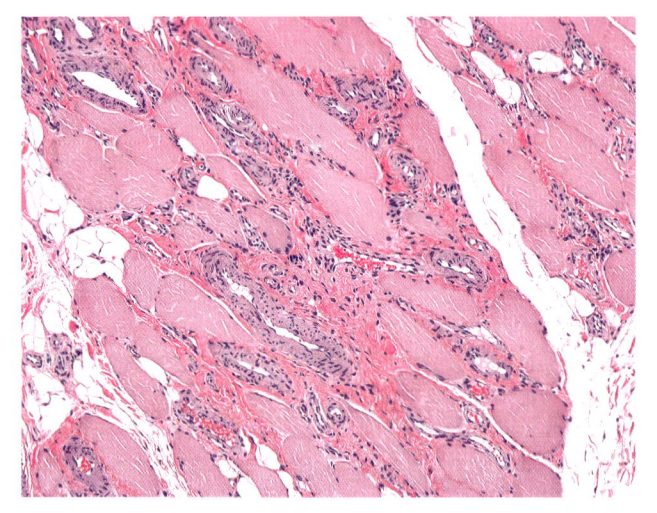

DEEPLY LOCATED HEMANGIOMAS INCLUDING ANGIOMATOSIS—PATHOLOGIC FEATURES

Gross Findings
- Large, poorly circumscribed
- Fatty
- Multiple large, abnormally configured vessels

Microscopic Findings
- May show principally features of capillary hemangioma or cavernous hemangioma
- Frequently show an admixture of both patterns, as well as larger, malformed vessels resembling both arteries and veins
- Splay apart skeletal muscle in a *checkerboard* pattern
- Abundant adipose tissue

Immunohistochemical Findings
- Endothelial cells express CD31, CD34, FLI-1 protein, and vWF

Differential Diagnosis
- Angiosarcoma
- Adipocytic tumors

FIGURE 9-23
Splaying apart of skeletal muscle by thick-walled blood vessels, a feature of intramuscular hemangioma.

such lesions have in the past been subclassified as, for example, *venous hemangioma* or *arteriovenous hemangioma*, lesions with overlapping histologic features seem to be the rule, rather than the exception, and subclassification does not appear to be clinically relevant. It has recently been suggested, particularly in the pediatric pathology literature, that all such lesions are better considered vascular malformations, rather than neoplasms. This has not, however, been universally accepted. Intramuscular hemangiomas of principally capillary type typically splay apart the skeletal muscle in a *checkerboard* pattern and usually contain abundant adipose tissue. This presence of this adipose tissue may make the determination of surgical margin status difficult.

ANCILLARY STUDIES

IMMUNOHISTOCHEMISTRY

Angiomatoses and deep hemangiomas contain mature endothelia, which express CD31, CD34, Fli-1, and vWf.

DIFFERENTIAL DIAGNOSIS

The extensive nature of angiomatoses and deep hemangiomas, and their infiltrative growth in the deep soft tissues, may raise concern for an angiosarcoma. Unlike angiosarcomas, angiomatoses and deep hemangiomas consist of uniformly well-formed vessels, which contain a muscular coat and bland, monolayered endothelial cells. Diffuse infiltration by irregular, elaborately anastomosing, poorly formed vessels, a characteristic feature of angiosarcoma, is not seen. Angiomatoses and deep hemangiomas with a prominent adipocytic component may be confused with both benign and malignant fatty tumors. Although lipomas and liposarcomas

CHAPTER 9 Vascular Tumors of Soft Tissue

are highly vascular, they do not show the gaping vascular channels or the lobular vascular proliferation generally present, at least focally, in angiomatosis/deep hemangioma. Atypical, hyperchromatic cells, a diagnostic feature of well-differentiated liposarcomas, are absent.

PROGNOSIS AND TREATMENT

Local recurrences are common in deep hemangiomas and angiomatoses, with up to 50% of patients with angiomatosis eventually suffering a local recurrence. These recurrences may be difficult to extirpate surgically but are usually nondestructive. Malignant transformation is essentially unheard of.

EPITHELIOID HEMANGIOMA (Angiolymphoid Hyperplasia with Eosinophilia)

CLINICAL FEATURES

Epithelioid hemangiomas usually present as small, superficial masses, most often in the head and neck region, in young to middle-aged adults. The tumors are more common in women than in men. Multiple lesions may be present. Although most epithelioid hemangiomas arise in the dermis or subcutis, deeply seated and intravascular cases may rarely occur (Figure 9-24).

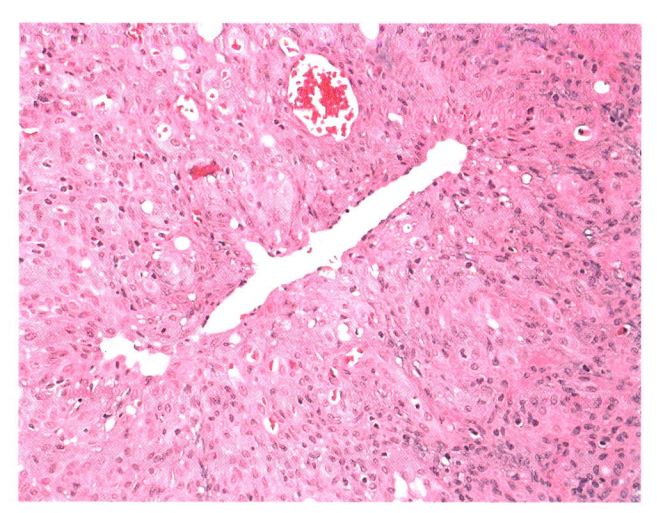

PATHOLOGIC FEATURES

GROSS FINDINGS

Epithelioid hemangiomas have a nonspecific gross appearance, although, rarely, attachment to or involvement of an artery may be apparent.

MICROSCOPIC FINDINGS

In more than 60% of cases, epithelioid hemangiomas will show a damaged, centrally located blood vessel, often lined, in part, by epithelioid endothelial cells (Figure 9-25). Typically, these epithelioid endothelial cells emanate through the wall of this vessel, forming numerous capillary-sized vessels in the surrounding soft tissues (Figure 9-26). A vaguely lobular growth

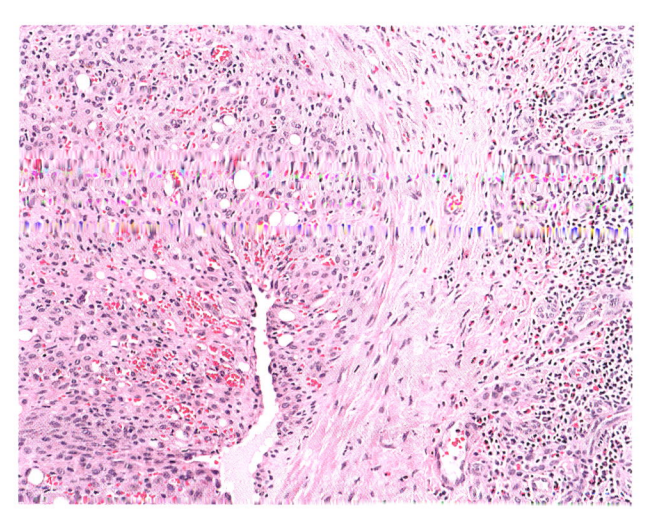

FIGURE 9-25
Proliferation of epithelioid endothelial cells in sheets and capillary-sized vessels, both within and without the wall of a damaged vessel.

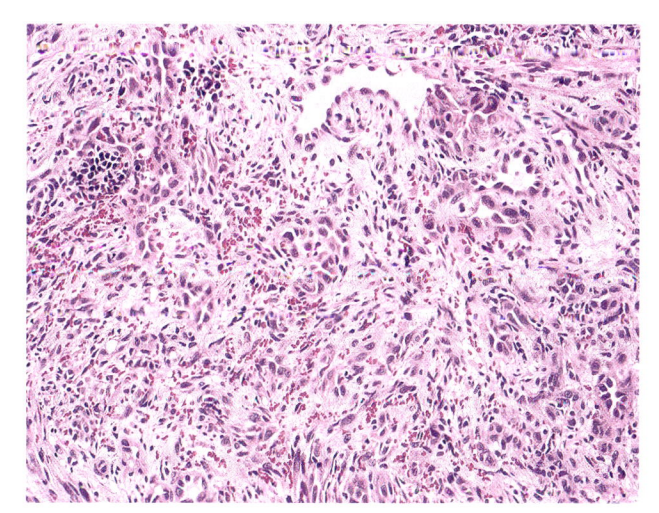

FIGURE 9-24
Central damaged blood vessel in epithelioid hemangioma, with a diffuse proliferation of epithelioid endothelial cells throughout the muscular wall.

FIGURE 9-26
Epithelioid endothelial cells with a "tombstone" configuration in epithelioid hemangioma. Note also the stromal eosinophils.

EPITHELIOID HEMANGIOMA—FACT SHEET

Definition
- Benign or possibly reactive endothelial tumor, frequently identified in association with a damaged vessel

Incidence and Location
- Uncommon
- Head and neck
- May be multiple
- Most often in dermis or subcutis; rarely in deeper locations

Morbidity and Mortality
- Benign

Sex, Race, and Age Distribution
- More common in women
- Young adults

Clinical Features
- Small subcutaneous mass

Prognosis and Treatment
- Benign
- Surgical excision

EPITHELIOID HEMANGIOMA—PATHOLOGIC FEATURES

Gross Findings
- Nonspecific
- Rarely, an attached artery may be seen

Microscopic Findings
- Organizing thrombi, calcifications, and phleboliths
- Damaged, centrally located blood vessel, often lined, in part, by epithelioid endothelial cells in 60% of cases
- Epithelioid endothelial cells emanate through the wall of the vessel, forming numerous capillary-sized vessels in the surrounding soft tissues
- Vaguely lobular growth pattern
- Accompanying eosinophil and lymphocyte-rich inflammatory infiltrate
- Epithelioid endothelial cells have abundant eosinophilic cytoplasm that may protrude into the lumen in a "tombstone" pattern
- Intracytoplasmic vacuoles
- Enlarged, normochromatic nuclei
- Mitotic figures may be present

Immunohistochemical Findings
- Endothelial cells express CD31, CD34, FLI-1 protein, and vWF
- May be low-molecular-weight cytokeratin positive

Differential Diagnosis
- EHE
- Epithelioid angiosarcoma

pattern may be appreciated at low-power magnification but is often to a degree obscured by the overall cellularity of the lesion, and by the accompanying eosinophil and lymphocyte-rich inflammatory infiltrate. The endothelial cells that line the proliferating vessels have abundant eosinophilic cytoplasm, reminiscent of epithelial cells, which may protrude into the lumen in a "tombstone" pattern. Intracytoplasmic vacuoles are frequently present. The nuclei of these epithelioid endothelial cells are typically enlarged but normochromatic, with finely dispersed chromatin and small nucleoli. Mitotic figures may be present, but atypical mitoses are not seen.

Ancillary Studies

Immunohistochemistry

Epithelioid hemangiomas express CD31, CD34, Fli-1, and vWF, and occasionally show anomalous expression of low-molecular-weight cytokeratins. This latter feature may result in confusion with an epithelial neoplasm, emphasizing the need to use a panel of immunostains. In particularly solid and cellular examples of epithelioid hemangioma, immunostaining for smooth muscle actin may be helpful for highlighting surrounding pericytes and vascular smooth muscle, revealing the well-formed and vaguely lobular nature of the proliferating vessels.

Differential Diagnosis

Epithelioid hemangiomas are typically confused with true epithelial neoplasms, such as metastatic carcinomas, and with other epithelioid vascular tumors, such as epithelioid hemangioendothelioma (EHE) and epithelioid angiosarcoma. Identification of a centrally located damaged blood vessel, when present, and recognition of the vaguely lobular growth pattern and associated eosinophilic infiltrate of epithelioid hemangioma are important in distinguishing it from carcinoma. In particularly difficult cases, immunohistochemistry for endothelial markers may be helpful.

Although epithelioid hemangiomas may show intracytoplasmic lumen formation, a hallmark of EHE, it lacks the distinctive myxochondroid matrix, single-file growth, and infiltration invariably present in EHE. Although EHEs may show origin from a larger blood vessel, they lack the lobular growth pattern and inflammatory cell infiltrate seen in epithelioid hemangioma. Epithelioid forms of angiosarcoma are much more extensive, obviously malignant-appearing tumors that typically grow in solid sheets and irregularly anastomosing vascular channels.

PROGNOSIS AND TREATMENT

Approximately 30% of epithelioid hemangiomas recur locally, but they have essentially no capacity for metastasis. Complete surgical resection is the therapy of choice.

VASCULAR TUMORS OF INTERMEDIATE (BORDERLINE) MALIGNANCY: HEMANGIOENDOTHELIOMAS

KAPOSIFORM HEMANGIOENDOTHELIOMA

CLINICAL FEATURES

KHE is a distinctive vascular neoplasm of childhood, which shows mixed features of a juvenile capillary hemangioma and KS. Unlike juvenile capillary hemangioma, KHE is frequently associated with the Kasabach-Merritt phenomenon (KMP; thrombocytopenia and hemorrhage) and does not spontaneously regress. KHE is not associated with immunosuppression.

KHE typically presents in early childhood, most often in the first year of life. Although it was previously thought to occur most often in the retroperitoneum, it is actually much more common in the skin and soft tissues of the extremities, where it presents as a large, vascular-appearing mass. Nearly 50% of patients with KHE will experience development of KMP. Conversely, most reported cases of KMP have occurred in association with KHE (often unrecognized).

PATHOLOGIC FEATURES

GROSS FINDINGS

In the skin, KHEs appear as large, violaceous plaques. In the deep soft tissues or retroperitoneum, they present as large, vascular-appearing tumors that may involve adjacent structures.

MICROSCOPIC FINDINGS

Both superficially located and deep KHEs grow in an infiltrative and nodular pattern, often with associated fibrosis (Figures 9-27 and 9-28). Frequently, dilated lymphatics are seen at the periphery of the tumor mass, sometimes resembling lymphangioma. Crescentic vascular spaces, identical to those seen in so-called tufted angioma, are frequently present (Figure 9-29).

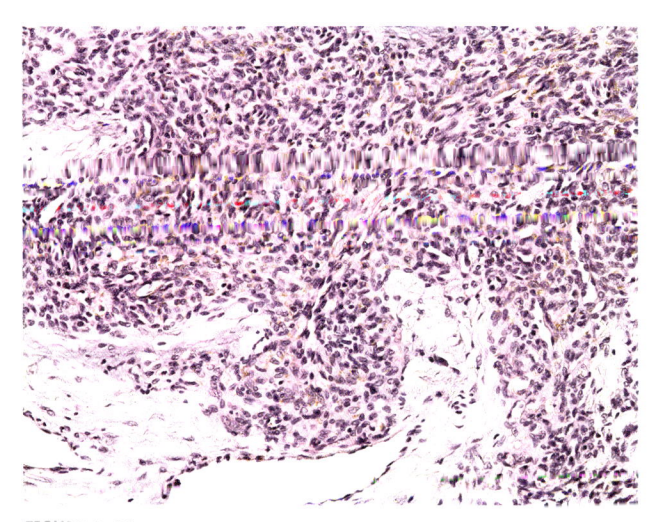

FIGURE 9-28
Stromal fibrosis, crescentic vascular spaces, and spindled endothelial proliferation in kaposiform hemangioendothelioma.

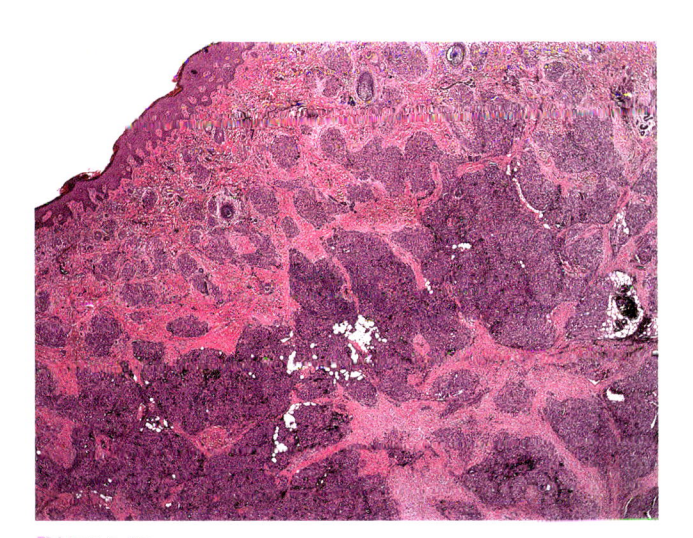

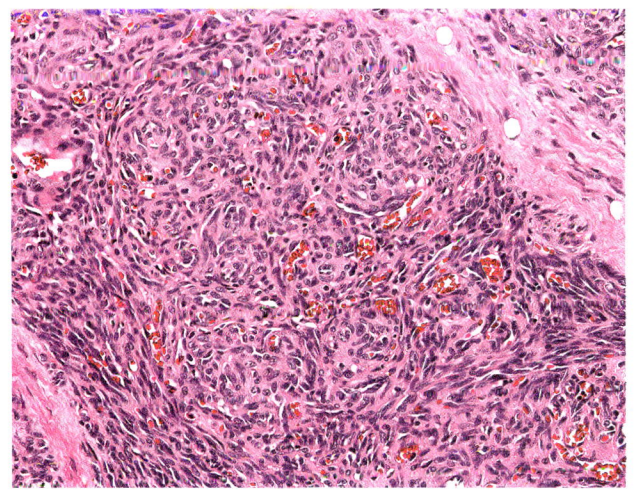

FIGURE 9-27
Kaposiform hemangioendothelioma: a large, infiltrative, dermal and subcutaneous mass in a very young child.

FIGURE 9-29
Nodule of kaposiform hemangioendothelioma, showing Kaposi sarcoma–like spindled cells and better formed small capillaries.

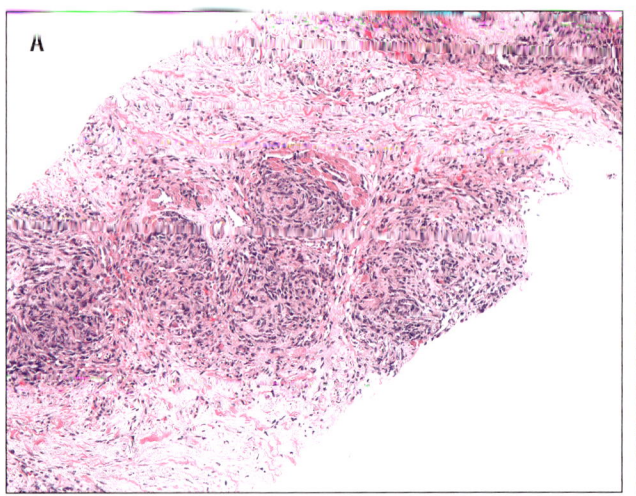

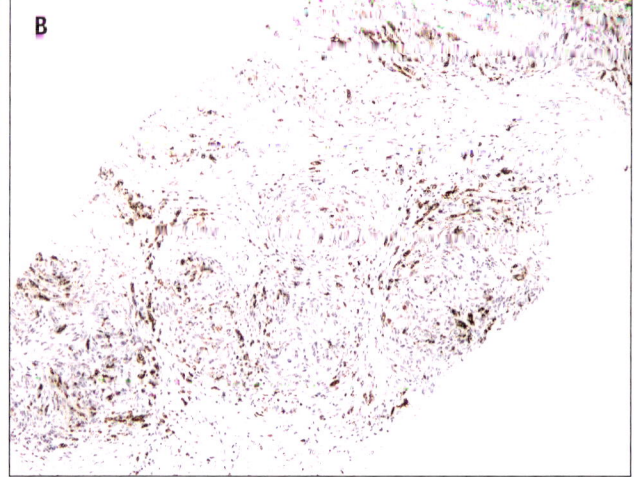

FIGURE 9-30
A, Kaposiform hemangioendothelioma. **B,** Negative for GLUT-1 protein. Absence of GLUT-1 expression is useful in distinguishing kaposiform hemangioendothelioma from capillary hemangioma.

KAPOSIFORM HEMANGIOENDOTHELIOMA—FACT SHEET

Definition
- Vascular tumor of intermediate malignancy, frequently associated with Kasabach–Merritt syndrome

Incidence and Location
- Rare
- Dermis and deep subcutis of extremities
- Retroperitoneum

Morbidity and Mortality
- Locally aggressive
- Little, if any, metastatic potential
- May result in death from disease if unresectable (retroperitoneal tumors) or from uncontrollable consumptive coagulopathy

Sex, Race, and Age Distribution
- Infants
- No sex or race predilection

Clinical Features
- Violaceous plaque when located in extremities
- Large, vascular-appearing mass when retroperitoneal

Prognosis and Treatment
- Locally aggressive
- May be difficult to completely resect
- Does not spontaneously regress or respond to interferons
- Little, if any, metastatic risk
- Kasabach–Merritt syndrome resolves with complete resection

KAPOSIFORM HEMANGIOENDOTHELIOMA—PATHOLOGIC FEATURES

Gross Findings
- Large violaceous plaque or mass

Microscopic Findings
- Infiltrative and nodular pattern, often with associated fibrosis
- Dilated lymphatics at periphery of tumor mass, resembling lymphangioma
- Crescentic vascular spaces
- Admixture of well-formed, capillary-sized vessels (resembling juvenile hemangioma) and solid-appearing foci, with spindled cells and slit-like vascular spaces (resembling KS)
- Glomeruloid foci that contain small fibrin/platelet thrombi

Immunohistochemical Findings
- Positive for CD31, CD34, and FLI-1 protein
- GLUT-1 negative

Differential Diagnosis
- Capillary hemangioma
- KS

The tumor nodules are composed of an admixture of well-formed, capillary-sized vessels (resembling juvenile hemangioma) and solid-appearing foci, with spindled cells and slit-like vascular spaces (resembling KS) (Figure 9-30). Epithelioid, or glomeruloid, foci that contain small fibrin/platelet thrombi are found scattered throughout the tumor.

ANCILLARY STUDIES

IMMUNOHISTOCHEMISTRY

By immunohistochemistry, the spindled and epithelioid cells express CD31, CD34, and FLI-1 protein, but not vWF. GLUT-1 protein, a sensitive marker of juvenile hemangiomas, is absent in KHE. KHEs are negative for the HHV-8–associated LANA protein, unlike KS, which is uniformly positive.

Differential Diagnosis

Although foci within KHE may closely resemble juvenile hemangioma, they differ significantly by virtue of their infiltrative growth, associated desmoplasia, absence of a uniform lobular architecture, and spindled and glomeruloid foci. In small biopsies, immunohistochemistry for GLUT-1 protein (positive in juvenile hemangioma, negative in KHE) may be helpful. The histologic features of tufted angioma (angioblastoma of Nakagawa) are essentially identical to those of KHE. Although tufted angioma was originally thought not to be associated with KMP, cases have now been reported. Most likely, tufted angioma and KHE are the same tumor, some of which occur in more superficial locations and are less often associated with KMP. KS typically occurs in much older patients than does KHE, and grows in a diffuse pattern, without the nodularity of KHE. The cells of KS are larger and more hyperchromatic than those of KHE, and glomeruloid foci and microthrombi are not seen. Immunohistochemical detection of HHV-8 LANA protein, specific for KS, may occasionally be of value in this differential diagnosis. SCH is a distinctive benign vascular lesion characterized by a well-circumscribed collection of thick-walled blood vessels, thrombi, phleboliths, and an admixture of spindled and vacuolated, epithelioid endothelial cells. It is frequently associated with Maffucci syndrome, and often recurs by propagation along a damaged blood vessel. It lacks the infiltrative growth and capillary hemangioma-like areas seen in KHE.

Prognosis and Treatment

Complete surgical resection is the therapy of choice for KHE, but it is not always possible because of the extent of local disease. Approximately 10% of patients with KHE will die either of local effects of the tumor or of complications related to KMP. KHE appears to be less responsive to interferons than are juvenile hemangiomas. Rare cases may metastasize to lymph nodes or perinodal soft tissue, although distant metastases have not yet been seen. Given the mortality associated with this tumor, and its low risk for metastasis, KHE is best considered a vascular tumor of intermediate malignancy, rather than benign, as has been suggested by some.

DABSKA-TYPE (PAPILLARY INTRALYMPHATIC ANGIOENDOTHELIOMA) AND RETIFORM HEMANGIOENDOTHELIOMAS

Dabska-type and retiform hemangioendotheliomas show significant histologic overlap, and are increasingly regarded as different manifestations of a single entity. They are discussed together here.

Clinical Features

Dabska-type hemangioendotheliomas occur almost exclusively in infants and young children, and present as ill-defined, sometimes violaceous lesions of the head, neck, and extremities. Retiform hemangioendothelioma typically presents as a slow-growing mass in the extremities, usually in older children and adults. Both Dabska-type and retiform hemangioendotheliomas have been associated with lymphedema and lymphatic proliferations.

Pathologic Features

Gross Findings

Dabska-type and retiform hemangioendotheliomas appear grossly as ill-defined, sometimes violaceous, plaque-like lesions.

Microscopic Findings

Dabska-type and retiform hemangioendotheliomas are fundamentally characterized by a proliferation of *hobnail-like* endothelial cells, showing cuboidal shape, scant cytoplasm, and irregular, hyperchromatic nuclei (Figure 9-31). In classic Dabska-type hemangioendotheliomas, these cells are found within relatively well-formed vessels that contain distinctive intraluminal papillations, consisting of hyaline cores with hobnailed endothelial lining (Figure 9-32). These vessels are often surrounded by dense fibrosis and a prominent lymphocytic infiltrate. Occasionally, dilated lymphatics are present adjacent to areas of typical Dabska-type hemangioendothelioma (Figure 9-33). Mitotic activity is usually sparse. Retiform hemangioendotheliomas consist of an infiltrative proliferation of elongated, branching vessels, reminiscent of the rete testis, which are lined by hobnailed endothelial cells (Figure 9-34). As in Dabska-type hemangioendotheliomas, hyaline fibrosis and chronic inflammation are commonly present. Occasional cases of retiform hemangioendothelioma may contain intraluminal papillae, identical to those seen in Dabska-type tumors.

Ancillary Studies

Immunohistochemistry

Both Dabska-type and retiform hemangioendotheliomas express common endothelial markers, such as CD31, CD34, and vWF, as well as putative lymphatic markers, such as vascular endothelial growth factor receptor 3 (VEGFR-3) and D2-40. This phenotype, as well as the association with lymphangiectasia, has led to the suggestion that both tumors show lymphatic endothelial differentiation.

Differential Diagnosis

Hobnail hemangiomas (targetoid hemosiderotic hemangiomas) differ from Dabska and retiform hemangioendotheliomas in that they are confined to the dermis and show a distinctive *biphasic* appearance, with a superficial portion showing dilated vessels lined by hobnail endothelial cells (occasionally with intraluminal papillae) and a deeper portion of slit-like capillaries, which infiltrate the dermal collagen. In general, the cells of hobnail hemangioma do not show the hyperchromatism of those seen in hobnailed hemangioendotheliomas, and hyaline

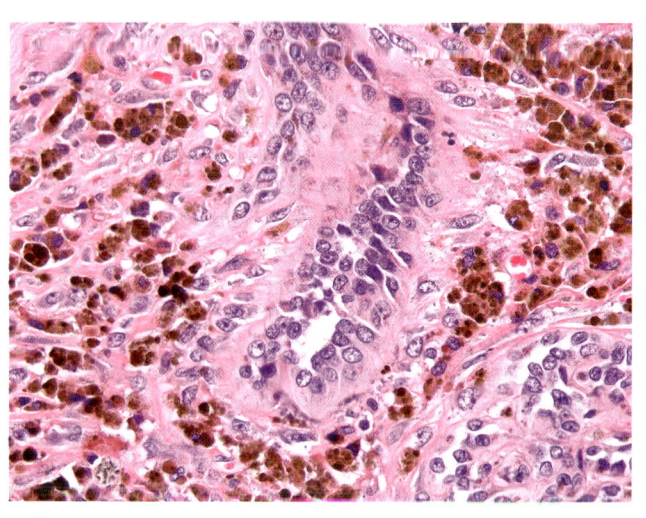

FIGURE 9-31
Hobnailed endothelial cells, the histologic hallmark of Dabska-type and retiform hemangioendotheliomas.

DABSKA-TYPE AND RETIFORM HEMANGIOENDOTHELIOMAS—FACT SHEET

Definition
- Vascular tumors of intermediate malignancy, defined by the presence of distinctive "hobnailed" endothelial cells, most likely showing lymphatic endothelial differentiation

Incidence and Location
- Rare
- Dermis and subcutis of head/neck and extremities

Morbidity and Mortality
- Locally aggressive; may be difficult to completely excise
- Low mortality rate

Sex, Race, and Age Distribution
- No sex or race predilection
- Dabska-type hemangioendothelioma occurs in infants and very young children
- Retiform hemangioendothelioma occurs in adults

Clinical Features
- Poorly demarcated violaceous plaque

Prognosis and Treatment
- Locally aggressive
- Extremely low metastatic risk
- Almost all patients are cured with wide excision

DABSKA-TYPE AND RETIFORM HEMANGIOENDOTHELIOMAS—PATHOLOGIC FEATURES

Gross Findings
- Ill-defined violaceous plaque that involves skin and subcutis

Microscopic Findings
- Infiltrative proliferation of "hobnailed" endothelial cells, showing cuboidal shape, scant cytoplasm, and irregular, hyperchromatic nuclei
- Dense fibrosis and prominent lymphocytic infiltrate
- Dabska-type hemangioendotheliomas show relatively well-formed vessels with intraluminal papillations composed of hyaline cores with hobnailed endothelial lining
- Retiform hemangioendotheliomas show an infiltrative proliferation of elongated, branching vessels (rete testis-like) lined by hobnailed endothelial cells
- Few mitotic figures
- Dilated lymphatics often present adjacent to areas of typical Dabska-type hemangioendothelioma
- Retiform hemangioendothelioma may contain intraluminal papillae, identical to Dabska-type tumors

Immunohistochemical Findings
- Both are positive for CD31, CD34, and FLI-1, and usually negative for vWF
- Both express lymphatic endothelial markers (VEGFR-3, D2-40)

Differential Diagnosis
- Hobnail hemangiomas
- Angiosarcomas with hobnailed endothelial cells
- Angiosarcomas and hemangioendotheliomas with intraluminal papillations

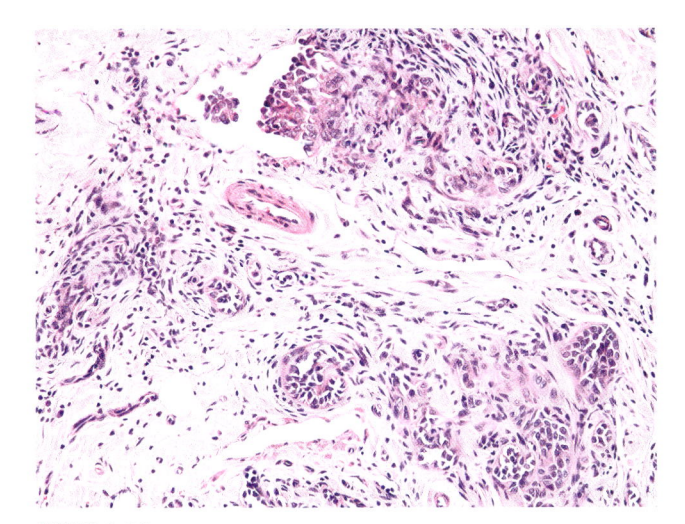

CHAPTER 9 Vascular Tumors of Soft Tissue   183

FIGURE 9-32
Dabska-type hemangioendothelioma, with fibrosis, chronic inflammation, and malignant hobnailed endothelial cells that form intravascular papillae.

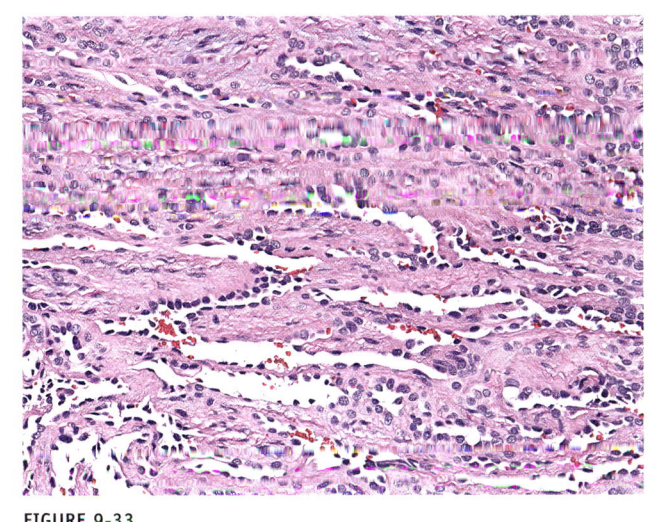

FIGURE 9-33
Retiform hemangioendothelioma, an infiltrative growth of hobnailed endothelial cells in a pattern reminiscent of the rete testis.

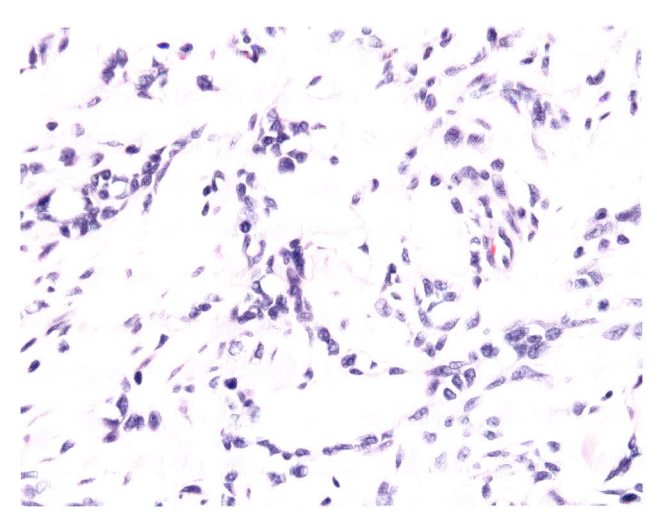

FIGURE 9-34
Hobnailed endothelial cells and fibrosis in retiform hemangioendothelioma.

fibrosis is not conspicuous. Intraluminal papillations are not specific to Dabska-type hemangioendotheliomas, and may be seen in otherwise conventional angiosarcomas and EHEs. Occasional fully malignant angiosarcomas are composed of *hobnailed* endothelial cells; such lesions typically show higher nuclear grade and more frequent mitotic activity, and are diffusely infiltrative lesions that lack the fibrosis typically seen in Dabska-type and retiform hemangioendotheliomas.

PROGNOSIS AND TREATMENT

Dabska-type and retiform hemangioendotheliomas are considered vascular neoplasms of intermediate malignancy, based on their limited capacity for lymph node metastasis and rarely distant metastasis. Only a single patient with a Dabska-type hemangioendothelioma has been reported to die of disease. Local recurrences are common in both tumors and may be aggressive. Wide excision is recommended for both tumors.

EPITHELIOID HEMANGIOENDOTHELIOMA

CLINICAL FEATURES

EHE is a rare, low-grade malignant, vascular tumor that most often occurs in adults but may also involve children. EHE involves the sexes equally. EHE may occur in the skin, deep soft tissues, bone, or viscera, in particular, the liver and lung (so-called intravascular bronchoalveolar tumor). Many cases arise from a small blood vessel, and EHE may rarely present as an entirely intravascular tumor. Pain is a frequent presenting symptom. Lesions in deep soft tissue may partially ossify and may be detectable on plain films or computed tomographic scans.

PATHOLOGIC FEATURES

EHE has a nonspecific, gross appearance. Microscopically, early lesions may show expansion of the affected blood vessel, with surrounding involvement of the adjacent soft tissues (Figure 9-35). Necrotic debris, hyaline collagen, and thrombotic material may be present within the vessel. EHE typically elaborates a dense, myxochondroid, or myxohyaline matrix, in which are embedded nests, cords, chains, and single-file arrays of small, uniform, epithelioid to slightly spindled cells with occasional intraluminal vacuoles (Figure 9-36). Multicellular vascular channels are uncommon. The

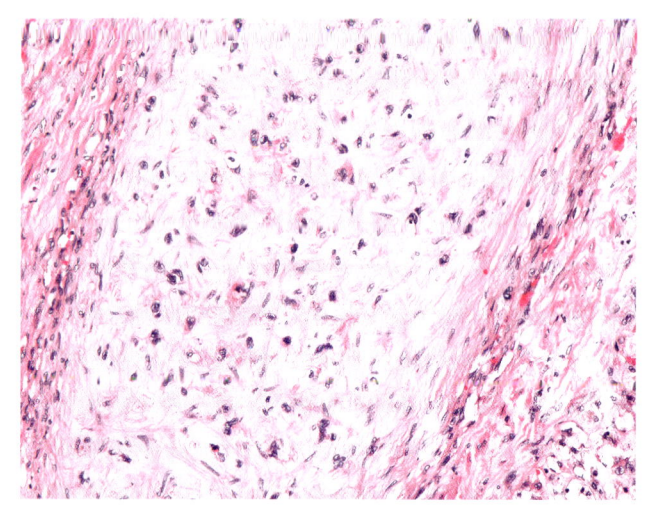

FIGURE 9-35
Intravascular epithelioid hemangioendothelioma, presenting as a thrombus. Note the distinctive myxochondroid matrix.

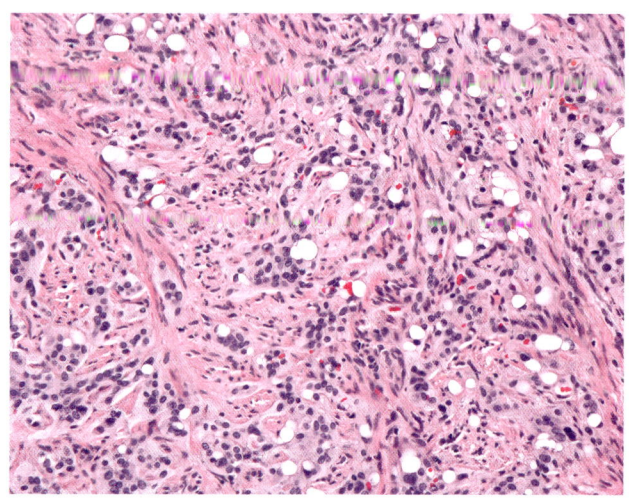

FIGURE 9-36
Epithelioid hemangioendothelioma, showing corded and single-file growth, bland, small cells, and prominent intracytoplasmic lumen formation.

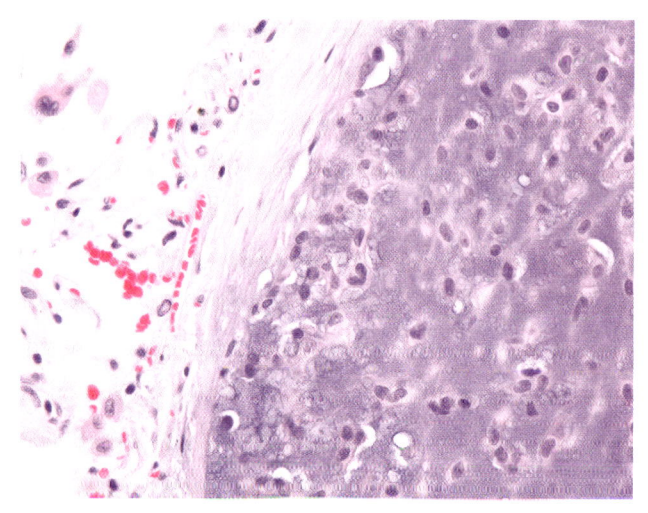

FIGURE 9-37
Myxochondroid matrix and small, bland cells in an epithelioid hemangioendothelioma of the lung.

EPITHELIOID HEMANGIOENDOTHELIOMA—FACT SHEET

Definition
- Low-grade malignant vascular tumor composed of bland epithelioid endothelial cells in a myxochondroid to hyalinized matrix

Incidence and Location
- Rare
- Skin, soft tissue, bone, lung, liver

Morbidity and Mortality
- Greater metastatic risk than other hemangioendotheliomas (10% for typical EHE, considerably greater for high-grade EHE), better considered a distinctive type of low-grade angiosarcoma

Sex, Race, and Age Distribution
- No sex or race predilection
- Adults, rarely in children

Clinical Features
- May present with pain and vascular thrombosis
- Soft tissue lesions usually present as nonspecific masses
- May present as lytic bone lesions
- Bone, liver, and lung lesions may be asymptomatic

Prognosis and Treatment
- Approximately 17% metastatic risk and 3% risk for mortality for classic EHE, lacking high-grade areas
- Inclusive of high-grade EHE, local recurrence risk rate is 10% to 15%, metastatic risk is approximately 25%, and mortality rate is 10% to 15%
- All should be treated with wide excision
- Adjuvant radiotherapy may be warranted in selected cases
- Liver transplantation has been successfully performed for extensive hepatic EHE

neoplastic cells are bland, with uniform nuclei and infrequent mitotic activity (Figure 9-37). Occasional EHE may show cytoplasmic spindling (Figure 9-38). Metaplastic bone may occasionally be present. Approximately one-third of EHEs show anaplastic features, including high nuclear grade, frequent mitotic activity, necrosis, and sheet-like growth; tumors with these features typically pursue a more aggressive clinical course, and have been referred to as *malignant* or *high-grade* EHE (Figure 9-39).

ANCILLARY STUDIES

IMMUNOHISTOCHEMISTRY

EHE shows a typical endothelial phenotype, with expression of vWF, CD31, CD34, and FLI-1 protein. Low-molecular-weight cytokeratins may be expressed in approximately 25% of cases.

CHAPTER 9 Vascular Tumors of Soft Tissue

EPITHELIOID HEMANGIOENDOTHELIOMA—PATHOLOGIC FEATURES

Gross Findings
- May be within a thrombosed blood vessel
- Firm, white mass, sometimes calcified

Microscopic Findings
- Early lesions may show expansion and occlusion of the affected blood vessel, with involvement of adjacent soft tissues
- Dense, myxochondroid or myxohyaline matrix
- Nests, cords, chains, and single-file arrays of small, uniform, epithelioid to slightly spindled cells with occasional intraluminal vacuoles
- Bland cells, with infrequent mitotic activity
- Multicellular vascular channels are uncommon
- Metaplastic bone may be present
- Approximately one-third of cases show anaplastic features, including high nuclear grade, frequent mitotic activity, necrosis, and sheet-like growth (high-grade or *malignant* EHE), associated with a more aggressive clinical course

Immunohistochemical Findings
- Positive for CD31, CD34, FLI-1 protein, and vWF
- Low-molecular-weight cytokeratin expression in 25% of cases

Differential Diagnosis
- Epithelioid hemangioma
- Epithelioid angiosarcoma
- Primary or metastatic carcinoma, especially lobular carcinoma of the breast

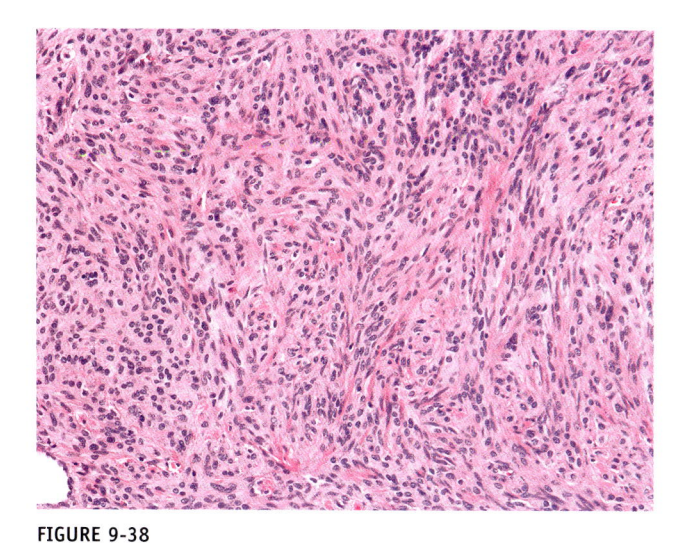

FIGURE 9-38
Cytoplasmic spindling may be seen on occasion in epithelioid hemangioendothelioma.

DIFFERENTIAL DIAGNOSIS

Epithelioid hemangioma lacks the distinctive myxochondroid matrix, single-file growth, and infiltration invariably present in EHE, and display a lobular growth pattern and a prominent inflammatory cell infiltrate. Epithelioid forms of angiosarcoma are much more extensive, obviously malignant-appearing tumors that typically grow in solid sheets and irregularly anastomosing vascular channels. The distinction of *high grade* forms of EHE from epithelioid angiosarcoma rests on identification of areas of more typical EHE.

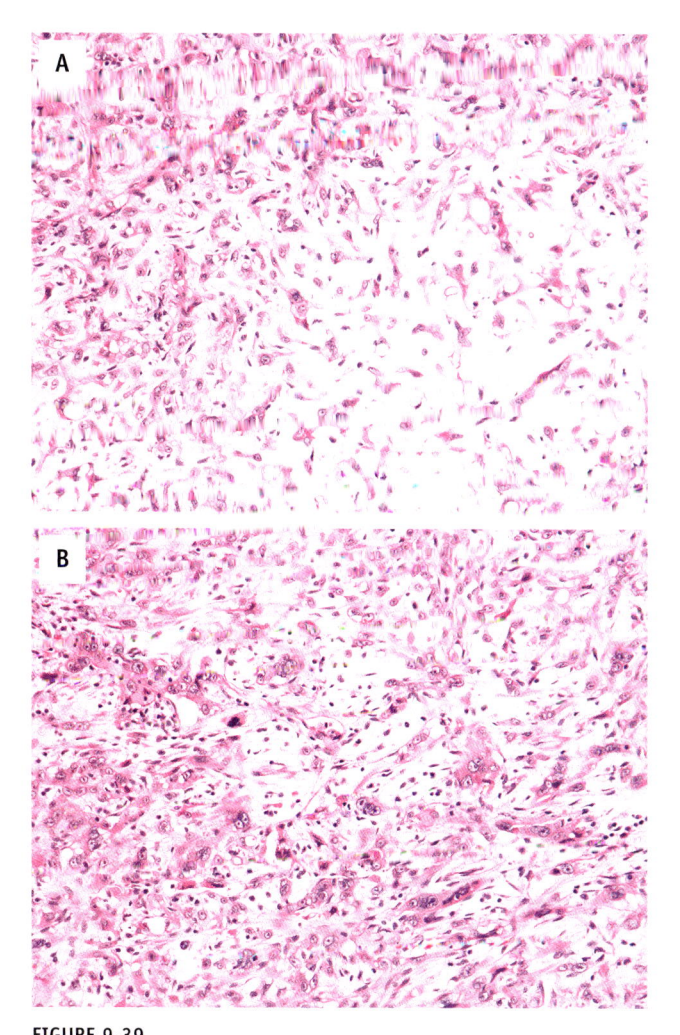

PROGNOSIS AND TREATMENT

Classic EHEs, lacking high-grade areas, have an approximately 17% metastatic risk and 3% risk for mortality. Studies of EHE that have not excluded high-grade EHE have documented a local recurrence risk rate of 10% to 15%, a metastatic risk of approximately 25%, and a mortality rate of 10% to 15%. Unlike many other sarcomas, EHEs may metastasize to lymph nodes (Figure 9-40). A risk stratification model for EHE based on a combination of cytology, mitotic rate, and size has been proposed but is not yet widely accepted. Although EHE is generally

FIGURE 9-39
High-grade ("malignant") epithelioid hemangioendothelioma showing a transition from more typical areas **(A)** to much more pleomorphic and mitotically active areas **(B)**. Such tumors have a greater risk for aggressive behavior.

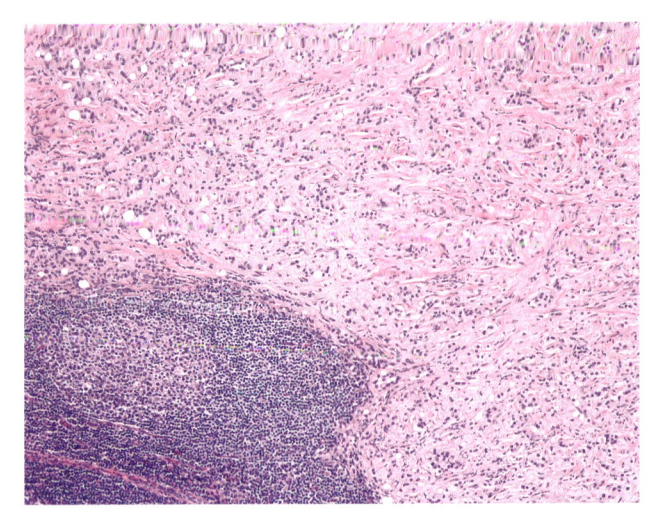

FIGURE 9-40
Metastasis of epithelioid hemangioendothelioma to a lymph node.

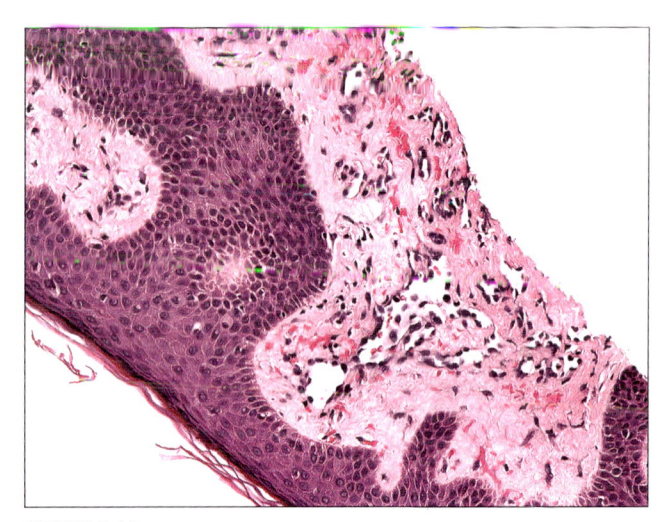

FIGURE 9-41
Relatively well-formed but clearly infiltrative vascular channels in a well-differentiated dermal angiosarcoma.

considered a vascular tumor of intermediate malignancy, it is perhaps better thought of as a low-grade form of angiosarcoma, given its much more aggressive behavior as compared with other hemangioendotheliomas.

FULLY MALIGNANT VASCULAR TUMORS

ANGIOSARCOMA

CLINICAL FEATURES

Angiosarcomas are rare sarcomas that occur in several different distinct clinical settings. The most common group of angiosarcomas is cutaneous, occurring most often in the head and neck region of elderly adults with significant solar damage. Angiosarcomas of deep soft tissue are uncommon and have no well-defined clinical associations. A significant number of angiosarcomas may be thought of as iatrogenic in nature, including lymphedema-associated angiosarcomas seen most often after radical and modified radical mastectomies *(Stewart–Treves angiosarcoma)*, postirradiation cutaneous angiosarcoma, frequently seen in patients who have received breast-conserving surgery and adjuvant irradiation, angiosarcomas associated with the use of Thorotrast contrast media, angiosarcomas associated with implanted Dacron vascular grafts, and angiosarcomas associated with arteriovenous fistulae. Angiosarcomas may also arise in association with implanted foreign material such as shrapnel, secondary to industrial vinyl chloride exposure, and in patients with syndromes associated with benign vascular proliferations, such as Klippel–Trenaunay syndrome. Finally, angiosarcomas may rarely arise within other soft tissue tumors, in particular, nerve sheath tumors.

Cutaneous angiosarcoma usually presents as a multifocal, erythematous or violaceous lesion. Postirradiation cutaneous angiosarcomas may arise in a short time after irradiation (median, 59 months), in contrast with other types of postirradiation sarcomas. Angiosarcomas of deep soft tissue present as large, hemorrhagic masses that may clinically be confused with hematomas.

PATHOLOGIC FEATURES

Angiosarcomas are extremely variable in appearance, ranging from well-differentiated lesions that may be difficult to distinguish from hemangiomas, to exclusively spindled lesions resembling fibrosarcoma or purely epithelioid lesions easily mistaken for carcinoma. Vasoformative growth, with production of highly infiltrative, irregularly configured vascular channels, often with intraluminal papillary projections, is frequently seen (Figure 9-41). The majority of angiosarcomas are high-grade lesions characterized by somewhat epithelioid cells having high nuclear grade and an architectural pattern that varies from sieve-like to solid (Figure 9-42). Necrosis and frequent mitotic figures including atypical forms are present. Well-differentiated lesions consist of highly differentiated, ramifying vessels composed of cells of low nuclear grade without mitotic activity, which dissect through the adjacent connective tissues (Figure 9-43). Epithelioid angiosarcomas are composed of sheets of epithelioid endothelial cells with abundant eosinophilic cytoplasm and uniformly high nuclear grade (Figures 9-44 and 9-45). Such lesions may show only focal vascular channel formation and are easily mistaken for carcinomas.

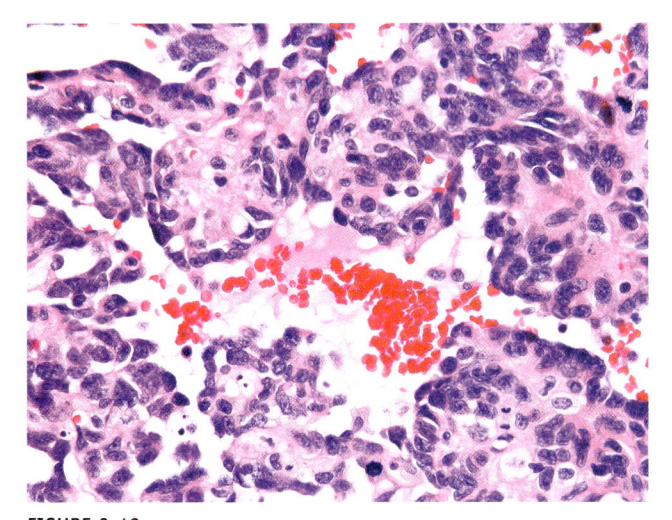

FIGURE 9-42
Most angiosarcomas show clear-cut vasoformation and clearly malignant endothelial cells.

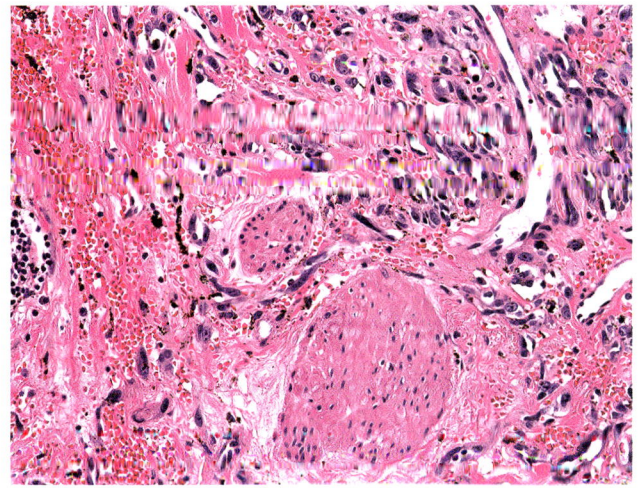

FIGURE 9-43
Diffuse infiltration around preexisting structures, a diagnostic feature of angiosarcoma.

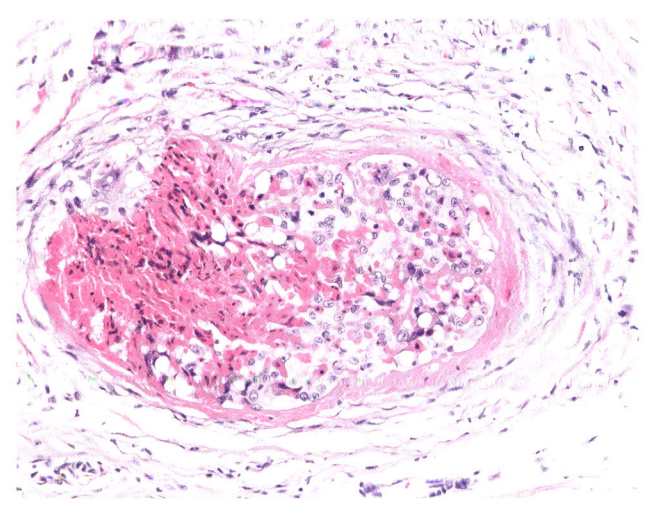

FIGURE 9-44
Intravascular epithelioid angiosarcoma, occurring in association with a Dacron vascular graft.

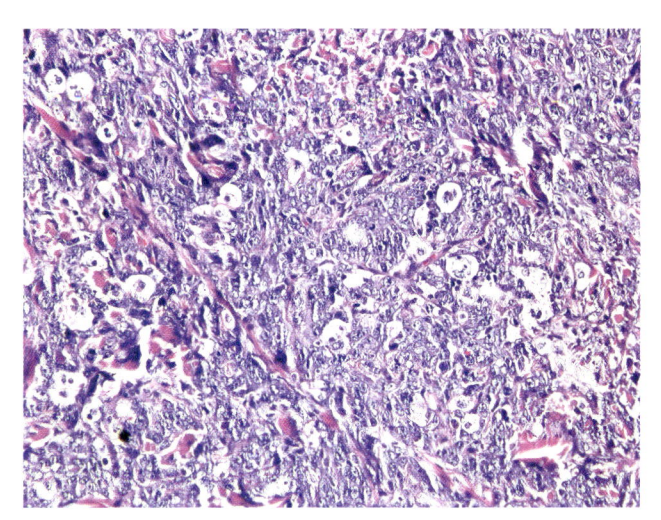

FIGURE 9-45
Epithelioid angiosarcoma, a sheet-like proliferation of highly malignant-appearing epithelioid cells, mimicking carcinoma.

ANCILLARY STUDIES

IMMUNOHISTOCHEMISTRY

The most sensitive markers of angiosarcoma are CD31 and FLI-1 protein, followed by CD34. vWF is the least sensitive marker of angiosarcomas, particularly poorly differentiated ones. Subsets of angiosarcomas express putative lymphatic markers, such as D2-40 and VEGFR-3; the specificity of these markers for lymphatic endothelial differentiation in malignant vascular tumors is questionable. All angiosarcomas may express low-molecular-weight cytokeratins; cytokeratin expression is particularly common in epithelioid angiosarcomas.

DIFFERENTIAL DIAGNOSIS

As noted earlier, angiosarcomas are notoriously protean tumors; thus, their differential diagnosis is wide. Well-differentiated angiosarcomas can be distinguished from benign vascular proliferations such as diffuse hemangioma, dermal angiomatosis, and postirradiation atypical vascular lesions by virtue of their infiltrative growth, absence of well-formed vessels with smooth muscle coats, endothelial stratification, presence of (sometimes subtle) nuclear atypia and hyperchromatism, and mitotic activity. Unlike carcinomas and epithelioid sarcomas, epithelioid angiosarcomas usually show at least focal vascular channel formation, a helpful clue. Immunohistochemistry may be valuable in this differential diagnosis; expression of high-molecular-weight cytokeratins is seen in many carcinomas and epithelioid sarcomas, but not in angiosarcomas.

ANGIOSARCOMA—FACT SHEET

Definition
▸▸ Fully malignant sarcoma showing endothelial differentiation

Incidence and Location
▸▸ Rare
▸▸ Cutaneous tumors related to sun exposure and therapeutic irradiation
▸▸ Deep soft tissue tumors of uncertain causative factor
▸▸ Iatrogenic tumors related to irradiation, Thorotrast, lymphedema, foreign materials
▸▸ Vinyl chloride in hepatic angiosarcomas

Morbidity and Mortality
▸▸ Local recurrences in 25% of cases, death from disease in > 50% of cases

Sex, Race, and Age Distribution
▸▸ No sex or race predilection
▸▸ Older adults with sun damage

Clinical Features
▸▸ Cutaneous tumors present as violaceous or erythematous plaque or nodule
▸▸ Deep soft tissue tumors present as hemorrhagic masses

Prognosis and Treatment
▸▸ Poor prognosis for all angiosarcomas
▸▸ Taxanes may be of value in cutaneous angiosarcomas related to sun damage

ANGIOSARCOMA—PATHOLOGIC FEATURES

Gross Findings
▸▸ Erythematous or violaceous plaque or nodule
▸▸ Large hemorrhagic deep soft tissue mass

Microscopic Findings
▸▸ Epithelioid cells forming primitive vascular channels
▸▸ Sieve-like and sheet-like patterns
▸▸ Necrosis, hemorrhage, and mitotic activity
▸▸ Diffuse infiltration of surrounding tissues by dissecting vascular channels
▸▸ Spindled and epithelioid variants

Immunohistochemical Findings
▸▸ Expression of CD31, CD34, FLI-1 protein, and vWF
▸▸ D2-40 and VEGFR-3 in some (lymphangiosarcoma)
▸▸ Low-molecular-weight cytokeratin expression in 25% of cases, particularly epithelioid tumors

Differential Diagnosis
▸▸ Hemangioma, diffuse angiomatosis, atypical vascular proliferations after irradiation
▸▸ Carcinoma
▸▸ EHE
▸▸ Spindle cell carcinoma and melanoma
▸▸ Other spindle cell sarcomas

Conversely, CD31 expression is seen in angiosarcomas, but not in carcinomas or epithelioid sarcomas. It is important to remember that many epithelioid sarcomas express CD34. Loss of INI-1 protein is seen in epithelioid sarcomas but not in angiosarcomas or carcinomas. EHEs produce distinctive myxochondroid matrix, lack formation of true vascular channels, and typically have low nuclear grade. The distinction of spindled angiosarcomas, particularly those arising in sun-damaged skin, from sarcomatoid carcinomas and melanomas may be difficult on purely histologic grounds. It is critically important to include angiosarcoma in this differential diagnosis, to avoid misdiagnosis and undertreatment. Again, immunohistochemistry for vascular markers, S-100 protein, and high-molecular-weight cytokeratins may be valuable. In deep soft tissue sites, other spindle cell sarcomas such as monophasic synovial sarcoma, fibrosarcoma, and leiomyosarcoma should be excluded through a combination of morphology (e.g., identification of occult glands and wiry collagen in synovial sarcoma and intersecting fascicles of eosinophilic cells in leiomyosarcoma) and immunohistochemistry for markers such as CD31, FLI-1 protein, cytokeratins, epithelial membrane antigen, smooth muscle actins, and desmin.

PROGNOSIS AND TREATMENT

Angiosarcomas in any location are aggressive sarcomas, with high rates of local recurrence, distant metastasis, and death from disease. The most common metastatic sites are the lungs, followed by soft tissue and skeleton. Approximately 35% of patients with angiosarcoma die of disease in less than 3 years. In general, angiosarcomas are resistant to all therapies, although there has been some recent success in the treatment of cutaneous angiosarcomas with taxane-based chemotherapy.

KAPOSI SARCOMA

CLINICAL FEATURES

KS occurs in four distinct clinical settings: (1) classic KS, typically occurring as lower extremity skin lesions in older men of Mediterranean, Central European, and African origin; (2) endemic KS, occurring in African young male individuals and very young children as bulky lymph node and soft tissue disease; (3) epidemic (AIDS-related) KS, occurring on the skin, mucosal surfaces, and viscera of HIV-infected patients (in particular, in homosexual male individuals); and (4) iatrogenic KS, occurring as cutaneous or visceral lesions in renal transplant patients. In any of these settings, cutaneous KS appears as a violaceous patch, plaque, papule, macule, or tumor, occasionally with associated limb edema. Visceral and lymph node involvement presents as a hemorrhagic mass. All forms of KS are now understood to be directly related to infection by HHV-8, which can be detected in essentially all cases of KS by reverse transcriptase polymerase chain reaction or with immunohistochemistry for HHV-8 LANA.

PATHOLOGIC FEATURES

The histologic appearance of KS is always the same, regardless of clinical scenario. The earliest patch lesions of KS appear as proliferations of small, infiltrative vessels surrounding larger, ectatic vessels, with associated chronic inflammation. In later plaque stage lesions, a proliferation of relatively bland, vaguely myoid spindled cells producing slit-like vascular channels is more prominent, with extravasated red blood cells and extracellular hyaline globules (Figure 9-46). Chronic inflammation is common and a helpful diagnostic clue (Figure 9-47). Papular or nodular lesions may have a polypoid growth pattern, mimicking pyogenic granuloma (Figure 9-48). The lesion may trap preexisting blood vessels, creating the so-called promontory sign. This spindle cell component predominates in later nodular or tumoral lesions of KS, mimicking fibrosarcoma (Figure 9-49). In lymph nodes, early lesions of KS are often visible as subtle spindle cell proliferations in the subcapsular sinus. Pleomorphism and mitotic activity are not generally features of classic, epidemic, or iatrogenic KS but may be seen in African endemic KS.

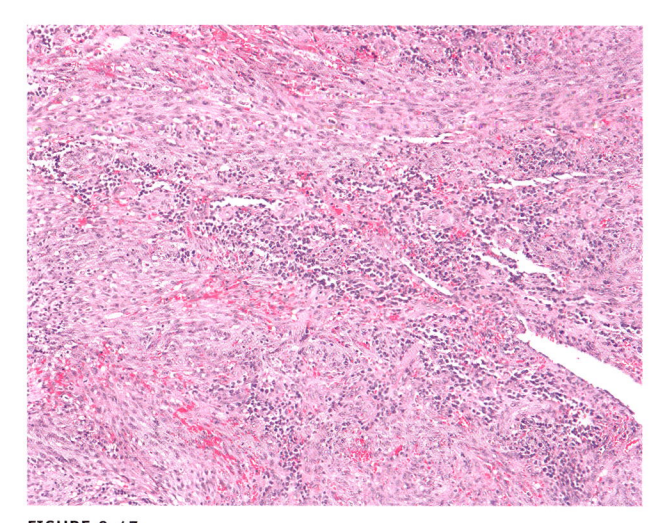

FIGURE 9-47
Chronic inflammatory cell aggregates, a clue to the diagnosis of Kaposi sarcoma.

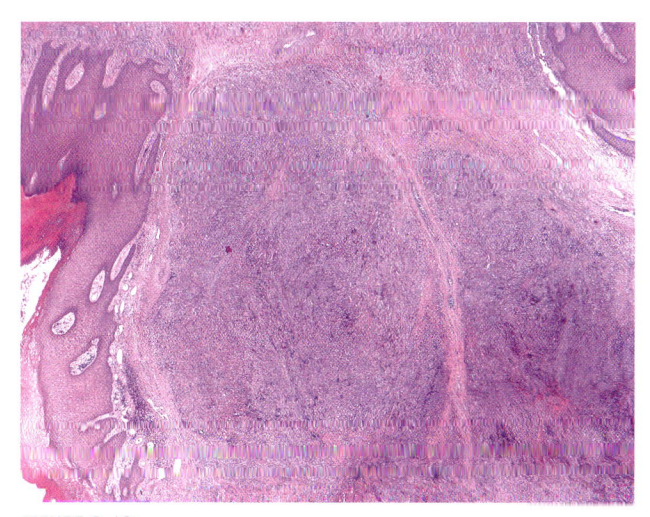

FIGURE 9-48
Nodular growth phase in Kaposi sarcoma.

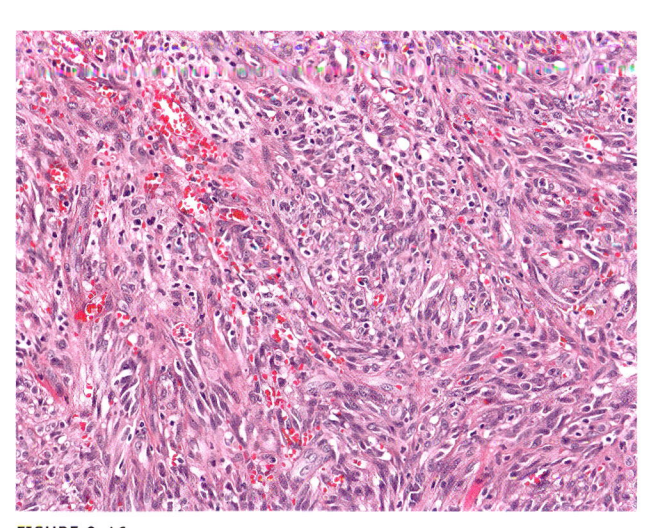

FIGURE 9-46
Vaguely myoid-appearing spindled cells forming slit-like vascular spaces in Kaposi sarcoma.

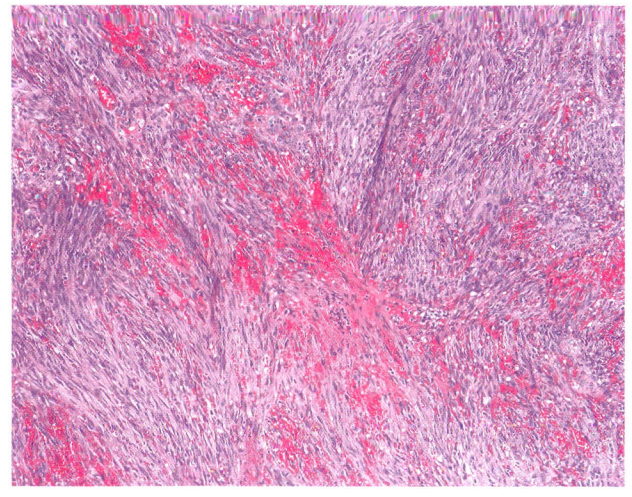

FIGURE 9-49
Fibrosarcomatous spindle cell proliferation in nodular Kaposi sarcoma.

KAPOSI SARCOMA—FACT SHEET

Definition
- Malignant vascular tumor caused by infection with HHV-8, most often in immunocompromised patients

Incidence and Location
- Classic KS: rare; skin of extremities
- Epidemic (AIDS-related) KS: extremely common in HIV-infected patients, particularly in homosexual male individuals; skin, mucosal and visceral locations
- Endemic (African) KS: rare; lymph node and soft tissue involvement
- Iatrogenic KS: rare, essentially only in kidney transplant patients; cutaneous and visceral locations

Morbidity and Mortality
- Low morbidity and mortality, and indolent clinical course in immunocompetent patients
- High morbidity and mortality rates (> 90%) in HIV-infected patients before highly active antiretroviral therapy (HAART), < 50% after development of HAART therapy

Sex, Race, and Age Distribution
- Classic KS: older men of Mediterranean, Central European, or African descent
- Endemic KS: children and young male individuals
- Epidemic KS: homosexual male individuals and intravenous drug abusers (United States), heterosexuals (Africa, India, Southeast Asia), recipients of infected transfusions or medical equipment (worldwide)
- Iatrogenic KS: kidney transplant recipients

Clinical Features
- Patch, plaque, papule, and tumor stages
- Violaceous appearance
- Hemorrhagic masses in viscera and lymph nodes

Prognosis and Treatment
- Good prognosis for cutaneous lesions in immunocompetent patients; may be treated with cryotherapy and radiotherapy
- Poor prognosis for KS in immunocompromised patients without HAART therapy; prognosis is improved with HAART therapy and systemic chemotherapy

KAPOSI SARCOMA—PATHOLOGIC FEATURES

Gross Findings
- Violaceous patch, plaque, papule, or tumor
- Large hemorrhagic deep soft tissue mass

Microscopic Findings
- Proliferating, infiltrative small vessels surrounding larger vessels, with associated chronic inflammation in earliest lesions
- Increased number of vaguely myoid, cytologically bland spindled cells forming slit-like vascular channels in later lesions
- Extravasated red blood cells, hemosiderin staining, and hyaline droplets
- Tumorous lesions may show pronounced fascicular growth (fibrosarcoma-like)

Immunohistochemical Findings
- Expression of CD31, CD34, and FLI-1 protein
- D2-40 and VEGFR-3 expression in most cases
- HHV-8 LANA protein expression is the most sensitive and specific marker of KS

Differential Diagnosis
- Stasis changes, angiosarcoma, SCH, various spindle cell sarcomas

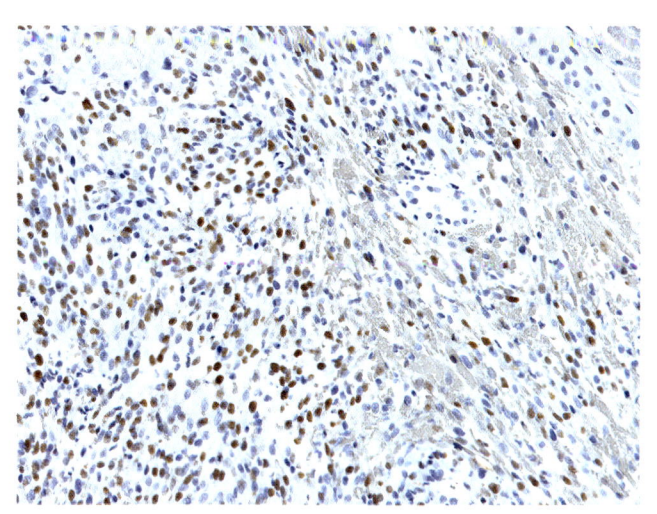

FIGURE 9-50
Nuclear expression of human herpes virus 8 latency-associated nuclear antigen (LANA) protein in Kaposi sarcoma. This finding is specific for Kaposi sarcoma, among vascular tumors.

ANCILLARY STUDIES

IMMUNOHISTOCHEMISTRY

CD31 and CD34 show approximately equal sensitivity in the diagnosis of KS, being positive in more than 90% of cases. FLI 1 protein is also expressed in a similar percentage of cases. vWF is the least sensitive marker of KS. The most specific marker of KS is LANA protein, which is positive in nearly 100% of KS lesions at all stages, but not in other types of vascular tumors (Figure 9-50). The cells of KS may also express putative markers of lymphatic differentiation, including VEGFR-3 and D2-40 (podoplanin).

DIFFERENTIAL DIAGNOSIS

Vascular proliferations associated with vascular stasis (acroangiodermatitis) may be difficult to distinguish from KS on histologic grounds alone. Correlation with clinical history and LANA immunostains may be valuable in making this distinction. Relatively low-grade–appearing angiosarcomas may mimic the earliest patch stage of KS but typically show greater cytologic atypia and more pronounced infiltrative growth. The absence of LANA expression may be helpful here as well. SCHs are well-circumscribed, typically subcutaneous lesions that contain phleboliths and calcifications, and consist of an admixture of cavernous hemangioma-like zones with cellular spindled zones, showing both spindle cells and vacuolated epithelioid cells. Highly cellular examples of KS may be confused with a variety of spindle cell sarcomas, including leiomyosarcoma and fibrosarcoma. Identification of the characteristic slit-like vascular spaces of KS and panel of immunostains to include epithelial markers, S-100 protein, muscle markers, and endothelial markers including LANA should allow this distinction without great difficulty.

PROGNOSIS AND TREATMENT

In immunocompetent patients with limited cutaneous disease, the disease-related mortality rate of KS is approximately 10% to 20%. In immunocompromised patients, treatment of KS is aimed first at elimination or amelioration of the underlying immune defect. Before the development of highly active antiviral therapy, the disease-specific mortality for KS in AIDS patients was close to 90%; with effective therapy, this has been reduced to less than 50%. Cryotherapy and radiotherapy have also been used successfully in patients with KS with limited cutaneous disease.

SUGGESTED READINGS

Papillary Endothelial Hyperplasia

1. Kuo T, Sayers CP, Rosai J: Masson's "vegetant intravascular hemangioendothelioma": A lesion often mistaken for angiosarcoma: Study of seventeen cases located in the skin and soft tissues. Cancer 1976;38:1227-1236.
2. Pins MR, Rosenthal DI, Springfield DS, et al: Florid extravascular papillary endothelial hyperplasia (Masson's pseudoangiosarcoma) presenting as a soft-tissue sarcoma. Arch Pathol Lab Med 1993;117:259-263.

Bacillary Angiomatosis

1. Calonje E, Fletcher CD: New entities in cutaneous soft tissue tumours. Pathologica 1993;85:1-15.
2. LeBoit PE: Bacillary angiomatosis: a systemic opportunistic infection with prominent cutaneous manifestations. Semin Dermatol 1991;10:194-198.
3. Nayler SJ, Allard U, Taylor L, et al: HHV-8 (KSHV) is not associated with bacillary angiomatosis. Mol Pathol 1999;52:345-348.
4. Spach DH, Koehler JE: Bartonella-associated infections. Infect Dis Clin North Am 1998;12:137-155.

Glomeruloid Hemangioma

1. Chan JK, Fletcher CD, Hicklin GA, et al: Glomeruloid hemangioma. A distinctive cutaneous lesion of multicentric Castleman's disease associated with POEMS syndrome. Am J Surg Pathol 1990;14:1036-1046.
2. Kingdon EJ, Phillips BB, Jarmulowicz M, et al: Glomeruloid haemangioma and POEMS syndrome. Nephrol Dial Transplant 2001;16:2105-2107.
3. Rongioletti F, Gambini C, Lerza R: Glomeruloid hemangioma. A cutaneous marker of POEMS syndrome. Am J Dermatopathol 1994;16:175-178.
4. Tsai CY, Lai CH, Chan HL, et al: Glomeruloid hemangioma—a specific cutaneous marker of POEMS syndrome. Int J Dermatol 2001;40:403-406.

Pyogenic Granuloma

1. Kapadia SB, Heffner DK: Pitfalls in the histopathologic diagnosis of pyogenic granuloma. Eur Arch Otorhinolaryngol 1992;249:195-200.
2. Patrice SJ, Wiss K, Mulliken JB: Pyogenic granuloma (lobular capillary hemangioma): a clinicopathologic study of 178 cases. Pediatr Dermatol 1991;8:267-276.
3. Requena L, Sangueza OP: Cutaneous vascular proliferation. Part II. Hyperplasias and benign neoplasms. J Am Acad Dermatol 1997;37:887-920.

Capillary Hemangioma

1. Coffin CM, Dehner LP: Vascular tumors in children and adolescents: a clinicopathologic study of 228 tumors in 222 patients. Pathol Annu 1993;28(pt 1):97-120.
2. Dadras SS, North PE, Bertoncini J, et al: Infantile hemangiomas are arrested in an early developmental vascular differentiation state. Mod Pathol 2004;17:1068-1079.
3. Drut RM, Drut R: Extracutaneous infantile haemangioma is also Glut1 positive. J Clin Pathol 2004;57:1197-1200.
4. North PE, Waner M, Buckmiller L, et al: Vascular tumors of infancy and childhood: beyond capillary hemangioma. Cardiovasc Pathol 2006;15:303-317.

Cavernous Hemangioma

1. Dehner LP, Ishak KG: Vascular tumors of the liver in infants and children. A study of 30 cases and review of the literature. Arch Pathol 1971;92:101-111.
2. Labauge P, Denier C, Bergametti F, et al: Genetics of cavernous angiomas. Lancet Neurol 2007;6:237-244.

Spindle Cell Hemangioma

1. Fletcher CD, Beham A, Schmid C: Spindle cell haemangioendothelioma: a clinicopathological and immunohistochemical study indicative of a non-neoplastic lesion. Histopathology 1991;18:291-301.
2. Perkins P, Weiss SW: Spindle cell hemangioendothelioma. An analysis of 78 cases with reassessment of its pathogenesis and biologic behavior. Am J Surg Pathol 1996;20:1196-1204.
3. Scott GA, Rosai J: Spindle cell hemangioendothelioma. Report of seven additional cases of a recently described vascular neoplasm. Am J Dermatopathol 1988;10:281-288.
4. Weiss SW, Enzinger FM: Spindle cell hemangioendothelioma. A low grade angiosarcoma resembling a cavernous hemangioma and Kaposi's sarcoma. Am J Surg Pathol 1986;10:521-530.

Deeply Located Hemangiomas Including Angiomatosis

1. Al-Adnani M, Williams S, Rampling D, et al: Histopathological reporting of paediatric cutaneous vascular anomalies in relation to proposed multidisciplinary classification system. J Clin Pathol 2006;59:1278-1282.
2. Buckmiller LM: Update on hemangiomas and vascular malformations. Curr Opin Otolaryngol Head Neck Surg 2004;12:476-487.
3. Hein KD, Mulliken JB, Kozakewich HP, et al: Venous malformations of skeletal muscle. Plast Reconstr Surg 2002;110:1625-1635.
4. Marler JJ, Mulliken JB: Vascular anomalies: Classification, diagnosis, and natural history. Facial Plast Surg Clin North Am 2001;9:495-504.
5. Morrison SC, Reid JR: Continuing problems with classifications of vascular malformations. Pediatr Radiol 2007;37:609.
6. Rao VK, Weiss SW: Angiomatosis of soft tissue. An analysis of the histologic features and clinical outcome in 51 cases. Am J Surg Pathol 1992;16:764-771.
7. Van Aalst JA, Bhuller A, Sadove AM: Pediatric vascular lesions. J Craniofac Surg 2003;14:566-583.

Epithelioid Hemangioma

1. Fetsch JF, Weiss SW: Observations concerning the pathogenesis of epithelioid hemangioma (angiolymphoid hyperplasia). Mod Pathol 1991;4:449–455.
2. O'Connell JX, Kattapuram SV, Mankin HJ, et al: Epithelioid hemangioma of bone. A tumor often mistaken for low-grade angiosarcoma or malignant hemangioendothelioma. Am J Surg Pathol 1993;17:610–617.
3. Olsen TG, Helwig EB: Angiolymphoid hyperplasia with eosinophilia. A clinicopathologic study of 116 patients. J Am Acad Dermatol 1985;12:781–796.
4. Weiss SW, Ishak KG, Dail DH, et al: Epithelioid hemangioendothelioma and related lesions. Semin Diagn Pathol 1986;3:259–287.

Kaposiform Hemangioendothelioma

1. Lyons LL, North PE, Mac-Moune Lai F, et al: Kaposiform hemangioendothelioma: A study of 33 cases emphasizing its pathologic, immunophenotypic, and biologic uniqueness from juvenile hemangioma. Am J Surg Pathol 2004;28:559–568.
2. Mentzel T, Mazzoleni G, Dei Tos AP, et al: Kaposiform hemangioendothelioma in adults. Clinicopathologic and immunohistochemical analysis of three cases. Am J Clin Pathol 1997;108:450–455.
3. North PE, Waner M, Mizeracki A, et al: GLUT1: A newly discovered immunohistochemical marker for juvenile hemangiomas. Hum Pathol 2000;31:11–22.
4. Zukerberg LR, Nickoloff BJ, Weiss SW: Kaposiform hemangioendothelioma of infancy and childhood. An aggressive neoplasm associated with Kasabach-Merritt syndrome and lymphangiomatosis. Am J Surg Pathol 1993;17:321–328.

Dabska-Type and Retiform Hemangioendothelioma

1. Calonje E, Fletcher CD, Wilson-Jones E, et al: Retiform hemangioendothelioma. A distinctive form of low-grade angiosarcoma delineated in a series of 15 cases. Am J Surg Pathol 1994;18:115–125.
2. Dabska M: Malignant endovascular papillary angioendothelioma of the skin in childhood. Clinicopathologic study of 6 cases. Cancer 1969;24:503–510.
3. Duke D, Dvorak A, Harris TJ, et al: Multiple retiform hemangioendotheliomas. A low-grade angiosarcoma. Am J Dermatopathol 1996;18:606–610.
4. Fanburg-Smith JC, Michal M, Partanen TA, et al: Papillary intralymphatic angioendothelioma (PILA): A report of twelve cases of a distinctive vascular tumor with phenotypic features of lymphatic vessels. Am J Surg Pathol 1999;23:1004–1010.
5. Sanz-Trelles A, Rodrigo-Fernandez I, Ayala-Carbonero A, et al: Retiform hemangioendothelioma. A new case in a child with diffuse endovascular papillary endothelial proliferation. J Cutan Pathol 1997;24:440–444.

Epithelioid Hemangioendothelioma

1. Bhagavan BS, Dorfman HD, Murthy MS, et al: Intravascular bronchiolo-alveolar tumor (IVBAT): a low-grade sclerosing epithelioid angiosarcoma of lung. Am J Surg Pathol 1982;6:41–52.
2. Deyrup AT, Tighiouart M, Montag AG, et al: Epithelioid hemangioendothelioma of soft tissue: a proposal for risk stratification based on 49 cases. Am J Surg Pathol 2008;32:924–927.
3. Mentzel T, Beham A, Calonje E, et al: Epithelioid hemangioendothelioma of skin and soft tissues: Clinicopathologic and immunohistochemical study of 30 cases. Am J Surg Pathol 1997;21:363–374.
4. Weiss SW, Enzinger FM: Epithelioid hemangioendothelioma: a vascular tumor often mistaken for a carcinoma. Cancer 1982;50:970–981.

Angiosarcoma

1. Aust MR, Olsen KD, Lewis JL, et al: Angiosarcomas of the head and neck: clinical and pathologic characteristics. Ann Otol Rhinol Laryngol 1997;106:943–951.
2. Billings SD, McKenney JK, Folpe AL, et al: Cutaneous angiosarcoma following breast-conserving surgery and radiation: An analysis of 27 cases. Am J Surg Pathol 2004;28:781–788.
3. Breiteneder-Geleff S, Soleiman A, Kowalski H, et al: Angiosarcomas express mixed endothelial phenotypes of blood and lymphatic capillaries: podoplanin as a specific marker for lymphatic endothelium. Am J Pathol 1999;154:385–394.
4. Brenn T, Fletcher CD: Postradiation vascular proliferations: an increasing problem. Histopathology 2006;48:106–114.
5. Deyrup AT, McKenney JK, Tighiouart M, et al: Sporadic cutaneous angiosarcomas: a proposal for risk stratification based on 69 cases. Am J Surg Pathol 2008;32:72–77.
6. Falk S, Krishnan J, Meis JM: Primary angiosarcoma of the spleen. A clinicopathologic study of 40 cases. Am J Surg Pathol 1993;17:959–970.
7. Fletcher CD, Beham A, Bekir S, et al: Epithelioid angiosarcoma of deep soft tissue: a distinctive tumor readily mistaken for an epithelial neoplasm. Am J Surg Pathol 1991;15:915–924.
8. Folpe AL, Chand EM, Goldblum JR, et al: Expression of Fli-1, a nuclear transcription factor, distinguishes vascular neoplasms from potential mimics. Am J Surg Pathol 2001;25:1061–1066.
9. Gray MH, Rosenberg AE, Dickersin GR, et al: Cytokeratin expression in epithelioid vascular neoplasms. Hum Pathol 1990;21:212–217.
10. Jennings TA, Peterson L, Axiotis CA, et al: Angiosarcoma associated with foreign body material. A report of three cases. Cancer 1988;62:2436–2444.
11. Kahn HJ, Bailey D, Marks A: Monoclonal antibody D2-40, a new marker of lymphatic endothelium, reacts with Kaposi's sarcoma and a subset of angiosarcomas. Mod Pathol 2002;15:434–440.
12. Lin BT, Colby T, Gown AM, et al: Malignant vascular tumors of the serous membranes mimicking mesothelioma. A report of 14 cases. Am J Surg Pathol 1996;20:1431–1439.
13. Maddox JC, Evans HL: Angiosarcoma of skin and soft tissue: A study of forty-four cases. Cancer 1981;48:1907–1921.
14. Meis-Kindblom JM, Kindblom LG: Angiosarcoma of soft tissue: a study of 80 cases. Am J Surg Pathol 1998;22:683–697.
15. Morgan MB, Swann M, Somach S, et al: Cutaneous angiosarcoma: a case series with prognostic correlation. J Am Acad Dermatol 2004;50:867–874.
16. Naka N, Ohsawa M, Tomita Y, et al: Angiosarcoma in Japan. A review of 99 cases. Cancer 1995;75:989–996.
17. Rossi S, Orvieto E, Furlanetto A, et al: Utility of the immunohistochemical detection of FLI-1 expression in round cell and vascular neoplasm using a monoclonal antibody. Mod Pathol 2004;17:547–552.
18. West JG, Qureshi A, West JE, et al: Risk of angiosarcoma following breast conservation: a clinical alert. Breast J 2005;11:115–123.

Kaposi Sarcoma

1. Babal P, Pec J: Kaposi's sarcoma—still an enigma. J Eur Acad Dermatol Venereol 2003;17:377–380.
2. Dorfman RF: Kaposi's sarcoma: evidence supporting its origin from the lymphatic system. Lymphology 1988;21:45–52.
3. Ensoli B, Sgadari C, Barillari G, et al: Biology of Kaposi's sarcoma. Eur J Cancer 2001;37:1251–1269.
4. Folpe AL, Veikkola T, Valtola R, et al: Vascular endothelial growth factor receptor-3 (VEGFR-3): a marker of vascular tumors with presumed lymphatic differentiation, including Kaposi's sarcoma, kaposiform and Dabska-type hemangioendotheliomas, and a subset of angiosarcomas. Mod Pathol 2000;13:180–185.
5. Fukunaga M: Expression of D2-40 in lymphatic endothelium of normal tissues and in vascular tumours. Histopathology 2005;46:396–402.
6. Hammock L, Reisenauer A, Wang W, et al: Latency-associated nuclear antigen expression and human herpesvirus-8 polymerase chain reaction in the evaluation of Kaposi sarcoma and other vascular tumors in HIV-positive patients. Mod Pathol 2005;18:463–468.
7. McNutt NS, Fletcher V, Conant MA: Early lesions of Kaposi's sarcoma in homosexual men. An ultrastructural comparison with other vascular proliferations in skin. Am J Pathol 1983;111:62–77.
8. O'Brien PH, Brasfield RD: Kaposi's sarcoma. Cancer 1966;19:1497–1502.
9. Verma SC, Robertson ES: Molecular biology and pathogenesis of Kaposi sarcoma-associated herpesvirus. FEMS Microbiol Lett 2003;222:155–163.

10 Nerve Sheath and Neuroectodermal Tumors

Julie C. Fanburg-Smith

- Traumatic Neuroma
- Mucosal Neuroma
- Pacinian Neuroma
- Palisaded Encapsulated Neuroma (Solitary Circumscribed Neuroma)
- Neurofibroma, Neurofibromatosis Type 1, and Early Malignant Change in Neurofibroma
- Schwannoma and Neurofibromatosis Type 2
- Psammomatous Melanotic Schwannoma
- Malignant Peripheral Nerve Sheath Tumor
- Granular Cell Tumor: Benign, Atypical, and Malignant
- Perineurioma: Intraneural, Soft Tissue, and Malignant
- Neurothekeoma: Nerve Sheath Myxoma
- Neuroblastoma, Ganglioneuroblastoma, and Ganglioneuroma
- Clear Cell Sarcoma

Nerve sheath and neuroectodermal tumors are derived from the neuroectoderm or neural crest tissue of the developing embryo. Neuromas are mainly reactive lesions of existing nerves. It is first important to understand *normal nerve architecture* (Figure 10-1). *Normal nerve* consists centrally of axons, surrounded by Schwann cells. The connective tissue of the axons, including the Schwann cells, fibroblasts, mast cells, capillaries, and collagen, is called the *endoneurium*. Groups of these axons with their Schwann cells are surrounded by perineurium, comprising a *fascicle*. Groups of fascicles are then surrounded by epineurium. Understanding normal nerve architecture helps to understand the specific derivation of nerve sheath lesions and tumors. *Neurofibromas* are neoplasms that arise from within the nerve or axon (demonstrating residual axons within neurofibroma), and the nerve must be taken to excise the lesion. *Schwannomas* are neoplasms that arise from the Schwann cells that encase the axon; therefore, the tumor can be extracted without damaging the involved nerve (axons are not usually found within schwannoma). Other variants of nerve sheath tumors, including *granular cell tumor, perineurioma*, and *neurothekeoma*, have specific clinicopathologic features. The most important aspect of making a diagnosis of nerve sheath tumors is to determine whether the lesion is benign or malignant, and in doing so, to determine whether the patient has an associated syndrome, neurofibromatosis type 1 (NF1) or NF2. *Neuroectodermal tumors* are usually malignant and have different treatment protocols from their tumor mimickers.

TRAUMATIC NEUROMA

CLINICAL FEATURES

Traumatic neuroma is a non-neoplastic lesion that occurs in response to injury or surgery. Usually nerves can repair themselves by proximal to distal proliferation of Schwann cells; when this reparation is interrupted or cannot occur in an orderly manner, the proximal aspect of the nerve creates a disorganized proliferation of nerves, that is, a neuroma. Traumatic neuromas can occur after amputation of a limb or autoamputation of a digit in utero. These lesions are often painful.

RADIOLOGIC FEATURES

When the patient has an obvious nerve terminating into a bulbous mass, a radiographic diagnosis can be made (Figure 10-2). It is more difficult to make a radiologic diagnosis if the neuroma shows only fusiform thickening of a small cutaneous nerve.

PATHOLOGIC FEATURES

GROSS FINDINGS

Traumatic neuroma can be a firm, white-gray nodule that measures less than 5 cm.

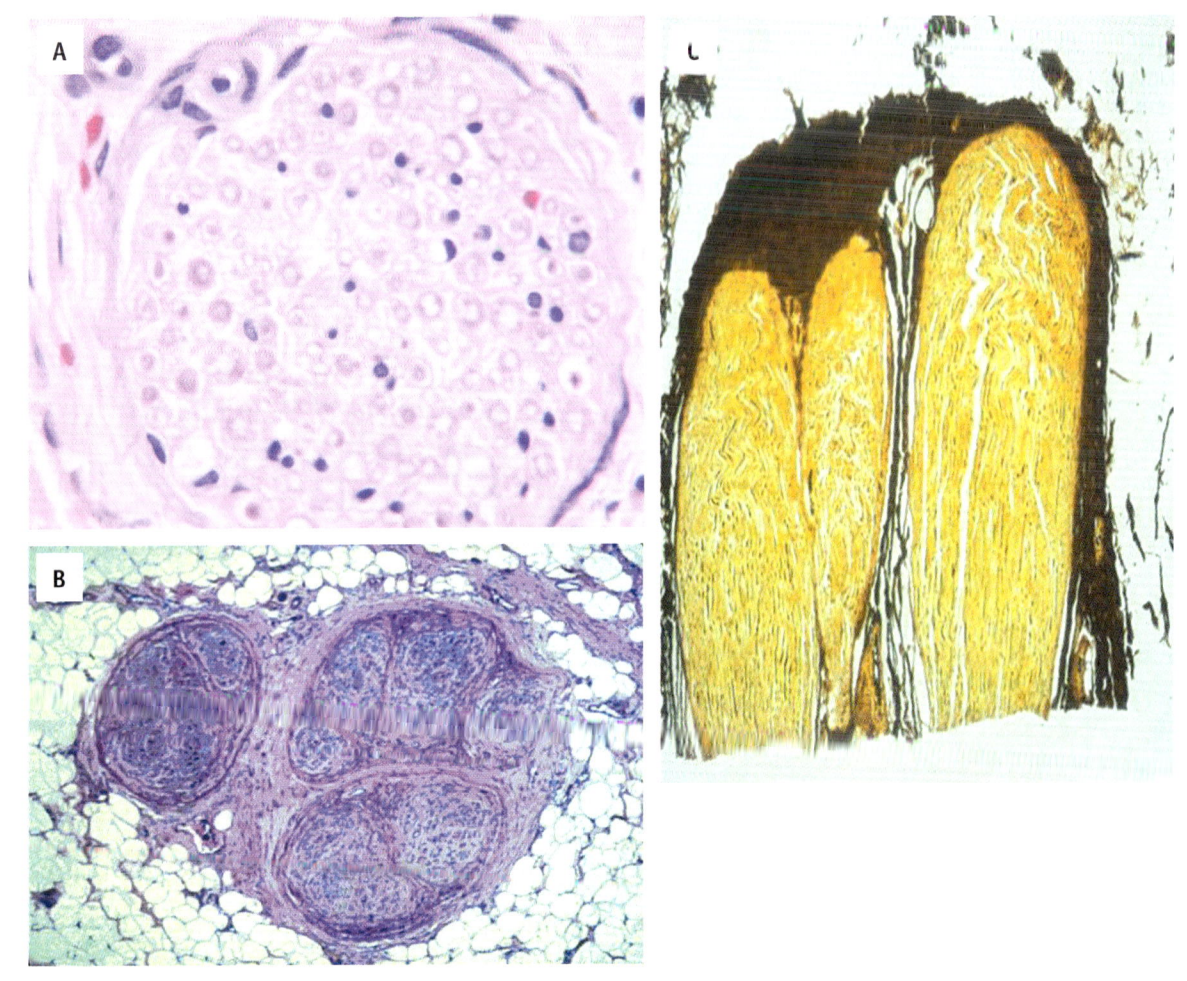

FIGURE 10-1
Normal nerve is composed of axons surrounded by Schwann cells (small circular structures) **(A)**, collagen fibers, capillaries, and a few mast cells, all comprising the connective tissue (stroma) called the *endoneurium*. Groups of axons, comprising a fascicle (**B** and **C**), are surrounded by perineurium. In turn, several fascicles of nerve are surrounded by epineurium.

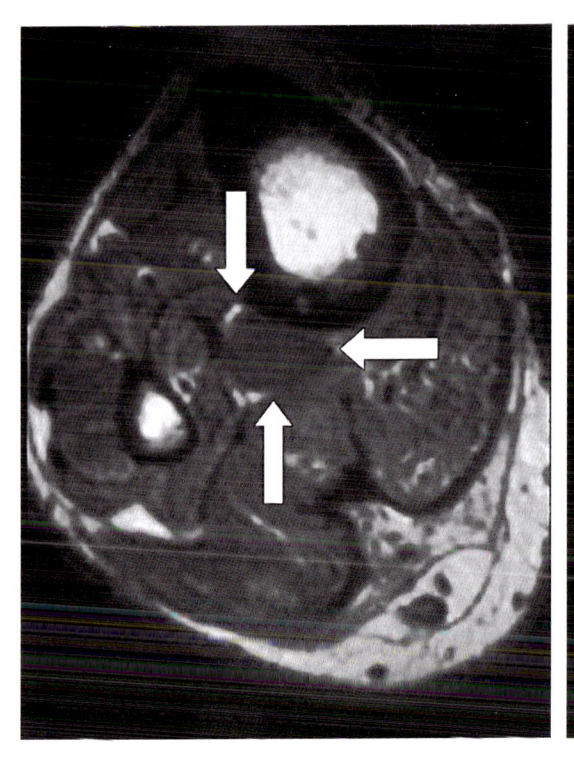

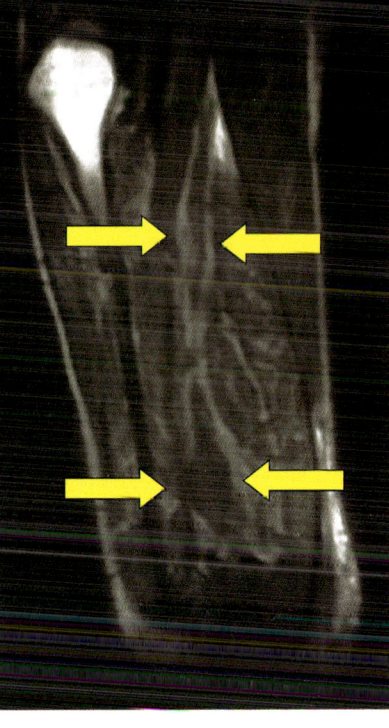

FIGURE 10-2
Postsurgical traumatic neuroma of tibial nerve after amputation. Computed tomographic scan (left) shows focal soft tissue mass with enlarged nerve ending *(white arrows)*. Magnetic resonance image (right) is a coronal t1-weighted image (500/16) showing the bulbous distal nerve ending, contiguous with the proximal tibial nerve *(yellow arrows)*. (Courtesy of Mark D. Murphey, MD)

TRAUMATIC NEUROMA—FACT SHEET

Definition
▸▸ Disorganized proliferation of nerve in response to injury or disruption

Incidence and Location
▸▸ Any nerve that has been surgically or autoamputated, especially the limbs and digits

Morbidity and Mortality
▸▸ None

Clinical Features
▸▸ Patient has firm, painful nodule

Radiologic Features
▸▸ Observation of bulbous end of truncated nerve

Prognosis and Treatment
▸▸ Benign reactive; treatments include prior reapproximation of nerve, removal, or re-embedding of proximal nerve stump

TRAUMATIC NEUROMA—PATHOLOGIC FEATURES

Gross Findings
▸▸ Small, firm, gray–white nodule at site of interrupted nerve

Microscopic Findings
▸▸ Proliferation of small nerve twigs with surrounding fibrosis

Differential Diagnosis
▸▸ PEN, mucosal neuroma, Morton's neuroma, and neurofibroma

MICROSCOPIC FINDINGS

Traumatic neuroma is a haphazard arrangement of small nerve fascicles, containing axons, Schwann cells, and perineurial cells, surrounded by fibrosis (Figure 10-3).

DIFFERENTIAL DIAGNOSIS

The differential diagnosis for traumatic neuroma includes palisaded encapsulated neuroma (PEN), mucosal neuroma, Morton's neuroma, or neurofibroma. However, the distinctive clinical history and solid growth pattern with small nerve twigs enwrapped in fibrosis helps to distinguish this from other entities. Mucosal neuroma also has a unique clinical setting with multiple endocrine neoplasia type 2b (MEN-2b), which is not associated with traumatic neuroma. Morton's neuroma is a variant of traumatic neuroma with distinctive clinical features and a slightly different morphologic appearance. Although myxoid traumatic neuromas may mimic neurofibroma, neurofibroma can be further distinguished by its characteristic collagen bundles, centrally cellular architecture, and scattered mast cells.

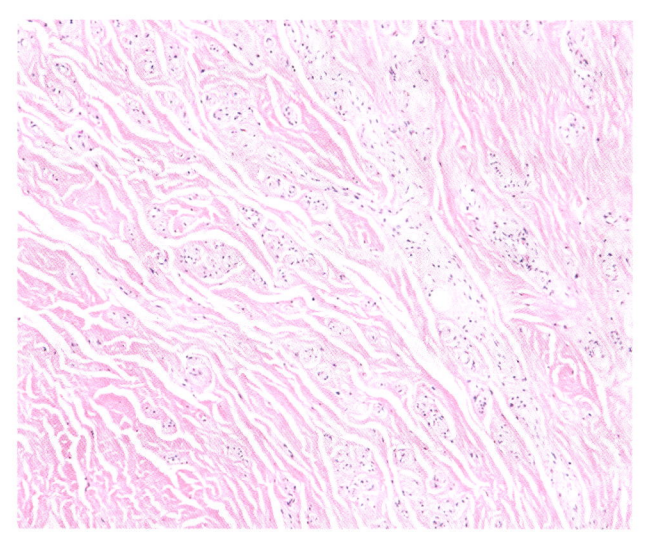

FIGURE 10-3
Traumatic neuroma is composed of bundles of disorganized axons surrounded by fibrosis.

PROGNOSIS AND TREATMENT

Traumatic neuroma is a non-neoplastic but painful lesion; its removal, prior reapproximation of nerve endings, or re-embedding of proximal nerve stump in an area away from scar are treatments of choice.

MUCOSAL NEUROMA

CLINICAL FEATURES

Mucosal neuroma (Figure 10-4) may occur during the first few decades of life in patients with and without MEN-2b syndrome (bilateral pheochromocytoma, C-cell hyperplasia of the thyroid or medullary thyroid carcinoma, and parathyroid hyperplasia). These are usually multiple and involve the mucosal surfaces of the lips, gingiva, tongue, eyelids, and intestines.

PATHOLOGIC FEATURES

GROSS FINDINGS

Mucosal neuroma is a firm, submucosal complex nodule.

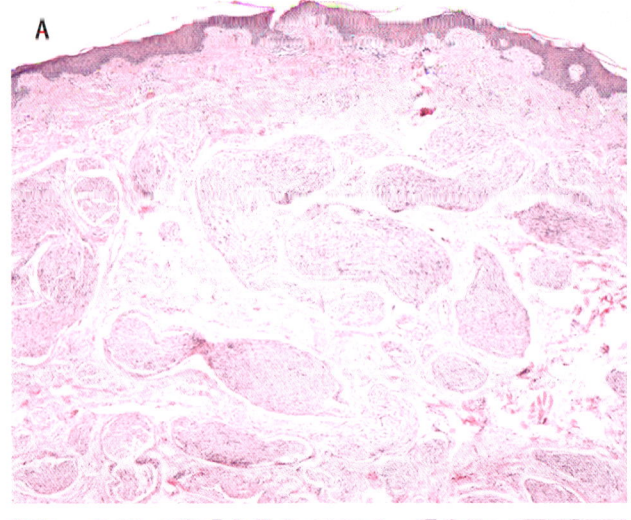

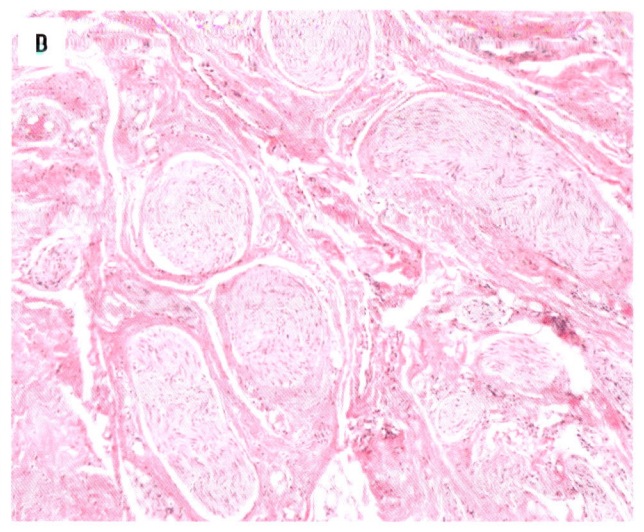

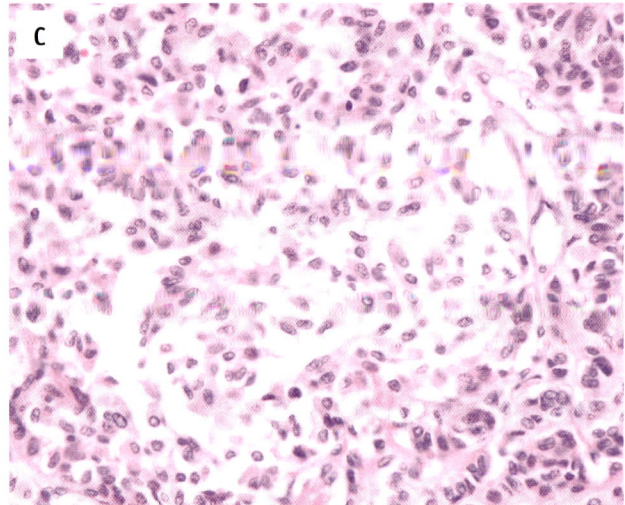

FIGURE 10-4
A, Mucosal neuroma in patient with multiple endocrine neoplasia type 2b syndrome, demonstrated by an increase in size and number of nerve in the oral submucosa. **B**, Neuroma is also adjacent to this patient's medullary carcinoma of the thyroid **(C)**.

MICROSCOPIC FINDINGS

Irregular bundles of nerve in the submucosa surrounded by prominent perineurium and myxoid change are classic histologic features (see Figure 10-4). In the gastrointestinal tract, these may include Schwann cells, neurons, and ganglion cells in a bandlike process of the submucous and myenteric plexuses, synonymous with ganglioneuroma.

DIFFERENTIAL DIAGNOSIS

The differential diagnosis would include other nerve sheath tumors such as palisading encapsulated neuroma, neurofibroma, and possibly ganglioneuroma, but the location and specific clinical associations would make it easy to distinguish from the other entities.

MUCOSAL NEUROMA—FACT SHEET

Definition
- Multiple submucosal convoluted nerves that may be associated with MEN-2b syndrome

Incidence and Location
- These are located on the mucosal surface of the lips, mouth, eyelids, and intestines

Morbidity and Mortality
- By itself, this is benign; however, if associated with MEN-2b, this lesion may indicate potential poor prognosis

Clinical Features
- Multiple submucosal lesions; potential association with MEN-2b syndrome

> **MUCOSAL NEUROMA—PATHOLOGIC FEATURES**
>
> **Gross Findings**
> ▸▸ Firm, submucosal complex nodule
>
> **Microscopic Findings**
> ▸▸ Multiple, irregular, convoluted submucosal nerves with prominent perineurium and focal myxoid change
>
> **Differential Diagnosis**
> ▸▸ Other neuromas, neurofibroma, ganglioneuroma

PROGNOSIS AND TREATMENT

The incidental finding of multiple mucosal neuromas may portend an underlying MEN-2b syndrome that can be life-threatening.

PACINIAN NEUROMA

CLINICAL FEATURES

Pacinian neuroma is a post-traumatic and painful lesion or lesions of the pressure receptors of the digit in middle-aged adults.

PATHOLOGIC FEATURES

GROSS FINDINGS

Pacinian neuroma has small to continuous subepineural nodule(s), attached to a nerve by stalk, and can be up to 1.5 cm.

MICROSCOPIC FINDINGS

Pacinian neuroma demonstrates mature Pacinian corpuscle(s) of increased size or number, associated with degenerative changes and fibrosis of the adjacent nerve.

DIFFERENTIAL DIAGNOSIS

Normal Pacinian corpuscle, Pacinian neurofibroma, neurothekeoma, and congenital nevi may be in the differential diagnosis; however, attention to increase in size and number of Pacinian corpuscles with history of trauma and pain is helpful.

> **PACINIAN NEUROMA—FACT SHEET**
>
> **Definition**
> ▸▸ Localized hyperplasia or hypertrophy of Pacinian corpuscles after trauma
>
> **Incidence and Location**
> ▸▸ Digits
>
> **Morbidity and Mortality**
> ▸▸ None
>
> **Clinical Features**
> ▸▸ Post-traumatic painful Pacinian corpuscles in digit of middle-aged adult
>
> **Prognosis and Treatment**
> ▸▸ Excision of benign process relieves pain completely, no recurrence

> **PACINIAN NEUROMA—PATHOLOGIC FEATURES**
>
> **Gross Findings**
> ▸▸ Single to multiple or contiguous subepineurial nodules attached to nerve
>
> **Microscopic Findings**
> ▸▸ Increase in number or size of Pacinian corpuscles with degeneration or fibrosis of adjacent nerve
>
> **Differential Diagnosis**
> ▸▸ Normal Pacinian corpuscle, other neuromas, neurofibroma, congenital nevi

PROGNOSIS AND TREATMENT

Complete excision of this benign mass arrests pain; no recurrence of this hyperplastic process occurs.

PALISADED ENCAPSULATED NEUROMA (SOLITARY CIRCUMSCRIBED NEUROMA)

CLINICAL FEATURES

PEN is probably better considered as a neoplastic process, a variant of neurofibroma unassociated with NF1, rather than a "neuroma." PEN affects middle-aged adults with no definite sex predilection. PEN is clinically a solitary, asymptomatic, skin-colored papule. The most common locations include the nose, cheek, and perioral region,

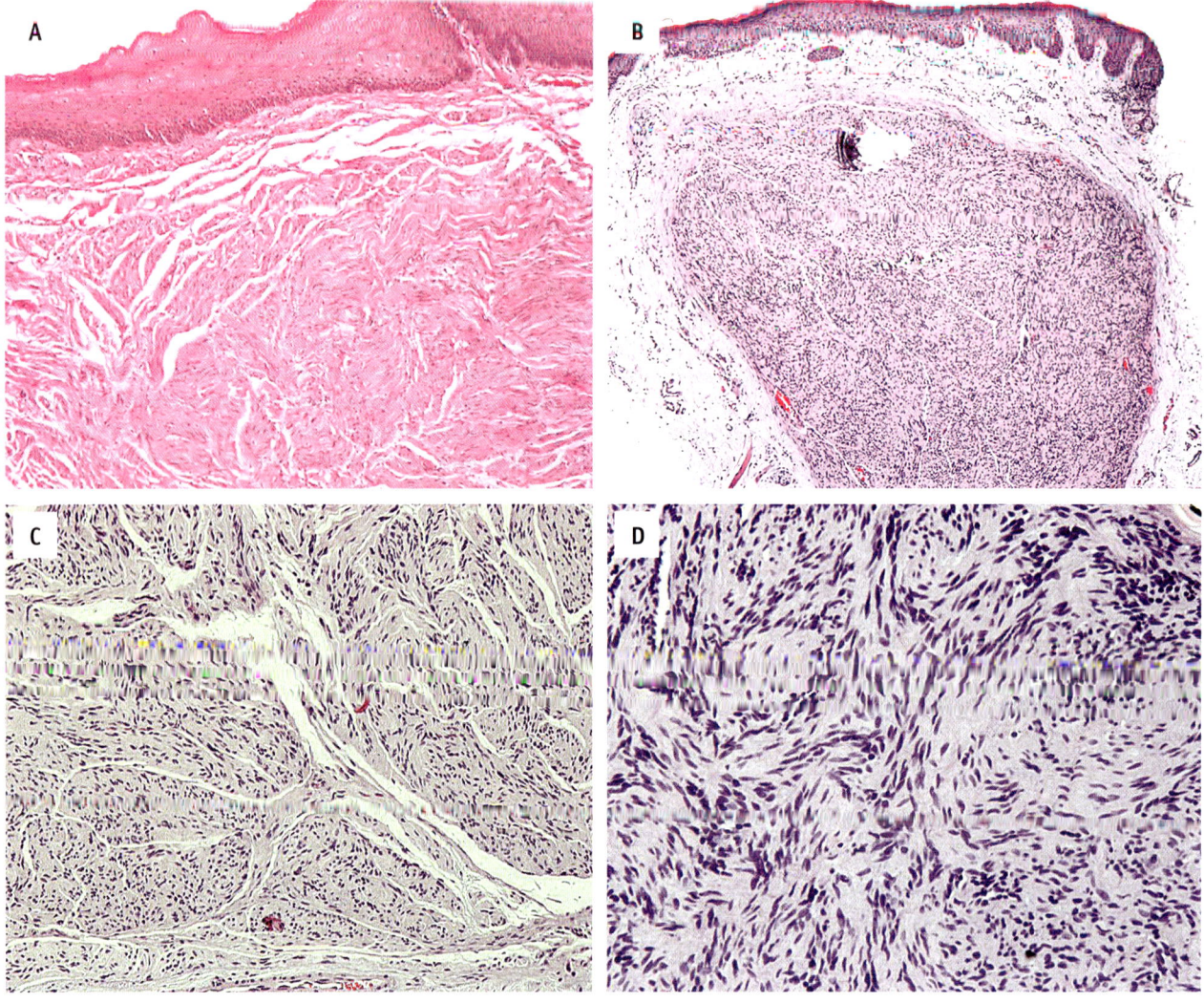

FIGURE 10-5

A, This palisading encapsulated neuroma (solitary circumscribed neuroma) is often found in the face and perioral region. **B,** It is usually well delineated. **C,** At low power it looks Schwannian with palisading of tumor cells. However, it is probably a neurofibroma variant but demonstrates spindled Schwann cells without well-formed Verocay bodies **(B–D).** The lesion has abundant axons like a neurofibroma but is not associated with neurofibromatosis type 1.

especially the palate. Occasionally, PEN can be plexiform or multinodular and associated with acne. PEN may be more common than neurofibroma or schwannoma in the maxillofacial region because it is possibly under-recognized. No association of PEN with NF1 or MEN-2b exists.

Pathologic Features

Gross Findings

PEN is a small, cutaneous, white, dome-shaped nodule(s), usually less than 5 mm.

Microscopic Findings

This Schwann cell tumor is not encapsulated but is circumscribed with one or more nodules and is ovoid to spheric in shape. Sometimes the normal adjacent tissue is compressed, giving the appearance of a capsule. PEN is predominantly dermal with spindled cells arranged in interlacing, compact fascicles (Figure 10-5), sometimes separated by narrow clefts. Palisading can be observed, but there are no well-formed Verocay bodies. An adjacent peripheral nerve can be identified in many cases.

Ancillary Studies

Immunohistochemistry

PEN has staining features similar to both neurofibroma and schwannoma: there is diffusely strong S-100 protein expression (as in schwannoma), neurofilament protein–positive axons (as in neurofibroma), and epithelial membrane antigen (EMA)–positive peripheral cells representing epineurial cells (as found in schwannoma and intraneural neurofibroma).

DIFFERENTIAL DIAGNOSIS

PEN can be separated from schwannoma, neurofibroma, spindled melanoma, and other neuromas by its anatomic location, compact appearance in the dermis, and immunophenotype (see earlier). Schwannoma lacks the neurofilament protein (NFP)-positive neurites within the lesion and usually demonstrates well-formed Verocay bodies. Spindled melanomas exhibit greater nuclear atypia and hyperchromatism, and may variably express specific melanocytic markers, such as HMB45. True neuromas resemble normal nerves and have more fibrosis and inflammation than PEN.

PROGNOSIS AND TREATMENT

PEN has benign behavior after simple excision; no association exists with NF1 or MEN-2b.

PALISADED ENCAPSULATED NEUROMA—FACT SHEET

Definition
- A Schwann cell tumor of the face and oral regions

Incidence and Location
- Probably more common than previously recognized; located in face and oral regions

Morbidity and Mortality
- Benign; no associated syndromes

Clinical Features
- Adult, male predominance; solitary flesh-colored, dome-shaped papule or nodule

Prognosis and Treatment
- Benign, simple excision

PALISADED ENCAPSULATED NEUROMA—PATHOLOGIC FEATURES

Gross Findings
- Small whitish nodule, less than 5 mm

Microscopic Findings
- One or more circumscribed nodules of spindled Schwann cells with focal palisading

Immunohistochemical Findings
- Diffuse S-100 reactivity, positive residual neurites, EMA in capsule, lack of CD34 and melanoma markers

Differential Diagnosis
- Other benign nerve sheath tumors, spindled melanoma

NEUROFIBROMA, NEUROFIBROMATOSIS TYPE 1, AND EARLY MALIGNANT CHANGE IN NEUROFIBROMA

CLINICAL FEATURES

Neurofibromas are relatively common. Solitary neurofibromas are almost never associated with NF1, whereas presentation with multiple neurofibromas should prompt consideration of possible NF1. NF1, von Recklinghausen disease, is a syndrome that arises from a germline mutation of the *NF1* gene, a tumor suppressor gene on chromosome 17. Fifty percent of NF1 cases are autosomal dominant, and the rest are a result of a new mutation of the *NF1* gene. The *NF1* gene encodes for a protein product called *neurofibromin*, homologous to the GAP protein that influences cell cycling by down-regulating the *p21 ras* gene. This product is present in neurofibromas of patients with NF1 and is absent when these undergo malignant transformation. Criteria for the diagnosis of NF1 are listed in Table 10-1. It is important to identify patients with NF1 because they are at risk for development of a malignant peripheral nerve sheath tumor (MPNST). Malignant transformation is most common in large, plexiform neurofibromas, followed by other deep neurofibromas associated with NF1, followed by cutaneous NF1-associated neurofibromas. The rate of malignant transformation is extremely low in non–NF1-associated neurofibromas.

TABLE 10-1
Criteria for Neurofibromatosis Type 1

The patient must have at least two or more of the following:
- Six or more café-au-lait macules > 5 mm (prepubertal) or > 15 mm (postpubertal)
- Two or more neurofibromas or one plexiform type
- Freckling in the axillary or inguinal regions
- Optic glioma
- Two or more Lisch nodules (iris hamartomas)
- Distinctive osseous lesion (e.g., sphenoid dysplasia or long-bone cortical thinning with or without pseudarthrosis)
- First-degree relative with neurofibromatosis type 1 by above criteria

From Enzinger and Weiss's Soft Tissue Tumors, 4th ed. SW Weiss, JR Goldblum, eds. Philadelphia, Mosby, 2000, by permission.

Both nonsyndromic and NF1-associated neurofibromas occur more often in men than in women. Non–NF1-associated neurofibromas typically occur between the ages of 20 and 40 years. In patients with NF1, café-au-lait spots appear shortly after birth, with Lisch nodules, axillary and inguinal freckles, and neurofibromas occurring in childhood before or around puberty. Solitary neurofibromas can arise in any location where there is a peripheral nerve, either as a superficial dermal or a deep soft tissue tumor. Diffuse neurofibromas, associated with NF1 in approximately 10% of cases, are often deeply situated and may occur in a variety of locations. The diagnosis of plexiform neurofibroma implies NF1, and it is important to emphasize that this diagnosis requires clinicopathologic correlation, inasmuch as these must be large, deeply seated tumors that expand and distort a large nerve, often with hypertrophy of the adjacent bone or soft tissue and overlying skin redundancy and hyperpigmentation.

Radiologic Features

Neurofibroma generally has a centrally located exiting or entering nerve that can be detected by radiologic methods. It is sometimes difficult to radiologically separate from schwannoma and even from MPNST. It is often difficult to determine whether the nerve is entering centrally or off center (the latter in schwannoma). The *target sign* is common in neurofibroma (Figure 10-6) but can also be seen in schwannoma.

Pathologic Features

Gross Findings

Solitary neurofibromas are fusiform shaped, rubbery, gray, and glistening, and usually measure approximately 1 to 2 cm. These are nonencapsulated and arise within the nerve, secondarily growing beyond the nerve sheath into the surrounding soft tissue. Diffuse neurofibroma demonstrates a plaque-like thickening of the dermis by a grayish firm tissue. Plexiform neurofibroma is often associated with overlying loose, redundant skin that may be hyperpigmented. The nerve is enlarged and distorted, and has a characteristic gross appearance, a *bag of worms*.

Microscopic Findings

Solitary neurofibromas are often relatively well delineated and zoned with cellular regions to the center, representing the residual nerve twigs, and myxoid to paucicellular regions at the periphery (Figure 10-7). The dermis, subcutis, or deeper soft tissue can be involved. A milieu of several cell types and stromal elements compose a neurofibroma: Schwann cells, hybrid perineurial cells, intraneural fibroblasts, bundles of collagen arrayed in a characteristic *shredded carrot* pattern, scattered mast cells, and myxoid change. The Schwann cells are spindled to ovoid and slender with characteristic *wavy* nuclei. Depending on which component predominates and the shape of the cells or possible pigmentation, neurofibroma can be further classified into various

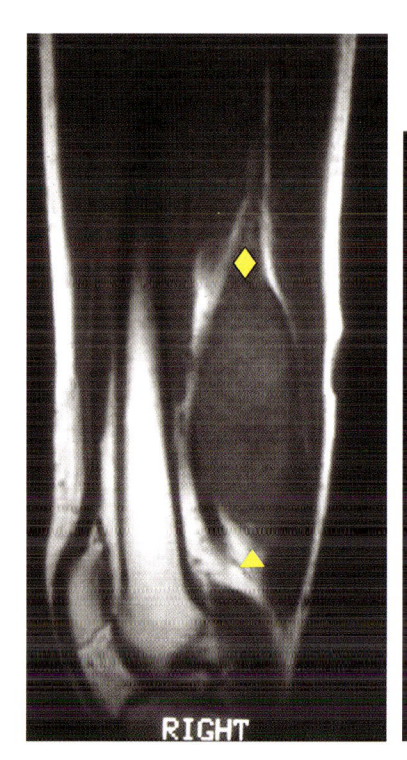

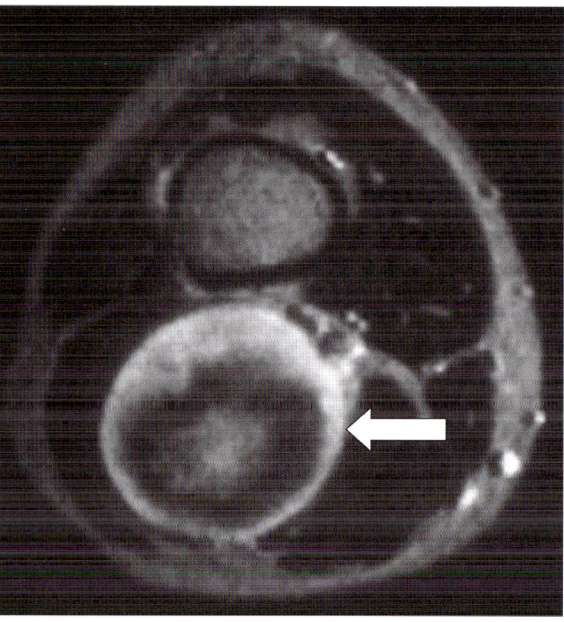

FIGURE 10-6

Magnetic resonance imaging (MRI) of neurofibroma. Left, Centrally entering *(yellow diamond)* and exiting *(yellow triangle)* nerve of neurofibroma on sagittal T1-weighted image. Right, *Target sign* radiologically of neurofibroma, axial T2-weighted MRI (right). This corresponds histologically to the more cellular central portion and more myxoid peripheral area of neurofibroma.

subtypes, including classic, myxoid, cellular, hyalinized, pigmented, or epithelioid. When solitary neurofibroma becomes cellular, it exhibits a swirling or storiform pattern, similar to fibrous histiocytoma. Diffuse neurofibroma consists of small round to spindled cells, with an associated fibrillar and myxoid background, which infiltrate subcutaneous fat in a honeycomb pattern, reminiscent of dermatofibrosarcoma protuberans (Figure 10-8). Wagner–Meissner bodies are the hallmark morphologic characteristic of diffuse neurofibroma (Figure 10-9). Plexiform neurofibroma demonstrates plexiform architecture radiologically, grossly, and microscopically (Figures 10-10 and 10-11), with multiple intraneural nodules of tumor separated by epineurium and stroma. It can involve the subcutis or skeletal structure, or both. Both plexiform and diffuse patterns of growth can be seen together. Although scattered enlarged, hyperchromatic cells, presumably representing degenerative

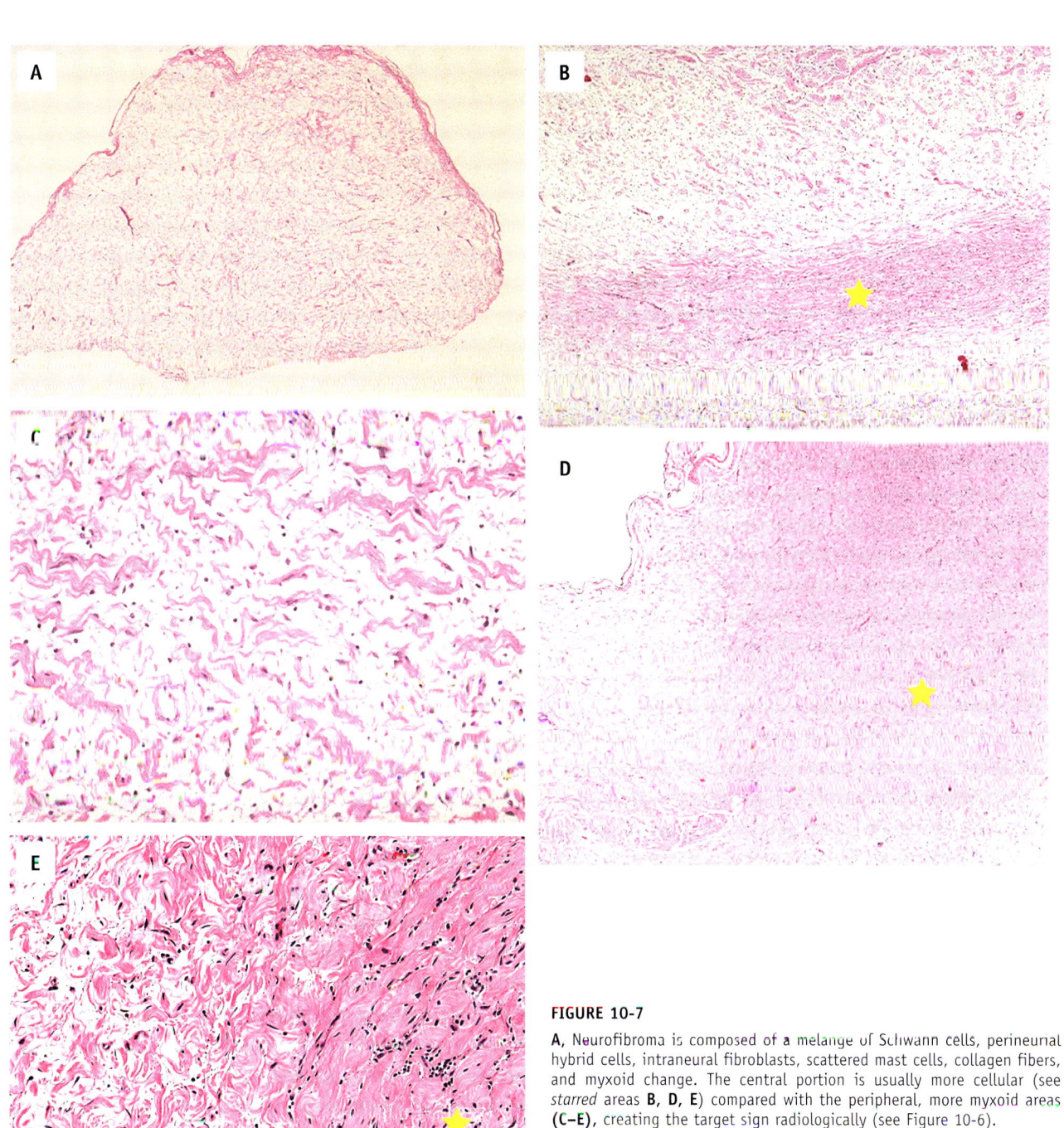

FIGURE 10-7

A, Neurofibroma is composed of a melange of Schwann cells, perineurial hybrid cells, intraneural fibroblasts, scattered mast cells, collagen fibers, and myxoid change. The central portion is usually more cellular (see *starred* areas **B, D, E**) compared with the peripheral, more myxoid areas (**C–E**), creating the target sign radiologically (see Figure 10-6).

NEUROFIBROMA—FACT SHEET

Definition
- Neurofibroma is a tumor arising from within a peripheral nerve; it can be associated with NF1

Incidence and Location
- The prevalence of NF1 is approximately 1:4000; solitary neurofibromas are relatively common; plexiform neurofibromas are relatively rare and are found only in patients with NF1; both can occur in any peripheral nerve; diffuse neurofibroma is quite rare, has a greater than 10% association with NF1, and is generally found in the scalp and lower extremity

Morbidity and Mortality
- Neurofibroma is benign but can undergo malignant transformation in approximately 3% to 22% of cases in patients with NF1, especially with deep or plexiform neurofibroma in NF1

Clinical Features
- Male sex predominance; age 20 to 40 years; childhood/puberty in NF1

Prognosis and Treatment
- Solitary, diffuse, and plexiform types are by themselves benign tumors and are excised for diagnosis, possible association with NF1, and to rule out early malignant change
- Diffuse type can be locally recurrent
- Solitary and diffuse type can be associated with NF1
- Plexiform type is associated with NF1
  - Solitary and especially plexiform have propensity to undergo malignant transformation
  - Complete local excision warranted for neurofibroma
  - Early malignant transformation is treated as a low-grade sarcoma
  - High-grade malignant transformation requires treatment as a high-grade sarcoma

NEUROFIBROMA—PATHOLOGIC FEATURES

Gross Findings
- Solitary: fusiform shaped, 1 to 2 cm
- Diffuse: gray, firm, plaquelike thickening of dermis
- Plexiform: large, grossly visible "bag of worms" appearance

Microscopic Findings
- Cellular and stromal milieu: Schwann, perineurial hybrid, intraneural fibroblasts, mast cells, collagen bundles, and myxoid change; increased cellularity at center of neurofibroma compared with edematous periphery
  - Solitary: well-delineated and intraneural to growth outside of nerve into surrounding tissue
  - Diffuse: infiltrative into subcutis and hallmark Wagner–Meissner bodies
  - Plexiform: tortuous distention of peripheral nerve cut tangentially, appearing plexiform, made as a clinicopathologic diagnosis with "bag of worms" appearance
  - Early malignant transformation of neurofibroma (low-grade MPNST): increased cellularity and fascicular growth, pleomorphism, and mitotic activity, especially atypical mitoses, particularly in center of deep neurofibroma or plexiform neurofibroma, in the setting of NF1

Immunohistochemical Findings
- Schwann cells: S-100 protein positive, diffusely throughout tumor but other cell types are negative
- Perineurium if still intraneural: EMA positive
- Intraneural fibroblasts: CD34 positive
- Residual neurites in center: NFP positive
- Other: glial fibrillary acidic protein (GFAP) occasionally positive

Differential Diagnosis
- Schwannoma, MPNST, benign fibrous histiocytoma, desmoplastic malignant melanoma

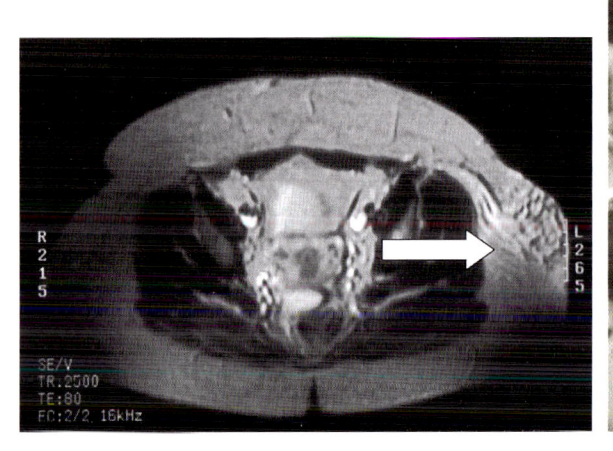

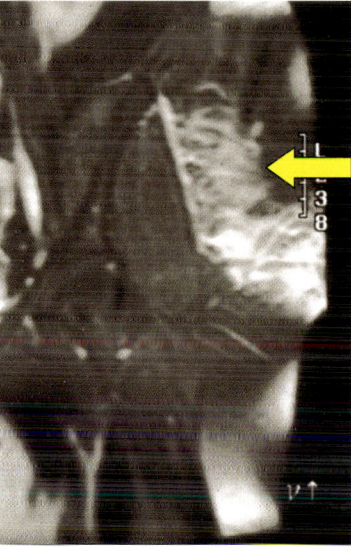

FIGURE 10-8

Radiologic imaging of diffuse neurofibroma in a patient who does not have neurofibromatosis type 1 (NF1). T2-weighted magnetic resonance imaging, axial, shows heterogeneous reticular growth pattern (*white arrow*, left). T2 post-gadolinium, fat suppressed (right) showing reticular growth along preexisting connective tissue septa (*yellow arrow*).

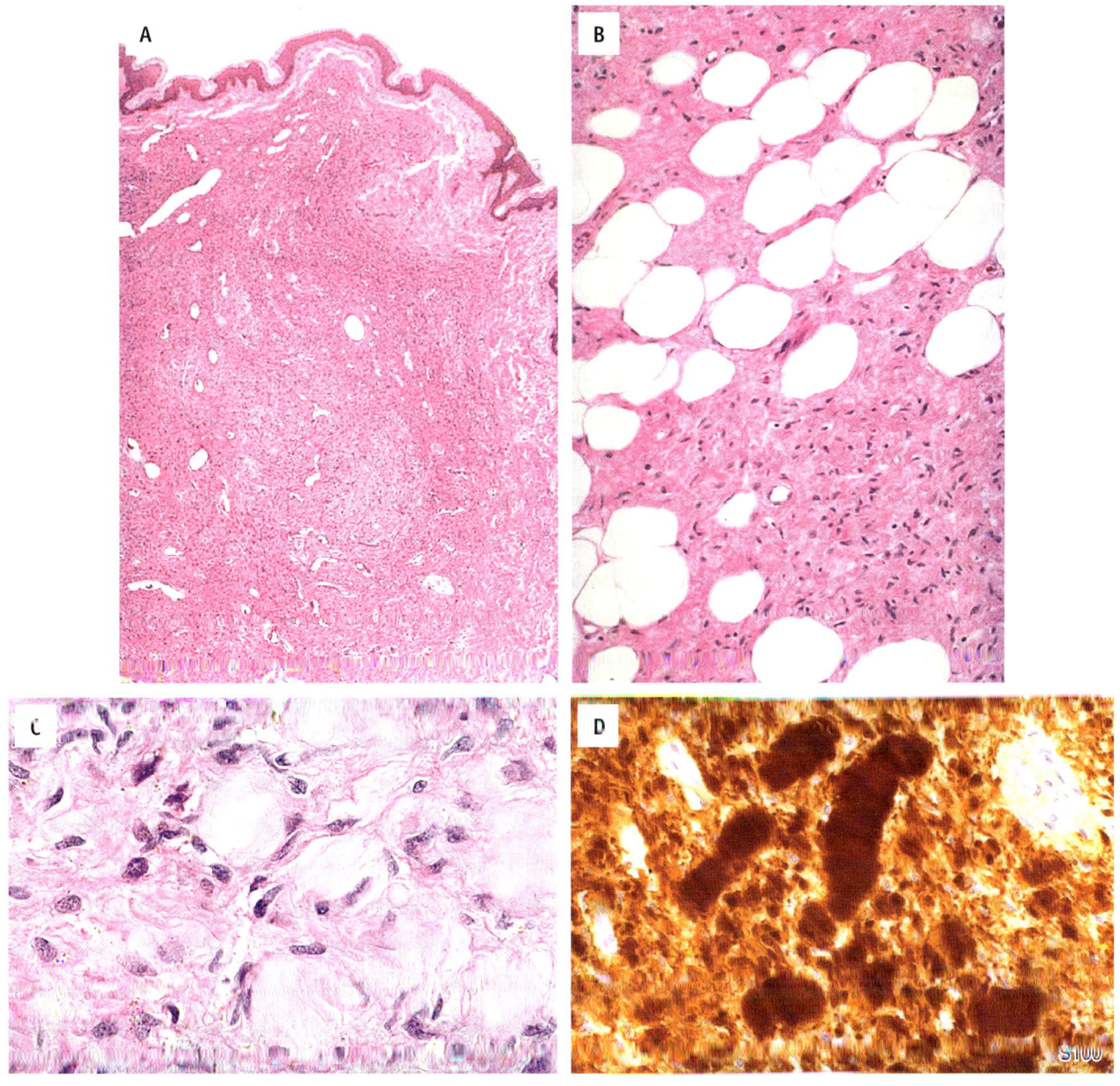

FIGURE 10-9
A, Diffuse neurofibroma involving dermis and subcutis, with honeycomb pattern of subcutis infiltration **(B)**. Hallmark Wagner-Meissner bodies **(B, C)** are positive for S-100 protein **(D)**.

change akin to that seen in *ancient* schwannoma, may be seen in all types of neurofibroma, features such as marked hypercellularity, pronounced fascicular growth, necrosis, and mitotic activity should prompt consideration of malignant change.

Early malignant transformation may be subtle and is to a degree subject to interobserver variation. Important clues to this diagnosis include the presence of areas of increased cellularity, particularly in association with fascicular growth and uniform cytologic atypia. Although rare mitotic figures may be found in ordinary neurofibromas, the finding of more than an occasional mitotic figure, and certainly atypical mitotic figures, is cause for concern. In general, mitotic figures are best searched for in areas showing increased cellularity and fascicular growth. Mitotic activity is best observed in the center of a neurofibroma, especially a deep or plexiform neurofibroma, where early malignant transformation is first apparent. One should be particularly alert for this possibility in NF1-associated neurofibromas, particularly in plexiform tumors (Figure 10-12). Diffuse neurofibromas only rarely undergo malignant transformation; in tumors with mixed diffuse and plexiform features that occur in patients with NF1, early malignant change occurs within the plexiform component.

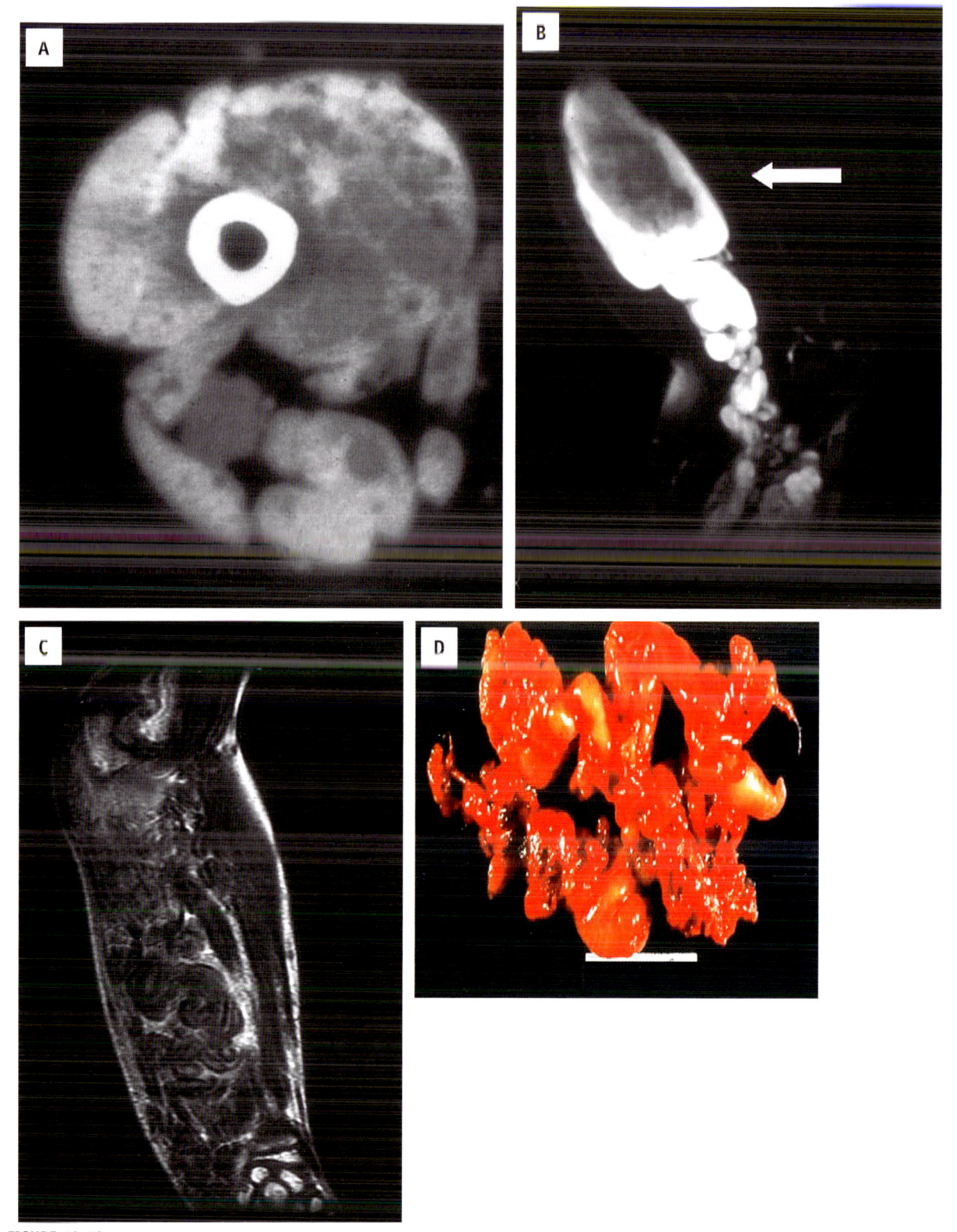

FIGURE 10-10

Radiologic images of plexiform neurofibroma in neurofibromatosis type 1 (NF1).
A, Multiple low-attenuation masses on computed tomography represent solitary and plexiform neurofibromas in NF1. B, Target sign of plexiform neurofibroma on T2 *(arrow)*, low central high periphery of plexiform neurofibroma on long axis, near elbow. C, Magnetic resonance imaging long-axis proximal forearm shows typical *bag of worms* that correlates with (D) gross findings.

(Continued)

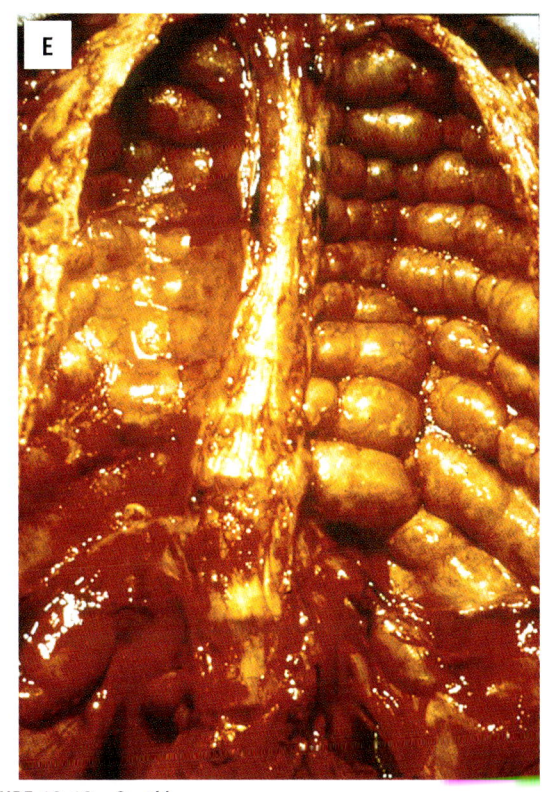

CHAPTER 10   Nerve Sheath and Neuroectodermal Tumors

FIGURE 10-10—Cont'd
E, Another example of NF1 multiple and plexiform neurofibromas.

ANCILLARY STUDIES

IMMUNOHISTOCHEMISTRY

Neurofibromas have a distinctive immunoprofile, with multiple cell populations. The majority of cells within a neurofibroma express S-100 protein (Schwann cells), with a minority of cells expressing CD34 (perineurial fibroblasts) and EMA (perineurial cells). Residual axons may be demonstrated, on occasion, with neurofilament protein immunostains (Figure 10-13). Expression of S-100 protein tends to be significantly diminished in MPNSTs (see later), and loss of S-100 protein expression in areas worrisome for malignant change may be a useful adjunctive finding on occasion.

DIFFERENTIAL DIAGNOSIS

Solitary neurofibromas may be distinguished from PENs and schwannomas by virtue of their distinctive collagen pattern, lack of encapsulation, and immunophenotype, with multiple cell populations. Although the Antoni-B areas of schwannoma may be indistinguishable from neurofibroma, identification of cellular Antoni A zones showing nuclear palisading and Verocay bodies should allow this distinction without undue trouble. Perineuriomas show a different pattern of collagenization and are EMA positive, S-100 protein

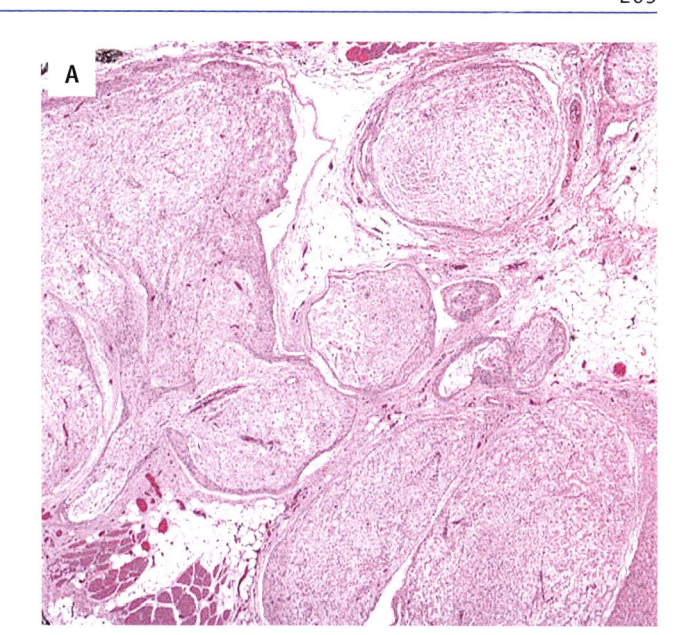

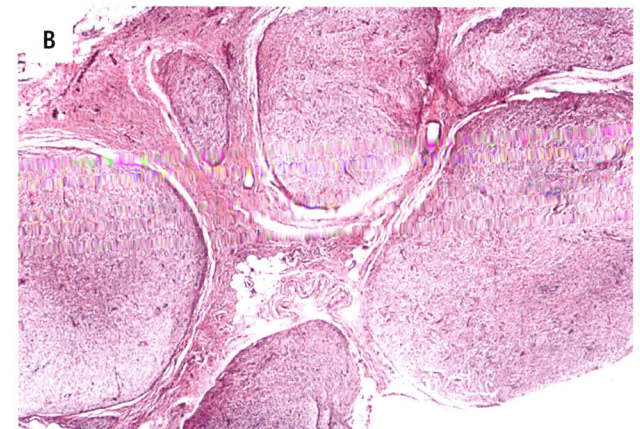

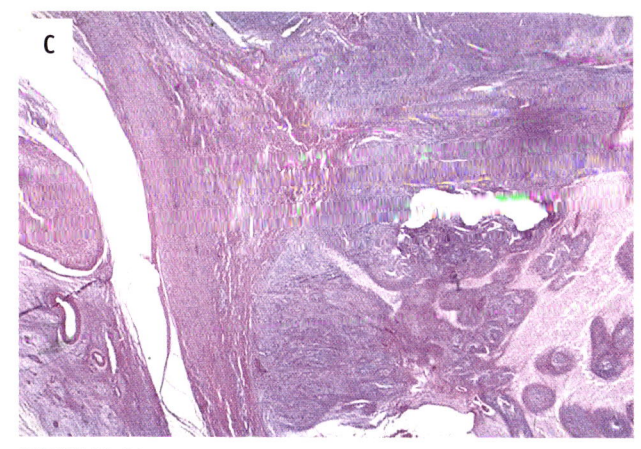

FIGURE 10-11
Plexiform neurofibroma must be a clinicopathologic diagnosis. It is a complex intraneural mass that involves (A) fat or skeletal muscle. B, Sometimes plexiform and diffuse forms coexist, yet it is the plexiform component that may undergo malignant transformation (C).

negative. Benign fibrous histiocytomas (dermatofibromas) show peripheral collagen trapping, contain secondary elements (giant cells, foamy macrophages), and are S-100 protein-negative. Desmoplastic malignant melanomas will often show an associated atypical junctional

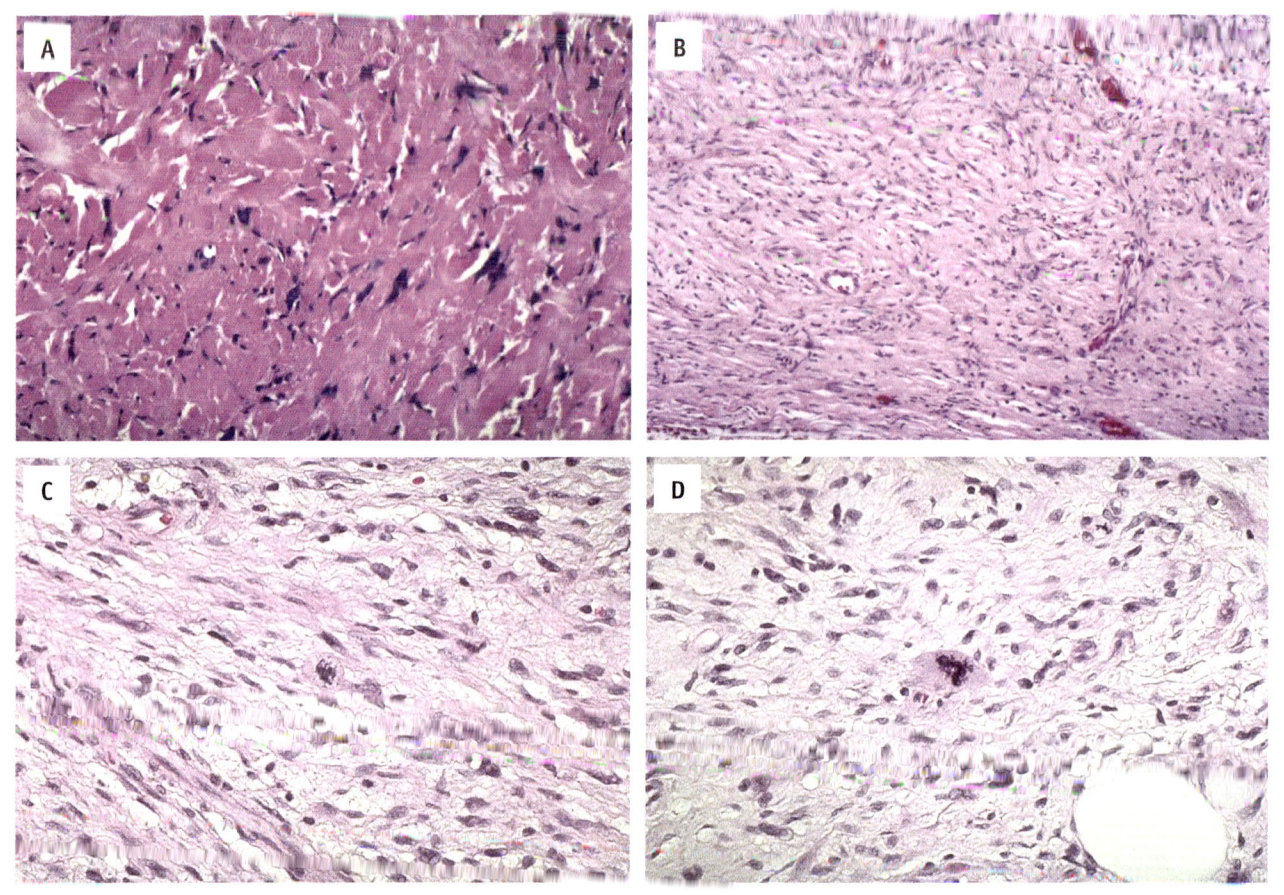

FIGURE 10-12
Early malignant transformation of neurofibroma.
A, Cytologic atypia by itself is not worrisome. **B,** Cellularity usually makes neurofibroma resemble the loose storiform pattern of fibrous histiocytoma but is not, by itself, diagnostic of malignant change. **C,** Fascicular growth and mitoses, especially atypical mitoses **(D)**, are the first signs of early malignant transformation, especially in a patient with neurofibromatosis type 1 (NF1). With these latter early changes, the tumors are treated as low-grade malignant.

melanocytic proliferation, frequently have an associated lymphocytic inflammatory response, and usually show enlarged, hyperchromatic spindled cells. Large, deep neurofibromas may occasionally be confused with low-grade fibromyxoid sarcoma but lack the whirling growth pattern, curvilinear vessels, and abrupt transition into myxoid nodules seen in the latter lesion. Diffuse neurofibromas should be distinguished from dermatofibrosarcoma protuberans, which is composed of slender CD34-positive, S-100 protein-negative, spindled cells arranged in a prominent storiform pattern. Plexiform neurofibromas may be confused with plexiform schwannomas; the latter lesions are typically much smaller, uniformly S-100 protein-positive, and contain areas of solid Antoni growth.

PROGNOSIS AND TREATMENT

Neurofibroma, by itself, is benign and is excised mainly for diagnosis and ruling out early malignant transformation in the setting of NF1. Early malignant change in neurofibroma is treated as a low-grade sarcoma, with wide excision and careful patient follow-up. Neurofibromas with flagrant malignant transformation should be treated as high-grade sarcomas, typically in a multidisciplinary fashion.

SCHWANNOMA AND NEUROFIBROMATOSIS TYPE 2

CLINICAL FEATURES

Schwannomas usually occur between the ages of 20 and 50 years without a sex predilection, except in the setting of NF2, where there is a slight female predominance. Schwannoma is a common tumor of peripheral nerves; it accounts for 8% of intracranial and 28% of primary spinal tumors. Most commonly located in the head and neck, it can also be located on the extensor areas of the extremities or centrally/axially located. In the head and neck, schwannoma

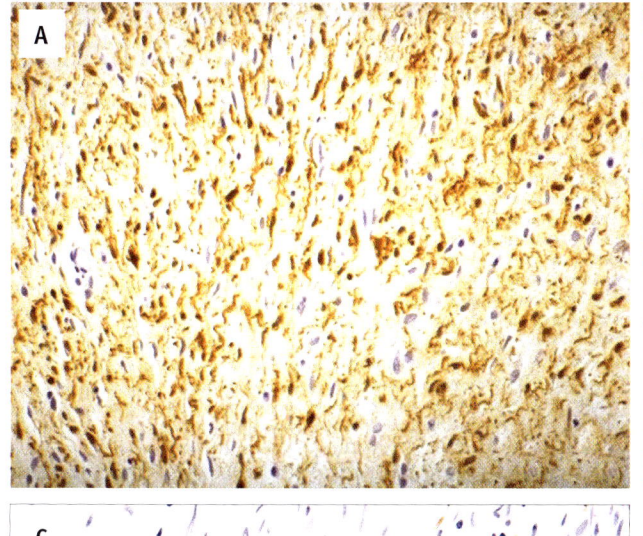

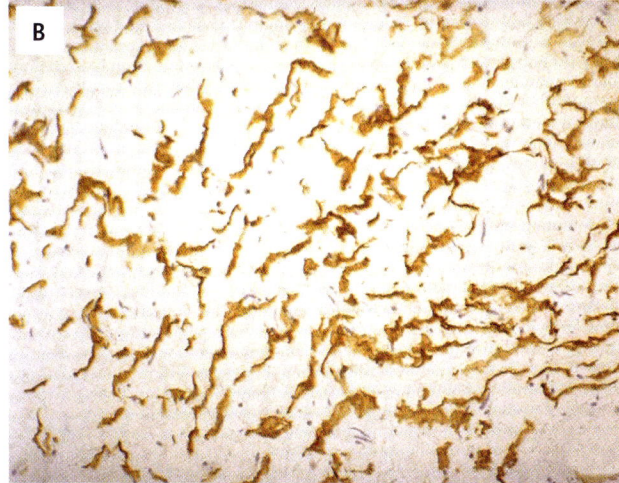

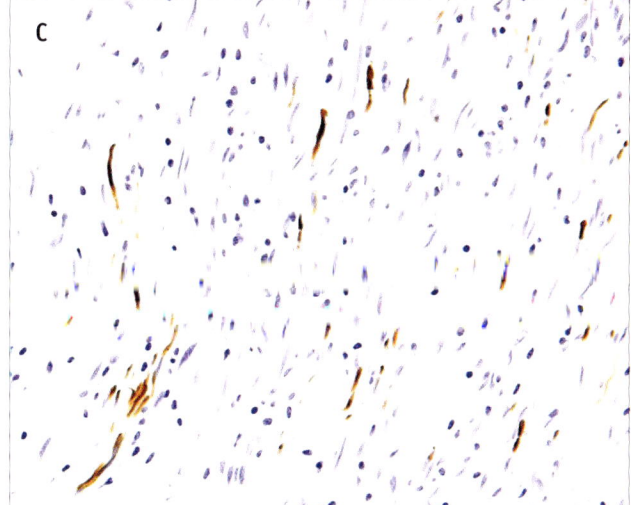

FIGURE 10-13

Immunohistochemistry of all neurofibroma subtypes: **A**, Diffuse S-100 protein, but only Schwann cells are positive so not every cell is staining. **B**, EMA is throughout the lesion, staining intraneural fibroblasts. Residual axons within the nerve are positive for neurofilament protein (**C**).

commonly involves the vestibular division of the eighth cranial nerve.

Bilateral vestibular schwannomas indicate NF2, a syndrome caused by germline mutation of the *NF2* gene, located on chromosome 22, with a protein product merlin. NF2 criteria are listed in Table 10-2. In addition to bilateral vestibular schwannoma, these patients may also have meningiomas, glial tumors, and posterior lens opacities and/or cerebral calcifications. Schwannomas can be multiple, nonacoustic, and associated with a somatic rather than a germline mutations of NF2. In addition, schwannoma can also be plexiform, associated with gliomas, meningiomas, and neural deficits but not associated with a germline or somatic mutation of NF2.

Schwannoma may be asymptomatic or cause tinnitus, hearing loss, and facial paresthesias when in the cerebellopontine angle. Peripheral schwannoma usually presents as an asymptomatic mass, favoring sensory nerves. The axial and retroperitoneal schwannomas are usually histologically found to be the cellular variant.

RADIOLOGIC FEATURES

The radiologic features for schwannoma are similar to features for neurofibroma, except the mass is eccentric to the nerve (Figure 10-14). Sometimes this is hard to appreciate. The target sign is less common for schwannoma than for neurofibroma. Degenerative features may create central necrosis or cyst formation and be radiologically detected in schwannoma. Intracranial calcifications can be detected radiologically in patients with NF2, particularly in the cerebral and cerebellar cortices, periventricular areas, and choroid plexus.

PATHOLOGIC FEATURES

GROSS FINDINGS

Because schwannomas arise from Schwann cells outside of the nerve, it can be surgically separated from the nerve, sparing the patient's nerve (Figure 10-15).

SCHWANNOMA—FACT SHEET

Definition
- A peripheral nerve sheath tumor arising eccentric to nerve

Incidence and Location
- Common; 8% of intracranial and 29% of primary spinal tumors; any peripheral or axial nerve may be involved, particularly in the head and neck, extremities, retroperitoneum

Morbidity and Mortality
- Generally none, but acoustic schwannomas can cause pain, hearing loss, face drop, and deformity, especially when excised; careful search for NF2 warranted with bilateral acoustic schwannomas

Clinical Features
- Affects mainly ages 20 to 50 years; female sex predilection only when associated with NF2; tinnitus, hearing loss, facial paresthesias with acoustic schwannoma; asymptomatic mass for peripheral schwannomas

Radiologic Features
- Mass eccentric to nerve, sometimes target sign, sometimes degenerative and cystic features observed

Prognosis and Treatment
- Benign, excision advised for diagnosis; exceedingly rare epithelioid malignant transformation from classic schwannoma; multiple non-acoustic schwannomas associated with somatic mutation of *NF2* gene; plexiform schwannoma may be associated with glioma, meningioma, neurologic deficit, without somatic or germline mutation of NF2

TABLE 10-2
Criteria for Neurofibromatosis Type 2

Definite Neurofibromatosis Type 2

- Bilateral vestibular schwannoma *or*
- Family history of neurofibromatosis type 2 (first-degree relative) *plus*
- Unilateral vestibular schwannoma at age < 30 years *or*
- Any **two** of the following: meningioma, glioma, schwannoma, juvenile posterior subcapsular lenticular opacities/juvenile cortical cataract

Presumptive or Probable Neurofibromatosis Type 2

- Unilateral vestibular schwannoma at age < 30 years plus at least **one** of the following: meningioma, glioma, schwannoma, or juvenile posterior subcapsular lenticular opacities/juvenile cortical cataract *or*
- Multiple meningiomas (two or more) plus unilateral vestibular schwannoma at age < 30 years or one of the following: meningioma, glioma, schwannoma, or juvenile posterior subcapsular lenticular opacities/juvenile cortical cataract

From Enzinger and Weiss's Soft Tissue Tumors, 4th ed. SW Weiss, JR Goldblum, eds. Philadelphia, Mosby, 2000, by permission.

SCHWANNOMA—PATHOLOGIC FEATURES

Gross Findings
- 2- to 10-cm, tan-yellow, firm-to-cystic mass

Microscopic Findings
- Classic: encapsulated; alternating Antoni A cellular (with Verocay) and Antoni B myxoid, hypocellular areas
- Cellular: encapsulated, pericapsular lymphocytic cuffing; all Antoni A, no Antoni B, or well-formed Verocay, more fascicular arrangement of tumor cells
- Immunohistochemical features: diffuse, strong S-100 protein expression; rarely cytokeratin positive

Differential Diagnosis
- Neurofibroma, nevomelanocytic lesions, leiomyosarcoma, gastrointestinal stromal tumor, MPNST

Schwannomas are tan-yellow, firm, and encapsulated (Figure 10-16), measuring 2 to 10 cm.

MICROSCOPIC FINDINGS

Classic schwannoma is encapsulated, except when in a sinonasal or intracranial location. Microscopically, classic schwannoma is composed of alternating Antoni A cellular areas with Verocay bodies (nuclear palisading around cell processes) and Antoni B hypocellular areas with myxoid change, a similar milieu to neurofibroma, and numerous thick-walled vessels with perivascular hyalinization (Figure 10-17). The spindled cells are deeply eosinophilic and have elongated nuclei. Schwannoma can frequently undergo cystic change and may, at times, resemble a thrombosed vessel with a thin rim of tumor at the periphery (Figure 10-18). Cellular schwannoma, usually found in an axially location, is defined by the presence of almost exclusive Antoni A pattern growth, fascicular architecture, and absent Verocay bodies. Frequently, the capsule of cellular schwannomas shows pericapsular lymphocytic cuffing (Figure 10-19). Lipid-laden histiocytes within the tumor may be a clue to the diagnosis of cellular schwannoma. *Degenerative cytologic atypia (ancient change)* and occasional mitotic figures may be seen in otherwise benign schwannomas. A plexiform growth pattern is observed in approximately 5% of schwannomas; this subtype is not associated with NF1 but may be occasionally associated with NF2, particularly when multiple. Occasionally, schwannomas are composed principally of epithelioid-appearing cells; recognition of more typical areas and strong S-100 protein expression should allow recognition of this unusual variant.

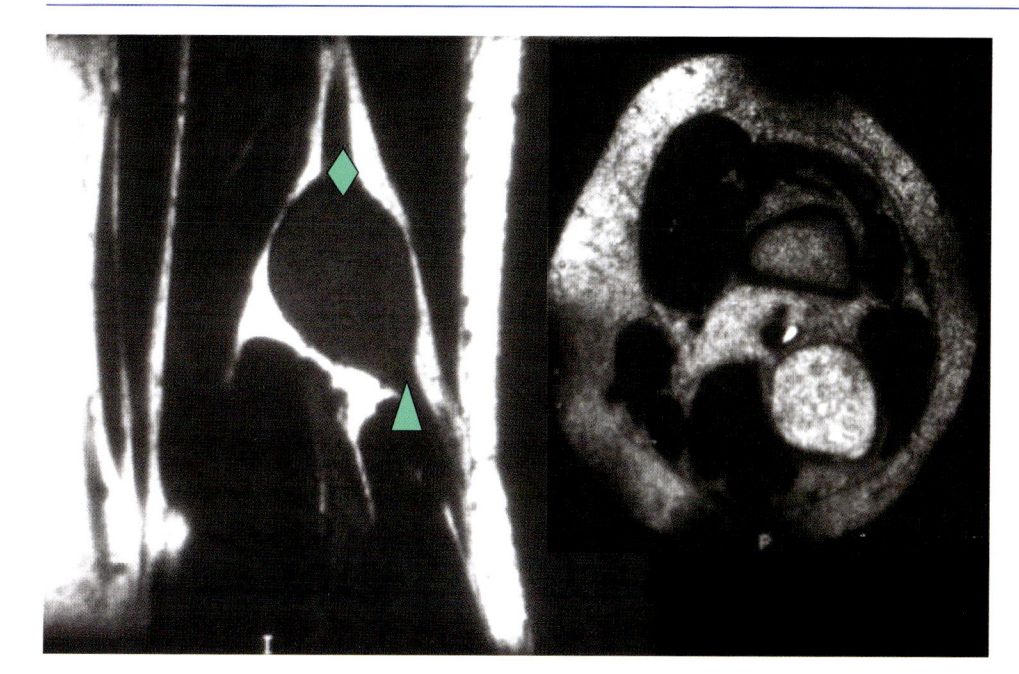

CHAPTER 10 Nerve Sheath and Neuroectodermal Tumors   209

FIGURE 10-14
Magnetic resonance image of schwannoma, coronal T1 (left), entering *(green diamond)* and exiting *(green triangle)* nerve is slightly eccentric to the intermuscular mass. On axial proton density T2, the mass is between the muscles in the distribution of the sciatic nerve and shows a *fascicular sign* with circular low-intensity areas, seen here in schwannoma but also noted in neurofibroma.

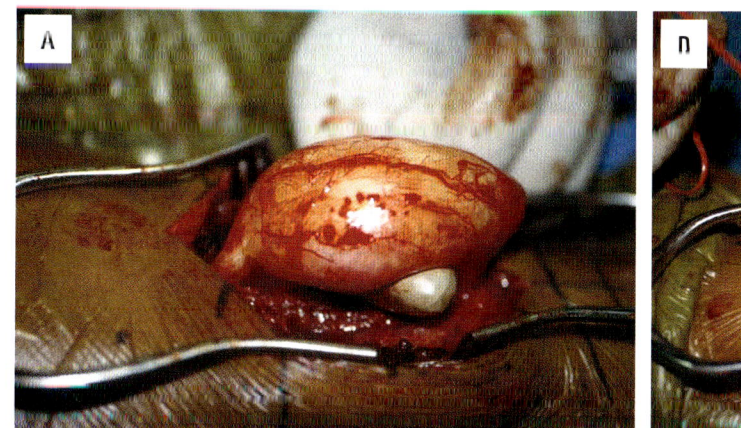

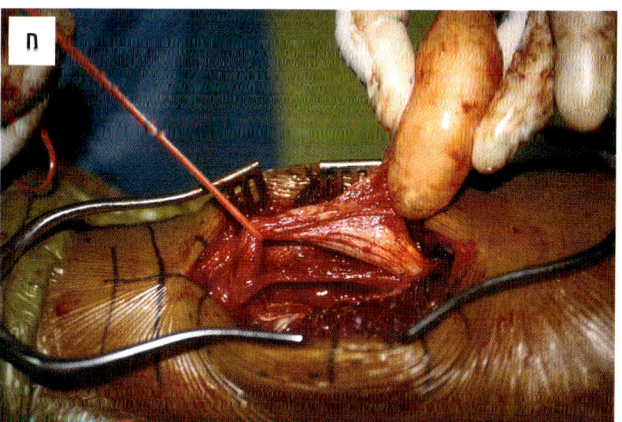

FIGURE 10-15
A, Intraoperative view of schwannoma with lesion adjacent to nerve but inside sheath. **B,** Tumor can be extracted from the nerve, leaving the patient's nerve intact.

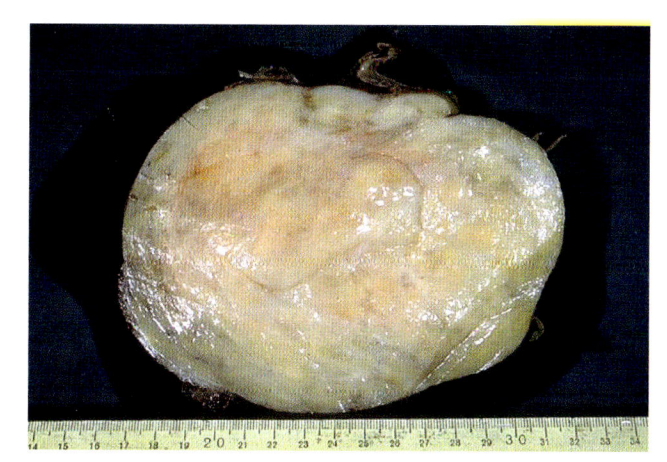

FIGURE 10-16
Gross photograph of a schwannoma with yellow color and firm consistency.

ANCILLARY STUDIES

IMMUNOHISTOCHEMISTRY

By immunohistochemistry, all schwannomas are uniformly and strongly S-100 protein positive. Occasional EMA-positive perineurial cells may be seen in the capsule or around blood vessels; axons are absent. Rare schwannomas may show significant cytokeratin immunopositivity, which most likely represents cross reactivity with GFAP rather than true expression (Figure 10-20).

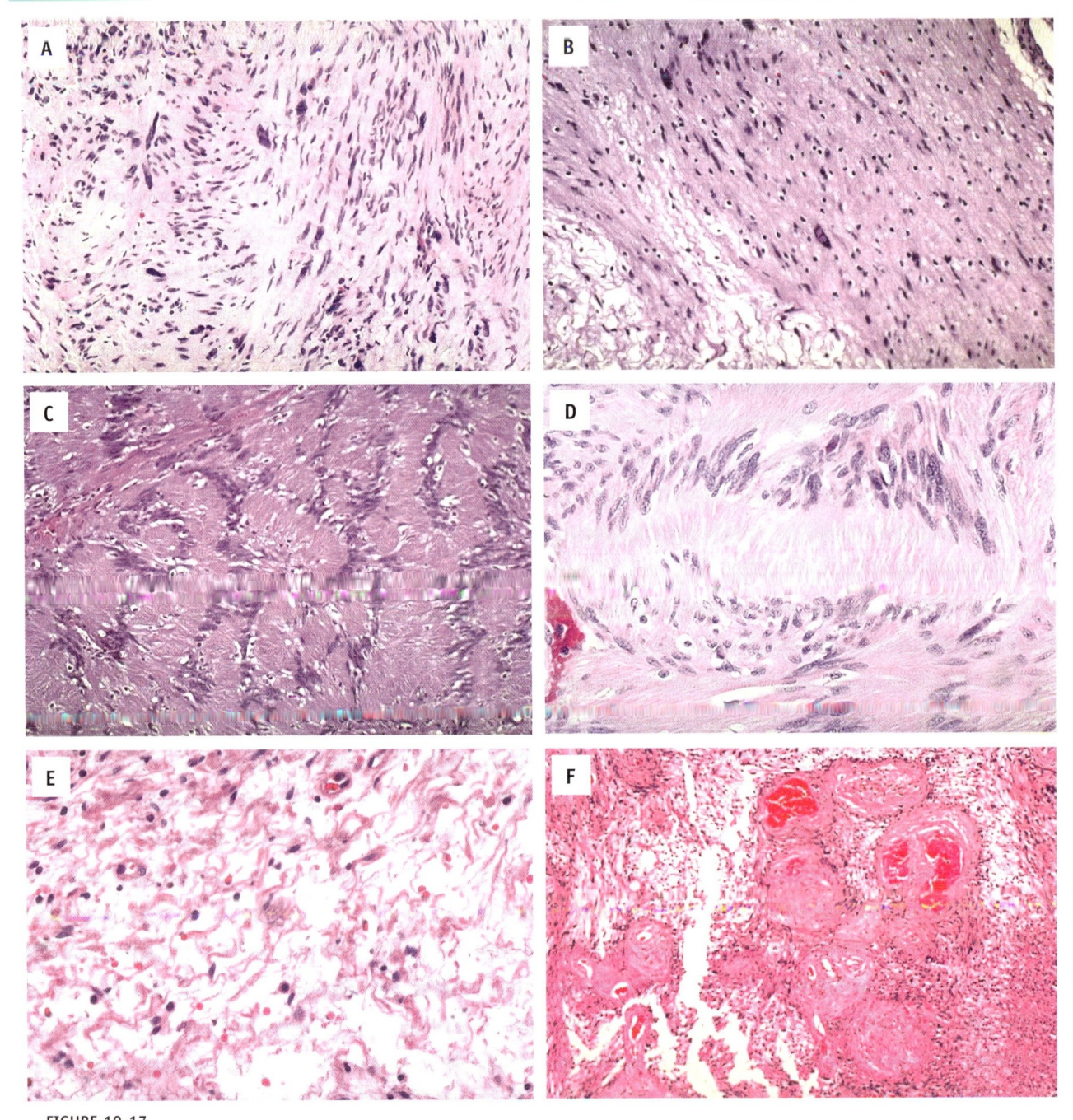

FIGURE 10-17

Microscopic appearance of classic schwannoma with cellular Antoni A areas **(A, B)** and well-defined Verocay bodies (nuclear palisading) **(C, D)** alternating with myxoid neurofibroma-like areas **(E)**, with typical perivascular hyalinization **(F)**.

DIFFERENTIAL DIAGNOSIS

Typical schwannomas are most often confused with neurofibromas; attention to the presence of both Antoni A and B zones, encapsulation, hyalinized blood vessels, and diffuse S-100 protein expression should allow this distinction without great difficulty. Epithelioid schwannomas may mimic nevomelanocytic tumors and true epithelial tumors; recognition of areas of more typical schwannoma, encapsulation, and immunohistochemistry for melanocytic markers (e.g., HMB45, Melan-A) and cytokeratins are the keys to eliminating this diagnosis. Cellular schwannomas are most often confused with leiomyosarcomas, gastrointestinal stromal tumors, and MPNST. The distinction from leiomyosarcoma and gastrointestinal stromal tumor is greatly facilitated by immunohistochemistry for

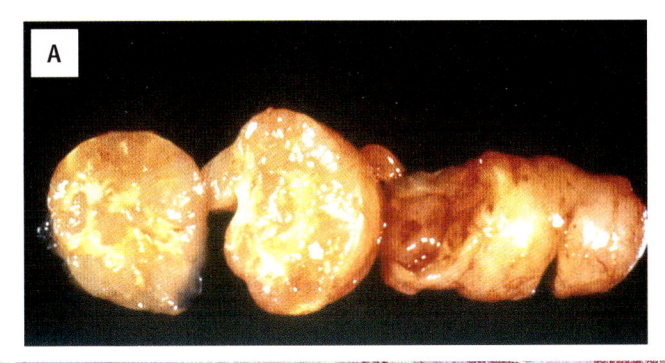

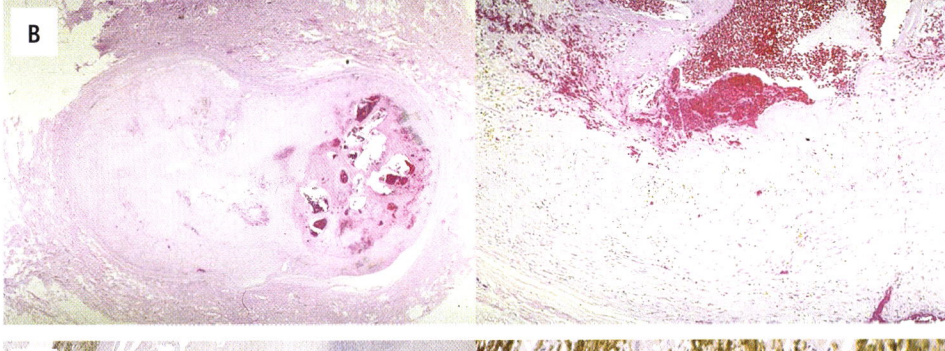

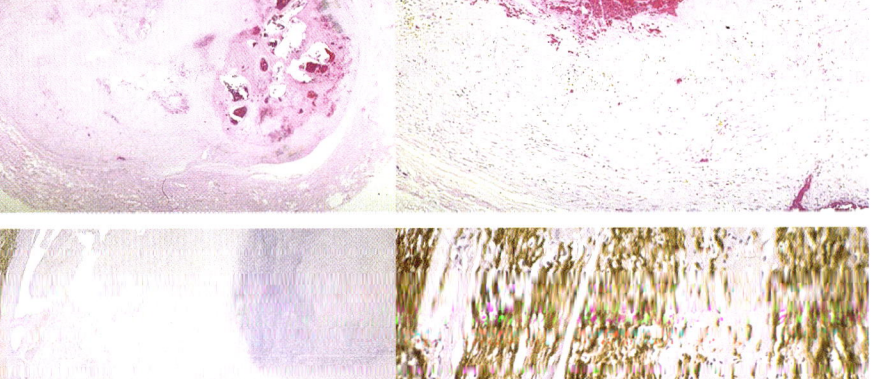

CHAPTER 10 Nerve Sheath and Neuroectodermal Tumors

FIGURE 10-18
Gross photograph of the cross section of a common occurrence in classic schwannoma: **(A)** central degeneration, which correlates microscopically with an appearance mimicking a thrombosed vessel **(B)** but showing positivity for S-100 protein by immunohistochemistry on the thin rim of residual schwannoma **(C)**.

S-100 protein, smooth muscle actin, desmin, and CD117 (c-kit), and these markers should be evaluated before the diagnosis of any of these tumors, particularly in the retroperitoneum. MPNSTs are unencapsulated, usually show clear-cut cytologic atypia, frequently contain necrosis, and are only focally and weakly S-100 protein-positive.

PROGNOSIS AND TREATMENT

Schwannomas are benign tumors that only infrequently recur. Exceptionally rare typical schwannomas may undergo malignant transformation, typically showing morphologic features of epithelioid MPNST. Curiously, angiosarcomas arising within schwannomas have been reported with sufficient frequency to suggest that this is more than a chance occurrence. Cellular schwannomas have not been reported to undergo malignant transformation.

PSAMMOMATOUS MELANOTIC SCHWANNOMA

CLINICAL FEATURES

Psammomatous melanotic schwannoma should be considered as a separate clinicopathologic entity from conventional or cellular schwannoma. Approximately 50% of patients with psammomatous melanotic schwannoma will have associated Carney's complex, an autosomal dominant syndrome characterized by spotty pigmentation (lentigines, blue nevus, epithelioid blue nevus), endocrine overactivity (Cushing disease, acromegaly, or sexual precocity), superficial angiomyxomas, and most importantly, atrial myxomas, which can cause patient mortality. Psammomatous melanotic schwannoma in the setting of Carney's complex occurs at a peak age one decade before those without Carney's complex. Most commonly,

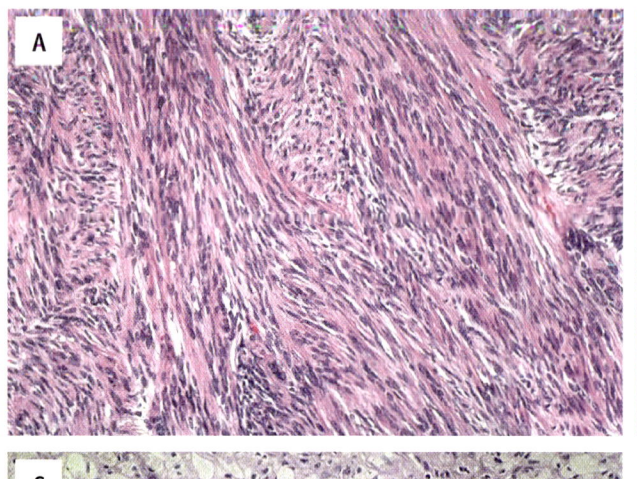

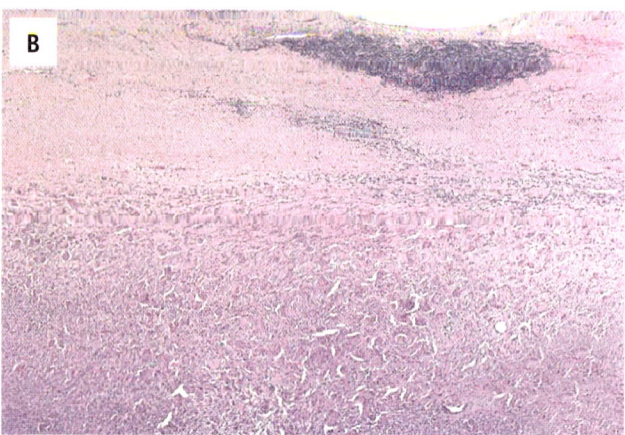

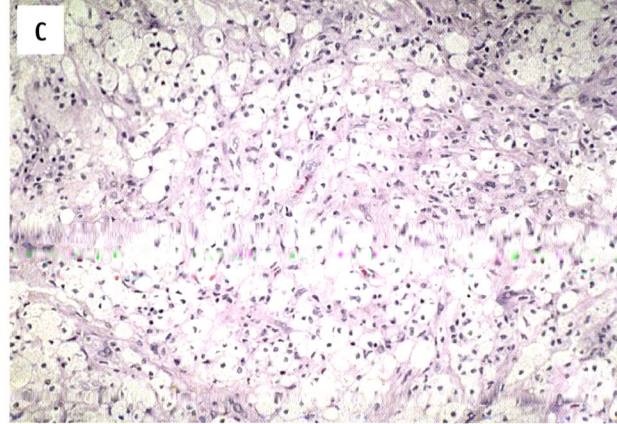

FIGURE 10-19
A, Histologic appearance of central, cellular schwannoma: fascicular growth pattern, only Antoni A, lack of Verocay bodies, and lack of Antoni B, as well as distinctive pericapsular lymphocytic cuffing (**B**) unlike classic schwannoma. **C,** Foam cells can be found in both cellular and classic schwannoma but mainly in the former.

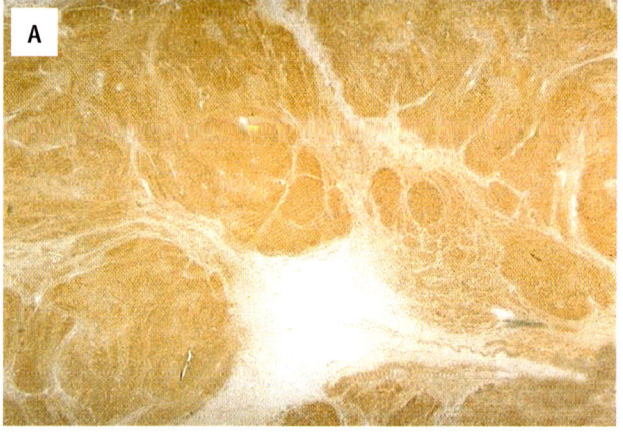

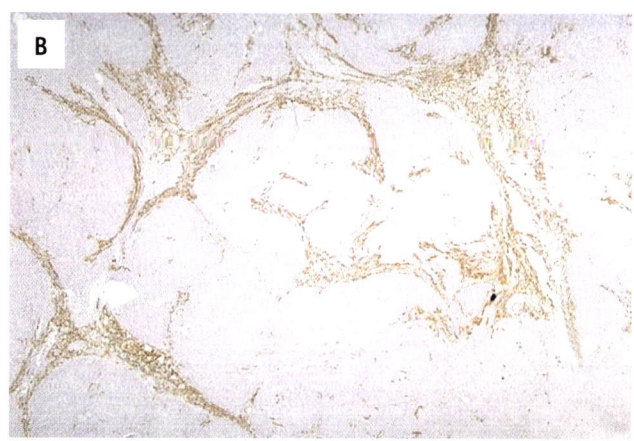

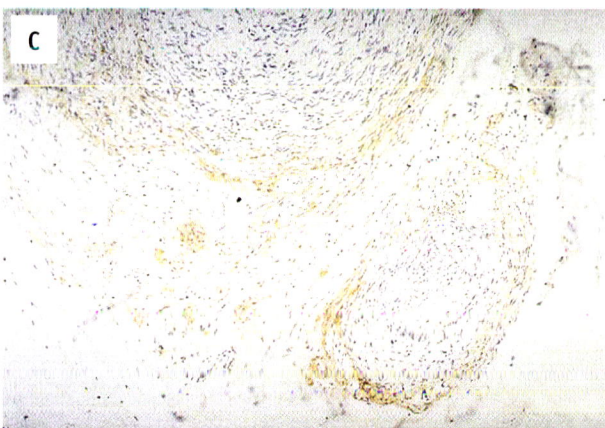

FIGURE 10-20
Immunohistochemistry of all schwannoma subtypes: **A,** Diffuse S-100 protein staining of Schwann cells in Antoni A areas; CD34 reactivity only in scant Antoni B areas. **B,** Epithelial membrane antigen stains perineurial cells around peripheral (capsule) of schwannoma (**C**).

the spinal nerve roots, soft tissues of the trunk and extremities, and intestinal tract nerves may be involved. The heart, bone, liver, bronchus, and skin may also be involved. This lesion, on occasion, can be multiple.

PATHOLOGIC FEATURES

GROSS FINDINGS

Psammomatous melanotic schwannoma forms a black–brown pigmented and circumscribed globoid to fusiform mass, ranging from 1 to 10 cm (mean, 5 cm). Cysts may be present.

MICROSCOPIC FINDINGS

Psammomatous melanotic schwannoma (Figure 10-21) is composed of tightly packed spindled cells with a solid, fascicular, or whorled growth pattern. The cells are deeply eosinophilic, and any nuclear atypia may be obscured by the dark brown melanin pigmentation. The cells are polygonal to spindled, and cytoplasmic borders are difficult to visualize. The nuclei are wavy and may have intracytoplasmic inclusions. Nuclear palisading may be present. Most nuclei are only mildly atypical. However, nucleoli may be prominent or nuclei may be hyperchromatic. Coarse pigment is found in tumor cells and melanophages. Calcified psammoma bodies are present in nearly all cases. Histologic features of marked nuclear atypia, mitotic activity, and necrosis have been associated with malignant behavior; however, melanotic schwannomas without these features may also behave in a malignant fashion.

ANCILLARY STUDIES

IMMUNOHISTOCHEMISTRY

The tumors strongly express schwannian markers, such as S-100 protein and GFAP, as well as melanocytic markers, such as HMB45. It may be necessary to bleach the sections to visualize this immunoreactivity.

DIFFERENTIAL DIAGNOSIS

Malignant melanoma is the most important tumor in the differential diagnosis; the absence of psammoma bodies may help separate it from psammomatous melanotic schwannoma. Blue nevi may also enter the differential diagnosis, and may be distinguished by the absence of psammoma bodies, generally smaller size and cutaneous location, and lesser degree of nuclear atypia.

PROGNOSIS AND TREATMENT

A careful search for other elements of Carney's complex is warranted when the diagnosis of melanotic schwannoma is made. The majority of psammomatous melanotic schwannomas are benign. Complete excision with tumor-free margin is the optimal treatment. Malignant behavior occurs in less than 10% of cases, with metastasis to lungs, pleura, liver, and spleen.

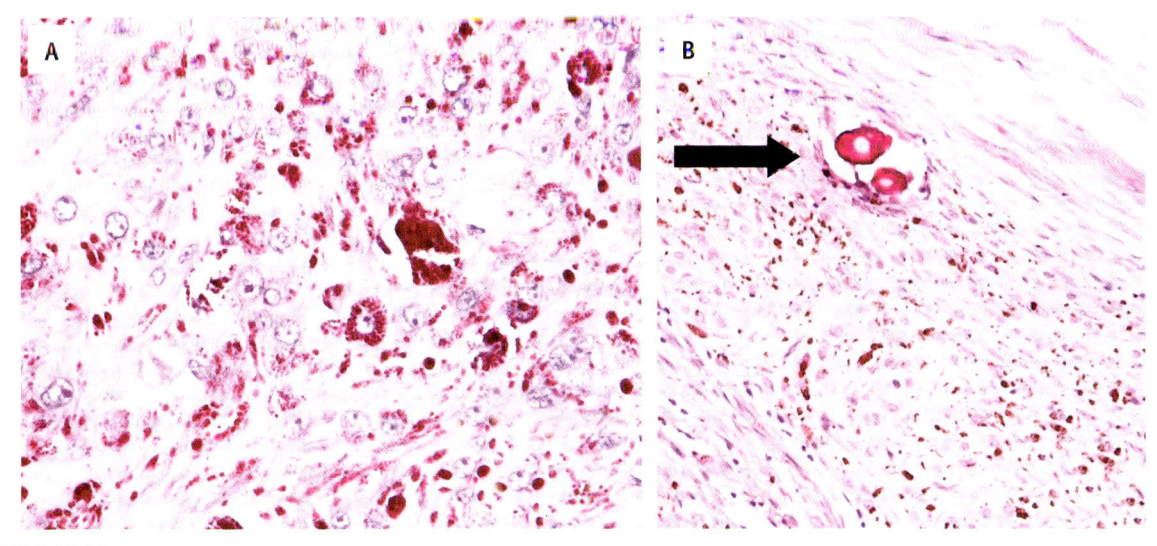

FIGURE 10-21

A, Typical morphologic appearance of psammomatous melanotic schwannoma: a spindle cell lesion with plump cells and heavy pigmentation obscuring morphologic detail. Melanophages (histiocytes that have engulfed melanin pigment from the tumor) are also present. **B**, The helpful additional diagnostic feature is the psammoma bodies *(arrow)*.

PSAMMOMATOUS MELANOTIC SCHWANNOMA—FACT SHEET

Definition
▸▸ Melanin pigmented neural tumor arising from sympathetic nervous system; differs substantially from typical schwannomas

Incidence and Location
▸▸ Rare; 14% of patients with Carney's complex have melanotic schwannomas; locations include spinal or autonomic nerves near the midline

Morbidity and Mortality
▸▸ Difficult to predict the biologic behavior from histology, but metastases may develop

Clinical Features
▸▸ Age range, 20 to 40 years; 50% of cases have associated Carney's complex (myxomas including atrial myxoma, endocrine overactivity, pigmented skin lesions)

Prognosis and Treatment
▸▸ The majority of tumors are benign; complete excision with tumor-free margin is optimal treatment; malignant behavior can occur in less than 10% of cases, with metastasis to lungs, pleura, liver, and spleen

PSAMMOMATOUS MELANOTIC SCHWANNOMA—PATHOLOGIC FEATURES

Gross Findings
▸▸ Mean size, 5 cm; circumscribed fusiform or sausage-shaped gray–black tumor

Microscopic Findings
▸▸ Spindled eosinophilic cells with wavy nuclei obscured by dense melanin pigment; psammoma bodies

MALIGNANT PERIPHERAL NERVE SHEATH TUMOR

CLINICAL FEATURES

MPNSTs, comprising about 5% to 10% of soft tissue sarcomas, can arise de novo from a nerve or in the setting of NF1 from a neurofibroma. When de novo, they most often occur in the fourth decade of life, although they may occur at any age. Patients with NF1 experience development of MPNSTs at earlier ages. NF1-associated MPNST accounts for between 50% and 67% of cases. A marked male predominance is seen with both sporadic and NF1-associated tumors. The most common sites of involvement include the buttocks or thigh, the brachial plexus and upper arm, and the paraspinal region.

RADIOLOGIC FEATURES

MPNST is difficult to separate radiologically from benign nerve sheath tumors. Potential clues include the presence of multiple associated neurofibromas, particularly a plexiform neurofibroma, size greater than 5 cm, an infiltrative appearance, and necrosis. Figures 10-22 and 10-23 demonstrate radiologic appearances of MPNST.

PATHOLOGIC FEATURES

GROSS FINDINGS

MPNST is a fusiform to globoid, pseudoencapsulated tumor with a firm-to-hard consistency, often with gross evidence of necrosis (Figure 10-24). An attached medium or large nerve is often evident, if the tumor is arising from a nerve. De novo MPNST is cream gray, with foci of necrosis and hemorrhage. MPNST arising in neurofibroma, in the setting of NF1, also shows necrosis and hemorrhage evident in an otherwise homogeneous rubbery gray lesion. Almost all MPNSTs are greater than 5 cm at presentation.

MICROSCOPIC FINDINGS

MPNST (Figure 10-25) can be spindled in 95% of cases and epithelioid in 5% of cases. At low power, spindled MPNSTs exhibit a *marbled* appearance, with alternating zones of hypercellularity and hypocellularity. The neoplastic cells grow in long fascicles and occasionally in storiform arrays, contain a moderate amount of lightly eosinophilic cytoplasm, and have wavy or buckled, hyperchromatic nuclei. Accentuated perivascular cellularity, often with herniation of the tumor into blood vessels, is a relatively characteristic feature of MPNST. A hemangiopericytoma-like vascular pattern may also be present. Wiry collagen, of the type seen in synovial sarcoma, is usually absent. Epithelioid MPNSTs show a distinctly nested appearance, with epithelioid to rhabdoid-appearing cells with prominent macronucleoli (reminiscent of melanoma). Divergent differentiation, in the form of rhabdomyoblasts (so-called *malignant Triton tumor*), mucinous glands, osteoid, and cartilage may be seen, typically in patients with NF1. It should be emphasized that there are no histologic features that are absolutely diagnostic of MPNST, and this diagnosis often requires clinical correlation for a history of NF1 and careful exclusions of other similar-appearing tumors, in particular, monophasic synovial sarcoma (MSS).

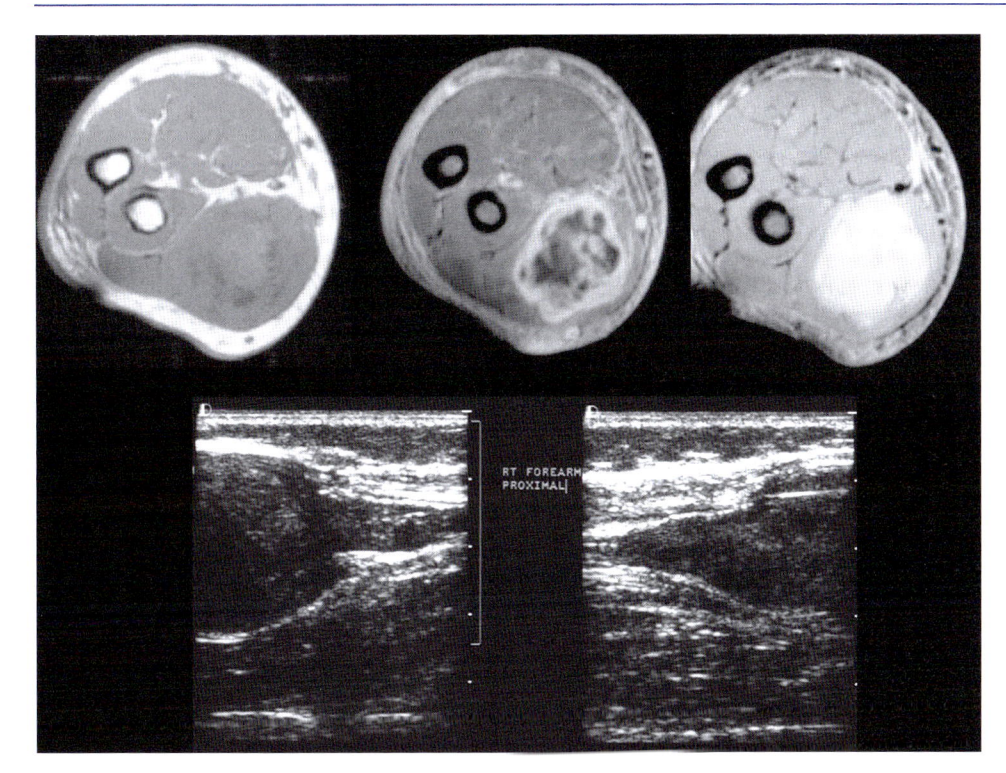

CHAPTER 10 Nerve Sheath and Neuroectodermal Tumors 215

FIGURE 10-22
Radiologic images of de novo malignant peripheral nerve sheath tumor (MPNST). T1 (top left), after gadolinium (middle), T2 (top right), and split-screen sonogram showing entering and exiting nerve of MPNST.

MALIGNANT PERIPHERAL NERVE SHEATH TUMOR—FACT SHEET

Definition
- A malignant tumor arising from peripheral nerve, a neurofibroma, or showing nerve sheath differentiation; half are associated with NF1

Incidence and Location
- Malignant transformation occurs in approximately 3% to 22% of neurofibromas; MPNST represents 5% to 10% of sarcomas; most common locations include the buttocks, thigh, brachial plexus, upper arm, and paraspinal region

Morbidity and Mortality
- Older studies report 5-year survival rate of 15% for MPNST in NF1; 5-year survival rate of 50% for de novo MPNST; newer studies support 5-year survival rate of 85% for both groups; best prognosis is for head and neck MPNST, which can be low grade

Clinical Features
- Second to fifth decade of life for sporadic tumors, and third to sixth decade in NF1-related tumors

Radiologic Features
- Difficult to separate from benign nerve sheath tumors, size greater than 5 cm, irregular borders, and necrosis are suggestive of malignancy

Prognosis and Treatment
- Most MPNSTs are high grade and require adjuvant therapy in addition to surgery

---

MALIGNANT PERIPHERAL NERVE SHEATH TUMOR—PATHOLOGIC FEATURES

Gross Findings
- Fusiform, cream gray, necrosis, hemorrhage, greater than 5 cm

Microscopic Findings
- Alternating hypocellularity and hypercellularity, fascicular growth, accentuated perivascular cellularity, wavy to buckled nuclei; may be purely epithelioid; heterologous differentiation (skeletal muscle, osteochondroid, glands) in a minority of NF1-related cases

Immunohistochemical Findings
- Weak and focal S-100 protein expression in spindled tumors; diffuse strong S-100 protein expression in epithelioid MPNST; desmin, myogenin and MyoD1 expression in MPNST with rhabdomyoblastic differentiation

Differential Diagnosis
- Synovial sarcoma, fibrosarcoma, malignant solitary fibrous tumor, melanoma

Ultrastructural Findings
- Varying stages of melanosomes combined with schwannian features of complex cell processes and well-developed basement membranes

Immunohistochemical Findings
- Strong S-100 protein and HMB45 expression, best seen on bleached sections

Differential Diagnosis
- Malignant melanoma, blue nevus

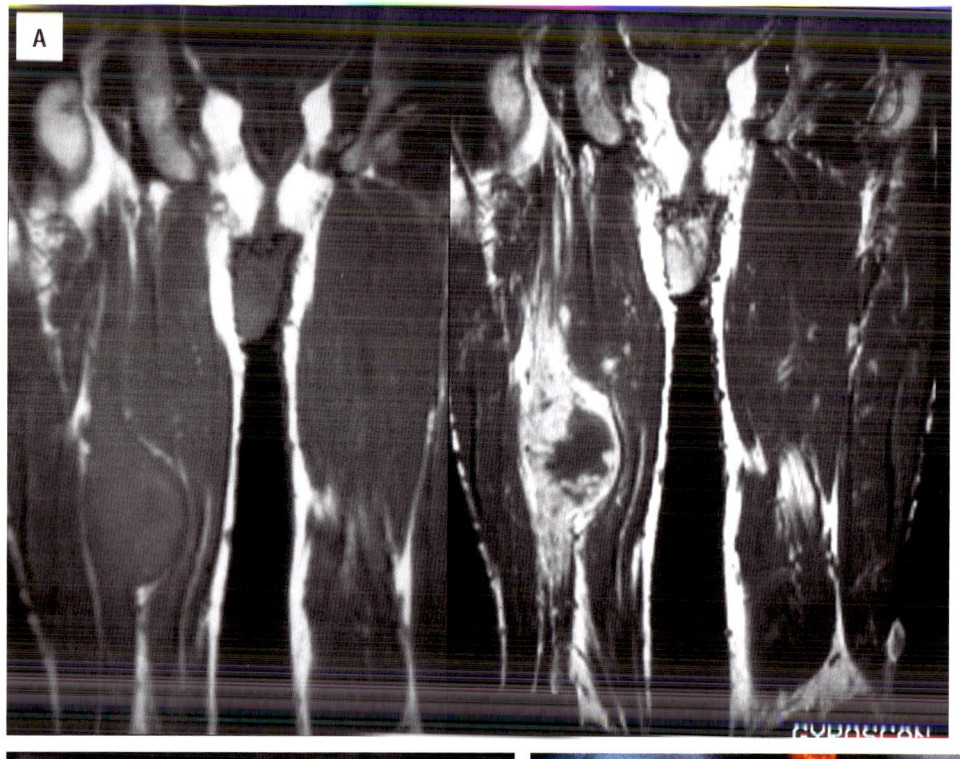

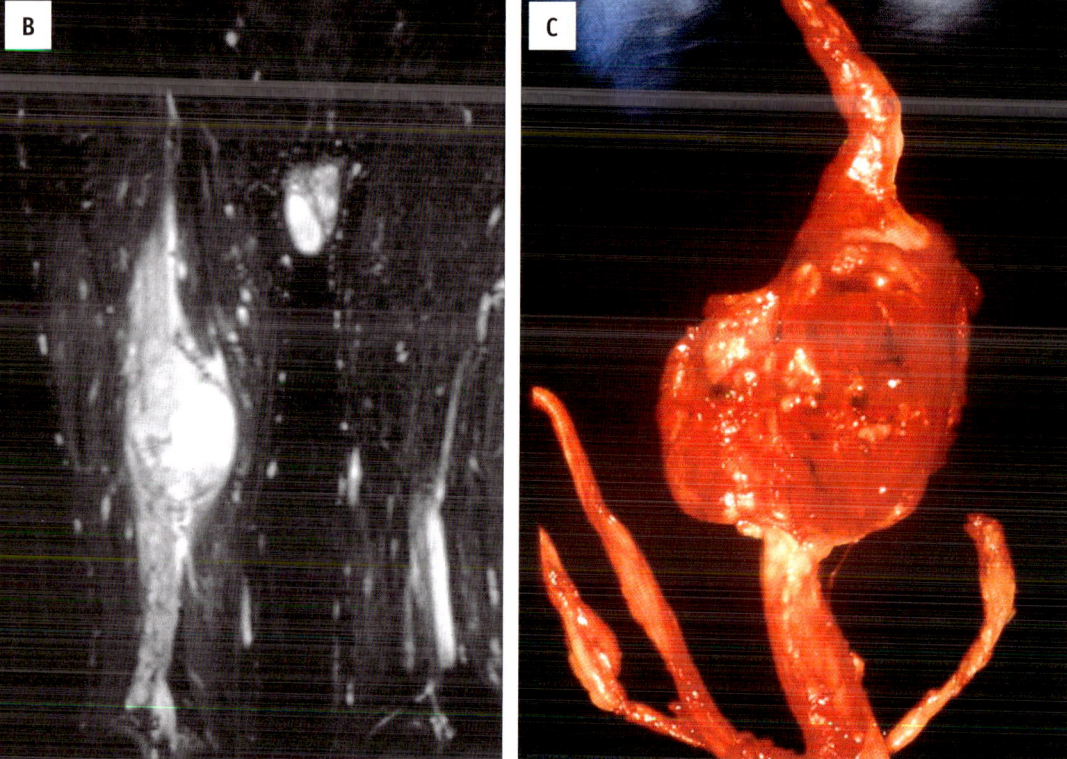

FIGURE 10-23

Coronal T1 and coronal T1 after gadolinium showing malignant peripheral nerve sheath tumor (MPNST) arising in plexiform neurofibroma of sciatic nerve in patient with neurofibromatosis type 1. Necrosis and invasion are present along nerve; the tumor has an infiltrative margin **(A)**. MPNST arising in neurofibromatosis demonstrates coronal short Tau inversion recovery **(B)** and gross correlation of nerve, branches, and tumor **(C)**.

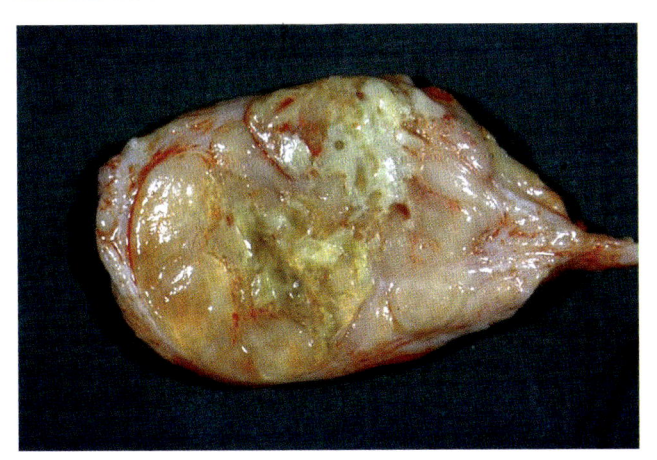

CHAPTER 10 Nerve Sheath and Neuroectodermal Tumors

FIGURE 10-24
Gross photograph of tan malignant peripheral nerve sheath tumor with areas of yellow–gray necrosis; nerve entering into lesion at right.

ANCILLARY STUDIES

IMMUNOHISTOCHEMISTRY

Spindled and epithelioid MPNSTs have different staining patterns (Figure 10-26). Spindled MPNST are generally only focally positive for S-100 protein, and are occasionally positive for GFAP and CD34. Although EMA-positive cells may be present, reflecting limited perineurial differentiation, cytokeratin-positive cells should not be seen, except in MPNST with glandular differentiation. MPNST with rhabdomyoblastic differentiation will show expression of desmin, myogenin, and MyoD1, often in many more cells than might be expected on routinely stained slides. Epithelioid MPNSTs, unlike spindled MPNSTs, are diffusely and strongly positive for S-100 protein. Melanocytic markers are negative in these tumors, assisting in their distinction from melanoma.

DIFFERENTIAL DIAGNOSIS

The differential diagnosis of spindled MPNST includes principally the other *monomorphic spindle cell sarcomas*, including MSS, fibrosarcoma, leiomyosarcoma, and malignant solitary fibrous tumor. The histologic features of spindled MPNST and MSS overlap to a significant degree, necessitating the routine use of immunostains to cytokeratins (positive scattered cell in nearly all MSSs, generally negative in MPNSTs), S-100 protein (weakly positive in almost all MPNSTs, weakly positive in ~20% of MSSs), and CD34 (variably positive in MPNST, invariably absent in MSS). In particularly difficult cases, such as MSS arising in association with nerves, cytogenetic, or molecular genetic analysis,

looking for the synovial sarcoma-associated t(X;18) (SYT-SSX) may be essential in arriving at a definitive diagnosis. Leiomyosarcoma and malignant solitary fibrous tumor may be excluded by a combination of morphologic and immunohistochemical findings, such as intersecting fascicles of eosinophilic, actin, and desmin-positive cells in leiomyosarcoma, and abundant collagen with cracking artifact and diffuse CD34 expression in malignant solitary fibrous tumor. Epithelioid MPNST may closely simulate malignant melanoma histologically; lack of expression of melanocytic markers may be helpful here.

PROGNOSIS AND TREATMENT

Most MPNSTs are high-grade sarcomas (Fédération Nationale des Centres de Lutte Contre le Cancer/National Federation for the Fight against Cancer [FNCLCC] or National Cancer Institute [NCI] grades 2 or 3), which metastasize to the lungs and bone. Those that occur in patients with NF1 have a greater morbidity and shorter 5-year survival rate (15%) as compared with sporadic MPNST (5-year survival, 50%). The epithelioid variant of MPNST can also metastasize to lymph nodes, and thus mimic malignant melanoma. Rare MPNST, particularly those tumors that occur in the head and neck, and "early" tumors arising in neurofibromas are histologically and clinically low grade.

GRANULAR CELL TUMOR: BENIGN, ATYPICAL, AND MALIGNANT

CLINICAL FEATURES

Granular cell tumors are schwannian tumors with granular eosinophilic cytoplasmic features, because of abundant lysosomes. These are usually benign tumors and can occur in almost any anatomic location, including the dermis, subcutis, submucosal, and even internal organs, including the larynx, bronchus, stomach, and bile duct. An individual may be affected at any age, but these tumors occur most commonly in adults between the ages of 40 and 60 years. A female sex and African American predominance exist. The lesions are usually painless and are of less than 6 months in duration. Although most are solitary lesions, about 15% to 25% of patients are found to have multiple lesions, either simultaneously or over time. When multiple lesions occur, they are usually either all dermal/subcutaneous (superficial) or all internal (organ related);

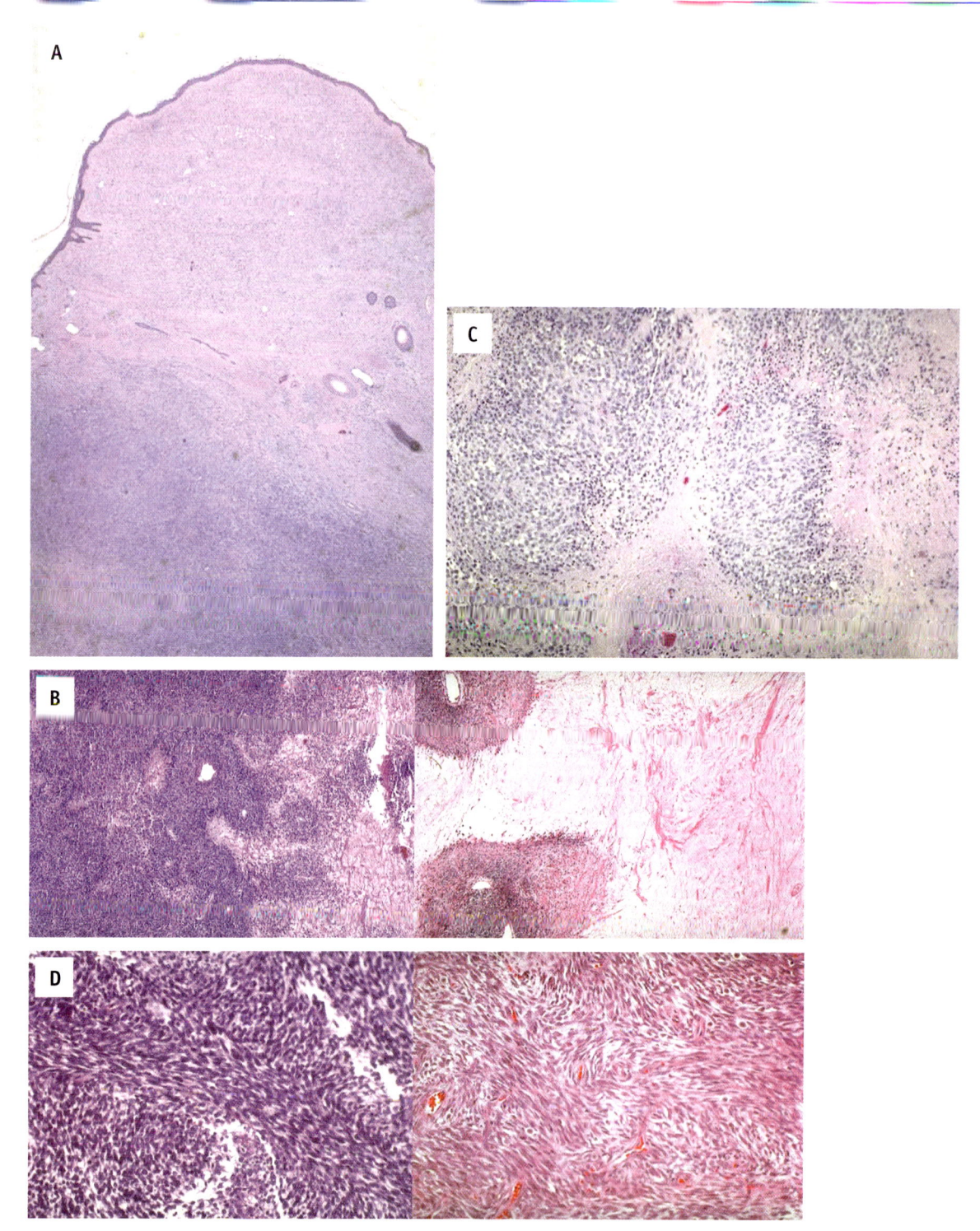

FIGURE 10-25

Microscopic images of malignant peripheral nerve sheath tumor. **A,** Patient with neurofibromatosis type 1 and malignant (blue, deep) transformation of cutaneous neurofibroma (pink, superficial). **B,** Typical histologic appearance of malignant peripheral nerve sheath tumor (MPNST) with perivascular tumor sparing and adjacent geographic necrosis of spindled MPNST and **(C)** epithelioid MPNST. **D,** Spindled bluish MPNST (left) compared with pinker synovial sarcoma (right).

rarely do patients with multiple granular cell tumors have extremity/trunk and internal organ involvement simultaneously. Although these are schwannian tumors, no association of multiple granular cell tumors with NF1 or NF2 exists. Malignant granular cell tumors are found de novo, not arising from a benign granular cell tumor, and usually occur in an older age population than benign granular cell tumors, most commonly in the superficial or deep soft tissue of the proximal upper extremity.

FIGURE 10-26

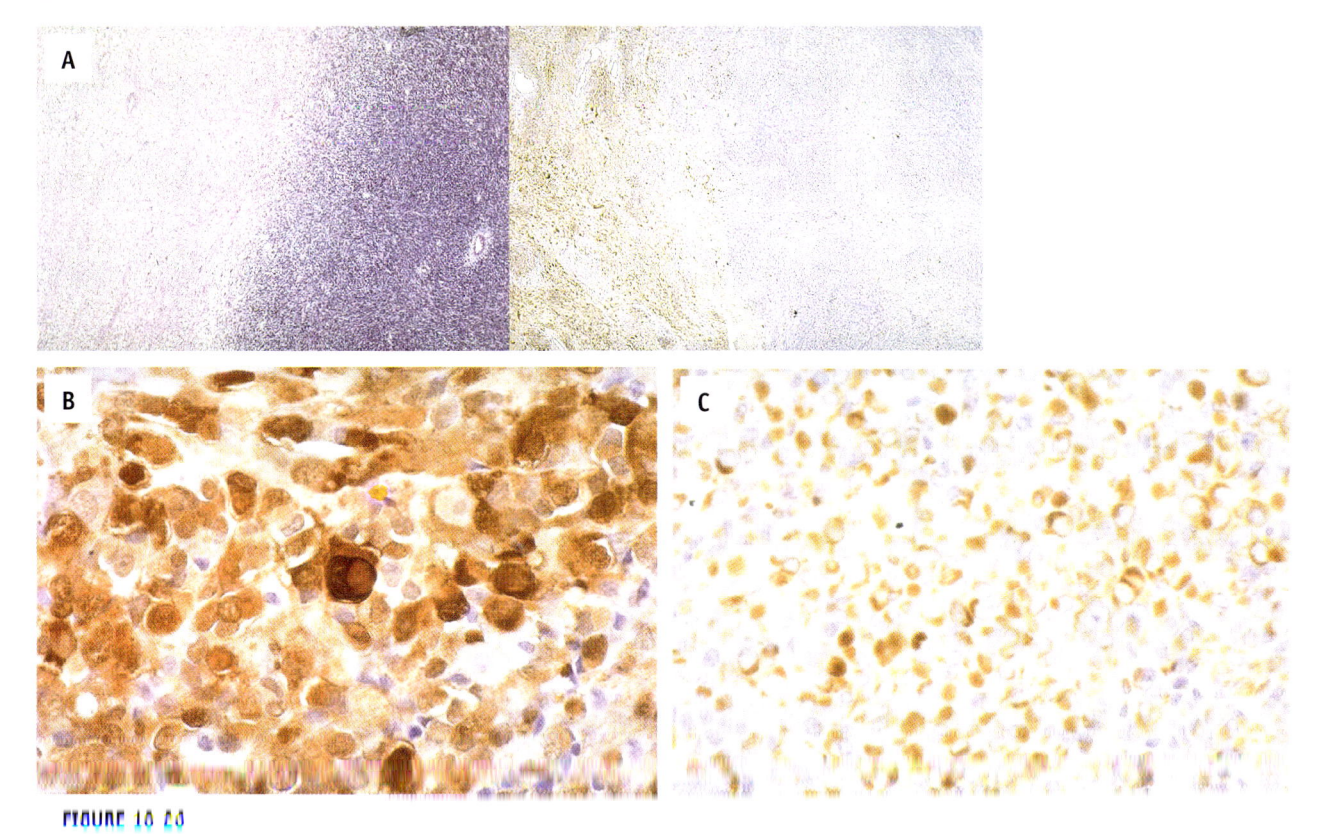

Typical immunohistochemistry for spindled malignant peripheral nerve sheath tumor (MPNST) arising in neurofibroma in patient with neurofibromatosis type 1. Diffuse S-100 protein of pink neurofibroma (left of both images) is decreased or absent with malignant transformation to spindled MPNST (right of both images, **A**), whereas epithelioid MPNST is diffusely strongly positive for S-100 protein **(B).** Both epithelioid and spindled MPNST can demonstrate glial fibrillary acidic protein **(C).**

PATHOLOGIC FEATURES

GROSS FINDINGS

Benign granular cell tumors are usually less than 3 cm, poorly delineated, and pale yellow-tan on cut surface. Malignant granular cell tumors have a similar gross appearance but tend to be larger, with a median size of 4 cm.

MICROSCOPIC FINDINGS

Most granular cell tumors are poorly circumscribed proliferations of large polygonal cells with eosinophilic, granular cytoplasm, and ovoid dark nuclei with inconspicuous nucleoli and minimal mitotic activity, which involves the dermis, subcutis, or submucosal area (Figure 10-27). Cytoplasmic aggregation of lysosomes yields a cytoplasmic globule surrounded by an artifactual halo, a diagnostically useful feature in separating true granular cell tumors from granular cell variants of other tumor types. The overlying epidermis may be acanthotic or show pseudoepitheliomatous hyperplasia, and the tumor is often found in close association with small peripheral nerves, often with perineurial growth. The diagnosis of malignant granular cell tumor is given to tumors that show at least three and usually five or six of the following six histologic features: pronounced spindling with fascicular growth, necrosis, mitotic activity greater than 2 in 10 high power fields (hpf), high nuclear to cytoplasmic ratio, diffuse nuclear pleomorphism, and vesicular nuclei with prominent macronucleoli (Figure 10-28). Tumors with only one or two of these features may be classified as *atypical;* such lesions appear to behave in a similar fashion to entirely benign-appearing tumors (Figure 10-29).

ANCILLARY STUDIES

IMMUNOHISTOCHEMISTRY

All granular cell tumors are intensely positive for S-100 protein and CD68, highlighting the characteristic cytoplasmic granular (Figure 10-30). Inhibin α subunit may be positive in benign granular cell tumors but has not been fully evaluated in malignant granular cell tumors. Basement membrane proteins such as collagen type IV and laminin are present.

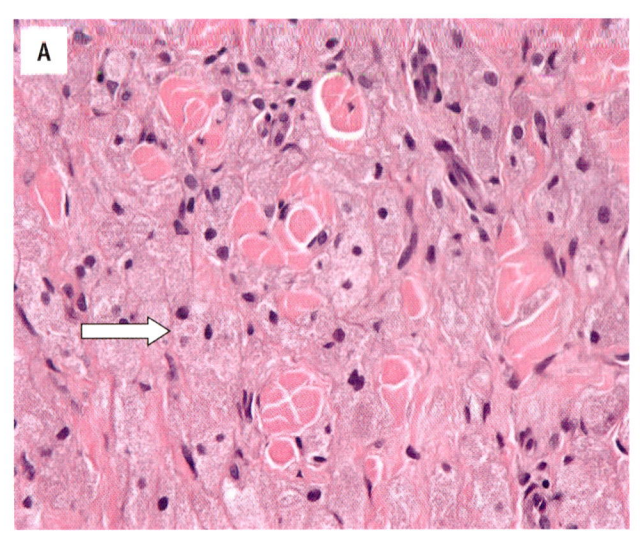

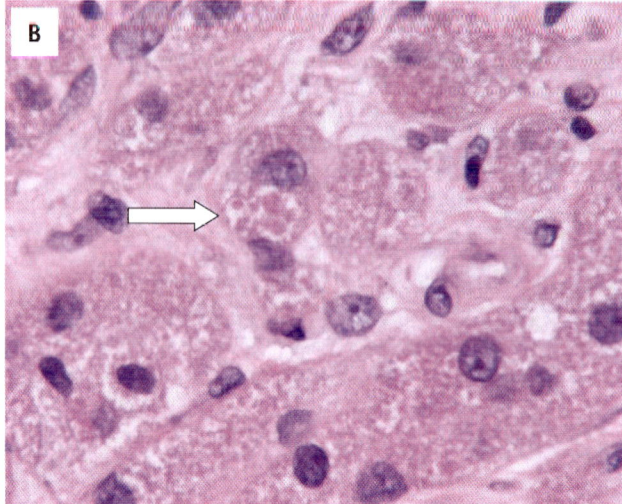

FIGURE 10-27
Microscopic appearance of benign granular cell tumor with large polygonal cells, small nuclei, absence of mitoses, infiltrative appearance, granular cytoplasm, and cytoplasmic lysosomal aggregates with clear halos (**A**, *arrow*; **B**, better demonstrated).

GRANULAR CELL TUMOR—FACT SHEET

Definition
- A Schwann cell tumor with cytoplasmic granules representing lysosomes and lysosomal aggregates

Incidence and Location
- Benign granular cell tumor is common, occurring in soft tissue, gastrointestinal tract, and respiratory tract; malignant granular cell tumor is rare and has been reported only in soft tissue, most commonly the proximal upper extremity

Morbidity and Mortality
- Benign granular cell tumor may recur locally and can be multiple in 15% to 25% of cases; malignant granular cell tumors have been reported to have a 50% distant metastatic rate, with associated poor prognosis and short survival

Clinical Features
- These tumors may occur in patients of any age but are most common in the second to fourth decades of life; a female sex and African American predominance exist

Prognosis and Treatment
- Benign granular cell tumors may recur locally if incompletely excised; histologically malignant granular cell tumors behave as high-grade sarcomas

GRANULAR CELL TUMOR—PATHOLOGIC FEATURES

Gross Findings
- Poorly delineated, pale yellow–tan, small (< 3 cm) tumors; malignant tumors may be larger

Microscopic Findings
- Sheets of infiltrative large granular cells, usually with small nuclei and indistinct nucleoli and low mitotic activity; distinctive cytoplasmic aggregations of lysosomes separated by a clear halo are found; atypical granular cell tumors have one or two of the following histologic features, and malignant granular cell tumors have at least three and usually five to six of the following histologic features: sarcomatoid spindling, necrosis, mitoses greater than 2 per 10 hpf, high nuclear-to-cytoplasmic ratio, diffuse pleomorphism, vesicular nuclei with macronucleoli

Ultrastructural Findings
- Granular cytoplasm contains numerous autophagic vacuoles; some cells have large boat-shaped cytoplasmic crystals (angulated bodies)

Immunohistochemical Findings
- S-100 protein, CD68, α inhibin positive

Differential Diagnosis
- Granular cell variants of many other types of neoplasm

DIFFERENTIAL DIAGNOSIS

Essentially any tumor type may show granular cell change, thus, the differential diagnosis of true granular cell tumors is quite broad. In general, granular cell variants of other tumor types lack the large, clumped granules surrounded by an artifactual halo seen in true granular cell tumors. Demonstration of intense S-100 protein in the absence of expression of other markers (e.g., factor XIIIa, actins, desmin) may be helpful in this differential diagnosis. It should be remembered that CD68 is a nonspecific marker of lysosomes, which may, therefore, be positive in any tumor with granular cell features.

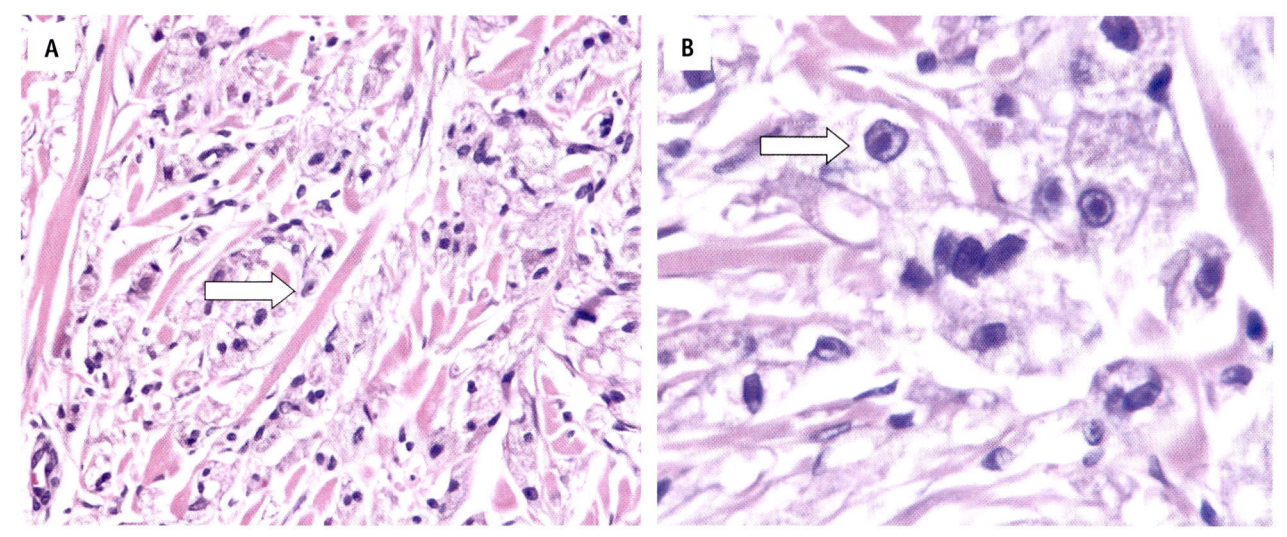

CHAPTER 10 Nerve Sheath and Neuroectodermal Tumors 221

FIGURE 10-28
Atypical granular cell tumor with focally enlarged nuclei and prominent nucleoli. **A,** Low-power view. **B,** Higher magnification of **A.**

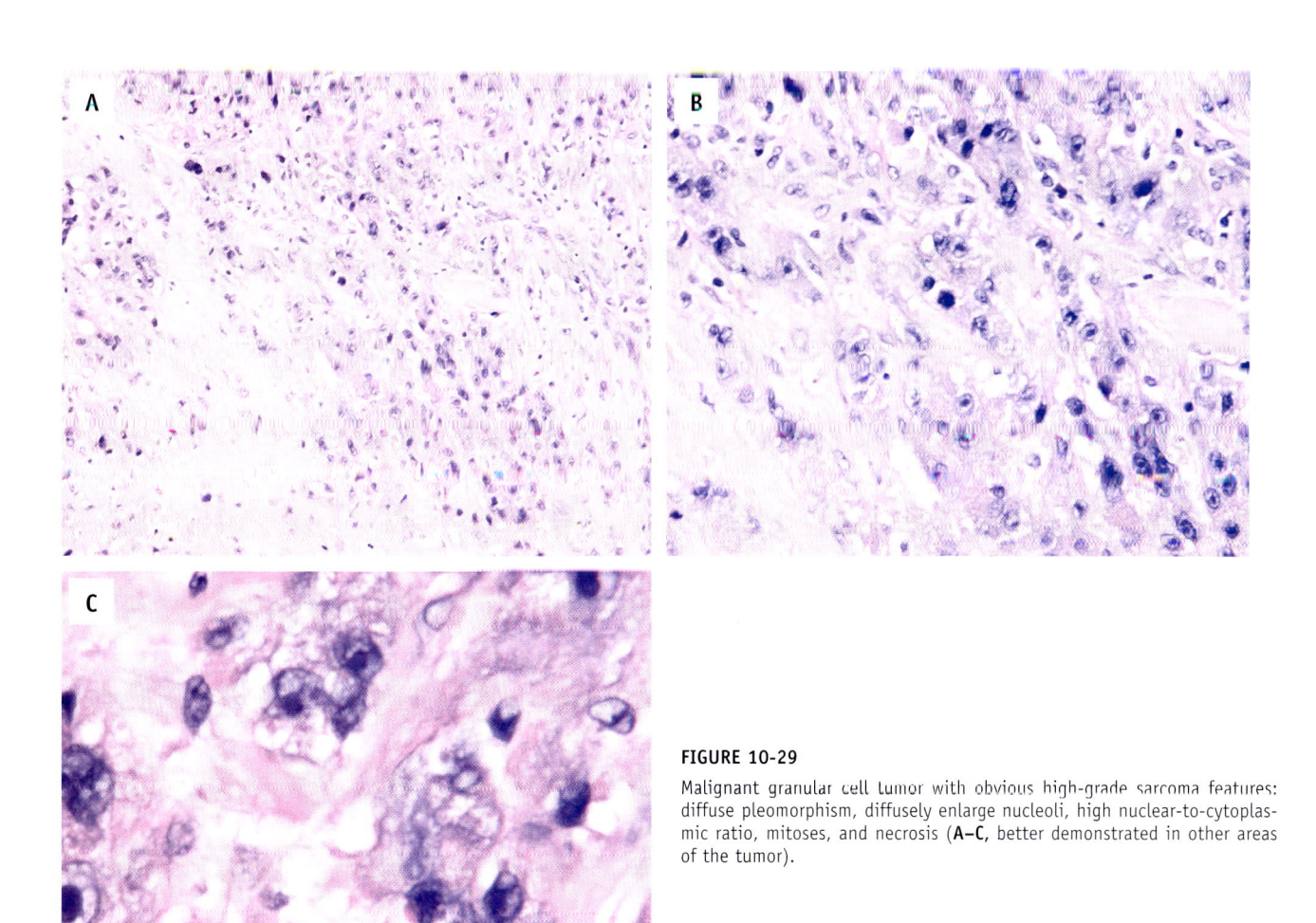

FIGURE 10-29
Malignant granular cell tumor with obvious high-grade sarcoma features: diffuse pleomorphism, diffusely enlarge nucleoli, high nuclear-to-cytoplasmic ratio, mitoses, and necrosis (**A–C,** better demonstrated in other areas of the tumor).

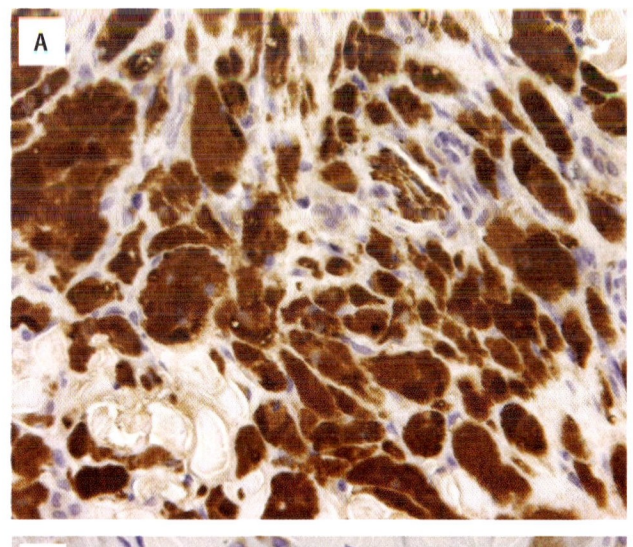

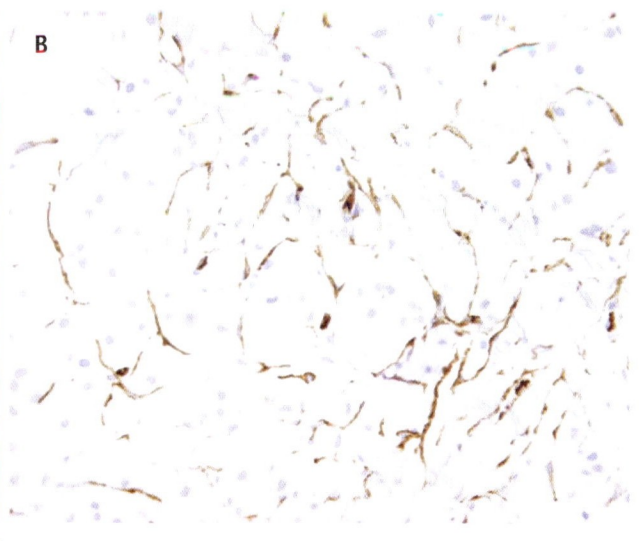

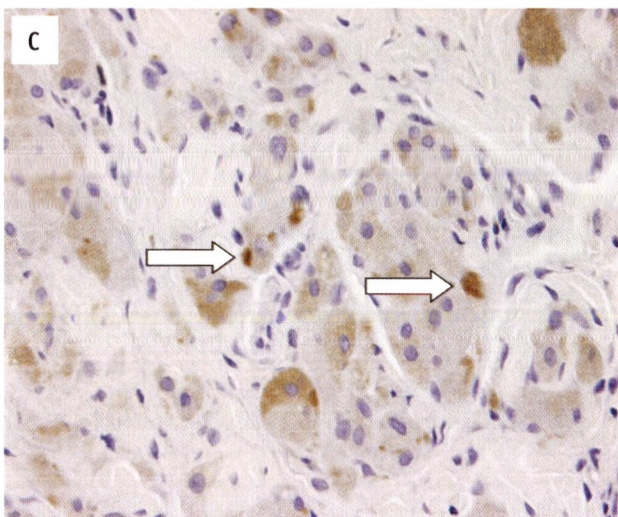

FIGURE 10-30

Immunohistochemistry of granular cell tumor: **A**, Diffuse S100 protein staining; **(B)** silhouette of clusters of tumor cells in benign granular cell tumor by CD34-positive fibroblasts; and **(C)** KP1 (CD68) highlighting cytoplasmic lysosomal aggregates, so characteristic for granular cell tumor and not identified in other tumors with granular cell features.

PROGNOSIS AND TREATMENT

Benign granular cell tumors are often relatively infiltrative tumors, which are commonly initially resected with positive surgical margins. Such tumors may recur locally, unless completely excised. Malignant granular cell tumors behave as high-grade sarcomas and should be treated as such.

PERINEURIOMA: INTRANEURAL, SOFT TISSUE, AND MALIGNANT

CLINICAL FEATURES

Perineurioma is generally a benign tumor composed of perineurial cells, the peripheral counterpart of meningeal cells from the intracranial pia-arachnoid membranes. Perineurioma involves mainly peripheral nerves of the extremities (intraneural type) or is unassociated with nerve (soft tissue type). Sclerosing perineurioma is the most common type of perineurioma, followed by typical soft tissue perineurioma, intraneural perineurioma, and rare reticular perineuriomas. Perineuriomas can be superficial or deep. Intraneural perineurioma most commonly occurs in adolescence with an equal sex distribution; soft tissue perineurioma occurs in adults with a female predominance, but children can also be affected. Symptoms of intraneural perineurioma include progressive muscle weakness and sometimes skeletal muscle atrophy. Soft tissue perineuriomas often present as an asymptomatic mass.

PATHOLOGIC FEATURES

GROSS FINDINGS

Intraneural manifestations include segmental or tubular enlargement of nerve, up to 10 cm or longer. *Soft tissue* involvement includes solitary, small, well-circumscribed

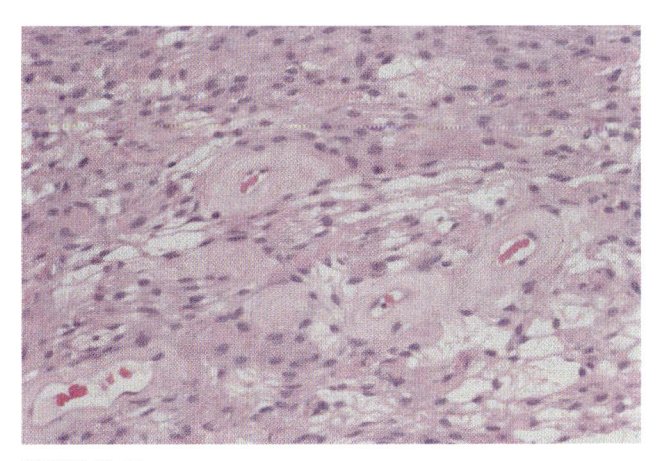

FIGURE 10-31
Soft tissue perineurioma demonstrating whorls of bland, ovoid perineurial cells embedded in a myofibrous matrix. *(Courtesy of John F. Fetsch, MD)*

mass, measuring 1.5 to up to 12 cm in greatest dimension. These can be firm to gelatinous and gray–white.

MICROSCOPIC FINDINGS

Intraneural findings include neoplastic perineurial cells seen throughout the endoneurium, forming concentric layers around nerve fibers, creating an *onion bulb*–like effect. The lesion may become progressively hyalinized.

Soft tissue perineuriomas are composed of spindled wavy cells with elongated cytoplasmic processes. In myxoid areas, these processes can be seen to overlap from cell to cell. The tumors typically grow in short fascicles and meningioma-like whorls (Figure 10-31). Although degenerative atypia may be observed in longstanding lesions, mitoses are generally rare and necrosis is absent.

Sclerosing perineuriomas display bland epithelioid to spindled cells arranged in concentric whorls, embedded in a distinctly sclerotic matrix (Figure 10-32).

Malignant perineurioma, also known as *perineurial MPNST*, displays greater cellularity, nuclear enlargement and hyperchromatism, mitotic activity, infiltrative growth, and necrosis. Ultrastructural or immunohistochemical study, or both, is typically necessary to distinguish malignant perineuriomas from other types of MPNST. This distinction currently is not known to be clinically significant.

ANCILLARY STUDIES

IMMUNOHISTOCHEMISTRY

Intraneural involvement shows EMA-positive perineurial cells surrounding S-100-protein–positive residual Schwann cells and NFP-positive residual axons of the nerve fibers.

Soft tissue perineuriomas (Figure 10-33), including sclerosing perineuriomas, are positive for EMA and negative for S-100 protein or CD34. All perineuriomas can be claudin-1 positive. Claudin-1, a tight junction-related protein, and GLUT-1, a glucose transporter protein, are frequently positive in perineurial tumors and not in the majority of tumors in the differential diagnosis. On occasion, claudin-1, GLUT-1, or both may be positive in tumors that lack or nearly lack EMA expression.

GENETIC FEATURES

Cytogenetic study of both intraneural and soft tissue perineuriomas has shown monosomy of chromosome 22.

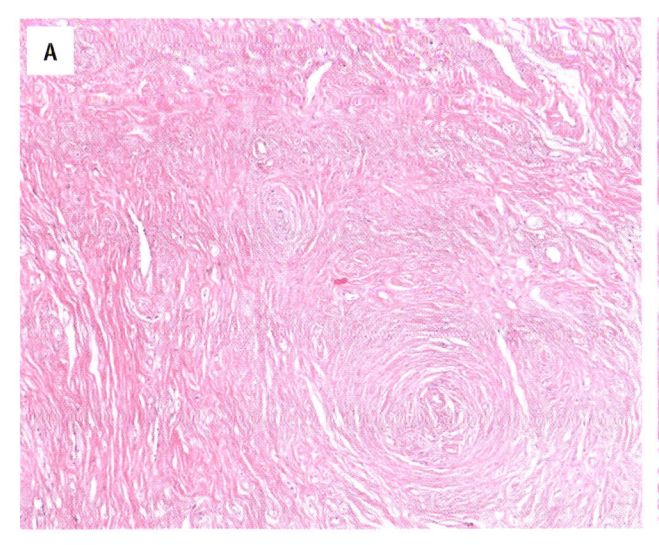

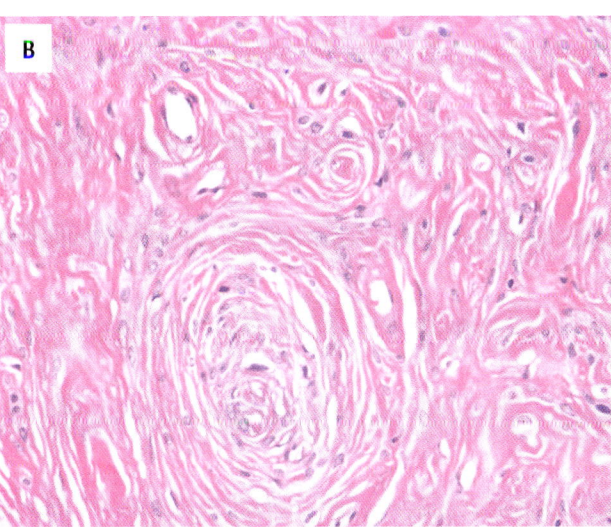

FIGURE 10-32
Sclerosing perineurioma is the most common type of soft tissue perineurioma, demonstrating whorls of uniform perineurial cells embedded in collagenized stroma **(A, B)**.

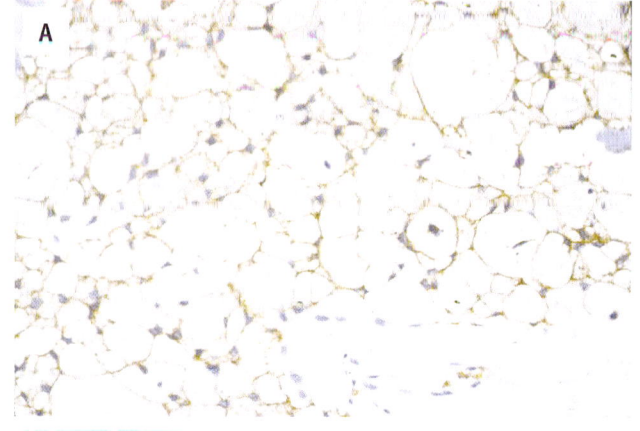

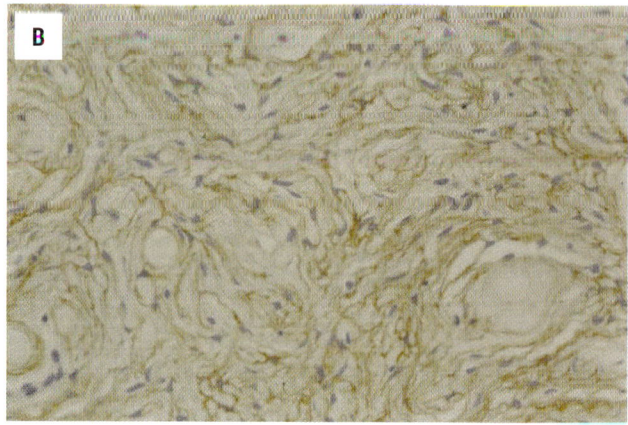

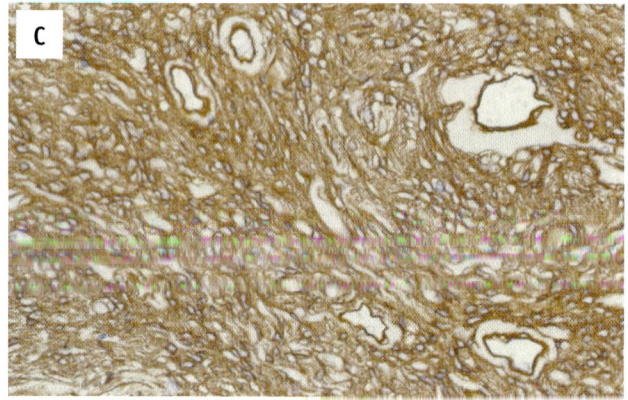

FIGURE 10-33

Immunohistochemistry of soft tissue perineurioma: **(A)** Glut-1, **(B)** epithelial membrane antigen, and **(C)** diffuse laminin. (C, Courtesy of John F. Fetsch, MD)

PERINEURIOMA—FACT SHEET

Definition
▸▸ A tumor of nerve or soft tissue composed mainly of perineurial cells

Incidence and Location
▸▸ Rare, located in peripheral extremity nerves for intraneural type and mainly in extremities for soft tissue type

Morbidity and Mortality
▸▸ Low for intraneural and benign soft tissue perineuriomas; greater for malignant perineuriomas

Clinical Features
▸▸ Intraneural perineurioma occurs in adolescents to young adults, with equal sex distribution, in peripheral extremity nerves, causing muscle weakness
▸▸ Soft tissue perineurioma occurs in adults with a female predilection, not arising within nerve

Prognosis and Treatment
▸▸ Intraneural tumors are benign and require only biopsy for diagnosis
▸▸ Most other perineuriomas are benign and require only local excision
▸▸ Malignant perineuriomas should be treated as sarcomas

PERINEURIOMA—PATHOLOGIC FEATURES

Gross Findings
▸▸ Intraneural perineurioma: thickening of nerve
▸▸ Soft tissue perineurioma: small, circumscribed mass

Microscopic Findings
▸▸ Intraneural perineurioma: concentric onion bulb–like perineurial cells around residual nerve twigs and fibrosis
▸▸ Soft tissue perineurioma: spindled, wavy, perineurial cells embedded in collagen with some whorls

Immunohistochemical Findings
▸▸ Intraneural perineurioma: residual S-100 protein-positive Schwann cells and NFP-positive axons surrounded by EMA-positive perineurial cells
▸▸ Soft tissue perineurioma: EMA reactivity, negative for S-100 protein; both can be claudin-1 and GLUT-1 positive

Genetic Findings
▸▸ Monosomy of chromosome 22

Differential Diagnosis
▸▸ Intraneural perineurioma: none
▸▸ Sclerosing perineurioma: glomus tumor, benign fibrous histiocytoma, myoepithelial tumors
▸▸ Soft tissue perineurioma: neurofibroma, low-grade fibromyxoid sarcoma, solitary fibrous tumor, dedifferentiated liposarcoma with meningothelial-like whorls, conventional MPNST

DIFFERENTIAL DIAGNOSIS

Intraneural perineuriomas are quite distinctive and unlikely to be confused with other tumors. Sclerosing perineuriomas, by virtue of their frequent location on the extremities, may be confused with hyalinized glomus tumors, benign fibrous histiocytoma and collagenous fibroma, and myoepithelial tumors. Identification of EMA expression, in the absence of expression of actins, desmin, S-100 protein, cytokeratin, or factor XIIIa, may be helpful. Deeply seated perineuriomas may be confused with a variety of collagenized or myxoid tumors, including neurofibroma, low-grade fibromyxoid sarcoma, solitary fibrous tumor, and rare variants of dedifferentiated liposarcoma with meningothelial-like whorls. Neurofibromas may be recognized by virtue of their distinctive *shredded carrot-like* collagen and S-100 protein expression. Low-grade fibromyxoid sarcomas show a characteristic abrupt transition from heavily collagenized zones into myxoid nodules and are EMA-negative. Solitary fibrous tumors typically show a more *patternless* pattern of growth, hemangiopericytoma-like blood vessels, and diffuse CD34 expression. Although the meningothelial-like whorls seen in rare cases of dedifferentiated liposarcoma may closely resemble perineurioma, they are seen in the context of areas of well-differentiated liposarcoma and are EMA negative.

PROGNOSIS AND TREATMENT

Intraneural perineuriomas are benign, without risk for local recurrence. Biopsy for diagnosis is sufficient because resection will result in loss of neurologic function. Soft tissue perineuriomas are generally benign and can be surgically excised without recurrence or postoperative morbidity. Malignant perineuriomas do have significant potential for local recurrences and some risk for metastasis; their biologic potential relative to other types of MPNST remains to be determined.

NEUROTHEKEOMA: NERVE SHEATH MYXOMA

Neurothekeoma was first described by Harkin and Reed in 1969. It is a benign myxoid tumor of nerve sheath origin. Although the tumor known as *cellular neurothekeoma* has traditionally been considered a variant of myxoid neurothekeoma, more recent evidence suggests this is an unrelated neoplasm of possible fibrohistiocytic derivation. Cellular neurothekeoma will not be discussed in this chapter.

CLINICAL FEATURES

Nerve sheath myxoma affects children and young adults with no definite sex predilection. The head and neck and extremities, especially the upper extremities, are the most common locations for this tumor. These are dermal and subcutaneous lesions that only rarely involve deep soft tissue. No known association exists with NF1 or NF2.

PATHOLOGIC FEATURES

GROSS FINDINGS

Nerve sheath myxoma is generally a multinodular mucoid mass in the dermis or subcutis that is small, 0.5 to 2.0 cm.

MICROSCOPIC FINDINGS

Nerve sheath myxoma is a highly distinctive neoplasm composed of well-demarcated, abundantly myxoid lobules of varying sizes, separated by fibrous septa (Figure 10-34). Within this myxoid stroma the tumor cells are stellate, spindled, and occasionally epithelioid, with lightly eosinophilic cell processes and small, darkly staining nuclei. Usually, little pleomorphism or mitotic activity is present, although occasional tumors may show scattered enlarged, hyperchromatic cells.

ANCILLARY STUDIES

IMMUNOHISTOCHEMISTRY

Myxoid neurothekeomas are strongly positive for S-100 protein and basement membrane proteins, such as collagen type IV. EMA-positive cells may occasionally be found around the periphery of the tumor, representing residual perineurial cells.

DIFFERENTIAL DIAGNOSIS

Myxoid neurothekeoma may be confused with other myxoid neoplasms of the skin and subcutis, such as cutaneous angiomyxoma and myxofibrosarcoma (myxoid malignant fibrous histiocytoma). Both cutaneous angiomyxoma and myxofibrosarcoma are more infiltrative lesions that lack the distinctly lobular growth pattern

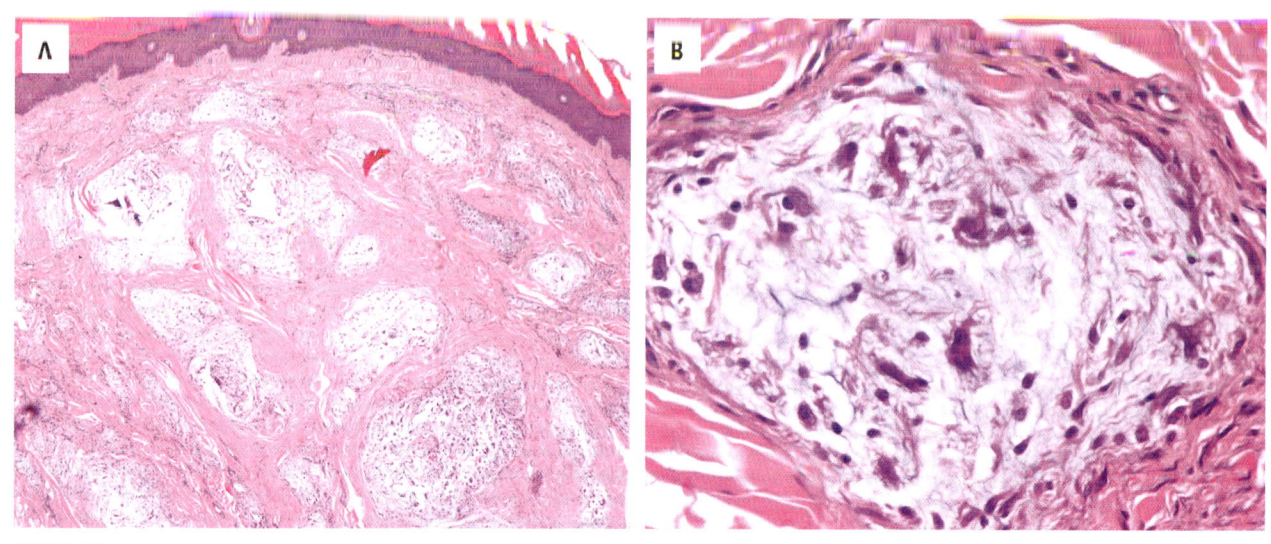

FIGURE 10-34

A, Nerve sheath myxoma (neurothekeoma) demonstrating lobules of myxoid change separated by fibrous septa and **(B)** higher magnification of stellate whorling cells in areas of myxoid change.

NEUROTHEKEOMA—FACT SHEET

Definition
- A peripheral, superficial, multiloculated nerve sheath tumor in young adults
- Incidence and location: typically extremities, not uncommon

Morbidity and Mortality
- None; benign; no association with NF1 or NF2

Clinical Features
- Young adults, equal sex distribution, extremity mass
- Prognosis and treatment: benign, simple excision

NEUROTHEKEOMA—PATHOLOGIC FEATURES

Gross Findings
- Dermal or subcutaneous multinodular mucoid mass, less than 2.0 cm

Microscopic Findings
- Nodules of myxoid change separated by fibrous septa with stellate, usually bland cells in a slight whorled pattern; sometimes hyperchromasia or multinucleation, rare mitoses

Immunohistochemical Findings
- S-100 protein-positive

Differential Diagnosis
- Angiomyxoma, myxofibrosarcoma, myxoid schwannoma, myxoid neurofibroma

---

of myxoid neurothekeoma and show other features not seen in neurothekeoma, such as stromal neutrophils in angiomyxoma and mitotically active, hyperchromatic, pleomorphic spindled cells in myxofibrosarcoma. These two lesions are also S-100 protein-negative. On occasion, both schwannoma and neurofibroma may show abundant myxoid change and mimic neurothekeoma. Clues to these diagnoses include the focal presence of Antoni A zones with Verocay bodies in myxoid schwannoma and the distinctive collagen pattern of neurofibroma.

PROGNOSIS AND TREATMENT

Myxoid neurothekeoma is a benign tumor that can be treated with local excision.

NEUROBLASTOMA, GANGLIONEUROBLASTOMA, AND GANGLIONEUROMA

CLINICAL FEATURES

Neuroblastoma is a tumor of the primitive migratory neural crest elements that normally invade the fetal adrenal gland and form the sympathetic nervous system. Neuroblastomas that occur along the sympathetic nervous system chain and adrenal gland are the most frequent of the pediatric neural tumors, 96% occurring in the first year of life, and almost all by 5 years of age. No sex predilection exists. The adrenals (40%) are the most common site, followed by the abdominal cavity (25%), thoracic cavity (15%), cervical region (5%), and pelvic sympathetic ganglia (5%). Patients present with a palpable abdominal mass, hepatomegaly, or a thoracic mass on routine chest radiograph. Secretion of vasoactive intestinal polypeptide by the tumor can cause the patient to have watery diarrhea and hypokalemia. Ganglioneuroma is a benign sympathetic nervous system tumor that occurs in children and young adults in the retroperitoneum, pelvis, adrenals, gastrointestinal tract, and posterior mediastinum, with a female sex predominance.

RADIOLOGIC FEATURES

Neuroblastoma can be detected on radiographic or CT scan, especially when demonstrating stippled calcifications, present in both ganglioneuroma and the less mature neuroblastoma variants. Magnetic resonance imaging (MRI) is generally nonspecific, demonstrating an intermediate or low intensity on T1-weighted images and a high signal on T2-weighted images. A radioisotope study using ^{131}I-meta-iodobenzylguanidine, a substance taken up by adrenergic secretory vesicles, can be used to demonstrate primary and metastatic tumors.

PATHOLOGIC FEATURES

GROSS FINDINGS

Neuroblastoma may present as a large (> 10 cm) mass and is lobulated, encapsulated, soft, tan–gray, hemorrhagic, sometimes cystic, and often calcified. Intraadrenal lesions may show a thin rim of residual adrenal gland flattened against the capsule of the neuroblastoma. Ganglioneuroblastoma and ganglioneuroma tumors are more firm and tan–white. Ganglioneuroblastomas often contain nodules of grossly different appearance and consistency.

MICROSCOPIC FINDINGS

The Shimada classification is used to separate four main *neuroblastoma* subtypes: (1) neuroblastoma (Schwannian stroma poor; Figure 10-35); (2) ganglioneuroblastoma (Schwannian stroma rich, > 50%, grossly intermingled areas); (3) ganglioneuroblastoma (Schwannian stroma-poor component and either Schwannian stroma-rich or

---

NEUROBLASTOMA—FACT SHEET

Definition
▸▸ Neuroblastoma is a spectrum of tumors from mature ganglioneuroma to ganglioneuroblastoma to undifferentiated neuroblastoma that arise from primitive neural crest cells

Incidence and Location
▸▸ Neuroblastoma is the third most common pediatric tumor and the most common tumor in patients younger than 5 years, usually in the adrenal or other retroperitoneal or posterior mediastinal site; ganglioneuroma is found in the retroperitoneum in older children

Morbidity and Mortality
▸▸ Prognosis depends on stage, patient age, location, histologic classification, and molecular findings; poor prognosis is associated with nodular ganglioneuroblastoma, high MKI, undifferentiated or poorly differentiated in a child between 1 and 5 years old, and deletions or loss of hybridization of 1p36, amplification or MYCN, or both; those with intermixed schwannian stroma, differentiating or low MKI, or ganglioneuroma have good prognosis; alternatively, neuroblastomas, even high stage, in very young (less than 1 year) patients may involute or spontaneously regress

Clinical Features
▸▸ Abdominal mass, child younger than 5 years, for neuroblastoma; older child or young adult, retroperitoneum, for ganglioneuroma

Radiologic Features
▸▸ Stippled calcification by X ray or CT, in patient younger than 5 years with midline or adrenal mass with high signal intensity on T2-weighted MRI, is suggestive of neuroblastoma; ganglioneuroma can also show calcification on radiograph or CT scan
▸▸ Prognosis and treatment: prognosis depends on type, staging, and above factors (see Morbidity and Mortality). Treatment is according to risk protocol, varying from no additional therapy to chemotherapy to myeloablative treatment with stem cell transplantation for high-stage, poor prognosis patients

---

NEUROBLASTOMA—PATHOLOGIC FEATURES

Gross Findings
▸▸ Hemorrhagic foci, stippled calcification, neuroblastoma. More firm, tan-white for ganglioneuroma

Microscopic Findings
▸▸ See earlier Shimada classification, separates neuroblastoma into four main subtypes; spectrum from primitive round cell embedded in neuropil stroma to tumor with schwannian features and mature ganglion cells

Immunohistochemical Findings
▸▸ Synaptophysin, chromogranin, neurofilament, NSE, and protein gene product 9.5 may be positive in neuroblastoma; CD99 is generally negative; CD44 expression may be a prognostic factor

Genetic Findings
▸▸ FISH: MYCN amplification; cytogenetics: deletion chromosome 1p, dm chromosomes, hsrs

Differential Diagnosis
▸▸ Other small blue cell tumors, including primitive neuroectodermal tumor, rhabdomyosarcoma, lymphoma, and desmoplastic small round cell tumor; ganglioneuroma: schwannoma and neurofibroma

FIGURE 10-35

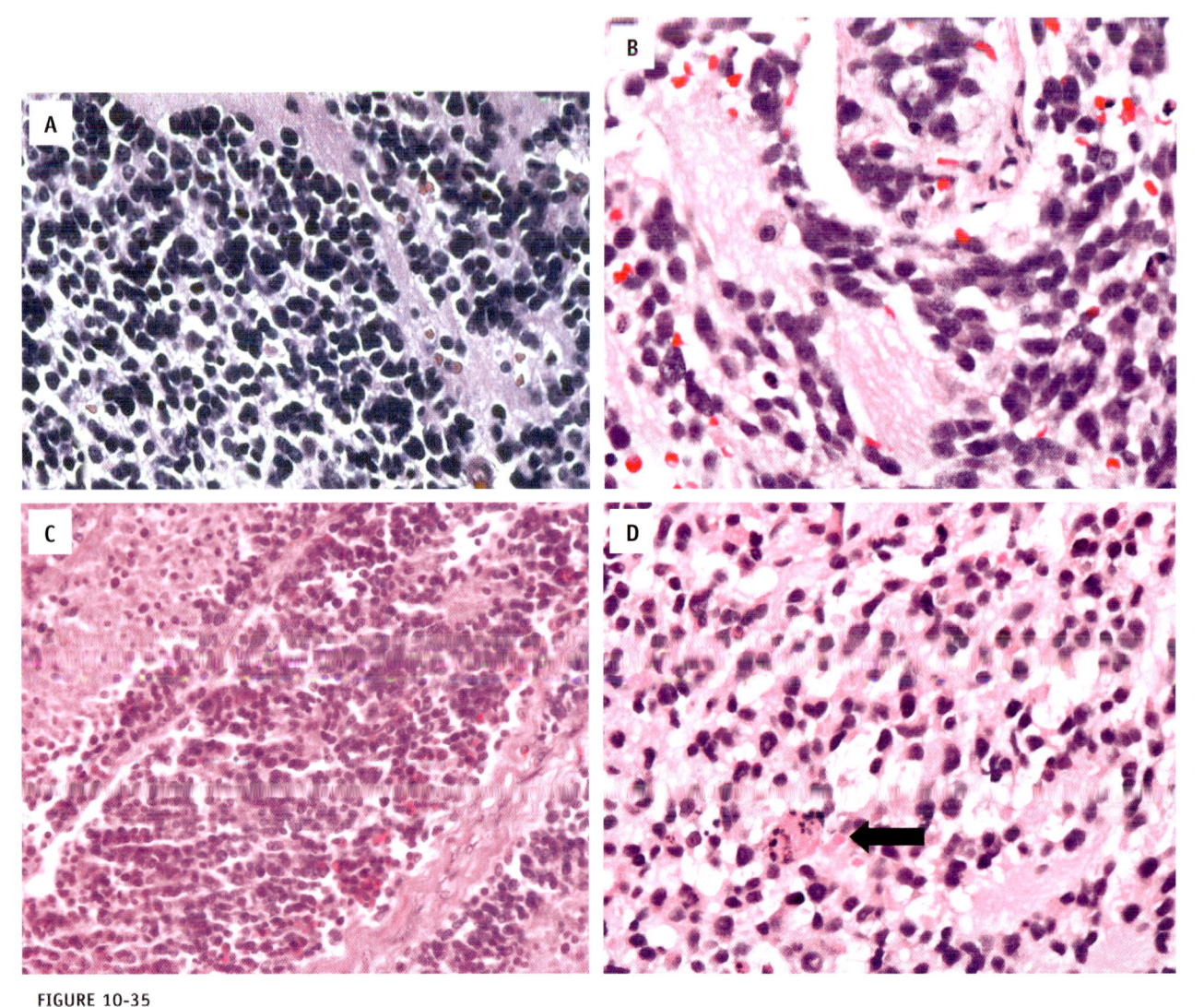

A, The spectrum of neurofibroma (Shimada classification) ranges from poorly or undifferentiated neuroblastoma with round blue cells sometimes identified in **(B)** a neuropil stroma, **(C)** often abundant necrosis, or **(D)** apoptosis, and

(Continued)

Schwannian stroma dominant component, grossly in separate nodules); and (4) ganglioneuroma (Schwannian stroma dominant). The first subtype is further separated into three variants. It can be fully undifferentiated, requiring ancillary studies for diagnosis, poorly differentiated with readily recognizable neuropil and Homer–Wright rosette formation, or differentiating (usually abundant neuropil and at least 5% of tumor cells maturing to ganglion cells). Neuroblasts are small, dark cells with high nuclear-to-cytoplasmic ratio and stippled chromatin. Neuroblastoma usually has high mitotic activity and karyorrhexis, and is often hemorrhagic. Ganglion cells maturing from neuroblasts are defined as having an enlarged, eccentrically located nucleus with a prominent nucleolus and synchronously abundant amphophilic cytoplasm that is twice or more the diameter of the nucleus (Figure 10-36). In the second subtype, the ganglioneuroblastoma has greater than 50% Schwannian stroma, neuropil, and neuroblasts in various stages of differentiation. The third subtype has grossly visible nodules (Figure 10-37), with coexistence of the first and third or first and fourth subtypes. The fourth subtype can be further subdivided into a Schwannian stroma-dominant tumor with maturing ganglion cells and that with fully mature ganglion cells (and small round satellite cells; Figure 10-38). Ganglioneuroma should, therefore, be well sampled to rule out areas of immature components, especially if neuropil is identified. Tumors that have a few immature cells in an otherwise ganglioneuroma-like tumor are considered *maturing ganglioneuroma*. Ganglion cells in ganglioneuroma may be multinucleated or may occasionally have satellite cells around them but are usually intermixed in a neurofibroma-like Schwannian tumor. The mitosis karyorrhexis index (MKI) is a semiquantitative valued derived from counting the number of mitoses and fragmented karyorrhectic nuclei in a 40X objective, high-power field.

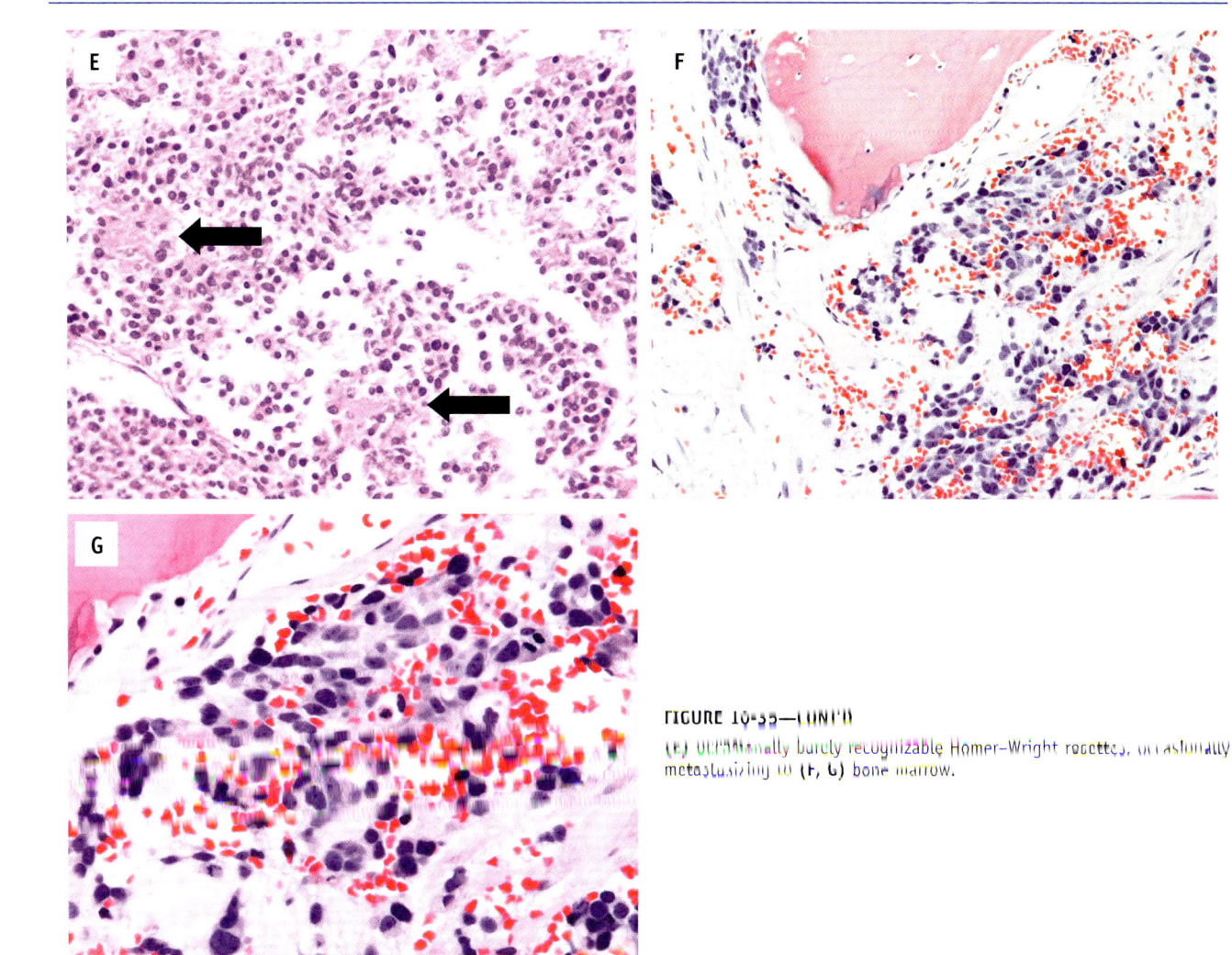

CHAPTER 10 Nerve Sheath and Neuroectodermal Tumors   229

FIGURE 10-35—CONT'D
(E) Occasionally barely recognizable Homer-Wright rosettes, occasionally metastasizing to (F, G) bone marrow.

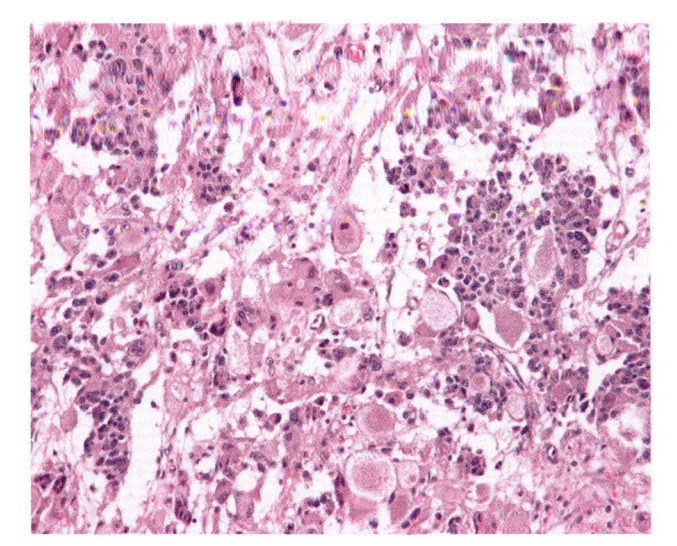

FIGURE 10-36
Neuroblastoma immature round cells can fully mature to ganglion cells. Depending on the percentage of ganglioneuroma (schwannian stroma), these can be then classified into ganglioneuroblastoma subtypes of diffuse, nodular when the stomal component reaches 50% and then final maturation without small round cells (ganglioneuroma).

ANCILLARY STUDIES

IMMUNOHISTOCHEMISTRY

Synaptophysin, chromogranin, neuron specific enolase (NSE) and protein gene product 9.5 may be positive in neuroblastoma. Used only for research, high levels of TrkA, one of the nerve growth factor receptors, have been found in 82% of neuroblastomas.

For any other ancillary method, MYC-related oncogene (MYCN), normally located on chromosome 2p24 and known to play a role in transcriptional activation, has been found to be amplified in 25% of primary untreated neuroblastomas by fluorescent in situ hybridization (FISH). Thirty to forty percent of cases may demonstrate deletion of chromosome 1p by DNA polymorphisms; allelic loss of chromosome 11q can be detected by DNA polymorphism and by comparative genomic hybridization in 30% to 50% of cases. Another karyotypic abnormality of neuroblastoma may be trisomy for chromosome 17q. In addition to loss of

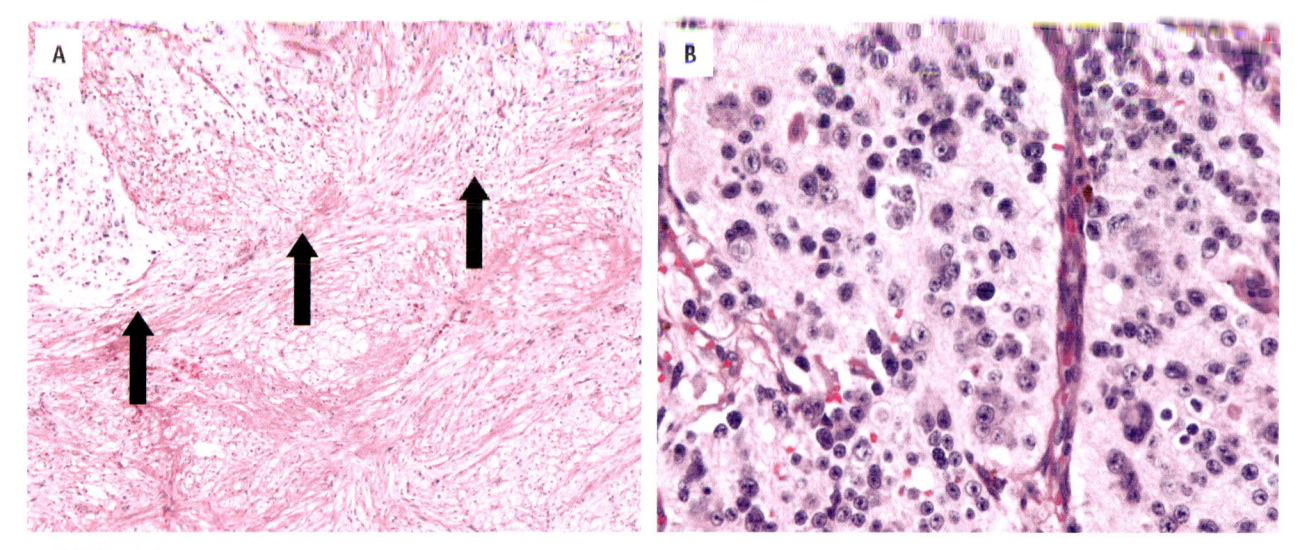

FIGURE 10-37
Ganglioneuroblastoma has greater than 50% ganglioneuroma (bottom pinkish portion) and either nodular or intermixed maturing neuroblastoma, in this case as separate nodules representing type 3 (**A,** above *arrows*); higher magnification of these immature areas (**B**). Ganglioneuroblastoma has a maturing neuroblastoma component that can be intermixed with the ganglioneuroma (**B**) or as separate nodules from ganglioneuroma.

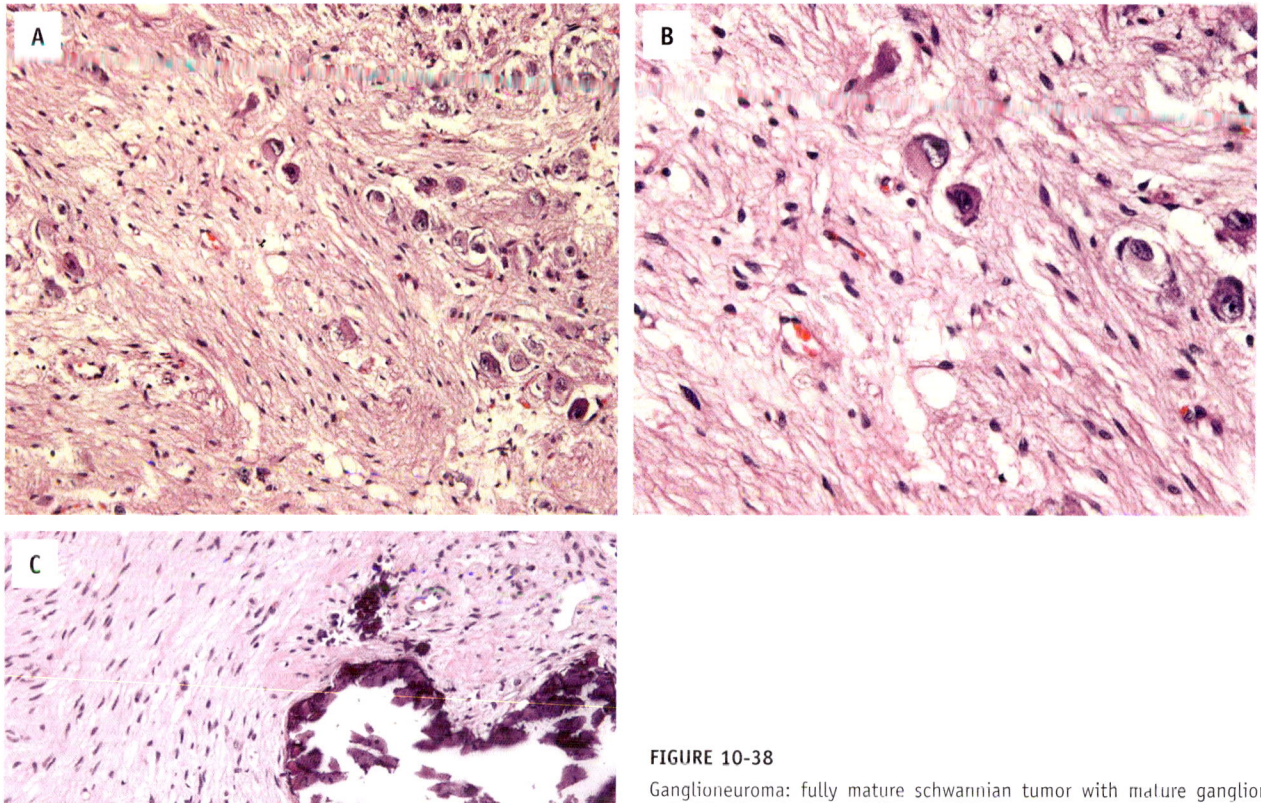

FIGURE 10-38
Ganglioneuroma: fully mature schwannian tumor with mature ganglion cells (**A, B**) and often calcification (**C**).

CHAPTER 10 Nerve Sheath and Neuroectodermal Tumors

1p, cytogenetics of neuroblastoma can also reveal a double-minute (dm) chromosome or homogenous staining regions (hsrs).

DIFFERENTIAL DIAGNOSIS

Other small round blue cell tumors, including rhabdomyosarcoma, Ewing sarcoma/primitive neuroectodermal tumor, desmoplastic round cell tumor, and lymphoma, may be considered in the differential diagnosis of neuroblastoma. Neuroblastoma usually occurs in a younger age and has catecholamine secretion, and does not usually express CD99 as does Ewing sarcoma/primitive neuroectodermal tumor or desmoplastic round cell tumor. The true rosettes of neuroblastoma are different from the pseudorosettes of primitive neuroectodermal tumor. Rhabdomyosarcoma can be separated by its morphology and reactivity with myoid (skeletal muscle–specific) markers. Desmoplastic small round cell tumor is generally desmin and keratin positive, and demonstrates stromal desmoplasia. Lymphoma can also be separated by hematopoietic immunostains specific to type. Ganglioneuroma can be separated from schwannoma and neurofibroma by its morphology and presence of ganglion cells.

PROGNOSIS AND TREATMENT

Tumor prognosis depends on stage, patient age, tumor location, histologic subtype, and laboratory genetic markers. Lower stage tumors (1 or 2) have a better prognosis than do those at higher stages (3 or 4), with the exception of 4S (stage 1 or 2 with liver, skin, or marrow involvement). Stage 1, for example, usually has an 80% survival rate compared with 47% survival rate in stage 4. Neuroblastoma can metastasize to bone marrow, lymph node, and rarely lung. Metastases to bone are a particular ominous sign. Younger patients, less than 1 year of age, have better prognosis than do older patients, because some of these tumors will involute on their own or spontaneously regress (and are usually associated with lack of 1p deletion, MYCN amplification, and near triploidy). Adrenal tumors have worse prognosis than extra-adrenal tumors, particularly thoracic tumors. Specific histologic features portend worse prognosis: mitotic rate greater than 10 mitoses per hpf, necrosis, and foam cells. Alternatively, calcification, S-100 reactivity, multinucleation, and ganglion cells are associated with better prognosis. The four subtypes have worse prognosis for the undifferentiated, poorly differentiated (first subtype), and composite (third subtype) than for the intermixed, maturing, and mature (second and fourth subtypes). Both MYCN amplification and 1p loss of heterozygosity have been correlated with poor outcome. Finally, lack of CD44 expression by immunohistochemistry may correlate with poor prognosis. PHOX2B is the first bona fide neuroblastoma predisposition gene identified but is mutated in only a small subset of cases. Somatically acquired alterations at chromosome arms 3p and 11q are highly correlated with acquisition of metastases in the absence of MYCN amplification and may be useful as prognostic markers. Much data exist on potential clinical and biologic markers in neuroblastoma that it is often difficult to decide which ones will be helpful in specific patient neuroblastoma cases. Treatment is by protocols according to risk, varying from no additional therapy besides surgery to chemotherapy to myeloablative treatment with stem cell transplantation for high stage and poor prognosis tumors.

CLEAR CELL SARCOMA

Clear cell sarcoma was originally described by Dr. Franz Enzinger in 1965. Although clear cell sarcoma shows melanocytic differentiation (see later), it differs from cutaneous malignant melanoma by virtue of its soft tissue location in association with tendons and aponeuroses, absent junctional changes, and specific t(12;22) with a EWS-ATF1 fusion transcript.

CLINICAL FEATURES

Clear cell sarcoma represents 1% of all sarcomas. It is generally a slowly enlarging and painful mass that usually does not ulcerate the skin surface. Clear cell sarcoma mainly affects adolescents and young adults, between the ages of 20 and 40 years, with a female sex predominance. It is actually the most common sarcoma of the foot and ankle; this location accounts for 50% of all clear cell sarcomas. Other sites of involvement include the knee, thigh, hand, neck, and trunk. Rarely, retroperitoneum and primary bone lesions exist. So-called clear cell sarcoma of the kidney is a different entity and should not be confused with this entity.

RADIOLOGIC FEATURES

Clear cell sarcoma frequently involves/invades the tendon sheath, and tendon (Figure 10-39) may be seen on either side of the tumor. The tumor may be slightly hyperintense on T1-weighted MRI.

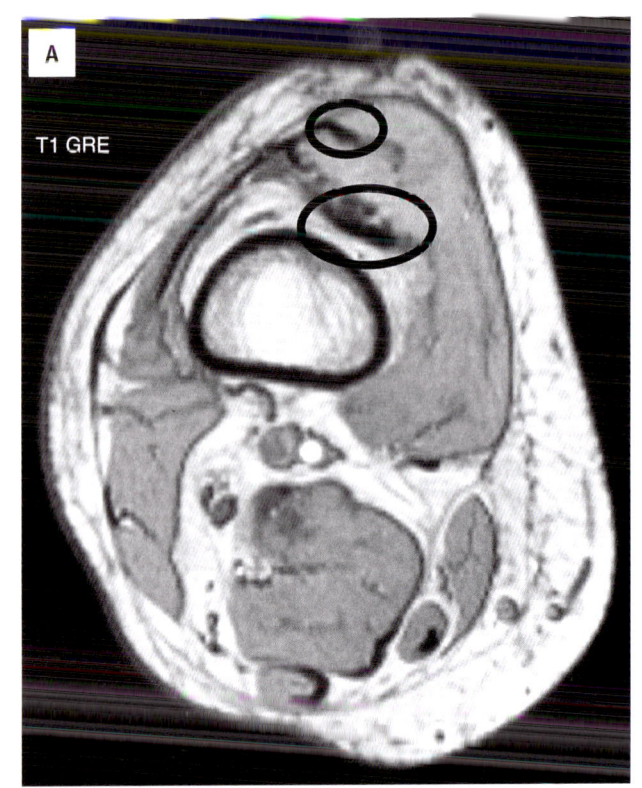

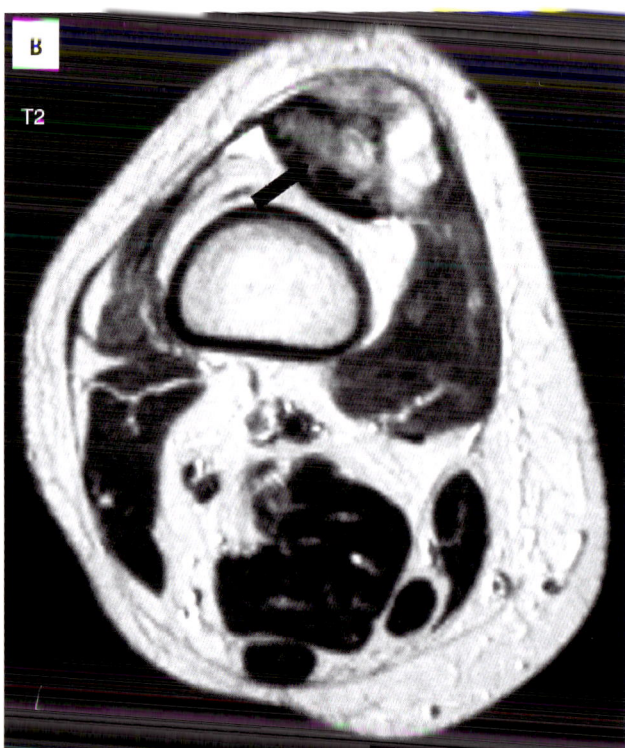

FIGURE 10-39

Clear cell sarcoma is a tumor that actually involves tendon, not just surrounds it, as noted on these T1- **(A)** and T2-weighted **(B)** images; the tendon (**A**, *circled*) is seen on either side of this 4-cm quadriceps tendon mass, and the mass is heterogeneous (**B**, *arrow*).

PATHOLOGIC FEATURES

GROSS FINDINGS

Clear cell sarcoma is generally lobulated or multinodular, gray-white, and involves the tendon or aponeuroses. Tumor sizes vary from 1 to 10 cm, with a mean of 4 cm.

MICROSCOPIC FINDINGS

Microscopically, the tumor can often be seen infiltrating into the dense fibroconnective tissue of the associated tendon (Figure 10-40). The tumor is usually at least focally separated into nests by variably thick fibrous bands (Figure 10-41). Melanin pigment may be found in up to 50% of cases. The neoplastic cells vary from epithelioid to spindled with clear-to-pale eosinophilic cytoplasm, vesicular nuclei, and prominent nucleoli (Figure 10-42). A characteristic feature is the presence of multinucleated, Touton-type tumor giant cells. Mitotic activity is minimal. Necrosis, when present, is a poor prognostic factor.

ANCILLARY STUDIES

IMMUNOHISTOCHEMISTRY

The neoplastic cells express a variety of melanocytic markers, including S-100 protein, gp100 (HMB45), Melan-A, tyrosinase, and MiTF. HMB45 and/or Melan-A expression may be stronger than S-100 protein expression (Figure 10-43).

Molecular findings are characterized by a reproducible t(12;22) (q13;q12), with an EWS-ATF1 fusion transcript. This fusion gene is specific for clear cell sarcoma and is not found in conventional malignant melanoma. Other molecular changes involve chromosome 8, sometimes with additional copies, but these are not found in every tumor.

DIFFERENTIAL DIAGNOSIS

The most important differential diagnostic consideration is conventional malignant melanoma, either metastatic or primary to the deep dermis/subcutis. No morphologic or immunohistochemical findings reliably separate these two entities, and clinical correlation and molecular testing for the EWS-ATF1 fusion gene may be necessary. As noted earlier, conventional melanoma does not contain this fusion gene. Epithelioid MPNST may closely resemble clear cell sarcoma. The presence of spindled zones resembling conventional MPNST and the absence of expression of specific markers of melanocytic differentiation (e.g., HMB45) may help to establish the correct diagnosis. Epithelioid sarcoma tends to involve the skin and expresses cytokeratins but not S-100 protein. Cellular blue nevus lacks cytologic

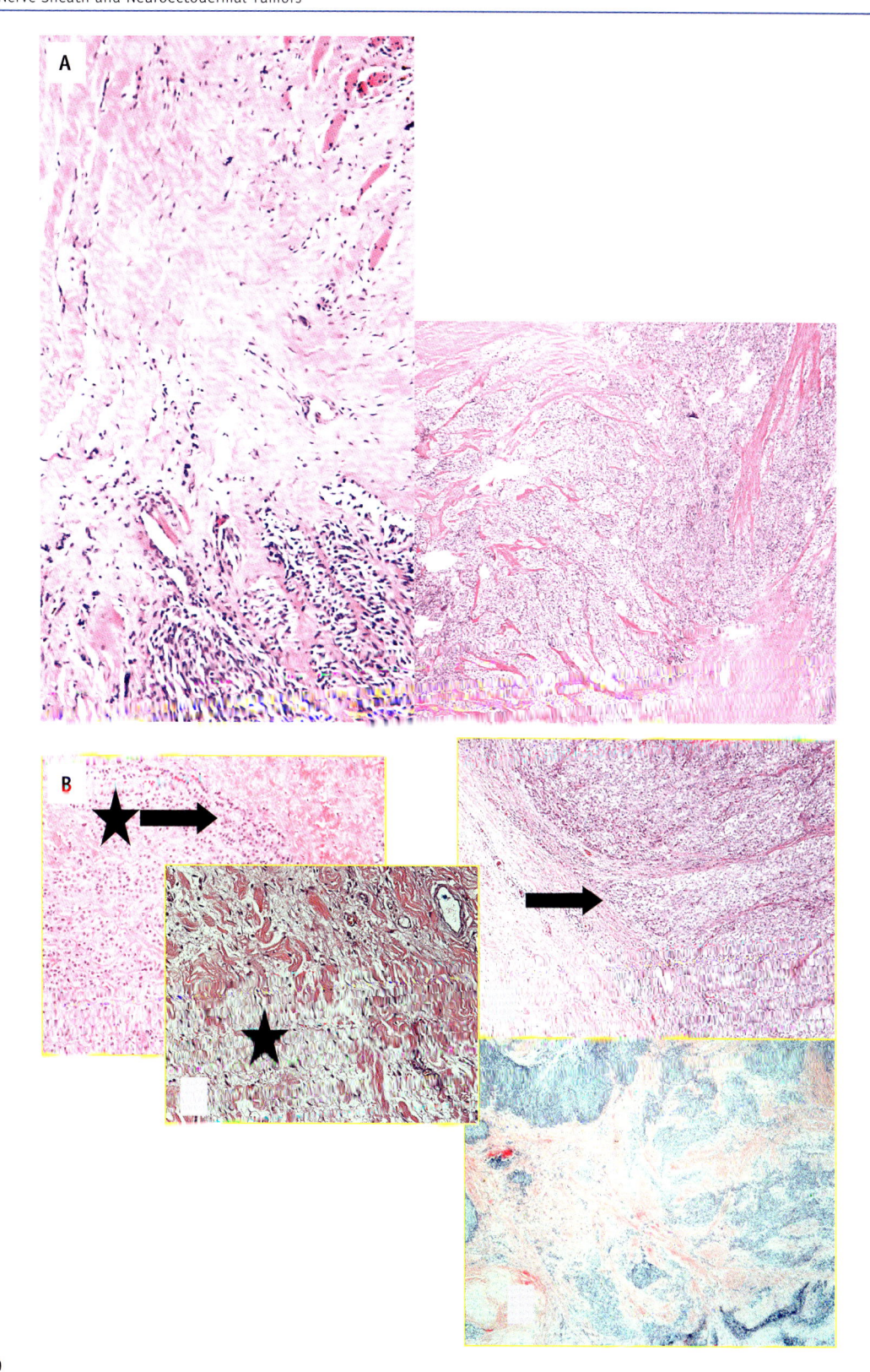

FIGURE 10-40
A, B, Microscopically, corresponding with the radiology, the tumor infiltrates dense fibroconnective tissue, representing tendon.

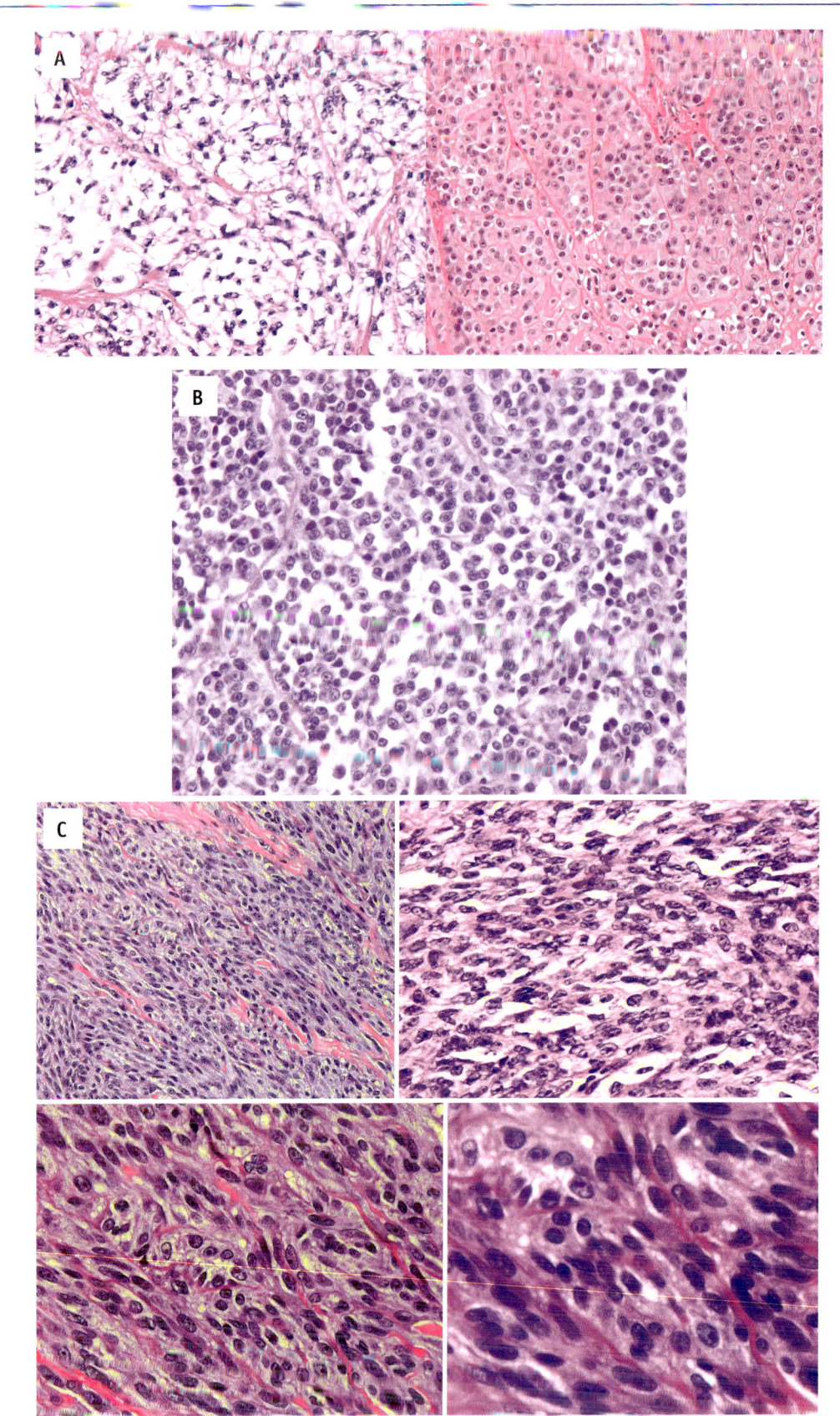

FIGURE 10-41

Clear cell sarcoma is often separated into nests by variably thick fibrous septa and demonstrates both clear cytoplasm (A, left, hence its name) and eosinophilic cytoplasm (A, right). Sometimes clear cell sarcoma has a more epithelioid appearance to tumor cells (B), and in other areas of the tumor it may be more spindled (C).

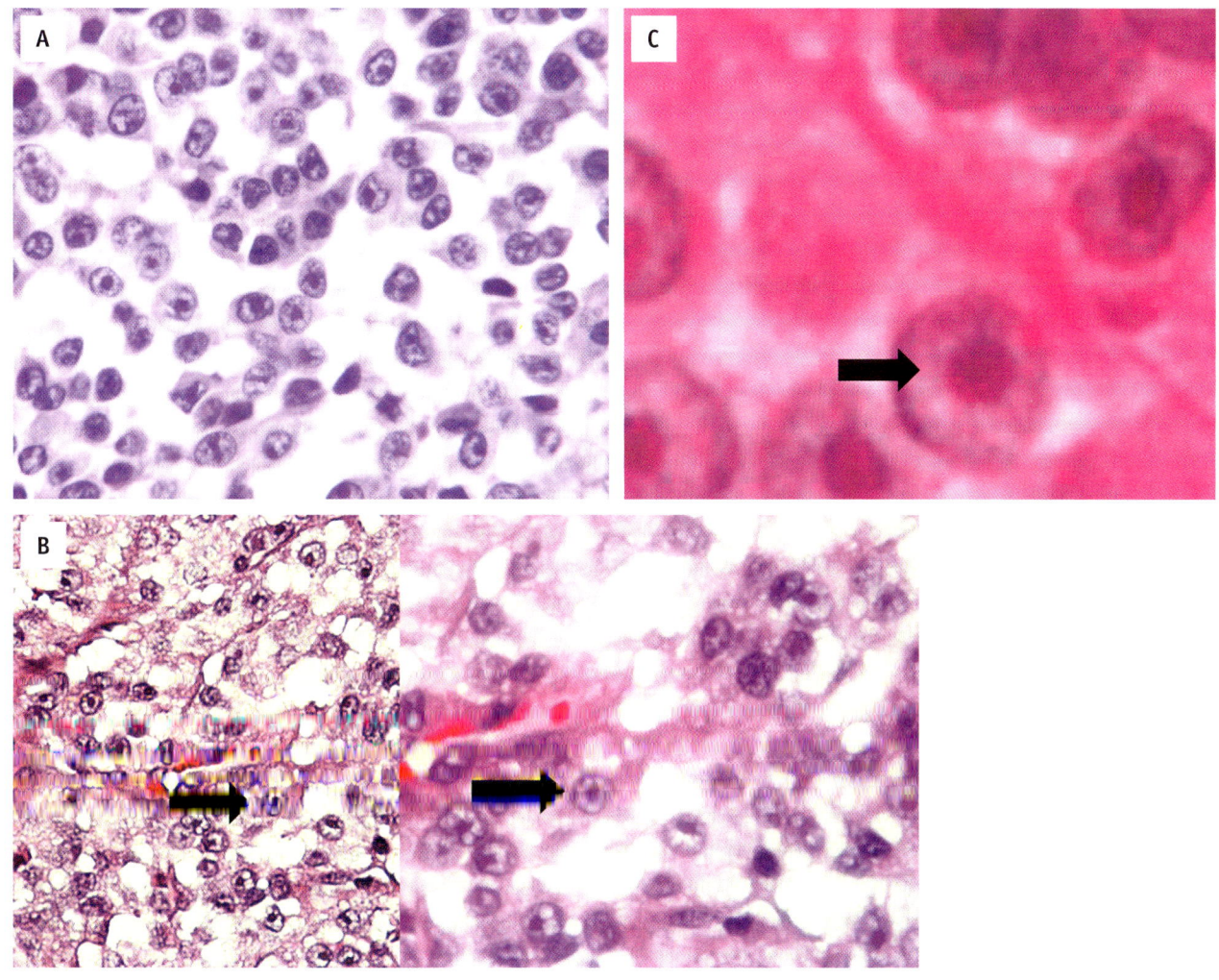

CHAPTER 10 Nerve Sheath and Neuroectodermal Tumors

FIGURE 10-42
Whether clear, eosinophilic, epithelioid, or spindled, clear cell sarcoma always has large eosinophilic prominent nucleoli **(A–C)**.

atypia, frequently grows in a *dumbbell-shaped* configuration, and is negative for the EWS-ATF1 gene fusion.

Prognosis and Treatment

Clear cell sarcoma has a poor prognosis. Approximately 50% or more patients die of metastatic disease to lung, lymph node, or bone. The 5-year survival rate is 50% to 65%, which decreases over time, with late metastases reported up to two to three decades after onset of disease. Recurrences occur in about 20% of patients, with an increased risk for metastasis after multiple recurrences. Unfavorable prognostic factors include tumor size larger than 5 cm, necrosis, and local recurrence. The most effective treatment for clear cell sarcoma is wide surgical resection. Although almost always radiation and sometimes chemotherapy are utilized, both and particularly chemotherapy are largely ineffective. It is unclear whether there is a role for sentinel lymph node biopsy in the management of patients with this disease.

CLEAR CELL SARCOMA—FACT SHEET

Definition
- A malignant melanocytic lesion that occurs within soft tissue, frequently in association with a tendon, differing from conventional malignant melanoma

Incidence and Location
- Lower extremity, relatively rare tumor

Morbidity and Mortality
- 50% metastatic potential with low long-term survival rate

Clinical Features
- 20 to 40 years, lower extremity tendinous painful mass with no overlying ulceration

Radiologic Features
- Intratendinous mass with possible hyperintensity on T1-weighted MRI

Prognosis and Treatment
- Poor; adjuvant therapy advocated but largely ineffective

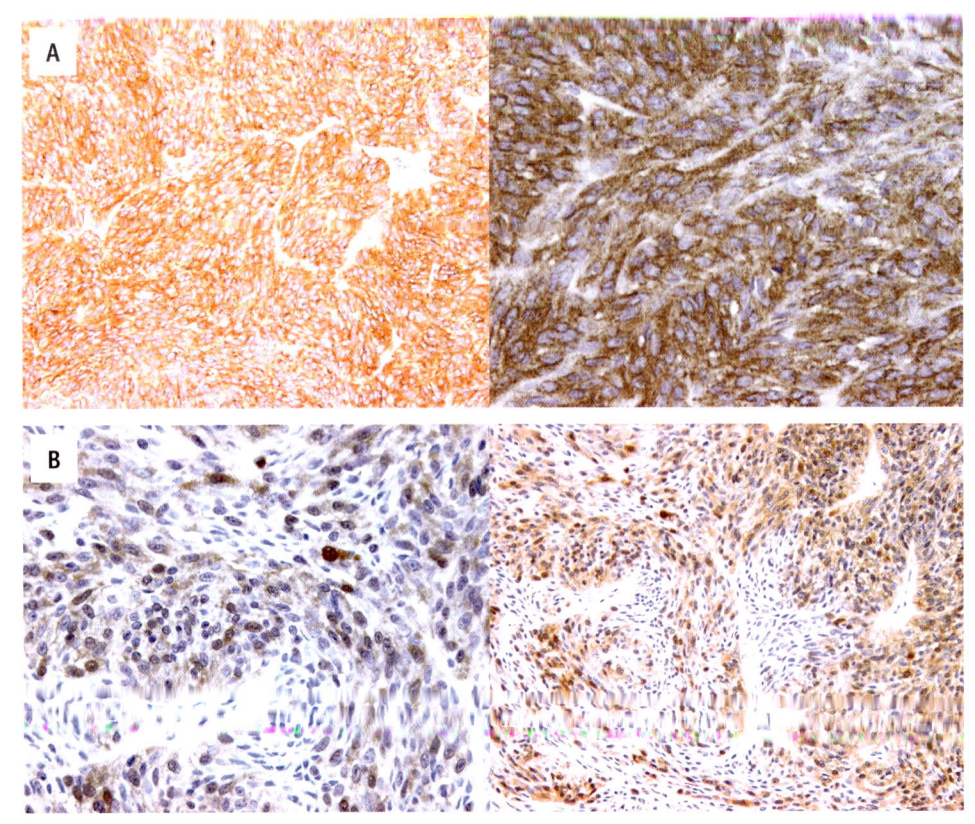

FIGURE 10-43
Helpful to separate clear cell sarcoma from malignant melanoma is that the HMB45 **(A)** is always stronger and more diffuse than the S-100 protein staining **(B)** in clear cell sarcoma, whereas the reverse is true for malignant melanoma.

CLEAR CELL SARCOMA—PATHOLOGIC FEATURES

Gross Findings

▸▸ Lobulated, gray-white, and involves the tendon; mean size, 4 cm
▸▸ Microscopic findings: infiltrates dense fibroconnective tissue, sheets or nests of tumor separated by variably thick fibrous band, melanin pigment in 50%, epithelioid to spindled tumor cells with variable clear-to-pale eosinophilic cytoplasm, vesicular nuclei with prominent eosinophilic nucleoli, low mitotic activity, Touton-type neoplastic giant cells

Immunohistochemical Findings

▸▸ Express S-100 protein, melanocytic markers
▸▸ Molecular features: t(12;22) (EWS-ATF1)

Differential Diagnosis

▸▸ Conventional malignant melanoma, epithelioid MPNST, epithelioid sarcoma, cellular blue nevus

---

SUGGESTED READINGS

Traumatic Neuroma

1. Garozzo D, Ferraresi S, Buffatti P: Surgical treatment of common peroneal nerve injuries: Indications and results. A series of 62 cases. J Neurosurg Sci 2004;48:105-112.
2. Haymaker W: The pathology of peripheral nerve injuries. Mil Surg 1948;102:448-459.

Mucosal Neuroma

1. Carney JA, Hayles AB: Alimentary tract manifestations of multiple endocrine neoplasia, type 2b. Mayo Clin Proc 1977;52:543.

Pacinian Neuroma

1. Fletcher CD, Theaker JM: Digital pacinian neuroma: A distinctive hyperplastic lesion. Histopathology 1989;15:249-256.
2. Kumar A, Darby AJ, Kelly CP: Pacinian corpuscles hyperplasia—an uncommon cause of digital pain. Acta Orthop Belg 2003;69:74-76.

Palisaded Encapsulated Neuroma

1. Argenyi ZB, Cooper PH, Santa Cruz D: Plexiform and other unusual variants of palisaded encapsulated neuroma. J Cutan Pathol 1993;20:34-39.
2. Chrysomali E, Papanicolaou SI, Dekker NP, et al: Benign neural tumors of the oral cavity: a comparative immunohistochemical study. Oral Surg Oral Med Oral Pathol Oral Radiol Endod 1997;84:381-390.
3. Dover JS, From L, Lewis A: Palisaded encapsulated neuromas. A clinicopathologic study. Arch Dermatol 1989;125:386-389.
4. Eckert F, Kutzner H: Palisaded encapsulated neuroma (solitary circumscribed neuroma). Am J Dermatopathol 1995;17:316.
5. Kossard S, Kumar A, Wilkinson B: Neural spectrum: Palisaded encapsulated neuroma and Verocay body poor dermal schwannoma. J Cutan Pathol 1999;26:31-36.
6. Megahed M: Palisaded encapsulated neuroma (solitary circumscribed neuroma). A clinicopathologic and immunohistochemical study. Am J Dermatopathol 1994;16:120-125.

Neurofibroma, Neurofibromatosis Type 1, and Early Malignant Change in Neurofibroma

1. Arun D, Gutmann DH: Recent advances in neurofibromatosis type 1. Curr Opin Neurol 2004;17:101–105.
2. Laskin WB, Fetsch JF, Lasota J, et al: Benign epithelioid peripheral nerve sheath tumors of the soft tissues: clinicopathologic spectrum of 33 cases. Am J Surg Pathol 2005;29:39–51.
3. Levy P, Bieche I, Leroy K, et al: Molecular profiles of neurofibromatosis type 1-associated plexiform neurofibromas: identification of a gene expression signature of poor prognosis. Clin Cancer Res 2004;10:3763–3771.
4. Melean G, Sestini R, Ammannati F, et al: Genetic insights into familial tumors of the nervous system. Am J Med Genet 2004;129C:74–84.
5. Scheithauer BW, Woodruff JM, Erlandson RA, et al: Tumors of the peripheral nervous system. Washington, DC, Armed Forces Institute of Pathology, 1999, p 421.
6. Stephens K: Genetics of neurofibromatosis 1-associated peripheral nerve sheath tumors. Cancer Invest 2003;21:897–914.
7. Upadhyaya M, Han S, Consoli C, et al: Characterization of the somatic mutational spectrum of the neurofibromatosis type 1 (NF1) gene in neurofibromatosis patients with benign and malignant tumors. Hum Mutat 2004;23:134–146.

Schwannoma and Neurofibromatosis Type 2

1. Baser ME, Evans DGR, Gutmann DH: Neurofibromatosis 2. Curr Opin Neurol 2003;16:27–33.
2. Baser ME, Kuramoto L, Joe H, et al: Genotype-phenotype correlations for nervous system tumors in neurofibromatosis 2: a population-based study. Am J Hum Genet 2004;75:231–239.
3. Feany MB, Anthony DC, Fletcher CD: Nerve sheath tumors with hybrid features of neurofibroma and schwannoma: a conceptual challenge. Histopathology 1998;32:405–410.
4. Ferner RE, O'Doherty MJ: Neurofibroma and schwannoma. Curr Opin Neurol 2002;15:679–684.
5. Kissil JL, Wilker EW, Johnson KC, et al: Merlin, the product of the NF2 tumor suppressor gene, is an inhibitor of the p21-activated kinase, Pak1. Mol Cell 2003;12:841–849.
6. Kurtkaya-Yapicier O, Scheithauer B, Woodruff JM: The pathobiologic spectrum of Schwannomas. Histol Histopathol 2003;18:925–934.
7. Lim HS, Jung J, Chung KY: Neurofibromatosis type 2 with multiple plexiform schwannomas. Int J Dermatol 2004;43:336–340.
8. McMenamin ME, Fletcher CD: Expanding the spectrum of malignant change in schwannomas: Epithelioid malignant change, epithelioid malignant peripheral nerve sheath tumor, and epithelioid angiosarcoma: a study of 17 cases. Am J Surg Pathol 2001;25:13–25.
9. Woodruff JM, Scheithauer BW, Kurtkaya-Yapicier O, et al: Congenital and childhood plexiform (multinodular) cellular schwannoma: a troublesome mimic of malignant peripheral nerve sheath tumor. Am J Surg Pathol 2003;27:1321–1329.

Psammomatous Melanotic Schwannoma

1. Carney JA: Psammomatous melanotic schwannoma. A distinctive, heritable tumor with special associations, including cardiac myxoma and the Cushing syndrome. Am J Surg Pathol 1990;14:206–222.
2. Carney JA: The Carney complex (myxomas, spotty pigmentation, endocrine overactivity, and schwannomas). Dermatol Clin 1995;13:19–26.
3. Utiger CA, Headington JT: Psammomatous melanotic schwannoma. A new cutaneous marker for Carney's complex. Arch Dermatol 1993;129:202–204.

Malignant Peripheral Nerve Sheath Tumor

1. Cashen DV, Parisien RC, Raskin K, et al: Survival data for patients with malignant schwannoma. Clin Orthop Relat Res 2004;(426):69–73.
2. Frahm S, Mautner VF, Brems H, et al: Genetic and phenotypic characterization of tumor cells derived from malignant peripheral nerve sheath tumors of neurofibromatosis type 1 patients. Neurobiol Dis 2004;16:85–91.
3. Kluwe L, Friedrich RE, Peiper M, et al: Constitutional NF1 mutations in neurofibromatosis 1 patients with malignant peripheral nerve sheath tumors. Hum Mutat 2003;22:420.
4. Perrone F, Tabano S, Colombo F, et al: p15INK4b, p14ARF, and p16INK4a inactivation in sporadic and neurofibromatosis type 1-related malignant peripheral nerve sheath tumors. Clin Cancer Res 2003;9:4132–4138.
5. Zhou H, Coffin CM, Perkins SL, et al: Malignant peripheral nerve sheath tumor: A comparison of grade, immunophenotype, and cell cycle/growth activation marker expression in sporadic and neurofibromatosis 1-related lesions. Am J Surg Pathol 2003;27:1337–1345.

Granular Cell Tumor

1. Brannon RB, Anand PM: Oral granular cell tumors: An analysis of 10 new pediatric and adolescent cases and a review of the literature. J Clin Pediatr Dent 2004;29:69–74.
2. Fanburg-Smith JC, Meis-Kindblom JM, Fante R, et al: Malignant granular cell tumor of soft tissue: Diagnostic criteria and clinicopathologic correlation. Am J Surg Pathol 1998;22:779–794.
3. Fine SW, Li M: Expression of calretinin and the alpha-subunit of inhibin in granular cell tumors. Am J Clin Pathol 2003;119:259–264.
4. Kindblom LG, Widehn S, Meis-Kindblom JM: The role of electron microscopy in the diagnosis of pleomorphic sarcomas of soft tissue. Semin Diagn Pathol 2003;20:72–81.
5. Le BH, Boyer PJ, Lewis JE, et al: Granular cell tumor: Immunohistochemical assessment of inhibin-alpha, protein gene product 9.5, S100 protein, CD68, and Ki-67 proliferative index with clinical correlation. Arch Pathol Lab Med 2004;128:771–775.
6. Ordoñez NG: Granular cell tumor: a review and update. Adv Anat Pathol 1999;6:186–203.
7. Ordoñez NG, Mackay B: Granular cell tumor: a review of the pathology and histogenesis. Ultrastruct Pathol 1999;23:207–222.

Perineurioma

1. Fetsch JF, Miettinen M: Sclerosing perineurioma: a clinicopathologic study of 19 cases of a distinctive soft tissue lesion with a predilection for the fingers and palms of young adults. Am J Surg Pathol 1997;21:1433–1442.
2. Folpe AL, Billings SD, McKenney JK, et al: Expression of claudin-1, a recently described tight junction-associated protein, distinguishes soft tissue perineurioma from potential mimics. Am J Surg Pathol 2002;26:1620–1626.
3. Giannini C, Scheithauer BW, Jenkins RB, et al: Soft-tissue perineurioma. Evidence for an abnormality of chromosome 22, criteria for diagnosis, and review of the literature. Am J Surg Pathol 1997;21:164–173.
4. Graadt van Roggen JF, McMenamin ME, Belchis DA, et al: Reticular perineurioma: A distinctive variant of soft tissue perineurioma. Am J Surg Pathol 2001;25:485–493.
5. Hirose T, Scheithauer BW, Sano T: Perineurial malignant peripheral nerve sheath tumor (MPNST): a clinicopathologic, immunohistochemical, and ultrastructural study of seven cases. Am J Surg Pathol 1998;22:1368–1378.
6. Rankine AJ, Filion PR, Platten MA, et al: Perineurioma: a clinicopathological study of eight cases. Pathology 2004;36:309–315.
7. Tsang WY, Chan JK, Chow LT, et al: Perineurioma: an uncommon soft tissue neoplasm distinct from localized hypertrophic neuropathy and neurofibroma. Am J Surg Pathol 1992;16:756–763.
8. Yamaguchi U, Hasegawa T, Hirose T, et al: Sclerosing perineurioma: a clinicopathological study of five cases and diagnostic utility of immunohistochemical staining for GLUT1. Virchows Arch 2003;443:159–163.
9. Zelger B, Weinlich G, Zelger B: Perineurioma. A frequently unrecognized entity with emphasis on a plexiform variant. Adv Clin Path 2000;4:25–33.

Neurothekeoma

1. Gallager RL, Helwig EB: Neurothekeoma—a benign cutaneous tumor of neural origin. Am J Clin Pathol 1980;74:759–764.

2. Laskin WB, Fetsch JF, Miettinen M: The neurothekeoma: immunohistochemical analysis distinguishes the true nerve sheath myxoma from its mimics. Hum Pathol 2000;31:1230-1241.
3. Scheithauer BW, Woodruff JM, Erlandson RA, et al: Tumors of the peripheral nervous system. Washington, DC, Armed Forces Institute of Pathology, 1999.

Neuroblastoma, Ganglioneuroblastoma, and Ganglioneuroma

1. Fritsch P, Kerbl R, Lackner H, et al: "Wait and see" strategy in localized neuroblastoma in infants: an option not only for cases detected by mass screening. Pediatr Blood Cancer 2004;43:679-682.
2. Gultekin M, Dursun P, Salman C, et al: Ganglioneuroma mimicking ovarian tumor: a report of a case and review of the ganglioneuromas. Arch Gynecol Obstet 2005;271:66-68.
3. Hicks MJ, Mackay B: Comparison of ultrastructural features among neuroblastic tumors: maturation from neuroblastoma to ganglioneuroma. Ultrastructural Pathol 1995;19:311-322.
4. Hsiao CC, Huang CC, Sheen JM, et al: Differential expression of delta-like gene and protein in neuroblastoma, ganglioneuroblastoma and ganglioneuroma. Mod Pathol 2005;18:656-662.
5. Hsu WM, Hsieh FJ, Jeng YM, et al: Calreticulin expression in neuroblastoma—a novel independent prognostic factor. Ann Oncol 2005;16:314-321.
6. Iwanaka T, Yamamoto K, Ogawa Y, et al: Maturation of mass-screened localized adrenal neuroblastoma. J Ped Surg 2001;36:1633-1636.
7. Kobayashi C, Monforte-Munoz HL, Gerbing RB, et al: Enlarged and prominent nucleoli may be indicative of MYCN amplification: a study of neuroblastoma (Schwannian stroma poor), undifferentiated/poorly differentiated subtype with high mitosis-karyorrhexis index. Cancer 2005;103:174-180.
8. Kushner BH, LaQuaglia MP, Kramer K, et al: Radically different treatment recommendations for newly diagnosed neuroblastoma: pitfalls in assessment of risk. J Pediatr Hematol Oncol 2004;26:35-39.
9. Limpt VV, Schramm A, Lakeman A, et al: The Phox2B homeobox gene is mutated in sporadic neuroblastomas. Oncogene 2004;23:9280-9288.
10. Maris JM: The biologic basis for neuroblastoma heterogeneity and risk stratification. Curr Opin Pediatr 2005;17:7-13.
11. Peuchmaur M, d'Amore ES, Joshi VV, et al: Revision of the International Neuroblastoma Pathology Classification: confirmation of favorable and unfavorable prognostic subsets in ganglioneuroblastoma, nodular. Cancer 2003;98:2274-2281.
12. Scaruffi P, Parodi S, Mazzocco K, et al: Detection of MYCN amplification and chromosome 1p36 loss in neuroblastoma by cDNA microarray comparative genomic hybridization. Mol Diagn 2004;8:93-100.
13. Shimada H, Ambros IM, Dehner LP, et al: Terminology and morphologic criteria of neuroblastic tumors. Recommendations by the International Neuroblastoma Pathology Committee. Cancer 1999;86:349-363.
14. Shimada H, Ambros IM, Dehner LP, et al: The International Neuroblastoma Pathology Classification (the Shimada system). Cancer 1999;86:364-372.
15. Spitz R, Hero B, Skowron M, et al: MYCN-status in neuroblastoma: characteristics of tumours showing amplification, gain, and non-amplification. Eur J Cancer 2004;40:2753-2759.
16. Shimada H, Nakagawa A, Peters J, et al: TrkA expression in peripheral neuroblastic tumors: Prognostic significance and biological relevance. Cancer 2004;101:1873-1881.
17. Wei JS, Greer BT, Westermann F, et al: Prediction of clinical outcome using gene expression profiling and artificial neural networks for patients with neuroblastoma. Cancer Res 2004;64:6883-6891.

Clear Cell Sarcoma

1. Antonescu CR, Tschernyavsky SJ, Woodruff JM, et al: Molecular diagnosis of clear cell sarcoma: detection of EWS-ATF1 and MITF-M transcripts and histopathological and ultrastructural analysis of 12 cases. J Mol Diagn 2002;4:44-52.
2. Choi JH, Gu MJ, Kim MJ, et al: Primary clear cell sarcoma of bone. Skeletal Radiol 2003;32:598-602.
3. Chung EB, Enzinger FM: Malignant melanoma of soft parts. A reassessment of clear cell sarcoma. Am J Surg Pathol 1983;7:405-413.
4. Enzinger FM: Clear-cell sarcoma of tendons and aponeuroses. An analysis of 21 cases. Cancer 1965;18:1163-1174.
5. Ferrari A, Casanova M, Bisogno G, et al: Clear cell sarcoma of tendons and aponeuroses in pediatric patients: a report from the Italian and German Soft Tissue Sarcoma Cooperative Group. Cancer 2002;94:3269-3276.
6. Jacobs IA, Chang CK, Guzman G, et al: Clear cell sarcoma: an institutional review. Am Surg 2004;70:300-303.
7. Kuiper DR, Hoekstra HJ, Veth RP, et al: The management of clear cell sarcoma. Eur J Surg Oncol 2003;29:568-570.
8. Langezaal SM, Graadt van Roggen JF, Cleton-Jansen AM, et al: Malignant melanoma is genetically distinct from clear cell sarcoma of tendons and aponeurosis (malignant melanoma of soft parts). Br J Cancer 2001;84:535-538.
9. Panagopoulos I, Mertens F, Isaksson M, et al: Absence of mutations of the BRAF gene in malignant melanoma of soft parts (clear cell sarcoma of tendons and aponeuroses). Cancer Genet Cytogenet 2005;156:74-76.
10. Panagopoulos I, Mertens F, Debiec-Rychter M, et al: Molecular genetic characterization of the EWS/ATF1 fusion gene in clear cell sarcoma of tendons and aponeuroses. Int J Cancer 2002;99:560-567.
11. Patel SR: Classification of clear-cell sarcoma. Curr Oncol Rep 2004;6:307.

11 Osteocartilaginous Tumors
John X. O'Connell

- Myositis Ossificans
- Fibro-Osseous Pseudotumor of Digits
- Soft Tissue Osteosarcoma
- Soft Tissue Chondroma
- Extraskeletal Myxoid Chondrosarcoma
- Mesenchymal Chondrosarcoma
- Aneurysmal Cyst of Soft Tissue

Normally, the somatic soft tissues do not contain mature osteoblasts or chondrocytes; therefore, these tissues do not typically contain bone or cartilage. However, under certain circumstances, undifferentiated mesenchymal cells are stimulated to develop into these specialized cells. This results in a variety of bone and cartilage matrix-producing "tumors." These span the spectrum from reactive conditions through benign and malignant neoplasms. This chapter deals with those lesions that present clinically as matrix-producing tumors of the soft tissues.

MYOSITIS OSSIFICANS

Myositis ossificans (MO) is a non neoplastic reactive bone and cartilage matrix-producing pseudotumor that develops in skeletal muscle after trauma. The clinical and pathologic appearance of MO will vary depending on the time after the injury at which the mass is discovered. Early lesions (within the first few weeks) can simulate spindle cell sarcomas of various types, whereas lesions examined later in their evolution consist of mature lamellar bone.

CLINICAL FEATURES

MO typically occurs in young adults. Male and female individuals are affected equally. Patients present with a short history (usually less than 3 months) of pain and swelling in the affected area. Greater than 75% of cases of MO occur in the large skeletal muscles of proximal extremities (the quadriceps and the brachialis muscles are the most common sites). Occasionally there may be localized erythema in the overlying skin. Although MO represents a peculiar reaction to trauma, not all patients recount a history of trauma to the site.

RADIOLOGIC IMAGES

The radiologic appearance of MO varies depending on its degree of "maturity." Early lesions (see earlier) exhibit a nonspecific soft tissue mass–type appearance. Later lesions appear as ossified soft tissue nodules (Figure 11-1).

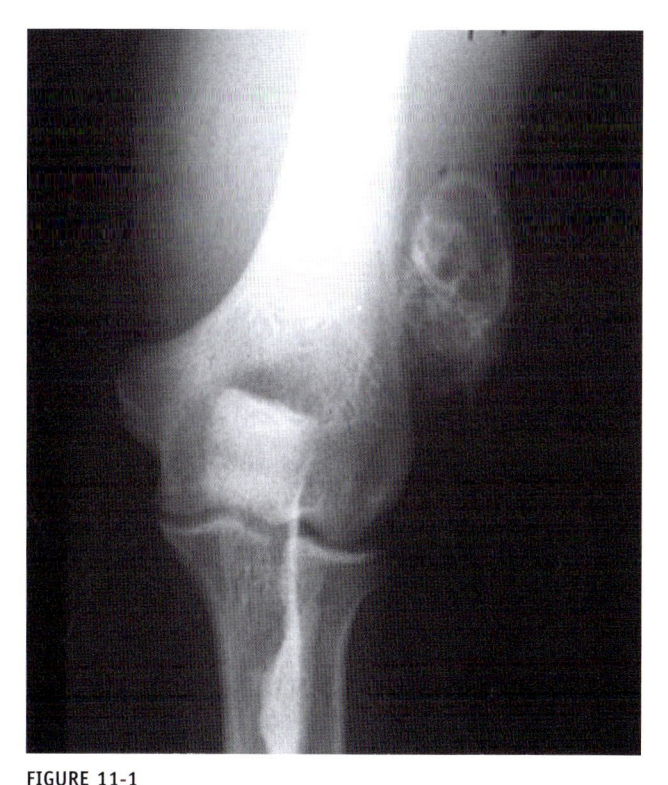

FIGURE 11-1

A mature mass of myositis ossificans within the Brachialis muscle. Note the well-formed shell of bone.

PATHOLOGIC FEATURES

GROSS FINDINGS

MO typically measures less than 5.0 cm. Lesions examined early in their evolution are solid gray and may exhibit gritty tan regions of mineralized bone. More mature MO has the appearance of a solid bone nodule that requires cutting with a saw (Figure 11-2).

MICROSCOPIC FINDINGS

In the early phase, MO demonstrates intense cellularity being composed of sheets and fascicles of plump spindled myofibroblastic cells (Figure 11-3). These cells have oval nuclei with vesicular chromatin and eosinophilic nucleoli. They are embedded within a myxoid to collagenous ground substance. Mitotic figures are usually readily found. They are all typical in type. Necrosis is usually not seen. Intersecting trabeculae of fibrillary eosinophilic osteoid appear to arise from the spindle cells (Figure 11-4). These immature foci of woven osteoid transition to thicker, more obvious, mineralized, woven bone trabeculae that show prominent osteoblastic rimming. These, in turn, become continuous with more mature lamellar bone trabeculae (Figure 11-5). This gradual evolution in the histologic appearance from plump spindle cells through immature woven bone to mature lamellar bone is referred to as a *zoning phenomenon*. This is one of the key histologic hallmarks of MO. Obviously, the degree to which this is identifiable will depend on

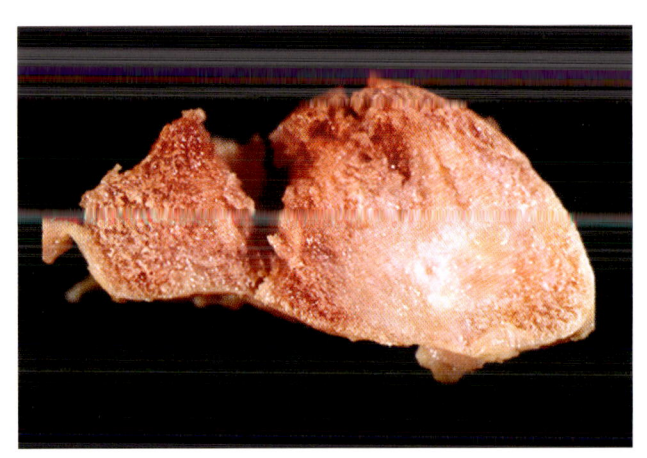

FIGURE 11-2
The mass from Figure 11-1 has been bisected with a saw. The center has the appearance of normal cancellous bone.

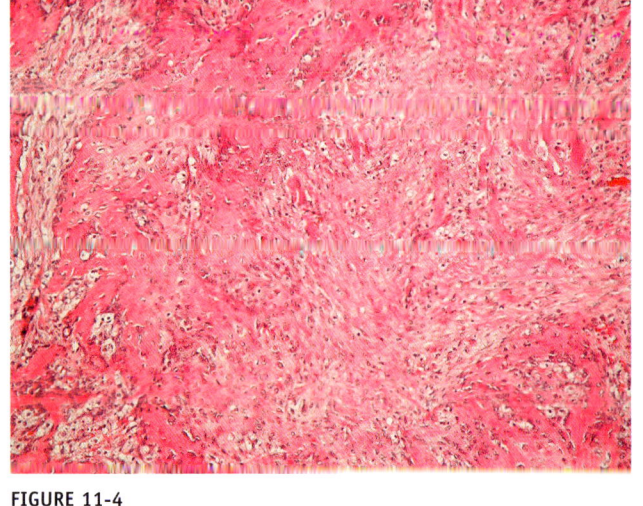

FIGURE 11-4
Woven bone with prominent *osteoblastic rimming* arises from the cellular spindle cell proliferation.

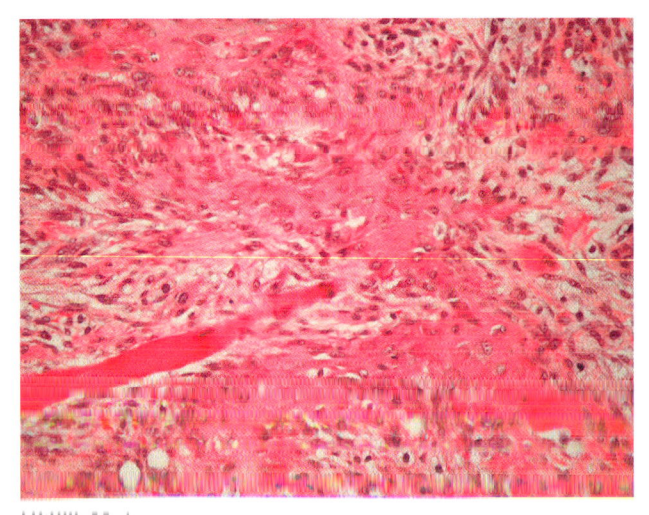

FIGURE 11-3
The center of an immature myositis ossificans. A residual skeletal myocyte is surrounded by a proliferation of plump myofibroblasts. Early woven bone formation is also evident.

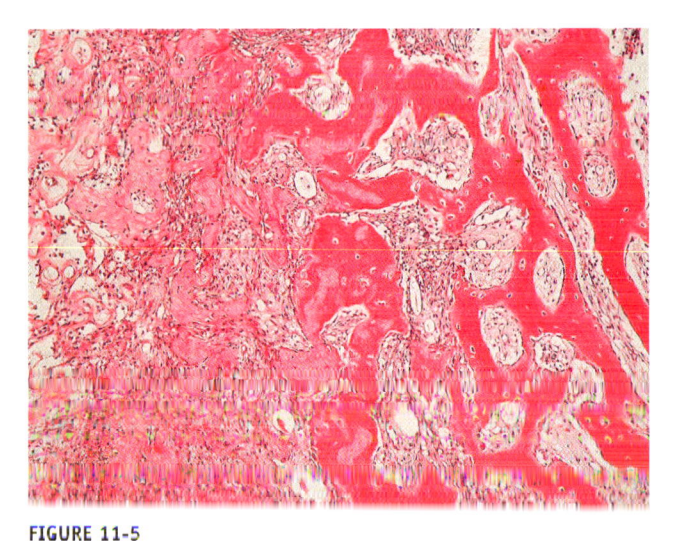

FIGURE 11-5
A transition from immature woven to mature lamellar type bone. This is the hallmark of myositis ossificans.

the type of surgical pathology specimen. In practical terms, although it is one of the most characteristic features of MO, it is not always perfectly represented on histologic materials.

Ancillary Studies

Immunohistochemistry

The spindle cells that comprise the early phases of MO stain positively for smooth muscle actin and muscle-specific actin consistent with their myofibroblastic phenotype.

Differential Diagnosis

MO is histologically virtually identical to so-called fibro-osseous pseudotumor of digits (FOPD). However, the latter entity (discussed in detail later), as is suggested by its name, occurs exclusively in the nonmuscular soft tissues of the digits. The central immature regions of MO closely resemble nodular fasciitis (NF). NF typically occurs in the superficial soft tissues and does not contain bone except in rare cases. These two lesions are easily differentiated on clinical grounds. The most important differential diagnostic consideration is soft tissue osteosarcoma (STO). STO also occurs in the deep soft tissues, but it most commonly arises in patients in the fifth and sixth decades of life. STO is usually larger than 5.0 cm, grossly heterogeneous with hemorrhagic and necrotic regions, and histologically demonstrates nuclear pleomorphism and cytologic atypia (see later).

Prognosis and Treatment

MO is a benign non-neoplastic condition that is treated by simple excision only. Recurrence is extremely uncommon, even when resection margins are positive.

MYOSITIS OSSIFICANS—FACT SHEET

Definition
- A non-neoplastic reactive bone- and cartilage-producing pseudotumor that develops in skeletal muscle after trauma

Incidence and Location
- Rare (annual incidence less than 1 per 1 million individuals)
- The large muscles of the proximal extremities are most commonly involved

Morbidity and Mortality
- Benign condition

Sex and Age Distribution
- Male and female sexes affected equally
- Most common in the second and third decades of life

Clinical Features
- Short history of pain and swelling at the affected site
- Uncommonly localized erythema

Radiologic Features
- With plain radiographs, initially only a soft tissue mass may be visible
- Lesions ossify as they mature
- Magnetic resonance imaging in early lesions shows an inhomogeneous soft tissue mass

Prognosis and Treatment
- Local excision results in cure
- Recurrence is extremely uncommon, even when excision margins are positive

---

MYOSITIS OSSIFICANS—PATHOLOGIC FEATURES

Gross Findings
- Most lesions measure 5.0 cm or less
- In early lesions, an ill-defined soft tissue mass may exhibit focal gritty calcifications
- In more mature examples, the mass is completely ossified and readily demarcated from the skeletal muscle

Microscopic Findings
- The morphology of the lesion depends on the time point in relation to the inciting injury at which it is examined
- In "early" lesions, sheets of plump "myofibroblast-like" spindle cells are arranged as sheets and fascicles associated with intersecting trabeculae of lace-like woven bone
- Cellular hyaline/fibrocartilage may be present
- Mitotic figures are readily found
- Necrosis is not present
- In "later" lesions, the bone is more mature and well organized
- Typically, a transition occurs from the sheets of spindled myofibroblastic cells at the center of the lesion to the bone-rich periphery; this is referred to as a *zoning phenomenon*
- Fully mature examples are composed of lamellar cortical and cancellous bone that may contain fatty and hematopoietic marrow

Immunohistochemical Features
- In the early lesions, the spindle cells express smooth muscle actin and muscle-specific actin reflecting their myofibroblastic morphology

Differential Diagnosis
- FOPD
- NF
- Extraskeletal osteosarcoma

FIBRO-OSSEOUS PSEUDOTUMOR OF DIGITS

FOPD is a non-neoplastic, reactive pseudotumor analogous to MO. Unlike MO, FOPD occurs in the nonmuscular soft tissues of the digits. Similar to MO, FOPD develops as a reaction to injury, although less than half of the affected patients are able to pinpoint a specific preceding injury.

CLINICAL FEATURES

FOPD usually occurs in young patients, with a peak incidence in the second and third decades of life. Male and female sexes are affected equally. Patients present with a short history of localized digital swelling that may be painful or painless.

RADIOLOGIC FEATURES

Plain radiographs show soft tissue swelling with or without linear periosteal type new bone formation.

PATHOLOGIC FEATURES

GROSS FINDINGS

FOPDs are firm, rubbery, tan nodules that typically measure less than 3.0 cm in maximum size (Figure 11-6).

MICROSCOPIC FINDINGS

The histologic features of FOPD are similar to MO (see earlier). Microscopically, the lesion consists of an admixture of plump spindle cells and cellular osteocartilaginous tissue. The "zoning phenomenon" that characterizes MO is usually not evident in FOPD. Cellular callus-like fibrocartilage is also a more prominent feature than in MO (Figures 11-7 and 11-8). Typical mitotic figures are found; however, high-grade nuclear atypia and necrosis are not present.

DIFFERENTIAL DIAGNOSIS

The differential diagnosis of FOPD includes MO, STO soft tissue chondroma (STC), and fracture callus. Although microscopically similar, MO is readily distinguished from FOPD on clinical grounds. Similarly, STO usually occurs in the deep soft tissues of the proximal

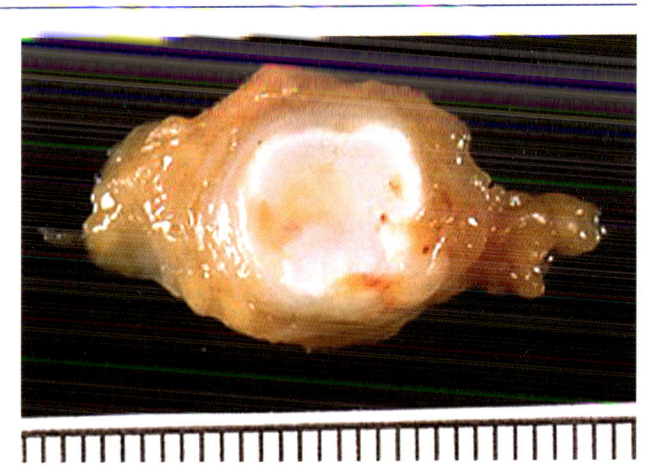

FIGURE 11-6
A small, circumscribed, rubbery nodule of fibro-osseous pseudotumor with adherent fat.

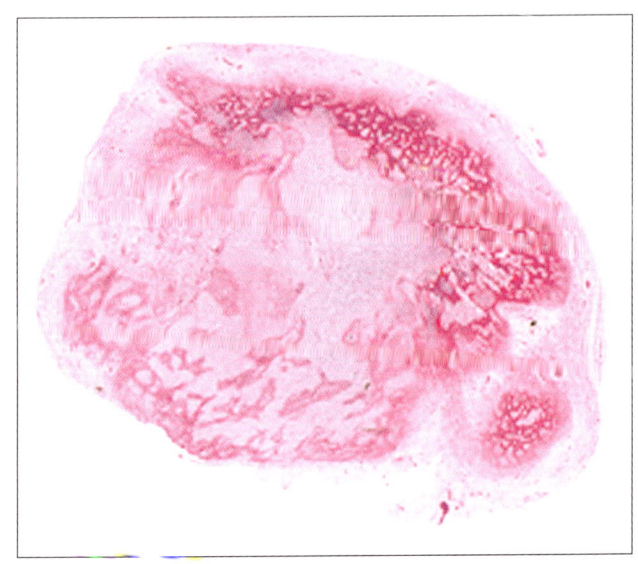

FIGURE 11-7
A *whole-mount* view of the specimen from Figure 11-6 demonstrating central cartilage and peripheral bone.

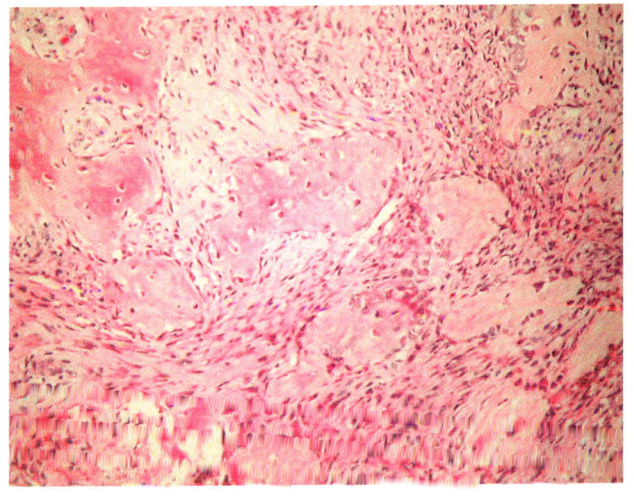

FIGURE 11-8
Plump spindle cells and spicules of woven bone, morphologically similar to myositis ossificans; however, note the absence of skeletal muscle fibers.

extremities, and it usually demonstrates high-grade nuclear atypia in comparison with FOPD. STC commonly occurs in the distal extremities, including the digits. In comparison with FOPD, STC is composed of plump chondrocytes embedded in a hyaline cartilage matrix. The cellular heterogeneity that is one of the features of FOPD is not seen in STC (see later). Fracture callus can appear histologically identical to FOPD. Despite the microscopic similarity, appropriate clinical and radiographic information should allow these two lesions to be readily distinguished.

FIBRO-OSSEOUS PSEUDOTUMOR OF DIGITS—FACT SHEET

Definition
- A non-neoplastic, reactive bone- and cartilage-producing pseudotumor that selectively occurs in the soft tissues of the digits; it is clinically and pathologically analogous to MO

Incidence and Location
- Rare (annual incidence less than 1 per 1 million individuals)
- The soft tissues adjacent to the small tubular bones of the hands (most commonly) and feet

Morbidity
- Benign condition

Sex and Age Distribution
- Male and female sexes affected equally
- Most common in the second and third decades of life

Clinical Features
- Short history of digital swelling
- Less than half of patients give a history of trauma

Radiologic Features
- Plain radiographs demonstrate soft tissue swelling with or without linear periosteal bone formation affecting the underlying bone

Prognosis and Treatment
- Local excision results in cure
- Recurrence is extremely uncommon, even when excision margins are positive

FIBRO-OSSEOUS PSEUDOTUMOR OF DIGITS—PATHOLOGIC FEATURES

Gross Findings
- Lesions typically measure less than 3.0 cm
- Lesions are firm, tan, and rubbery

Microscopic Findings
- Plump spindle cells similar to MO
- Visible mitotic activity
- Bone formation that varies from immature woven in type to mature lamellar
- Cellular, callus-like cartilage
- No necrosis or high-grade nuclear atypia
- The zoning phenomenon of MO is typically not apparent

Differential Diagnosis
- MO
- STO
- STC
- Fracture callus

PROGNOSIS AND TREATMENT

FOPD is treated by simple excision. Recurrence is extremely uncommon, even when initial resection margins are positive. Aggressive, destructive growth does not occur.

SOFT TISSUE OSTEOSARCOMA

STOs arise in extraskeletal sites and are defined by the manufacture of bone/osteoid by the tumor cells. Most of these tumors are histologically high grade and clinically aggressive.

CLINICAL FEATURES

STO occurs in adults with a peak incidence in the fifth and sixth decades of life. This is in contrast with skeletal osteosarcoma that most commonly occurs in younger patients. The tumors typically arise in the deep soft tissues of the proximal extremities where they present as a painless mass. Rarely, patients may have a history of prior therapeutic irradiation at the site of the tumor. Male individuals are affected approximately twice as frequently as female individuals.

RADIOLOGIC FEATURES

Usually the tumors present nonspecific imaging characteristics that appear only as soft tissue masses. Radiographically detectable mineralization is uncommon.

PATHOLOGIC FEATURES

GROSS FINDINGS

STOs are usually large (often > 10 cm), grossly heterogeneous tumors that exhibit regions of hemorrhage, necrosis, or both (Figure 11-9). Like most soft tissue sarcomas, they may appear grossly circumscribed;

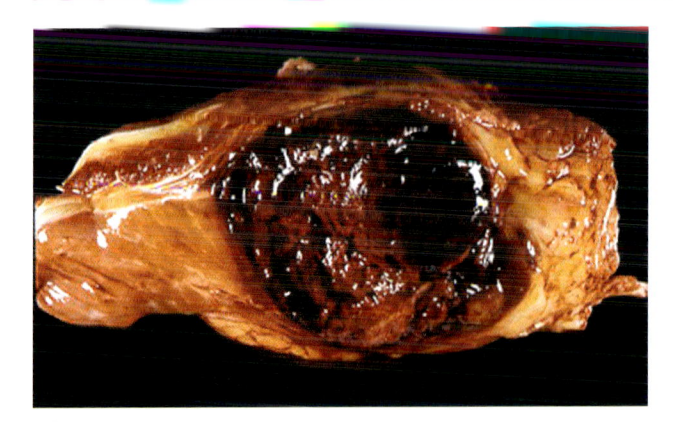

FIGURE 11-9
A large hemorrhagic and necrotic soft tissue mass without grossly apparent bone formation, as is typically seen in soft tissue osteosarcoma.

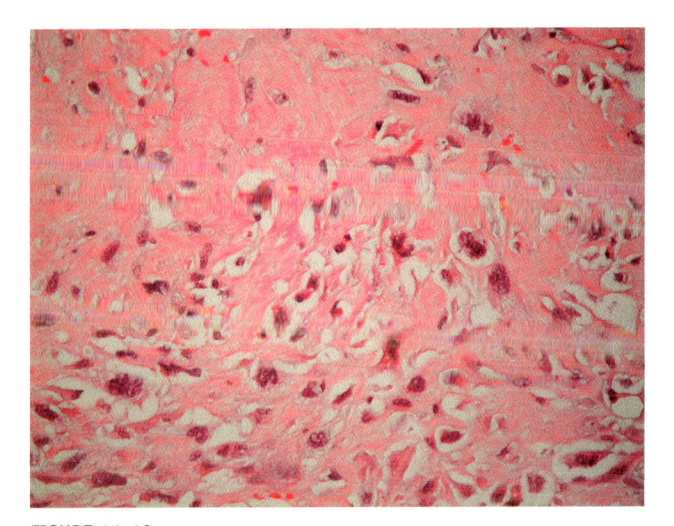

FIGURE 11-10
Coarse, irregular neoplastic osteoid outlines highly pleomorphic sarcoma cells in a typical *lace-like* manner.

SOFT TISSUE OSTEOSARCOMAS—FACT SHEET

Definition
▸▸ A sarcoma arising in extraskeletal somatic soft tissue in which the neoplastic cells produce osteoid or bone matrix, or both

Incidence and Location
▸▸ Rare; STOs account for between 1% and 2% of soft tissue sarcomas
▸▸ The most common locations for these tumors are the deep soft tissues of the thigh and buttocks

Morbidity and Mortality
▸▸ High rate of metastases, and up to 75% of patients die of disease within 5 years of diagnosis
▸▸ The rare examples of low-grade STO have a much better prognosis

Sex and Age Distribution
▸▸ Male individuals are affected approximately twice as often as female individuals
▸▸ Most common in the fifth and sixth decades of life

Clinical Features
▸▸ As with most soft tissue sarcomas, patients present with a painless mass

Radiologic Features
▸▸ Most of the tumors have nonspecific imaging features similar to other high-grade soft tissue sarcomas
▸▸ Mineralization, if radiologically detectable, tends to be minimal

Prognosis and Treatment
▸▸ High-grade tumors, which form the majority, have a poor prognosis because of the high rate of metastases
▸▸ Treatment is by wide surgical excision, with systemic chemotherapy

however, they are microscopically infiltrative. Grossly detectable mineralized bone is not usually present.

MICROSCOPIC FINDINGS

STOs are highly cellular, cytologically pleomorphic sarcomas. Most tumor cells are spindled to epithelioid in shape. The defining feature is the presence of neoplastic osteoid or bone production, or both. This usually outlines individual cells or clusters of cells in a "lace-like" manner; however, solid sheets of amorphous osteoid may also be found (Figure 11-10). Usually, the bone/osteoid matrix is found in a minority of the tumor, and often much of the neoplasm has a nonspecific, undifferentiated, spindle cell sarcoma appearance (Figure 11-11). Lobules of highly cellular atypical hyaline/fibrocartilage may also be present. In essence, any of the microscopic patterns of high-grade intraosseous osteosarcoma may be seen in STO. This means that foci of small-cell and telangiectatic osteosarcoma may also be encountered. Usually, the tumors demonstrate a high mitotic rate, including atypical mitotic figures. Necrosis may be prominent.

IMMUNOHISTOCHEMISTRY

The STO tumor cells have an identical pattern of staining to skeletal osteosarcoma. Diffuse strong vimentin staining occurs. Focal staining for S-100, desmin, and smooth muscle actin may also be present. Early experience suggests that antibodies to the bone matrix protein osteocalcin may have good specificity for both tumor cells and bone/osteoid matrix.

DIFFERENTIAL DIAGNOSIS

Most STOs are high-grade tumors, and because the bone/osteoid production may be a focal finding, only the differential diagnosis will include other high-grade

CHAPTER 11 Osteocartilaginous Tumors

SOFT TISSUE OSTEOSARCOMAS—PATHOLOGIC FEATURES

Gross Findings
- Most tumors measure between 5 and 15 cm
- Their cut surface is tan/hemorrhagic with focal regions of necrosis
- Focal calcification may be present but is often indistinct
- As with many soft tissue sarcomas, they may appear grossly well circumscribed

Microscopic Findings
- Highly cellular mitotically active tumors
- Usually considerable nuclear pleomorphism with necrosis
- Lace-like eosinophilic osteoid outlines individual cells or clusters of cells
- Mineralized osteoid (bone) is relatively uncommon
- Lobules of cellular atypical hyaline cartilage may be present
- All histologic patterns of osseous osteosarcoma including small-cell, telangiectatic, and undifferentiated spindle cell sarcoma patterns may be seen

Immunohistochemical Features
- Similar to osseous osteosarcoma
- Vimentin-positive with focal positive staining for smooth muscle actin, desmin, and S-100 protein (cartilage cells and some non-cartilaginous cells)
- Osteocalcin stains both tumor cells and the neoplastic matrix (Fanburg-Smith and colleagues, 1999)

Differential Diagnosis
- Other nonmatrix-producing, high-grade soft tissue sarcomas
- MO
- Osseous osteosarcoma (primary or metastatic/recurrent)

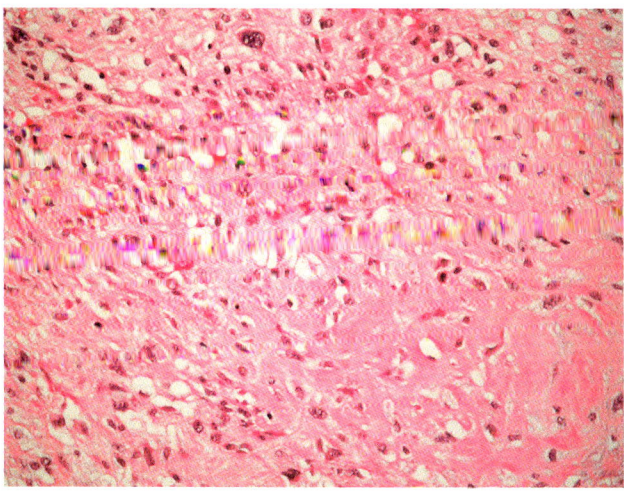

FIGURE 11-11
A transition between an undifferentiated spindle cell sarcoma region of a tumor and an area that demonstrates clear neoplastic osteoid production.

spindle cell sarcomas. The key to the diagnosis is identifying the matrix surrounding the tumor cells. Antibodies to osteocalcin have shown some promise in providing positive identification of this bone matrix. MO, particularly in its early cellular phase, when the bone production is scant and somewhat "lace-like," is usually readily distinguished from STO by the uniform reactive appearance to the proliferating myofibroblastic and osteoblastic cells. High-grade nuclear atypia, which is present in virtually all STOs, is not seen in MO. Clinical features (see earlier) also are usually of help in the distinction of the two entities. Soft tissue recurrence or metastasis of skeletal osteosarcoma will appear histologically identical to STO and can be recognized only by history.

PROGNOSIS AND TREATMENT

STOs are high-grade tumors. Patients commonly present with metastatic disease, which accounts for the high mortality rate with these tumors. Treatment involves wide surgical resection and systemic chemotherapy.

SOFT TISSUE CHONDROMA

STCs are benign tumors composed of mature chondrocytes associated with hyaline cartilage matrix. They are histologically similar to the osseous enchondroma.

CLINICAL FEATURES

STCs are relatively uncommon tumors that usually present as painless masses that involve the distal extremities. The soft tissues about the wrist and fingers represent the most commonly affected site. The tumors occur in male and female individuals with equal frequency, with most being diagnosed in adults in the fourth through seventh decades of life. Although most of these tumors are composed of well-formed hyaline cartilage, a recently recognized variant tends to exhibit greater cellularity, have less matrix, and may resemble osseous chondroblastoma.

RADIOLOGIC FEATURES

Often, no imaging studies are performed in affected patients because the tumors present as small, superficial masses. If radiographs have been done, the tumor may either appear as a nonspecific soft tissue mass, or on occasion, typical "rings and arcs" of mineralization characteristic of cartilage matrix may be present.

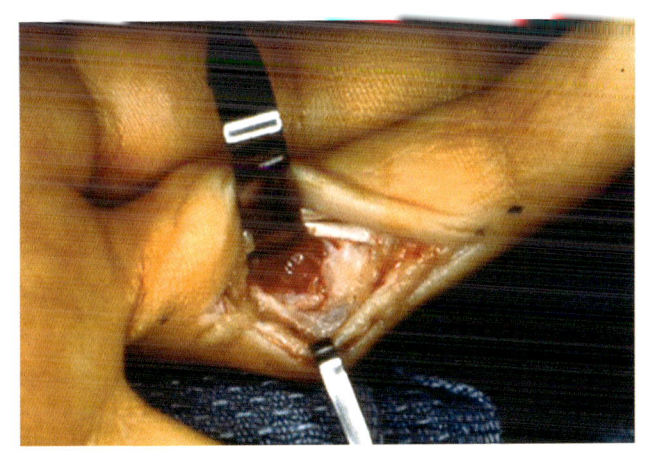

FIGURE 11-12
Intraoperative image showing a glistening red–gray soft tissue chondroma adjacent to a tendon and tendon sheath.

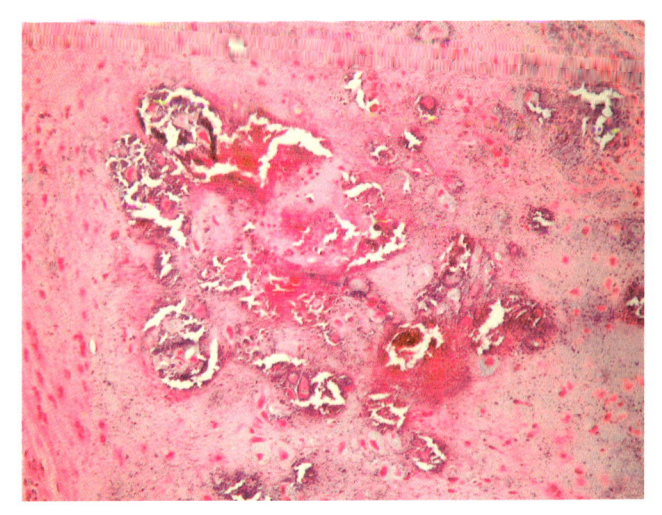

FIGURE 11-14
Punctate stromal calcification.

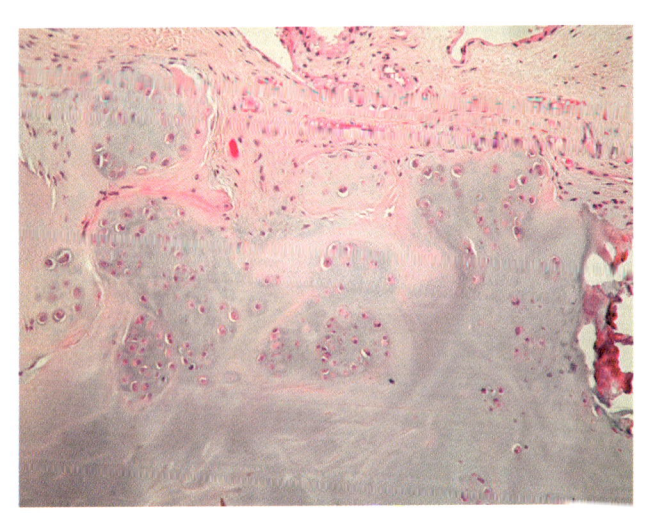

FIGURE 11-13
Lobule of moderately cellular hyaline cartilage with the typical clustering of chondrocytes.

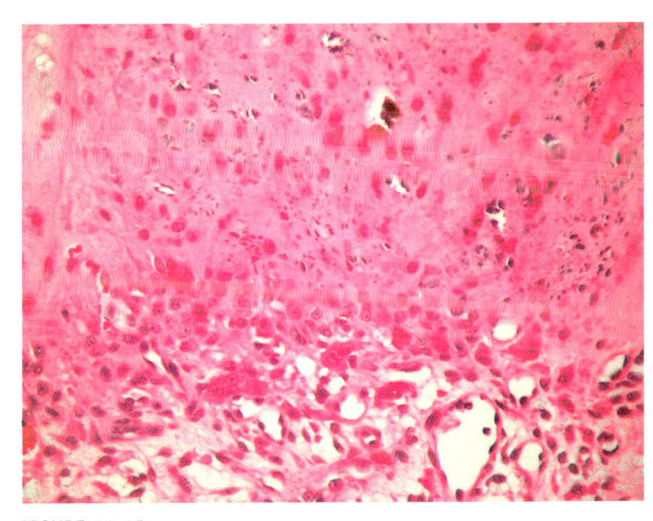

FIGURE 11-15
Cellular region of a soft tissue chondroma, chondroblastoma-like, with larger plump chondrocytes and osteoclast-like giant cells.

PATHOLOGIC FEATURES

GROSS FINDINGS

Most STCs measure less than 2.0 cm. Usually, they are readily separable from the adjacent soft tissues and commonly are described as "popping out" at the time of surgical removal (Figure 11-12). The tumors are usually lobulated and gray-white. Gritty regions of calcification may be present.

MICROSCOPIC FINDINGS

Most STCs are composed of mature chondrocytes arranged in a clustered pattern embedded within well-formed hyaline cartilage (Figure 11-13). The lesional cells may demonstrate mild nuclear irregularity and visible nucleoli, but mitotic figures are only rarely encountered. The overall cellularity of these tumors is greater than normal hyaline articular cartilage and may resemble or exceed that of low-grade osseous chondrosarcoma. The tumors are lobulated, and although well demarcated from the adjacent soft tissues, they are nonencapsulated. Microscopic stromal calcification, with or without enchondral ossification, is commonly found (Figure 11-14). A minority of STCs exhibit greater cellularity, have less extracellular matrix, and are composed of more plump epithelioid chondrocytes. These tumors may also show clusters of multinucleated osteoclast-like giant cells and have been designated as "chondroblastoma-like" STCs (Figure 11-15).

SOFT TISSUE CHONDROMA—FACT SHEET

Definition
▸▸ Benign soft tissue tumor composed of mature chondrocytes, typically associated with well-formed hyaline cartilage matrix

Incidence and Location
▸▸ Rare
▸▸ Tumors characteristically occur in the distal extremities, particularly involving the fingers and wrist region

Morbidity and Mortality
▸▸ Benign tumor

Sex and Age Distribution
▸▸ Slightly more common in male individuals
▸▸ Predominantly in adults, with most cases in the fourth through seventh decades of life

Clinical Features
▸▸ Usually a painless soft tissue mass

Radiologic Features
▸▸ Usually a nonspecific appearance
▸▸ No attachment to the underlying skeleton

Prognosis and Treatment
▸▸ Benign tumor treated by local excision only
▸▸ Recurrence in less than 20% of cases

SOFT TISSUE CHONDROMA—PATHOLOGIC FEATURES

Gross Findings
▸▸ Usually less than 2.0 cm
▸▸ Well-circumscribed and easily removed from the surrounding structures
▸▸ Pearly white with "chalk-like" areas of calcification

Microscopic Findings
▸▸ Cellular lobules of hyaline cartilage
▸▸ Clustered chondrocytes with pale nuclei and small nucleoli
▸▸ Infrequent mitotic figures
▸▸ Stromal calcification
▸▸ A minority resemble osseous chondroblastoma

Immunohistochemical Features
▸▸ Vimentin and S-100-positive

Differential Diagnosis
▸▸ Synovial chondromatosis
▸▸ FOPD
▸▸ Soft tissue chondrosarcoma

DIFFERENTIAL DIAGNOSIS

STC shows many histologic similarities to synovial chondromatosis, a condition characterized by the formation of well formed lobules of hyaline cartilage within intra-articular or extra-articular synovial membranes. Because the individual nodules of cartilage are histologically identical in both entities, the association with a synovial surface is crucial in establishing the correct diagnosis. In addition, extra-articular synovial chondromatosis usually forms a larger mass. FOPD (see earlier), although occurring in a similar location to many STC, is microscopically more varied. The cartilage present in the former is characteristically less well organized and more resembles fracture callus. Soft tissue chondrosarcomas (see later) are usually larger, exhibit more varied cellularity, and typically occur more centrally as opposed to the acral location for most STCs.

PROGNOSIS AND TREATMENT

STC is managed by simple local excision. Recurrence develops in about 20% of cases.

EXTRASKELETAL MYXOID CHONDROSARCOMA

Extraskeletal myxoid chondrosarcoma (EMC) is a soft tissue sarcoma composed of spindle and epithelioid tumor cells associated with extracellular matrix that histologically and histochemically resembles cartilage. The majority of tumors exhibit the t(9;22)(q22;q12) translocation involving the *EWS* and *CHN* genes. These tumors are histologically, immunohistochemically, and genotypically distinct from osseous chondrosarcoma.

CLINICAL FEATURES

EMC typically presents as a painless mass occurring in the deep soft tissues of adults in the fourth through seventh decades of life. Male individuals are more commonly affected than female individuals. The original descriptions of EMCs suggested that they were low-grade tumors; however, as greater numbers of patients with this tumor have been identified, treated, and followed up for longer periods, it has become apparent that distant metastases and aggressive clinical behavior are more common than originally thought.

RADIOLOGIC FEATURES

EMCs present as nonspecific soft tissue masses. They are virtually always unmineralized.

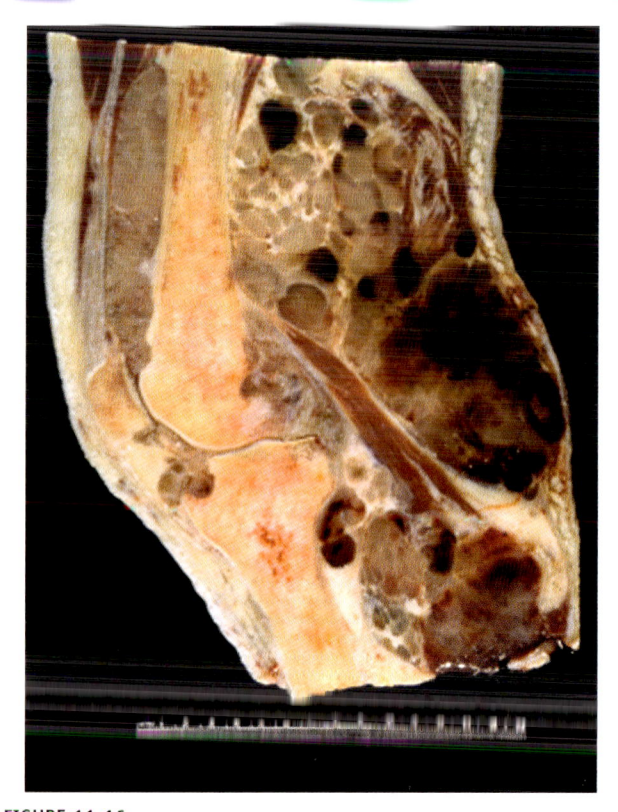

248　　　BONE AND SOFT TISSUE PATHOLOGY

FIGURE 11-16
A massive extraskeletal myxoid chondrosarcoma extensively involving the thigh and knee joint, demonstrating the typical lobulated gelatinous tumor nodules.

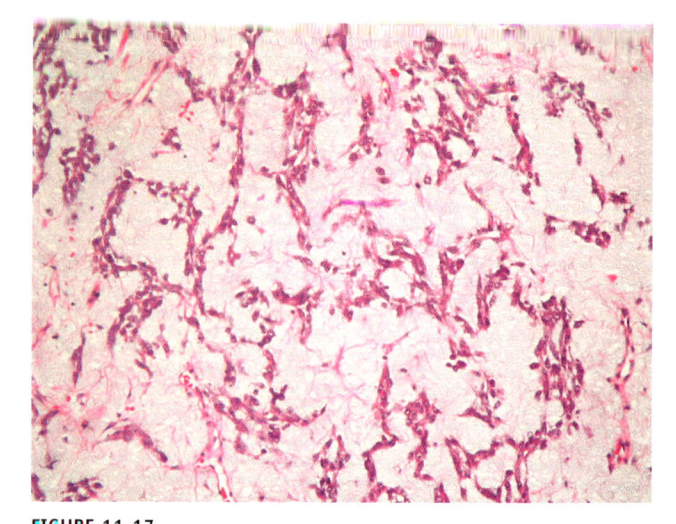

FIGURE 11-17
Cords of uniform oval spindle cells within flocculent myxoid ground substance.

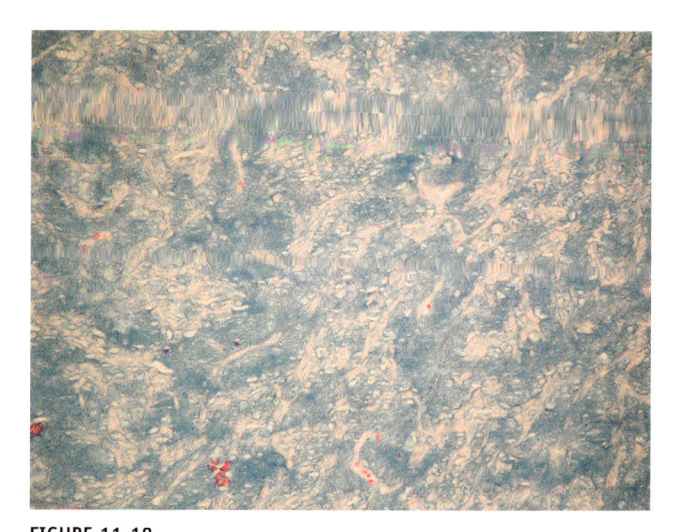

FIGURE 11-18
An Alcian blue stain showing strong positive staining of the tumor extracellular matrix.

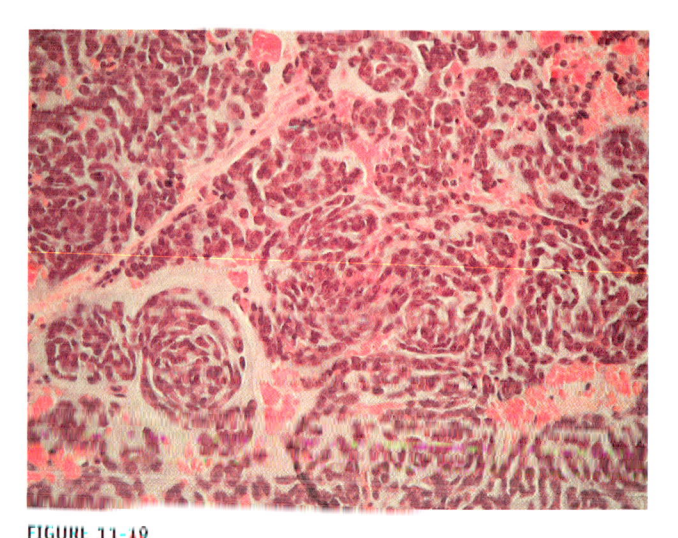

FIGURE 11-19
A high-grade tumor exhibiting greater cellularity and relatively scant extracellular matrix.

PATHOLOGIC FEATURES

GROSS FINDINGS

EMCs typically measure greater than 5.0 cm. Like many soft tissue sarcomas, they appear grossly lobulated. The cut surface of the tumors is typically gray, soft, and gelatinous (Figure 11-16).

MICROSCOPIC FINDINGS

EMCs demonstrate a lobular growth pattern at low-power examination. Typically, these are composed of cords, clusters, and nests of uniform oval to spindled cells embedded within flocculent basophilic matrix (Figure 11-17). Blood vessels are indistinct, and individual lobules of tumor are separated by fibrous bands. The tumor cells have uniform dark staining nuclei with indistinct nucleoli. Alcian blue histochemical staining is positive at pH 4.0 and 1.0, suggesting the presence of chondroitin sulphates (Figure 11-18). In recent years, the existence of cellular matrix–poor regions of EMC has been recognized. In these areas, often a sheet-like growth of tumor cells with relatively little intervening extracellular matrix is present (Figure 11-19). The tumor cells in these areas are larger, have higher nuclear/

cytoplasmic ratios, and demonstrate diffuse nuclear atypia with hyperchromatism and visible eosinophilic nucleoli. Mitotic figures are readily found in these areas but are usually infrequent in the conventional matrix-rich areas.

ANCILLARY STUDIES

IMMUNOHISTOCHEMISTRY

EMC tumor cells usually demonstrate diffuse positive staining for vimentin. Early reports suggested S-100 staining in more than half of these tumors, although as experience with these lesions has accumulated, it has become apparent that S-100 staining occurs in a minority (<20%) of tumors. Positive staining for neuron specific enolase (NSE) and synaptophysin commonly occurs, particularly in the more cellular regions of the tumor.

DIFFERENTIAL DIAGNOSIS

Differential diagnoses of EMC include STC, STO, and osseous chondrosarcoma with soft tissue extension. The first two entities were discussed in detail earlier. The essential histologic difference pertains to the nature of the cartilage-like matrix. In both STC and STO, bone fide hyaline cartilage matrix occurs; however, in EMC, the matrix is only cartilage-like. Osseous chondrosarcoma with soft tissue extension, particularly when myxoid, may be confused with EMC; however, appropriate clinical and radiologic information should readily clarify the issue. Myoepithelioma/mixed tumor of soft tissue and ossifying fibromyxoid tumor are rare soft tissue tumors of uncertain histogenesis that may exhibit focal areas that are microscopically similar to EMC. These are discussed in detail in another chapter.

PROGNOSIS AND TREATMENT

Treatment of EMC is principally by wide surgical excision. Five-year survival rates are high (>80%); however, 10- and 15-year disease-free survival rates are considerably lower, primarily because of a high metastatic rate.

EXTRASKELETAL MYXOID CHONDROSARCOMA—FACT SHEET

Definition
- A soft tissue sarcoma composed of uniform spindle and epithelioid cells in which the extracellular matrix exhibits some histologic and histochemical characteristics of cartilage; the majority exhibits the t(9;22)(q22;q12) translocation involving the *EWS* and *CHN* genes

Incidence and Location
- The tumors are rare, comprising approximately 2.5% of soft tissue sarcomas
- They primarily occur in the deep soft tissues of the proximal extremities and trunk, although any site may be affected

Morbidity and Mortality
- The tumors have a high rate of metastasis (approximately 50%), although long-term survival after diagnosis, even in the presence of metastasis, is characteristic

Sex and Age Distribution
- Male individuals are affected more commonly than female individuals
- Tumors occur throughout adulthood, with most in the fourth through seventh decades of life

Clinical Features
- Most tumors present as a painless soft tissue mass
- Rare cases may present with lung metastases and an occult primary

Prognosis and Treatment
- Treatment is principally by surgical excision
- Five-year survival rates are high (>80%); however, late lung metastases occur, and 10- and 15-year disease-free survivals are considerably lower

---

EXTRASKELETAL MYXOID CHONDROSARCOMA—PATHOLOGIC FEATURES

Gross Findings
- Most tumors measure greater than 5.0 cm
- They are typically lobulated, tan-gray, and gelatinous

Microscopic Findings
- Cytologically uniform oval and spindle cells embedded in flocculent myxoid ground substance
- Fibrous bands dividing individual lobules of tumor
- Hypovascular
- The cells may be arranged as cords, strands, nests, and sheets
- Typically uniform dark staining nuclei with indistinct nucleoli
- In hypercellular matrix-poor regions, the tumor cells often display larger, more vesicular nuclei with visible nucleoli; some tumor cells may have a distinctly rhabdoid morphology
- Alcian blue–positive staining of matrix at pH 4.0 and 1.0 (chondroitin sulfate positive)

Immunohistochemical Features
- Uniformly vimentin positive
- Focal positivity for S-100 (less than 50%), NSE, and synaptophysin

Differential Diagnosis
- STC
- Osseous chondrosarcoma with soft tissue extension
- STO
- Myoepithelioma/mixed tumor of soft tissue
- Ossifying fibromyxoid tumor

MESENCHYMAL CHONDROSARCOMA

Mesenchymal chondrosarcomas (MCs) are high-grade, biphasic sarcomas composed of an admixture of small, blue, undifferentiated cells and islands of well-formed hyaline cartilage.

CLINICAL FEATURES

MCs are uncommon tumors that account for less than 1% of soft tissue sarcomas. Male and female individuals are affected equally. The tumors may occur at any age, although most cases are diagnosed in adults within the second through fourth decades of life. The tumors may occur at diverse locations, although they most commonly arise in the soft tissues adjacent to the craniospinal axis including the paraspinal musculature. The meninges are one of the most common extraskeletal sites for these tumors. As with most soft tissue sarcomas, the patients usually present with a painless mass. Patients with meningeal tumors commonly present with focal neurologic signs depending on their intracranial location.

RADIOLOGIC FEATURES

Typically, MC has the appearance of a soft tissue mass that shows focal cartilaginous-type calcification.

PATHOLOGIC FEATURES

GROSS FINDINGS

MCs have a wide range in size from less than 5.0 to greater than 20.0 cm. The tumors appear grossly well defined and have a tan–gray cut surface. Focal hemorrhage or necrosis is commonly present. Gritty areas representing the calcified cartilage are often present (Figure 11-20).

MICROSCOPIC FINDINGS

Typically, the majority of the tumor consists of the undifferentiated "small blue cell" component. These cells are usually arranged as sheets, vague nests, or both (Figure 11-21). A characteristic feature is the presence of a supporting capillary network that has acute angle branching, resulting in a "hemangiopericytoma-like" growth pattern (Figure 11-22). The blue cells often are associated with bands of hyalinized eosinophilic collagen that may resemble the "rope-like" collagen of solitary fibrous tumor. The defining light microscopic feature is the presence of island of hyaline cartilage. These typically form only a minority of the tumor and show an abrupt separation from the blue cell regions (Figure 11-23). Focal coarse purple deposits of calcification may occur on the hyaline matrix. Mitotic activity is variable but often high within the blue cell regions. Similarly, necrosis usually involved this component of the tumor.

IMMUNOHISTOCHEMISTRY

Vimentin labels the small blue cells and the chondrocytes. CD99 is positive within the blue cell component, whereas S-100 labels the chondrocytes.

MESENCHYMAL CHONDROSARCOMA—FACT SHEET

Definition
- High grade biphasic sarcoma composed of undifferentiated small blue cells and islands of well-formed hyaline cartilage

Incidence and Location
- These tumors are rare, comprising less than 1% of soft tissue sarcomas
- The most common location is within the soft tissues of the craniospinal axis, including the paraspinal musculature; the meninges represent the most common extraskeletal site for this tumor

Morbidity and Mortality
- These are aggressive malignant neoplasms that have a high rate of metastases and tumor-related mortality
- Metastases may occur as late as 20 years after the initial presentation

Sex and Age Distribution
- Male and female individuals are affected equally
- Tumors occur at all ages; however, the majority occur in the second through the fourth decades of life

Clinical Features
- Patients present with a soft tissue mass similar to other soft tissue sarcomas
- Because of their association with the craniospinal axis, focal neurologic signs or symptoms, or both, may occur

Radiologic Features
- Cartilaginous-type calcification is often present on plain radiographs that otherwise show a nonspecific appearance

Prognosis and Treatment
- Treatment involves a combination of surgical excision and systemic chemotherapy
- Prognosis is determined by the location and stage at presentation
- Up to 50% of patients succumb to disease within 5 years of diagnosis

MESENCHYMAL CHONDROSARCOMA—PATHOLOGIC FEATURES

Gross Findings

- Soft gray-tan tumors that are well delineated from the surrounding tissues
- Focal gritty calcification may be evident within the cartilaginous areas
- Necrosis may be present
- There is a wide range in size from less than 5 cm to more than 20 cm

Microscopic Findings

- Most of the tumor is composed of undifferentiated "small blue" cells arranged as sheets and nests
- Well-formed acute angle branching capillary vasculature between "blue cells" producing a "hemangiopericytoma" appearance
- Highly variable mitotic rate
- Necrosis often present
- Focal aggregates of hyalinized eosinophilic collagen
- Microscopic islands of well-formed, hyaline-type cartilage matrix with embedded well-differentiated chondrocytes; typically, these islands exhibit granular purple mineralization of the matrix
- Cartilage islands may be extremely few (this must be considered in core needle biopsy or small incisional biopsy specimens)

Immunohistochemical Features

- Vimentin staining in the small blue cells and the chondrocytes
- CD99 staining in the blue cell regions
- S-100 staining in the cartilaginous regions but not in the blue cell areas

Differential Diagnosis

- Ewing sarcoma/PNET
- STO (small cell variant)
- Solitary fibrous tumor
- Synovial sarcoma

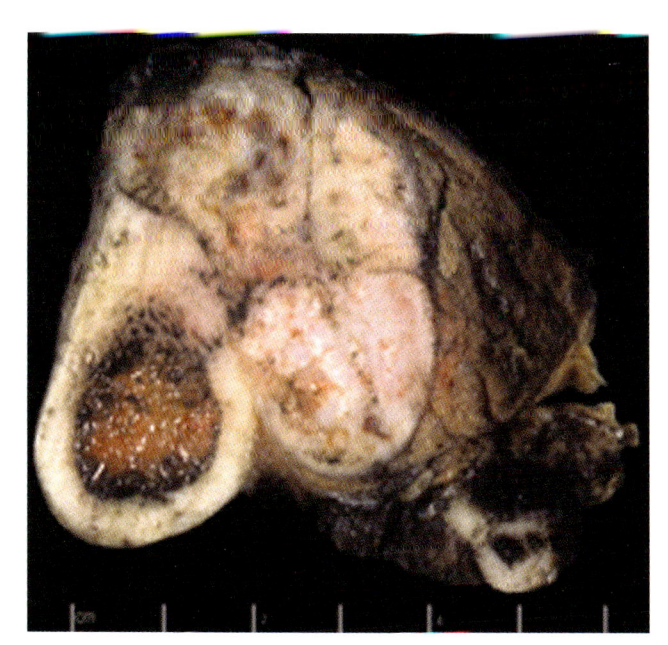

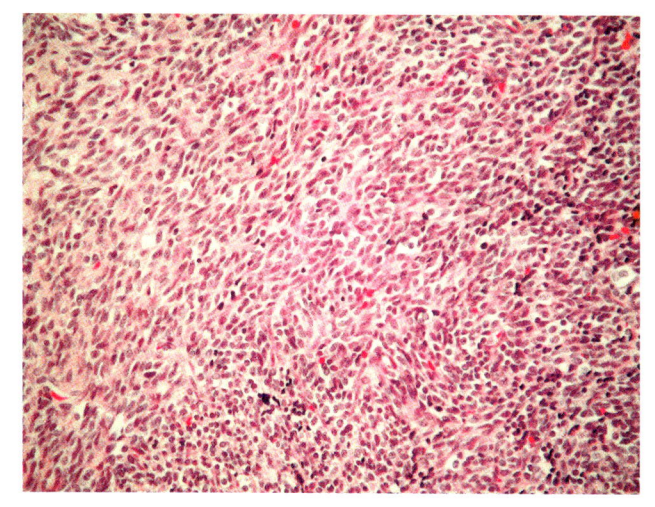

FIGURE 11-21
Sheets of undifferentiated small blue cells.

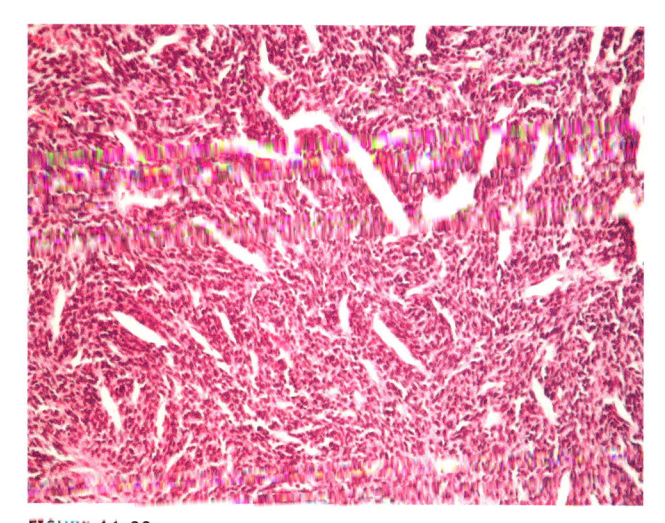

FIGURE 11-20
Large soft tissue mesenchymal chondrosarcoma of the anterior lower leg. Note the yellow calcification within the tan tumor mass.

FIGURE 11-22
Typical irregular acute angle branching so-called hemangiopericytoma-like vascular pattern.

DIFFERENTIAL DIAGNOSIS

Other small blue cell sarcomas such as Ewing sarcoma/primitive neuroectodermal tumor (PNET) and small-cell osteosarcoma may histologically closely resemble MC. Because the islands of cartilage, which allow distinction of MC from Ewing sarcoma/PNET, are often few, this differential may be extremely difficult on small biopsy samples. Molecular genetic examination for the translocation associated with Ewing sarcoma/PNET (t[11;22]) is extremely helpful in resolving this differential. Small-cell osteosarcoma may demonstrate sheets and nests of blue cells similar to MC; however, lace-like osteoid outlining individual cells or clusters of cells is present in the former tumor and not found in the latter. Solitary fibrous tumor and synovial sarcoma are two tumors that may

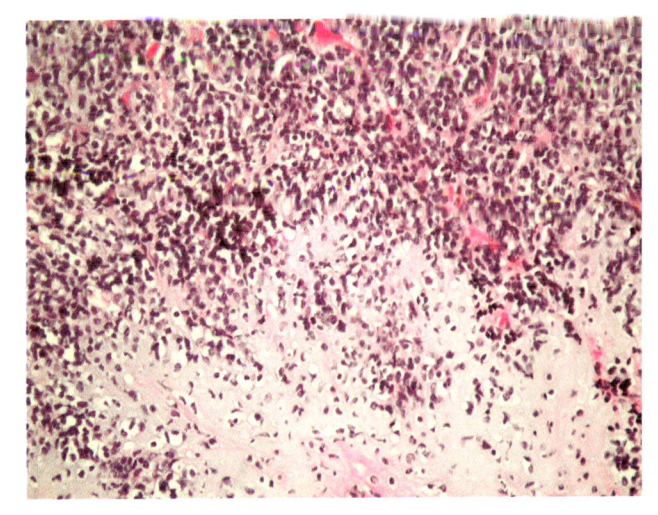

FIGURE 11-23
Abrupt transition between small blue cell tumor and an island of hyaline cartilage.

exhibit sheets of small, rather undifferentiated appearing cells often associated with a hemangiopericytoma-like vascular pattern. These tumors do not show islands of hyaline cartilage, however.

PROGNOSIS AND TREATMENT

MCs are high-grade, clinically aggressive tumors that are treated by a combination of surgery and systemic chemotherapy. Up to 50% of patients have died of disease at 5-year follow up.

ANEURYSMAL CYST OF SOFT TISSUE

ACSTs are benign soft tissue tumors that are histologically identical to aneurysmal bone cyst, but that show no association with the skeleton.

CLINICAL FEATURES

ACSTs are exceptionally rare soft tissue tumors that arise in the deep soft tissues of the extremities of adults. Male and female individuals are affected equally. Patients typically present with a history of a painless soft tissue mass. Some patients report rapid growth.

RADIOLOGIC FEATURES

Plain radiographs demonstrate a soft tissue mass with focal linear ossification. Computed tomographic imaging demonstrates a well-formed shell of bone at the periphery of the mass. Magnetic resonance imaging shows the multinodular pattern of growth with blood-filled cystic spaces.

PATHOLOGIC FEATURES

GROSS FINDINGS

ACSTs usually measure less than 10.0 cm and are well circumscribed within the affected muscle. The peripheral shell of well-formed bone is readily apparent. The cut surface of the mass demonstrates its center to consist of blood-filled spaces separated by thin strands of red–gray soft tissues (Figure 11-24).

MICROSCOPIC FEATURES

The cystic spaces do not have an endothelial lining. Rather, the walls of the spaces are composed of a population of reactive fibroblasts and myofibroblastic cells that often exhibit a fasciitis-like arrangement. Clusters of osteoclast-like multinucleated giant cells are usually present, although these do not form the majority of the mass (Figure 11-25). Hemosiderin-laden macrophages are present. Mitotic figures are found within the mononuclear spindle cell population; however, atypical mitoses or high-grade nuclear atypia is not a feature. At the periphery of the tumor, a shell of well-formed lamellar and woven bone is found. Infiltration of cells into the surrounding skeletal muscle is not present.

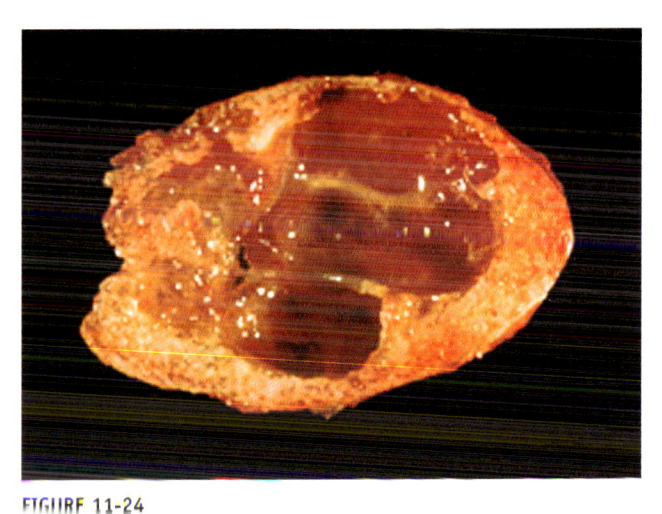

FIGURE 11-24
Soft tissue aneurysmal cyst with a shell of bone and central hemorrhagic cystic cavities.

CHAPTER 11 Osteocartilaginous Tumors

DIFFERENTIAL DIAGNOSIS

The differential diagnosis of ACST includes giant cell tumor of soft tissue, MO, and STO. Giant cell tumor of soft tissue may show focal cystic change but not to the degree seen in ACST. In addition, the fasciitis-like spindle cell population dominates in ACST but does not form a significant component of giant cell tumor of soft tissue. MO, although exhibiting a reactive fasciitis-like appearance, does not demonstrate blood-filled cystic spaces that dominate the morphology of ACST. Finally, STO rarely can exhibit a telangiectatic appearance, and thus grossly simulate ACST. The distinction is readily apparent microscopically because of the high-grade nuclear morphology that the cells in STO exhibit.

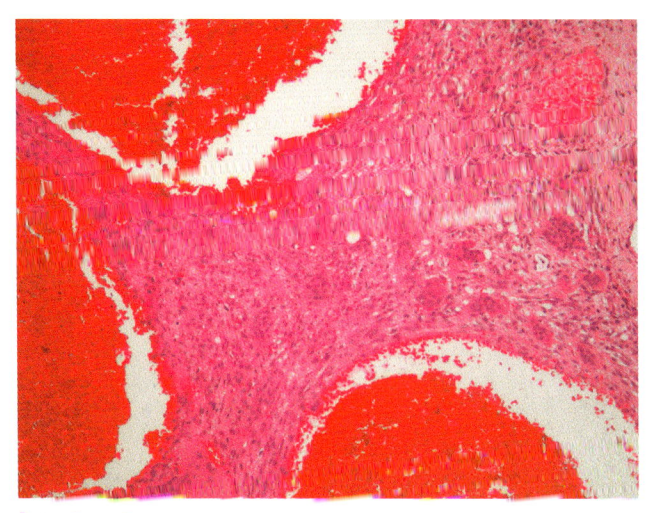

FIGURE 11-25
Blood-filled cystic spaces divided by nonendothelial lined septae composed of a mixture of mononuclear spindle cells and osteoclast-like giant cells.

PROGNOSIS AND TREATMENT

ACSTs are benign tumors that are managed by local excision. If the surgical excision is incomplete, then local recurrence may develop, but aggressive local growth or metastases do not occur.

ANEURYSMAL CYST OF SOFT TISSUE—FACT SHEET

Definition
- A tumor occurring in soft tissue that is histologically identical to aneurysmal bone cyst

Incidence and Location
- These tumors are exceptionally rare
- Aneurysmal cysts predominantly arise in the skeletal muscles of the extremities

Morbidity and Mortality
- Benign tumors

Sex and Age Distribution
- Male and female sexes are affected equally
- Wide age range of affected patients; most are in the third through fifth decades of life

Clinical Features
- Presents as a painless soft tissue mass
- Some patients give a history of rapid growth

Radiologic Features
- Plain radiographs demonstrate a soft tissue mass with focal ossification
- Computed tomographic images show a well-formed peripheral shell of bone
- Magnetic resonance images show a multinodular tumor with blood-filled cystic spaces

Prognosis and Treatment
- Treatment is by local excision only
- Local recurrence may occur in incompletely excised cases
- Metastasis or aggressive local growth does not occur

ANEURYSMAL CYST OF SOFT TISSUE—PATHOLOGIC FEATURES

Gross Findings
- Tumors typically measure less than 10 cm
- Tumors are well circumscribed within the affected skeletal muscle
- A peripheral shell of bone is present
- The center of the tumor is composed of hemorrhagic cystic spaces separated by thin strands of soft tissue

Microscopic Findings
- The blood-filled cystic spaces are nonendothelial lined
- The "walls" of the cysts are composed of plump, spindled, fibroblastic cells arranged as fascicles and storiform aggregates
- Clusters of multinucleated osteoclast-like giant cells are present
- Hemosiderin granules are present
- A peripheral shell of mixed woven and lamellar bone is present

Differential Diagnosis
- Giant cell tumor of soft tissue
- MO
- STO

SUGGESTED READINGS

Myositis Ossificans

1. Ackerman LC: Extra-osseous localized non-neoplastic bone and cartilage formation (so-called myositis ossificans). Clinical and pathological confusion with malignant neoplasms. J Bone Joint Surg Am 1958;40:278-298.
2. Angervall L, Stener B, Stener I, et al: Pseudomalignant osseous tumour of soft tissue. A clinical, radiological, and pathological study of five cases. J Bone Joint Surg Br 1969;51:654-663.
3. Kransdorf JM, Meis JM, Jelinek JS: Myositis ossificans. MR appearance with radiologic-pathologic correlation. AJR Am J Roentgenol 1991;157:1243-1248.
4. Lagier R, Cox JN: Pseudomalignant myositis ossificans. A pathological study of eight cases. Hum Pathol 1975;6:653-665.
5. Nuovo MA, Norman A, Chumas J, et al: Myositis ossificans with atypical clinical, radiographic, or pathologic findings: A review of 23 cases. Skeletal Radiol 1992;21:87-101.
6. Shirkhoda A, Armin A, Bis KG, et al: MR imaging of myositis ossificans: Variable patterns at different stages. J Magn Reson Imaging 1995;5:287-292.

Fibro-Osseous Pseudotumor of Digits

1. Craver RD, Correa-Gracian H, Heinrich S: Florid reactive periostitis. Hum Pathol 1997;28:745-747.
2. De Silva MV, Reid R: Myositis ossificans and fibroosseous pseudotumor of digits: A clinicopathological review of 64 cases with emphasis on diagnostic pitfalls. Int J Surg Pathol 2003;11:187-195.
3. Dupree WB, Enzinger FM: Fibro-osseous pseudotumor of the digits. Cancer 1986;58:2103-2109.
4. Ostrowski ML, Spjut HJ: Lesions of the bones of the hands and feet. Am J Surg Pathol 1997;21:676-690.
5. Sleater J, Mullins D, Chun K, et al: Fibro-osseous pseudotumor of the digit: a comparison to myositis ossificans by light microscopy and immunohistochemical methods. J Cutan Pathol 1995;23:373-377.
6. Spjut HJ, Dorman HD: Florid reactive periostitis of the tubular bones of the hands and feet: a benign lesion which may resemble osteosarcoma. Am J Surg Pathol 1981;5:423-433.

Soft Tissue Osteosarcomas

1. Chung EB, Enzinger FM: Extraskeletal osteosarcoma. Cancer 1987;60:1132-1142.
2. Bane BL, Evans HL, Ro JY, et al: Extraskeletal osteosarcoma: a clinicopathologic review of 26 cases. Cancer 1990;66:2762-2770.
3. Dubec JJ, Munk PL, O'Connell JX, et al: Soft tissue osteosarcoma with telangiectatic features: MR imaging findings in two cases. Skeletal Radiol 1997;26:732-736.
4. Fanburg-Smith JC, Bratthauer GL, Miettinen M: Osteocalcin and osteonectin immunoreactivity in extraskeletal osteosarcoma: A study of 28 cases. Hum Pathol 1999;30:32-38.
5. Jensen ML, Schumacher B, Jense OM, et al: Extraskeletal osteosarcomas: a clinicopathologic study of 25 cases. Am J Surg Pathol 1998;22:588-594.
6. Okada K, Ito H, Miyakoshi N, et al: A low-grade extraskeletal osteosarcoma. Skeletal Radiol 2002;32:165-169.
7. Sordillo PP, Hajdu SI, Magil GB, et al: Extraosseous osteogenic sarcoma: A review of 48 patients. Cancer 1983;51:727-734.
8. Yi ES, Shmookler BM, Malawer MM, et al: Well-differentiated extraskeletal osteosarcoma: a soft tissue homologue of parosteal osteosarcoma. Arch Pathol Lab Med 1991;115:906-909.

Soft Tissue Chondroma

1. Bansal M, Goldman AB, DiCarlo EJ, et al: Soft tissue chondromas: Diagnosis and differential diagnosis. Skeletal Radiol 1993;22:309-315.
2. Cates JM, Rosenberg AE, O'Connell JX, et al: Chondroblastoma-like chondroma of soft tissue: an underrecognized variant and its differential diagnosis. Am J Surg Pathol 2001;25:661-666.
3. Chung EB, Enzinger FM: Chondroma of soft parts. Cancer 1978;41:1414-1424.
4. Dahlin DC, Salvador AH: Cartilaginous tumors of the soft tissues of the hands and feet. Mayo Clin Proc 1974;49:721-726.
5. Deisignore JL, Torre BA, Miller AJ: Extraskeletal chondroma of the hand: case report and review of the literature. Clin Orthop Relat Res 1990;254:147-152.
6. Fletcher CDM, Krausz T: Cartilaginous tumours of the soft tissue. Appl Pathol 1988;6:208-220.

Extraskeletal Myxoid Chondrosarcoma

1. Abromovici LC, Steiner GC, Bonar F: Myxoid chondrosarcoma of soft tissue and bone: a retrospective study of 11 cases. Hum Pathol 1995;26:1215-1220.
2. Antonescu CR, Argani P, Erlandson RA, et al: Skeletal and extraskeletal myxoid chondrosarcoma: A comparative clinicopathologic, ultrastructural, and molecular study. Cancer 1998;83:1504-1521.
3. Brody RI, Ueda T, Hamelin A, et al: Molecular analysis of fusion of EWS to an orphan nuclear receptor gene in extraskeletal myxoid chondrosarcoma. Am J Pathol 1997;150:1049-1058.
4. Enzinger FM, Shiraki M: Extraskeletal myxoid chondrosarcoma: an analysis of 34 cases. Hum Pathol 1972;3:421-435.
5. Goh YW, Spagnolo DV, Platten M, et al: Extraskeletal myxoid chondrosarcoma: a light microscopic, immunohistochemical, ultrastructural and immuno-ultrastructural study indicating neuroendocrine differentiation. Histopathology 2001;39:514-524.
6. Jambhekar NA, Baraniya J, Baruah R, et al: Extraskeletal myxoid chondrosarcoma: clinicopathologic, histochemical and immunohistochemical study of 10 cases. Int J Surg Pathol 1997;5:77-82.
7. Meis-Kindblom JM, Bergh P, Gunterberg B, et al: Extraskeletal myxoid chondrosarcoma: a reappraisal of its morphologic spectrum and prognostic factors based on 117 cases. Am J Surg Pathol 1999;23:636-650.
8. Saleh G, Evans HL, Ro JY, Ayala AG: Extraskeletal myxoid chondrosarcoma: a clinicopathologic study of ten patients with long term follow-up. Cancer 1992;70:2827-2830.
9. Sciot R, Dal Cin P, Fletcher C, et al: t(9;22)(q22-31;q11-12) is a constant marker of extraskeletal myxoid chondrosarcoma: evaluation of three cases. Mod Pathol 1995;8:765-768.

Mesenchymal Chondrosarcomas

1. Bagachi M, Husain N, Goel MM, et al: Extraskeletal mesenchymal chondrosarcoma of orbit. Cancer 1993;72:2224-2226.
2. Granter SR, Renshaw AA, Fletcher CDM, et al: CD99 reactivity in mesenchymal chondrosarcoma. Hum Pathol 1996;27:1273-1276.
3. Jacobs JL, Merriam JC, Chadburn A, et al: Mesenchymal chondrosarcoma of the orbit: report of three new cases and review of the literature. Cancer 1994;73:399-405.
4. Kransdorf MJ, Meis JM: Extraskeletal osseous and cartilaginous tumors of the extremities. Radiographics 1993;13:853-884.
5. Nakashima Y, Unni KK, Shives TC, et al: Mesenchymal chondrosarcoma of bone and soft tissue: a review of 111 cases. Cancer 1986;57:2444-2453.
6. Rushing J, Armonda RA, Ansari Q, et al: Mesenchymal chondrosarcoma: a clinicopathologic and flow cytometric study of 13 cases presenting in the central nervous system. Cancer 1996;77:1884-1891.

Aneurysmal Cyst of Soft Tissue

1. Lopez-Barea F, Rodriguez-Peralto JL, Burgos-Lizaldez E, et al: Primary aneurysmal cyst of soft tissue. Report of a case with ultrastructural and MRI studies. Virchows Arch 1996;428:125-129.
2. Nielsen GP, Fletcher CDM, Smith MA, et al: Soft tissue aneurysmal bone cyst. A clinicopathologic study of five cases. Am J Surg Pathol 2002;26:64-69.
3. Petrik PK, Findlay JM, Sherlock RA: Aneurysmal cyst, bone type, primary in an artery. Am J Surg Pathol 1993;17:1062-1066.
4. Rodriguez Peralto JL, Lopez-Barea F, Sanchez-Herrera S, et al: Primary aneurysmal cyst of soft tissues (extraosseous aneurysmal cyst). Am J Surg Pathol 1994;18:632-636.
5. Shannon P, Bedard Y, Bell R, et al: Aneurysmal cyst of soft tissue: Report of a case with serial magnetic resonance imaging and biopsy. Hum Pathol 1997;28:255-257.

12

Tumors of Synovial Tissue

G. Petur Nielsen · John X. O'Connell

TENOSYNOVIAL GIANT CELL TUMOR
- Pigmented Villonodular Synovitis
- Localized Giant Cell Tumor of Tendon Sheath
- Hemosiderotic Synovitis
- Villous Lipomatous Proliferation of Synovial Membrane (Lipoma Arborescens)
- Fibroma of Tendon Sheath
- Primary Synovial Chondromatosis
- Loose Bodies
- Malignant Tumors of the Joint

MALIGNANT TENOSYNOVIAL GIANT CELL TUMOR
- Synovial Reaction to Loosened Joint Arthroplasties

The synovium is one of the more recent phylogenetic developments of the vertebrate locomotor system, with the first synovial joints appearing in the piscine jaw of ancestors of the modern lungfish. Embryologically, synovium is derived from specialized mesoderm termed *interzonal mesenchyme*, which differentiates from the primitive mesenchyme that lies between and connects the developing mobile cartilaginous anlage of the skeleton (Figure 12-1). In a specific sequence controlled genetically, the mesenchyme around the joint cavity subsequently cavitates, and forms the joint space and synovial membrane. The synovium helps generate synovial fluid, which nourishes the articular cartilage and helps reduce the friction associated with articulation. It also has the capacity to remove small particles from the joint space. Tumors of the synovium can be divided into those that are primary or arise de novo within the joint and those that are secondary and access the joint by invading from neighboring bones and soft tissues or by spreading from distant sites via the vascular system. Primary joint neoplasms are the more common tumor and tend to recapitulate the phenotype of tissues that normally construct the joint, namely, synovium, fat, blood vessels, fibrous tissue, and cartilage. Regardless of the histologic type, the benign variants greatly outnumber their malignant counterparts, and as a group, these tumors tend to develop in the synovium, not the other periarticular structures.

Normal Anatomy

The synovial intima is composed of two to three layers of specialized connective tissue cells named *synoviocytes* that form the lining of joints, tendons, and bursae. These cells overlay loose connective tissue that contains variable elements of fat, collagen, and blood vessels. By light microscopy, quiescent synoviocytes are relatively indistinct, appearing as flattened oval dark staining nuclei with indistinct cytoplasmic borders; however, when they are stimulated, as in reaction to some form of injury, they enlarge and acquire abundant eosinophilic cytoplasm and have a more epithelioid morphology (Figure 12-2).

Ultrastructurally, the cells lining the luminal aspect of the synovial cavity have ovoid nuclei, inconspicuous nucleoli, and long cytoplasmic processes that radiate in a tendril-like fashion from the cell body. The cytoplasmic processes contain flattened endoplasmic reticulum, ribosomes, a well-developed Golgi apparatus, and numerous subplasmalemmal pinocytotic vesicles. Although the processes interdigitate extensively, cell junctions are not present. These cells have traditionally been termed B cells. The so-called type A cells lack cytoplasmic processes, but they have short filopodia. The A cells have a similar complement of cytoplasmic organelles as the B cells, as well as harbor occasional lysosomes. Transitional forms between A and B cells are also present. The synovial cells adhere directly to the underlying connective tissue; no basement membrane is present. This absence of basement membrane facilitates the transport of material into and out of the synovial fluid (Figure 12-3).

Immunohistochemically, synoviocytes stain positively for vimentin and may express CD68 (KP1). However, they are negative for cytokeratin, S-100 protein, actins, desmin, CD34, and leukocyte common antigen.

TENOSYNOVIAL GIANT CELL TUMOR

Based on the growth characteristic, tenosynovial giant cell tumor can be divided into two categories, *localized* (giant cell tumor of tendon sheath [GCTTS]) and *diffuse*

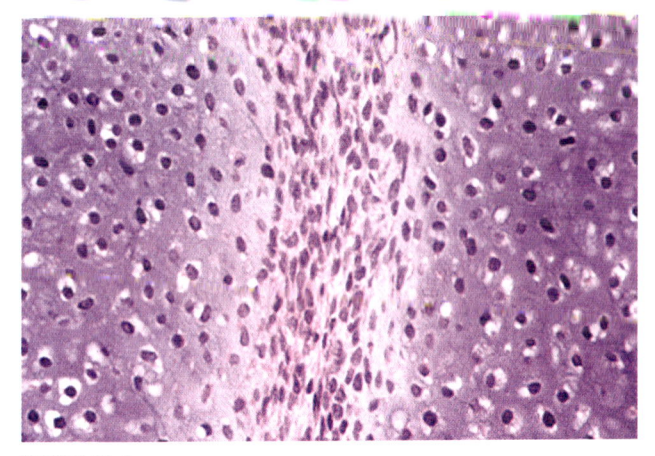

FIGURE 12-1
Interzonal mesenchyma connecting cartilaginous anlage of the skeleton.

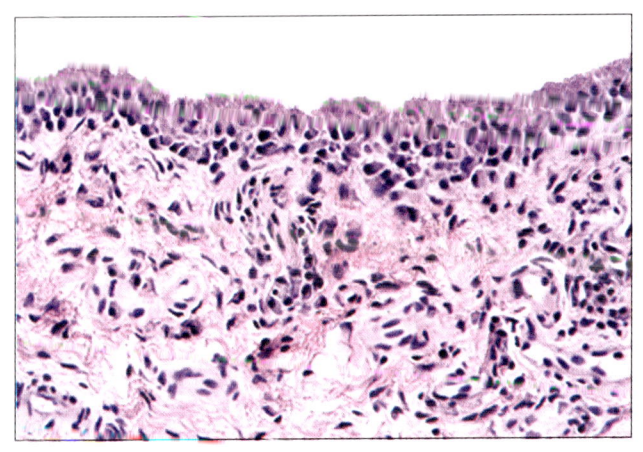

FIGURE 12-2
Normal synoviocytes overlying loose connective tissue.

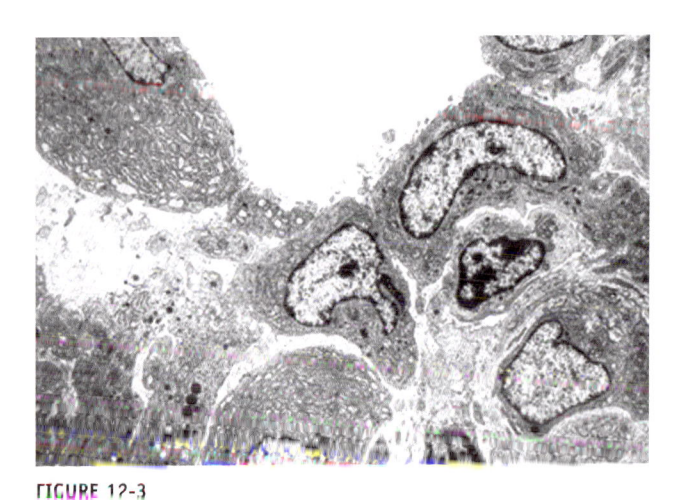

FIGURE 12-3
Electron microscopy.
Synoviocytes adhere directly to the underlying connective tissue without any basement membrane.

(pigmented villonodular synovitis [PVNS]). The localized one forms a discrete nodule and primarily affects the tenosynovium of the hand, whereas the diffuse form diffusely involves the synovium, usually of large weight-bearing joints. These two tumors are closely related to one another and are thought to recapitulate synoviocytes (hence the old term *synovioma*). Once considered a reactive process, possibly in response to repeated hemorrhage, many tenosynovial giant cell tumors have now been shown to result from a translocation between chromosomes 1p13 and 2q35 in which the gene encoding colony-stimulating factor-1 (CSF1) is fused to collagen VI α-3 *(COL6A3)* gene. Consequently, overexpression of CSF1 exists in the neoplastic cells, which account for only 2% to 16% of the cells in mass. The remaining cells largely represent non-neoplastic inflammatory cells that are recruited into the tumor because they contain the receptor for CSF. This phenomenon has been termed a *landscape effect* and is also observed in certain types of lymphomas.

PIGMENTED VILLONODULAR SYNOVITIS

PVNS produces widespread thickening of the synovium. Any synovial-lined structure may be affected, although the large joints, especially the knee, are most commonly involved, followed by the hip, ankle, and foot. Rare locations include the temporomandibular joint and the posterior element of the spine. Extra-articular involvement is uncommon and usually arises in tendon sheaths proximal to the ankle and wrist, and produces a periarticular soft tissue mass. Bursal involvement is rare, but when it does occur, it usually involves popliteal and iliopectineal bursa and the bursa anserina.

CLINICAL FEATURES

PVNS affects male and female individuals equally and has its greatest incidence in the second to fourth decades of life. PVNS is slow growing and typically produces pain, swelling, or limitation of movement of the affected joint. Bilateral or involvement of separate joints has infrequently been reported.

RADIOLOGIC FEATURES

Plain radiographs are often normal or show only a soft tissue density. Computed tomography (CT) scans and magnetic resonance imaging (MRI) may be helpful in that they can demonstrate the extent of the tumor and

CHAPTER 12 Tumors of Synovial Tissue

presence of intralesional lipid and iron (hemosiderin). A minority of tumors erode into adjacent bones, in which case multiple well-marginated, subchondral, cyst-like lucencies or pressure erosions are seen (Figures 12-4 and 12-5).

PATHOLOGIC FEATURES

GROSS FINDINGS

PVNS forms a diffuse villous and nodular red–brown thickening of the synovium and contains finger-like excrescences admixed with 0.5- to 2.0-cm round nodules. Scattered areas of grossly uninvolved synovium are invariable present. On cross section, the tumor is solid, rusty brown and yellow with white gray foci (Figures 12-6 and 12-7).

MICROSCOPIC FINDINGS

The synovium has a prominent papillary, villous, and nodular architecture. The preexisting synoviocytes overlie sheet-like proliferation of mononuclear cells, multinucleated osteoclast-like giant cells, and lipid or hemosiderin-rich cells. It is the mononuclear cells that are thought to be the neoplastic cells (Figure 12-8). The

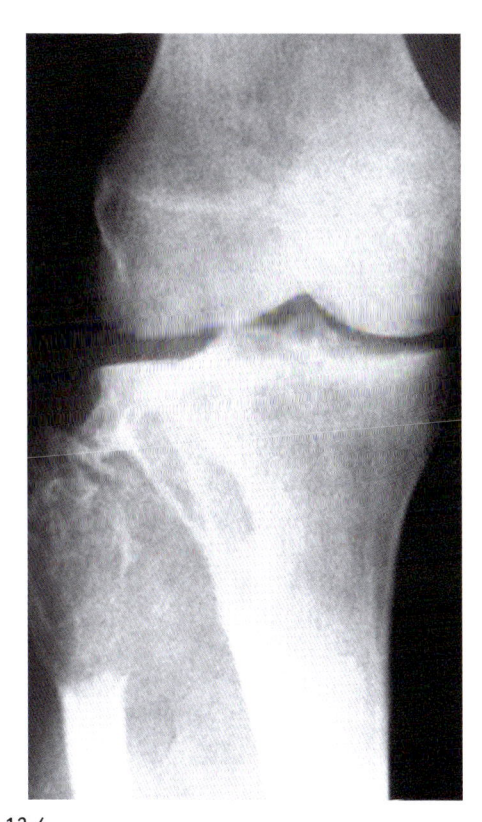

FIGURE 12-5
Intra-articular pigmented villonodular synovitis (PVNS).
Gross photo showing diffuse nodularity and discoloration of the synovium.

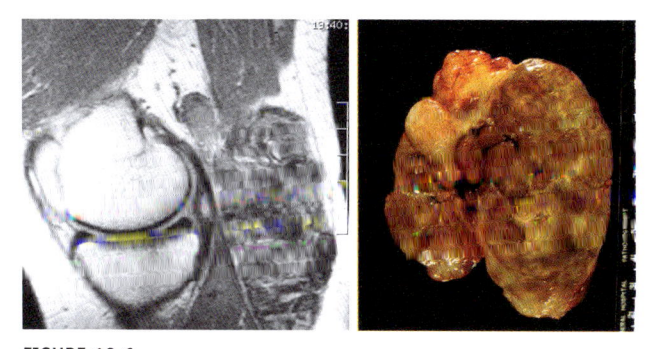

FIGURE 12-6
Pigmented villonodular synovitis.
Magnetic resonance imaging and gross picture of a pigmented villonodular synovitis involving the knee joint with extension into a Baker's cyst. On cross section, it is has the characteristic brown, fibrous, and yellow areas similar to giant cell tumor of tendon sheath (see Figure 12-9).

FIGURE 12-4
Pigmented villonodular synovitis (PVNS).
Plain radiograph showing destructive changes of fibula and tibia from a PVNS arising in the tibiofibular joint.

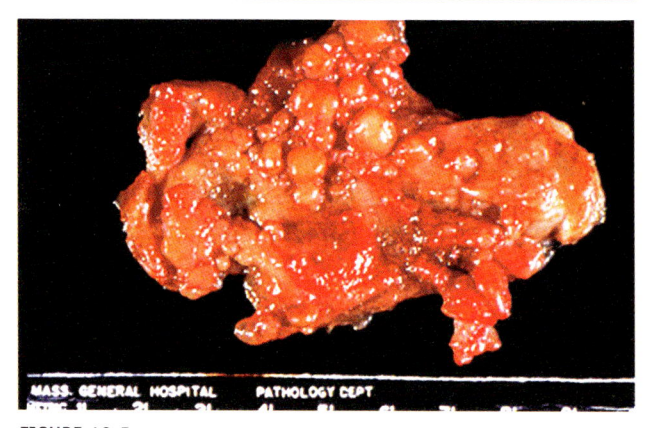

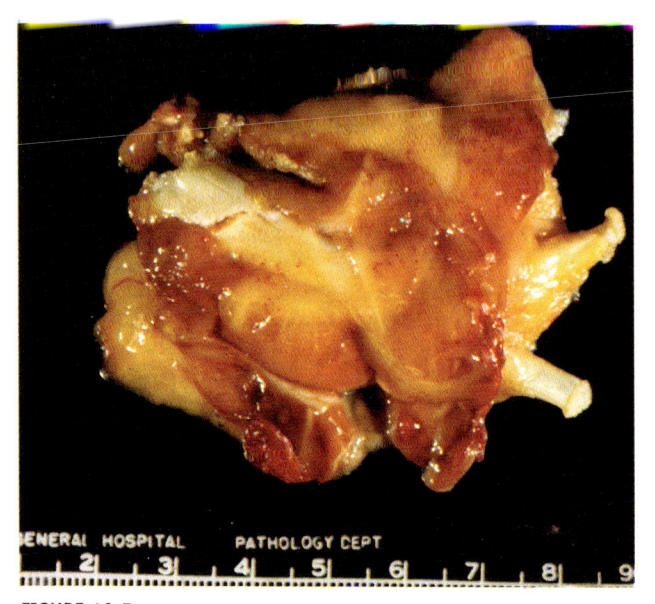

FIGURE 12-7
Extra-articular pigmented villonodular synovitis involving tenosynovium.

PIGMENTED VILLONODULAR SYNOVITIS—FACT SHEET

Definition
- Proliferative disorder of the synovial lining of joints that results in diffuse papillary and nodular thickening of the synovium

Incidence and Location
- Any synovial joint may be affected; most commonly, PVNS affects the knee joint

Morbidity and Mortality
- PVNS is a benign condition that does not metastasize

Sex, Race, and Age Distribution
- Male and female sexes are affected with equal frequency
- Most common in the second through fourth decades of life

Clinical Features
- Symptoms are related to mechanical disruption of the affected joint; typically, pain, swelling, and limitation of movement; rarely, PVNS may result in erosion of one or more of the bones comprising the articulation

Radiologic Features
- Plain radiographs may show soft tissue mass or bone erosion if present
- MRI accurately defines the extent of the lesion and is able to positively identify lipid and iron deposits that are characteristically present

Prognosis and Treatment
- Treatment is primarily surgical excision
- Low-dose radiation therapy may be used in cases refractory to surgery
- Local recurrence rates after surgical excision are high (> 50%) because of the diffuse involvement of the synovial membrane that makes complete excision difficult

PIGMENTED VILLONODULAR SYNOVITIS—PATHOLOGIC FEATURES

Gross Findings
- Diffuse thickening of the synovial membrane with villous-like excrescences and nodules up to 2.0 cm
- Golden yellow to dark brown

Microscopic Findings
- Intact enlarged cuboidal surface synovial cells
- Underlying sheets and nodules of epithelioid cells, multinucleated osteoclast-like giant cells, lipid-rich cells, and lymphocytes
- Hemosiderin granules within deeper located mononuclear cells
- Mitoses usually less than 6/10 hpf
- Relatively scant intercellular hyalinized collagen

Immunohistochemical Features
- The mononuclear cells demonstrate a mixed histiocyte and fibroblastic/myofibroblastic immunophenotype (CD68, smooth muscle actin (SMA) positive)
- The giant cells stain intensely and strongly for CD68

Differential Diagnosis
- Localized GCTTS (extra-articular)
- Localized nodular synovitis (intra-articular)
- Giant cell tumor of bone with extraosseous extension
- Lipoma arborescens
- Rhabdomyosarcoma (when strongly desmin positive and arising in an extra-articular location)
- Acral myxoinflammatory fibroblastic sarcoma (can involve or arise from synovium)
- Hemosiderotic synovitis

---

mononuclear cells are round or polygonal and have eosinophilic cytoplasm and frequently eccentric nuclei. The osteoclast-like giant cells are not as numerous as in giant cell tumor of tendon sheath and the collagenous or hyalinized matrix are usually less prominent. The mononuclear cells may demonstrate mild nuclear pleomorphism and prominent nucleoli. Mitotic counts rarely exceed 5 per 10 high-power fields (hpf). Necrosis is rare, and when present, it is usually of the infarct type. The surface synoviocytes are hyperplastic and may contain phagocytized hemosiderin, mimicking hemosiderotic synovitis.

PROGNOSIS AND TREATMENT

PVNS is treated by surgical excision, however, the diffuse involvement of the synovium makes complete excision difficult, resulting in a high local recurrence rate (> 50%). PVNS that is refractory to repeated surgical excisions has been managed by low-dose radiation therapy in some cases.

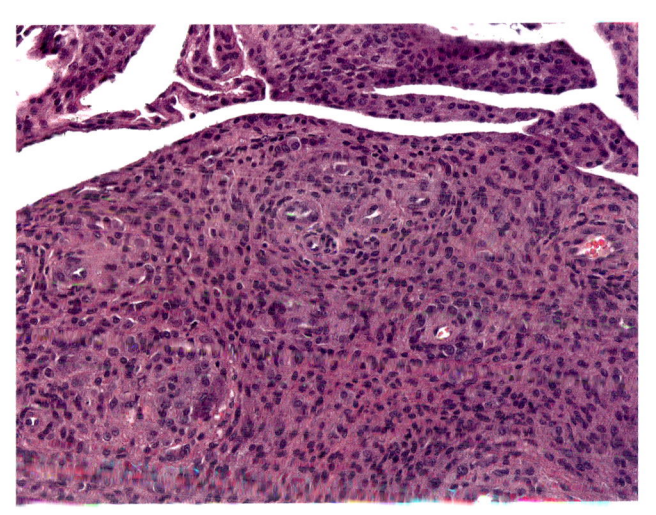

FIGURE 12-8
Pigmented villonodular synovitis.
Microscopically, the tumor cells diffusely infiltrate the subsynovial connective tissue. Otherwise, the morphology is identical to giant cell tumor of tendon sheath.

LOCALIZED GIANT CELL TUMOR OF TENDON SHEATH

Localized GCTTS contains the same cell population as PVNS, but unlike PVNS, it has a tendency to arise in extra-articular locations and grow as a well-defined nodule.

CLINICAL FEATURES

GCTTS may occur at any age but is usually diagnosed in patients between 30 and 50 years of age, and is more common in women. It may arise in any synovial sheath; however, those of the hands are preferentially affected, usually close to the interphalangeal joint. In fact, GCTTS is the most common soft tissue tumor of the hand. The tumor is slow growing and produces a firm nodule that is usually less than 2.0 cm in diameter.

RADIOLOGIC FEATURES

GCTTS appears as a circumscribed soft tissue mass that may be associated with bony erosions of the adjacent bone. The erosions are well defined and have sclerotic margins, and are due to the direct pressure of the lesion on the underlying bone (Figure 12-9).

PATHOLOGIC FEATURES

GROSS FINDINGS

GCTTS is well circumscribed and lobulated. They are usually small, and on cross sections are gray-tan with brown and yellow areas, depending on the amount of hemosiderin and lipid-laden macrophages (Figure 12-10).

MICROSCOPIC FINDINGS

GCTTS is well demarcated, encapsulated, and attached to the adjacent tendon sheath. Fibrous septae transverse the tumor, giving it a lobulated appearance (Figure 12-11). In general, GCTTS contains less hemosiderin than PVNS and more extracellular collagen. GCTTS is basically identical to the individual lobules of PVNS; however, the amount of sclerosis and number of mononuclear cells, osteoclast-type giant cells, hemosiderin, and foamy macrophages vary (see Figures 12-11A, 12-12, 12-13, and 12-14). Mitoses and vascular invasion may be seen, but these features usually do not indicate a more aggressive behavior.

PROGNOSIS AND TREATMENT

The tumor is treated with surgical excision, preferentially with a rim of normal tissue. The local recurrence rate is approximately 10% to 20%.

ANCILLARY STUDIES

IMMUNOHISTOCHEMISTRY

Immunohistochemically, PVNS and GCTTS exhibit a similar staining reaction as normal and reactive synovium; that is, the mononuclear cells and multinucleated osteoclast-like giant cells stain positively with

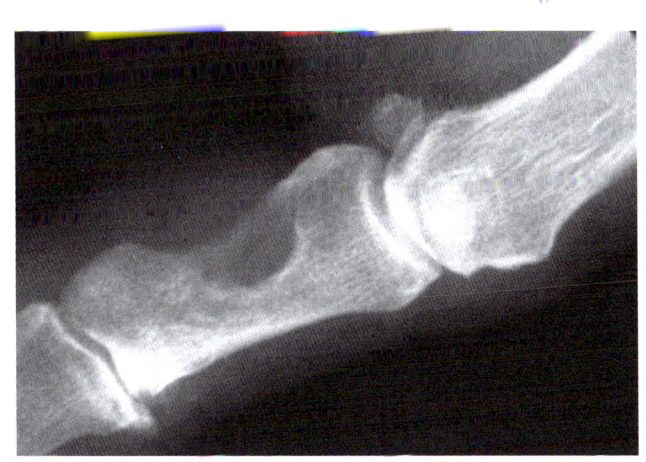

FIGURE 12-9
Giant cell tumor of tendon sheath.
Plain radiograph shows a soft tissue mass and scalloping of the underlying bone.

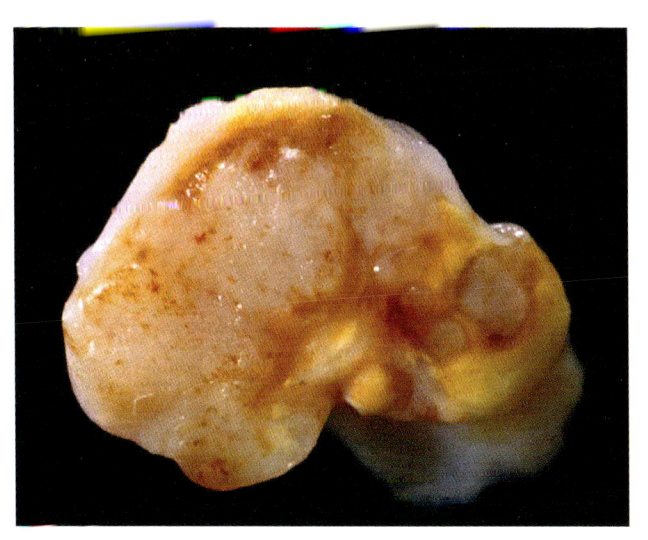

FIGURE 12-10
Giant cell tumor of tendon sheath.
Cross sections showing brown, gray, and yellow areas.

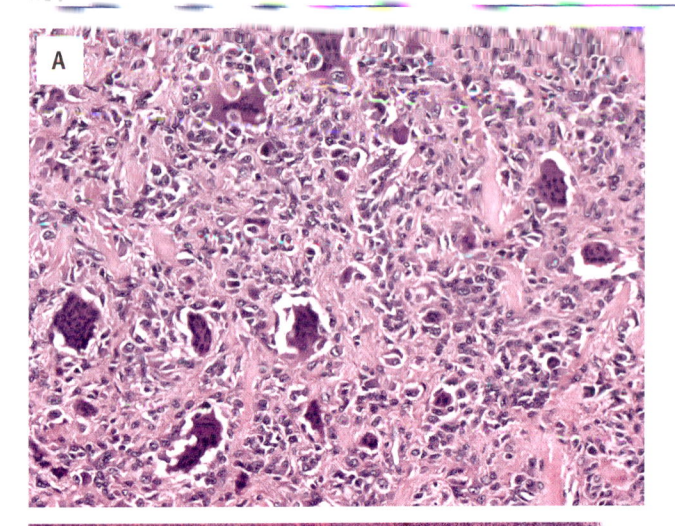

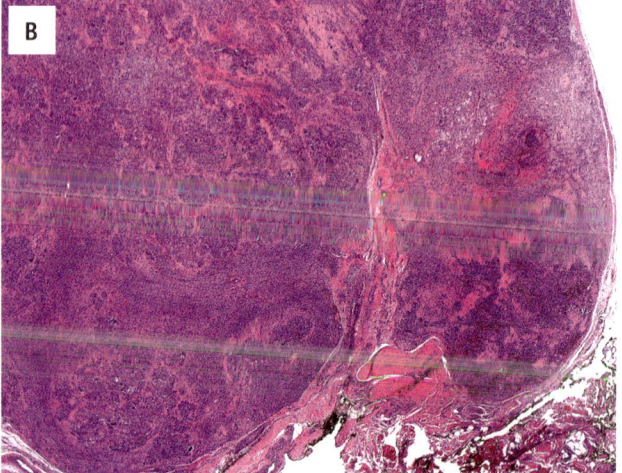

FIGURE 12-11

A, B, Giant cell tumor of tendon sheath, lobulated and composed of an admixture of osteoclast-type giant cells and mononuclear cells in a collagenous stroma.

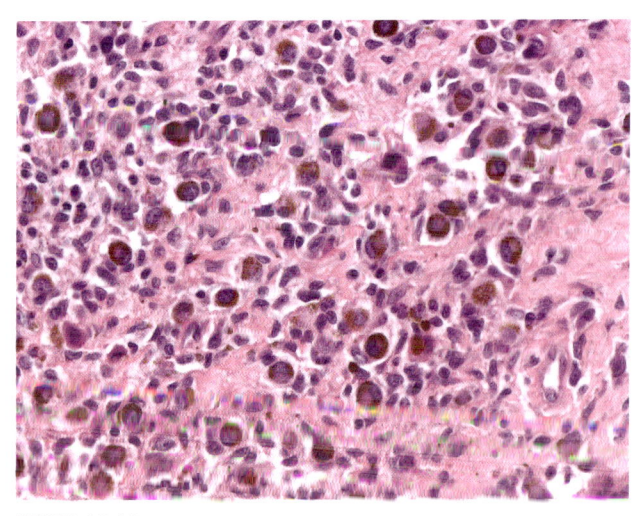

FIGURE 12-12

Giant cell tumor of tendon sheath. Hemosiderin deposition is seen in the mononuclear cells often peripherally in the cytoplasm.

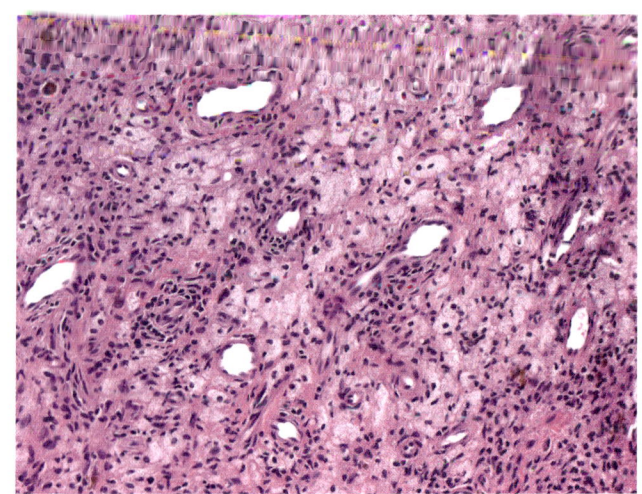

FIGURE 12-13

Giant cell tumor of tendon sheath showing aggregates of foamy histiocytes.

antibodies to CD68 and vimentin. Some tumors may also show staining for desmin that sometimes may be strong and diffuse (Figure 12-15). The mononuclear cells have also been shown to stain for Ham56, PGM1, and MAC387.

DIFFERENTIAL DIAGNOSIS

The distinction between GCTTS and PVNS can be difficult to make on a small biopsy, and the histologic features have to be correlated with the clinical or radiographic findings. The diagnosis can also be difficult in cases where the needle biopsy samples areas of sclerosis or

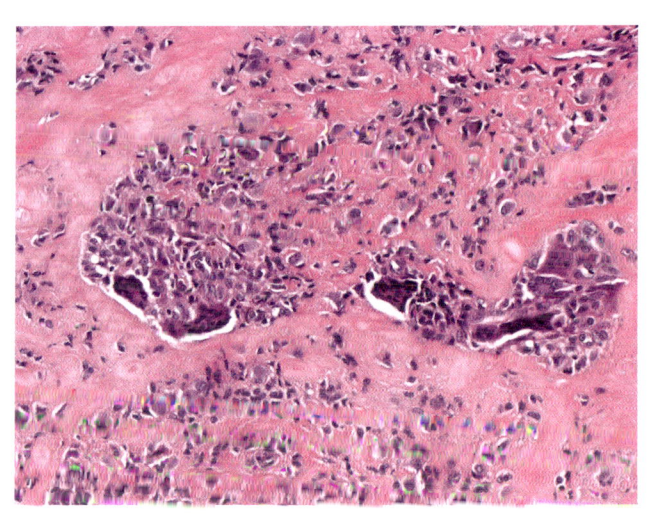

FIGURE 12-14

Giant cell tumor of tendon sheath showing extensive sclerosis.

CHAPTER 12 Tumors of Synovial Tissue

LOCALIZED GIANT CELL TUMOR OF TENDON SHEATH—FACT SHEET

Definition
›› Localized proliferation of extra-articular synovial cells that results in a well-circumscribed soft tissue tumor

Incidence and Location
›› GCTTS is uncommon
›› Any tendon sheath may be affected; by far the most common site is the tendon sheaths of the digits of the hand

Morbidity and Mortality
›› Benign condition

Sex, Race, and Age Distribution
›› More common in female than male individuals
›› Adults in fourth through sixth decades of life most commonly affected

Clinical Features
›› Typically presents as a painless or minimally painful lump in the hand or digits
›› Usually measures less than 3.0 cm in maximum size

Radiologic Features
›› Because of its location in the hands and digits, GCTTS may result in bone erosion of the adjacent small bones
›› Erosions are usually well defined

Prognosis and Treatment
›› Simple local excision usually results in cure
›› Recurrence occurs in 10% to 20% of patients after incomplete excision

LOCALIZED GIANT CELL TUMOR OF TENDON SHEATH—PATHOLOGIC FEATURES

Gross Findings
›› A well-circumscribed, usually firm nodule
›› Variegated cut surface with tan, brown, and yellow areas

Microscopic Findings
›› Similar to the nodules of PVNS (see earlier)
›› Usually no villous projections
›› Smaller amounts of hemosiderin compared with PVNS
›› Often more hyalinized collagen present that may outline individual cells or groups of cells
›› Rare cases have few giant cells and are recognized based on the mononuclear cellular component and architecture

Immunohistochemical Findings
›› Same as PVNS (see earlier)

Differential Diagnosis
›› PVNS, diffuse GCTTS (histologically identical to the localized type but characterized by larger size and less well-defined growth characteristics)
›› Diffuse GCTTS demonstrates many of the gross and microscopic features of PVNS albeit in an extra-articular location

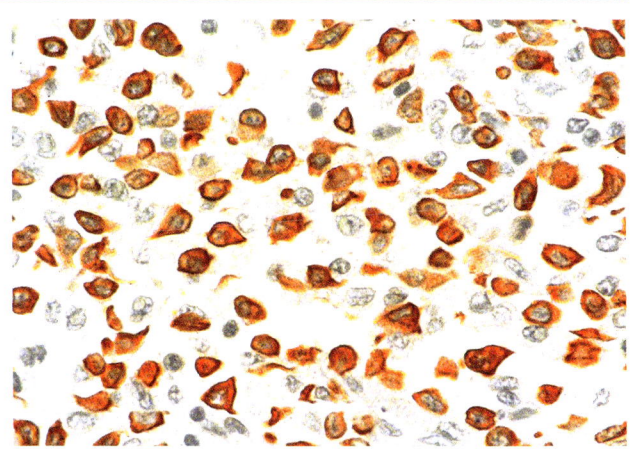

FIGURE 12-15
Pigmented villonodular synovitis.
Immunohistochemical stain for desmin shows numerous positive cells.

cellular areas devoid of multinucleated giant cells. A diffuse desmin stain of the mononuclear cells may suggest the diagnosis of a rhabdomyosarcoma. Also, acral myxoinflammatory fibroblastic sarcoma can have a similar growth pattern as PVNS, however, a closer inspection shows a different histologic appearance.

HEMOSIDEROTIC SYNOVITIS

Hemosiderotic synovitis develops as a result of chronic intra-articular hemorrhage. This usually occurs in patients with hemophilia who are predisposed to hemarthrosis, especially of the knees, elbows, and ankles. Hemosiderotic synovitis is rarely caused by a synovial hemangioma. An as indistinguishable from hemosiderotic synovitis may also be seen in synovium affected by PVNS.

CLINICAL FEATURES

Patients with hemosiderotic synovitis report pain and stiffness of the involved joint. This is almost invariably caused by secondary osteoarthritis, developing in association with chronic intra-articular hemorrhage.

RADIOLOGIC FEATURES

Radiologic features that may be seen are juxtaepiphyseal osteoporosis and subperiosteal hemorrhage. During arthroscopy or surgery, diffuse discoloration of the synovium is present.

PATHOLOGIC FEATURES

GROSS FINDINGS

The synovium shows a diffuse brown–rust discoloration. In early hemosiderotic synovitis, fine villous projections are present, but the larger nodules and thickened fronds of PVNS do not occur. In the later stages, after chronic repeated hemorrhage, the synovium becomes thickened and opaque because of intrasynovial and subsynovial fibrosis. The adjacent articular cartilage may show a greenish-black discoloration.

MICROSCOPIC FINDINGS

The synovium is hyperplastic and contains yellow–brown hemosiderin granules. Within the subsynovial connective tissue, hemosiderin-laden macrophages are present, often in association with small blood vessels (Figure 12-16). Sheets of mononuclear synovial cells, lipid-laden cells, or multinucleated osteoclast-like giant cells as seen in PVNS are not a feature of hemosiderotic synovitis. The articular cartilage may show hemosiderin deposition within chondrocyte lacunae and necrosis of the chondrocytes.

PROGNOSIS AND TREATMENT

Hemosiderotic synovitis is often associated with severe degenerative changes of the articular cartilage, and hence the treatment revolves around surgical and conservative management of the arthritis.

DIFFERENTIAL DIAGNOSIS

A subset of hemosiderotic synovitis is caused by *intrasynovial hemangiomas*. These are rare tumors. Any joint may be affected, although the knee joint is the most frequent site. Intrasynovial hemangiomas are localized tumors that occur within the subsynovial supporting connective tissue. Patients describe pain or a mass, which diminishes in size when the affected limb is elevated to allow the blood to drain out of the lesion. Radiographic studies show a vague soft tissue swelling. These hemangiomas are classified as capillary, cavernous, and arteriovenous types. Occasionally, thrombosed large vascular spaces with papillary endothelial hyperplasia (Masson's lesion) may be found. Intra-articular hemorrhage may cause acute pain and swelling of the involved joint and, if repeated, may produce the histologic features of hemosiderotic synovitis. The hemorrhage is rarely as progressive as that in the bleeding diatheses, and accelerated osteoarthritis is usually not a feature. Synovial

HEMOSIDEROTIC SYNOVITIS—FACT SHEET

Definition
» Proliferation of synovial tissue accompanied by variable fibrosis caused by repeated episodes of intra-articular hemorrhage

Incidence and Location
» Hemosiderotic synovitis occurs most commonly in the knee joints of patients with hemophilia
» Other causes include recurrent joint trauma or bleeding from synovial hemangioma
» Condition is rare

Morbidity and Mortality
» Condition is benign, but when progressive and long standing, it results in severe degenerative arthritis of the affected joint

Sex, Race, and Age Distribution
» Predominantly affects male sex
» Usually occurs in the second through fourth decades of life

Clinical Features
» Acute hemarthrosis presents with abrupt painful swollen joints
» Chronic hemosiderosis results in chronic pain, swelling, and limitation in joint movement

Prognosis and Treatment
» Prognosis is determined by the treatment of the underlying condition that is resulting in the recurrent hemorrhage
» Chronic hemosiderotic synovitis may require joint replacement surgery because of the severe osteoarthritis

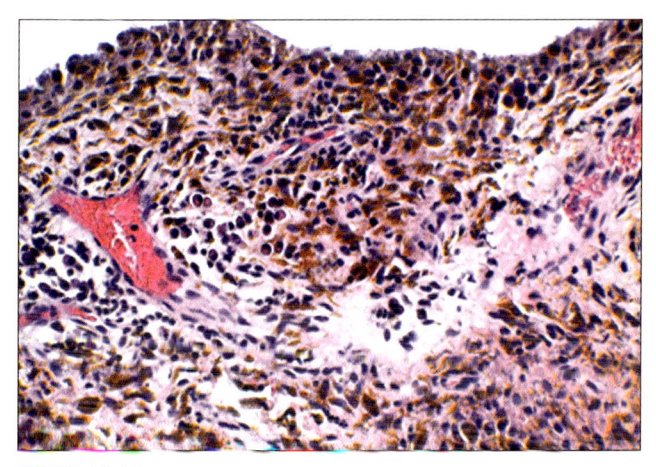

FIGURE 12-16
Hemosiderotic synovitis showing hemosiderin deposition within synoviocytes and subsynovial tissue.

hemangiomas are managed by local excision and recurrence is uncommon. *Ochronosis* (when fragments of articular cartilage become embedded in the synovium) and *metallosis* (secondary to prosthesis) can cause diffuse discoloration of the synovium.

CHAPTER 12 Tumors of Synovial Tissue

HEMOSIDEROTIC SYNOVITIS—PATHOLOGIC FEATURES

Gross Findings

- Brown–rust discoloration of the synovial membrane
- Early cases have thin villous excrescences that extend into the joint space
- Established/chronic cases have a flattened atrophic appearance

Microscopic Findings

- Surface synovial cells are plump cuboidal and have abundant readily found intracytoplasmic hemosiderin granules
- Hemosiderin-laden macrophages are present with the subsynovial connective tissue
- Nodular thickening of the synovial membrane in the manner that occurs in PVNS does not occur in hemosiderotic synovitis

Differential Diagnosis

- PVNS
- Synovial hemangioma
- Metallosis
- Ochronosis

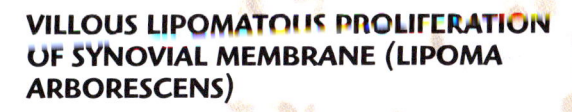

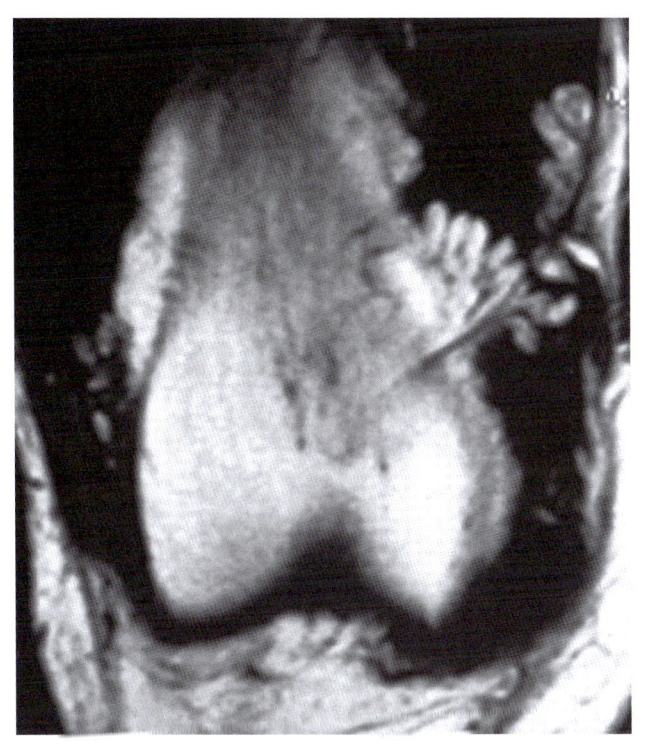

FIGURE 12-17
Lipoma arborescens.
Magnetic resonance image showing diffuse fatty infiltration of the synovium.

VILLOUS LIPOMATOUS PROLIFERATION OF SYNOVIAL MEMBRANE (LIPOMA ARBORESCENS)

Lipoma arborescens, which is characterized by diffuse fatty infiltration of the subsynovial connective tissue, is one of the rarest of the synovial proliferative lesions.

CLINICAL FEATURES

Lipoma arborescens preferentially affects adult men and presents as a slowly developing swelling of the affected joint. Any synovial-lined joint may be involved, although once more the knee is the favored site. Lipoma arborescens is thought to be non-neoplastic, probably a reactive process, and to represent an excessive accumulation of fat in the subsynovial space secondary to trauma or chronic synovitis.

RADIOLOGIC FEATURES

Plain radiograph usually shows joint fullness and osteoarthritic changes. CT and MRI show a low-density thickening of the synovium that has the characteristic features of fat (Figure 12-17).

PATHOLOGIC FEATURES

GROSS FINDINGS

The entire synovium has a bright yellow nodular and papillary appearance. On cross section, the subsynovial connective tissue is replaced by yellow adipose tissue (Figure 12-18).

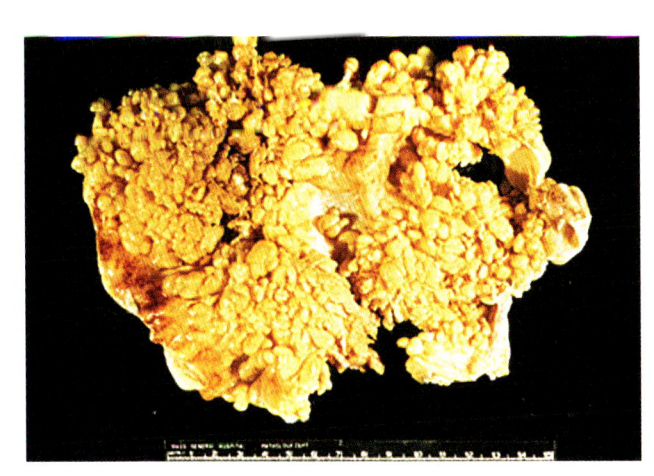

FIGURE 12-18
Lipoma arborescens.
Grossly, the synovium is yellow nodular and papillary.

LIPOMA ARBORESCENS—FACT SHEET

Definition
- Diffuse infiltration of the synovial connective tissue by mature fat, resulting in a villous and nodular thickening of the synovial membrane

Incidence and Location
- Lipoma arborescens is an extremely uncommon condition
- Any synovial joint may be affected, although the knee is by far the most commonly involved

Morbidity and Mortality
- Condition is benign but is often associated with coexistent osteoarthritis

Sex, Race, and Age Distribution
- Adult men predominantly affected

Clinical Features
- Patients have swelling, pain, or both

Radiologic Features
- Plain films show osteoarthritis of the involved joint
- CT and MRI show thickening of the synovial membrane with expansion by tissue with fat signal characteristics

Prognosis and Treatment
- Synovectomy is the treatment of choice
- Recurrence is uncommon

LIPOMA ARBORESCENS—PATHOLOGIC FEATURES

Gross Findings
- The synovial membrane is diffusely papillary/nodular and bright yellow

Microscopic Findings
- Surface synovial cells are enlarged cuboidal and reactive in appearance
- The subsynovial tissue is massively infiltrated by mature adipocytes
- Increased deposits of hemosiderin or inflammatory cells are not present

Differential Diagnosis
- Nonspecific focal accumulation of fat in synovial connective tissue in osteoarthritic joints
- PVNS
- Rheumatoid arthritis
- Hoffa's disease (a condition of irritation, inflammation, and hyperplasia of the synovial lining in regions where fat is normally present, such as adjacent to the patella or patellar ligament)

MICROSCOPIC FINDINGS

The subsynovial connective tissue is thickened and replaced by mature adipocytes. The surface synovial cells typically appear reactive and epithelioid. Chronic inflammation is invariably seen admixed with the fat (Figure 12-19).

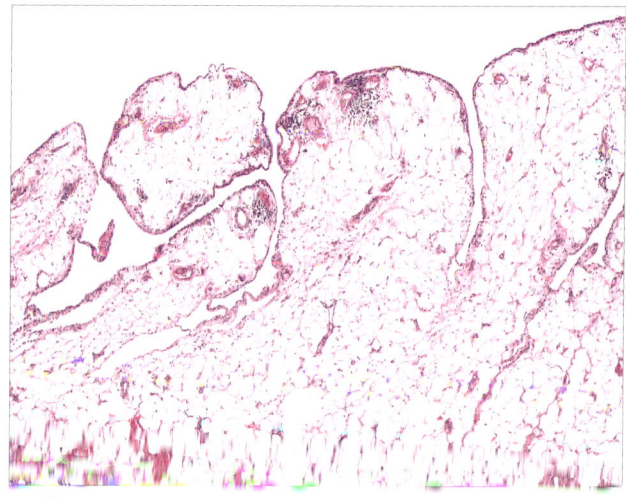

FIGURE 12-19
Lipoma arborescens.
Microscopically, the subsynovial connective tissue is replaced by mature adipocytes.

PROGNOSIS AND TREATMENT

Treatment of lipoma arborescens is synovectomy or treatment of the underlying condition. Recurrence is rare.

DIFFERENTIAL DIAGNOSIS

Minor degrees of fatty infiltration of the subsynovial space are normal in certain parts of the synovial membrane, particularly in the knee joint, and similarly, slight nodular thickening is a nonspecific finding in the synovium of osteoarthritic joints. Although in a single microscopic field these may simulate lipoma arborescens, this diagnosis should be suggested only when there is an appropriate diffuse villous and nodular involvement of the synovium.

FIBROMA OF TENDON SHEATH

CLINICAL FEATURES

Fibroma of tendon sheath (FTS) is an uncommon benign lesion that clinically mimics GCTTS. It usually arises from the tendon sheaths of the flexor surfaces of the distal extremities, and approximately 70% of cases involve the hand or fingers. Large joints are rarely affected. It usually arises in adults 20 to 50 years of age and is more

CHAPTER 12 Tumors of Synovial Tissue

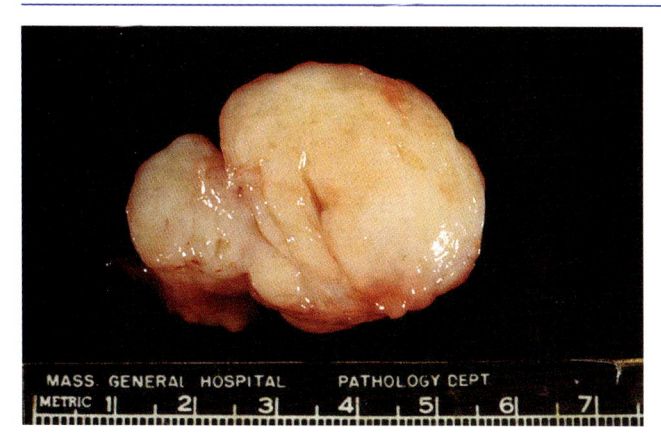

FIGURE 12-20
Fibroma of tendon sheath.
Grossly, it is uniform and tan-yellow with characteristic *clefting*.

common in male than female individuals. The patients have a slow-growing lesion, usually less than 2 cm in diameter. Recent cytogenetic studies suggest that FTS is neoplastic and not a reactive process.

RADIOLOGIC FEATURES

Radiographically, soft tissue fullness is present, the underlying bone rarely shows any changes. MRI and CT show a well-circumscribed lesion.

PATHOLOGIC FEATURES

GROSS FINDINGS

Grossly, FTS is nodular or multinodular with intervening *cleft*-like spaces, has a rubbery consistency, and has a tan-white cut surface (Figure 12-20).

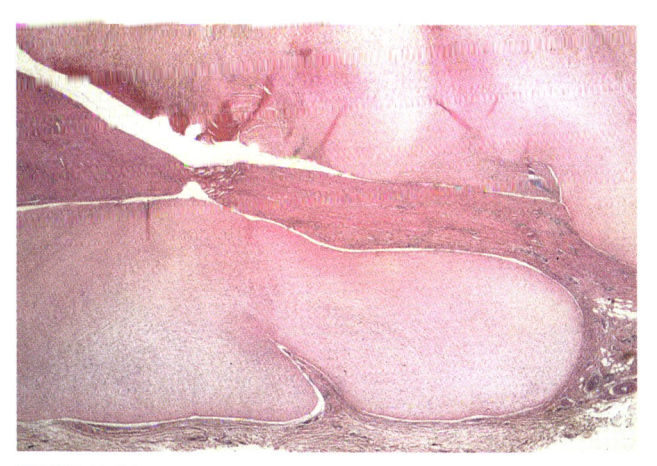

FIGURE 12-21
Fibroma of tendon sheath.
Low-power view shows that the tumor is hypocellular and collagenous with clefting or pseudovascular spaces.

FIBROMA OF TENDON SHEATH—FACT SHEET

Definition
- A circumscribed, benign, soft tissue tumor arising in tendon sheaths

Incidence and Location
- Uncommon lesion
- Most lesions arise in the tendon sheaths of the digits of the hand

Morbidity and Mortality
- Benign condition that has limited growth potential

Sex, Race, and Age Distribution
- Most common in adult men

Clinical Features
- Patients describe a slowly enlarging mass, usually involving the flexor surfaces of the digits of the hands

Prognosis and Treatment
- Simple excision results in cure; recurrence is rare

MICROSCOPIC FINDINGS

FTS is multinodular with clefts between lobules (Figure 12-21). These lobules are composed of spindle and stellate fibroblasts embedded in a collagenous and sometimes myxoid stroma (Figure 12-22). Cellular areas mimicking nodular fasciitis may be present especially in the early phase of the lesion. Prominent cytologic degenerative cytologic atypia is seen in the rare examples of the *pleomorphic fibroma* of the tendon sheath.

PROGNOSIS AND TREATMENT

Treatment of FTS is surgical excision, which is associated with an approximately 20% local recurrence rate.

FIBROMA OF TENDON SHEATH—PATHOLOGIC FEATURES

Gross Findings
- Small (usually less than 3.0 cm), tan, rubbery nodular tumor

Microscopic Findings
- Variable cellularity
- Most lesions are hypocellular and richly collagenous
- A minority can show hypercellularity with a tissue culture-like appearance resembling nodular fasciitis
- Aggregated nodules of tissue are often separated from adjacent nodules by cleft-like spaces that may show a synovial lining

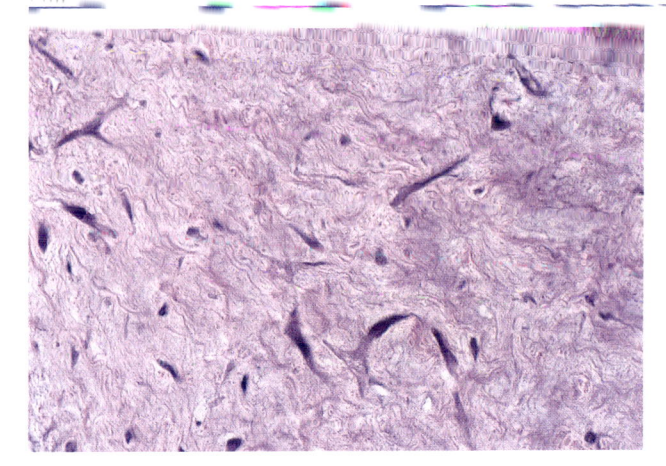

FIGURE 12-22
Fibroma of tendon sheath.
High-power view shows bland spindle and stellate cells embedded in abundant extracellular collagenous matrix.

ANCILLARY STUDIES

Immunohistochemical findings and electron microscopy show features to suggest fibroblastic and myofibroblastic differentiation.

PRIMARY SYNOVIAL CHONDROMATOSIS

Synovial chondromatosis is an uncommon condition characterized by the formation of multiple nodules of hyaline cartilage within the subsynovial connective tissue. If the nodules undergo enchondral ossification, then the term *synovial osteochondromatosis* is appropriate. It is unclear whether the proliferating cartilage is metaplastic or neoplastic; however, recent cytogenetic abnormalities involving chromosome 6 support a neoplastic process.

CLINICAL FEATURES

Synovial chondromatosis affects patients in a wide age range from childhood to late adult life without any sex preference. Patients report pain and swelling related to the involved joint. Any synovial-lined structure can be affected, although the large joints are the most frequent location; the knee is affected in more than 50% of cases. Other common sites include the hip, elbow, shoulder, and ankle. Infrequently, it can affect the small joints of the hand and foot, and the temporomandibular joint. Outside the joints, the term *extra-articular synovial chondromatosis* is used.

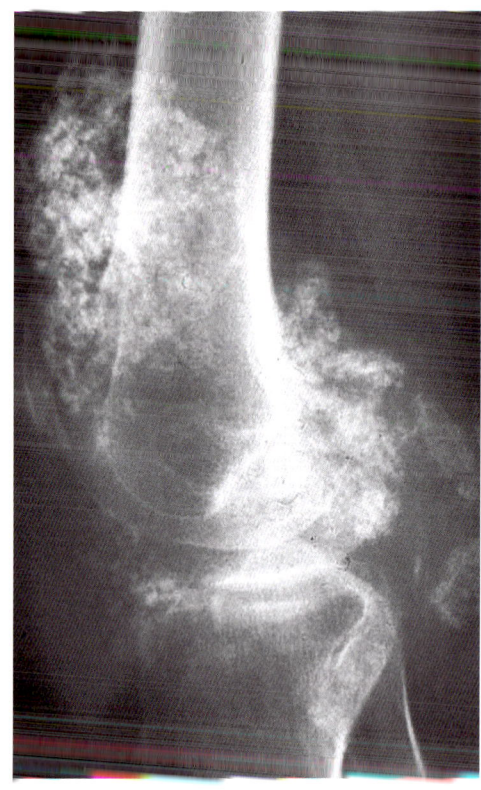

FIGURE 12-23
Synovial chondromatosis.
Intra-articular synovial chondromatosis showing numerous mineralized nodules within the joint.

RADIOLOGIC FEATURES

Plain radiographic findings depend on whether the nodules are mineralized or ossified, in which case multiple nodules are seen within joints tendon sheaths (Figures 12-23 and 12-24). CT and MRI scans are also helpful in diagnosing the lesion, in addition to identifying the intra-articular locations of the lesion and its anatomic extent.

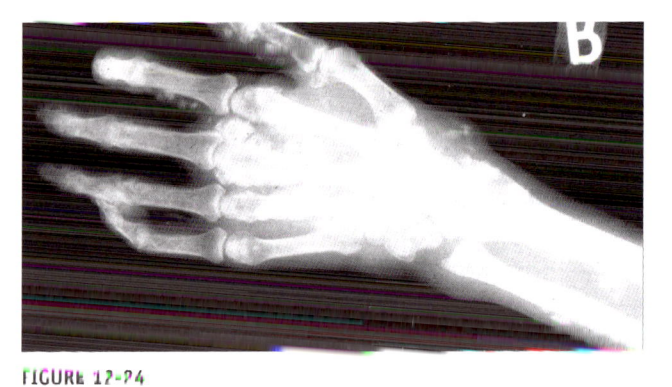

FIGURE 12-24
Synovial chondromatosis.
Extra-articular synovial chondromatosis involving the synovium of the hand and arm.

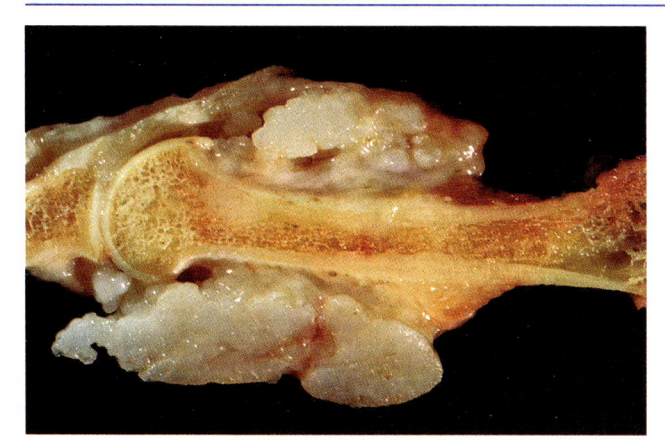

CHAPTER 12 Tumors of Synovial Tissue

FIGURE 12-25
Synovial chondromatosis.
Multiple gray, glistening nodules involving extra-articular synovium.

PATHOLOGIC FEATURES

GROSS FINDINGS

Synovial chondromatosis appears as numerous glistening gray–blue nodules within the synovial membrane (Figure 12-25). The nodules range from 2.0 mm to more than 1.0 cm in size and are firm on cut section. They often demonstrate chalky yellow regions that represent calcification or foci of enchondral ossification, in which case the term *synovial osteochondromatosis* is used.

MICROSCOPIC FINDINGS

Nodules of hypercellular hyaline cartilage are embedded within the subsynovial connective tissue (Figure 12-26). Individual nodules are circumscribed, round, and demonstrate greater cellularity than normal hyaline articular cartilage. Chondrocytes are typically clustered rather than being evenly distributed throughout the matrix (Figure 12-27). The individual cells exhibit

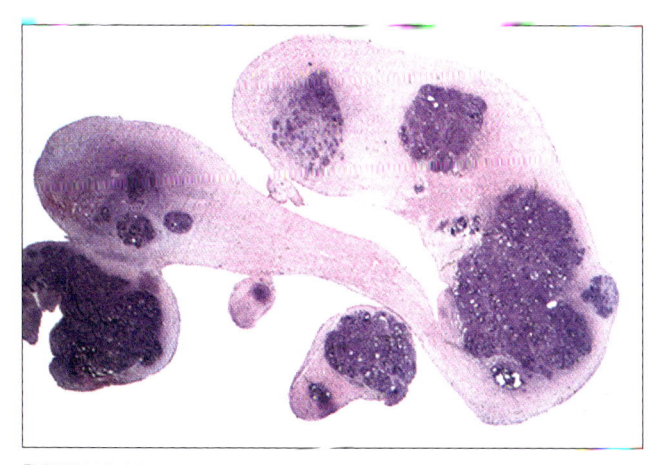

FIGURE 12-26
Synovial chondromatosis.
Multiple cartilaginous nodules involving the subsynovial connective tissue.

PRIMARY SYNOVIAL CHONDROMATOSIS—FACT SHEET

Definition
- Condition in which multiple benign nodules of hyaline cartilage develop in synovial membranes

Incidence and Location
- Condition is rare
- Any synovial lined joint may be affected
- Large joints such as the knee are most commonly involved; exceptionally, the condition may involve extra-articular synovial sheaths

Morbidity and Mortality
- Condition is benign; sarcomatous transformation may occur, but it is uncommon

Clinical History
- Patients describe pain and swelling of the affected joint
- Joint *locking* may also occur

Radiologic Features
- Plain radiographs may show typical cartilage-type calcifications if present
- CT and MRI accurately delineate the location and extent of the disease

Prognosis and Treatment
- Treatment is synovectomy
- After surgery, recurrence develops in approximately 15% of cases

---

PRIMARY SYNOVIAL CHONDROMATOSIS—PATHOLOGIC FEATURES

Gross Findings
- Numerous nodules of gray glistening cartilage embedded within the synovial membrane
- Nodules range in size from 0.2 to greater than 1.0 cm
- Chalky yellow calcified/ossified foci may be evident

Microscopic Findings
- The hyaline cartilage nodules exhibit "relative hypercellularity" and clustering of chondrocytes
- Individual chondrocytes demonstrate mild variability in nuclear size chromaticity
- Small nucleoli may be evident
- Mitotic figures are infrequent
- High-grade nuclear pleomorphism is not present

Differential Diagnosis
- Loose bodies
- Soft tissue/articular invasion by osseous chondrosarcoma
- Soft tissue chondrosarcoma

---

a considerable range in size. Most have pyknotic dark staining nuclei; however, many cells exhibit atypical features, including larger nuclei, dispersed chromatin, and visible nucleoli. Occasional mitoses may be found. The degree of cellularity and nuclear atypia found in synovial chondromatosis is, in most cases, equal to or

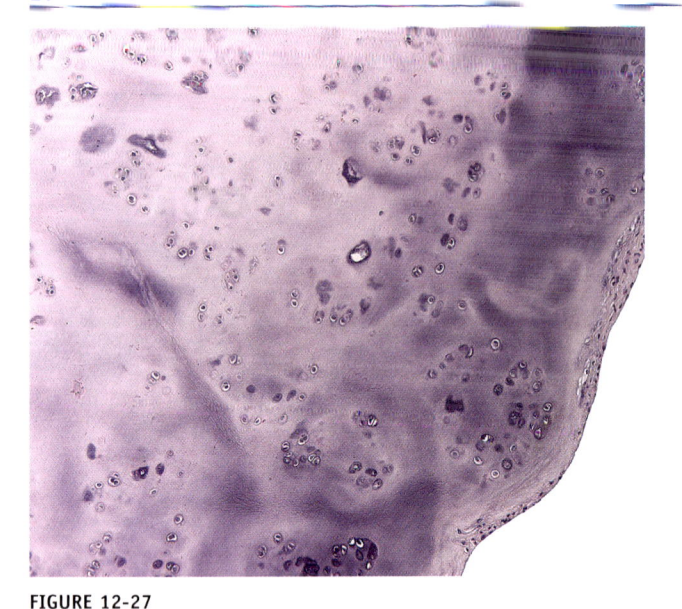

FIGURE 12-27
Synovial chondromatosis.
Clustering of chondrocytes is seen; synovial lining (bottom right) is present.

exceeds that seen in low- to intermediate-grade intraosseous chondrosarcoma. Hence, care must be taken not to overdiagnose malignancy in this setting. Knowledge of the radiographic and clinical features is, therefore, essential. Enchondral ossification, when present, proceeds from the periphery toward the center of the lobules (Figure 12-28).

PROGNOSIS AND TREATMENT

Synovial chondromatosis is managed by synovectomy of the involved joint. Recurrence develops in up to 15% of cases. Rare cases of malignant transformation have been reported.

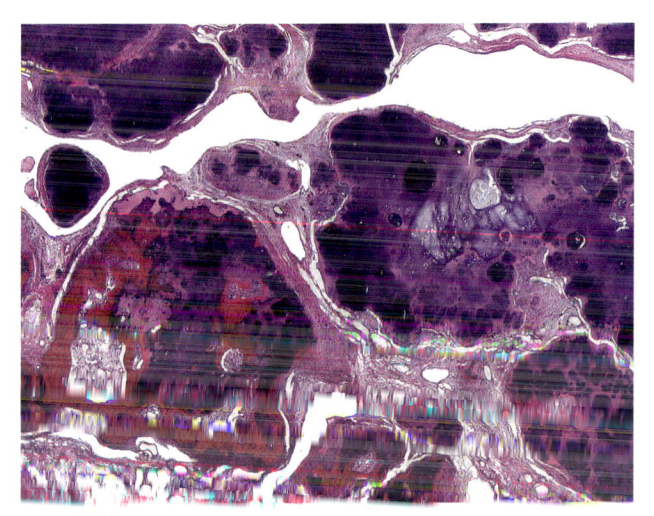

FIGURE 12-28
Synovial chondromatosis showing endochondral ossification.

LOOSE BODIES

Loose bodies or *joint mice* are generic terms for any free-floating structures within a joint cavity. They develop when intra-articular fragments of bone or hyaline articular cartilage come to lie free within the joint. Conditions resulting in loose body formation include idiopathic epiphyseal osteonecrosis, osteochondral fracture, and osteochondritis dissecans. The sloughed articular cartilage remains viable because it receives its nutrition from the synovial fluid, whereas the bone dies because of lack of blood supply. These fragments reside in the joint for some time, and its edges become round and smooth. Eventually, they become embedded in the synovium. Joint locking is the cardinal symptom of intra-articular loose bodies. Other symptoms include pain and swelling.

PATHOLOGIC FEATURES

GROSS FINDINGS

Loose bodies may be single or multiple, and often are larger than individual nodules of synovial chondromatosis, measuring in excess of 1.5 cm each (Figure 12-29). The external aspect of an individual loose body is hard, white, and typically nodular and bosselated. Sectioning the nodule sometimes demonstrates within its center the fragment that initiated the process surrounded by linear deposition of cartilage.

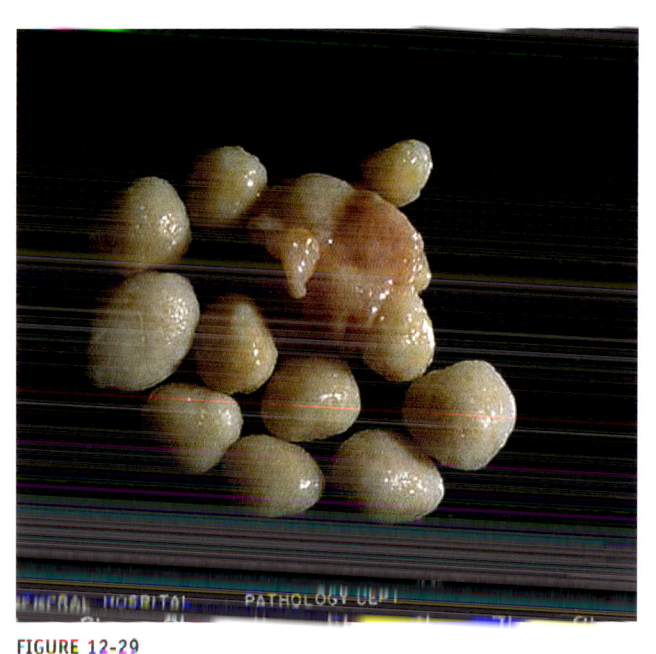

FIGURE 12-29
Loose bodies.
Numerous smooth and rounded loose bodies from the knee joint.

CHAPTER 12 Tumors of Synovial Tissue

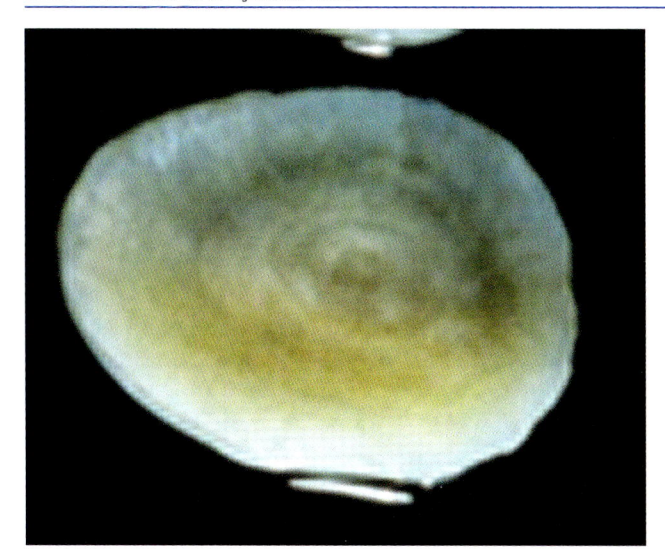

FIGURE 12-30
Loose body.
Cross section of a loose body shows the characteristic *cambium* layering.

MICROSCOPIC FINDINGS

After loose bodies become embedded in the synovium, they may either be resorbed or stimulate a proliferative response in which the loose body fragments serve as a nidus for the deposition of newly formed fibrocartilage and hyaline cartilage, which may undergo enchondral ossification. The newly formed cartilage and bone surround the loose bodies like a cambium layers of a tree (Figures 12-30 and 12-31). As the fragments become larger, the central portion can no longer be supplied by diffusion of synovial fluid and undergoes necrosis and becomes calcified. This explains the speckled and ring-like calcifications seen radiographically.

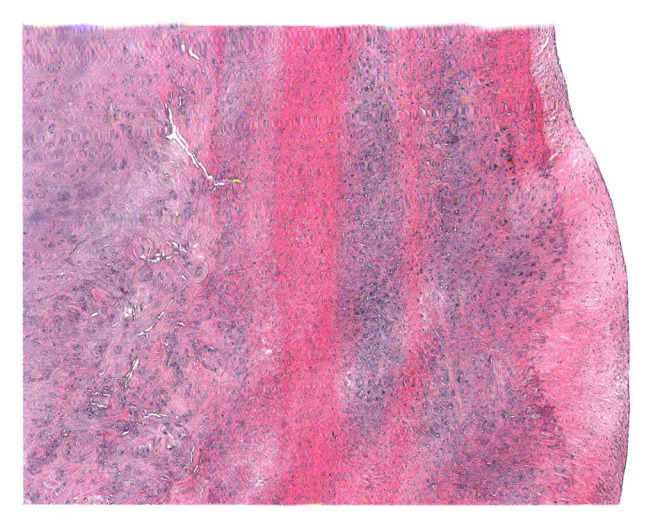

FIGURE 12-31
Loose body.
Cartilaginous nidus (top upper) surrounded by layers of fibrocartilage.

DIFFERENTIAL DIAGNOSIS

The main differential diagnosis of loose bodies includes synovial chondromatosis. In contrast with synovial chondromatosis, loose bodies are predominantly composed of reactive/metaplastic cartilage, which is usually nonlobular and exhibits features intermediate between hyaline cartilage and fibrocartilage. The matrix typically stains eosinophilic in hematoxylin and eosin sections, and exhibits a more uniform cellularity than primary synovial chondromatosis in addition to a distinctly laminar arrangement of cells and matrix. Loose bodies rarely demonstrate the range of chondrocyte pleomorphism, atypia, and mitotic activity that is a feature of synovial chondromatosis.

PROGNOSIS AND TREATMENT

Loose bodies are managed by local excision only; total synovectomy is not necessary. Recurrences are less common than primary synovial chondromatosis and depend on the underlying disease process.

LOOSE BODIES—FACT SHEET

Definition
- Condition in which one or more osteocartilaginous fragments come to reside either free within joint space or embedded within the synovial membrane

Incidence and Location
- The most commonly affected synovial joint is the knee

Morbidity and Mortality
- Condition is benign

Sex, Race, and Age Distribution
- Both sexes are affected equally; the condition is most common in adults

Clinical Features
- Patients report pain and/or swelling of the affected joint
- Because the fragments are mobile within the joint, locking may also occur
- Preexisting skeletal conditions that result in epiphyseal bone necrosis such as idiopathic epiphyseal osteonecrosis, osteochondritis dissecans, and osteochondral fracture may be present

Radiologic Features
- If the fragment is ossified or mineralized, it may be visible on plain radiographs

Prognosis and Treatment
- Treatment is surgical removal
- Recurrence may occur, particularly in the setting of one of the above listed conditions

LOOSE BODIES—PATHOLOGIC FINDINGS

Gross Findings
- Loose bodies that have become embedded in the synovium have a bosselated white bone-like appearance
- Nodules frequently are larger than 1.5 cm
- The synovial membranous layer is often indistinct and often is not grossly apparent when the specimen is received in the laboratory

Microscopic Findings
- The nodule is formed of concentric layers of moderately cellular fibrocartilage centered on piece of necrotic bone or hyaline articular cartilage

Differential Diagnosis
- Synovial chondromatosis

MALIGNANT TUMORS OF THE JOINT

CLINICAL FEATURES

Malignant tumors of joints are uncommon and are classified into primary and secondary types. Primary malignancies are virtually always sarcomas and usually arise within the synovium of large diarthrodial joints, especially the knee. Patients are adults who have chronic symptoms of pain, swelling, and effusion, and most of the tumors are either chondrosarcomas or synovial sarcomas. Rarely, other sarcomas originate within a joint such as intra-articular myxoinflammatory fibroblastic sarcoma, pleomorphic fibrosarcoma, synovial sarcoma, conventional chondrosarcoma, extraskeletal myxoid chondrosarcoma, and angiosarcoma. Secondary malignant tumors of joints, by definition, originate beyond the confines of the joint and most are sarcomas that extend from neighboring bones or surrounding soft tissues. Although synovial tissue is vascular, metastases or involvement of the synovium by carcinoma, lymphoma, or leukemia is relatively uncommon.

PATHOLOGIC FEATURES

Bona fide *chondrosarcomas* of synovium are rare; currently, less than 50 cases have been reported in the English language literature. In approximately 50% of cases, the chondrosarcoma arises in association with preexisting synovial chondromatosis. In patients who have preexisting synovial chondromatosis, the duration of symptoms is usually longstanding and, in some instances, may be present for as many as 25 years. Patients with chondrosarcoma of the joint are usually in their fifth to seventh decade of life, and chondrosarcoma has an equal sex distribution. The tumors are frequently large, being bigger than synovial chondromatosis, and more consistently present as a soft tissue mass. Bone destruction adjacent to the joint is a suspicious feature, although this may also be seen in minority of examples of synovial chondromatosis. Most chondrosarcomas arise in the knee joint, followed by the hip and elbow joints. Radiographic studies usually demonstrate a periarticular soft tissue mass that may have dense irregular or ring-like calcifications. Grossly, the involved joint is filled with one to many nodules of firm, opalescent, blue–white cartilage. Histologically, synovial chondrosarcomas exhibit diffuse hypercellularity and usually lack the clustering of chondrocytes that is typically seen in synovial chondromatosis. Nuclear atypia is usually prominent, with the chondrocytes nuclei being large, irregular, hyperchromatic, and contain prominent nucleoli. Multinucleated chondrocytes, some having three or more nuclei, are commonplace. Mitoses and myxoid change of the stroma are other frequent findings. An important indicator of malignancy is destructive invasion and permeation of the marrow of the adjacent bone. This is in contrast with synovial chondromatosis, which grows into bone with a *pushing* border. Treatment is usually surgical and may necessitate amputation. Chemotherapy may be given in high-grade lesions or those that have metastasized. Metastases occur in approximately one-third of patients, with the lung being the most common site for systemic spread.

MALIGNANT TENOSYNOVIAL GIANT CELL TUMOR

Primary malignant tenosynovial giant cell tumor or malignant transformation in a preexisting benign tumor is rare. One of the larger series is by Bertoni and coworkers, who reported eight cases of what they considered malignant tenosynovial giant cell tumor. Five tumors were primary and three secondary, arising in patients with a previous diagnosis of diffuse tenosynovial giant cell tumor. The histologic features of malignancy were a nodular, solid, infiltrative pattern; large, atypical plump, round, or oval cells with deep eosinophilic cytoplasm and indistinct borders; large nuclei with prominent nucleoli; and areas of necrosis. Four patients died with pulmonary metastasis.

SYNOVIAL REACTION TO LOOSENED JOINT ARTHROPLASTIES

Large Joint Detritic Synovitis

Large joint arthroplasty is one of the most common elective orthopedic surgical procedures performed today. Complications are few; however, because arthroplasties are being performed on younger and more physically active patients, an increased incidence of aseptic loosening of the prostheses has occurred. This is because the materials used in large joint reconstruction (i.e., polyethylene, metal alloys, and methyl methacrylate [bone cement]) do have a tendency to undergo mechanical failure over time, particularly with excessive use. The mechanical failure is usually manifested by progressive fragmentation of the components. This occurs at the interface between moving parts of the artificial joint or between host tissue and foreign material. The net result is that microscopic fragments of the arthroplasty components are extruded into the joint cavity where they elicit an inflammatory reaction. This is usually accompanied by osteolysis of the involved bones, producing clinical loosening of the arthroplasty. The cardinal symptom of loosened prostheses is progressive pain.

Detritic synovitis is the descriptive term applied to the constellation of changes seen in the synovium and soft tissue that surrounds these loose large joint arthroplasties. The most commonly involved joints are the hips and knees. Detritic synovitis presents as red–tan nodular thickening of the synovium. In a minority of cases, the synovium may be black because of the extensive deposition of metal debris.

In detritic synovitis, particles of synthetic material embedded within the synovium are associated with a histiocytic and foreign body giant cell reaction (Figures 12-32 and 12-33). The histiocytes are oval and rounded, and have abundant eosinophilic foamy to granular cytoplasm (Figure 12-34). Nuclei are central, round, and lack nucleoli. Mitoses are not seen. Three types of foreign material are recognizable. Methyl methacrylate (bone cement) is dissolved in tissue processing. It elicits a foreign body giant cell reaction and surrounds large oval and rounded defects, which appear empty but often contain fine yellow–green granules of refractile nonpolarizable barium (Figure 12-35). Needle-shaped fragments of *polyethylene* are also found within foreign body giant cells. These are typically small and may be overlooked without examining slides under polarized light (Figure 12-36). The *metal debris* is the most inconspicuous and, therefore, most easily overlooked of the foreign material, and is evenly dispersed as single fragments within the cytoplasm of histiocytes (Figure 12-37). Additional histologic findings include

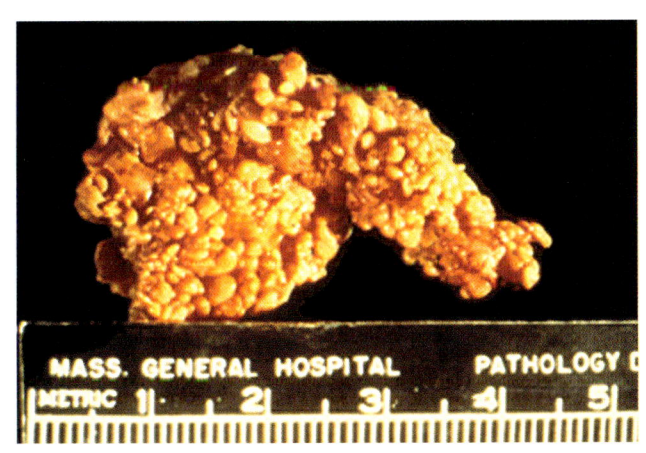

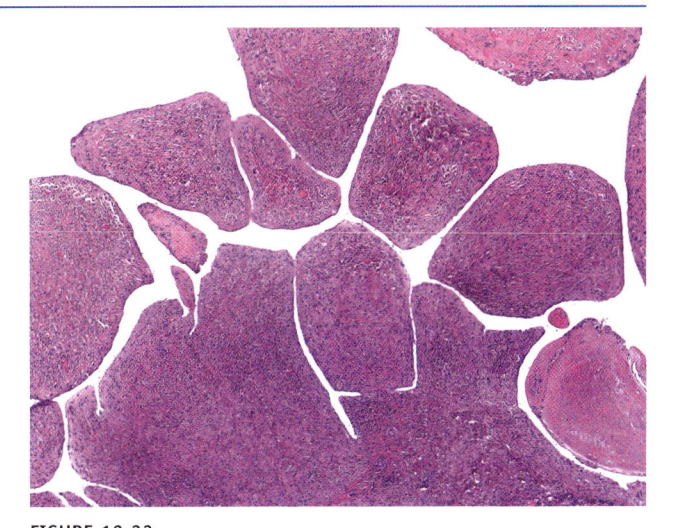

FIGURE 12-33
Low-power view showing diffuse histiocytic infiltrate of the subsynovial connective tissue.

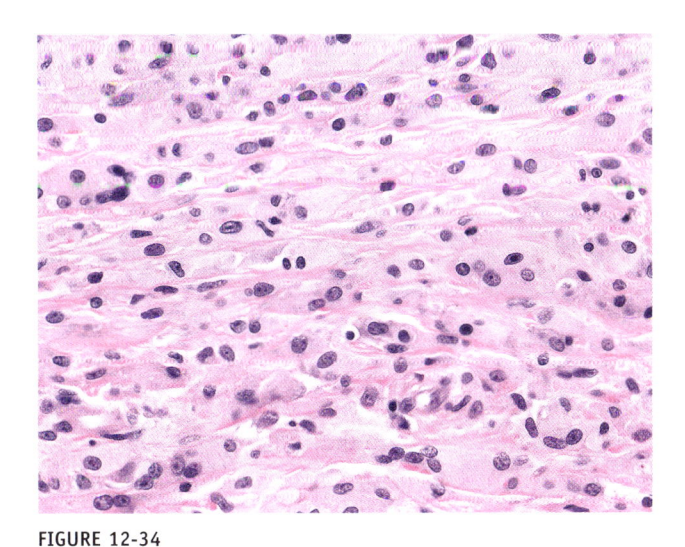

FIGURE 12-32
Detritic synovitis.
Diffuse nodular thickening of the synovium.

FIGURE 12-34
Detritic synovitis.
Diffuse histiocytic reaction to prosthetic material. The histiocytes have a granular, gray–blue cytoplasm.

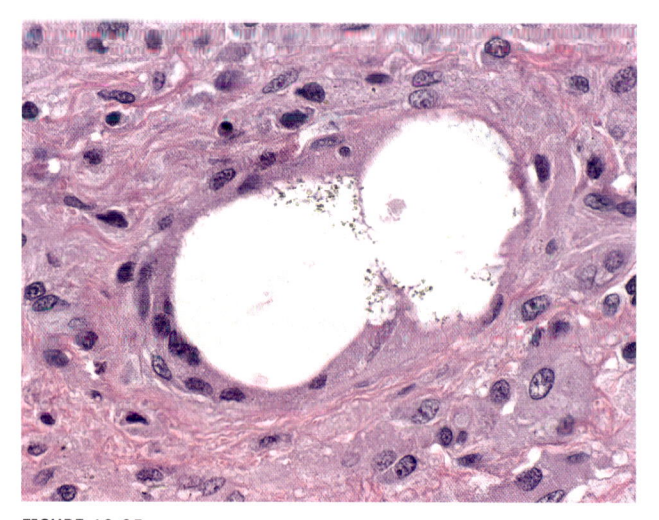

FIGURE 12-35
Detritic synovitis.
Giant cell reaction to methyl methacrylate. The methyl methacrylate is dissolved during processing, leaving behind the fine yellow barium granules.

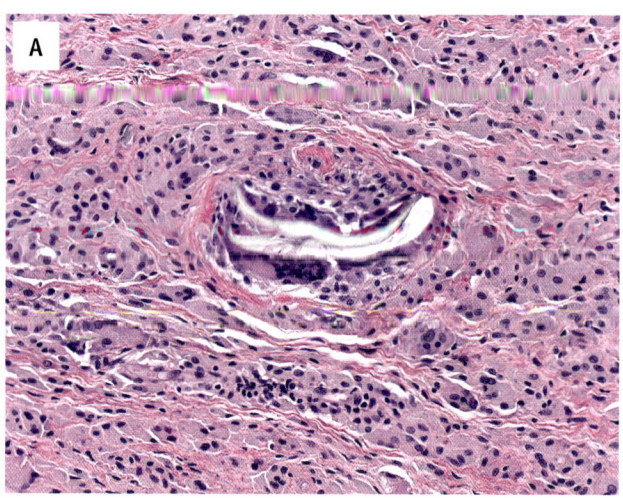

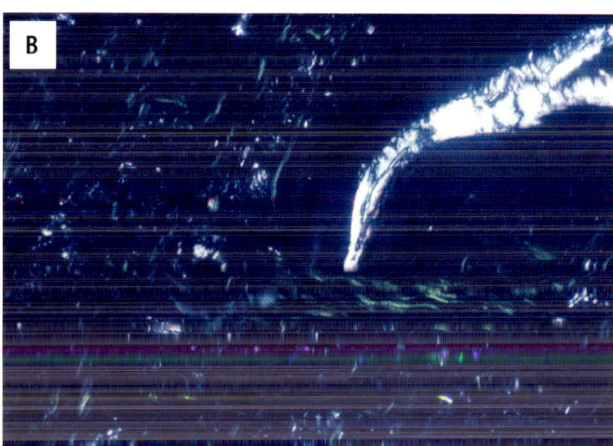

papillary fibrocartilaginous metaplasia of the synovial surface, sheets of coagulative necrosis without inflammation, aggregates of hemosiderin-laden macrophages, and in a minority of cases, reactive myofibroblastic proliferation that resembles nodular/proliferative fasciitis. The presence of stromal infiltrates of neutrophils is strongly correlated with bacterial infection surrounding the prosthesis. It is worth noting that particles of metal, polyethylene, and the typical histiocytic reaction that accompanies them can also be found in regional lymph nodes (Figure 12-38). These lymph nodes are often enlarged and may be suspicious for involvement by a malignant tumor. This can result in confusion at the time of staging procedures performed during treatment of pelvic malignancies, usually prostatectomy in male individuals and hysterectomy and/or oophorectomy in female individuals.

Detritic synovitis occurs on the background of loose large joint prostheses, and hence its management revolves around reconstruction of the affected joint. This is frequently troublesome because of the severe localized osteoporosis that usually accompanies loosening of the prosthesis.

Sarcoma arising in association with a metallic prosthesis or hardware is uncommon but is a recognized complication. The material used in these prostheses is generally considered to be nontoxic; however, some of the constituents have been shown to be potentially carcinogenic in animal studies. These sarcomas are of different types but are usually osteosarcoma or malignant fibrous histiocytoma, although a variety of other sarcomas have also been reported (Figure 12-39). In a study by Keel and colleagues on 12 cases, the patients ranged in age from 18 to 85 (mean, 55) years, and the time interval between the placement of hardware and diagnosis of sarcoma ranged from 2.5 to 33 (mean, 11) years. The patients described pain, swelling, or loosening of hardware, and were found to have a destructive bone or soft tissue mass radiographically. Of eight patients with follow-up, five died of disease. Although the possibility of a sarcoma arising in association with an implant is small,

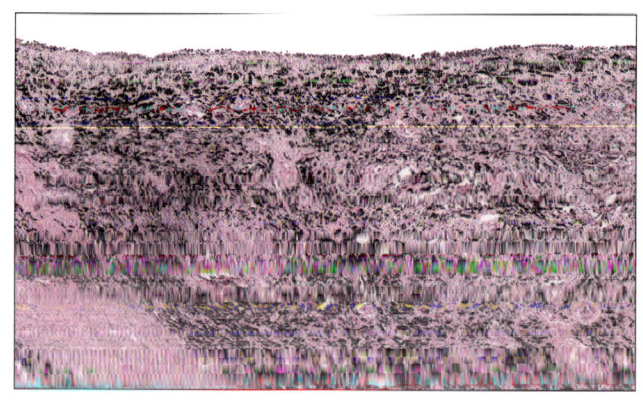

FIGURE 12-36
A, B, Detritic synovitis.
Histiocytic reaction to prosthetic material (A), with focal giant cell reaction to polarizable polyethylene fibers (B).

FIGURE 12-37
Draining lymph node of a prosthetic joint showing florid histiocytic reaction.

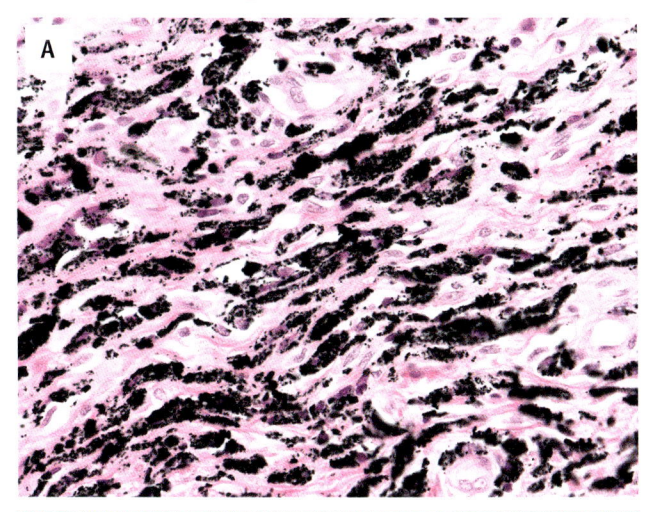

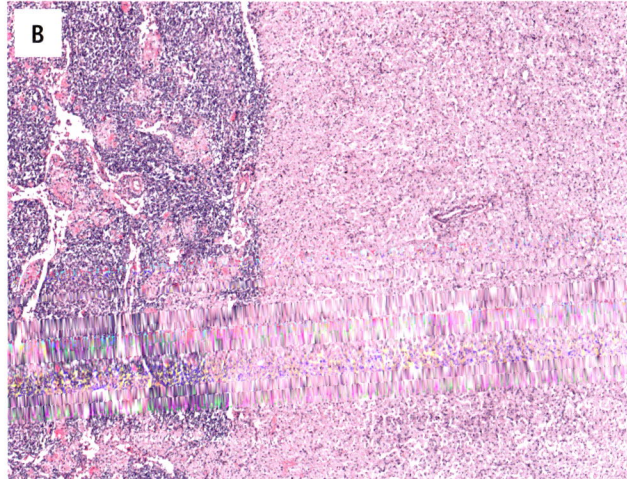

CHAPTER 12 Tumors of Synovial Tissue   273

FIGURE 12-38
A, B, Detritic synovitis.
Black metal particles are seen within synoviocytes and subsynovial connective tissue.

It should be considered when pain or other new findings develop in patients with metallic orthopedic hardware. One should, however, also be aware that destructive tumoral reaction *(tumoral detritic synovitis)* can occur around a prosthesis (Figure 12-40).

SMALL JOINT DETRITIC SYNOVITIS

The prostheses used to replace damaged small synovial joints such as those in the hands and feet are different from the ones that are used for large joint arthroplasty. Small joint prostheses are composed of silicone polymers. Silicone (dimethyl siloxane) is composed of carbon, oxygen, hydrogen, and silica. The solid silicone prostheses, which are often referred to by their proprietary name as *silastic prostheses,* have been used extensively for small joint reconstruction, and like their large joint counterparts, have for the most part been extremely successful in alleviating pain and dysfunction. Unfortunately, as

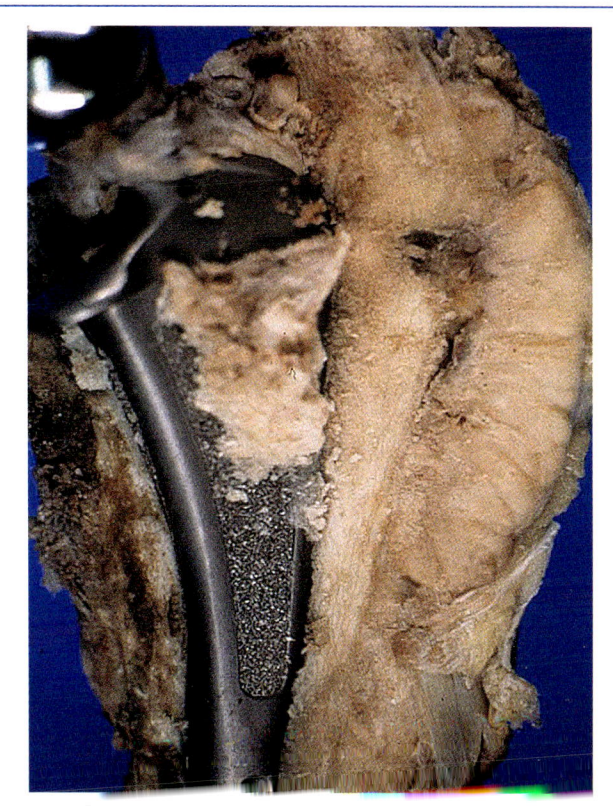

FIGURE 12-39
Sarcoma arising in association with a metal prosthesis.

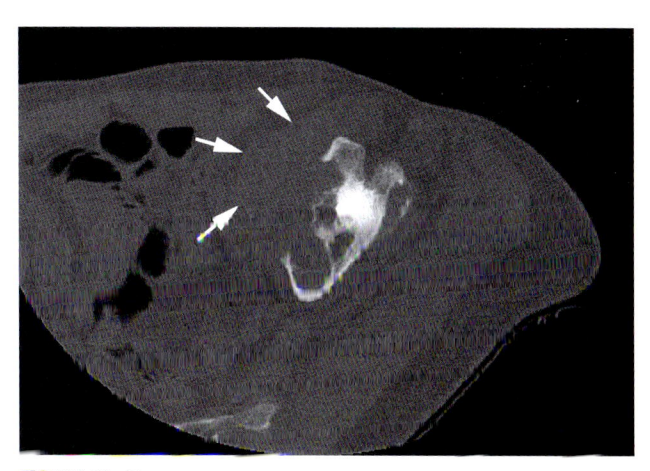

FIGURE 12-40
Tumoral detritic synovitis.
Destructive lesion is seen around a prosthesis. A biopsy showed that this tumor was composed of histiocytic reaction to the prosthesis.

with large joint arthroplasties, a minority of patients encounter problems because of mechanical failure, particularly in joints that are subjected to greater degrees of stress and activity, such as the thumb and hallux. The abraded silicone particles are capable of eliciting an inflammatory reaction that differs somewhat from large joint detritic synovitis.

Small joint detritic synovitis produces a nodular thickening of the synovial membrane similar to its large joint counterpart. Blackening of the membrane does not occur because metal alloys are not a part of these prostheses. Microscopically, the subsynovial space is expanded by a histiocytic and multinucleated giant cell infiltrate that surrounds small fragments of yellow-green lobulated foreign material (the fragmented solid phase silicone) (Figure 12-41). This material predominantly occurs within the cytoplasm of mononuclear histiocytes, synovial cells, and multinucleated giant cells; however, small pieces may be found in an entirely extracellular location. Solid silicone is refractile but not birefringent, and hence is not visible when viewed with polarized light. Neutrophils are not typically found unless there is a coexistent bacterial infection. Other changes in the synovial membrane include scattered lymphocytes and plasma cells, strands of fibrosis, and embedded shards of bone. The latter probably arise from the adjacent bones, which may also contain large amounts of silicone particles. In a minority of cases, the intraosseous silicone elicits intense osteoclastic resorptive activity that may produce radiographically and surgically detectable cystic defects. Silicone synovitis is managed by thorough curettage and reconstruction of the affected joint if possible.

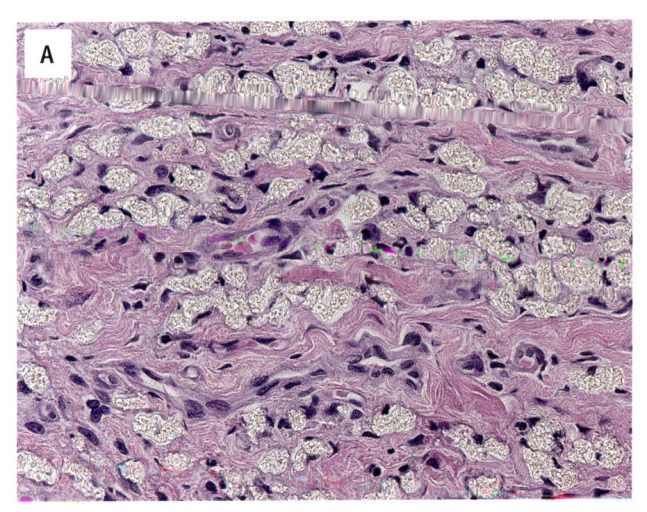

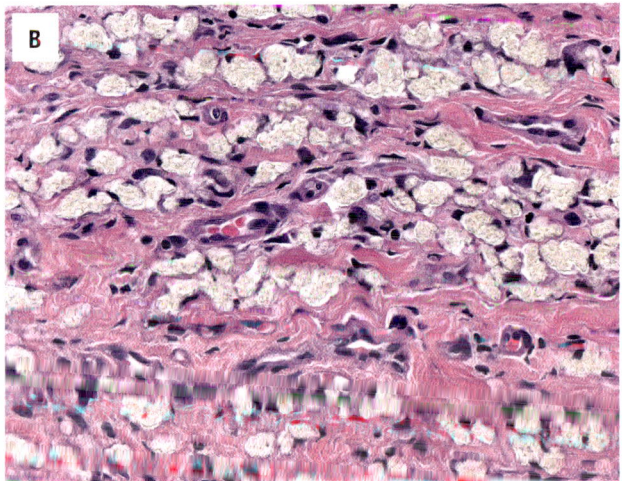

FIGURE 12-41

A, Histiocytic reaction to silicone prosthesis, which is refractile **(B).**

SUGGESTED READINGS

Pigmented Villonodular Synovitis

1. Alguacil-Garcia A, Unni KK, Goellner JR: Giant cell tumor of tendon sheath and pigmented villonodular synovitis. An ultrastructural study. Am J Clin Pathol 1978;69:6-17.
2. Folpe AL: Tenosynovial giant cell tumor and pigmented villonodular synovitis. Skeletal Radiol 2007;36:899-900.
3. Jaffe HL, Lichtenstein L, Sutro CJ: Pigmented villonodular synovitis, bursitis and tenosynovitis. Arch Pathol 1941;31:731-765.
4. O'Connell JX, Fanburg JC, Rosenberg AE: Giant cell tumor of tendon sheath and pigmented villonodular synovitis: immunophenotype suggests a synovial cell origin. Hum Pathol 1995;26:771-775.
5. Oda Y, Izumi T, Harimaya K, et al: Pigmented villonodular synovitis with chondroid metaplasia, resembling chondroblastoma of the bone: a report of three cases. Mod Pathol 2007;20:545-551.
6. Rao AS, Vigorita VJ: Pigmented villonodular synovitis (giant cell tumor of tendon sheath and synovial membrane). A review of eighty one cases. J Bone Joint Surg Am 1984;66-A:76-94.
7. Ray RA, Morton CC, Lipinski KK, et al: Cytogenetic evidence of clonality in a case of pigmented villonodular synovitis. Cancer 1991;67:121-125.
8. Rubin PB: Reply to Dr. Folpe's comments on the article "Tenosynovial giant cell tumor and pigmented villonodular synovitis: a proposal for unification of these clinically distinct but histologically and genetically identical lesions." Skeletal Radiol 2007;36:901.
9. Rubin PB: Tenosynovial giant cell tumor and pigmented villonodular synovitis: a proposal for unification of these clinically distinct but histologically and genetically identical lesions. Skeletal Radiol 2007;36:267-268.
10. Schwartz HS, Unni KK, Pritchard DJ: Pigmented villonodular synovitis. A retrospective review of affected large joints. Clin Orthop Relat Res 1989;247:243-255.
11. Sciot R, Rosai J, Dal Cin P, et al: Analysis of 35 cases of localized and diffuse tenosynovial giant cell tumor. A report from the Chromosomes and Morphology (CHAMP) study group. Mod Pathol 1999;12:676-674.
12. Somerhausen NS, Fletcher CD: Diffuse type giant cell tumor: clinicopathologic and immunohistochemical analysis of 50 cases with extraarticular disease. Am J Surg Pathol 2000;24:479-492.
13. Vogrincic GS, O'Connell JX, Gilks CB: Giant cell tumor of tendon sheath is a polyclonal cellular proliferation. Hum Pathol 1997;28:815-819.
14. West RB, Rubin BP, Miller MA, et al: A landscape effect in tenosynovial giant-cell tumor from activation of CSF1 expression by a translocation in a minority of tumor cells. Proc Natl Acad Sci USA 2006;103:690-695.

Hemosiderotic Synovitis

1. Devaney K, Vinh TN, Sweet DE: Synovial hemangioma: a report of 20 cases with differential diagnostic considerations. Hum Pathol 1993;24:737-745.
2. Greenspan A, Azouz EM, Matthews J II, et al: Synovial hemangioma: Imaging features in eight histologically proven cases, review of the literature, and differential diagnosis [review]. Skeletal Radiol 1995;24:583-590.
3. Luck JV, Kasper CK: Surgical management of advanced hemophilic arthropathy: an overview of 20 years experience. Clin Orthop Relat Res 1989;242:60-82.
4. Stein H, Duthie RB: The pathogenesis of chronic haemophilic arthropathy. J Bone Joint Surg Br 1981;63B:601-609.

Villous Lipomatous Proliferation of Synovial Membrane (Lipoma Arborescens)

1. Chikura B, Bucknall R: Clinical Image: lipoma arborescens: a rare cause of recurrent knee effusion. Arthritis Rheum 2008;58:1881.
2. Grieten M, Buckwalter KA, Cardinal E, et al: Case report 873: lipoma arborescens (villous lipomatous proliferation of the synovial membrane). Skeletal Radiol 1994;23:652-655.
3. Hallel T, Lew S, Bansal M: Villous lipomatous proliferation of the synovial membrane (lipoma arborescens). J Bone Joint Surg Am 1988;70-A:264-270.

4. Hirano K, Deguchi M, Kanamono T: Intra-articular synovial lipoma of the knee joint (located in the lateral recess): a case report and review of the literature [review]. Knee 2007;14:63–67.
5. Hubscher O, Costanza E, Elsner B: Chronic monoarthritis due to lipoma arborescens. J Rheumatol 1990;17:861–862.
6. Martin S, Hernández L, Romero J, et al: Diagnostic imaging of lipoma arborescens. Skeletal Radiol 1998;27:325–329.

Fibroma of Tendon Sheath

1. Chung EB, Enzinger FM: Fibroma of tendon sheath. Cancer 1979;44:1945–1954.
2. Dal Cin P, Sciot R, De Smet L, et al: Translocation 2;11 in fibroma of tendon sheath. Histopathology 1998;32:433–435.
3. Lamovec J, Bracko M, Voncina D: Pleomorphic fibroma of tendon sheath. Am J Surg Pathol 1991;15:1202–1205.
4. Pulitzer DR, Martin PC, Reed RJ: Fibroma of tendon sheath. A clinicopathologic study of 32 cases. Am J Surg Pathol 1989;13:472–479.

Primary Synovial Chondromatosis

1. Apte SS, Athanasou NA: An immunohistological study of cartilage and synovium in primary synovial chondromatosis. J Pathol 1992;166:277–281.
2. Davis RI, Hamilton A, Biggart JD: Primary synovial chondromatosis: a clinicopathologic review and assessment of malignant potential. Hum Pathol 1998;29:683–688.
3. Sah AP, Geller DS, Mankin HJ, et al: Malignant transformation of synovial chondromatosis of the shoulder to chondrosarcoma. A case report. J Bone Joint Surg Am 2007;89:1321–1328.
4. Sciot R, Dal Cin P, Samson I, et al: Synovial chondromatosis. Clonal chromosome changes provide further evidence for a neoplastic disorder. Virchows Arch 1998;433:189–191.
5. Sim FH, Dahlin DC, Ivins JC: Extra-articular synovial chondromatosis. J Bone Joint Surg Am 1977;59A:492–495.
6. Villacin AB, Brigham LN, Bullough PG: Primary and secondary synovial chondrometaplasia: histopathologic and clinicoradiologic differences. Hum Pathol 1979;10:439–451.
7. Xu WH, Ma XC, Guo CB, et al: Synovial chondromatosis of the temporomandibular joint with middle cranial fossa extension [review]. Int J Oral Maxillofac Surg 2007;36:652–655.

Loose Bodies

1. Milgram JW: The classification of loose bodies in human joints. Clin Orthop Relat Res 1977;124:282–291.
2. Milgram JW: The development of loose bodies in human joints. Clin Orthop Relat Res 1977;124:292–303.

Malignant Tumors of the Joint

1. Case 4-1980-An 82-year-old woman was admitted to the hospital because of a mass in the left shoulder. N Engl J Med 1980;302:83–89.
2. Case 45-1991-An 84-year-old man with a slowly enlarging mass in the left popliteal space. N Engl J Med 1991;325:361–367.
3. Bertoni F, Unni KK, Beabout JW, et al: Chondrosarcomas of the synovium. Cancer 1991;67:155–162.
4. Bukawa H, Kawabata A, Murano A, et al: Monophasic epithelial synovial sarcoma arising in the temporomandibular joint. Int J Oral Maxillofac Surg 2007;36:762–765.
5. Einhorn TA, Nielsen GP: Case 1-2001 - A 26-year-old man with a mass in the knee. N Engl J Med 2001;344:124–131.
6. Fetsch JF, Meis JM: Intra-articular synovial sarcoma. Mod Pathol 1992;5:6A.
7. Gebhardt MC, Parekh SG, Rosenberg AE, et al: Extraskeletal myxoid chondrosarcoma of the knee. Skeletal Radiol 1999;28:354–358.
8. Goldman RL, Lichenstein L: Synovial chondrosarcoma. Cancer 1964;17:1233–1240.
9. Hurtado RM, McCarthy E, Frassica F, et al: Intraarticular epithelioid sarcoma. Skeletal Radiol 1998;27:453–456.
10. Ishida T, Iijima T, Moriyama S, et al: Intra-articular calcifying synovial sarcoma mimicking synovial chondromatosis. Skeletal Radiol 1996;25:766–769.
11. Kenan S, Abdelwahab IF, Klein MJ, et al: Case report 817: synovial chondrosarcoma secondary to synovial chondromatosis. Skeletal Radiol 1993;22:623–626.
12. Kindblom LG, Angervall L: Myxoid chondrosarcoma of the synovial tissue. A clinicopathologic, histochemical, and ultrastructural analysis. Cancer 1983;52:1886–1895.
13. King JW, Spjut HJ, Fechner RE, et al: Synovial chondrosarcoma of the knee joint. J Bone Joint Surg Am 1967;49:1389–1396.
14. Li C-F, Wang J-W, Huang WW, et al: Malignant diffuse-type tenosynovial giant cell tumors. a series of 7 cases comparing with 24 benign lesions. With review of the literature. Am J Surg Pathol 2008;32:587–599.
15. Manivel JC, Dehner LP, Thompson R: Case report 460: synovial chondrosarcoma of left knee. Skeletal Radiol 1988;17:66–71.
16. Nielsen AL, Kiaer T: Malignant giant cell tumor of synovium and locally destructive pigmented villonodular synovitis: ultrastructural and immunohistochemical study and review of the literature. Hum Pathol 1989;20:765–771.
17. Okamoto S, Hisaoka M, Ishida T, et al: Extraskeletal myxoid chondrosarcoma: a clinicopathologic, immunohistochemical, and molecular analysis of 18 cases. Hum Pathol 2001;32:1116–1124.
18. Taconis WK, van der Heul RO, Taminiau AM: Synovial chondrosarcoma: report of a case and review of the literature. Skeletal Radiol 1997;26:682–685.
19. Thunold J, Bang G: Synovial sarcoma: a case report. Acta Orthop Scand 1976;47:231–235.
20. Ushijima M, Hashimoto H, Tsuneyoshi M, et al: Malignant giant cell tumor of tendon sheath. Report of a case. Acta Pathol Jpn 1985;35:699–709.
21. Wright PH, Sim FH, Soule EH, et al: Synovial sarcoma. J Bone Joint Surg Am 1982;64:112–122.

Synovial Reaction to Loosened Joint Arthroplasties

1. Chiyule AJ, Pforret C, Levison J: Silicone synovitis. Semin Arthritis Rheum 1989;19:166–171.
2. Christie AJ, Weinberger KA, Dietrich M: Silicone lymphadenopathy and synovitis. Complications of silicone elastomer finger joint prostheses. JAMA 1977;237:1463–1464.
3. Harboldt SL, Gumley GJ, Balogh K: Osteolysis after silicone arthroplasty. Am J Clin Pathol 1992;98:594–597.
4. Keel SB, Jaffe KA, Nielsen GP, Rosenberg AE: Orthopedic implant related sarcoma. A study of twelve cases. Mod Pathol 2001;12:969–977.
5. Mirra JM, Marder RA, Amstutz HC: The pathology of failed large joint arthroplasty. Clin Orthop Relat Res 1982;170:175–183.
6. Shokeir MO, Duncan CP, O'Connell JX: Revision hip arthroplasty: a histologic review. Int J Surg Pathol 1996;3:247–256.

13 Tumors of Miscellaneous Type or Uncertain Lineage

Andrew L. Folpe

- Myxoma
- Intramuscular Myxoma
- Juxta-Articular Myxoma
- Cutaneous Myxoma
- Angiomyofibroblastoma and Related Tumors (Cellular Angiofibroma, Angiomyofibroblastoma-like Tumor of the Male Genital Tract)
- Aggressive Angiomyxoma
- Ossifying Fibromyxoid Tumor of Soft Parts
- Pleomorphic Hyalinizing Angiectatic Tumor
- Phosphaturic Mesenchymal Tumor
- Perivascular Epithelioid Cell Neoplasms
- Epithelioid Sarcoma
- Alveolar Soft Part Sarcoma
- Ewing Family of Tumors (Ewing Sarcoma and Primitive Neuroectodermal Tumor)
- Synovial Sarcoma
- Desmoplastic Small Round Cell Tumor

A significant number of soft tissue tumors either show no clear line of differentiation or appear to differentiate along the lines of a cell type with no known normal counterpart. Some of these tumors, for example, myxoma, appear to show principally fibroblastic differentiation but have not traditionally been included among the fibroblastic tumors of soft tissue. As with all other soft tissue tumors, the tumors of uncertain lineage span a spectrum from benign to intermediate malignancy to fully malignant sarcomas.

MYXOMA

The myxomas are a group of relatively common, probably unrelated lesions, which most commonly involve large muscles (intramuscular myxoma) but may also occur around large joints (juxta-articular myxoma) or in the skin (cutaneous myxoma). All are characterized by abundant myxoid matrix, bland stellate to spindled cells, and hypovascularity.

INTRAMUSCULAR MYXOMA

CLINICAL FEATURES

Intramuscular myxomas occur almost exclusively in middle-aged to older adults, more often in women than in men. A strong association exists between the presence of multiple intramuscular myxomas and fibrous dysplasia, typically of the monostotic type (Mazabraud syndrome). The large muscle of the buttocks, thigh, shoulder, and upper arm are most commonly involved, although rare cases have been reported in almost any location. These tumors usually present as a nonspecific soft tissue mass, without characteristic clinical or radiographic features. Most are between 5 and 10 cm, although occasional cases can be considerably larger.

PATHOLOGIC FEATURES

GROSS FINDINGS

Intramuscular myxomas are almost always well-delineated, gelatinous-appearing masses, which may show cystic change.

MICROSCOPIC FINDINGS

Despite their gross appearance of circumscription, intramuscular myxomas typically extend into muscle to a limited extent, splaying apart individual skeletal muscle fibers; this finding is a helpful clue to their diagnosis (Figure 13-1). Microscopically, they contain abundant myxoid matrix, which typically shows multifocal microcystic change (Figure 13-2). The tumor cells are spindled to stellate in appearance, with darkly staining, pyknotic-appearing nuclei and a small amount of eosinophilic cytoplasm (Figure 13-3). Myxomas lack the well-developed, arborizing vasculature seen in myxoid liposarcoma. Occasionally, a myxoma may show greater cellularity and focal areas of fascicular growth, sometimes accompanied by slightly greater number of blood vessels (*cellular myxoma*).

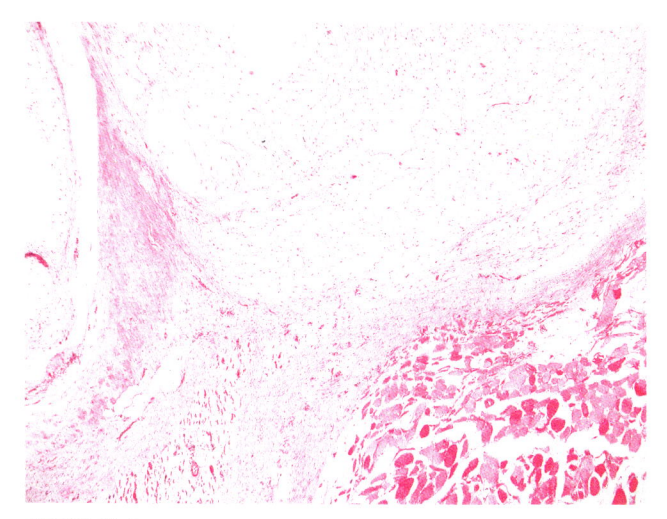

FIGURE 13-1
Intramuscular myxoma, a uniformly myxoid, hypocellular lesion with characteristic splaying apart of skeletal muscle.

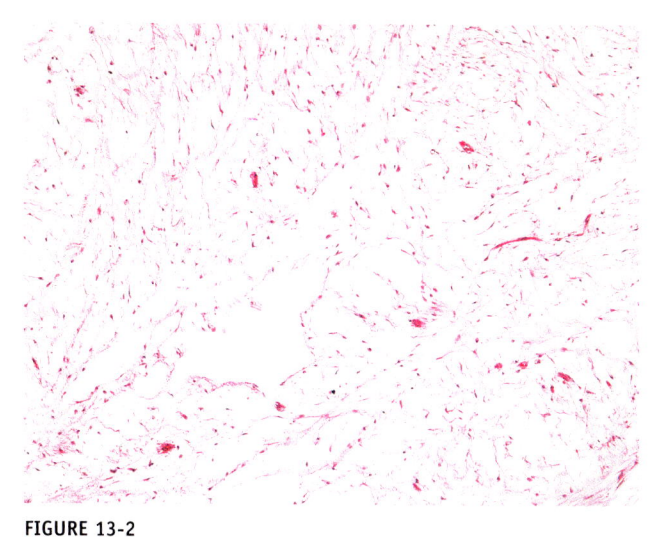

FIGURE 13-2
Myxoid matrix, relative hypovascularity without arborizing vessels, and microcystic change in intramuscular myxoma.

Identification of areas of more typical myxoma is the key to recognizing such *cellular myxomas*. The matrix of myxomas is Alcian blue positive, hyaluronidase sensitive.

ANCILLARY STUDIES

IMMUNOHISTOCHEMISTRY

The cells of intramuscular myxoma usually express only vimentin but may rarely express smooth muscle actin in a myofibroblastic, *tram-track* pattern.

DIFFERENTIAL DIAGNOSIS

Intramuscular myxomas are commonly confused with a wide variety of both benign and malignant myxoid tumors. Myxoid nodular fasciitis is usually much smaller, more often superficially located, and shows at least focal areas of increased cellularity, with short, randomly arranged fascicles of bland myofibroblasts. Myxoid variants of desmoid fibromatosis more often occur within the abdomen, and contain a well-developed, thin-walled, nonarborizing vasculature and at least focal areas of typical fibromatosis. Myxoid liposarcoma contains an extremely well-developed, arborizing, capillary-sized vasculature and easily identifiable lipoblasts. Myxofibrosarcoma (myxoid malignant fibrous histiocytoma) has a well-developed, thick-walled vasculature and contains hyperchromatic, pleomorphic tumor cells. Extraskeletal myxoid chondrosarcoma is composed of cords and chains of small eosinophilic cells, embedded in a *dense*-appearing myxoid matrix, often with abundant hemorrhage, but with relatively few blood vessels.

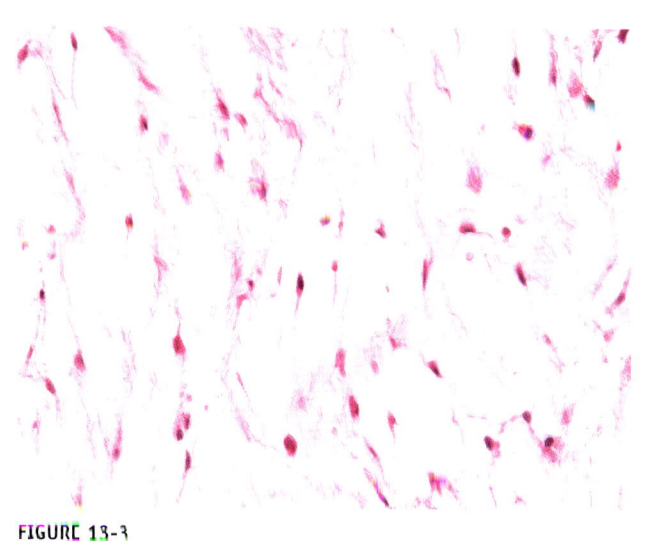

FIGURE 13-3
The cells of intramuscular myxoma are bland, with scant eosinophilic cytoplasm and pyknotic nuclei.

PROGNOSIS AND TREATMENT

Intramuscular myxomas are entirely benign lesions that require only simple excision.

JUXTA-ARTICULAR MYXOMA

CLINICAL FEATURES

As indicated by their name, juxta-articular myxomas occur in direct association with large joints. By far the most common location is adjacent to the knee joint,

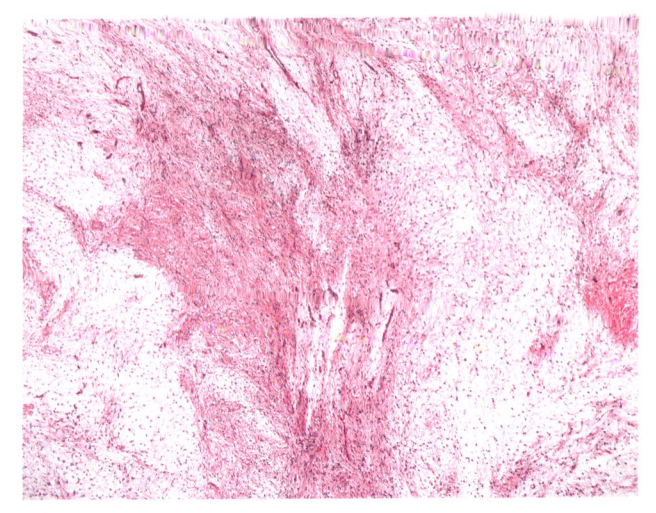

FIGURE 13-4
Juxta-articular myxomas are frequently more cellular and vascular than are other myxomas, and may mimic various myxoid sarcomas.

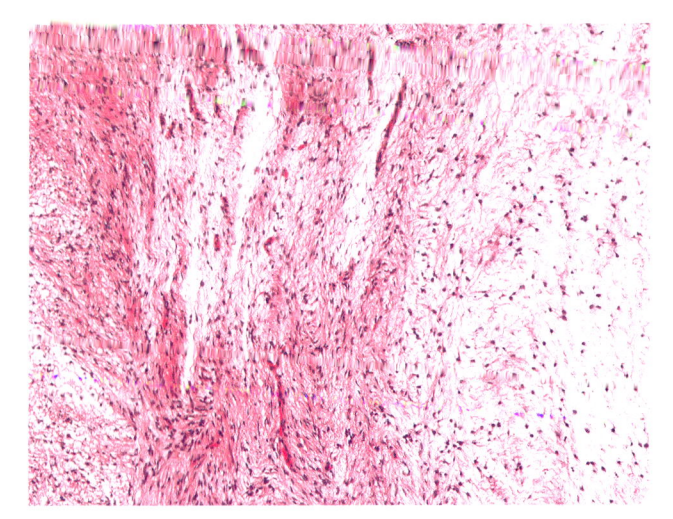

FIGURE 13-5
Fascicular, cellular growth in juxta-articular myxoma.

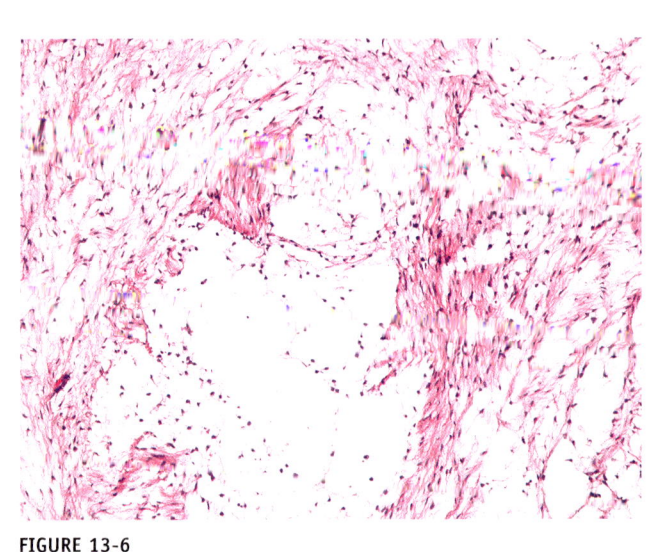

FIGURE 13-6
Careful inspection of juxta-articular myxomas, and other cellular myxomas, will invariably reveal small areas of more typical myxoma, with cystic change.

followed by the shoulder, hip, and ankle. Most patients are older men, frequently with a history of osteoarthritis. The tumors are usually 2 to 6 cm at the time of diagnosis, although some may be significantly larger.

PATHOLOGIC FEATURES

GROSS FINDINGS

Juxta-articular myxomas are grossly identical to intramuscular myxomas.

MICROSCOPIC FINDINGS

In general, juxta-articular myxomas closely recapitulate the histologic features of intramuscular myxoma. However, a significant subset of these lesions may show features of cellular myxoma, with fascicular growth, areas of well-developed vasculature, and mild pleomorphism (Figures 13-4 and 13-5). As with cellular intramuscular myxomas, identification of areas of typical myxoma is the key to correct diagnosis (Figure 13-6).

ANCILLARY STUDIES

ULTRASTRUCTURAL FEATURES

Ultrastructural features of juxta-articular myxoma are identical to those seen in intramuscular myxoma.

IMMUNOHISTOCHEMISTRY

Juxta-articular myxomas show the same immunophenotype as intramuscular myxomas, with expression of vimentin and occasionally smooth muscle actin.

DIFFERENTIAL DIAGNOSIS

The differential diagnosis of juxta-articular myxoma is essentially the same as that of intramuscular myxoma. Although particularly cellular, juxta-articular myxomas may mimic myxofibrosarcoma, among others; the characteristic location around the knee joint and the frequent history of osteoarthritis should point one in the correct direction. In this location adjacent to the knee, a myxoid monophasic fibrous synovial sarcoma (MSS) may also be a diagnostic consideration. Myxoid change in synovial sarcomas is almost always focal rather than diffuse, and identification of areas of more typical synovial sarcoma, characterized by hyperchromatic nuclei, alternating hypocellular and hypercellular zones, wiry collagen, and focal keratin immunoreactivity, is diagnostic.

CHAPTER 13 Tumors of Miscellaneous Type or Uncertain Lineage

PROGNOSIS AND TREATMENT

Juxta-articular myxomas are entirely benign, but may recur locally in up to 30% of cases, particularly if incompletely excised.

MYXOMA (INTRAMUSCULAR AND JUXTA-ARTICULAR)—FACT SHEET

Definition
- Benign, mesenchymal tumor composed of bland spindled cells embedded in hypovascular, frequently cystic, myxoid matrix

Incidence and Location
- Relatively common
- Intramuscular myxoma: large muscles of thigh and buttock
- Juxta-articular myxoma: near knees, shoulders, hips

Morbidity and Mortality
- None

Sex, Race, and Age Distribution
- Intramuscular myxoma is more common in women, may be associated with fibrous dysplasia (Mazabraud syndrome)
- Juxta-articular myxoma is most common in men with degenerative joint disease

Clinical Features
- Painless soft tissue mass

Prognosis and Treatment
- Cured with complete excision

MYXOMA (INTRAMUSCULAR AND JUXTA-ARTICULAR)—PATHOLOGIC FEATURES

Gross Findings
- Well-circumscribed mass, myxoid appearing, cystic

Microscopic Findings
- Abundant Alcian blue–positive, hyaluronidase-sensitive myxoid matrix
- Splaying apart of skeletal muscle
- Hypovascular, without well-developed arborizing vessels
- Slender spindled cells with pyknotic nuclei
- Juxta-articular myxomas often show areas of increased cellularity, with partial fascicular growth pattern

Immunohistochemical Findings
- Typically express only vimentin, occasionally show limited smooth muscle actin expression

Differential Diagnosis
- Myxofibrosarcoma, myxoid liposarcoma, myxoid chondrosarcoma, myxoid nodular fasciitis, myxoid desmoid-type fibromatosis

---

CUTANEOUS MYXOMA

CLINICAL FEATURES

Cutaneous myxoma, also known as *superficial myxoma* or *superficial angiomyxoma,* is a rare myxoid tumor of the skin and subcutis. Cutaneous myxomas are histologically identical to the cutaneous myxoid tumors seen in patients with Carney's syndrome, although most occur sporadically. Men are affected slightly more often than women, and the typical patient is a middle-aged adult. The most common locations for sporadic cutaneous myxomas are the trunk, lower extremities, and head and neck; Carney's syndrome–associated myxomas are more often multiple, and involve the eyelids and ear.

PATHOLOGIC FEATURES

GROSS FINDINGS

Cutaneous myxomas are typically small, sometimes polypoid tumors that have a gelatinous appearance. These lesions are often poorly circumscribed, and may involve the subcutis and occasionally deeper muscle.

MICROSCOPIC FINDINGS

Cutaneous myxomas are considerably more vascular than other myxomas, as reflected in the alternative term, *superficial angiomyxoma* (Figure 13-7). This vasculature may be well developed and arborizing, reminiscent of myxoid liposarcoma. However, the overall

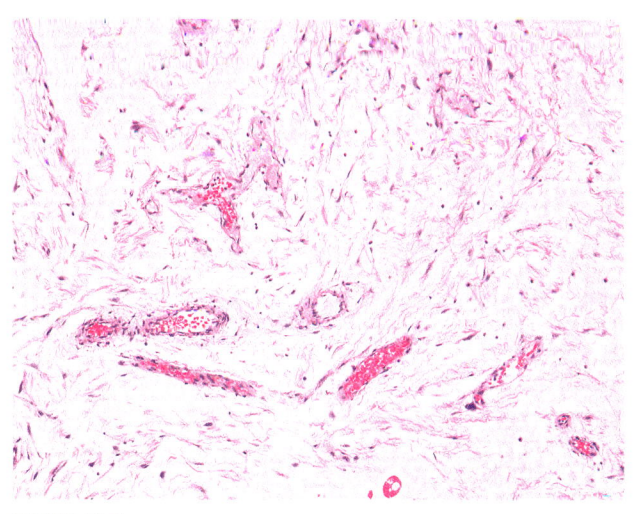

FIGURE 13-7

Cutaneous myxoma (angiomyxoma), a highly vascularized myxoid tumor of the skin and subcutis.

cellularity of the lesion is quite low, and the lesional cells are small, cytologically bland, and spindled to stellate in shape. A prominent neutrophilic infiltrate is often present and is a helpful clue to this diagnosis (Figure 13-8). Epithelioid structures, probably representing entrapped adnexal glands, are seen in roughly one-third of cases. A vaguely lobular growth pattern is often present.

ANCILLARY STUDIES

The ultrastructural and immunohistochemical features of cutaneous myxoma are identical to those of the other myxomas.

DIFFERENTIAL DIAGNOSIS

Focal cutaneous mucinosis lacks the neutrophils, lobular growth pattern, and elaborate vasculature seen in cutaneous myxoma. Digital mucinous cyst occurs exclusively in the digits and lacks a well-developed vasculature. Aggressive angiomyxoma is a deeply seated tumor of the genital region, which only focally involves the skin (if at all), lacks neutrophils, and contains ectatic, nonarborizing vessels. Neurothekeoma is more distinctly lobular and is composed of plumper, occasional pleomorphic, S-100 protein–positive cells. Myxoid neurofibromas lack the well-developed vasculature of myxoma and contain wavy, *comma-shaped* cells that express S-100 protein. Myxoid dermatofibrosarcoma protuberans are much more infiltrative, CD34-positive lesions that typically show at least small areas of more typical dermatofibrosarcoma.

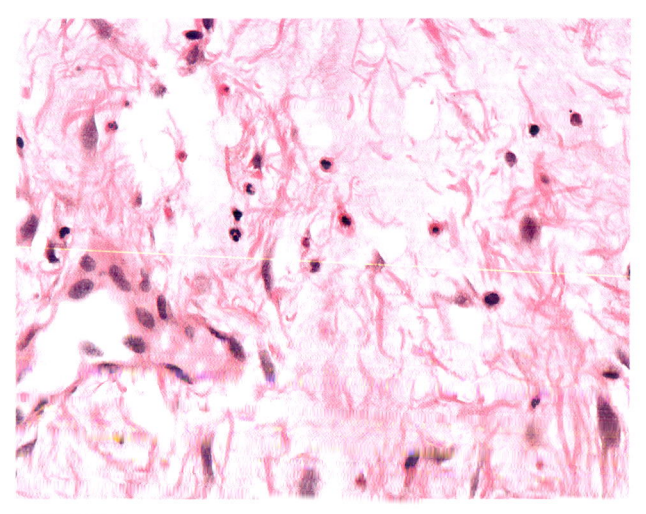

PROGNOSIS AND TREATMENT

Local, complete excision is adequate treatment, and no malignant behavior is documented.

CUTANEOUS MYXOMA—FACT SHEET

Definition
- Benign myxoid mesenchymal tumor of the skin and subcutis

Incidence and Location
- Rare
- Sporadic cutaneous myxoma: trunk, legs, head and neck
- Carney syndrome–associated myxomas: eyelids and ear, may be multiple

Morbidity and Mortality
- None

Sex, Race, and Age Distribution
- Most often occur in middle-aged men

Clinical Features
- Polypoid or papular skin lesion

Prognosis and Treatment
- May recur locally
- Complete excision

CUTANEOUS MYXOMA—PATHOLOGIC FEATURES

Gross Findings
- Poorly circumscribed, gelatinous, small

Microscopic Findings
- Vaguely lobular
- Much more vascular than other myxomas; may show well-developed arborizing vasculature
- Bland spindled cells
- Abundant myxoid matrix
- Stromal neutrophils and entrapped adnexal units in some

Immunohistochemical Findings
- Typically express only vimentin

Differential Diagnosis
- Cutaneous mucinosis, digital mucinous cyst, aggressive angiomyxoma, nerve sheath myxoma (neurothekeoma), myxoid neurofibroma, myxoid dermatofibrosarcoma protuberans

---

FIGURE 13-8
The cells of cutaneous myxoma are uniformly normochromatic, assisting in its distinction from superficially located myxofibrosarcomas. Note also the presence of stromal neutrophils, a useful clue.

ANGIOMYOFIBROBLASTOMA AND RELATED TUMORS (Cellular Angiofibroma, Angiomyofibroblastoma-like Tumor of the Male Genital Tract)

CLINICAL FEATURES

Angiomyofibroblastoma is an uncommon, benign, non-recurring myofibroblastic lesion of the vulva and pelviperineal region. So-called *cellular angiofibroma* appears to represent a morphologic variant of angiomyofibroblastoma, and these two tumors will be considered together. Most cases are observed in the vulva of middle-aged women, and less frequently in the vagina (10%–15% of cases), perineum, or inguinal region. Rare tumors essentially identical to cellular angiofibroma have been reported in men as *angiomyofibroblastoma-like tumors of the male genital tract*; such lesions typically involve the scrotum, spermatic cord, or inguinal region. Angiomyofibroblastomas present as slow-growing, painless masses, which are usually considered clinically to be Bartholin gland cysts.

ANGIOMYOFIBROBLASTOMA AND RELATED TUMORS (Cellular Angiofibroma)—FACT SHEET

Definition
- Benign myofibroblastic lesions of the vulva, inguinoscrotal, and pelviperineal regions

Incidence and Location
- Angiomyofibroblastoma
  - Rare
  - Mostly observed in the vulva, less frequent in the vagina
  - Rare cases in men (scrotum, spermatic cord, inguinal region)
- Cellular angiofibroma
  - Rare
  - Found in the vulva, and in the inguinoscrotal region in male individuals

Morbidity and Mortality
- Benign, nonrecurring neoplasms
- Malignant angiomyofibroblastoma exceptional

Sex, Race, and Age Distribution
- Middle-aged women and men

Clinical Features
- Slow-growing painless nodule

Prognosis and Treatment
- Benign, nonrecurring neoplasms

PATHOLOGIC FEATURES

GROSS FINDINGS

Angiomyofibroblastomas are well circumscribed but usually nonencapsulated lesions, 1 to 10 cm (4 cm on average). The consistency is soft, and the cut section of the lesion is gray–pink with a glistening appearance. Cellular angiofibromas tend to be larger in men (2.5–14 cm).

ANGIOMYOFIBROBLASTOMA AND RELATED TUMORS (Cellular Angiofibroma)—PATHOLOGIC FEATURES

Gross Findings
- Well circumscribed
- Small (2–3 cm on average)
- Cellular angiofibroma in male individuals tend to be larger (5–10 cm)

Microscopic Findings
- Angiomyofibroblastoma
  - Numerous small- to medium-sized vessels
  - Round to spindle-shaped myofibroblasts concentrated around vessels
  - Epithelioid appearing, plasmacytoid, binucleate, and multinucleate cells frequent
  - Loose edematous stroma
  - Mitotic figures rare
  - Intralesional mature adipocytes in about 10% of cases
- Cellular angiofibroma
  - Numerous spindle cells (strong resemblance to spindle cell lipoma)
  - Numerous small- to medium-sized hyalinized vessels
  - Fibrinoid deposits around small vessels/organizing intraluminal thrombi
  - Mitoses often numerous in vulvar lesions, rare in lesions in male individuals
  - Intralesional mature adipocytes in about 50% of cases

Immunohistochemical Findings
- Angiomyofibroblastoma
  - Strong positivity for desmin
  - Focal reactivity for smooth muscle actin
  - Occasional reactivity for CD34
  - Positivity for estrogen and progesterone receptors in women
  - Negativity for S-100 protein, keratins, and EMA
- Cellular angiofibroma in female individuals
  - Frequent negativity for smooth muscle actin and desmin
  - Variable positivity for CD34
  - Positivity for estrogen and progesterone receptors
- Cellular angiofibroma in male individuals
  - Frequent positivity for smooth muscle actin, desmin, and/or CD34
  - Positivity for estrogen and progesterone receptors

Differential Diagnosis
- Angiomyofibroblastoma
  - Aggressive angiomyxoma, epithelioid smooth muscle tumors
- Cellular angiofibroma
  - Spindle cell lipoma, solitary fibrous tumor

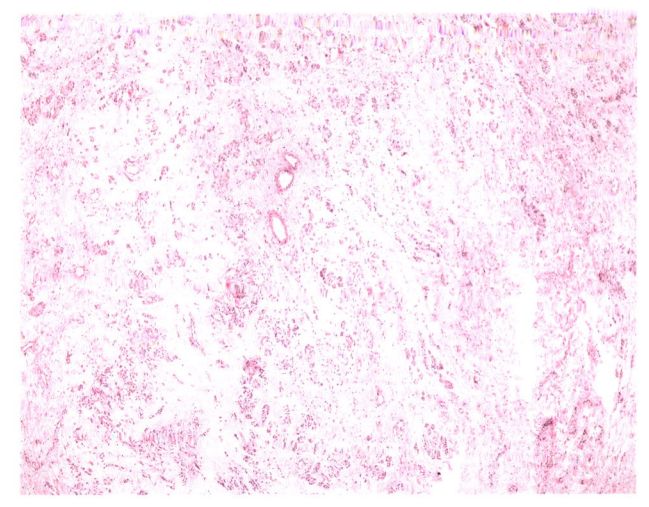

FIGURE 13-9
Angiomyofibroblastoma, showing abundant myxohyaline stroma and clusters of epithelioid genital-type myofibroblasts surrounding blood vessels.

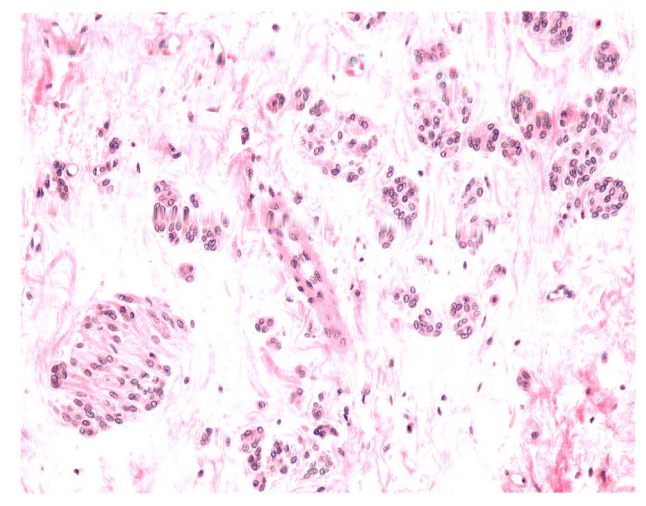

FIGURE 13-11
Cellular angiofibroma is closely related to angiomyofibroblastoma but consists of more spindled cells arrayed about thicker, hyalinized blood vessels.

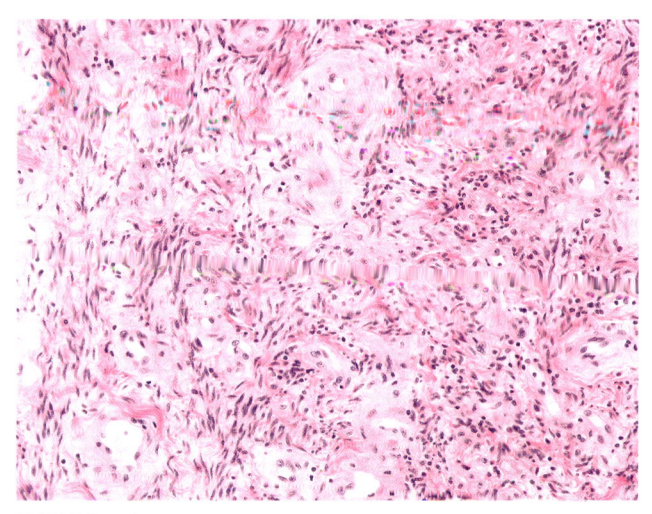

FIGURE 13-10
Clusters of bland epithelioid cells arrayed about a small blood vessel in angiomyofibroblastoma.

FIGURE 13-12
Bland spindled cells, wiry collagen, and hyalinized blood vessels in cellular angiofibroma.

MICROSCOPIC FINDINGS

Angiomyofibroblastoma, which develops in the pelviperineal subcutaneous tissue, is composed of small- to medium-sized, well-formed vessels, round to spindled myofibroblasts arranged around the vessels, and loose edematous stroma in varying proportions (Figure 13-9). The tumor cells have an eosinophilic cytoplasm and bland nuclei, occasionally with smudged chromatin. Epithelioid to plasmacytoid neoplastic cells may be present, as well as binucleate or multinucleate cells (Figure 13-10). Mitotic figures are rare, and no tumor necrosis is present. Interstitial mast cells are commonly observed. About 10% of cases also contain mature adipocytes. Fibrosis and perivascular hyalinization are common in longstanding lesions. Some cases show considerable morphologic overlap with cellular angiofibroma, and these are best thought of as morphologic variants of the same lesion.

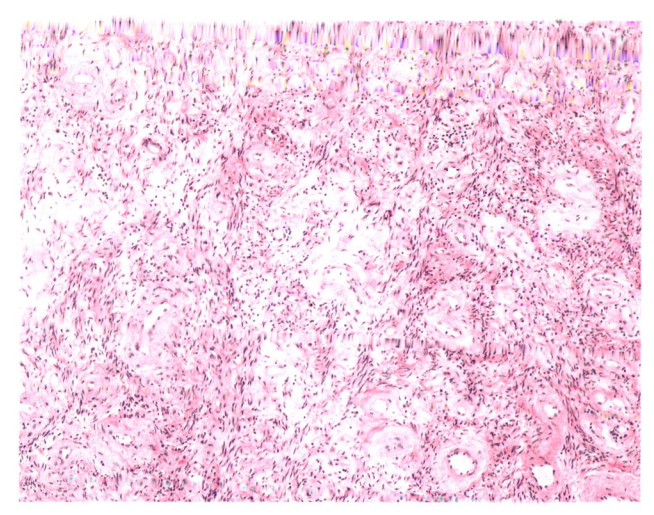

Cellular angiofibroma is generally well circumscribed and is composed of proliferating bland spindle cells. In addition, the lesion contains numerous small- to medium-sized vessels with hyalinized walls, perivascular fibrinoid deposits, and/or intraluminal thrombi (Figures 13-11 and 13-12). Atypical mitotic figures and necrosis are absent. As in angiomyofibroblastoma, intralesional fat can be observed in cellular angiofibroma, as well as interstitial mast cells.

ANCILLARY STUDIES

IMMUNOHISTOCHEMISTRY

Most angiomyofibroblastomas are strongly positive for desmin and focally positive for smooth muscle actin and CD34. Desmin staining may be reduced or absent in postmenopausal cases. Positivity for estrogen and progesterone receptors is the rule. S-100 protein, keratins, and epithelial membrane antigen (EMA) are not expressed. Smooth muscle actin, desmin, and CD34 are variably expressed in cellular angiofibroma. In contrast with lesions in male individuals, vulvar cellular angiofibromas tend to be negative for smooth muscle actin and desmin but positive for estrogen and progesterone receptors.

DIFFERENTIAL DIAGNOSIS

Angiomyofibroblastoma is a small, cellular, superficially located lesion with numerous small vessels, unlike aggressive angiomyxoma, a large, deeply situated, hypocellular myxoid lesion with gaping vessels. Epithelioid smooth muscle tumors are more solid, eosinophilic tumors that typically show at least small areas of more typical smooth muscle, and are diffusely smooth muscle actin and desmin positive. The *cellular angiofibroma* end of this morphologic spectrum may closely resemble spindle cell lipoma but tends to lack bundles of refractile collagen and a *packeted* pattern of growth. Solitary fibrous tumors (SFTs) show more abundant collagen, a pronounced *hemangiopericytoma-like* vascular pattern, and have a *patternless* growth pattern.

PROGNOSIS AND TREATMENT

Angiomyofibroblastoma and cellular angiofibromas are benign nonrecurring lesions. Simple excision is curative. Malignant angiomyofibroblastomas have been reported but are exceptional.

AGGRESSIVE ANGIOMYXOMA

CLINICAL FEATURES

Most aggressive angiomyxomas occur in the genital, perineal, and pelvic regions of women of reproductive age, although rare cases also occur in the pelvis, spermatic cord, or scrotum of men (female/male ratio, 6:1). These tumors typically present as slowly growing, deeply situated masses that may infiltrate adjacent structures, including the soft tissues surrounding the rectum and vagina. Because of their infiltrative growth and myxoid nature, aggressive angiomyxomas may be difficult to completely excise, and recur in up to 30% of cases. More recent series have, however, emphasized that correctly diagnosed and appropriately treated angiomyxomas have a much lower rate of local recurrence (< 10%). Metastases are not seen.

PATHOLOGIC FEATURES

GROSS FINDINGS

Aggressive angiomyxomas typically appear as soft, myxoid, variably circumscribed masses of up to 60 cm. Some tumors may be polypoid.

MICROSCOPIC FINDINGS

Aggressive angiomyxomas are composed of bland, spindled to stellate cells widely dispersed in a myxoid matrix (Figure 13-13). A characteristic feature is the presence of numerous blood vessels, ranging from capillaries up to large, gaping vessels with hyalinized walls. In general, these vessels tend to be nonarborizing. Small aggregates of conventional-appearing smooth muscle cells often are seen in close proximity to the blood vessels. Cellularity is typically low, mitotic figures are rare, and necrosis is absent (Figure 13-14). Mast cells and lymphoid aggregates may be present. Occasional tumors show areas reminiscent of angiomyofibroblastoma, including aggregates of epithelioid cells arrayed about blood vessels, suggesting a possible link between these two genital tumors.

ANCILLARY STUDIES

IMMUNOHISTOCHEMISTRY

Most angiomyxomas express both desmin and smooth muscle actins, with some also expressing CD34. S-100 protein and cytokeratins are absent. Estrogen and progesterone receptors are positive.

GENETIC STUDIES

Aggressive angiomyxomas are typified by clonal aberrations involving the *HMGA2* gene, located at 12q13-15.

DIFFERENTIAL DIAGNOSIS

Extensively myxoid leiomyomas may closely mimic aggressive angiomyxoma but are typically better circumscribed, contain larger areas of more typical smooth muscle, and have larger, thick-walled blood vessels. Angiomyofibroblastomas are superficially located and smaller, and consist of epithelioid cells arranged in a perivascular distribution. Myxoid change is unusual in angiomyofibroblastoma. Fibroepithelial polyps of the genital region blend into the overlying epidermis or mucosa, without a Grenz zone, and are usually much more cellular and cytologically variable than are angiomyxomas. Myxofibrosarcomas show much greater cytological atypia and have a well-developed, arborizing, thick-walled vasculature. Myxomas, including cutaneous myxoma, are unusual in the genital region and have distinctive histologic features, as described earlier in this chapter.

PROGNOSIS AND TREATMENT

Despite its name, aggressive angiomyxoma is not an especially aggressive lesion. It does, however, have significant potential for local recurrence, because of its infiltrative growth pattern and the difficulty of completely resecting extensively myxoid tumors. As noted earlier, incompletely excised aggressive angiomyxomas have a roughly 30% risk for recurrence; this risk decreases with more complete initial resection. Aggressive angiomyxoma has no potential for distant metastasis or malignant transformation.

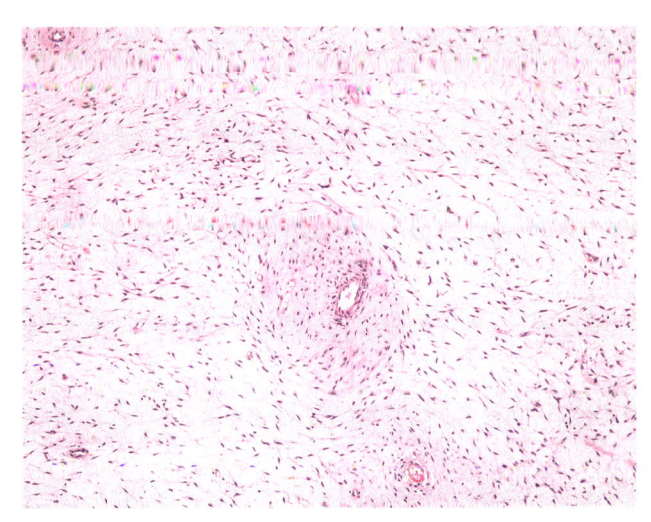

FIGURE 13-13
Aggressive angiomyxoma, a deeply situated, uniformly myxoid tumor, with low cellularity and numerous thin-walled, nonarborizing vessels.

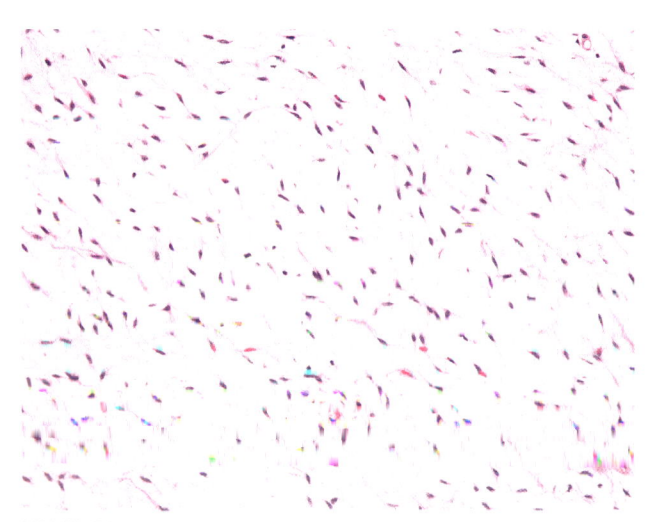

FIGURE 13-14
Spindled to stellate tumor cells in aggressive angiomyxoma.

AGGRESSIVE ANGIOMYXOMA—FACT SHEET

Definition
▸▸ Distinctive myxoid tumor of the genital region, most often seen in women of reproductive age

Incidence and Location
▸▸ Rare
▸▸ Perineum, pelvis, and genital region in women
▸▸ Scrotum, spermatic cord, and pelvis in men

Morbidity and Mortality
▸▸ Benign neoplasm with significant potential for local recurrence

Sex, Race, and Age Distribution
▸▸ Much more common in women than in men (6:1)
▸▸ Reproductive-aged women and adult men
▸▸ No race predilection

Clinical Features
▸▸ Slow-growing, deeply situated mass

Prognosis and Treatment
▸▸ Significant potential for local recurrence if incompletely excised
▸▸ Requires wide excision
▸▸ No known role for adjuvant therapies

AGGRESSIVE ANGIOMYXOMA—PATHOLOGIC FEATURES

Gross Findings
▸▸ Variably circumscribed but infiltrative
▸▸ Large (up to 60 cm)
▸▸ Myxoid

Microscopic Findings
▸▸ Infiltrative
▸▸ Grenz zone present if near skin/mucosa
▸▸ Abundant myxoid matrix
▸▸ Bland spindled to stellate cells
▸▸ Prominent vasculature: capillaries and dilated, hyalinized larger vessels
▸▸ Small smooth muscle aggregates near blood vessels
▸▸ Lymphoid aggregates and mast cells

Immunohistochemical Findings
▸▸ Positive for desmin, smooth muscle actins, often CD34
▸▸ S-100 protein and cytokeratins negative

Differential Diagnosis
▸▸ Angiomyofibroblastoma, myxoid leiomyoma, other myxomas, myxofibrosarcoma, fibroepithelial polyp

OSSIFYING FIBROMYXOID TUMOR OF SOFT PARTS

CLINICAL FEATURES

Ossifying fibromyxoid tumor of soft parts (OFMT) is an extremely rare mesenchymal tumor that may occur in essentially any location, usually in adults. Although OFMTs were initially believed to be benign, they are better classified as mesenchymal tumors of intermediate (borderline) malignancy, because even histologically benign OFMTs may produce distant metastases in up to 6% of cases. Histologically malignant OFMT are high-grade sarcomas, with distant metastases and adverse patient outcome in nearly 60% of cases.

PATHOLOGIC FEATURES

GROSS FINDINGS

OFMTs present as relatively small, painless masses, often with a radiographically apparent shell of bone.

MICROSCOPIC FINDINGS

Typical OFMTs are characterized by a peripheral shell of bone in 70% of cases, lobulated growth, and small, bland cells arranged in cords and nests within a fibromyxoid stroma (Figure 13-15). The stroma of OFMTs varies from highly myxoid to fibrous, and may, on occasion, be hyalinized and calcify. A characteristic feature of OFMT is its even and regular cell-cell spacing (Figure 13-16). Mitotic activity is usually low. Hyalinized blood vessels are often present. Malignant OFMTs maintain the overall cytoarchitectural features of benign OFMT but show accentuated lobularity, greatly increased cellularity with nuclear overlapping, coarse chromatin and prominent nucleoli, necrosis, vascular invasion, and mitotic activity of more than 2 per 50 high-power fields (hpf) (Figures 13-17 and 13-18). Prominent spindling or extensive stromal hyalinization may be present. Bone production may be either absent or increased, sometimes within the center of the lesion.

ANCILLARY STUDIES

IMMUNOHISTOCHEMISTRY

S-100 protein is expressed by more than 70% of typical OFMTs and by a smaller percentage of atypical or malignant OFMTs, or both. A minority of OFMTs will show focal expression of cytokeratins, smooth muscle actin, or desmin. Some OFMTs may also express other markers of putative nerve sheath differentiation, such as CD57 (Leu 7), *neuron-specific* enolase, and glial fibrillary acidic protein.

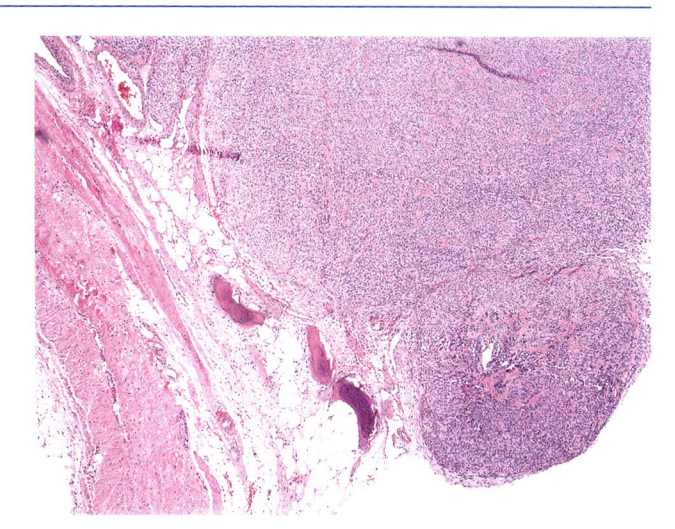

FIGURE 13-15
Typical ossifying fibromyxoid tumor of soft parts, with a peripheral shell of bone surrounding a lobulated, moderately cellular proliferation of uniform cells in a fibromyxoid background.

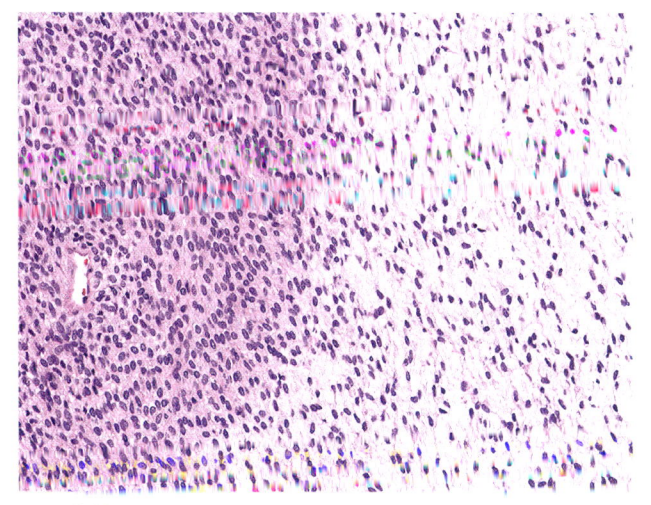

FIGURE 13-16
Uniform cell-cell spacing, cytologically bland, amitotic round to ovoid cells, and fibromyxoid matrix in ossifying fibromyxoid tumor.

GENETIC STUDIES

No consistent genetic abnormality for OFMT has been reported, although occasional cases have been reported to show various translocations.

DIFFERENTIAL DIAGNOSIS

Epithelioid schwannomas lack the bone shell and extremely uniform cell-cell spacing seen in OFMT, and often arise adjacent to a nerve. Epithelioid malignant

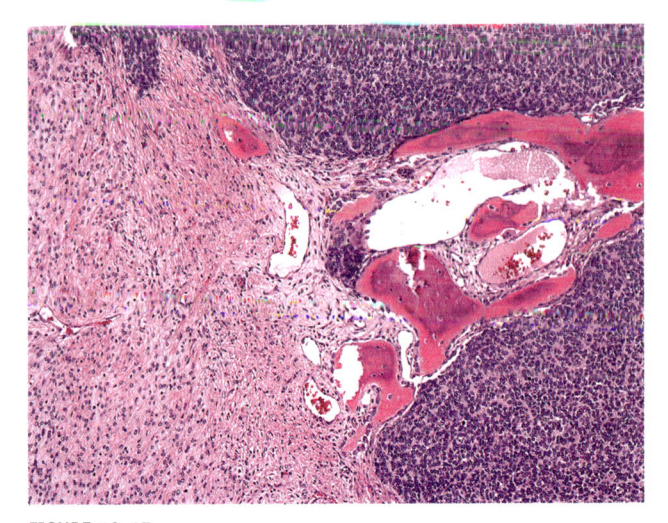

FIGURE 13-17
Area of transition from typical to malignant ossifying fibromyxoid tumor.
Note retention of the bone shell and maintenance of the overall cytoarchitectural pattern in the much more cellular malignant zone.

peripheral nerve sheath tumors show much greater cytologic atypia than do OFMT, resembling melanoma. Mixed tumors/myoepitheliomas do not produce a bone shell, usually show epithelial differentiation, and express epithelial markers, such as cytokeratins, much more often than do OFMTs. Extraskeletal myxoid chondrosarcomas contain distinctly eosinophilic cells that grow in nests, cords, and chains, often with abundant associated hemorrhage and hemosiderin deposition. Osteosarcomas lack a lobular growth pattern, show much greater cytologic atypia and pleomorphism than do even malignant OFMTs, and often produce abundant lace-like osteoid, as well as malignant-appearing chondroid matrix.

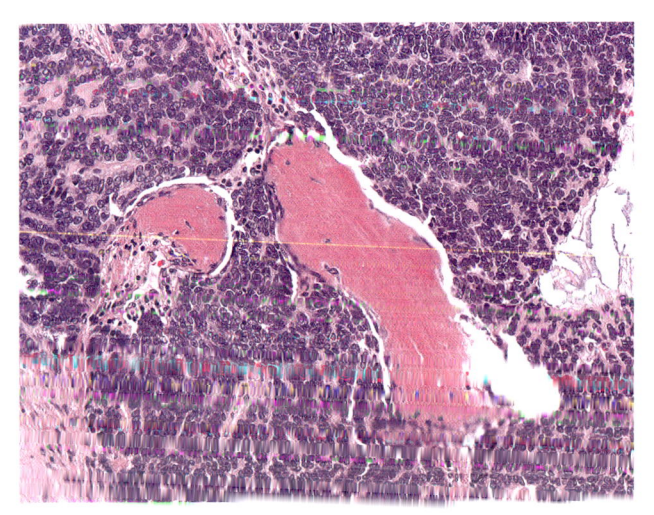

FIGURE 13-18
Malignant ossifying fibromyxoid tumor, showing high cellularity, high nuclear grade, and brisk mitotic activity.

OSSIFYING FIBROMYXOID TUMOR OF SOFT PARTS—FACT SHEET

Definition
▸▸ Mesenchymal tumor of intermediate (borderline) malignancy and an uncertain line of differentiation, characterized by a shell of bone and bland, round cells in a fibromyxoid matrix

Incidence and Location
▸▸ Rare
▸▸ Any soft tissue location including head and neck

Morbidity and Mortality
▸▸ None

Sex, Race, and Age Distribution
▸▸ Adults
▸▸ No sex or race predilection

Clinical Features
▸▸ Small, painless soft tissue mass, often with a shell of bone

Prognosis and Treatment
▸▸ More than 90% of histologically typical tumors are cured with complete excision
▸▸ Local recurrences and distant metastases in approximately 10% and 6% of histologically typical tumors, respectively
▸▸ Histologically malignant ossifying fibromyxoid tumors have an approximately 60% risk for distant metastases and death from disease

OSSIFYING FIBROMYXOID TUMOR OF SOFT PARTS—PATHOLOGIC FEATURES

Gross Findings
▸▸ Small, nonspecific mass, often with a visible shell of bone

Microscopic Findings
▸▸ Shell of woven bone in 70% of cases
▸▸ Bland, round to ovoid cells with uniform cell-cell spacing in a fibromyxoid to hyalinized matrix
▸▸ Lobulated
▸▸ May entrap adnexal glands if superficially located
▸▸ Rare mitotic figures and absent necrosis
▸▸ Malignant examples show accentuated lobularity, increased cellularity, high nuclear grade, high mitotic activity, increased intralesional bone/osteoid and necrosis; bone shell is less frequent

Immunohistochemical Findings
▸▸ S-100 protein expression in 70% of typical and 30% of malignant ossifying fibromyxoid tumors, respectively
▸▸ Desmin expression in approximately 10%
▸▸ Rare cases with smooth muscle actin or cytokeratin expression, or both
▸▸ May express CD57, neuron specific enolase, and glial fibrillary acidic protein

Differential Diagnosis
▸▸ Epithelioid schwannoma, epithelioid malignant peripheral nerve sheath tumor, osteosarcoma, mixed tumor/myoepithelioma, extraskeletal myxoid chondrosarcoma

PLEOMORPHIC HYALINIZING ANGIECTATIC TUMOR

CLINICAL FEATURES

Pleomorphic hyalinizing angiectatic tumor (PHAT) is an extremely rare mesenchymal tumor that typically occurs in the subcutaneous tissues of the distal extremities, usually the ankles and feet. PHATs typically present as slow-growing masses, thought clinically to represent hematomas or Kaposi sarcoma. These tumors are slightly more common in women than in men. Although PHATs were initially believed to be benign, they are better classified as mesenchymal tumors of intermediate (borderline) malignancy, because they frequently recur locally (50% local recurrence rate) and may necessitate amputation. Extraordinarily rare examples have been reported to progress histologically to myxoid sarcoma (myxofibrosarcoma-like).

PATHOLOGIC FEATURES

GROSS FINDINGS

PHATs most often present as 5- to 7-cm masses, with a variably myxoid, cystic, fibrous, or hemorrhagic appearance.

MICROSCOPIC FINDINGS

PHATs are circumscribed but nonencapsulated masses composed of numerous ectatic, partially thrombosed, fibrin-filled, thin-walled blood vessels, surrounded by a sheet-like to fascicular proliferation of pleomorphic but largely amitotic cells, with bizarre-appearing hyperchromatic nuclei, containing pseudonuclear inclusions (Figures 13-19 to 13-21). Intracytoplasmic hemosiderin is often conspicuous within the neoplastic cells. A mixed chronic inflammatory cell infiltrate is often present. The periphery of PHAT often shows a distinctive pattern, descriptively termed *early PHAT*, of relatively uniform spindled cells, with intracytoplasmic hemosiderin and rare enlarged cells, which infiltrate adipose tissue and surround small capillaries and blood vessel aggregates (Figure 13-22). Occasional damaged vessels with intraluminal thrombotic material can often be found in these peripheral zones as well, suggesting that these areas represent the earlier stage of PHAT.

ANCILLARY STUDIES

IMMUNOHISTOCHEMISTRY

PHAT are typically CD34 positive and negative for all other markers except vimentin.

PLEOMORPHIC HYALINIZING ANGIECTATIC TUMOR—FACT SHEET

Definition
- Mesenchymal tumor of intermediate (borderline) malignancy, characterized by angiectasia and largely amitotic, pleomorphic tumor cells

Incidence and Location
- Rare
- Distal extremities, particularly foot and ankle

Morbidity and Mortality
- Local recurrences in up to 50% of cases
- Recurrences may be extensive and require amputation
- Metastases and death from disease have not been reported

Sex, Race, and Age Distribution
- Older adults
- No sex or race predilection

Clinical Features
- Slow-growing mass resembling hematoma or Kaposi sarcoma

Prognosis and Treatment
- 50% local recurrence rate
- Requires wide excision
- No known role for adjuvant therapies

PLEOMORPHIC HYALINIZING ANGIECTATIC TUMOR—PATHOLOGIC FEATURES

Gross Findings
- Variably sized soft tissue mass, occasionally with myxoid, cystic, or hemorrhagic appearance

Microscopic Findings
- Circumscribed but nonencapsulated
- Clusters of ectatic, thin-walled vessels filled with thrombotic material and fibrin
- Sheets and fascicles of pleomorphic but largely amitotic cells with bizarre appearing nuclei, pseudonuclear inclusions, and intracytoplasmic hemosiderin
- Chronic inflammation
- Peripheral zone *(early PHAT)* consisting of relatively monomorphic spindled cells infiltrating though fat and around clusters of damaged blood vessels

Immunohistochemical Findings
- CD34 positive in most cases

Differential Diagnosis
- Schwannoma, undifferentiated pleomorphic sarcoma, so-called *hemosiderotic fibrohistiocytic lipomatous lesion*

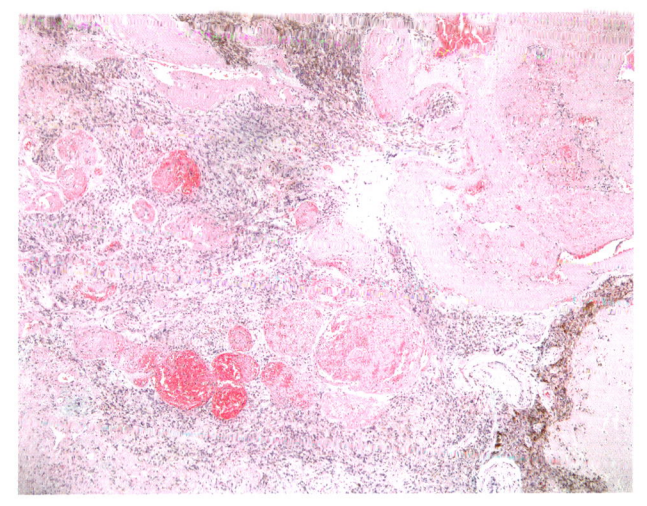

FIGURE 13-19
At low power, pleomorphic hyalinizing angiectatic tumors are most notable for large congeries of dilated, thrombosed, thick- and thin-walled blood vessels. Note prominent hemosiderin staining in surrounding cells.

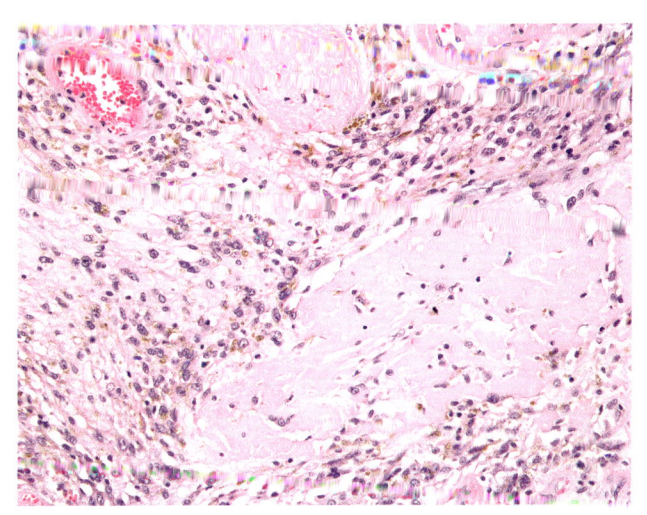

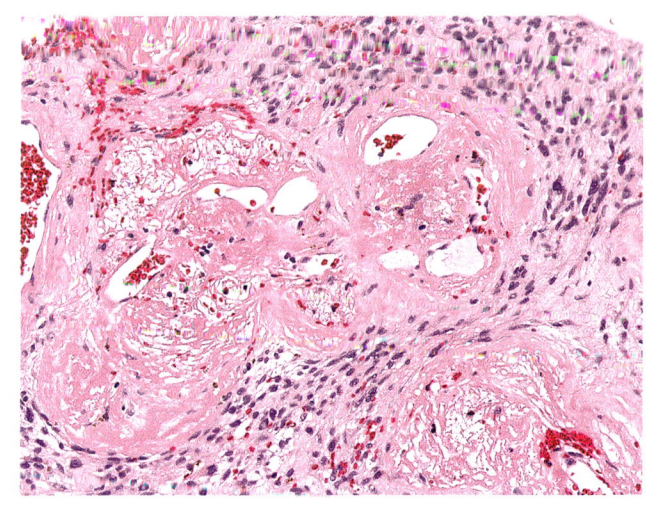

FIGURE 13-21
Thrombosed, fibrin-filled vessels in pleomorphic hyalinizing angiectatic tumor.

FIGURE 13-20
Pleomorphic hyalinizing angiectatic tumor, with a sheet-like proliferation of pleomorphic cells with rare intranuclear pseudoinclusions and abundant intracytoplasmic hemosiderin.

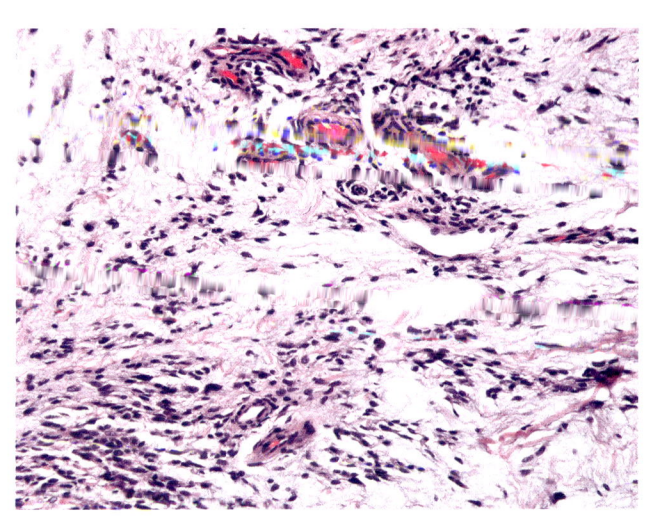

FIGURE 13-22
The periphery of pleomorphic hyalinizing angiectatic tumor (PHAT) often shows a distinctive spindle cell proliferation, descriptively termed *early PHAT*. These spindled cells appear to surround and damage small vessels, a phenomenon that likely leads to the development of classic PHAT over time.

GENETIC STUDIES

No consistent genetic abnormality has been reported.

DIFFERENTIAL DIAGNOSIS

Unlike schwannomas, PHATs are nonencapsulated, contain intracytoplasmic hemosiderin, and are S-100 protein negative. Undifferentiated pleomorphic sarcomas may at times show vascular changes identical to PHAT but show far greater mitotic activity and lack intranuclear pseudoinclusions. The histologic features of early PHATs and so-called *hemosiderotic fibrohistiocytic lipomatous lesions* are identical, and these almost certainly represent the same entity.

PHOSPHATURIC MESENCHYMAL TUMOR

CLINICAL FEATURES

Phosphaturic mesenchymal tumors are rare mesenchymal tumors that result in systemic osteomalacia through secretion of a phosphaturic hormone, recently identified as fibroblast growth factor 23 (FGF-23). Most

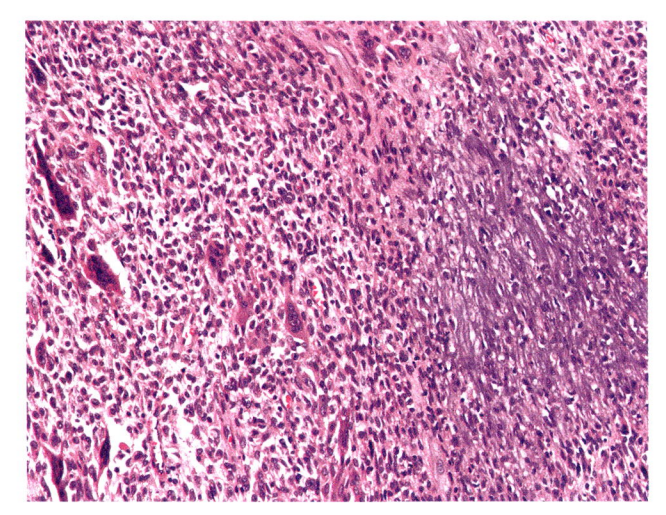

CHAPTER 13 Tumors of Miscellaneous Type or Uncertain Lineage

FIGURE 13-23
Phosphaturic mesenchymal tumor, mixed connective tissue variant, showing a characteristic admixture of calcified matrix, small vessels, innocuous spindled cells, and osteoclast-like giant cells.

phosphaturic mesenchymal tumors comprise a single histologic entity, designated *phosphaturic mesenchymal tumor, mixed connective tissue type* (PMTMCT). PMTMCTs are rare tumors, which most often occur in middle aged adults, either in soft tissue or bone. Most PMTMCTs present as small, inapparent lesions that may require careful clinical examination and radionuclide scans for localization in some cases. A long history of osteomalacia is almost always present. The overwhelming majority of PMTMCTs are histologically and clinically benign, with complete excision resulting in dramatic improvement of phosphate wasting and osteomalacia. Rare PMTMCTs are histologically and clinically malignant.

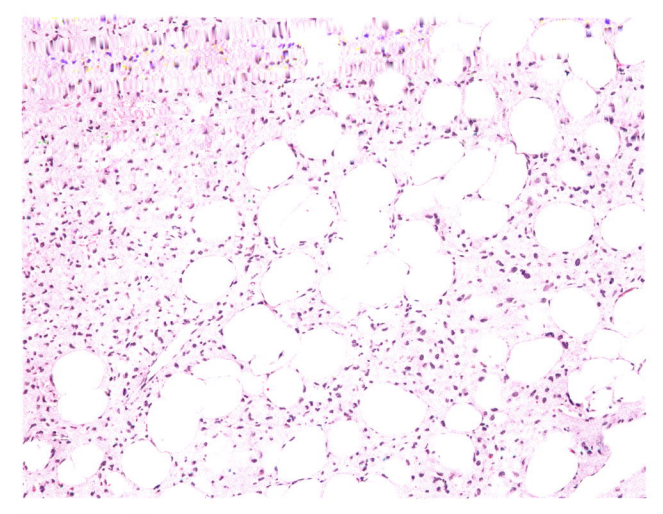

PATHOLOGIC FEATURES

GROSS FINDINGS

Most PMTMCTs present as nonspecific soft tissue or bone masses. Some tumors may be highly calcified.

MICROSCOPIC FINDINGS

PMTMCTs are variable in their appearance but often show an admixture of calcified matrix, mature fat, bland spindled cells, and osteoclast-like giant cells (Figure 13-23). The neoplastic component of PMTMCT is characterized by a proliferation of small, innocuous-appearing, round to spindled cells embedded in a highly vascular, myxochondroid matrix, with a variable component of mature adipose tissue (Figure 13-24). This matrix commonly calcifies in an unusual, *grungy* fashion, inciting an osteoclast-rich and fibrohistiocytic response (Figure 13-25). Malignant PMTMCTs contain obviously sarcomatous foci, resembling an undifferentiated pleomorphic sarcoma or fibrosarcoma.

ANCILLARY STUDIES

IMMUNOHISTOCHEMISTRY

By immunohistochemistry (IHC), the cells of PMTMCTs express FGF-23 and vimentin, in the absence of other markers.

GENETIC STUDIES

A specific genetic event has not been identified in PMTMCTs. Reverse transcriptase-polymerase chain reaction (RT-PCR) can confirm that the tumor cells are producing FGF-23.

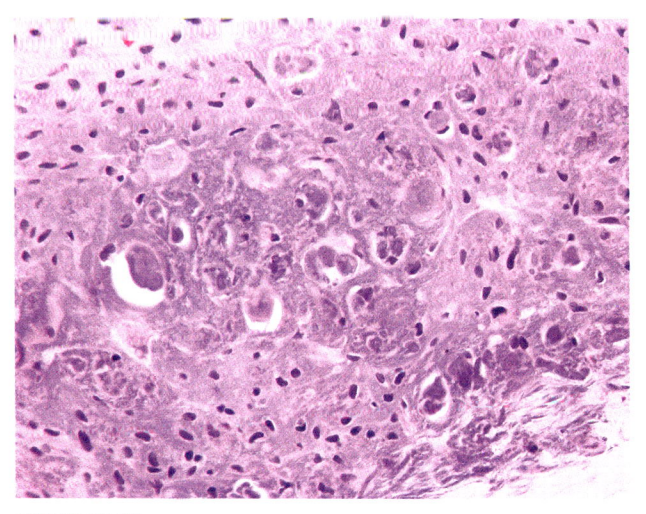

FIGURE 13-24
Unusual hyalinized, partially calcified matrix and fat in phosphaturic mesenchymal tumor, mixed connective tissue variant.

FIGURE 13-25
Phosphaturic mesenchymal tumor, mixed connective tissue variant, showing distinctive *grungy* pattern of matrix calcification.

PHOSPHATURIC MESENCHYMAL TUMORS—FACT SHEET

Definition
- Usually benign, distinctive mesenchymal tumor that produces oncogenic osteomalacia through elaboration of a phosphaturic hormone, FGF-23

Incidence and Location
- Rare
- Roughly equal incidence in bone and soft tissue locations; tend to involve extremities rather than trunk
- May involve head and neck, particularly the sinuses

Morbidity and Mortality
- Tumor-induced osteomalacia may be extremely debilitating and does not resolve without complete tumor resection
- Rare malignant examples may metastasize and kill patients

Sex, Race, and Age Distribution
- Usually occur in middle-aged to older adults
- No sex or race predilection

Clinical Features
- Presents in almost all cases with long-standing osteomalacia
- Usually a small and difficult to find mass in soft tissues or bone
- Octreotide nuclear medicine study may be extremely valuable in finding occult tumors

Prognosis and Treatment
- Almost all PMTMCTs are cured with complete excision, phosphaturia resolves with complete tumor removal
- Patients with incompletely resected tumors may be successfully managed medically in some instances, but resection should always be the goal
- Rare malignant examples behave as sarcomas and require wide resection
- No known role for adjuvant therapies

PHOSPHATURIC MESENCHYMAL TUMORS—PATHOLOGIC FEATURES

Gross Findings
- Partially fatty-appearing mass, sometimes calcified

Microscopic Findings
- Small round to spindled cells embedded in a distinctive myxochondroid matrix, with *grungy* calcification
- Variable amount of mature fat
- Highly vascular; may show capillary or *hemangiopericytoma-like* pattern
- Chondroid- or osteoid-like matrix
- Aggregates of osteoclast-like giant cells and associated fibrohistiocytic proliferation
- Malignant examples resemble undifferentiated pleomorphic sarcoma or fibrosarcoma

Immunohistochemical Findings
- Typically express only vimentin
- FGF-23 production may be identified by IHC; however, the antibody is not commercially available (may also be detected by RT-PCR)

Differential Diagnosis
- Hemangiopericytoma, hemangioma, chondrosarcoma, osteosarcoma, chondromyxoid fibroma, spindle cell lipoma, giant cell tumor

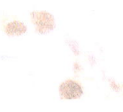

PERIVASCULAR EPITHELIOID CELL NEOPLASMS

CLINICAL FEATURES

The perivascular epithelioid cell neoplasms (PEComas) are a group of related tumors, the members of which include angiomyolipoma of the kidney (and other locations), clear cell *sugar* tumor of the lung, lymphangioleiomyomatosis, and rare tumors that occur in the soft tissues, bone, skin, abdominal cavity, and gynecologic tract, among other locations. This family of tumors is defined by the presence of distinctive perivascular epithelioid cells with a *myomelanocytic* immunophenotype (see later), and by an association with tuberous sclerosis complex in subsets of patients. Angiomyolipoma, clear cell sugar tumor, and lymphangioleiomyomatosis are covered in depth in the textbooks in this series on tumors of the kidney and lung, and will not be covered in this chapter. The term *PEComa*, as used later, refers only to PEComas other than these three entities.

PEComas are far more common in women than in men (female/male ratio, 7:1) and most often occur in middle-aged adults, although they may be seen in very

DIFFERENTIAL DIAGNOSIS

In most cases of PMTMCT, a clinical history of osteomalacia will be available, and the tumor will have been resected specifically for treatment of tumor-induced osteomalacia, greatly simplifying the diagnosis of PMTMCT. Unsuspected PMTMCT may be confused with hemangiopericytomas/SFTs, hemangiomas, giant cell tumors, spindle cell lipomas, and various cartilaginous tumors, among others. Recognition of the unique constellation of histologic features shown by PMTMCT, in particular, the distinctive *grungy*-appearing calcified matrix, is the best way to distinguish it from other tumors. The histologic features of PMTMCT overlap considerably with those of chondromyxoid fibroma of bone, and radiographic studies and clinical/laboratory correlation may be required to make this distinction.

young and old patients. They most commonly involve the gynecologic tract, in particular the uterus, but are also relatively common in intra-abdominal locations including the falciform ligament and omentum. Tumors in somatic soft tissue, bone, and cutaneous locations have been reported but are rare. PEComas present as nonspecific masses with symptoms referable to impingement of local anatomic structures. Most PEComas behave in a benign fashion and require only complete excision. Rare PEComas are clinically malignant, with aggressive local recurrences and distant metastases. Little, if any, data have been reported on the role of adjuvant therapies in the management of malignant PEComas. Only a small minority of soft tissue, bone, intra-abdominal, or gynecologic PEComas occur in patients with known tuberous sclerosis complex.

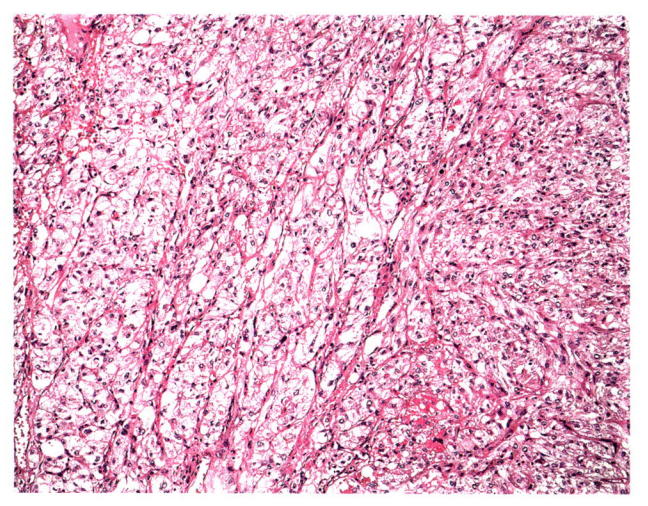

Pathologic Features

Gross Findings

PEComas appear grossly as nonspecific soft tissue masses.

Microscopic Findings

Perivascular epithelioid cells are characterized by spindled to epithelioid morphology, clear to lightly eosinophilic, somewhat *stringy*-appearing cytoplasm, and round to ovoid nuclei with small, visible nucleoli. These tumors may grow in principally a spindled and partially nested pattern in association with an elaborate renal cell carcinoma–like capillary network (clear cell myomelanocytic pattern) (Figure 13-26), as sheets of epithelioid cells (epithelioid angiomyolipoma pattern) (Figure 13-27), or with prominent perivascular and stromal hyalinization (sclerosing pattern) (Figure 13-28). Combinations of these three patterns are common, and there do not appear to be any clinical differences between tumors showing one or the other growth pattern. Hemosiderin-laden macrophages are commonly present, and calcifications may be seen. Occasional tumors show multinucleated tumor giant cells or giant cells resembling the *spider cells* of rhabdomyoma, with central cytoplasmic eosinophilia and peripheral clearing. Rare tumors show striking degenerative cytological atypia, similar to that seen in symplastic uterine leiomyomas. Malignant PEComas show high nuclear grade,

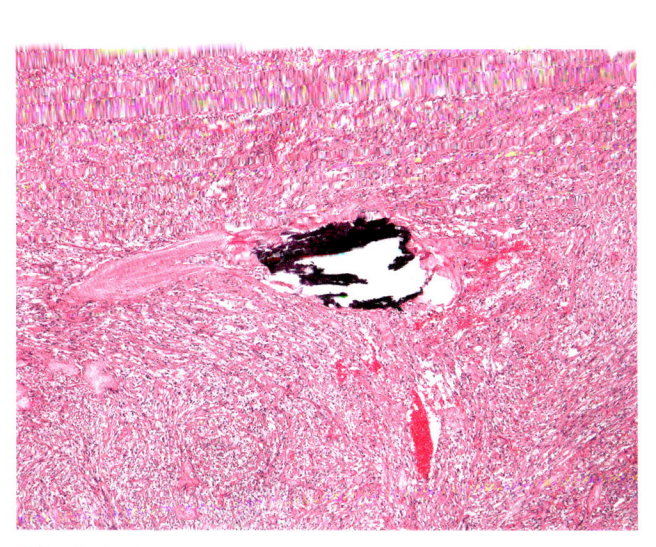

FIGURE 13-27
Nested proliferation of spindled to epithelioid cells with clear cytoplasm and round to ovoid nuclei in perivascular epithelioid cell neoplasm of the omentum.

FIGURE 13-26
Perivascular epithelioid cell neoplasm of the thigh with an elaborate capillary vasculature *(renal cell carcinoma-like)*, stromal calcification, and fascicles of clear to lightly eosinophilic spindled cells.

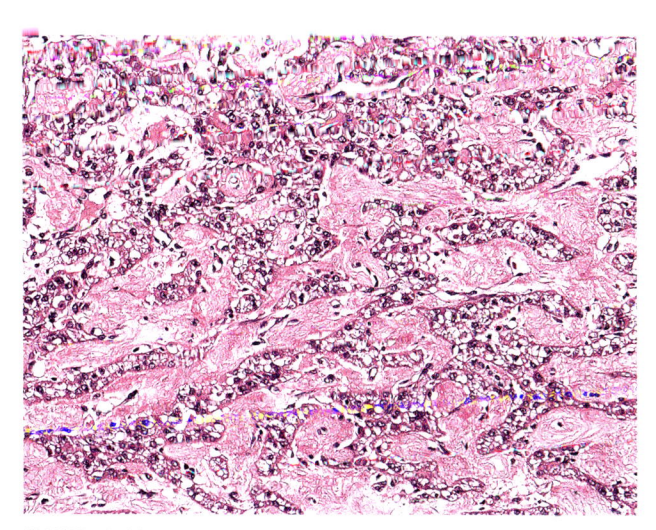

FIGURE 13-28
Mesenteric perivascular epithelioid cell neoplasm with stromal and perivascular sclerosis.

high cellularity, frequent mitotic activity with atypical forms, and necrosis.

ANCILLARY STUDIES

IMMUNOHISTOCHEMISTRY

PEComas are, in part, defined by their *myomelanocytic* immunophenotype, with coexpression of melanocytic markers such as HMB45, Melan-A, and tyrosinase with muscle markers, such as smooth muscle actin. Expression of these melanocytic markers in PEComas is believed to represent true melanocytic differentiation, as reflected in the presence of premelanosomes on ultrastructural study. A minority of cases may show expression of S-100 protein or desmin, potentially resulting in confusion with melanocytic tumors and true smooth muscle tumors, respectively. Expression of cytokeratins, CD34, and CD117 (c-kit) is rare. Loss of tuberin expression has been demonstrated in a small number of studied PEComas. Estrogen and progesterone receptors may be expressed.

GENETIC STUDIES

PEComas show frequent deletions of one of the tuberous sclerosis–associated genes, *TSC2*, with activation of the mammalian target of rapamycin pathway.

DIFFERENTIAL DIAGNOSIS

Malignant melanocytic tumors, including melanoma, clear cell sarcoma, and gastrointestinal clear cell sarcoma-like tumor, show uniform strong S-100 protein expression and lack expression of smooth muscle actin. Melanocytic tumors also tend to lack the distinctive clear to lightly eosinophilic cytoplasm of PEComas and show much more prominent nucleoli. Smooth muscle tumors are composed of fascicles of eosinophilic spindled cells with *cigar shaped* nuclei and perinuclear vacuoles, show strong desmin expression in most cases, and lack expression of Melan-A and tyrosinase. It is important to remember that some conventional smooth muscle tumors may show positivity with HMB45, thought to represent a cross-reactivity, rather than true melanocytic differentiation. Clear cell carcinomas of renal or adrenal origin almost always show strong expression of cytokeratins, using modern immunohistochemical technique. Alveolar soft part sarcoma (ASPS) lacks expression of myomelanocytic markers and shows much higher nuclear grade. Gastrointestinal stromal tumors are negative for myomelanocytic markers and positive for CD117 in more than 90% of cases.

PERIVASCULAR EPITHELIOID CELL NEOPLASMS—FACT SHEET

Definition
- Family of related tumors, defined by the presence of morphologically and immunohistochemically distinctive perivascular epithelioid cells

Incidence and Location
- Rare
- Most commonly involve gynecologic tract and intra-abdominal locations such as falciform ligament, but may involve any soft tissue, bone, cutaneous, or visceral location

Morbidity and Mortality
- Great majority of PEComas are histologically and clinically benign
- Malignant PEComas behave as high-grade sarcomas, with significant potential for aggressive growth and distant metastasis

Sex, Race, and Age Distribution
- Far more common in women than in men (7:1)
- Usually occur in middle-aged patients, but may affect children and older adults

Clinical Features
- Mass, with symptoms depending on location and extent of disease
- Infrequent association with known tuberous sclerosis complex

Prognosis and Treatment
- Benign PEComas require only complete excision
- Malignant PEComas should be treated surgically as high-grade sarcomas
- Little or no data on the role of adjuvant therapies in malignant PEComa exist

---

PERIVASCULAR EPITHELIOID CELL NEOPLASMS—PATHOLOGIC FEATURES

Gross Findings
- Nonspecific mass

Microscopic Findings
- Clear to lightly eosinophilic, spindled to epithelioid cells with round to ovoid nuclei and small nucleoli
- Elaborate vasculature, ranging from capillary sized to large and hyalinized
- Three main patterns: spindled, epithelioid, and sclerosing
- Multinucleated giant cells and "spider cell"–like giant cells in some

Immunohistochemical Findings
- *Myomelanocytic* immunophenotype, with coexpression of smooth muscle actin and HMB45/Melan-A/tyrosinase
- May show limited S-100 protein or desmin expression in a minority of cases

Differential Diagnosis
- Melanoma, clear cell sarcoma, gastrointestinal clear cell sarcoma-like tumor, gastrointestinal stromal tumor, ASPS, clear cell carcinoma, true smooth muscle tumors

EPITHELIOID SARCOMA

CLINICAL FEATURES

Epithelioid sarcomas most commonly occur in the hands, fingers, and lower arm of adolescents and young adults but may occur in essentially any location and any age group. Many occur in association with a tendon or aponeurosis; however, they may involve skin away from such structures. Epithelioid sarcomas recur in more than 70% of cases, often as multiple subcutaneous nodules in the more proximal extremity. Nearly 50% of epithelioid sarcomas will eventually metastasize distantly, most often to lymph nodes and the lungs, but also to skin and soft tissue sites. Metastatic epithelioid sarcomas are almost uniformly fatal. Epithelioid sarcomas are not graded; adverse prognostic features include male sex, proximal location, size larger than 5 cm, deep location, high mitotic rate, necrosis, and vascular invasion.

PATHOLOGIC FEATURES

GROSS FINDINGS

Epithelioid sarcomas typically present as relatively small, ulcerated, firm, single or multiple nodules that may mimic nonspecific ulcers.

MICROSCOPIC FINDINGS

Epithelioid sarcomas typically grow as nodular, vaguely circumscribed, infiltrative masses, often with central necrosis (Figure 13-29). Fusion of individual tumor nodules and extension along tendons may create a garland-like appearance. The relatively bland nuclear features of the neoplastic cells in association with central necrosis may closely mimic a granulomatous process, such as a necrobiotic granuloma. The neoplastic cells range from small epithelioid cells, to larger rhabdoid cells, to elongated and distinctly spindled forms (Figure 13-30). The nuclei of epithelioid sarcomas are relatively uniform appearing but hyperchromatic. Some epithelioid sarcomas consist almost entirely of spindled cells, mimicking benign fibrous histiocytoma or fibrosarcoma. Epithelioid sarcomas in more proximal locations are typically composed of more pleomorphic, rhabdoid cells *(proximal variant)* (Figure 13-31). Rare epithelioid sarcomas may show prominent hemorrhage and pseudovascular space formation, mimicking angiosarcoma (Figure 13-32), or may contain calcifications or bone, or both, suggesting synovial sarcoma or calcifying aponeurotic fibroma.

EPITHELIOID SARCOMA—FACT SHEET

Definition
▸▸ Malignant mesenchymal tumor showing epithelial differentiation

Incidence and location
▸▸ Rare
▸▸ Fingers, hands, and lower arm
▸▸ May occur in more proximal locations

Morbidity and Mortality
▸▸ Local recurrences in 70% of cases
▸▸ Recurrences often involve more proximal soft tissues
▸▸ Eventual metastases in 50% of patients
▸▸ Almost all patients with metastases die of disease

Sex, Race, and Age Distribution
▸▸ Most common in adolescent and young adults of both sexes
▸▸ May involve patients of any age

Clinical Features
▸▸ Small ulcerated nodule, may be multiple

Prognosis and Treatment
▸▸ Local recurrences and metastases in 70% and 50% of patients, respectively
▸▸ Requires aggressive surgical management, often including amputation
▸▸ Radiotherapy and chemotherapy may be indicated but are not known to be highly effective

---

EPITHELIOID SARCOMA—PATHOLOGIC FEATURES

Gross Findings
▸▸ Single or multiple nodules involving the skin and subcutis
▸▸ May be ulcerated or show necrosis on cut section
▸▸ Proximal lesions appear as nonspecific, often necrotic large masses

Microscopic Findings
▸▸ Deceptively bland epithelioid cells growing in nodules, sheets, chains, and garlands
▸▸ Central necrosis (granuloma-like)
▸▸ May modulate between epithelioid and spindled forms, or rarely be predominantly spindled (fibroma-like variant)
▸▸ May contain rhabdoid cells, particularly in larger, proximal lesions
▸▸ Pseudovascular changes in some
▸▸ Rarely, metaplastic bone

Immunohistochemical Findings
▸▸ Coexpression of cytokeratins (low and high molecular weight) and vimentin
▸▸ CD34 expression in 50%
▸▸ Loss of INI-1 expression in 90%

Differential Diagnosis
▸▸ Necrobiotic granulomas, cutaneous carcinomas (squamous cell and adnexal), metastatic carcinoma, benign fibrous histiocytoma (fibroma-like variants), epithelioid angiosarcoma (pseudovascular variants)

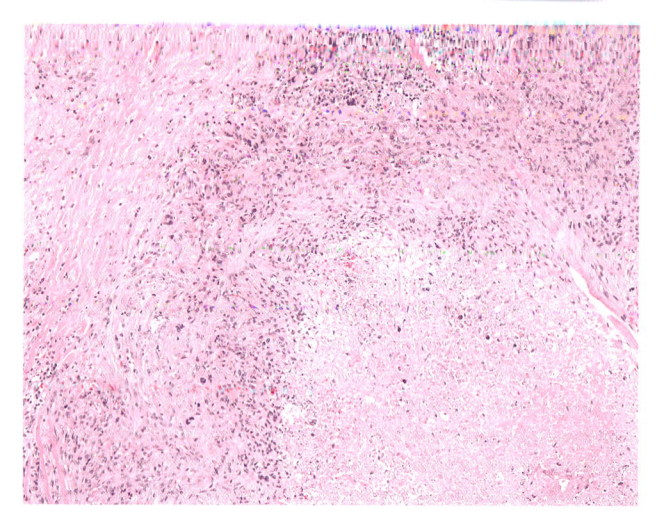

FIGURE 13-29
Epithelioid sarcoma, with a garland-like proliferation of malignant epithelioid cells around a central focus of necrosis.

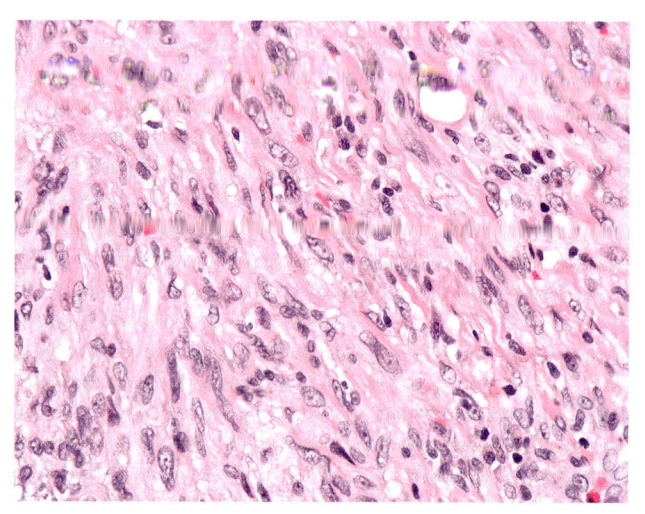

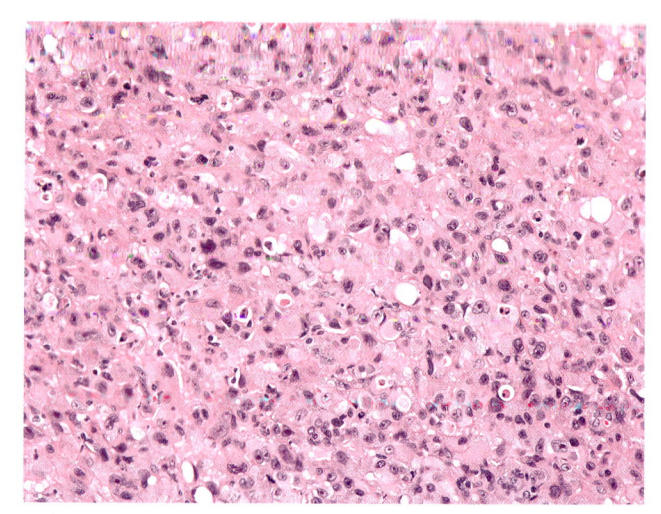

FIGURE 13-31
Proximal-type epithelioid sarcoma, with greater pleomorphism and many rhabdoid cells.

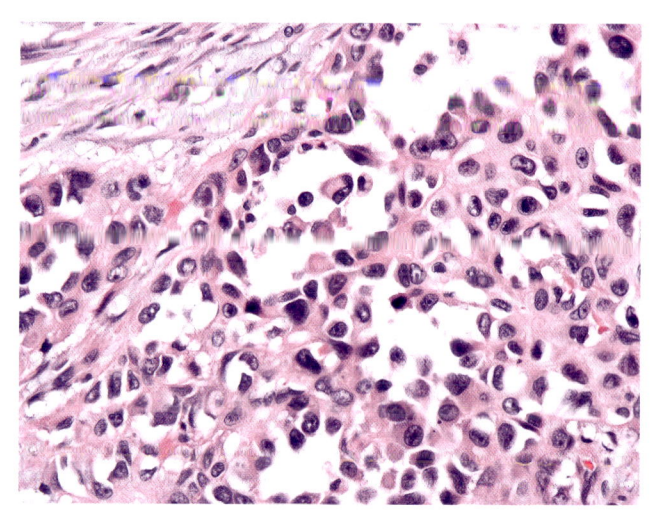

FIGURE 13-30
Relatively bland, but hyperchromatic, epithelioid to spindled cells in epithelioid sarcoma.

FIGURE 13-32
Pseudovascular or pseudoglandular change in epithelioid sarcoma.

ANCILLARY STUDIES

IMMUNOHISTOCHEMISTRY

By IHC, epithelioid sarcomas coexpress cytokeratins (including both low and high molecular weights isoforms) and vimentin, and express CD34 in roughly 50% of cases. In general they do not express cytokeratins 5/6, a finding that may help to distinguish them from squamous cell carcinomas. A small number of epithelioid sarcomas are cytokeratin negative. Epithelioid sarcomas do not express other vascular markers, such as CD31, FLI-1, or von Willebrand factor (vWF). Recent studies have shown loss of INI-1 protein in more than 90% of epithelioid sarcomas, a finding that may be useful in their distinction from carcinomas and other sarcomas, which essentially always show retained INI-1 expression.

DIFFERENTIAL DIAGNOSIS

Epithelioid sarcomas can be distinguished from granulomatous inflammation by virtue of its infiltrative growth, true tumor cell necrosis, and typical admixture of hyperchromatic epithelioid and spindled cells. Pseudovascular epithelioid sarcomas may be distinguished from angiosarcoma by positive staining for high-molecular-weight cytokeratins and negative staining for CD31, FLI-1 protein, vWF, and INI-1. Unlike most squamous cell carcinomas, epithelioid sarcomas lack associated in situ carcinoma, do not show squamous pearl formation, and often appear to blend into the surrounding collagen. IHC for CD34 (positive in epithelioid sarcoma but not squamous cell carcinoma), and p63, CK5/6, and INI-1 (positive in squamous cell carcinoma but not in epithelioid sarcoma) may be helpful. Spindled epithelioid sarcomas are deceptively bland appearing, often contain hyalinized collagen, and may closely simulate benign fibrous histiocytoma (dermatofibroma), particularly in unusual locations where clinical suspicion for epithelioid sarcomas may be low. Epithelioid sarcomas do not contain the foamy macrophages and siderophages seen in fibrous histiocytomas, and show a greater degree of nuclear hyperchromatism. Cytokeratin immunostains are critical in making this crucial distinction. Epithelioid sarcomas may be factor XIIIa positive, and this marker is not helpful in this situation.

ALVEOLAR SOFT PART SARCOMA

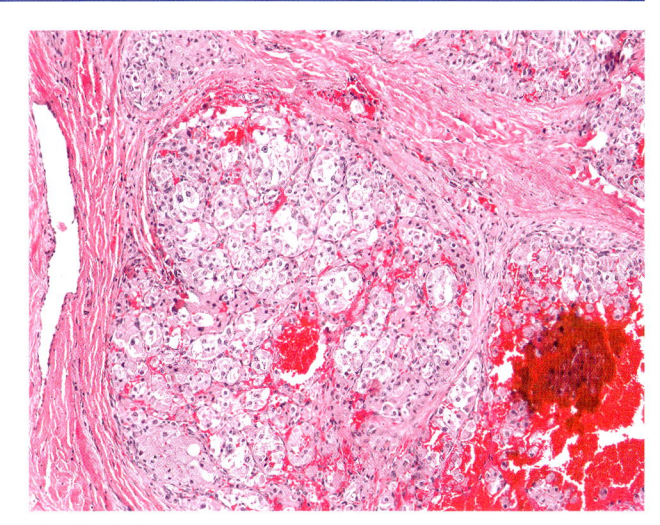

FIGURE 13-33
Alveolar soft part sarcoma with hemorrhage and prominent nested growth.

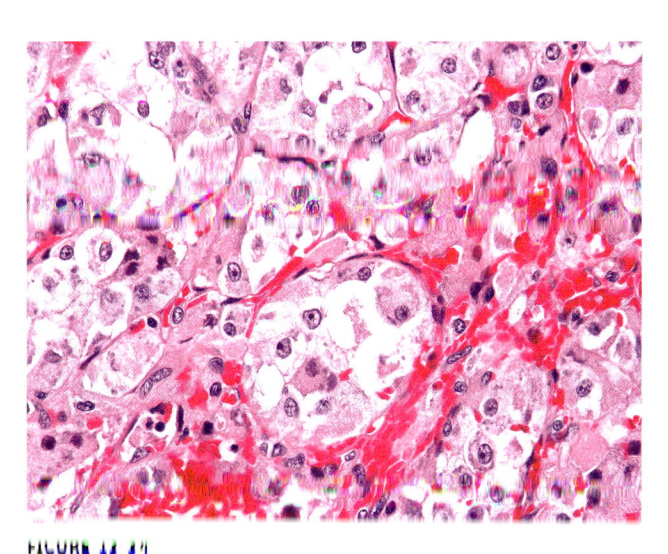

Clinical Features

Most cases of ASPS occur in the deep soft tissues of the extremities. A substantial percentage occurs in the head and neck, particularly in children, often involving the orbit and tongue. ASPS is extremely rare, accounting for less than 1% of soft tissue tumors overall. Approximately 60% of ASPSs occur in women. ASPSs are relatively indolent but relentless sarcomas, characterized by late metastases and an extended clinical course. ASPSs are not graded. Reported survival rates are 77% at 2 years, 60% at 5 years, 38% at 10 years, and only 15% at 20 years. ASPSs most frequently metastasize to lungs, brain, and bone. No effective systemic therapy exists for ASPS.

Pathologic Features

Gross Findings

ASPSs usually present as painless masses, which may be highly vascular on imaging studies.

Microscopic Findings

ASPSs are characterized by uniform, organoid nests of polygonal tumor cells, separated by fibrovascular septa and delicate capillary-sized vascular channels (Figure 13-33). Within these nests, there is prominent cellular dyshesion, imparting the characteristic pseudoalveolar pattern. Intravascular tumor extension is usually present. The cells of ASPS have distinct cell borders and abundant eosinophilic to clear, somewhat granular cytoplasm (Figure 13-34). A characteristic finding is the presence of PAS-positive, diastase-resistant crystalline structures, which may be rhomboid, rod-like, or spiked. The nuclei of ASPS are round, regular, and eccentrically placed with vesicular chromatin and a prominent central nucleolus. Mitotic activity is usually low, and necrosis is infrequent.

FIGURE 13-34
Tumor cells with abundant eosinophilic cytoplasm and prominent nucleoli in alveolar soft part sarcoma.

Ancillary Studies

Immunohistochemistry

IHC plays a limited role in the diagnosis of ASPS. ASPSs are negative for cytokeratins, EMA, chromogranin A, synaptophysin, HMB45, and Melan-A. Nonspecific markers such as neuron-specific enolase and vimentin may be present in roughly 30% to 50% of cases. Antibodies to pan-muscle actins, smooth muscle actins, and skeletal muscle actins are occasionally positive. Focal desmin expression may be seen in some ASPSs, typically only in a small number of cells. ASPSs are consistently negative for specific markers of skeletal muscle differentiation, such as myogenin and MyoD1. Nuclear expression of TFE3 is a highly sensitive and specific marker of ASPS.

ALVEOLAR SOFT PART SARCOMA—FACT SHEET

Definition
- Malignant mesenchymal tumor characterized by large eosinophilic cells with an alveolar growth pattern

Incidence and Location
- Rare, < 1% of soft tissue tumors
- Deep soft tissues of extremities
- Head and neck
- Oral cavity in children

Morbidity and Mortality
- Relatively indolent with extended clinical course
- Late metastases in many, with 5-year survival rate of 60% but only 15% at 20 years

Sex, Race, and Age Distribution
- 60% of cases occur in women

Clinical Features
- Painless soft tissue mass, often highly vascular

Prognosis and Treatment
- Good short-term survival (77% at 2 years) but poor long-term survival
- Aggressive surgical management
- No proven role for chemotherapy or radiotherapy

ALVEOLAR SOFT PART SARCOMA—PATHOLOGIC FEATURES

Gross Findings
- Large, hemorrhagic, soft tissue mass

Microscopic Findings
- Uniform, organoid nests of large, dyshesive, eosinophilic tumor cells with prominent nucleoli
- PAS-positive, diastase-resistant intracytoplasmic crystals
- Intravascular extension
- Mitoses are rare, and necrosis is uncommon
- Rare cases with pleomorphism, spindling, or both

Immunohistochemical Findings
- Vimentin positive; negative for epithelial and melanocytic markers
- May show limited desmin expression; usually negative for actins
- Negative for nuclear expression of myogenin/MyoD1
- Nuclear TFE3 expression

Differential Diagnosis
- Carcinoma (renal, adrenal, hepatocellular), melanoma, paraganglioma, granular cell tumor

GENETIC STUDIES

At the genetic level, ASPS is characterized by an unbalanced translocation: der(17)t(X;17)(p11;p25), resulting in the fusion of a gene of unknown function, ASPL (alveolar soft part sarcoma locus), on chromosome 17 to the TFE3 (transcription factor 3) transcription factor gene on the X chromosome. This fusion gene may be detected by RT-PCR or fluorescent in situ hybridization (FISH) for TFE3.

DIFFERENTIAL DIAGNOSIS

The differential diagnosis of ASPS includes other tumors with nested/organoid patterns of growth and cells with abundant eosinophilic cytoplasm, such as metastatic carcinoma (renal, adrenal, hepatocellular), paraganglioma, melanoma, and granular cell tumor. Positive immunostaining for TFE3 and negative immunostaining for cytokeratins, melanocytic markers (e.g., HMB45), and chromogranin/synaptophysin distinguish ASPS from carcinomas, melanomas, and paragangliomas, respectively. Although granular cell tumors may express TFE3, they lack the striking cytologic atypia seen in ASPS, in most instances, and show strong S-100 protein expression.

EWING FAMILY OF TUMORS (Ewing Sarcoma and Primitive Neuroectodermal Tumor)

CLINICAL FEATURES

Ewing sarcoma (ES) and primitive neuroectodermal tumor (PNET) are rare sarcomas of bone and soft tissue, which may involve any location. ES/PNETs most often occur in children and young adolescents, with a male sex predilection. ES/PNET is extremely rare in African American patients, for unknown reasons. Although ES and PNET were originally regarded as distinct entities, it is now known that they are ends along the histologic spectrum of a single neoplasm, sharing in more than 90% of cases a balanced translocation (11;22) (q24;q12) (513). The term *Ewing family of tumors* (EFT) comprises both ES and PNET. EFTs are high-grade sarcomas, with a 10-year survival rate of just greater than 60% reported in patients treated with modern multimodality therapy. EFT is not graded.

PATHOLOGIC FEATURES

In its classic form, ES shows a sheet-like to vaguely lobular growth pattern (Figure 13-35), a well-developed capillary vasculature, and uniform cell population of round cells with small amounts of clear to lightly eosinophilic cytoplasm, regular nuclear contours, finely dispersed

FIGURE 13-35
Ewing sarcoma/primitive neuroectodermal tumor, showing a vaguely lobular to sheetlike proliferation of uniform small blue round cells.

FIGURE 13-36
The cells of Ewing sarcoma/primitive neuroectodermal tumor are typically regular, with small amounts of clear to lightly eosinophilic cytoplasm, finely dispersed chromatic, and small nucleoli.

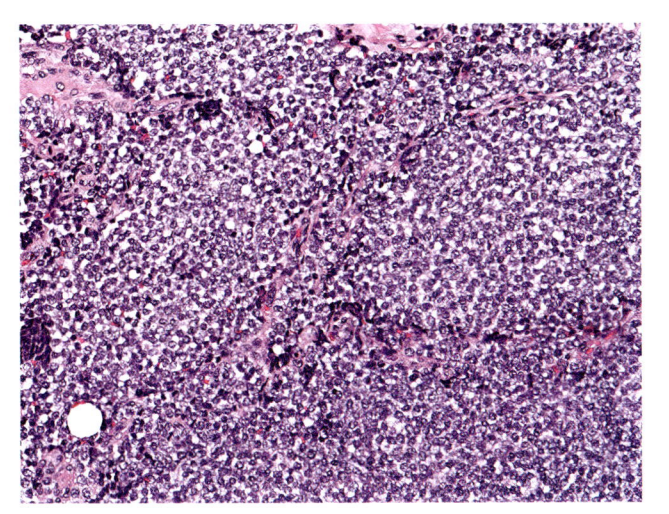

chromatin, and inapparent or small nucleoli (Figure 13-36). Geographic necrosis and individual degenerating cells are frequently present. Features suggesting more complete neuroectodermal differentiation (i.e., PNET) include pseudorosette formation and a mild-to-moderate degree of spindling. Rare histologic variants of ES/PNET may be seen, including large-cell (atypical), adamantinoma-like, sclerosing, and extensively spindled tumors.

ANCILLARY STUDIES

IMMUNOHISTOCHEMISTRY

By IHC, the overwhelming majority of ES/PNET shows intense membranous expression of CD99 (p30/32, MIC2). CD99 expression is, however, not specific for ES/PNET, being present in lymphoblastic lymphomas, poorly differentiated synovial sarcomas (PDSSs), a subset of rhabdomyosarcomas, and many other *small blue round cell tumors*. IHC for FLI1 protein is positive in close to 90% of histologically typical ES/PNETs and is useful in confirming this diagnosis in difficult cases. Approximately 25% of ES/PNETs may show focal anomalous expression of low-molecular-weight cytokeratins. Anomalous desmin expression may be seen in a small minority of cases (<3%), typically limited to only a few cells. Other markers such as CD56, S-100 protein, chromogranin A, or synaptophysin are only rarely positive.

GENETIC FINDINGS

At the genetic level, more than 90% of EFTs harbor the t(11;22)(q24;q12) *(EWS-FLI1)*, with approximately 5% of cases showing t(21;22)(q22;q12) *(EWS-ERG)*, and less than 1% of cases harboring rare translocations,

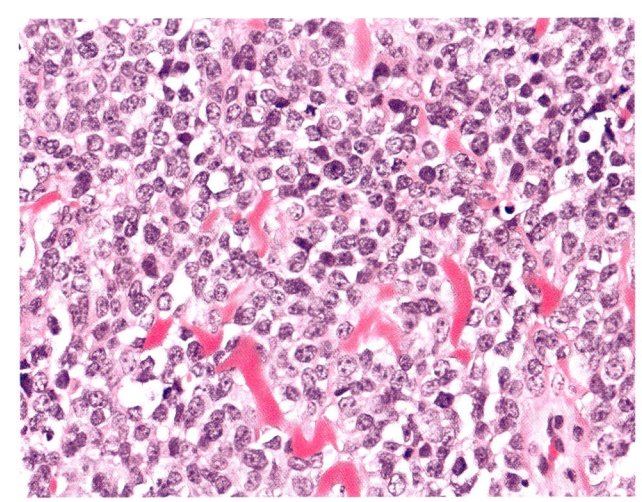

such as t(7;22)(p22;q12) *(EWS-ETV1)*, t(17;22)(q12;q12) *(EWS-E1AF)*, and t(2;22)(q33;q12) *(EWS-FEV)* (513). The identification of these translocations is generally regarded as highly specific for the diagnosis of EFT. These genetic events may be identified by traditional cytogenetic study, or by molecular genetic study with RT-PCR or FISH.

DIFFERENTIAL DIAGNOSIS

The differential diagnosis of EFT includes other round blue cell tumors, including lymphoblastic lymphoma, esthesioneuroblastoma/neuroblastoma, PDSS, alveolar rhabdomyosarcoma, mesenchymal chondrosarcoma, small-cell osteosarcoma, small-cell carcinoma, and small-cell variants of melanoma. Lymphoblastic lymphoma may occur in both bone and soft tissue locations, invariably expresses both CD99 and FLI1, and is commonly CD45 (common leukocyte antigen) negative. IHC for terminal deoxynucleotide transferase, CD43, and CD10 (CALLA) helps to distinguish lymphoblastic lymphoma from EFT. Esthesioneuroblastomas and neuroblastomas generally consist of more uniform-appearing cells within a neurofibrillary background and are CD99 negative/CD56 positive. PDSSs almost always show at least focal areas of more typical monophasic or biphasic synovial sarcoma (BSS), and although they are CD99 positive, usually show greater cytokeratin expression, including high-molecular-weight cytokeratins, and lack FLI-1 expression. Alveolar rhabdomyosarcomas show greater nuclear variability than do EFTs, often contain multinucleated tumor giant cells, and show diffuse expression of desmin and myogenin. Mesenchymal chondrosarcomas and small-cell osteosarcomas contain chondroid or osteoid, respectively. Small-cell carcinomas generally lack

CD99 expression, and show much stronger expression of cytokeratins and neuroendocrine markers. Small-cell variants of melanoma, which may be only focally S-100 protein positive, are usually strongly positive for HMB45, Melan-A, or both.

EWING FAMILY OF TUMORS—FACT SHEET

Definition
▸▸ Highly malignant *small blue round cell tumor* of bone or soft tissue

Incidence and Location
▸▸ Rare
▸▸ Any soft tissue or bone location

Morbidity and Mortality
▸▸ 10-year survival rate of 60% with modern treatment regimens

Sex, Race, and Age Distribution
▸▸ Most common in children and young adolescents but may occur at any age
▸▸ Uncommon in African Americans for unknown reasons

Clinical Features
▸▸ Large, destructive mass of bone or soft tissue

Prognosis and Treatment
▸▸ 10-year survival rate of 60%
▸▸ Requires modern multimodality therapy (chemotherapy and radiotherapy)

EWING FAMILY OF TUMORS—PATHOLOGIC FEATURES

Gross Findings
▸▸ Large, destructive mass involving soft tissue or bone, frequently with necrosis and hemorrhage

Microscopic Findings
▸▸ Vaguely lobular
▸▸ Uniform, malignant-appearing round blue cells with clear to lightly eosinophilic cytoplasm, fine chromatin, and small nucleoli
▸▸ "Light and dark cell" pattern
▸▸ Pseudorosettes and mild spindling in some (PNET)
▸▸ Rare variants with more extensive spindling, hyalinization, pleomorphism, or epithelial differentiation

Immunohistochemical Findings
▸▸ Membranous CD99 expression in 100%
▸▸ FLI-1 expression in 90%
▸▸ Anomalous low molecular weight cytokeratin expression in 25%
▸▸ < 5% with anomalous desmin expression
▸▸ Typically negative for chromogranin, synaptophysin, CD56

Differential Diagnosis
▸▸ Alveolar rhabdomyosarcoma, lymphoblastic lymphoma, neuroblastoma, olfactoneuroblastoma, desmoplastic small round cell tumor (DSRCT), mesenchymal chondrosarcoma, small-cell osteosarcoma, small-cell carcinoma

---

SYNOVIAL SARCOMA

CLINICAL FEATURES

Synovial sarcomas are relatively common, accounting for approximately 10% of soft tissue sarcomas. Synovial sarcomas usually occur in young adults, although they may be seen in patients of any age. The most common location for synovial sarcoma is adjacent to the knee, although this tumor may occur in any somatic soft tissue location, as well as rarely within the viscera. For unknown reasons, synovial sarcomas are rare in the retroperitoneum. Calcifications may be present radiographically. By definition, synovial sarcomas are at least grade II sarcomas under the National Cancer Institute (NCI) or French sarcoma grading systems, with cases showing poorly differentiated histology having the worst prognosis. Tumors that occur in patients younger than 15 years, are less than 5 cm in dimension, and contain massive calcification with relatively few tumor cells appear to have the best prognosis. Although one large study has suggested a significant difference in the outcome of synovial sarcomas that contain the SYT/SSX1 or SYT/SSX2 gene fusions, this has not been confirmed by other studies. Synovial sarcomas are treated with aggressive multimodality therapy, with a 5-year survival rate of approximately 55%.

PATHOLOGIC FEATURES

GROSS FINDINGS

Most synovial sarcomas appear as relatively nonspecific soft tissue masses. Calcified examples may have a gritty texture.

MICROSCOPIC FINDINGS

Monophasic synovial sarcomas account for approximately 70% of synovial sarcomas, and are characterized by uniform, hyperchromatic spindled cells, with *carrot-shaped* nuclei, arranged in moderately long fascicles, with alternating zones of hypercellularity and hypocellularity (Figure 13-37). Other typical features of MSS include abundant wiry collagen, a hemangiopericytoma-like vascular pattern, and stromal calcification (Figure 13-38). BSSs show foci of glandular differentiation, frequently containing necrotic debris, alongside spindled areas identical to MSS (Figure 13-39). These glands are lined by low cuboidal to columnar epithelium, rarely with extensive squamous differentiation. Glandular differentiation may be focal (occult glandular differentiation) (Figure 13-40). PDSSs may arise from either MSS or BSS, and are characterized by round cell differentiation, rhabdoid features, geographic necrosis, and increased

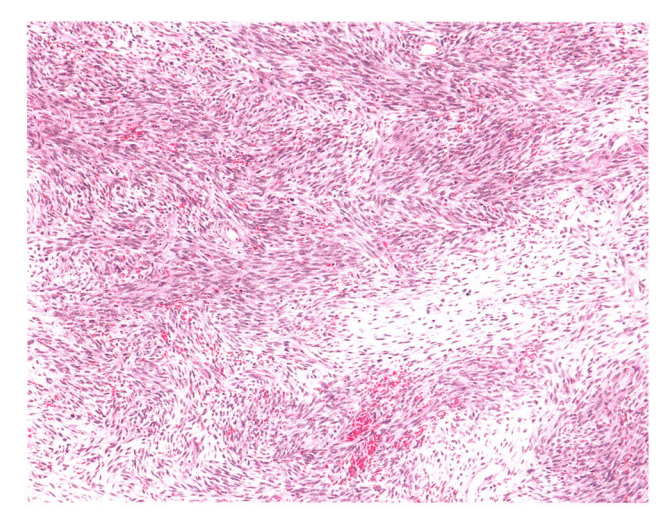

FIGURE 13-37
Monophasic synovial sarcoma, with alternating areas of hypercellularity and hypocellularity, moderately long fascicles, wiry collagen, and uniform hyperchromatic spindled cells.

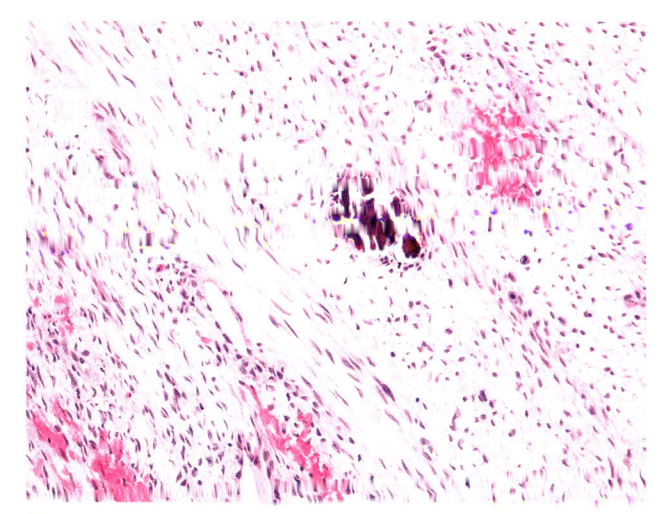

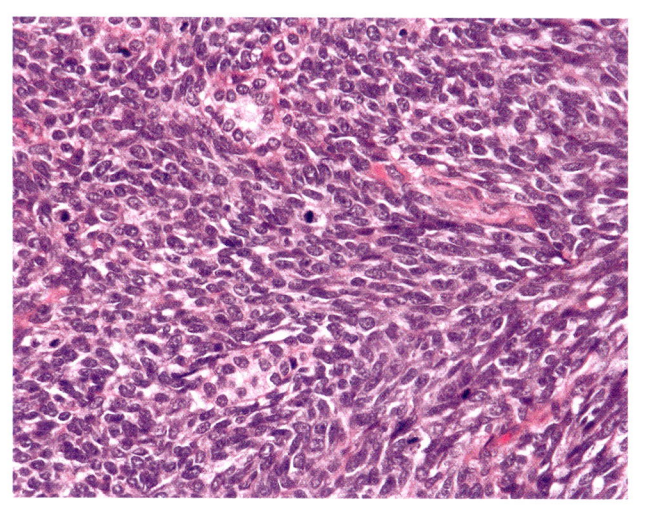

FIGURE 13-40
Biphasic synovial sarcoma with *occult* glandular differentiation. Immunostains for cytokeratins may be helpful in identifying small, inapparent foci of glandular differentiation.

FIGURE 13-38
Stromal calcification should always suggest the possibility of synovial sarcoma in a small spindle cell tumor of the hands and feet.

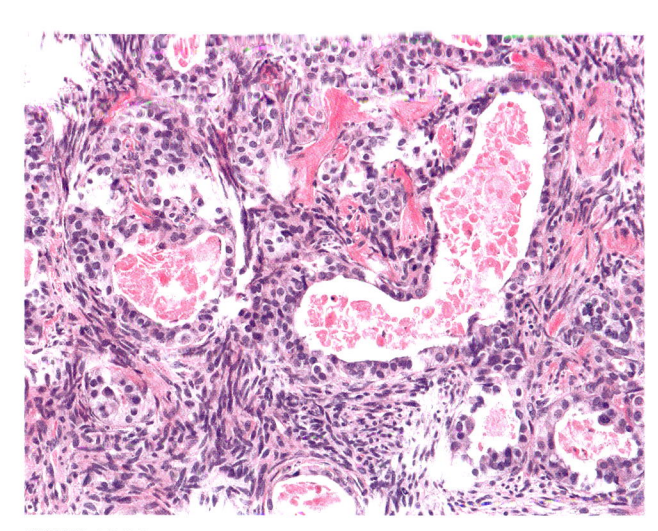

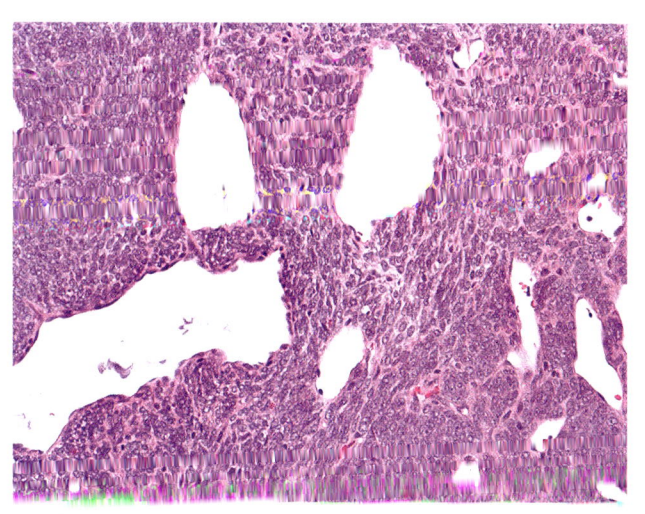

FIGURE 13-41
Poorly differentiated synovial sarcoma, showing a *malignant hemangiopericytoma* growth pattern.

mitotic activity. The hemangiopericytoma-like vascular pattern is often accentuated in PDSS (Figure 13-41).

ANCILLARY STUDIES

IMMUNOHISTOCHEMISTRY

BSS does not require IHC for diagnosis, although occasionally a cytokeratin immunostain may reveal *occult* glandular differentiation in a tumor previously regarded as MSS. MSSs express both low- and high-molecular-weight cytokeratins, and antibodies to high-molecular-weight cytokeratins may be somewhat more sensitive in the diagnosis of PDSS. Cytokeratin expression is typically quite focal in MSS and PDSS, and may be confined to only rare cells in an entire section. EMA may be positive in some cytokeratin-negative MSSs and PDSSs. S-100

FIGURE 13-39
Biphasic synovial sarcoma, with overt glandular differentiation.

protein expression is present in close to 30% of synovial sarcomas, but CD34 expression is not seen. More than 70% of synovial sarcomas are CD99 positive, particularly PDSS. Nuclear expression of TLE-1 protein has recently been reported to be a sensitive and specific marker of synovial sarcoma, although data are limited.

GENETIC FINDINGS

The balanced, reciprocal translocation t(X; 18) (p11.2; q11.2) is found in more 90% of synovial sarcomas of all types, resulting in fusion of the *SYT* gene on chromosome 18 with the *SSX1*, *SSX2*, or rarely, *SSX4* gene on the X chromosome. These translocations may be detected by traditional cytogenetics, RT-PCR, or FISH (571) (572). To date, no credible evidence exists to suggest that this translocation may be seen in nonsynovial sarcomas.

DIFFERENTIAL DIAGNOSIS

MSS should be distinguished from MPNST, fibrosarcoma, and SFTs. The histologic features of MSS and MPNST overlap significantly, and it may be impossible to distinguish these two entities by light microscopy alone. Although both MSS and MPNST may occur within nerves, occurrence in a patient with known NF1 or clear cut origin from a neurofibroma strongly favors MPNST. Expression of cytokeratins, in the absence of S-100 protein and CD34, is most characteristic of MSS, although up to 20% may show S-100 protein expression. Cytogenetic or molecular genetic evidence of the t(X;18) is the *gold standard* for this distinction. Fibrosarcoma is a diagnosis of exclusion. Although the wiry collagen and hemangiopericytomatous areas seen in SFT may suggest MSS, SFTs lack the fascicular arrangement, alternating hypocellularity and hypercellularity, and hyperchromatism exhibited by MSS, and are CD34 positive. PDSS may be distinguished from other round cell sarcomas by identification of areas of more typical MSS or BSS. Molecular genetic testing may be valuable in the distinction of PDSS from cytokeratin-positive EFT. Small synovial sarcomas of the hands and feet may be deceptively bland-appearing and confused with benign fibrous histiocytomas. The presence of calcifications should always suggest synovial sarcoma. Immunostains for epithelial markers assist in this differential diagnosis.

SYNOVIAL SARCOMA—FACT SHEET

Definition
- Malignant mesenchymal tumor showing epithelial differentiation, either overtly (BSS) or by IHC alone (monophasic synovial sarcoma)

Incidence and Location
- 10% of soft tissue sarcomas
- Most common near the knees
- May occur in any soft tissue location, although retroperitoneal lesions are extremely rare

Morbidity and Mortality
- High-grade sarcoma with significant potential for metastases and adverse outcome

Sex, Race, and Age Distribution
- Most common in young adults but may be seen at any age
- No sex or race predilection

Clinical Features
- Soft tissue mass, occasionally painful
- Small lesions on hands and feet may be present for many years before diagnosis
- Calcifications may be present on radiographic studies and are highly suggestive of this diagnosis

Prognosis and Treatment
- 5-year survival of approximately 55%
- Requires modern multimodality therapy

SYNOVIAL SARCOMA—PATHOLOGIC FEATURES

Gross Findings
- Synovial sarcomas of the hands and feet may be small
- Usually appears as nonspecific soft tissue mass
- Calcified lesions may have a gritty texture

Microscopic Findings
- Alternating zones of hypercellularity and hypocellularity
- Wiry collagen
- Moderately long fascicles of hyperchromatic spindled cells with "carrot-shaped" nuclei
- Hemangiopericytoma-like vascular pattern
- Scattered calcifications
- Mitoses and necrosis are infrequent in typical monophasic and BSSs but are common in poorly differentiated tumors
- Biphasic tumors show a variable degree of glandular differentiation, often with intraluminal necrotic debris
- Glands are lined by cuboidal to columnar cells, rarely with squamous differentiation

Immunohistochemical Findings
- Limited expression of low- and high-molecular-weight cytokeratins and EMA, often confined to individual cells
- S-100 protein expression in 20% of cases
- CD34 negative
- CD99 expression is common, particularly in poorly differentiated tumors
- Nuclear expression of TLE-1

Genetic Features
- t(X; 18) (p11.2, q11.2) (SYT-SSX1/2)

Differential Diagnosis
- Malignant peripheral nerve sheath tumor, fibrosarcoma, solitary fibrous tumor, benign fibrous histiocytoma, various small blue round cell tumors (PDSS)

DESMOPLASTIC SMALL ROUND CELL TUMOR

CLINICAL FEATURES

DSRCTs are relatively rare sarcomas that almost always involve the peritoneum of the pelvis or peritoneum, typically in male individuals between the ages of 15 and 35. Extraordinarily rare examples of DSRCT have, however, been reported in locations such as the hand and parotid gland (among others) and in very young and very old patients. DSRCT is far more common in men than in women (male/female ratio, 4:1). Most patients have a large intra-abdominal mass, with symptoms attributable to mass effect. The prognosis for patients with DSRCT is extremely poor, with most series reporting more than 75% of patients dead of disease in less than 5 years from metastases and uncontrollable local disease. Improved progression-free survival has been reported in patients who underwent extensive tumor debulking surgery and showed a good response to multiagent chemotherapy.

PATHOLOGIC FEATURES

GROSS FINDINGS

DSRCT typically present as a large, solid, fibrous-appearing mass, sometimes with areas of necrosis and hemorrhage.

MICROSCOPIC FINDINGS

DSRCTs are relatively stereotypical tumors, almost always consisting of small nests of highly malignant-appearing round blue cells, in a highly vascular, desmoplastic stroma (Figure 13-42). The neoplastic cells usually have little cytoplasm and hyperchromatic nuclei with inapparent nucleoli, although examples with greater pleomorphism and rhabdoid morphology have been reported (Figure 13-43). Occasional cases may show formation of glandular or papillary structures.

ANCILLARY STUDIES

IMMUNOHISTOCHEMISTRY

DSRCTs have a unique immunophenotype, with coexpression of vimentin, desmin, and cytokeratins, often in a dot-like pattern. Other markers of epithelial differentiation, such as EMA and Ber-Ep4, are also typically expressed. Myogenin and MyoD1 are negative. CD99 expression may be seen in approximately one-third of cases but is typically not as diffusely positive as in ES/PNET. Antibodies directed to the carboxy-terminus of WT 1 are frequently positive in DSRCT, reflecting the presence of the diagnostic translocation t(11;22)(p13;q12)(EWS-WT1). Other markers of mesothelial differentiation, such as calretinin and CK5/6, are negative. DSRCT express neuron-specific enolase but are negative for specific markers of neuroendocrine differentiation, such as chromogranin A and synaptophysin.

GENETIC FINDINGS

DSRCTs are characterized in almost all instances by the specific translocation t(11;22)(p13; q12), which results in fusion of the EWS and WT1 genes and formation of

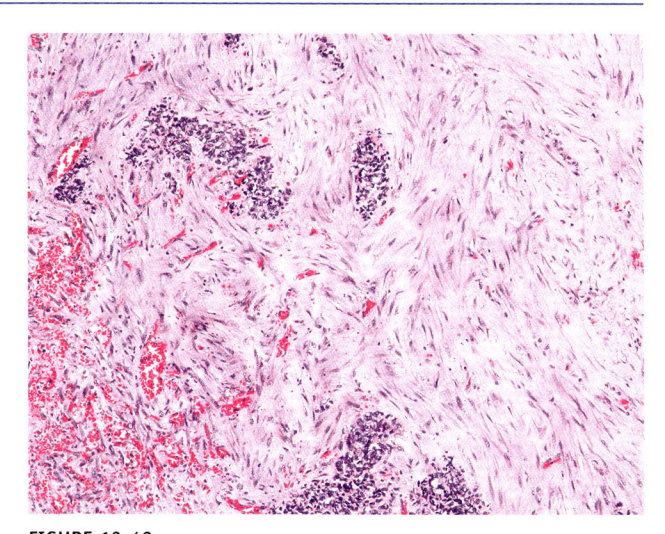

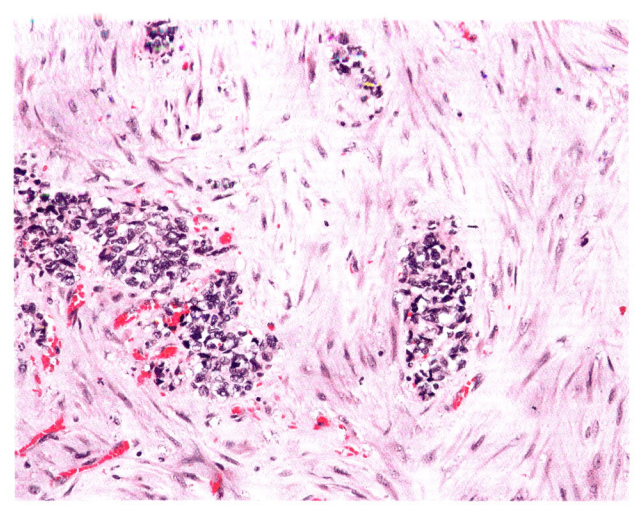

FIGURE 13-42
Desmoplastic small round cell tumor, with nests of malignant cells in a highly vascular, desmoplastic stroma.

FIGURE 13-43
In most instances, the cells of desmoplastic round cell tumor are relatively small and monotonous, although rare examples with pleomorphic and rhabdoid features may be seen.

DESMOPLASTIC SMALL ROUND CELL TUMOR—FACT SHEET

Definition
- Malignant small blue round cell tumor typified by striking desmoplasia and a unique immunophenotype, with coexpression of cytokeratins, desmin, and vimentin

Incidence and Location
- Rare
- Almost always occurs in mesothelial lined spaces, particularly the abdomen and pelvis, but may rarely occur in other locations

Morbidity and Mortality
- Highly aggressive sarcoma with poor outcome

Sex, Race, and Age Distribution
- Males individuals 15 to 35 years of age
- Rare cases in young children and older adults

Clinical Features
- Large intra-abdominal or pelvic mass

Prognosis and Treatment
- > 75% of patients dead of disease in < 5 years
- Progression-free survival may be increased with aggressive debulking, in patients whose tumors have responded to multiagent chemotherapy

DESMOPLASTIC SMALL ROUND CELL TUMOR—PATHOLOGIC FEATURES

Gross Findings
- Large, fibrous mass, often with necrosis and hemorrhage

Microscopic Findings
- Nests of malignant round blue cells in a highly vascular, desmoplastic stroma
- Occasional cases with pleomorphism and rhabdoid cells
- Glandular and papillary structures may rarely be seen

Immunohistochemical Findings
- Coexpression of desmin, cytokeratins, and vimentin, often in a dot-like pattern
- Positivity with antibody to carboxyl-terminal WT1, reflecting presence of EWS-WT1 fusion protein
- Positive for CD99 in up to one-third of cases
- Positive for epithelial markers such as EMA and Ber-Ep4; negative for mesothelial markers such as calretinin and CK5/6
- Neuron-specific enolase positive; negative for chromogranin A and synaptophysin

Genetic Features
- t(11;22)(p13; q12)(EWS-WT1)

Differential Diagnosis
- Alveolar rhabdomyosarcoma, ES/PNET, small-cell carcinoma, small-cell mesothelioma

---

a EWS-WT1 fusion protein. This fusion protein appears to act, in part, by causing upregulation in expression of platelet-derived growth factor A. This translocation can be detected by traditional cytogenetics and by molecular methods, such as RT-PCR and FISH. Rare cases of DSRCT have been reported to contain ES/PNET-associated fusion genes such as *EWS-FLI1* and *EWS-ERG*; the exact nature of these cases is controversial.

DIFFERENTIAL DIAGNOSIS

DSRCT's should be distinguished from other small round blue cell tumors, including alveolar rhabdomyosarcoma, ES/PNET, small-cell carcinoma, and small-cell variants of mesothelioma. Alveolar rhabdomyosarcoma is uncommon in the abdomen, typically lacks prominent desmoplasia, and expresses myogenin/MyoD1, in addition to desmin. It is important to remember that cytokeratins are frequently expressed in alveolar rhabdomyosarcoma. Although ES/PNET may show expression of either cytokeratin or desmin, coexpression of these markers is rare. ES/PNET also typically shows uniform CD99 expression and is FLI1 positive but carboxyl-terminal WT1 negative. In problematic cases, RT-PCR for the *EWS-WT1* and *EWS-FLI1/EWS-ERG* fusions may be helpful. Small cell carcinomas tend to occur in much older patients, lack desmin expression, and are positive for chromogranin, synaptophysin, or both. Small-cell mesotheliomas also occur in older patients, often with a history of asbestos exposure, and express other mesothelial markers, such as calretinin and CK5/6.

SUGGESTED READINGS

Myxoma (Including Juxta-Articular Myxoma)

1. Kindblom LG, Stener B, Angervall L: Intramuscular myxoma. Cancer 1974;34:1737–1744.
2. Meis JM, Enzinger FM: Juxta-articular myxoma: a clinical and pathologic study of 65 cases. Human Pathol 1992;23:639–646.
3. Wirth WA, Leavitt D, Enzinger FM: Multiple intramuscular myxomas. Another extraskeletal manifestation of fibrous dysplasia. Cancer 1971;27.1167–1173.

Cutaneous Myxoma

1. Allen PW, Dymock RB, MacCormac LB: Superficial angiomyxomas with and without epithelial components. Report of 30 tumors in 28 patients. Am J Surg Pathol 1988;12.519–530.
2. Calonje E, Guerin D, McCormick D, et al: Superficial angiomyxoma: clinicopathologic analysis of a series of distinctive but poorly recognized cutaneous tumors with tendency for recurrence. Am J Surg Pathol 1999;23:910–917.
3. Carney JA: The Carney complex (myxomas, spotty pigmentation, endocrine overactivity, and schwannomas). Dermatol Clin 1995;13: 19–26.
4. Carney JA, Gordon H, Carpenter PC, et al: The complex of myxomas, spotty pigmentation, and endocrine overactivity. Medicine (Baltimore) 1985;64:270–283.

Angiomyofibroblastoma and Related Tumors (Cellular Angiofibroma, Angiomyofibroblastoma-like Tumor of the Male Genital Tract)

1. Fletcher CD, Tsang WY, Fisher C, et al: Angiomyofibroblastoma of the vulva. A benign neoplasm distinct from aggressive angiomyxoma. Am J Surg Pathol 1992;16:373–382.
2. Laskin WB, Fetsch JF, Mostofi FK: Angiomyofibroblastomalike tumor of the male genital tract: analysis of 11 cases with comparison to female angiomyofibroblastoma and spindle cell lipoma. Am J Surg Pathol 1998;22:6–16.
3. Nucci MR, Fletcher CD: Vulvovaginal soft tissue tumours: update and review. Histopathology 2000;36:97–108.
4. Nucci MR, Granter SR, Fletcher CD: Cellular angiofibroma: a benign neoplasm distinct from angiomyofibroblastoma and spindle cell lipoma. Am J Surg Pathol 1997;21:636–644.
5. Silverman JS, Albukerk J, Tamsen A: Comparison of angiomyofibroblastoma and aggressive angiomyxoma in both sexes: four cases composed of bimodal CD34 and factor XIIIa positive dendritic cell subsets. Pathol Res Pract 1997;193:673–682.
6. Zamecnik M, Michal M: Comparison of angiomyofibroblastoma and aggressive angiomyxoma in both sexes: four cases composed of bimodal CD34 and factor XIIIa positive dendritic cell subsets [Letter]. Pathol Res Pract 1998;194:736–738.

Aggressive Angiomyxoma

1. Fetsch JF, Laskin WB, Lefkowitz M, et al: Aggressive angiomyxoma: a clinicopathologic study of 29 female patients. Cancer 1996;78:79–90.
2. Iezzoni JC, Fechner RE, Wong LS, et al: Aggressive angiomyxoma in males. A report of four cases. Am J Surg Pathol 1995;104:391–396.
3. Nucci MR, Fletcher CD: Vulvovaginal soft tissue tumours: Update and review. Histopathology 2000;36:97–108.
4. Steeper TA, Rosai J: Aggressive angiomyxoma of the female pelvis and perineum. Report of nine cases of a distinctive type of gynecologic soft tissue neoplasm. Am J Surg Pathol 1983;7:463–475.
5. Tsang WY, Chan JK, Lee KC, et al: Aggressive angiomyxoma. A report of four cases occurring in men. Am J Surg Pathol 1992;16:1059–1065.

Ossifying Fibromyxoid Tumor of Soft Parts

1. Enzinger FM, Weiss SW, Liang CY: Ossifying fibromyxoid tumor of soft parts. A clinicopathological analysis of 59 cases. Am J Surg Pathol 1989;13:817–827.
2. Folpe AL, Weiss SW: Ossifying fibromyxoid tumor of soft parts: a clinicopathologic study of 70 cases with emphasis on atypical and malignant variants. Am J Surg Pathol 2003;27:421–431.
3. Kilpatrick SE, Ward WG, Mozes M, et al: Atypical and malignant variants of ossifying fibromyxoid tumor. Clinicopathologic analysis of six cases. Am J Surg Pathol 1995;19:1039–1046.
4. Miettinen M, Finnell V, Fetsch JF: Ossifying fibromyxoid tumor of soft parts—a clinicopathologic and immunohistochemical study of 104 cases with long-term follow-up and a critical review of the literature. Am J Surg Pathol 2008;32:996–1005.
5. Zamecnik M, Michal M, Simpson RH, et al: Ossifying fibromyxoid tumor of soft parts: a report of 17 cases with emphasis on unusual histological features. Ann Diagn Pathol 1997;1:73–81.

Pleomorphic Hyalinizing Angiectatic Tumor

1. Folpe AL, Weiss SW: Pleomorphic hyalinizing angiectatic tumor: analysis of 41 cases supporting evolution from a distinctive precursor lesion. Am J Surg Pathol 2004;28:1417–1425.
2. Marshall-Taylor C, Fanburg-Smith JC: Hemosiderotic fibrohistiocytic lipomatous lesion: ten cases of a previously undescribed fatty lesion of the foot/ankle. Mod Pathol 2000;13:1192–1199.
3. Smith ME, Fisher C, Weiss SW: Pleomorphic hyalinizing angiectatic tumor of soft parts. A low-grade neoplasm resembling neurilemoma. Am J Surg Pathol 1996;20:21–29.

Phosphaturic Mesenchymal Tumor

1. Folpe AL, Fanburg-Smith JC, Billings SD, et al: Most osteomalacia-associated mesenchymal tumors are a single histopathologic entity: an analysis of 32 cases and a comprehensive review of the literature. Am J Surg Pathol 2004;28:1–30.
2. Shimada T, Mizutani S, Muto T, et al: Cloning and characterization of FGF23 as a causative factor for tumor-induced osteomalacia. Proc Natl Acad Sci U S A 2001;98:6500–6505.
3. Weidner N, Santa Cruz D: Phosphaturic mesenchymal tumors. A polymorphous group causing osteomalacia or rickets. Cancer 1987;59:1442–1454.
4. Williams K, Flanagan A, Folpe A, et al: Lymphatic vessels are present in phosphaturic mesenchymal tumours. Virchows Arch 2007;451:871–875.

Perivascular Epithelioid Cell Neoplasms

1. Bonetti F, Martignoni G, Colato C, et al: Abdominopelvic sarcoma of perivascular epithelioid cells. Report of four cases in young women, one with tuberous sclerosis. Mod Pathol 2001;14:563–568.
2. Bonetti F, Pea M, Martignoni G, et al: Clear cell tumor of the lung is a lesion strictly related to angiomyolipoma—the concept of a family of lesions characterized by the presence of the perivascular epithelioid cells (PEC). Pathology 1994;26:230–236.
3. Folpe AL, McKenney JK, Li Z, et al: Clear cell myomelanocytic tumor of the thigh: report of a unique case. Am J Surg Pathol 2002;26:809–812.
4. Folpe AL, Mentzel T, Lehr HA, et al: Perivascular epithelioid cell neoplasms of soft tissue and gynecologic origin: a clinicopathologic study of 26 cases and review of the literature. Am J Surg Pathol 2005;29:1558–1575.
5. Hornick JL, Fletcher CD: PEComa: what do we know so far?. Histopathology 2006;48:75–82.
6. Hornick JL, Fletcher CD: Sclerosing PEComa: clinicopathologic analysis of a distinctive variant with a predilection for the retroperitoneum. Am J Surg Pathol 2008;32:493–501.
7. Kenerson H, Folpe AL, Takayama TK, et al: Activation of the mTOR pathway in sporadic angiomyolipomas and other perivascular epithelioid cell neoplasms. Hum Pathol 2007;38:1361–1371.
8. Lehman NL: Malignant PEComa of the skull base. Am J Surg Pathol 2004;28:1230–1232.
9. Mentzel T, Reisshauer S, Rutten A, et al: Cutaneous clear cell myomelanocytic tumour: a new member of the growing family of perivascular epithelioid cell tumours (PEComas). Clinicopathological and immunohistochemical analysis of seven cases. Histopathology 2005;46:498–504.
10. Pea M, Martignoni G, Bonetti F, et al: Tumors characterized by the presence of HMB45-positive perivascular epithelioid cell (PEC): a novel entity in surgical pathology. Electron J Pathol Histol 1997;3:28–40.
11. Pea M, Martignoni G, Zamboni G, et al: Perivascular epithelioid cell [Letter]. Am J Surg Pathol 1996;20:1149–1153.
12. Tazelaar HD, Batts KP, Srigley JR: Primary extrapulmonary sugar tumor (PEST): a report of four cases. Mod Pathol 2001;14:615–622.
13. Vang R, Kempson RL: Perivascular epithelioid cell tumor (PEComa) of the uterus: a subset of HMB-45-positive epithelioid mesenchymal neoplasms with an uncertain relationship to pure smooth muscle tumors. Am J Surg Pathol 2002;26:1–13.
14. Weinreb I, Howarth D, Latta E, et al: Perivascular epithelioid cell neoplasms (PEComas): four malignant cases expanding the histopathological spectrum and a description of a unique finding. Virchows Arch 2007;450:463–470.
15. Zamboni G, Pea M, Martignoni G, et al: Clear cell *sugar* tumor of the pancreas. A novel member of the family of lesions characterized by the presence of perivascular epithelioid cells. Am J Surg Pathol 1996;20:722–730.

Epithelioid Sarcoma

1. Chase DR, Enzinger FM: Epithelioid sarcoma. Diagnosis, prognostic indicators, and treatment. Am J Surg Pathol 1985;9:241–263.
2. Chase DR, Enzinger FM, Weiss SW, et al: Keratin in epithelioid sarcoma. An immunohistochemical study. Am J Surg Pathol 1984;8:435–441.
3. Enzinger FM: Epithelioid sarcoma: a sarcoma simulating a granuloma or a carcinoma. Cancer 1970;26:1029–1041.
4. Guillou L, Wadden C, Coindre JM, et al: *Proximal-type* epithelioid sarcoma, a distinctive aggressive neoplasm showing rhabdoid features. Clinicopathologic, immunohistochemical, and ultrastructural study of a series. Am J Surg Pathol 1997;21:130–146.
5. Halling AC, Wollan PC, Pritchard DJ, et al: Epithelioid sarcoma: a clinicopathologic review of 55 cases. Mayo Clin Proc 1996;71:636–642.
6. Hoot AC, Russo P, Judkins AR, et al: Immunohistochemical analysis of hSNF5/INI1 distinguishes renal and extra-renal malignant rhabdoid tumors from other pediatric soft tissue tumors. Am J Surg Pathol 2004;28:1485–1491.

7. Laskin WB, Miettinen M: Epithelioid sarcoma: new insights based on an extended immunohistochemical analysis. Arch Pathol Lab Med 2003;127:1161–1168.
8. Lin L, Skacel M, Sigel JE, et al: Epithelioid sarcoma: an immunohistochemical analysis evaluating the utility of cytokeratin 5/6 in distinguishing superficial epithelioid sarcoma from spindled squamous cell carcinoma. J Cutan Pathol 2003;30:114–117.
9. Miettinen M, Fanburg-Smith JC, Virolainen M, et al: Epithelioid sarcoma: an immunohistochemical analysis of 112 classical and variant cases and a discussion of the differential diagnosis. Hum Pathol 1999;30:934–942.
10. Modena P, Lualdi E, Facchinetti F, et al: SMARCB1/INI1 tumor suppressor gene is frequently inactivated in epithelioid sarcomas. Cancer Res 2005;65:4012–4019.

Alveolar Soft Part Sarcoma

1. Argani P, Lal P, Hutchinson B, et al: Aberrant nuclear immunoreactivity for TFE3 in neoplasms with TFE3 gene fusions: a sensitive and specific immunohistochemical assay. Am J Surg Pathol 2003;27:750–761.
2. Christopherson WM, Foote FW Jr, Stewart FW: Alveolar soft-part sarcomas; structurally characteristic tumors of uncertain histogenesis. Cancer 1952;5:100–111.
3. Evans HL: Alveolar soft-part sarcoma. A study of 13 typical examples and one with a histologically atypical component. Cancer 1985;55:912–917.
4. Folpe AL, Deyrup AT: Alveolar soft-part sarcoma: a review and update. J Clin Pathol 2006;59:1127–1132.
5. Font RL, Jurco S 3rd, Zimmerman LE: Alveolar soft-part sarcoma of the orbit: a clinicopathologic analysis of seventeen cases and a review of the literature. Hum Pathol 1982;13:569–579.
6. Ladanyi M, Antonescu CR, Drobnjak M, et al: The precrystalline cytoplasmic granules of alveolar soft part sarcoma contain monocarboxylate transporter 1 and CD147. Am J Pathol 2002;160:1215–1221.
7. Ladanyi M, Lui MY, Antonescu CR, et al: The der(17)t(X;17)(p11;q25) of human alveolar soft part sarcoma fuses the TFE3 transcription factor gene to ASPL, a novel gene at 17q25. Oncogene 2001;20:48–57.
8. Lieberman PH, Brennan MF, Kimmel M, et al: Alveolar soft-part sarcoma. A clinico-pathologic study of half a century. Cancer 1989;63:1–13.
9. Lieberman PH, Foote FW Jr, Stewart FW, et al: Alveolar soft-part sarcoma. JAMA 1966;198:1047–1051.
10. Matsuno Y, Mukai K, Itabashi M, et al: Alveolar soft part sarcoma. A clinicopathologic and immunohistochemical study of 12 cases. Acta Pathol Jpn 1990;40:199–205.
11. Sciot R, Dal Cin P, De Vos R, et al: Alveolar soft-part sarcoma: evidence for its myogenic origin and for the involvement of 17q25. Histopathology 1993;23:439–444.
12. Wang NP, Bacchi CE, Jiang JJ, et al: Does alveolar soft-part sarcoma exhibit skeletal muscle differentiation? An immunocytochemical and biochemical study of myogenic regulatory protein expression. Mod Pathol 1996;9:496–506.

Ewing Family Tumors

1. Collini P, Sampietro G, Bertulli R, et al: Cytokeratin immunoreactivity in 41 cases of ES/PNET confirmed by molecular diagnostic studies. Am J Surg Pathol 2001;25:273–274.
2. de Alava E, Gerald WL: Molecular biology of the Ewing's sarcoma/primitive neuroectodermal tumor family. J Clin Oncol 2000;18:204–213.
3. de Alava E, Pardo J: Ewing tumor: tumor biology and clinical applications. Int J Surg Pathol 2001;9:7–17.
4. Ewing J: Diffuse endothelioma of bone. Proc NY Soc Pathol 1921;21:17–24.
5. Folpe AL, Goldblum JR, Rubin BP, et al: Morphologic and immunophenotypic diversity in Ewing family tumors: a study of 66 genetically confirmed cases. Am J Surg Pathol 2005;29:1025–1033.
6. Folpe AL, Hill CE, Parham DM, et al: Immunohistochemical detection of FLI-1 protein expression: a study of 132 round cell tumors with emphasis on CD99-positive mimics of Ewing's sarcoma/primitive neuroectodermal tumor. Am J Surg Pathol 2000;24:1657–1662.
7. Gu M, Antonescu CR, Guiter G, et al: Cytokeratin immunoreactivity in Ewing's sarcoma: prevalence in 50 cases confirmed by molecular diagnostic studies. Am J Surg Pathol 2000;24:410–416.
8. Hisaoka M, Tsuji S, Morimitsu Y, et al: Molecular detection of EWS-FLI1 chimeric transcripts in Ewing family tumors by nested reverse transcription-polymerase chain reaction: application to archival paraffin embedded tumor tissues. APMIS 1999;107:577–584.
9. La TH, Meyers PA, Wexler LH, et al: Radiation therapy for Ewing's sarcoma: results from Memorial Sloan Kettering in the modern era. Int J Radiat Oncol Biol Phys 2006;64:544–550.
10. Nascimento AG, Unni KK, Pritchard DJ, et al: A clinicopathologic study of 20 cases of large-cell (atypical) Ewing's sarcoma of bone. Am J Surg Pathol 1980;4:29–36.
11. Parham DM, Hijazi Y, Steinberg SM, et al: Neuroectodermal differentiation in Ewing's sarcoma family of tumors does not predict tumor behavior. Hum Pathol 1999;30:911–918.
12. Raney RB, Asmar L, Newton WA Jr, et al: Ewing's sarcoma of soft tissues in childhood: a report from the Intergroup Rhabdomyosarcoma Study, 1972 to 1991. J Clin Oncol 1997;15:574–582.
13. Rossi S, Orvieto E, Furlanetto A, et al: Utility of the immunohistochemical detection of FLI-1 expression in round cell and vascular neoplasm using a monoclonal antibody. Mod Pathol 2004;17:547–552.
14. Shing DC, McMullan DJ, Roberts P, et al: FUS/ERG gene fusions in Ewing's tumors. Cancer Res 2003;63:4568–4576.
15. Soule EH, Newton W Jr, Moon TE, et al: Extraskeletal Ewing's sarcoma: a preliminary review of 26 cases encountered in the Intergroup Rhabdomyosarcoma Study. Cancer 1978;42:259–264.
16. Verrill MW, Judson IR, Harmer CL, et al: Ewing's sarcoma and primitive neuroectodermal tumor in adults: are they different from Ewing's sarcoma and primitive neuroectodermal tumor in children? J Clin Oncol 1997;15:2611–2621.
17. Wilkins RM, Pritchard DJ, Burgert EO Jr, et al: Ewing's sarcoma of bone. Experience with 140 patients. Cancer 1986;58:2551–2555.
18. Zucman J, Delattre O, Desmaze C, et al: Cloning and characterization of the Ewing's sarcoma and peripheral neuroepithelioma t(11;22) translocation breakpoints. Genes Chromosomes Cancer 1992;5:271–277.

Synovial Sarcoma

1. Albritton KH, Randall RL: Prospects for targeted therapy of synovial sarcoma. J Pediatr Hematol Oncol 2005;27:219–222.
2. an de Rijn M, Barr FG, Xiong QB, et al: Poorly differentiated synovial sarcoma: an analysis of clinical, pathologic, and molecular genetic features. Am J Surg Pathol 1999;23:106–112.
3. Bergh P, Meis-Kindblom JM, Gherlinzoni F, et al: Synovial sarcoma. Identification of low and high risk groups. Cancer 1999;85:2596–2607.
4. Coindre JM, Hostein I, Benhattar J, et al: Malignant peripheral nerve sheath tumors are t(X;18)-negative sarcomas. Molecular analysis of 25 cases occurring in neurofibromatosis type 1 patients, using two different RT-PCR-based methods of detection. Mod Pathol 2002;15:589–592.
5. Crew AJ, Clark J, Fisher C, et al: Fusion of SYT to two genes, SSX1 and SSX2, encoding proteins with homology to the Kruppel-associated box in human synovial sarcoma. EMBO J 1995;14:2333–2340.
6. Fisher C: Synovial sarcoma: ultrastructural and immunohistochemical features of epithelial differentiation in monophasic and biphasic tumors. Human Pathol 1986;17:996–1008.
7. Folpe AL, Schmidt RA, Chapman D, et al: Poorly differentiated synovial sarcoma: immunohistochemical distinction from primitive neuroectodermal tumors and high-grade malignant peripheral nerve sheath tumors. Am J Surg Pathol 1998;22:673–682.
8. Guillou L, Benhattar J, Bonichon F, et al: Histologic grade, but not SYT-SSX fusion type, is an important prognostic factor in patients with synovial sarcoma: a multicenter, retrospective analysis. J Clin Oncol 2004;22:4040–4050.
9. Guillou L, Wadden C, Kraus MD, et al: S-100 protein reactivity in synovial sarcomas: a potentially frequent diagnostic pitfall. Immunohistochemical analysis of 100 cases. Applied Immunohistochemistry 1996;4:167–175.
10. Krane JF, Bertoni F, Fletcher CD: Myxoid synovial sarcoma: an underappreciated morphologic subset. Mod Pathol 1999;12:456–462.
11. Ladanyi M: Fusions of the SYT and SSX genes in synovial sarcoma. Oncogene 2001;20:5755–5762.
12. Ladanyi M, Antonescu CR, Leung DH, et al: Impact of SYT-SSX fusion type on the clinical behavior of synovial sarcoma: a multi-institutional retrospective study of 243 patients. Cancer Res 2002;62:135–140.
13. Mirra JM, Wang S, Bhuta S: Synovial sarcoma with squamous differentiation of its mesenchymal glandular elements. A case report with light-microscopic, ultramicroscopic, and immunologic correlation. Am J Surg Pathol 1984;8:791–796.
14. Pappo AS, Fontanesi J, Luo X, et al: Synovial sarcoma in children and adolescents: The St Jude Children's Research Hospital experience. J Clin Oncol 1994;12:2360–2366.

15. Pelmus M, Guillou L, Hostein I, et al: Monophasic fibrous and poorly differentiated synovial sarcoma: immunohistochemical reassessment of 60 t(X;18)(SYT-SSX)-positive cases. Am J Surg Pathol 2002;26:1434–1440.
16. Smith TA, Machen SK, Fisher C, et al: Usefulness of cytokeratin subsets for distinguishing monophasic synovial sarcoma from malignant peripheral nerve sheath tumor. Am J Clin Pathol 1999;112:641–648.
17. Surace C, Panagopoulos I, Palsson E, et al: A novel FISH assay for SS18-SSX fusion type in synovial sarcoma. Lab Invest 2004;84:1185–1192.
18. Terry J, Saito T, Subramanian S, et al: TLE1 as a diagnostic immunohistochemical marker for synovial sarcoma emerging from gene expression profiling studies. Am J Surg Pathol 2007;31:240–246.

Desmoplastic Small Round Cell Tumor

1. Adsay V, Cheng J, Athanasian E, et al: Primary desmoplastic small cell tumor of soft tissues and bone of the hand. Am J Surg Pathol 1999;23:1408–1413.
2. Barnoud R, Sabourin JC, Pasquier D, et al: Immunohistochemical expression of WT1 by desmoplastic small round cell tumor: a comparative study with other small round cell tumors. Am J Surg Pathol 2000;24:830–836.
3. Bertoldin R, Drei N, D'Inca G, et al: A paratesticular localization of desmoplastic small cell tumor. A case report. Tumori 1996;82:497–498.
4. Charles AK, Moore IE, Berry PJ: Immunohistochemical detection of the Wilms' tumour gene WT1 in desmoplastic small round cell tumour. Histopathology 1997;30:312–314.
5. Cummings OW, Ulbright TM, Young RH, et al: Desmoplastic small round cell tumors of the paratesticular region. A report of six cases. Am J Surg Pathol 1997;21:219–225.
6. de Alava E, Ladanyi M, Rosai J, et al: Detection of chimeric transcripts in desmoplastic small round cell tumor and related developmental tumors by reverse transcriptase polymerase chain reaction. A specific diagnostic assay. Am J Pathol 1995;147:1584–1591.
7. Dorsey BV, Benjamin LE, Rauscher F 3rd, et al: Intra-abdominal desmoplastic small round-cell tumor: expansion of the pathologic profile. Mod Pathol 1996;9:703–709.
8. Gerald WL, Ladanyi M, de Alava E, et al: Clinical, pathologic, and molecular spectrum of tumors associated with t(11;22)(p13;q12): desmoplastic small round-cell tumor and its variants. J Clin Oncol 1998;16:3028–3036.
9. Gerald WL, Miller HK, Battifora H, et al: Intra-abdominal desmoplastic small round-cell tumor. Report of 19 cases of a distinctive type of high-grade polyphenotypic malignancy affecting young individuals. Am J Surg Pathol 1991;15:499–513.
10. Gerald WL, Rosai J: Desmoplastic small cell tumor with multi-phenotypic differentiation. Zentralblatt fur Pathologie 1993;139:141–151.
11. Gerald WL, Rosai J, Ladanyi M: Characterization of the genomic breakpoint and chimeric transcripts in the EWS-WT1 gene fusion of desmoplastic small round cell tumor. Proc Natl Acad Sci U S A 1995;92:1028–1032.
12. Hill DA, Pfeifer JD, Marley EF, et al: WT1 staining reliably differentiates desmoplastic small round cell tumor from Ewing sarcoma/primitive neuroectodermal tumor. An immunohistochemical and molecular diagnostic study. Am J Clin Pathol 2000;114:345–353.
13. Ladanyi M, Gerald W: Fusion of the EWS and WT1 genes in the desmoplastic small round cell tumor. Cancer Res 1994;54:2837–2840.
14. Ordi J, de Alava E, Torne A, et al: Intraabdominal desmoplastic small round cell tumor with EWS/ERG fusion transcript. Am J Surg Pathol 1998;22:1026–1032.
15. Ordonez NG: Desmoplastic small round cell tumor: I: a histopathologic study of 39 cases with emphasis on unusual histological patterns. Am J Surg Pathol 1998;22:1303–1313.
16. Ordonez NG: Desmoplastic small round cell tumor: II: an ultrastructural and immunohistochemical study with emphasis on new immunohistochemical markers. Am J Surg Pathol 1998;22:1314–1327.
17. Schwarz RE, Gerald WL, Kushner BH, et al: Desmoplastic small round cell tumors: prognostic indicators and results of surgical management. Ann Surg Oncol 1998;5:416–422.
18. Sebire NJ, Gibson G, Rampling D, et al: Immunohistochemical findings in embryonal small round cell tumors with molecular diagnostic confirmation. Appl Immunohistochem Mol Morphol 2005;13:1–5.
19. Tison V, Cerasoli S, Morigi F, et al: Intracranial desmoplastic small-cell tumor. Report of a case. Am J Surg Pathol 1996;20:112–117.

Section III

BONE PATHOLOGY

14 Bone-Forming Tumors
G. Petur Nielsen · Andrew E. Rosenberg

15 Cartilage-Forming Tumors
Andrew Horvai

16 Fibroblastic and Fibrohistiocytic Tumors
Edward F. McCarthy

17 Ewing Sarcoma
Michael J. Klein

18 Hematopoietic Tumors
Edward F. McCarthy

19 Vascular Tumors of Bone
Andrew Horvai

20 Giant Cell Tumor of Bone
Patrizia Bacchini · Franco Bertoni

21 Notochordal Tumors
Andrew Horvai

22 Adamantinoma
Leonard B. Kahn

23 Bone Tumors of Miscellaneous Type or Uncertain Lineage
S. Fiona Bonar

24 Metastases Involving Bone
Yasuaki Nakashima

14

Bone-Forming Tumors

G. Petur Nielsen · Andrew E. Rosenberg

- Bone Island
- Osteoma
- Osteoid Osteoma
- Osteoblastoma
- Osteosarcoma

Bone-forming tumors of the skeletal system represent a broad spectrum of neoplasms that vary significantly in their morphology and biology. They are defined as neoplasms that arise within or on the surface of a bone in which the neoplastic cells synthesize and secrete the organic components of bone matrix that may or may not mineralize. The neoplastic cells have the phenotype of osteoblasts, and in lesions in which the cells are rapidly synthesizing matrix, the cells are large, polyhedral, and have a moderate to abundant amount of eosinophilic cytoplasm that is intimately associated with the newly formed matrix. The nuclei tend to be eccentric in location and polarized away from the bone-forming surface, and have fine chromatin and prominent nucleoli. Tumor cells entrapped within the matrix are frequently smaller than those lining the surfaces and appear similar in appearance to non-neoplastic osteocytes, a phenomenon known as *normalization*. This compilation of cytologic features, however, varies with the biological potential of the tumor.

The growth pattern of the bone-forming tumor (circumscribed vs infiltrative) and the architecture of the neoplastic bone (cortical vs trabecular and woven vs lamellar) also correlates with the nature of the tumor. Benign tumors are usually well circumscribed, and the bone matrix is typically deposited as trabeculae of woven or lamellar bone, whereas osteosarcoma grows with an infiltrative pattern, and the bone is woven in architecture and deposited in a coarse, lace-like pattern. Cortical type bone is distinctly uncommon in bone tumors, except in osteomas and bone islands, and lamellar bone is rarely present in osteosarcoma.

The morphologic heterogeneity of bone-forming tumors has made them notorious for causing diagnostic difficulties. Because treatment may vary from observation to en bloc excision with neoadjuvant therapy, careful correlation of the tumor morphology with their radiographic features is required for their accurate diagnosis.

BONE ISLAND

CLINICAL FEATURES

Bone island (enostosis) is a benign, bone-forming tumor composed of cortical type bone that involves the medullary cavity. The frequency is unknown because it is usually detected as an incidental radiographic finding. Its prevalence in pelvic bones and ribs has been reported to be 1.08% and 0.43%, respectively. Bone islands have been identified in all age groups, are uncommon in children, and occur equally in male and female individuals. The pelvis, proximal femur, and ribs are the most frequently involved sites. Within tubular bones, they usually involve the epiphyses. Clinically, bone islands are asymptomatic, with only exceptional cases causing pain.

Osteopoikilosis is a syndrome that may be inherited in an autosomal dominant fashion and is caused by a loss of function mutation in LEMD3. Some patients may also have melorheostosis and Buschke-Ollendorff syndrome. Clinically, the disorder is characterized by the presence of innumerable bone islands. The enostoses are bilateral and symmetric, but unequal in distribution, and are most numerous in the metaphyseal and epiphyseal regions of tubular bones, carpal and tarsal bones, and the flat bones of the proximal limb girdles. Radiographically, macroscopically, and histologically, they are identical to sporadic, solitary bone islands.

RADIOLOGIC FEATURES

Bone islands have characteristic radiographic features. On plain films they appear as small, round, single or multiple, homogeneously radiodense lesions that have spiculated margins that merge with the surrounding cancellous bone (Figure 14-1). The lesions, especially larger

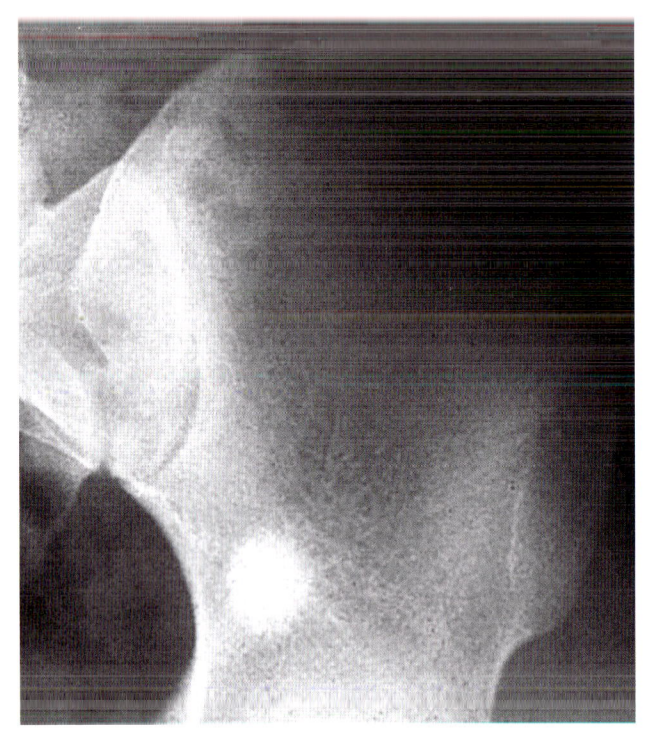

FIGURE 14-1
Bone island involving the wing of the sacrum. The lesion is small, round, and radiodense.

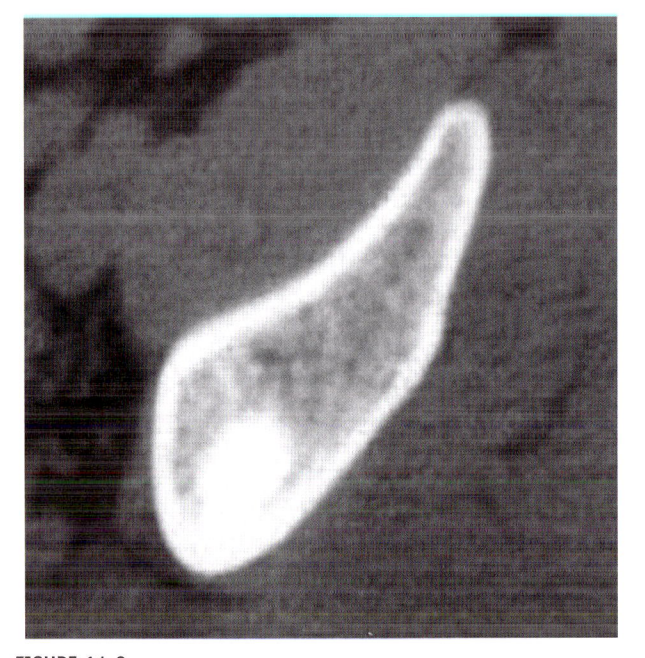

FIGURE 14-2
Axial computed tomographic scan of a bone island in the ilium. Note the speculated margin and homogeneous radiodensity.

FIGURE 14-3
Bone island composed of cortical-type bone merging with the surrounding bony trabeculae.

PATHOLOGIC FEATURES

Bone islands arise in the medullary cavity, are generally not much larger than 1 cm in diameter, and are hard, solid, and tan–white. Their periphery blends into the surrounding cancellous trabeculae.

Bone islands consist of cortical-type bone that is predominately lamellar but may be focally woven, which contains haversian-like canals (Figure 14-3). The osteoblasts lining the surfaces are flat and quiescent, and the osteocytes are small and cytologically banal. The periphery of lesion blends with the surrounding cancellous bone.

DIFFERENTIAL DIAGNOSIS

The most important tumor to distinguish a bone island from is well-differentiated intramedullary osteosarcoma. In contrast with bone island, well-differentiated osteosarcoma is infiltrative, the bone is usually trabecular and not cortical in pattern, and the neoplastic matrix is surrounded by groups of proliferating spindle cells and not a single layer of quiescent surface osteoblasts.

Another lesion that may enter into consideration is an osteoblastic metastasis. In contrast with an enostosis, the newly formed bone in an osteoblastic metastasis is trabecular and generally surrounds islands of carcinoma cells that are cytologically malignant and not present in a bone island.

variants, may abut or be based on the endosteal surface; however, they do not involve the cortex and do not elicit a periosteal reaction. On computed tomographic (CT) scans, bone islands have the same characteristics as cortical bone (Figure 14-2). On magnetic resonance imaging (MRI), they are dark; on bone scan, they are cold.

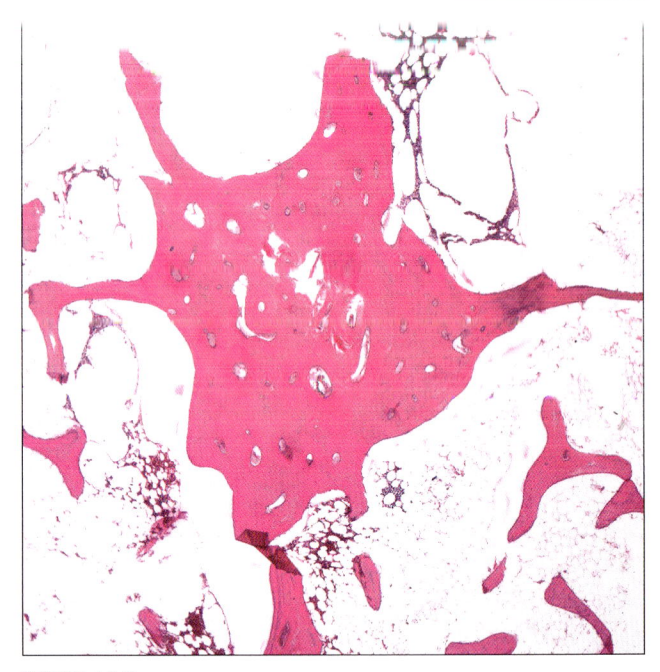

PROGNOSIS AND TREATMENT

Bone islands usually do not need any type of treatment because they are indolent and typically asymptomatic. Occasional cases, particularly larger variants, may require a biopsy to exclude a more aggressive neoplasm such as well-differentiated osteosarcoma and sclerotic metastases.

BONE ISLAND—FACT SHEET

Definition
- Benign bone-forming tumor composed of cortical-type bone
- Osteopoikilosis is a syndrome characterized by innumerable bone islands

Incidence and Location
- Frequency is unknown because it is a frequent incidental finding
- Pelvis, proximal femur, and ribs are most common locations

Morbidity and Mortality
- Bone Island is benign

Sex, Race, and Age Distribution
- Male and female sexes are affected with equal frequency
- Identified in all age groups but rare in children

Clinical Features
- Usually asymptomatic and incidental finding
- Rarely causes pain

Radiologic Features
- Radiodense lesion(s) that are spiculated and merge with the surrounding cancellous bone

Prognosis and Treatment
- No treatment necessary
- Biopsy sometimes performed on large bone islands to exclude a low-grade osteosarcoma or sclerotic metastases

---

BONE ISLAND—PATHOLOGIC FEATURES

Gross Findings
- Spiculated, dense, solid, and tan–white

Microscopic Findings
- Cortical-type bone that is spiculated and blends with the surrounding cancellous bone

Immunohistochemical Findings
- Not helpful

Differential Diagnosis
- Well-differentiated intramedullary osteosarcoma
- Osteoblastic metastasis

OSTEOMA

CLINICAL FEATURES

Osteoma is a benign, bone-forming tumor that arises on the surface of the cortex. The majority of tumors are composed of mature, dense, compact, cortical-like bone; however, some may be composed of cancellous bone. They usually develop on the surfaces of the craniofacial skeleton and have a propensity to involve the bones of the paranasal and frontal sinuses and the orbit where they are found in 1% to 3% of the adult population. Rarely, osteomas are located in the vertebral column and the appendicular skeleton where they develop on the surfaces of long tubular bones. They affect male individuals a little more frequently than female individuals and are typically diagnosed during midadulthood. Osteoma is usually solitary but may be multiple in a minority of cases. Importantly, a diagnosis of osteoma in a young patient or multiple osteomas should raise the suspicion of Gardner syndrome (autosomal dominant intestinal polyposis that progresses to adenocarcinoma, osteomas, dental anomalies, epidermal inclusion cysts, and soft tissue tumors).

Craniofacial osteomas are commonly asymptomatic and detected as an incidental radiographic finding. Larger tumors, however, may cause swelling, facial asymmetry, and symptoms secondary to sinus obstruction, including discharge and mucocele formation. Orbital osteomas can produce a variety of problems including dacryocystitis and exophthalmos. Tumors that involve the spine can be complicated by spinal cord or nerve compression, and those developing in the extremities can present as a palpable mass that may be painful.

RADIOLOGIC FEATURES

Osteomas are usually round or ovoid, uniformly radiodense, sharply demarcated from the surrounding soft tissue, and have a broad base of attachment to the cortical surface with which it merges (Figures 14-4 and 14-5). On CT and MRI, an osteoma manifests as a well-delineated surface-based mass of cortical-type bone; however, the cancellous variant has the characteristics of trabecular bone with intervening fat (Figure 14-6).

PATHOLOGIC FEATURES

Most osteomas are 0.5 to 2 cm in diameter, round to oval, hard, tan–white, and resemble and merge with the cortical bone from which they arise. Large lesions in the

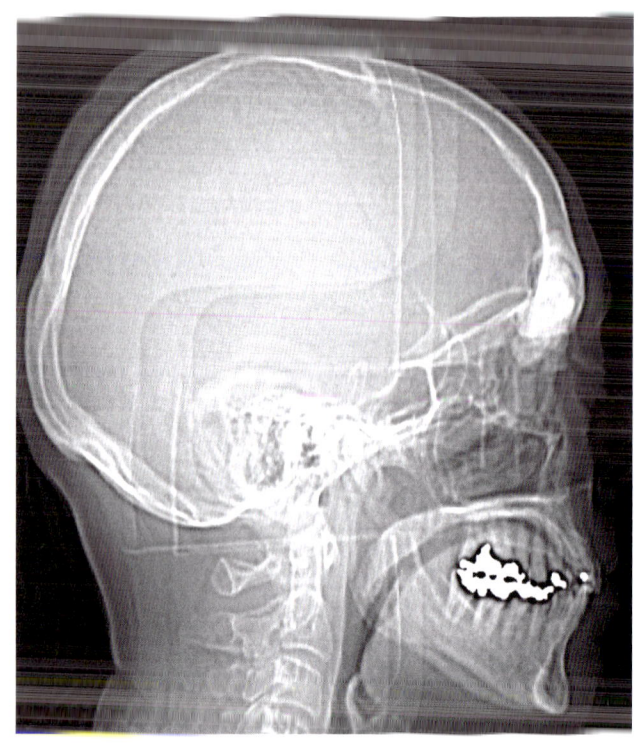

312   BONE AND SOFT TISSUE PATHOLOGY

FIGURE 14-4
Osteoma arising on the surface and filling the frontal sinus on lateral radiograph.

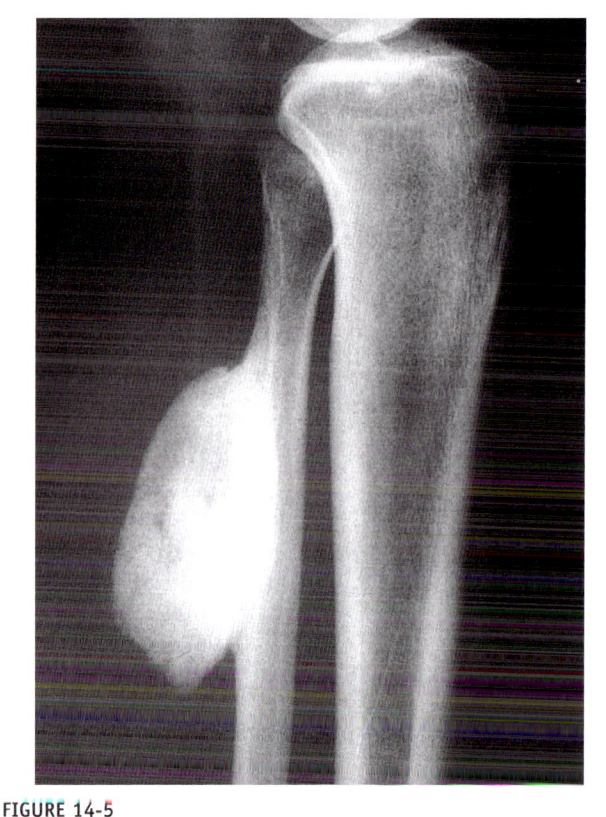

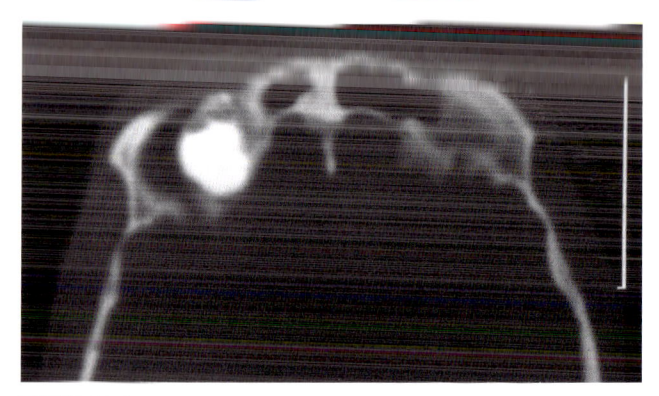

FIGURE 14-6
Axial computed tomography of osteoma involving frontal sinus.

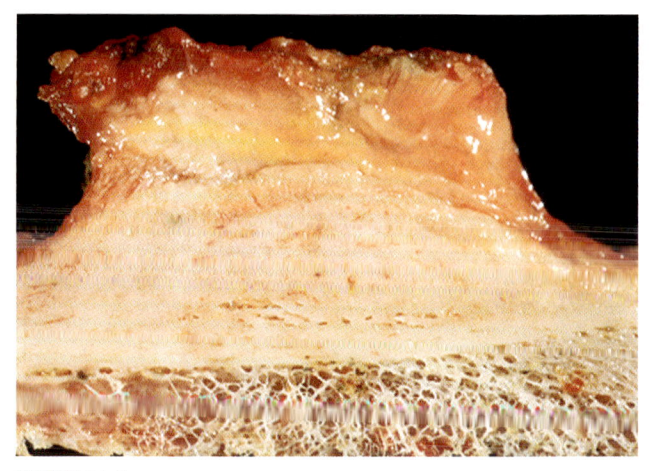

FIGURE 14-7
Gross image of osteoma of long bone.
The tumor is dense, tan-white, and merges with the underlying cortex.

appendicular skeleton are frequently sessile and elongate (Figure 14-7).

The bone in osteomas is cortical-like in appearance with vascular channels similar to haversian systems, and is usually composed of lamellar or an admixture of lamellar and woven bone (Figure 14-8). In the cancellous variant, the core of the lesion consists of interconnecting broad trabeculae of bone that is surrounded by fatty marrow. The cells that line the surfaces of the bone are flattened osteoblasts with small elongate nuclei and sparse amounts of eosinophilic cytoplasm. The osteocytes are also small and quiescent in appearance. Infrequently, however, especially in lesions that are in a stage of more rapid growth, the osteoblasts are large and polyhedral with prominent nuclei, and a layer of loose fibrous tissue cuffs the adjacent bone.

DIFFERENTIAL DIAGNOSIS

Parosteal osteosarcoma can be clinically confused with osteoma, especially those that are large and arising in the appendicular skeleton. Histologically, parosteal

FIGURE 14-5
Osteoma arising on the surface of the fibula. The tumor is ovoid, well circumscribed, and radiodense.

osteosarcoma is characterized by long trabeculae of woven bone surrounded by sheets of proliferating spindle cells that are absent in osteoma. Also, parosteal osteosarcoma may contain neoplastic cartilage that is not present in osteoma.

Melorheostosis can resemble osteoma radiographically; however, in melorheostosis, the thickened cortex has the appearance of *flowing wax* rather than a discrete ovoid or mushroom-shaped cortically based mass, although exceptions occur. Also, melorheostosis frequently involves more than one bone and may be associated with localized sclerotic lesions of the skin. Histologically, in our experience, the bone in a bona fide osteoma and melorheostosis are similar and cannot confidently be distinguished from one another.

PROGNOSIS AND TREATMENT

Osteomas are slow growing and indolent. Only symptomatic lesions need to be treated, which should consist of simple excision. Large osteomas of the long tubular bones may mimic low-grade surface osteosarcoma (parosteal osteosarcoma), and require diagnostic biopsy and excision. Malignant transformation of osteoma does not occur.

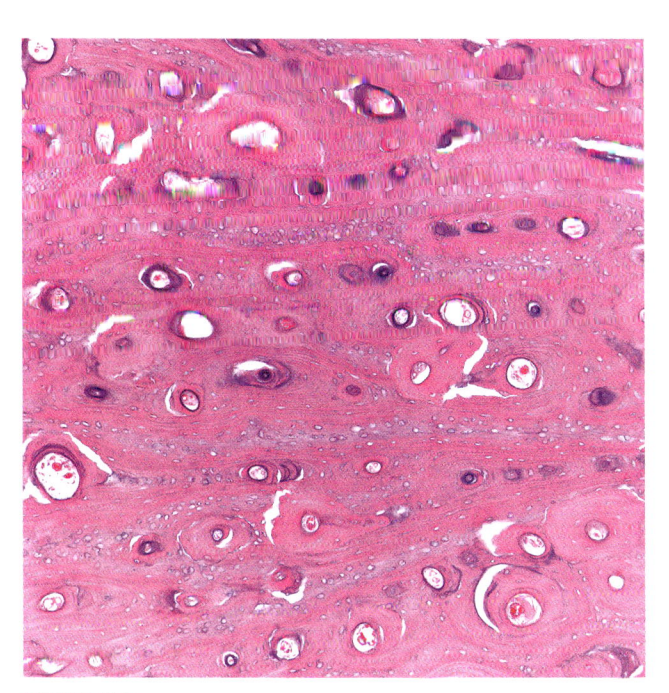

OSTEOMA—FACT SHEET

Definition
- Benign bone-forming tumor composed of cortical and less frequently cancellous bone

Incidence and Location
- 1% to 3% of adult population; true incidence unknown as many are incidental findings
- Craniofacial skeleton especially around sinuses; rarely affects the spine or long bones
- Usually solitary but may be multiple in patients with Gardner syndrome

Morbidity and Mortality
- Slow growing and benign

Sex, Race, and Age Distribution
- Slight male predominance and diagnosed in midadulthood

Clinical Features
- Commonly asymptomatic and incidental finding
- Can produce a variety of symptoms depending on location

Radiologic Features
- Surface based, homogeneously radiodense, and well demarcated

Prognosis and Treatment
- No treatment unless symptomatic
- Symptomatic tumors are conservatively excised
- Large osteomas of long tubular bones may require biopsy and excision to exclude a low-grade surface osteosarcoma

---

OSTEOMA—PATHOLOGIC FEATURES

Gross Findings
- Hard, tan-white, mimicking normal bone

Microscopic Findings
- Admixture of lamellar and woven bone mimicking compact cortical or trabecular bone

Immunohistochemical Findings
- Not applicable

Differential Diagnosis
- Low-grade surface osteosarcoma

FIGURE 14-8
Osteoma composed of an admixture of woven and lamellar bone deposited in a cortical-type pattern.

OSTEOID OSTEOMA

CLINICAL FEATURES

Osteoid osteoma is a benign, bone-forming tumor characterized by its small size, morphologic and radiographic features, and classic symptomatology. Although its neoplastic nature has been debated, cytogenetic studies have revealed clonal chromosomal abnormalities involving 22q in several cases, which supports the concept that osteoid osteoma is likely a neoplasm. Responsible for approximately 11% of benign bone tumors and 3% of all primary bone tumors, osteoid osteoma is usually diagnosed during the second and third decades of life, and is associated with a male-to-female predominance of 3:1. Osteoid osteoma commonly causes significant localized pain that is most severe at night and that is alleviated by aspirin and nonsteroidal anti-inflammatory drugs (NSAIDs). Tumors that arise in periarticular sites may elicit joint pain, swelling, effusions, and limited range of motion, which can cause confusion with an inflammatory arthritis. Lesions that involve the spine can produce painful scoliosis secondary to spasm of paravertebral muscles, whereas lesions of the small bones of the hand and feet may produce marked soft tissue swelling mimicking infection. Tumors in the vicinity of a growth plate may cause increased growth and bone length discrepancy.

Osteoid osteoma most frequently arises in the diaphyseal and metaphyseal regions of long tubular bones, especially the femur, and the posterior elements of vertebrae. The tumor frequently originates in the cortex and less commonly the medullary canal. By definition, osteoid osteoma is 1 to 2 cm in diameter, as morphologically similar tumors larger than 2 cm are classified as osteoblastomas. Most tumors are solitary, with rare cases being multicentric in the same bone.

RADIOLOGIC FEATURES

Osteoid osteoma is round and radiolucent with frequent central patchy mineralization (Figure 14-9A). The lesion or nidus has well-defined margins and is often surrounded by a zone of sclerosis (reactive zone) that may be so extensive that it obscures the underlying lesion and even simulates an aggressive tumor. Tumors of the cortex are more commonly associated with prominent reactive bone formation than those arising within the medullary canal. Thinly sliced CT scans may be invaluable in identifying a tumor that is obscured by sclerosis, and in contrast, MRI is of limited utility and generally reveals edema in the marrow and soft tissues adjacent to the nidus (see Figure 14-9B). Technetium bone scan shows that the tumor is avid and exquisitely hot.

PATHOLOGIC FEATURES

Osteoid osteoma is round, 1 to 2 cm in diameter, dark red with central tan-white speckled gritty mineralization and is well delineated from the surrounding reactive bone, which is often sclerotic and ivory white (Figure 14-10).

Haphazard interanastomosing trabeculae of woven bone rimmed prominently by osteoblasts with intervening

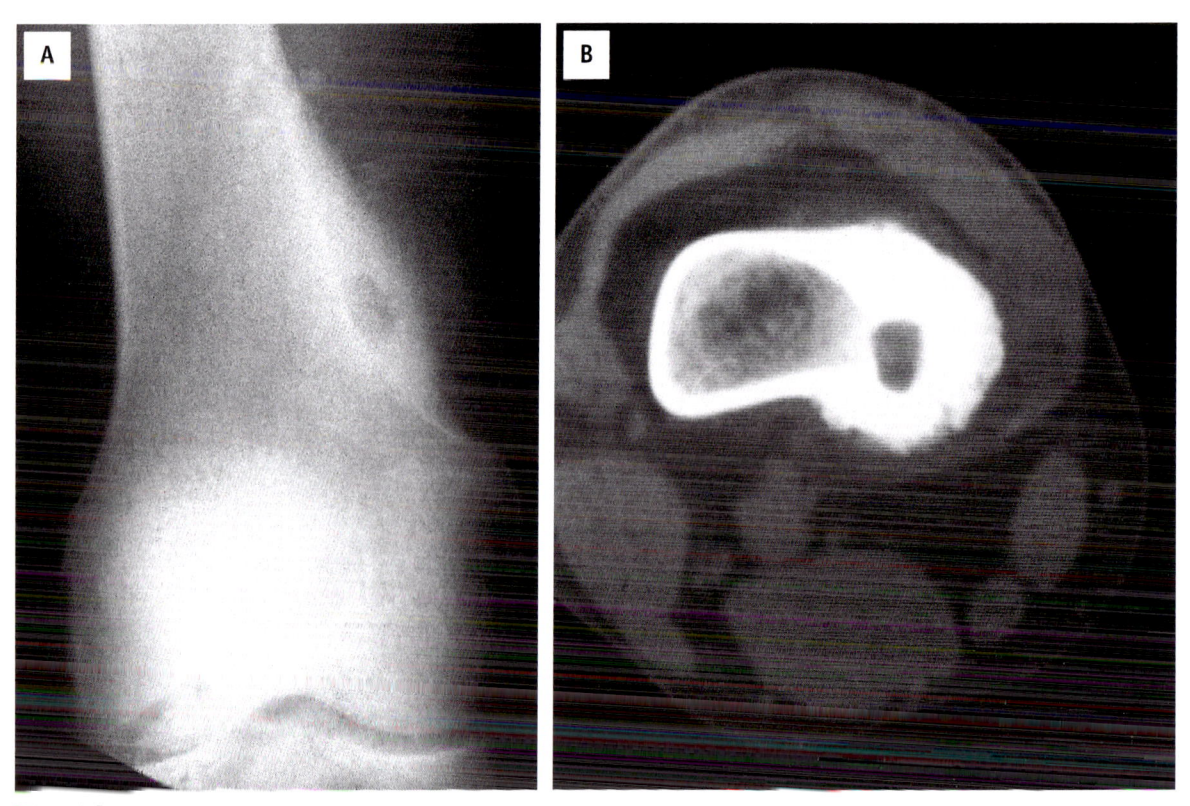

FIGURE 14-9

A, Anteroposterior radiograph and **B**, axial computed tomography of osteoid osteoma arising beneath the periosteum of the femur. The tumor is small, radiolucent, and surrounded by a prominent rim of reactive woven bone.

CHAPTER 14 Bone-Forming Tumors 315

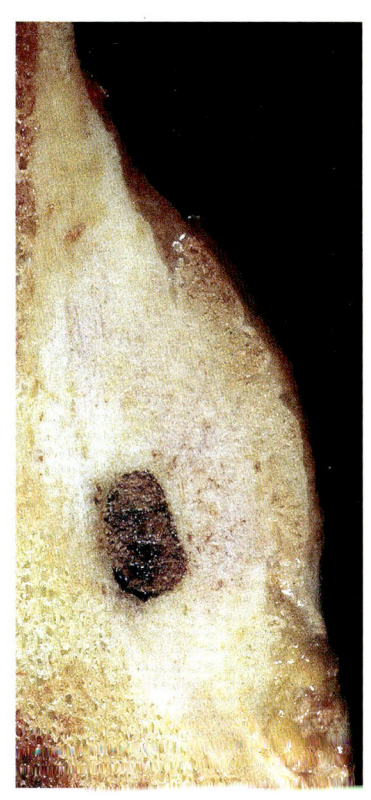

FIGURE 14-10
Gross image of osteoid osteoma. The small round red tan tumor is surrounded by dense reactive bone.

richly vascularized loose connective tissue characterize osteoid osteoma (Figure 14-11). Also present are scattered osteoclasts on some of the trabecular surfaces. Occasionally, the bone is sheet-like in architecture, and in our experience, chondroid areas are rarely seen and, when present, should raise the possibility of other types of tumors. The synovium in juxta-articular tumors may

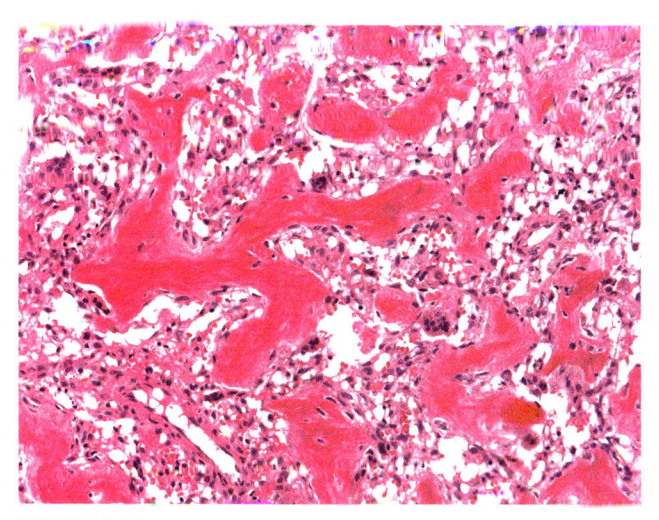

FIGURE 14-11
Osteoid osteoma composed of haphazardly interconnecting trabeculae of woven bone that are lined prominently by osteoblasts. The intervening loose connective tissue is vascular.

resemble rheumatoid arthritis with papillary hyperplasia and lymphoid follicles.

Immunohistochemistry generally does not have a role in diagnosing osteoid osteoma. However, antibodies to S-100 and neurofilament demonstrate nerve fibers within the tumor and the surrounding reactive zone. The presence of nerve fibers in primary bone tumors is uncommon and is usually seen only in osteoid osteoma. These nerve fibers, as well as high levels of prostaglandin E2 and prostacyclins within the nidus, are likely responsible for the pain associated with this tumor.

DIFFERENTIAL DIAGNOSIS

The histologic differential diagnosis of osteoid osteoma is largely with osteoblastoma. Because of their morphologic similarity, tumors larger than 2 cm are considered osteoblastomas. This distinction usually correlates with the characteristic clinical symptoms of osteoid osteoma, which include significant pain that is most severe at night, and sensitive to aspirin and related anti-inflammatory agents. Other findings such as cystic change or the presence of cartilage supports the diagnosis of osteoblastoma.

Lesions such as an abscess and Langerhans cell histocytosis are excluded by virtue of the prominent inflammatory cell infiltrate seen in both, and fracture callus is distinguished by the haphazard arrangement of the bony trabeculae in osteoid osteoma and its sharply demarcated round shape.

PROGNOSIS AND TREATMENT

Osteoid osteoma has limited growth potential. Some patients treated medically have their symptoms disappear over a period of months to a number of years. In these patients, the lesion may persist or eventually undergo mineralization and merge with the surrounding zone of sclerosis so it is not longer visible as a discrete mass. Many patients, however, have severe symptoms and require some form of eradication of the tumor. In the past, the treatment of osteoid osteoma was frequently burring down and curettage and *en bloc* resection. These invasive procedures are expensive, require hospitalization, and frequently weaken the underlying bone, requiring the insertion of metal hardware or bone grafts. In recent years, percutaneous ablations of the nidus by CT-guided core-drill excision and obliteration of the tumor by thermocoagulation, radiofrequency, or laser have become the treatment of choice. These techniques have a reported success rate of 80% to 100%.

OSTEOID OSTEOMA—FACT SHEET

Definition
- Benign, bone-forming tumor characterized by a central nidus surrounded by sclerotic bone
- The nidus is smaller than 2 cm

Incidence and Location
- Accounts for approximately 11% of benign bone tumors
- Diaphysis of long bones, especially the femur, but can affect any bone

Morbidity and Mortality
- Osteoid osteoma is benign, but painful

Sex, Race, and Age Distribution
- More common in male individuals at a ratio of 3:1
- Children and young adults

Clinical Features
- Localized pain most severe at night and relieved by NSAIDs
- Lesions close to joints can cause symptoms mimicking arthritis
- Lesion involving vertebrae can cause painful scoliosis

Radiologic Features
- Well-demarcated radiolucency with central mineralization surrounded by dense sclerosis

Prognosis and Treatment
- Treated with aspirin and related analgesics, surgical resection, or percutaneous ablation
- Local recurrence rate around 5%

OSTEOID OSTEOMA—PATHOLOGIC FEATURES

Gross Findings
- The nidus is well-demarcated, dark red and gritty, and is surrounded by dense sclerotic bone

Microscopic Findings
- The nidus is composed of interanastomosing woven bone with prominent osteoblastic rimming, with intervening fibrovascular stroma

Immunohistochemical Findings
- Immunohistochemical stains show nerve fibers within the tumor and surrounding reactive zone

Differential Diagnosis
- Osteoblastoma

OSTEOBLASTOMA

CLINICAL FEATURES

Osteoblastoma is a rare, benign, bone-forming tumor that by definition is larger than 2 cm in greatest dimension and is composed of neoplastic osteoblasts that deposit trabecular woven bone. It is uncommon and accounts for only approximately 1% of primary bone tumors. Osteoblastomas have been reported to arise in most bones of the body, but approximately 32% develop in the posterior elements of the spine, 12% in the femur, 10% in the tibia, and 9% in the bones of the foot and ankle. In the long bones, they usually originate within the medullary canal of the metadiaphyseal region but may also be juxtacortical or subperiosteal. In most instances, the tumor is diagnosed during the second to fourth decades of life, and male individuals are affected approximately twice as frequently as female individuals. Most osteoblastomas are solitary; however, rare cases of multifocal disease have been documented.

RADIOLOGIC FEATURES

On imaging studies, osteoblastoma is greater than 2 cm in size, oval to round, radiolucent with scattered areas of mineralization that have the density of trabecular bone, especially in the center, and has well-defined margins (Figure 14-12). Some cases may be extensively mineralized, whereas others may be almost completely radiolucent. The tumors are hot on bone scan, and a minority may contain areas of cystic degeneration and hemorrhage that is best appreciated on MRI.

PATHOLOGIC FEATURES

Dark red with speckled white areas, round to ovoid, osteoblastoma is well delineated from the surrounding cancellous and cortical bone, and expansile lesions are demarcated from the neighboring soft tissues by a layer of reactive subperiosteal bone. Cystic elements are hemorrhagic and blood filled, and they may involve small to large portions of the tumor (Figure 14-13).

Histologically, osteoblastoma has a sharp margin with the adjacent bone (Figure 14-14). It is composed of haphazardly interconnecting trabeculae of woven bone of variable mineralization that are surfaced by prominent osteoblasts and scattered osteoclasts (Figure 14-15). The intertrabecular spaces are filled with loose connective

CHAPTER 14 Bone-Forming Tumors 317

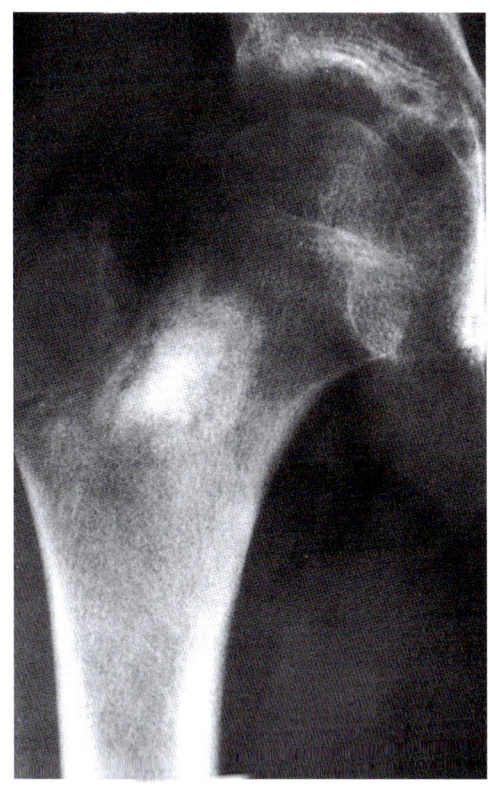

FIGURE 14-12
Osteoblastoma of the femoral neck. The tumor is oval, well defined, and radiodense.

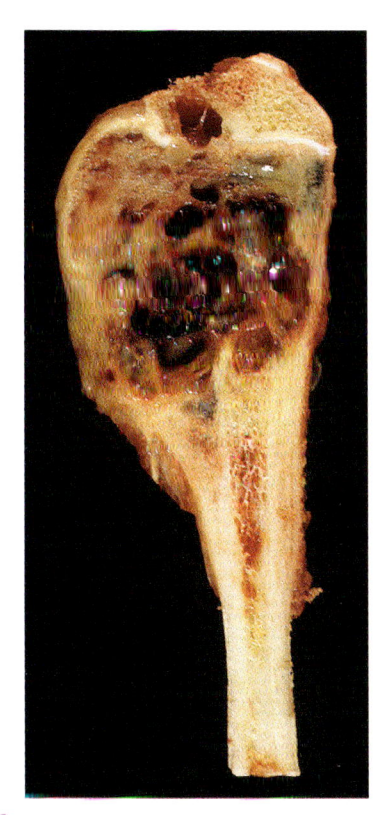

FIGURE 14-13
Resected osteoblastoma of the proximal fibula. The tumor is large, hemorrhagic, and cystic, and has extended into the adjacent soft tissue.

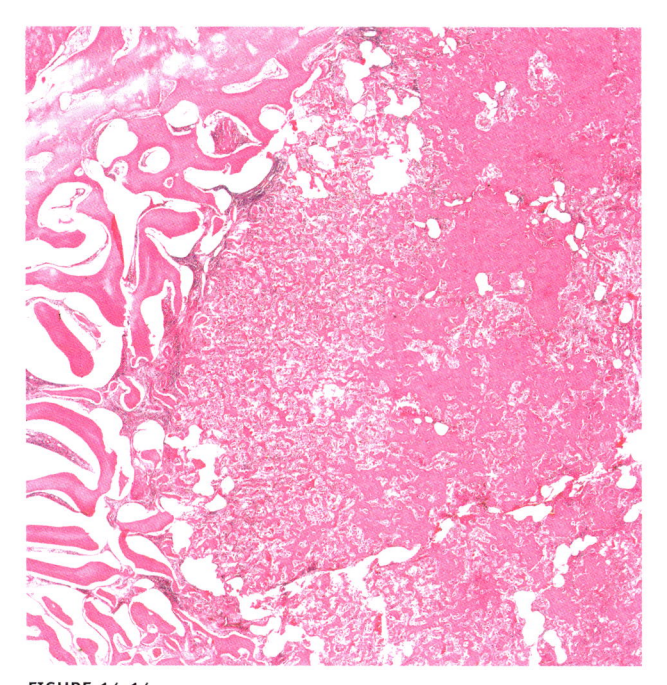

FIGURE 14-14
Osteoblastoma with well-circumscribed margin from the surrounding bone.

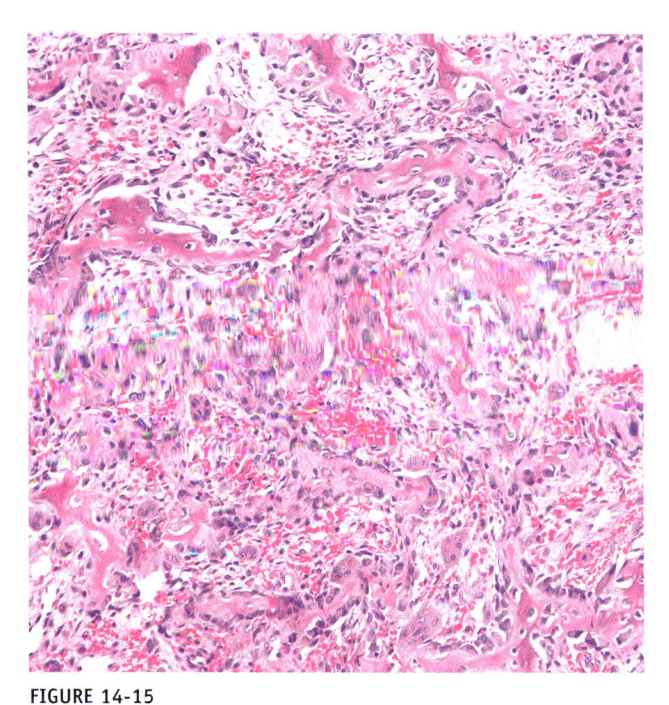

FIGURE 14-15
Interanastomosing trabeculae of osteoblastoma are rimmed by osteoblasts.

tissue that contains many thin-walled vascular spaces. In some cases, the bone is sheet-like or coarse and lace-like in appearance. The osteoblasts are large, ovoid, or round with eccentric nuclei and moderate amounts of eosinophilic or purple cytoplasm (Figure 14-16). Mitoses may be present but are not numerous, and necrosis

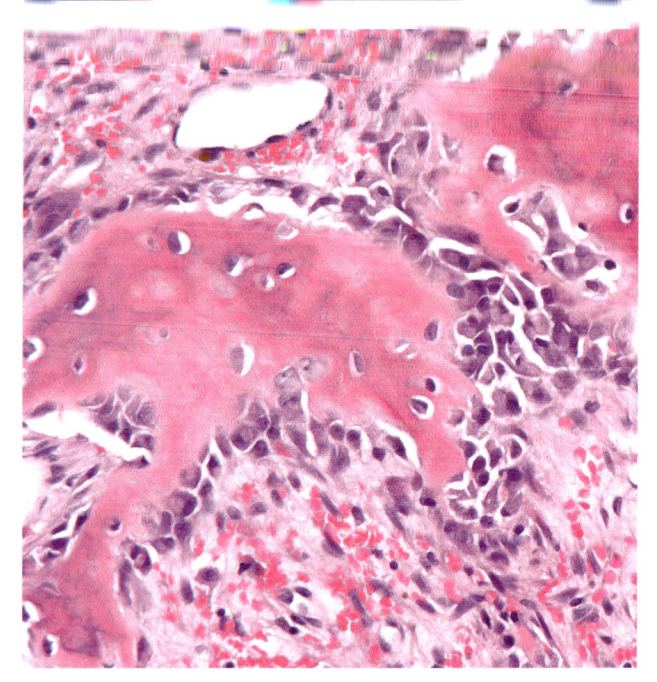

FIGURE 14-16
Osteoblasts in osteoblastoma are prominent.

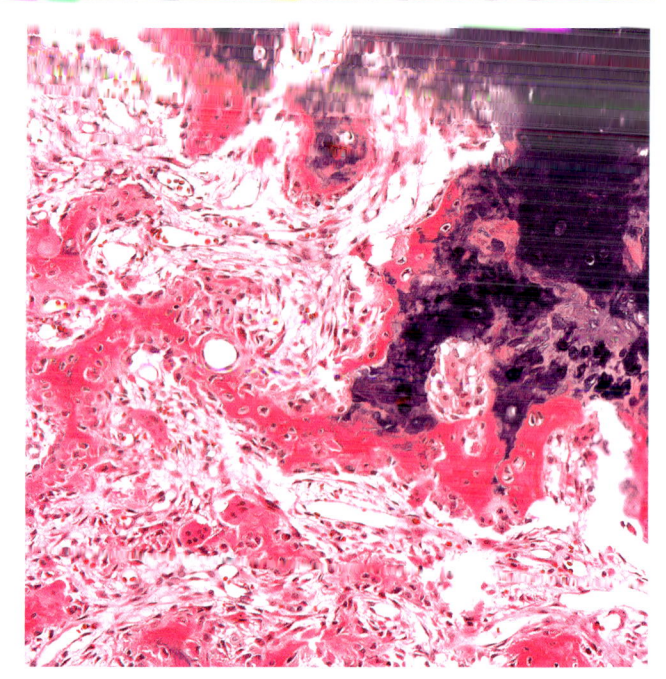

FIGURE 14-18
Osteoblastoma with hyaline-type cartilage.

is absent or limited in quantity unless there has been a pathologic fracture.

A variety of histologic variants of osteoblastoma is recognized and includes those with cystic change, cartilage matrix, epithelioid osteoblasts, and osteoblasts with so-called *pseudomalignant* malignant change. In cystic osteoblastoma, the cyst walls are composed of fibroblasts, collagen, extravasated red blood cells, scattered osteoclast-type giant cells, and trabeculae of woven bone that are deposited in a fashion that follows the contours of the wall (Figure 14-17). Areas diagnostic of osteoblastoma can be found in the solid components of the mass. In the cartilaginous variant, the chondrocytes are cytologically banal and the matrix is hyaline or chondro-osseous in appearance, with varying degrees of calcification and enchondral ossification (Figure 14-18). The cartilage may merge or be sharply demarcated from the adjacent tumor bone. Aggressive osteoblastoma is characterized by osteoblasts that are epithelioid, being two to three times larger than conventional osteoblasts, and have abundant eosinophilic cytoplasm and large vesicular nuclei with prominent nucleoli (Figure 14-19). The neoplastic bone may be trabecular or coarse and lace-like in appearance. This type of osteoblastoma can be confused with osteosarcoma, but the sharp margin of the tumor and the presence of osteoblastic rimming are helpful features in making this distinction. Pseudomalignant osteoblastoma is a rare variant and contains neoplastic cells with large, bizarre, and degenerative nuclei. This finding has no clinical significance except that the unusual pathology may be misinterpreted as representing osteosarcoma (Figure 14-20).

DIFFERENTIAL DIAGNOSIS

Osteoblastoma is in the differential diagnosis of a variety of benign and malignant bone tumors. Of these, the most important is osteosarcoma because of the drastic differences in treatment and prognosis. Notable distinguishing features are the infiltrative growth pattern

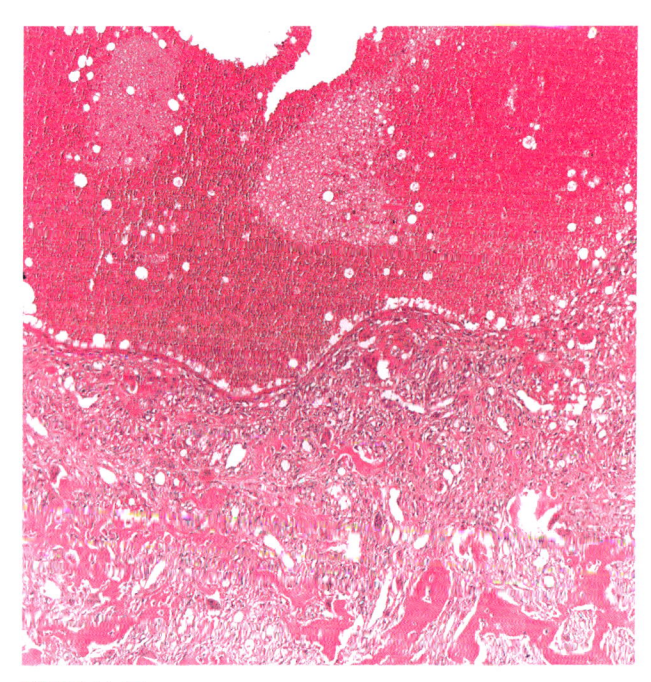

FIGURE 14-17
Osteoblastoma with large hemorrhagic cystic component.

CHAPTER 14 Bone-Forming Tumors

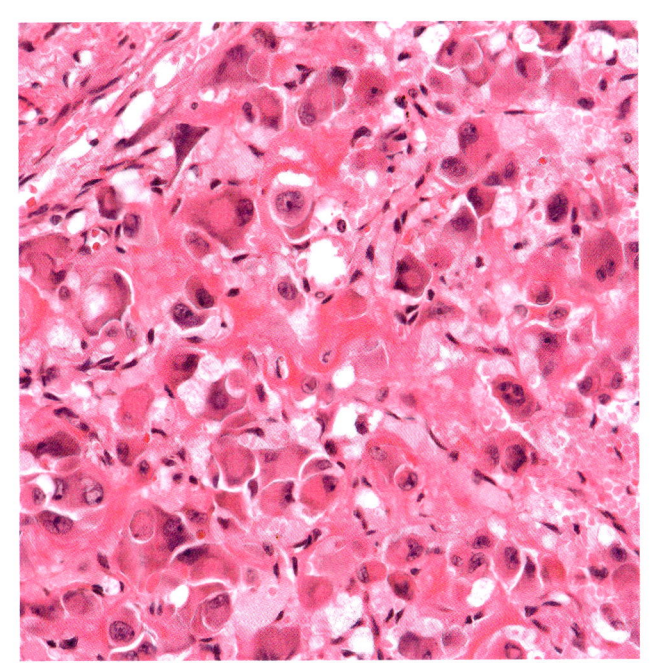

FIGURE 14-19
So-called aggressive osteoblastoma composed of epithelioid osteoblasts associated with coarse lace-like bone.

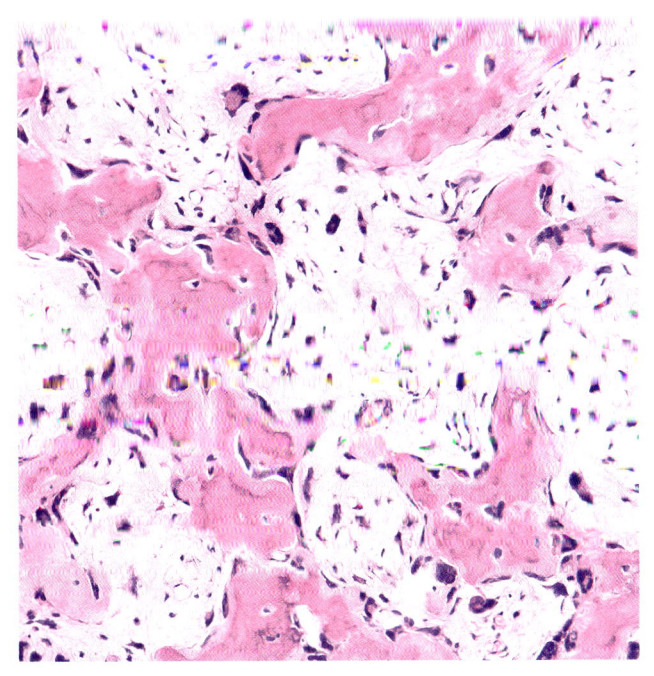

FIGURE 14-20
Pseudomalignant osteoblastoma.
Osteoblasts and some stromal cells demonstrate marked degenerative nuclear atypia.

OSTEOBLASTOMA—FACT SHEET

Definition
- Benign, bone-forming tumor that is histologically similar to osteoid osteoma but larger and does not contain the surrounding sclerotic bone

Incidence and Location
- Accounts for approximately 1% of primary bone tumors
- Vertebrae, femur, tibia bones of the foot and ankle

Sex, Race, and Age Distribution
- More common in male sex (M:F ratio, 2:1)
- Second to fourth decades of life

Clinical Features
- Pain

Radiologic Features
- Well-defined, mixed lytic, and mass greater than 2 cm

Prognosis and Treatment
- Curettage or en bloc resection
- Local recurrence rate after curettage is 10% to 20%

OSTEOBLASTOMA—PATHOLOGIC FEATURES

Gross Findings
- Well circumscribed, dark red and gritty

Microscopic Findings
- Sharp margin and composed of trabeculae of woven bone with prominent osteoblastic rimming and richly vascularized stroma
- Variants contain aneurysmal bone cyst like changes, cartilage matrix, epithelioid osteoblasts, and degenerative nuclear atypia

Immunohistochemical Findings
- Not helpful

Differential Diagnosis
- Osteoid osteoma
- Aneurysmal bone cyst
- Fibro-osseous lesions
- Osteosarcoma

and lack of osteoblastic rimming of the neoplastic bone in osteosarcoma, because osteoblastoma is well circumscribed and the tumor matrix is cuffed prominently by osteoblasts, which, in turn, is surrounded by vascular loose connective tissue. Also, many osteosarcomas show significant nuclear atypia in the form of hyperchromasia, distorted nuclear-to-cytoplasmic ratios, and abundant mitoses including atypical forms, which are absent in osteoblastoma.

Cystic osteoblastoma can be confused with aneurysmal bone cyst. Generally, the trabeculae of reactive bone in aneurysmal bone cyst are deposited in an organized fashion such that they follow the contours of the cyst wall. In comparison, the bone in osteoblastoma is haphazard in arrangement and lacks a pattern of organization. Fibrous dysplasia differs from osteoblastoma in that the bone lacks osteoblastic rimming and the stroma is more collagenous. In osteofibrous dysplasia, the stroma is also more collagenous, the spindle cells often are arranged in a storiform pattern and also focally express keratin, features not observed in osteoblastoma.

PROGNOSIS AND TREATMENT

The various histologic subtypes of osteoblastoma behave in a similar fashion, although there has been some controversy regarding the aggressive type. In essence, osteoblastoma is a benign tumor that can grow, become large, and produce bone destruction and pain. It does not have the capacity to metastasize; accordingly, its treatment is surgical and depends on the location and size of the mass. Curettage is a common mode of therapy and is associated with local recurrence in approximately 10% to 20% of cases. En bloc resection, which is usually curative, can be performed on tumors located in expendable bones or cortically based masses. Malignant transformation is exceptionally rare.

OSTEOSARCOMA

Osteosarcoma of bone is a primary malignancy of any part of the skeleton in which the neoplastic cells manufacture and deposit the organic constituents of bone matrix, which may undergo mineralization. No minimal amount of bone matrix is necessary to consider a tumor as osteosarcoma; therefore, the presence of any neoplastic bone, even if only minute in amount, is reason enough to categorize the tumor as an osteosarcoma.

Osteosarcoma has been recognized for almost two centuries and is the most common primary nonhematopoietic malignancy of the skeletal system. It accounts for approximately 20% of all primary malignant bone tumors, and its incidence in the United States is 4 to 5 per 1 million individuals, with 1000 to 1500 new cases diagnosed annually. Osteosarcoma has a bimodal age distribution and a propensity to develop in adolescents and young adults, with 60% of tumors occurring in patients younger than 25 years and only 13% to 30% in persons older than 40 years. Male individuals are affected more frequently than female individuals at a ratio of 1.3 to 1.6:1, with equal distribution among races. Osteosarcoma can arise in any bone of the body, but most tumors originate in the long bones of the appendicular skeleton, especially the distal femur, followed by the proximal tibia and proximal humerus, sites that contain the most proliferative growth plates. In the long bones, the tumor is most frequently centered in the metaphysis (90%), infrequently in the diaphysis (9%), and rarely in the epiphysis.

The clinicopathologic features of osteosarcoma form the basis of its classification, and important among them include the histologic features, biologic potential (grade), relation to bone (surface or intramedullary), multiplicity (solitary and multifocal), and the pre-existing state of underlying bone (primary or secondary). Most osteosarcomas can be categorized into four important groups: (1) conventional high-grade osteosarcoma and its histologic subtypes (75%–85%), (2) high-grade secondary osteosarcoma that arises in a diseased bone (10%), (3) intramedullary well-differentiated osteosarcoma (1%), and (4) surface osteosarcomas (5%–10%).

Conventional osteosarcoma, namely, garden-variety osteosarcoma, is solitary, arises in the medullary cavity of an otherwise normal bone, is high-grade, and produces neoplastic bone with or without cartilaginous or fibroblastic components. *Surface* osteosarcoma includes well-differentiated juxtacortical osteosarcoma also known as parosteal osteosarcoma (3%–5%), juxtacortical intermediate-grade chondroblastic osteosarcoma, which is known as periosteal osteosarcoma (2%–4%), and high grade surface (1%). Juxtacortical well differentiated osteosarcoma usually arises during the third decade of life, whereas juxtacortical intermediate-grade chondroblastic osteosarcoma and high-grade osteoblastic osteosarcoma (*high-grade surface* osteosarcoma) commonly develop in the second decade of life. Parosteal and periosteal osteosarcomas have a predilection for female individuals, whereas *high-grade surface* osteosarcomas more frequently affect male individuals. *Parosteal* osteosarcoma is most commonly based on the posterior femoral cortex in the metaphyseal-diaphyseal area of the popliteal region, followed by the metaphyseal-diaphyseal zone of the proximal tibia. *Periosteal* osteosarcoma originates from the cortex of the diaphysis or metaphysis of the tibia, followed in frequency by the femur. *High-grade surface* osteosarcoma arises on the metaphyseal surface of long bones in a distribution similar to conventional osteosarcoma, and most frequently involves the distal femur or proximal humerus. *Intramedullary well-differentiated* osteosarcoma is uncommon, most tumors develop during the second to fifth decades of life, and almost 50% of affected individuals are in their 20s at the time of diagnosis.

The cause of osteosarcoma is unknown; however, a variety of agents and disease states are associated with its development. The best-known causative association with osteosarcoma is radiation. Its causal relation was first documented in the radium dial painters. Since that time, numerous studies have evaluated the minimum dosage, the accumulated dosage, and the rate of delivery of the dosage of radiation necessary to induce an osteosarcoma. Osteosarcoma after therapeutic irradiation is an uncommon complication and usually develops after approximately 15 (range, 3–55) years.

Osteosarcoma is associated with a variety of genetic syndromes (Table 14-1). Information derived from these relations has provided insight into the molecular

TABLE 14-1
Genetic Syndromes Associated with Osteosarcoma

Syndrome	Mutation	Molecule Function
Rothmund–Thompson	Chromosome 8q24.3	DNA helicase
Bloom	Chromosome 15q26.1	DNA helicase
Werner	Chromosome 8p11	DNA helicase
Li–Fraumani	Chromosome 17p13	DNA repair
Bilateral retinoblastoma	Chromosome 13q14	Cell-cycle regulator

pathogenesis of sporadic osteosarcoma, which appears to result from the accrual of complex genetic alterations, usually involving the inactivation of tumor-suppressor genes and the overexpression of oncogenes.

Cytogenetic abnormalities are found in approximately 70% of osteosarcomas and are frequently complex. Unfortunately, they have proved to be of little importance in diagnosing, predicting prognosis, and understanding the molecular pathogenesis of these tumors. Some of the more frequent numeric chromosomal abnormalities involve gain of chromosome 1 and losses of genetic material on chromosomes 6, 9, 10, 13, and 17. Some recurring structural rearrangements are found in regions of chromosomes 1p11-13, 1q11-12, 1q21-22, 11p14-15, 14p11-13, 15p1-13, 17p, and 19q13. Comparative genomic hybridization studies have shown DNA sequence copy-number changes involving 1q21, 3q26, 6p, 8q, 12q12-q13, 14q24-qter, 17p11.2 p12, and 19q12-q13. Amplification of genes in the form of ring chromosomes, double minutes, and homogeneously staining regions are commonplace. Tumors with chromosomal abnormalities limited mainly to ring chromosomes, however, almost always parosteal osteosarcomas (low-grade surface osteosarcomas), and the ring chromosomes are composed of amplified regions of 12q13-15. Low-grade intramedullary osteosarcomas possess similar ring chromosomes, as well as abnormalities in chromosome 6p.

Osteosarcoma is known to affect approximately 1% of patients with Paget disease of bone, which reflects a several thousand-fold increase in risk in comparison with that of the general population. The tumor usually develops in patients with severe disease and arises in an affected site; histologically, it has the appearance of conventional high-grade osteosarcoma. The underlying genetic abnormalities linking the two disorders have yet to be identified with certainty.

Osteosarcoma may also arise in sites of previous bone infarction, chronic osteomyelitis, preexisting primary benign bone tumors (osteochondroma, enchondroma, fibrous dysplasia, giant cell tumor, osteoblastoma, aneurysmal bone cyst, and unicameral bone cyst), and adjacent to metallic implants. These secondary osteosarcomas account for only a small percentage of osteosarcomas, and their pathogenesis is likely related to chronic cell turnover that is associated with the underlying disease states.

CLINICAL FEATURES

Pain associated with a progressively enlarging mass is the typical manifestation of conventional osteosarcoma. The pain is often noted months before diagnosis, is deep seated, boring in nature, increases in intensity over time, and eventually produces unremitting discomfort. The skin overlying the tumor is hyperemic, warm, edematous, and cartographed by prominent engorged veins. Range of motion and musculoskeletal function is compromised by large tumors that may also cause joint effusions and, in far advanced cases, weight loss and cachexia. In 5% to 10% of cases, the heralding event is a sudden, devastating pathologic fracture through the destructive mass.

Surface osteosarcomas may or may not be associated with pain but usually present as an enlarging, firm, fixed mass. The low-grade variants are slow growing, may be painless, and are often of long duration.

Well-differentiated intramedullary osteosarcomas frequently cause pain that persists for months to years before diagnosis. In some instances, the tumor may be first detected as an enlarging palpable mass. Infrequently, we have seen cases that have been discovered as an incidental finding.

Laboratory studies are usually not helpful in assessing osteosarcoma. However, the serum alkaline phosphatase level is increased in many cases, and extremely high levels are associated with the presence of metastatic disease.

RADIOLOGIC FEATURES

Osteosarcoma has an extremely variable appearance on imaging studies. A conventional tumor is typically a large, destructive, poorly defined, mixed lytic, and blastic mass that transgresses the cortex and forms a large soft tissue component (Figure 14-21A). Some tumors are entirely lytic, a feature often seen in the telangiectatic variant, whereas others are diffusely mineralized producing a densely sclerotic mass. The periphery of the lesion is the least radiodense, and the soft tissue component may have a fine *cloud-like* pattern of radiodensity. As the enlarging mass destroys and invades beyond the cortex, it physically increases the periosteum, which

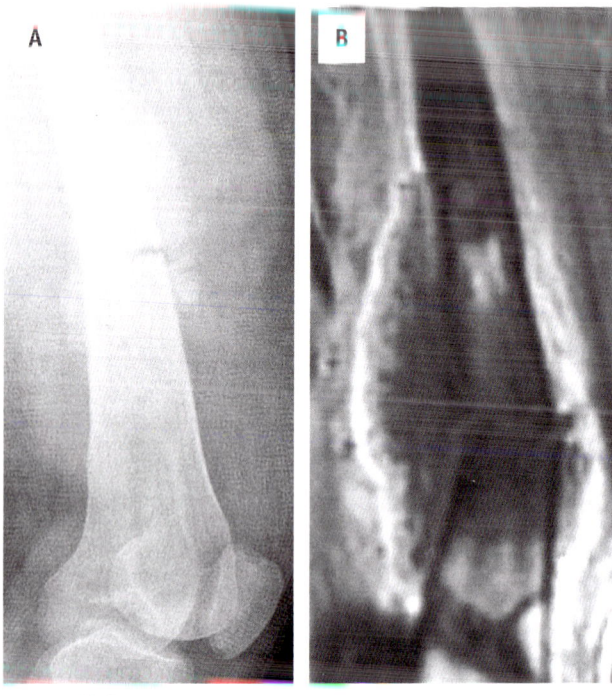

FIGURE 14-21
Large, poorly defined osteosarcoma of the distal diaphysis of the femur associated with a pathologic fracture. **A,** The tumor is poorly defined, and contains fine cloud-like mineralization on radiograph. **B,** Magnetic resonance imaging shows the extent of the neoplasm.

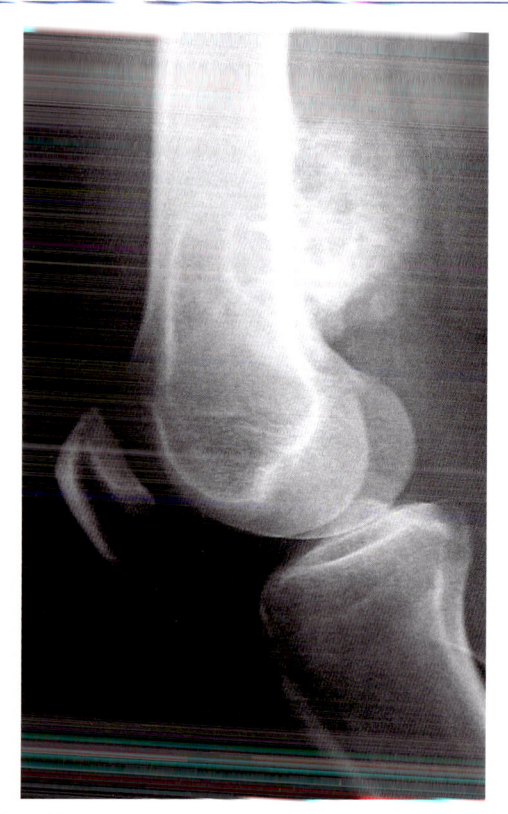

FIGURE 14-22
Juxtacortical low-grade osteosarcoma (parosteal osteosarcoma) arising on the posterior surface of the distal femur. The tumor is large and ovoid, and irregularly mineralized.

deposits layers of reactive bone at the proximal and distal extent of the tumor forming so-called Codman's triangle. In addition, reactive bone is deposited in a sunburst or onion skin-like pattern along the bulk of the length of the tumor. Conventional osteosarcoma is heterogeneous on CT and MRI, and these modalities provide valuable information regarding the overall dimensions of the tumor, its extent within the medullary cavity and soft tissue, and its relation to important neighboring anatomic structures (see Figure 14-21B). This type of information is essential in planning successful limb salvage surgical resection.

Surface osteosarcomas have a broad base of attachment to the underlying cortex. *Parosteal* tumors may be circumferential or mushroom shaped, and usually have large areas that are radiodense (Figure 14-22). Periosteal reaction is minimal. Sometimes present is a radiolucent line that separates the base of the tumor from the adjacent cortex. *Periosteal* osteosarcomas are fusiform, predominately lucent, and are frequently associated with a periosteal reaction in the form of Codman's triangle and perpendicular linear striae that radiate from the underlying bone and course through the tumor. *High-grade surface* osteosarcoma is similar in appearance to periosteal osteosarcoma but, in addition, tends to have fine cloud-like radiopacities. CT is helpful in assessing invasion of the cortex and medullary canal. MRI facilitates the identification of cartilage, which may be in the form of a peripheral cap in parosteal osteosarcoma or scattered throughout the mass in cases of periosteal or high-grade surface osteosarcoma.

Intramedullary well-differentiated osteosarcomas have heterogeneous radiographic findings. The tumors are poorly demarcated, contain lytic and densely mineralized regions, and may expand the underlying bone with little periosteal reaction (Figure 14-23). A soft tissue component, if present, is relatively small compared with the extent of intramedullary involvement.

PATHOLOGIC FEATURES

Conventional osteosarcoma manifests as a large, metaphyseal, intramedullary, and tan–gray–white, gritty mass (Figure 14-24). Tumors that contain abundant mineralized bone are tan–white and hard, whereas nonmineralized, cartilaginous components are glistening, gray, and may be mucinous if the matrix is myxoid or more rubbery if hyaline in nature. Areas of hemorrhage and cystic change are commonplace and, when extensive, produce a friable, bloody, and spongy mass (telangiectatic osteosarcoma). Intramedullary involvement is often considerable, and the tumor usually destroys the overlying cortex and forms an eccentric or circumferential soft tissue component that displaces the periosteum

CHAPTER 14 Bone-forming Tumors

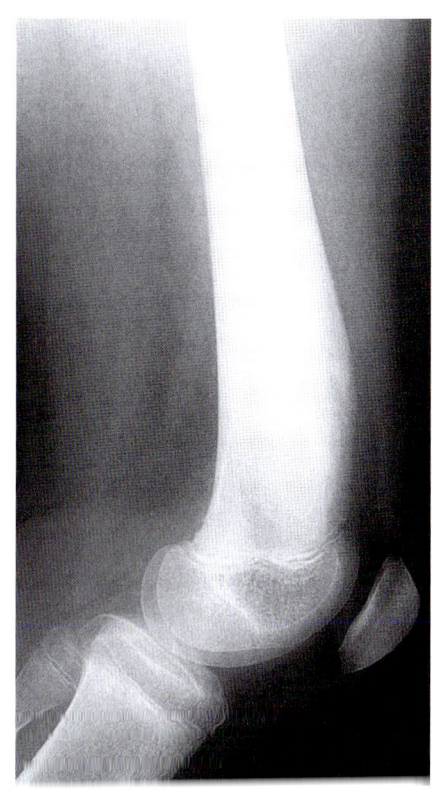

FIGURE 14-23
Intramedullary well differentiated osteosarcoma involving the distal femur. Although relatively large, the ill-defined radiodense tumor does not extend into the soft tissues.

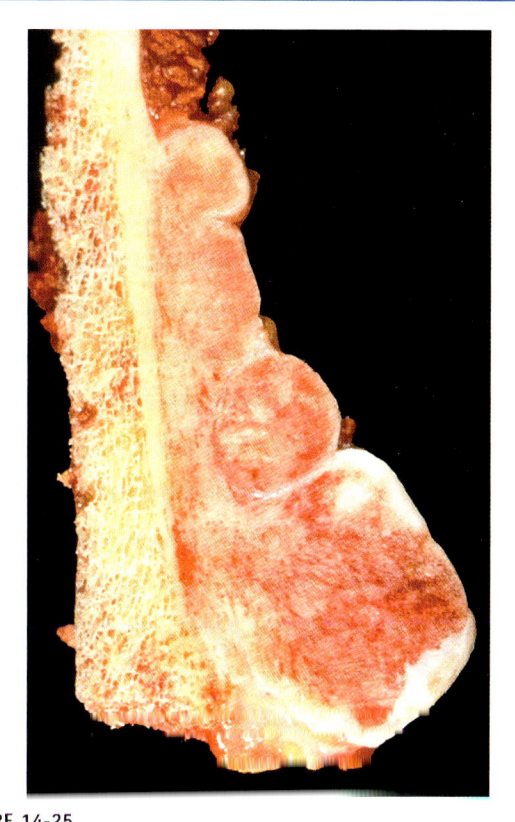

FIGURE 14-25
Juxtacortical low grade osteosarcoma (parosteal osteosarcoma) arising on the cortex. The tumor is homogenous pink–tan and solid. The surface is covered by a layer of neoplastic cartilage.

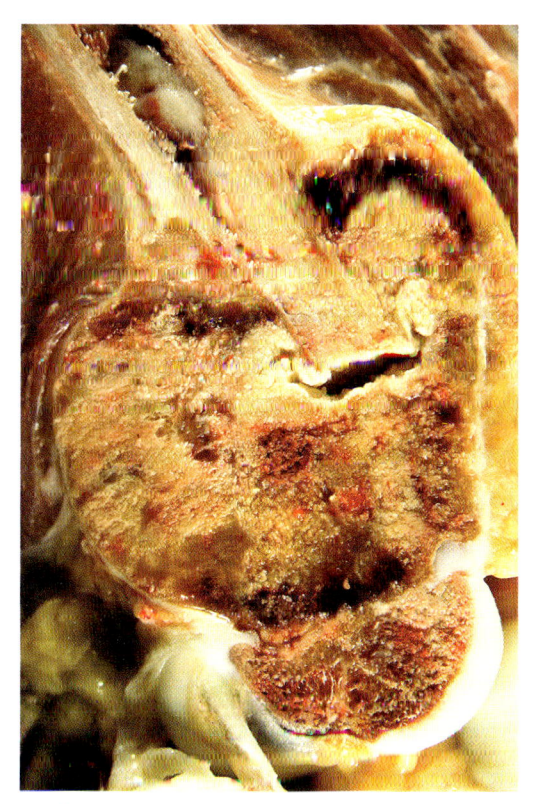

FIGURE 14-24
Gross specimen of osteosarcoma in Figure 14-21. The large tumor is solid tan–white and hemorrhagic.

peripherally. The dislodged periosteum becomes a sharp interface between the mass and the bordering skeletal muscle and fat. In addition, in the proximal and distal regions of the tumor, the raised periosteum deposits a layer of reactive bone known as Codman's triangle. In some cases, the tumor grows into the joint space via pathways offering little resistance to spread, such as tracking along the cortical surface and entering the joint beneath the synovium, or through tendoligamentous and joint capsule insertion sites. This phenomenon may be associated with coating of the peripheral portions of the articular cartilage by the sarcoma. Advancing tumors may be halted by an open growth plate; however, penetration of the physis and invasion into the epiphysis to the base of the articular surface occasionally occurs. Solitary or multiple skip metastases appear as intramedullary, firm, ovoid, tan–white nodules located in the vicinity of or far from the main mass.

Rigidly attached to the underlying cortex, surface osteosarcomas are broad based and demarcated from the surrounding soft tissues. Well-differentiated juxtacortical tumors *(parosteal osteosarcoma)* are solid, tan–white, hard, and gritty, and may have a gray, firm, glistening, hyaline cartilage cap or areas that are softer and fish flesh-like, representing elements that are fibrosarcomatous in appearance (Figure 14-25). High-grade juxtacortical osteosarcomas *(periosteal* and *high-grade*

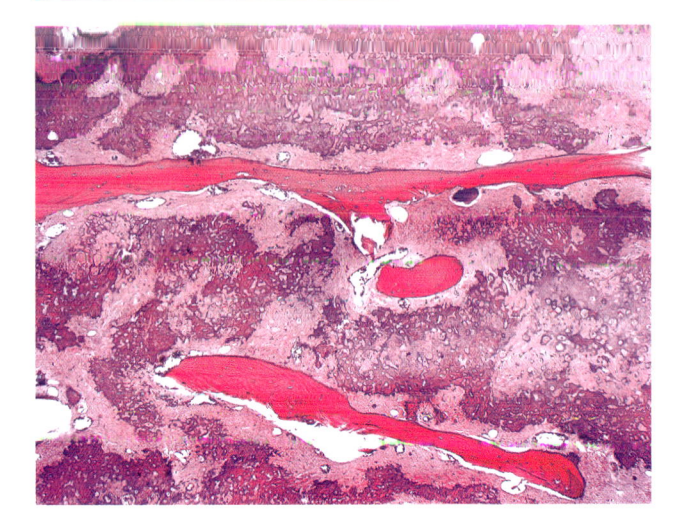

FIGURE 14-26
Osteosarcoma growing with a permeative pattern. The tumor replaces the marrow and surrounds the preexisting bone trabeculae.

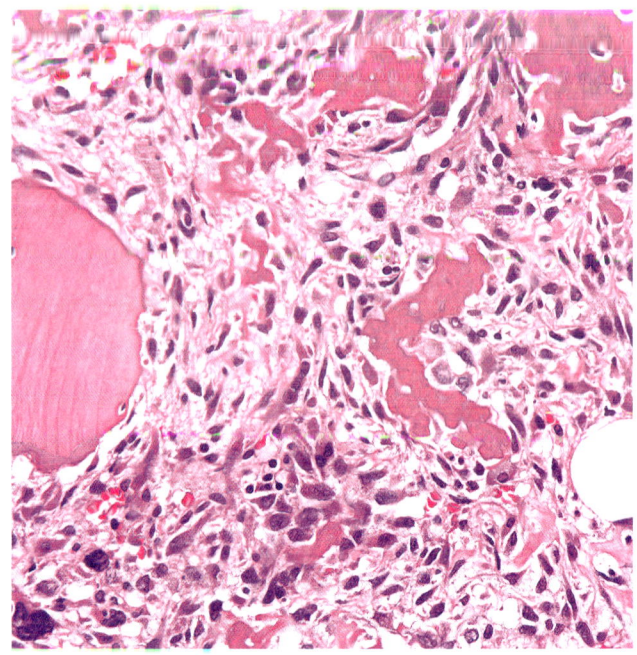

FIGURE 14-27
Osteoblastic osteosarcoma containing pleomorphic malignant cells and coarse neoplastic woven bone.

surface) may be dominated by cartilaginous tissue, or be composed of hard, tan–white areas admixed with fish flesh-like regions. Cortical destruction and invasion into the medullary canal is often absent, but when present, is only focal. If extensive, it becomes difficult, if not impossible, to distinguish an intramedullary tumor with an eccentric soft tissue component from a surface neoplasm with extensive invasion of the medullary canal.

Intramedullary well-differentiated osteosarcoma is typically centered in the medullary cavity of the metaphysis or metaphyseal-diaphyseal region. The tumor is hard, gritty, tan–white, and has poorly defined margins. Cortical destruction and an associated small soft tissue mass may be present.

By light microscopy, high-grade osteosarcoma permeates the marrow space, surrounds and erodes preexisting bony trabeculae, and fills and expands haversian systems (Figure 14-26). The *conventional* type can be subclassified into *osteoblastic, chondroblastic, fibroblastic,* and *mixed* types, by virtue of the predominance of the neoplastic component. The malignant cells in the osteoblastic variant have hyperchromatic nuclei that are central or eccentric in position, and frequently contain prominent nucleoli and eosinophilic cytoplasm that varies in volume according to cell size (Figure 14-27). The tumor cells are intimately related to the surface of the neoplastic bone, which is woven in architecture, varies in quantity, and is deposited as primitive, disorganized trabeculae that produce a coarse lace-like pattern or broad, large sheets fashioned by coalescing trabeculae as seen in the sclerosing variant. Depending on its state of mineralization, the bone is eosinophilic or basophilic and may have a pagetoid appearance caused by haphazardly deposited cement lines. Tumor cells surrounded and imprisoned by the matrix appear smaller and less atypical. Chondroblastic components are usually hyaline in appearance but may be predominately myxoid, particularly in tumors arising in jaw bones (Figure 14-28). Severe cytologic atypia characterize the neoplastic chondrocytes, which reside in lacunar spaces in hyaline matrix, or float singly or in cords in myxoid matrix. Fibroblastic foci manifest as cytologically malignant spindle cells arranged in a herringbone of storiform pattern (Figure 14-29). The degree of atypia is variable but is frequently severe. Mitoses are numerous, and structurally abnormal forms are common.

High-grade tumors that contain numerous blood-filled cystic spaces comprising the majority of the tumor are known as *telangiectatic* osteosarcoma. Lining the

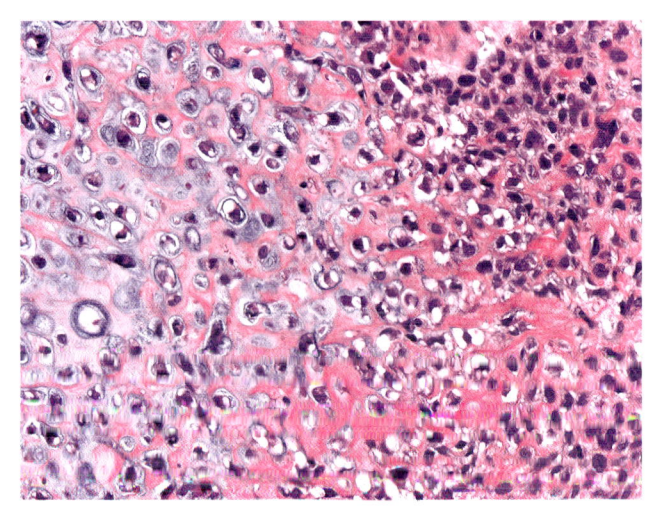

FIGURE 14-28
Chondroblastic osteosarcoma with neoplastic cartilage merging with tumor bone.

CHAPTER 14 Bone-Forming Tumors

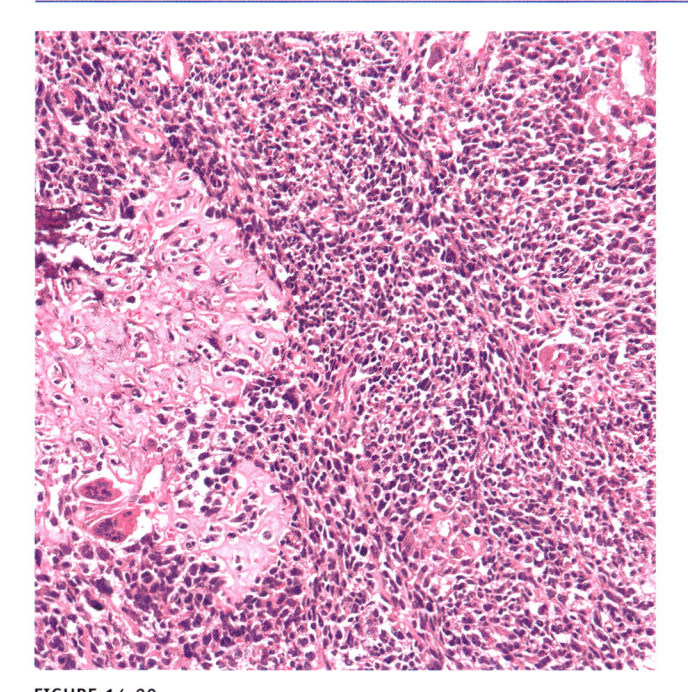

FIGURE 14-29
Fibroblastic osteosarcoma containing fascicles of malignant spindle cells adjacent to deposits of neoplastic bone.

cyst walls and percolating throughout them are malignant cells that produce variable amounts of neoplastic bone (Figure 14-30). The neoplastic cells in *small-cell* osteosarcoma are uniform, small, round, or spindle shaped and contain little cytoplasm. In the *giant-cell–rich* variant, numerous non-neoplastic osteoclast-type giant cells are present throughout the tumor, whereas large polyhedral tumor cells typify the *epithelioid* variant. Deceptively banal tumor cells in the *osteoblastoma-like* variant rim neoplastic bony trabeculae in a pattern that imitates osteoblastoma. Distinguishing features are the permeative growth pattern and solid cellular intertrabecular tissue that are found in osteosarcoma.

The presence of streamers of relatively well-formed trabeculae of woven bone surrounded by a mildly to moderately cellular spindle cell proliferation entangled in collagen fibers is the hallmark of *parosteal* osteosarcoma (Figure 14-31). The spindle cells have elongate nuclei with pointed ends and demonstrate limited degrees of cytologic atypia (Figure 14-32). The nuclei in deceptively bland-appearing cases have finely stippled chromatin, small nucleoli, poorly defined eosinophilic cytoplasm, and few mitoses, thereby simulating fibromatosis. Tumor cells with hyperchromatic nuclei are present in higher-grade tumors, and are frequently arranged in a herringbone pattern and exhibit a greater degree of mitotic activity. Malignant hyaline cartilage may be present in parosteal osteosarcoma, and when present, grows as a cap covering the periphery of the tumor and contains mildly to moderately atypical chondrocytes. This composition and configuration can cause confusion with osteochondroma. Rarely, parosteal osteosarcoma undergoes dedifferentiation that manifests as foci of pleomorphic spindle cell sarcoma or even high-grade osteosarcoma.

A grade 2/3 chondroblastic osteosarcoma arising on the cortical surface defines *periosteal* osteosarcoma. The lobules of neoplastic hyaline cartilage contain mitotically active chondrocytes that show moderate-to-severe cytologic atypia. The neoplastic bone usually has a coarse lace-like pattern and either merges with or is surrounded by the cartilage, or is enveloped by significantly atypical proliferating spindle or polyhedral-shaped tumor cells.

A *high-grade surface* osteosarcoma is a conventional osteoblastic osteosarcoma originating on the surface of the cortex. The tumor is densely cellular, and the neoplastic cells demonstrate severe cytologic atypia, mitotic activity, and areas of necrosis. Foci of neoplastic cartilage and fibroblastic components may be present as well.

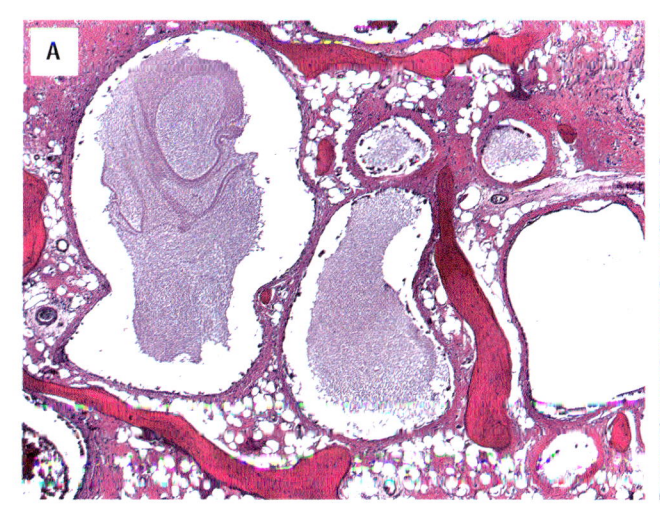

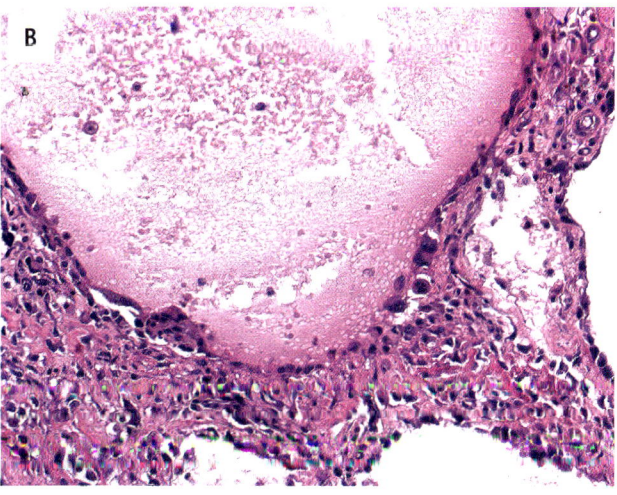

FIGURE 14-30
A, Telangiectatic osteosarcoma with numerous large cystic spaces filled with blood and fibrinous material. **B,** Malignant tumor cells associated with neoplastic bone comprise the cyst wall.

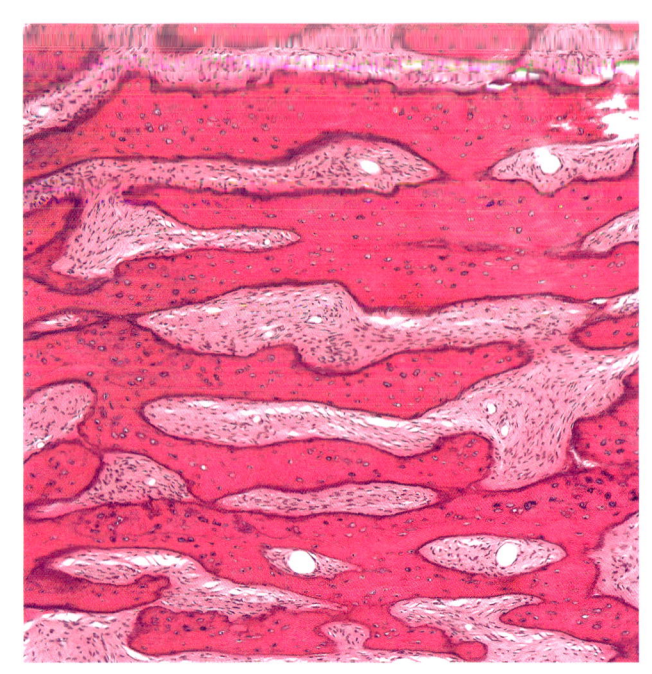

FIGURE 14-31
Streamers of woven bone surrounded by relatively bland spindle cells in parosteal osteosarcoma.

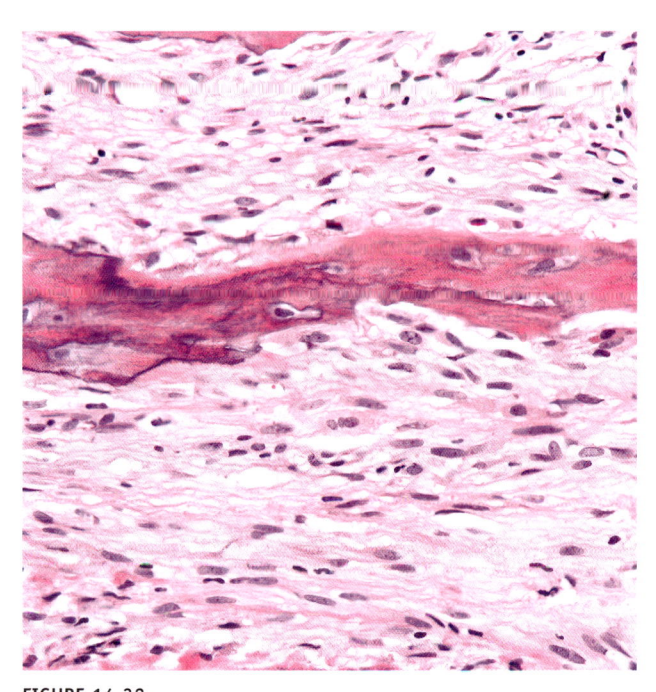

FIGURE 14-32
Sometimes the spindle cells can grow in sheets in parosteal osteosarcoma.

FIGURE 14-33
A, Intramedullary well-differentiated osteosarcoma permeates the medullary cavity, and **B,** the trabeculae of neoplastic woven bone are surrounded by minimally atypical spindle cells.

Similar to its juxtacortical counterpart, *Intramedullary well-differentiated* osteosarcoma contains long trabeculae or round islands of woven bone intimately associated with a mildly to moderately cellular population of cytologically bland neoplastic spindle cells (Figure 14-33). The neoplastic matrix may have a pagetoid appearance and is frequently deposited on the surfaces of the preexisting bony trabeculae.

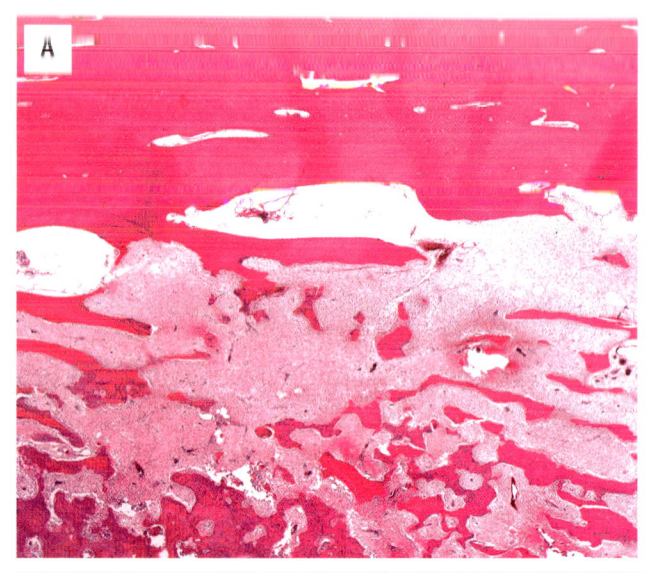

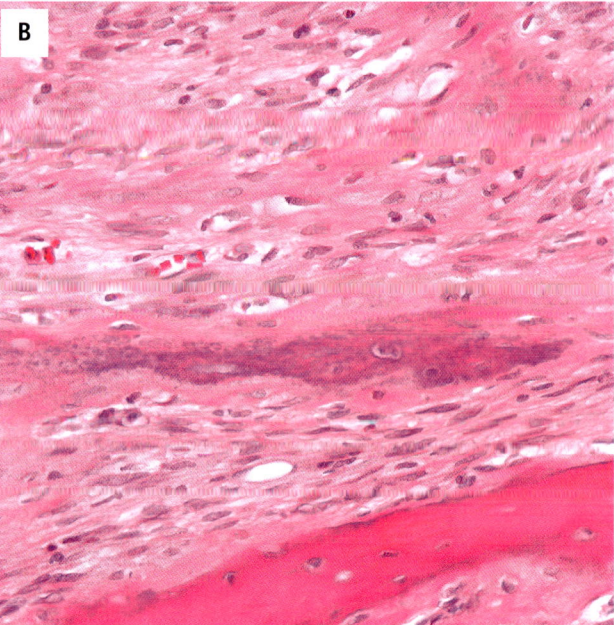

Ancillary Studies

Ancillary studies have a limited role in diagnosing osteosarcoma, as the tumor is recognized largely by its morphologic features. In problematic cases, where Ewing sarcoma/primitive neuroectodermal tumor, metastatic carcinoma, and melanoma, as well as lymphoma, are in the histologic differential diagnosis, however, immunohistochemical analysis, electron microscopic evaluation, and molecular studies may be helpful. Unlike those tumors, osteosarcoma cells have the features of mesenchymal cells with abundant dilated rough endoplasmic reticulum, and the matrix contains collagen fibers, which may show calcium hydroxyapatite crystal deposition.

Unfortunately, osteosarcoma has a broad immunoprofile that lacks diagnostic specificity. Vimentin, osteocalcin, osteonectin, S-100 protein, actin, smooth muscle actin, neuron-specific enolase, and CD99 are some of the antigens that are commonly expressed. Importantly, some tumors also stain with antibodies to keratin and epithelial membrane antigen. Also, it is worthy to note that osteosarcoma usually does not stain with antibodies to factor VIII, CD31, and leukocyte common antigen. Biopsies of osteosarcoma that lack neoplastic bone can be problematic because its immunophenotype can generate a broad list of differential diagnoses that includes Ewing sarcoma/primitive neuroectodermal tumor, metastatic carcinoma and melanoma, leiomyosarcoma, and malignant peripheral nerve sheath tumor. In this circumstance, ultrastructural analysis provides information regarding the phenotype of the tumor. Molecular analysis, such as karyotyping and fluorescent in situ hybridization (FISH), can be used in selective cases, especially when small-cell osteosarcoma and Ewing sarcoma are being considered. The presence of the t(11;22) translocation or one of its variants is diagnostic of Ewing sarcoma and is not present in any type of osteosarcoma.

Differential Diagnosis

The many varieties of osteosarcoma introduce diverse tumors in its histologic differential diagnosis. Osteosarcoma is distinguished from benign tumors and fibro-osseous lesions by virtue of its infiltrative growth pattern, with the tumor replacing the marrow space and surrounding preexisting bony trabeculae, which may also serve as scaffolding for the deposition of neoplastic bone. Telangiectatic osteosarcoma differs from aneurysmal bone cyst because it contains cytologically malignant cells within the cyst walls, whereas the cells in aneurysmal bone cyst are banal in appearance. Small-cell osteosarcoma is distinguished from Ewing sarcoma by the presence of neoplastic bone, and dilated rough endoplasmic reticulum by electron microscopy, and the absence of the t(11;22) translocation.

Stress fracture and accompanying callus can sometimes be confused with osteosarcoma because the reactive bone and cartilage is deposited around pre-existing bony trabeculae, which mimics an infiltrative pattern of growth. However, the cells in reactive tissues are banal, and osteoblastic rimming is usually present.

Prognosis and Treatment

The treatment of osteosarcoma is tailored to the age and medical condition of the patient and the location, size, grade, and stage of the tumor. Eradication of the primary tumor and the elimination of any metastases is the goal of therapy. The local disease is managed by limb salvage, wide surgical resection for appendicular tumors, and surgical excision in combination with radiation for tumors that are not resectable in their entirety with negative margins (such as those involving the spine or large areas of the pelvis). Preoperative adjuvant chemotherapy is now standard and is usually employed for all high-grade intramedullary and surface osteosarcomas, and continues after the surgical resection has been completed and wound healing has begun. The low-grade tumors such as intramedullary well-differentiated osteosarcoma and parosteal osteosarcoma are usually treated by surgery alone, because the risk of dissemination is very low.

A number of factors influence the prognosis of patients with osteosarcoma, including patient age, gender, tumor size, location, stage and response to chemotherapy,

---

OSTEOSARCOMA—FACT SHEET

Definition
- Malignant, bone-forming tumor in which the neoplastic cells form bone

Incidence and Location
- Account for approximately 20% of primary malignant bone tumors, representing the most common primary (nonhematopoietic) malignancy of the skeletal system
- Long bones commonly affected, although any bone may be involved

Morbidity and Mortality
- High-grade osteosarcoma is aggressive, and 80% of untreated patients die of disease

Sex, Race, and Age Distribution
- Slightly more common in male individuals
- Bimodal age distribution with 60% occurring before age 25, and 13% to 30% occurring in individuals older than 40 years

Clinical Features
- Localized pain with or without a mass
- Pathologic fracture
- Low-grade surface osteosarcoma may present as a painless mass

Radiologic Features
- Radiographic appearance is extremely variable
- High-grade osteosarcomas are usually large, poorly defined, destructive, mixed lytic, and blastic, and often have a soft tissue mass
- Low-grade osteosarcomas are sclerotic and frequently arise on the cortical surface

Prognosis and Treatment
- Combination of surgery and chemotherapy
- Prognosis is dependent of a variety of factors
- Survival rate for localized conventional high-grade osteosarcoma is 50% to 80%
- Low-grade surface osteosarcoma has a 90% to 100% survival rate

OSTEOSARCOMA—PATHOLOGIC FEATURES

Gross Findings

- Variable depending on the amount of bone and other components present
- Conventional osteosarcoma is large, destructive, necrotic, hemorrhagic, and cystic

Microscopic Findings

- Composed of malignant cells depositing coarse lace-like bone; other components include malignant-appearing cartilage and fibroblastic elements; the microscopic appearance is variable and depends on the type of osteosarcoma

Immunohistochemical Findings

- Variable and usually not helpful in diagnosing osteosarcoma

Differential Diagnosis

- Variety of benign and malignant bone tumors
- Fibrous dysplasia may mimic well-differentiated intramedullary osteosarcoma
- Osteoblastoma-like osteosarcoma can be confused with osteoblastoma
- Aneurysmal bone cyst needs to be distinguished from telangiectatic osteosarcoma
- Small-cell osteosarcoma can mimic Ewing sarcoma and other malignant small round cell tumors
- Stress fracture

---

multidrug resistance status, loss of heterozygosity of the retinoblastoma gene, and HER2/erbB-2 expression. Factors associated with a poor outcome are proximal location in an extremity or in the axial skeleton, large tumor size, detected metastases at the time of diagnosis, and poor response of the tumor to preoperative chemotherapy. Chemotherapy-induced tumor necrosis as measured histologically is believed to be one of the most important prognostic features for localized appendicular high-grade osteosarcoma (most of the tumors): good response is 90% or greater necrosis, and poor response is less than 90% necrosis. The histologic assessment of tumor necrosis requires extensive sampling and evaluation of the treated neoplasm.

Patients with a fatal outcome usually die from unrelenting disease progression (90%), whereas the remainder succumb to treatment-related complications (cardiomyopathy, pancytopenia, or the development of secondary malignancies).

Survival rates for relapse-free patients with localized conventional high-grade osteosarcoma of the extremity vary from 50% to 80%, which is a marked improvement from the pre-chemotherapy era when only 10% to 20% of patients were cured. Actuarial 10-year survival rates for patients with axial tumors are approximately 27% for patients with metastatic disease, 53% for patients with large tumors (greater than one-third length of involved bone), 47% for patients with tumors with a poor response, and 73% for patients with tumors with a good response. The chondroblastic variant of conventional osteosarcoma has been shown to be associated with a poor preoperative chemotherapy response and, in some studies, has a worse prognosis than other variants. Tumors with dismal prognoses include Paget osteosarcoma (approximately 10% survival rate) and radiation-induced osteosarcomas (long-term survival rate of 30–35%).

Patients with parosteal osteosarcoma have an excellent prognosis, with survival rates ranging from 91% to 100%. The outcome for periosteal osteosarcoma is not as good, with approximately a 75% survival rate, although a recent study utilizing chemotherapy achieved a 10-year metastasis-free survival rate of 100%. The prognosis of high-grade surface osteosarcoma is similar to that of conventional intramedullary osteosarcoma.

Intramedullary well-differentiated osteosarcoma is an indolent tumor and is associated with a metastatic rate of approximately 15%. Tumors that are associated with metastases have usually undergone dedifferentiation.

SUGGESTED READINGS

Bone Islands

1. Greenspan A, Steiner G, Knutzon R: Bone island (enostosis): clinical significance and radiologic and pathologic correlations. Skeletal Radiol 1991;20:85–90.
2. Hellemans J, Preobrazhenska O, Willaert A, et al: Loss-of-function mutations in LEMD3 result in osteopoikilosis, Buschke-Ollendorff syndrome and melorheostosis. Nat Genet 2004;36:1213–1218.
3. Park HS, Kim JR, Lee SY, et al: Symptomatic giant (10-cm) bone island of the tibia. Skeletal Radiol 2005;34:347–350.
4. White LM, Kandel R: Osteoid-producing tumors of bone. Semin Musculoskelet Radiol 2000;4:25–43.

Osteoma

1. Alexander AA, Patel AA, Odland R: Paranasal sinus osteomas and Gardner's syndrome. Ann Otol Rhinol Laryngol 2007;116:658–662.
2. Bertoni F, Unni KK, Beabout JW, et al: Parosteal osteoma of bones other than of the skull and face. Cancer 1995;75:2466–2473.
3. Sayan NB, Uçok C, Karasu HA, et al: Peripheral osteoma of the oral and maxilla facial region: a study of 35 new cases. J Oral Maxillofac Surg 2002;60:1299–1301.
4. Sundaram M, Falbo S, McDonald D, et al: Surface osteomas of the appendicular skeleton. AJR Am J Roentgenol 1996;167:1529–1533.

Osteoid Osteoma

1. Byers PD: Solitary benign osteoblastic lesions of bone. Osteoid osteoma and benign osteoblastoma. Cancer 1968;22:43–57.
2. Lee EH, Shafi M, Hui JH: Osteoid osteoma: a current review. J Pediatr Orthop 2006;26:695–700.
3. O'Connell Nanthakumar SS, Nielsen GP, et al: Osteoid osteoma: The uniquely innervated bone tumor. Mod Pathol 1998;11:175–180.
4. Rosenthal DI: Radiofrequency treatment. Orthop Clin North Am 2006;37:475–484.

Osteoblastoma

1. Bertoni F, Unni KK, Lucas DR, et al: Osteoblastoma with cartilaginous matrix. An unusual morphologic presentation in 18 cases. Am J Surg Pathol 1993;17:69–74.

2. Dorfman HD, Weiss SW: Borderline osteoblastic tumors: problems in the differential diagnosis of aggressive osteoblastoma and low-grade osteosarcoma. Semin Diagn Pathol 1984;1:215-234.
3. Kan P, Schmidt MH: Osteoid osteoma and osteoblastoma of the spine. Neurosurg Clin N Am 2008;19:65-70.
4. Lucas DR, Unni KK, McLeod RA, et al: Osteoblastoma: clinicopathologic study of 306 cases. Hum Pathol 1994;25:117-134.

Osteosarcoma

1. Campanacci M, Giunti A: Periosteal osteosarcoma. Review of 41 cases, 22 with long-term follow-up. Ital J Orthop Traumatol 1976;2:23-35.
2. Deyrup AT, Montag AG, Inwards CY, et al: Sarcomas arising in Paget disease of bone: a clinicopathologic analysis of 70 cases. Arch Pathol Lab Med 2007;131:942-946.
3. Kansara M, Thomas DM: Molecular pathogenesis of osteosarcoma. DNA Cell Biol 2007;26:1-18.
4. Mankin HJ, Hornicek FJ, Rosenberg AE, et al: Survival data for 648 patients with osteosarcoma treated at one institution. Clin Orthop Relat Res 2004;429:286-291.
5. Okada K, Frassica FJ, Sim FH, et al: Parosteal osteosarcoma. A clinicopathological study. J Bone Joint Surg Am 1994;76:366-378.
6. Raymond AK, Simms W, Ayala AG: Osteosarcoma. Specimen management following primary chemotherapy. Hematol Oncol Clin North Am 1995;9:841-867.
7. Unni KK, Dahlin DC: Osteosarcoma: pathology and classification. Semin Roentgenol 1989;24:143-152.

15 Cartilage-Forming Tumors
Andrew Horvai

BENIGN
- Osteochondroma
- Periosteal Chondroma
- Chondroblastoma
- Chondromyxoid Fibroma
- Enchondroma

MALIGNANT
- Conventional Chondrosarcoma

CHONDROSARCOMA VARIANTS
- Clear Cell Chondrosarcoma
- Dedifferentiated Chondrosarcoma
- Mesenchymal Chondrosarcoma

Cartilage is an extracellular matrix rich in aggrecan, a proteoglycan that serves to retain a large amount of water. The matrix consists of approximately 65% water, 15% proteoglycan, 15% collagen (predominantly type II), and less than 5% cells. Cartilage is unique in that it receives nutrients and oxygen by simple diffusion rather than a capillary network, thus limiting the extent of growth of native cartilaginous structures to, at most, 1 to 2 cm. The assessment of the presence of cartilage matrix is best made on hematoxylin-and-eosin (H&E)–stained sections where hyaline cartilage has a smooth basophilic quality with clearing around individual tumor cells (Figure 15-1). Fibrocartilage tends to be richer in collagen, imparting a pinker fibrillary quality on H&E. Some authors have used the term *chondroid* matrix interchangeably with *cartilage* matrix, but chondroid, strictly defined, is the putatively immature matrix with intermediate histologic features between osteoid and cartilage.

Chondrocytes are round with indistinct cytoplasmic borders and small, dark nuclei with perinuclear clearing (Figure 15-2). Benign chondrocytes typically demonstrate regular, albeit darkly staining, nuclei that are too small to make out nuclear detail at intermediate (200X) magnification. Nuclear atypia in chondrocytes is generally defined as the ability to detect nuclear detail, vesicular chromatin, or macronucleoli especially at intermediate magnification. Although cellularity and cytologic atypia are not typical of benign cartilage tumors, enchondromas located in the small bones of the hands and feet can show increased cellularity and slight atypia. Periosteal chondromas and enchondromas of Ollier disease also characteristically show more cytologic atypia and hypercellularity when compared with other benign cartilage tumors. Although binucleation of chondrocytes has historically been correlated with cytologic atypia, this finding is quite nonspecific for malignancy. Many benign tumors (e.g., synovial chondromatosis, periosteal chondroma, enchondroma) frequently demonstrate binucleated chondrocytes. Mature chondrocytes have little to no proliferative capacity, but it is thought that undifferentiated mesenchymal stem cells can undergo chondrocyte differentiation given the correct signals.

As for all bone tumors, evaluation of a cartilage lesion requires adequate correlation with radiographic findings. Oftentimes plain films (two views) of the lesion are sufficient to guide the diagnosis. Computed tomography (CT) and magnetic resonance imaging (MRI) are useful adjuncts to further evaluate the pattern of mineralization, cortical involvement, and presence or absence of soft tissue involvement.

BENIGN

OSTEOCHONDROMA

CLINICAL FEATURES

Osteochondroma is a benign cartilaginous tumor most commonly located in the distal femoral, proximal tibial, or proximal humeral metaphysis of adolescents and young adults (peak incidence in second decade of life). The lesion is more frequently seen in men than in women (2:1). Osteochondromas may present as a symptomatic, slow-growing mass as an incidental finding by radiography. It may be a mass lesion of long duration,

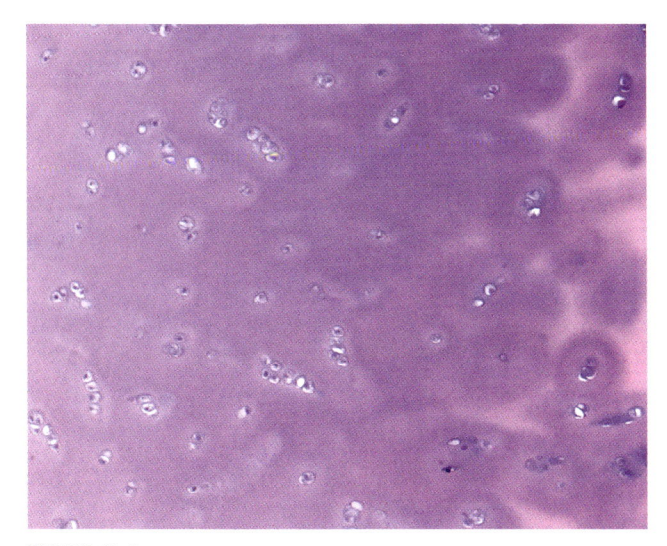

CHAPTER 15 Cartilage-Forming Tumors

FIGURE 15-1
Normal cartilage demonstrates the amphophilic quality of hyaline cartilage matrix and pericellular clearing around chondrocytes in lacunae.

with pain caused by compression of nearby structures or, less commonly, pain from fracture of the stalk. Recent and rapid growth of a preexisting osteochondroma, especially in a proximal skeletal location, can raise suspicion of malignant transformation.

The majority of patients will have a solitary osteochondroma. Less commonly, it occurs as multiple lesions in patients with the autosomal dominant disorder *multiple osteochondromas* or *hereditary multiple exostoses*. In almost 90% of multiple osteochondroma patients, germline mutations in the tumor-suppressor genes *EXT1* or *EXT2* are found. Moreover, *EXT1* appears to function as a classic tumor-suppressor gene in the cartilage cap of solitary nonhereditary osteochondromas. The rate of malignant transformation for solitary osteochondromas

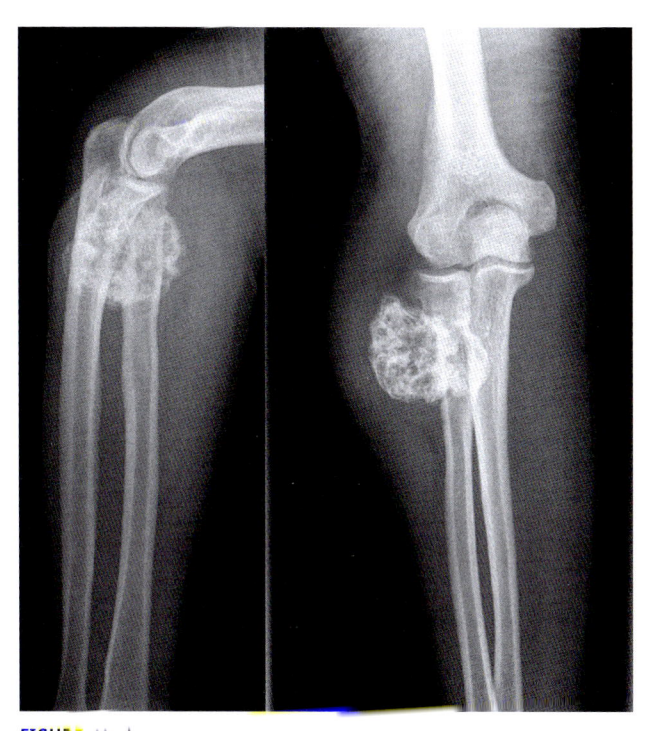

FIGURE 15-3
Osteochondroma is a relatively small, purely extraosseous tumor that is well circumscribed.

is approximately 1% to 3%. This is in contrast with patients with multiple osteochondromas who have greater rates of malignant transformation (between 5% and 25%). However, these data are from large referral centers and may overestimate the true incidence secondary to selection bias.

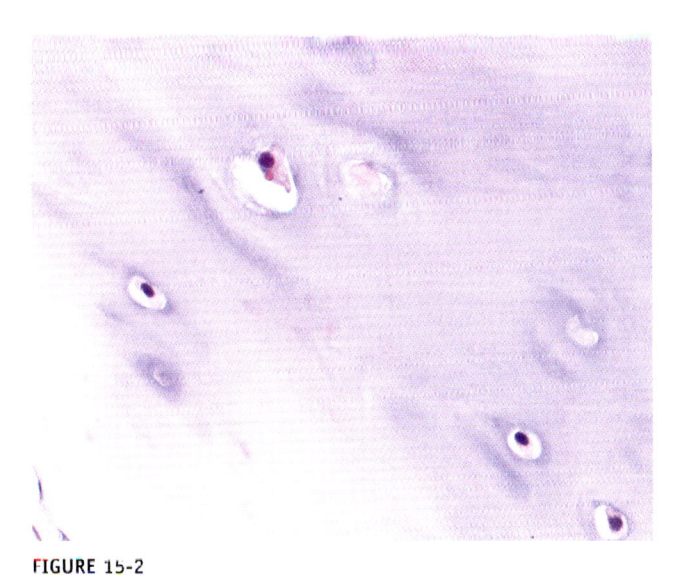

RADIOLOGIC FEATURES

An osteochondroma presents as an exophytic, sessile, or pedunculated projection of bone capped by cartilage (Figure 15-3). Importantly, the osteochondroma demonstrates both medullary and cortical components that are contiguous with the medulla and cortex, respectively, of the underlying native bone. Features that have been associated with malignant transformation include irregularity of the margin, inhomogeneous mineralization (Figure 15-4), and an associated soft tissue mass.

PATHOLOGIC FEATURES

GROSS FINDINGS

If resected intact, the lesion shows a thin (1-2 cm), pale blue, smooth cartilage cap overlying cortical and medullary bone (Figure 15-5). A pedunculated osteochondroma demonstrates a prominent stalk, whereas

FIGURE 15-2
High power view of benign chondrocytes has small, dark nuclei with smooth contours.

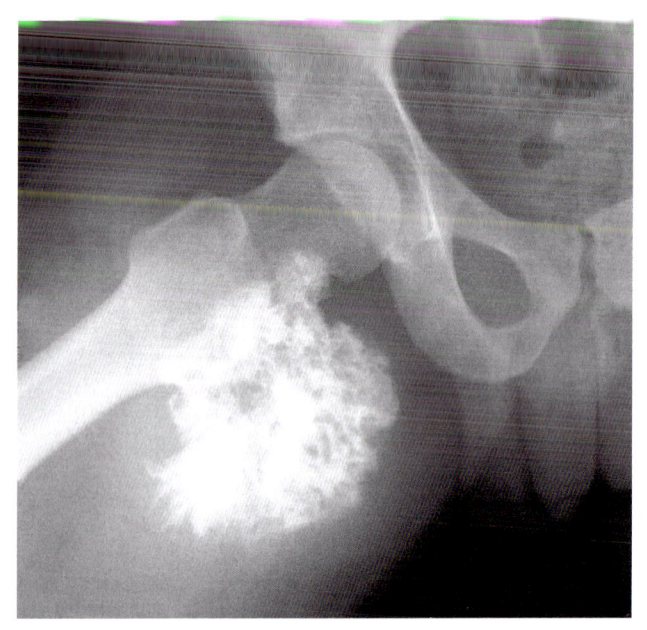

FIGURE 15-4
Malignancy in osteochondroma may be suggested by large size, irregular mineralization, and poor circumscription.

FIGURE 15-6
Low-power view of osteochondroma shows a thin cartilage cap and an orderly arrangement of chondrocytes undergoing endochondral ossification to create trabecular bone separated by marrow fat.

the sessile form shows a broad attachment to underlying normal bone.

MICROSCOPIC FINDINGS

In general, osteochondroma mimics an epiphyseal growth plate beginning with a thin (usually < 1 cm) cartilaginous cap superficially, a zone of endochondral ossification followed by regular trabecular bone surrounded by fatty, hematopoietic marrow as one scans proximally (Figure 15-6). The chondrocytes may be somewhat haphazard superficially but are arranged in orderly columnar growth at the ossification zone. Scattered zones of residual cartilage may be seen among the trabeculae. Occasionally, degenerative change and calcification are seen in the cartilage cap.

DIFFERENTIAL DIAGNOSIS

Rarely, secondary chondrosarcoma can arise from osteochondroma. The distinction between these entities requires clinical, radiographic, and pathologic correlation. Clinical or radiographic evidence of recent growth, pain, involvement of the proximal skeleton, irregular mineralization, or soft tissue destructive growth are concerning features. The thickness of the cartilage cap (normally < 1 cm) has long been reported as an indicator of potential malignancy. However, in skeletally immature individuals, a cartilage cap of up to 2 cm may be identified. One of the best criterion for confirming a diagnosis of malignancy is histologic evidence of permeative growth pattern into surrounding soft tissue. Other helpful microscopic features that suggest malignant change include prominent myxoid cystic change in the matrix, increased cellularity, and loss of the normal columnar arrangement of chondrocytes at the ossification zone.

Parosteal osteosarcoma may also demonstrate a superficial cap of cartilage with underlying bone. However, radiographically and grossly, the bone is not contiguous with the medullary cavity of the native bone. Most importantly, the intertrabecular space within parosteal osteosarcoma is occupied by a spindle cell proliferation with minimal nuclear atypia rather than fat and hematopoietic marrow, as is typically seen in osteochondroma.

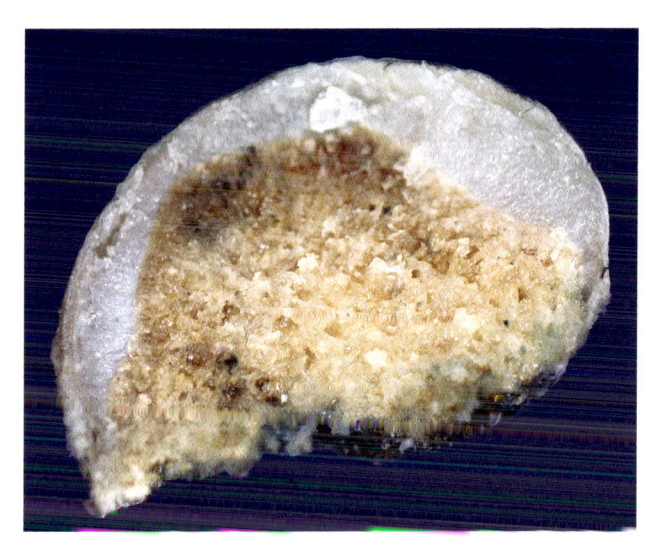

FIGURE 15-5
Gross photograph of osteochondroma demonstrates a thin, pale blue cartilage cap covering cancellous bone. In sessile examples, such as this, the attachment to the cortex (base) is relatively broad.

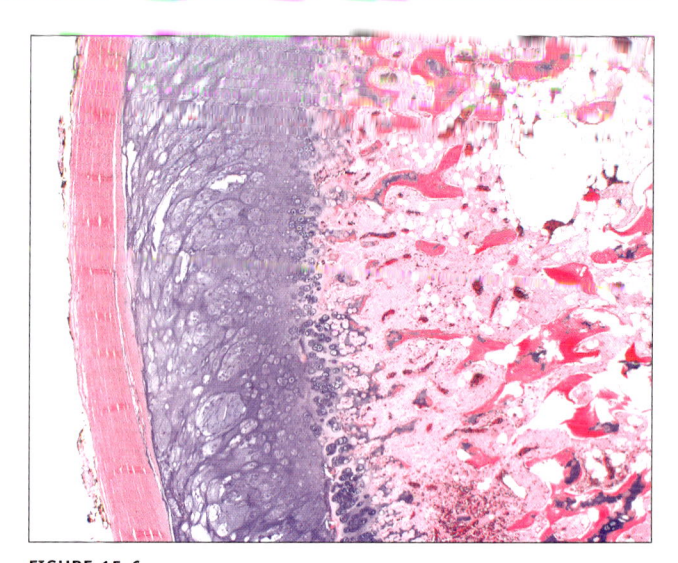

OSTEOCHONDROMA—FACT SHEET

Definition
- Benign, exophytic tumor of cartilage and bone that recapitulates a growth plate

Incidence and Location
- Syndromic form (multiple osteochondromas) estimated at 1 in 50,000
- Sporadic form (solitary) six times more common than those in the setting of multiple osteochondromas
- Most common in metaphysis of long bones, especially distal femur, proximal tibia, and proximal humerus
- Pelvic bones and scapula are uncommon sites

Sex, Race, and Age Distribution
- More common in male than female sex (2:1); peak in second decade of life

Clinical Features
- Asymptomatic or painless mass of long duration
- May be found incidentally on imaging for unrelated complaints
- Pain may be a feature because of local effects or fracture of lesion

Prognosis and Treatment
- Asymptomatic lesions can be observed
- Surgical excision is curative for symptomatic lesions
- Malignant transformation < 1% (sporadic form) and 5% to 25% (multiple osteochondroma syndrome)

OSTEOCHONDROMA—PATHOLOGIC FEATURES

Gross Findings
- Thin (< 2 cm), pale blue, firm cartilage cap overlying a stalk composed of hard bone
- Cut surface reveals medullary and cortical bone contiguous with underlying native bone

Microscopic Findings
- Cartilage cap undergoing endochondral ossification with orderly arrangement of chondrocytes
- Cancellous bone beneath the cartilage cap
- Intertrabecular spaces filled by fat and hematopoietic marrow
- Occasionally, degenerative changes in cartilage cap

Differential Diagnosis
- Chondrosarcoma arising in osteochondroma
- Parosteal osteosarcoma
- Bizarre parosteal osteochondromatous proliferation (Nora's lesion)

Bizarre parosteal osteochondromatous proliferation (Nora's lesion) differs clinically in the age of presentation (adults) and location (hands). Although the lesion is composed of a mixture of bone and cartilage, it is not contiguous with the underlying medullary cavity, nor does it show the organization of a growth plate.

PROGNOSIS AND TREATMENT

Surgical excision should be curative treatment for osteochondromas. Wide surgical margins are indicated when the tumor has undergone malignant transformation into chondrosarcoma.

PERIOSTEAL CHONDROMA

CLINICAL FEATURES

Periosteal chondroma is a benign cartilage tumor that grows in the periosteal region, frequently eroding the underlying cortex. These tumors present in the second and third decades of life with a male predilection (2:1), are usually asymptomatic, and are found incidentally on radiographs obtained for other reasons. However, a painful, palpable mass involving the femur or humerus (metaphysis or diaphysis) may bring the lesion to clinical attention.

RADIOGRAPHIC FEATURES

Periosteal chondromas are small (1-3 cm), infrequently calcified masses attached to the cortex with cortical erosion (saucerization) and cortical sclerosis underlying the base of the lesion. Periosteal reaction with peripheral buttressing may be seen.

PATHOLOGIC FEATURES

GROSS FINDINGS

The mass is firm, translucent, and pale blue, indicative of hyaline cartilage. The interface between the tumor and the underlying cortex is sharp with a zone of sclerotic bone. The medullary cavity is not involved.

MICROSCOPIC FINDINGS

The tumor consists of lobules of hyaline cartilage of moderate-to-high cellularity. The tumor does not permeate Haversian canals or the medulla. Binucleated chondrocytes are common (Figure 15-7), and rare examples can be hypercellular.

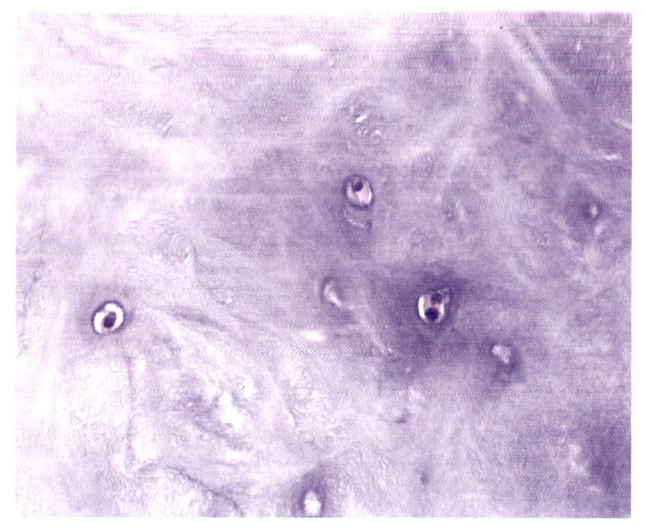

FIGURE 15-7
Periosteal chondroma can demonstrate binucleated chondrocytes, but chondrocytes do not have increased nuclear size, and nuclear detail is visible only at high power.

PERIOSTEAL CHONDROMA—PATHOLOGIC FEATURES

Gross Findings
- Small (1-4 cm), pale blue, firm cartilage attached to cortical surface
- Sclerotic interface with cortex, no medullary involvement

Microscopic Findings
- Lobular cartilage of moderate cellularity, variable nuclear atypia

Differential Diagnosis
- Synovial chondromatosis
- Periosteal chondrosarcoma
- Periosteal osteosarcoma

DIFFERENTIAL DIAGNOSIS

Synovial chondromatosis may be a consideration if the lesion is near a joint but can be distinguished radiographically by the presence of a solitary mass attached to the cortex with cortical sclerosis. Periosteal (juxtacortical) chondrosarcoma and periosteal osteosarcoma are tumors with some clinical and morphologic overlap. Like periosteal chondroma, periosteal chondrosarcomas arise from the surface of bone and may erode the cortex but do not involve the medulla. However, these tumors are typically large (>5 cm) with poorly defined margins. Periosteal osteosarcoma is also in the differential diagnosis because it is a surface lesion that contains cartilage. However, it also contains osteoid production typically found in the center of the cartilage lobules that are surrounded by a proliferation of atypical spindle cells.

PROGNOSIS AND TREATMENT

Surgical removal is the treatment of choice. Local recurrence is rare.

PERIOSTEAL CHONDROMA—FACT SHEET

Definition
- Benign tumor of cartilage that involves the surface of the bone

Incidence and Location
- Most common in metaphysis and diaphysis of long bones, especially femur and humerus

Sex, Race, and Age Distribution
- More common in male than female sex (2:1); peak in second and third decades of life

Clinical Features
- Painless mass present for years
- May be found incidentally on imaging for unrelated complaints

Prognosis and Treatment
- Asymptomatic lesions can be observed
- Surgical excision or curettage is curative for symptomatic lesions

CHONDROBLASTOMA

CLINICAL FEATURES

Chondroblastoma is a benign chondroid-producing tumor that affects the epiphyses of adolescents and young adults with a slight male predominance (3:2). The most common complaint is a several months to years history of pain involving a joint that may be accompanied by gait abnormality, swelling, or decreased mobility. Recurrence in chondroblastoma has been estimated at 15% for long bones. It should be noted that although most chondroblastomas occur in the epiphyses of long bones, the temporal bone and calcaneus are also common sites (5–10% of cases), and recurrence risk is generally greater in these "unusual" sites. Malignant transformation is the subject of case reports only.

RADIOGRAPHIC FEATURES

The lesion is sharply marginated, predominantly lytic, and rimmed by sclerotic bone. In long bones, it involves the epiphysis but may cross the physis into the metaphysis. Periosteal reaction is uncommon. Matrix calcifications within the tumor may be seen in 25% of cases (Figure 15-8).

PATHOLOGIC FEATURES

GROSS FINDINGS

Because these lesions are most often curetted, the material usually consists of fragmented, gray–pink firm tissue notably without the pale blue material of hyaline cartilage. Gritty calcifications and hemorrhage may be present. If resected, the tumor is usually smaller than 5 cm, sharply marginated from the surrounding bone, and often encapsulated with a thin rim of sclerotic bone.

MICROSCOPIC FINDINGS

The matrix of chondroblastoma has an amphophilic or eosinophilic quality that has been described as fibrochondroid (Figure 15-9). True hyaline cartilage is almost never present. Approximately 35% of chondroblastomas demonstrate delicate stippled calcifications that surround individual tumor cells in the so-called *chicken wire* pattern, although denser zones of calcification may be present (Figure 15-10). The cellular component consists of mononuclear cells and multinucleated giant cells. The mononuclear cells are predominantly ovoid with pale eosinophilic cytoplasm, relatively well-defined plasma membranes, and eccentric nuclei with nuclear grooves (Figure 15-11). Mitotic activity is often present but low. The osteoclast-like giant cells are irregularly scattered and demonstrate fewer than 10 nuclei with fine chromatin and prominent nucleoli. It is important to recognize that chondroblastoma can show varying degrees of the *typical* histologic findings, and only a minority of cases demonstrate all of the characteristic features (fibrochondroid matrix, chicken wire calcifications, and nuclear grooves). Secondary aneurysmal bone cyst is a common feature of chondroblastoma (30% of cases) and can, in fact, predominate on small biopsies that do not adequately sample the epiphyseal component of a chondroblastoma. Some chondroblastomas, particularly those located in

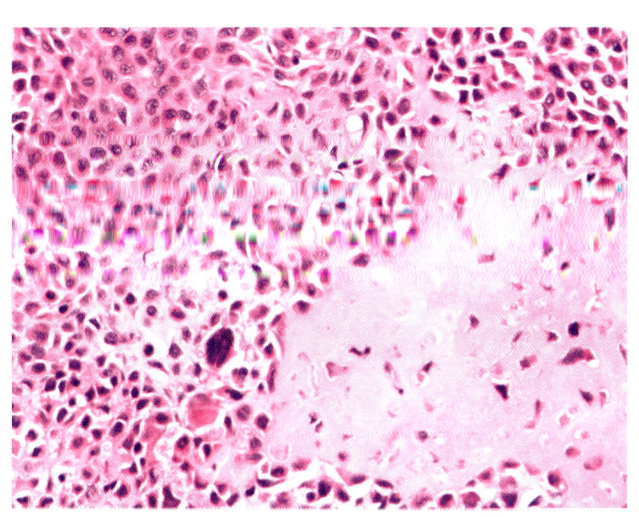

FIGURE 15-9
The cartilage matrix in chondroblastoma typically stains pink.

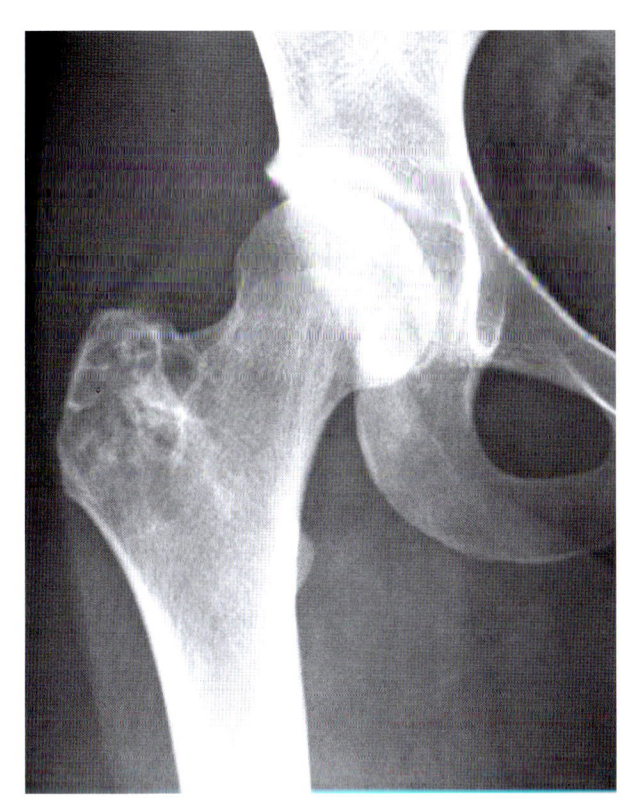

FIGURE 15-8
Chondroblastoma typically affects the epiphysis or, as in this case, the apophysis (greater trochanter of the femur). The lesion is well circumscribed, predominantly lytic, but with matrix calcifications.

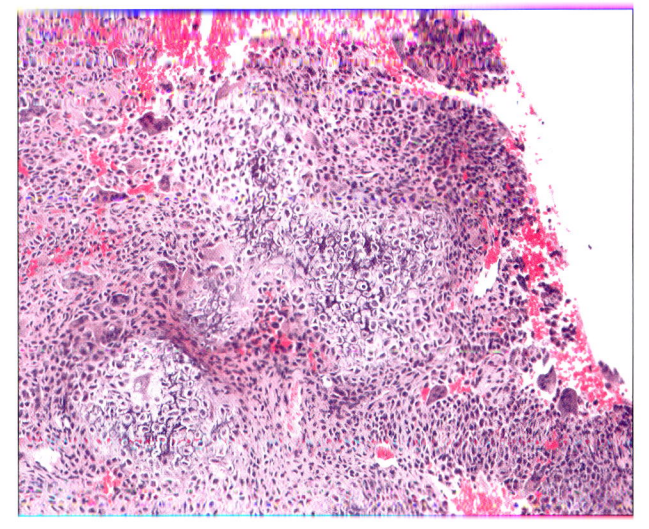

FIGURE 15-10
Chondroblastoma demonstrates sheets of round to ovoid cells admixed with osteoclast-like giant cells. The delicate pericellular calcification of the matrix has been described as *chicken wire*.

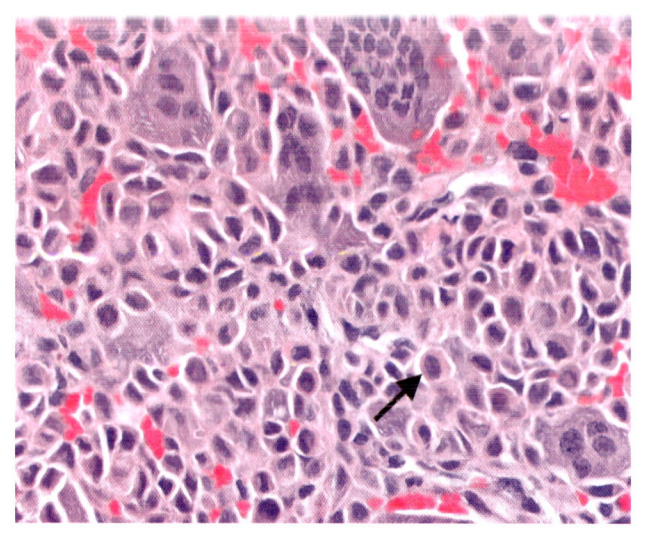

FIGURE 15-11
The mononuclear cells in chondroblastoma show eccentric, round to ovoid nuclei with occasional nuclear grooves *(arrow)*.

CHONDROBLASTOMA—FACT SHEET

Definition
▸▸ Benign, amphophilic or eosinophilic matrix-producing tumor that commonly involves the ends of long bones

Incidence and Location
▸▸ Rare (< 1% of bone tumors)
▸▸ Most common in epiphysis of long bones, rarely in flat bones of cranium or pelvis

Sex, Race, and Age Distribution
▸▸ More common in male than female sex (3:2); peak in second decade of life

Clinical Features
▸▸ Pain common, present for months to years, associated with limp

Prognosis and Treatment
▸▸ Curettage and bone graft are curative in almost all cases with rare (< 15%) recurrence

---

the craniofacial bones, contain plump epithelioid stromal cells with abundant eosinophilic cytoplasm with or without hemosiderin deposition. Immunohistochemistry for S-100 is positive in about 75% of chondroblastomas. Whether chondroblastoma is truly a chondrogenic neoplasm has been challenged using biochemical studies of the matrix proteins. Furthermore, histologically, chondroblastoma almost never demonstrates conventional hyaline cartilage but rather a fibrochondroid matrix.

DIFFERENTIAL DIAGNOSIS

The epiphyseal location and relative circumscription combined with the presence of osteoclast-type giant cells raises the possibility of giant cell tumor of bone. Clinically, giant cell tumor is unusual in skeletally immature individuals, and although both lesions can be circumscribed, the presence of a sclerotic rim radiographically points to chondroblastoma. Microscopically, the presence of fibrochondroid matrix, chicken wire calcifications, smaller, unevenly distributed giant cells, and mononuclear cells with nuclear grooves support chondroblastoma.

Aneurysmal bone cyst may also contain abundant osteoclast-like giant cells and basophilic calcifications. Primary aneurysmal bone cyst, however, typically does not involve the epiphysis and demonstrates collagenous, fibrous septae with hemosiderin and lacks the ovoid cells with nuclear grooves. As mentioned earlier, aneurysmal bone cyst can be seen as a secondary process in chondroblastoma. At times, secondary aneurysmal bone cyst is the predominate finding and, therefore, overshadows an underlying chondroblastoma. Care should be taken to exclude the possibility of chondroblastoma when an aneurysmal bone cyst is found centered in the epiphysis.

The matrix of chondromyxoid fibroma may sometimes resemble chondroblastoma, and both lesions can contain numerous osteoclast-like giant cells. However, chondromyxoid fibroma is almost never epiphyseal and demonstrates more prominent lobular growth pattern. The tumor cells of chondromyxoid fibroma grow in a sieve-like pattern, have stellate cytoplasm, and lack nuclear grooves.

Clear cell chondrosarcoma may enter the radiologic differential diagnosis of an epiphyseal lesion with calcifications and relative circumscription. However, the histologic picture of clear cell chondrosarcoma (described later) of large, clear cells with well-defined cytoplasmic borders, prominent macronucleoli, and delicate osteoid matrix distinguishes this tumor from chondroblastoma.

CHONDROBLASTOMA—PATHOLOGIC FEATURES

Gross Findings
▸▸ Curettage fragments of tan-pink firm tissue with calcifications without typical pale blue hyaline cartilage

Microscopic Findings
▸▸ Amphophilic or eosinophilic fibrochondroid matrix; no mature hyaline cartilage
▸▸ Chicken wire calcifications
▸▸ Ovoid to round, mononuclear cells with nuclear grooves
▸▸ Irregularly distributed osteoclast-like giant cells
▸▸ Aneurysmal bone cyst features may be secondary

Differential Diagnosis
▸▸ Giant cell tumor
▸▸ Aneurysmal bone cyst
▸▸ Chondromyxoid fibroma

CHONDROMYXOID FIBROMA

CLINICAL FEATURES

Chondromyxoid fibroma is a rare, benign, intramedullary tumor with a peak in the second and third decades of life, but with a wide age range. Pain is common, but usually mild and of long duration. Swelling and tenderness are less common features, typically seen if the small bones of the distal extremities are affected. The proximal tibia is the most common site, followed by the distal femur. However, the distribution is widespread including the pelvis, cranium, and the bones of the feet.

RADIOGRAPHIC FEATURES

Chondromyxoid fibroma lesions are typically eccentrically located in the metaphysis, predominantly lucent, and only rarely contain matrix calcification. Typical cases show sclerotic margins with scalloping (Figure 15-12). Especially in small tubular bones, soft tissue extension may be present, but the periosteum is intact.

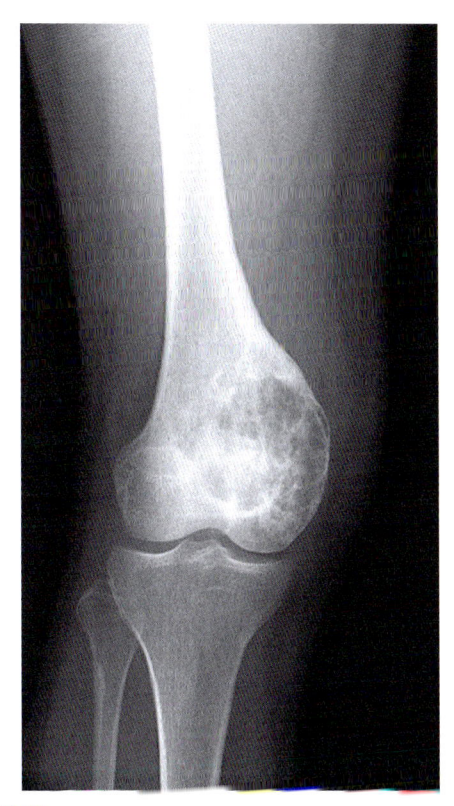

FIGURE 15-12
Chondromyxoid fibroma is marginated, lytic, and trabeculated.

PATHOLOGIC FEATURES

GROSS FINDINGS

In curettage specimens, chondromyxoid fibroma is composed of pale blue cartilage that may be softer than typical hyaline cartilage but not the viscous liquid of myxoid areas in chondrosarcoma. In a resection specimen, the tumor demonstrates lobulated architecture with a rim of sclerotic bone.

MICROSCOPIC FINDINGS

Chondromyxoid fibromas grow in a micro-lobular or macro-lobular pattern (Figure 15-13), with a tendency for increased cellularity at the periphery of individual lobules

---

CHONDROMYXOID FIBROMA—FACT SHEET

Definition
- Benign neoplasm composed of nodules with myxoid matrix and spindled to stellate spindle cells

Incidence and Location
- Rare (< 1% of bone tumors); proximal tibia, distal femur, and bones of foot are common locations

Sex, Race, and Age Distribution
- Male sex predominance (2:1); wide age range with peak in second and third decades of life

Clinical Features
- Pain is common; a mass may be present if small bones are involved

Prognosis and Treatment
- Curettage and bone grafting is curative in most cases with rare recurrences (15%)

CHONDROMYXOID FIBROMA—PATHOLOGIC FEATURES

Gross Findings
- Pale blue, matrix softer than hyaline cartilage but not liquid
- Well marginated with sclerotic rim

Microscopic Findings
- Lobular growth pattern with increased cells and giant cells at periphery of lobules
- Tumor cells within lobules are spindled to stellate with long cytoplasmic processes
- Occasional cells with larger, smaller hyperchromatic nuclei but preserved nuclear-to-cytoplasmic ratio

Differential Diagnosis
- Chondroblastoma
- Enchondroma
- Chondroblastic osteosarcoma
- Chondrosarcoma

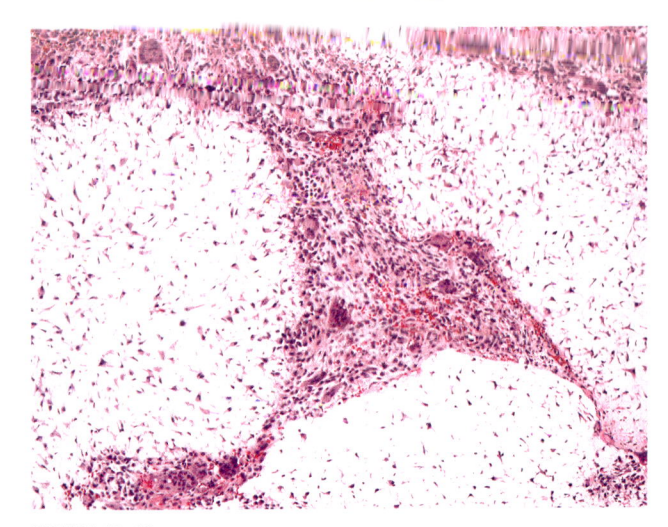

FIGURE 15-13
At low power, chondromyxoid fibroma has a lobulated growth pattern.

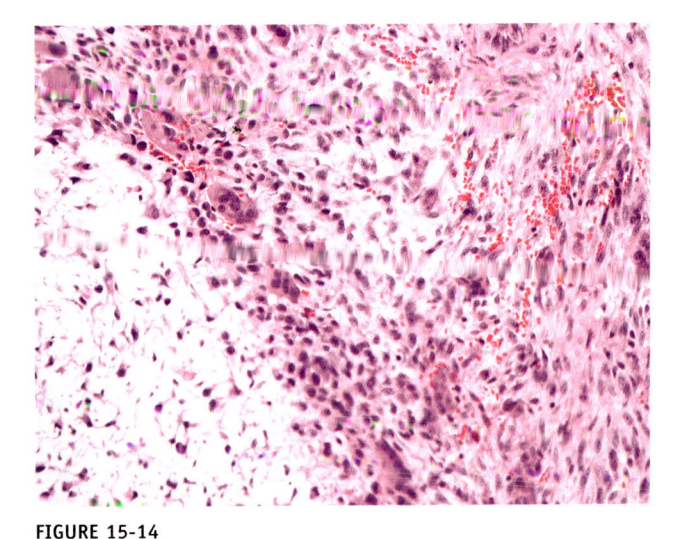

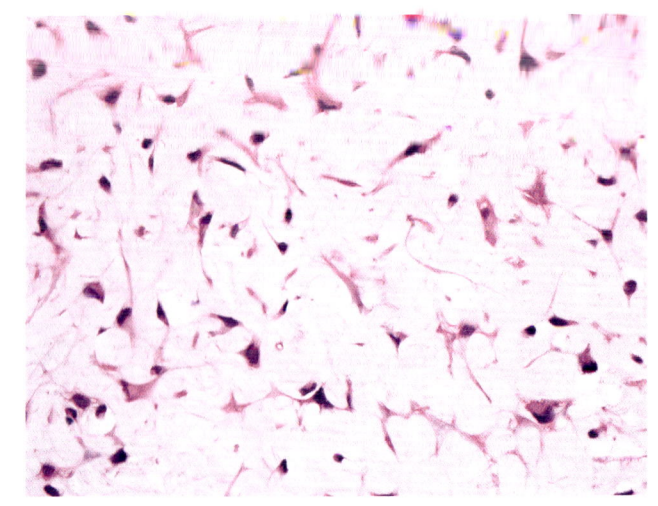

FIGURE 15-15
The cells of chondromyxoid fibroma within the lobules have spindled to stellate cytoplasm and small round to polygonal nuclei with fine chromatin and eosinophilic cytoplasmic extensions.

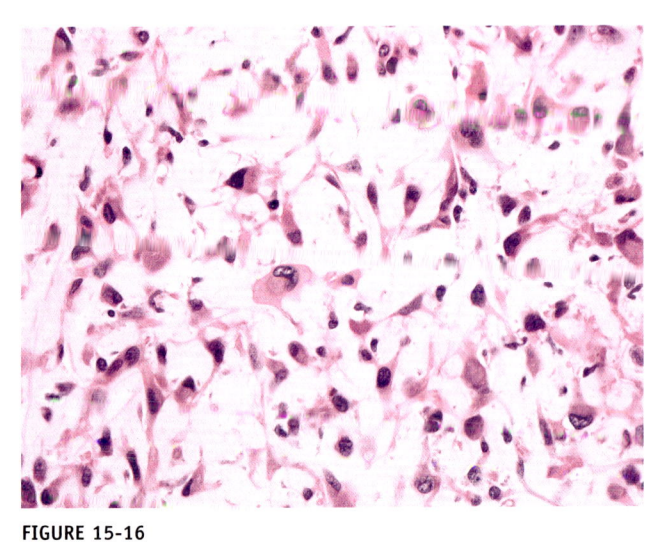

FIGURE 15-14
Lobules of chondromyxoid fibroma have increased cellularity at the periphery and loose myxoid stroma centrally.

FIGURE 15-16
Occasional cells may show nuclear atypia with larger nuclei with smudgy chromatin. Cytoplasm is abundant so that the nuclear-to-cytoplasmic ratio is not increased.

(Figure 15-14). The matrix is myxoid, lacking true hyaline cartilage in most cases. The tumor cells consist of small, delicate spindled to stellate cells with long processes that appear to interconnect, forming a reticular pattern (Figure 15-15). Occasional cells with larger, hyperchromatic, though smudgy, nuclei may be seen (so-called *pseudomalignant* cells because the nuclear/cytoplasmic ratio is preserved) (Figure 15-16). Osteoclast-like giant cells may be present at the periphery of lobules. Necrosis and prominent mitotic activity are not typically observed in chondromyxoid fibroma.

DIFFERENTIAL DIAGNOSIS

Chondromyxoid fibroma can, focally, demonstrate ovoid to round cells with similar cytomorphology to chondroblastoma. However, chondroblastoma is almost exclusively an epiphyseal lesion and does not demonstrate the lobular growth pattern with increased cellularity at the periphery of lobules. Enchondroma can be excluded by the presence of true hyaline cartilage and predominantly round rather than stellate cells. Chondroblastic osteosarcoma is an important consideration because of overlap in both the quality of the matrix and cytomorphology. However, chondroblastic osteosarcoma will demonstrate, at least focally, hyaline cartilage, as well as cells with dense, sheet-like growth associated with osteoid (Figure 15-17) and atypical spindle cells. Furthermore, osteosarcoma usually has a malignant radiographic appearance, whereas chondromyxoid fibroma looks benign. Finally, chondrosarcoma demonstrates a permeative pattern, both radiographically and

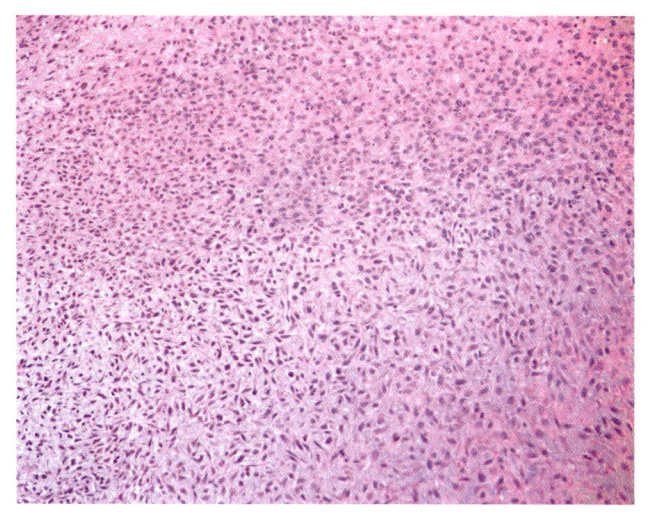

CHAPTER 15 Cartilage-Forming Tumors

FIGURE 15-17
Chondroblastic osteosarcoma may demonstrate stellate cells in a myxoid stroma similar to chondromyxoid fibroma. However, the sheet-like growth, absence of lobular architecture, and diffuse cytologic atypia are features of osteosarcoma.

microscopically, hyaline cartilage, and pools of cystic spaces with viscous liquid myxoid matrix.

ENCHONDROMA

CLINICAL FEATURES

Enchondroma, or simply *chondroma*, is the prototypical benign intraosseous tumor of hyaline cartilage. These tumors, by definition, are benign, and other than rare case reports, do not recur. They are often discovered incidentally because they are usually painless. Consequently, the exact incidence of enchondromas in the general population is not known. Pain, when present, may be related to pathologic fracture and is more common in small tubular bones of the hands and feet. Enchondromas demonstrate a wide age range (most common in third to fourth decades of life) and approximately equal sex distribution.

A small percentage of patients with enchondroma will have multiple tumors. Maffucci and Ollier syndromes are both sporadic and present with multiple enchondromas of the metaphyseal regions of tubular, and less commonly, flat bones. Maffucci differs from Ollier in the presence of cavernous hemangiomas in the former. Although various incidences have been reported for progression to chondrosarcoma for the two syndromes, the range of lifetime risk in Ollier syndrome is slightly greater, approaching 30% to 50%. Regardless of the exact lifetime risk, patients with these syndromes need to be carefully managed clinically and radiographically.

RADIOGRAPHIC FEATURES

Typically, enchondroma is a centrally placed intramedullary lesion with rarification and variable amounts of mineralization. Perhaps the most classic finding on plain films of enchondromas, and a prime example of radiopathologic correlation, is the presence of so-called *ring* calcifications. Although not invariably present, the radiographic finding of such rings correlates with the peripheral ossification and subsequent mineralization of individual lobules of cartilage as seen histologically (Figure 15-18). Expansile growth, but with an intact cortex and sclerotic rim, is typical. Transcortical spread, soft tissue extension, or permeative growth is generally incompatible with the diagnosis of enchondroma.

PATHOLOGIC FEATURES

GROSS FINDINGS

Curettage specimens will demonstrate firm to rubbery pale blue translucent hyaline cartilage without gross hemorrhage or necrosis. Small spicules of white-tan hard bone may represent endochondral ossification. In a resection specimen, a rim of sclerotic bone will surround the tumor.

MICROSCOPIC FINDINGS

Pale blue hyaline cartilage will dominate the histologic picture. The interface between the cartilage and the surrounding bone is sharp (Figure 15-19), and tight permeation of trabeculae or invasion within the Haversian canals is absent. Chondrocytes in lacunae are haphazardly scattered without obvious columnar or nested distribution. Individual chondrocytes are round with pale-eosinophilic cytoplasm and small, central dark nuclei (Figure 15-20). Nuclear detail is difficult to discern except at high magnification (400X) (Figure 15-21). Mitotic activity is almost invariably absent. Although cellularity and cytologic atypia are not features of enchondroma, some sites, particularly the small bones of the hands and feet, can show increased cellularity and slight atypia (Figure 15-22). Enchondromas of Ollier disease also characteristically show more cytologic atypia and hypercellular areas with clustering, but these are usually focal findings.

DIFFERENTIAL DIAGNOSIS

A cartilage tumor with increased cellularity and atypia in the long bones raises the possibility of a low-grade chondrosarcoma. Various guidelines, based on histology

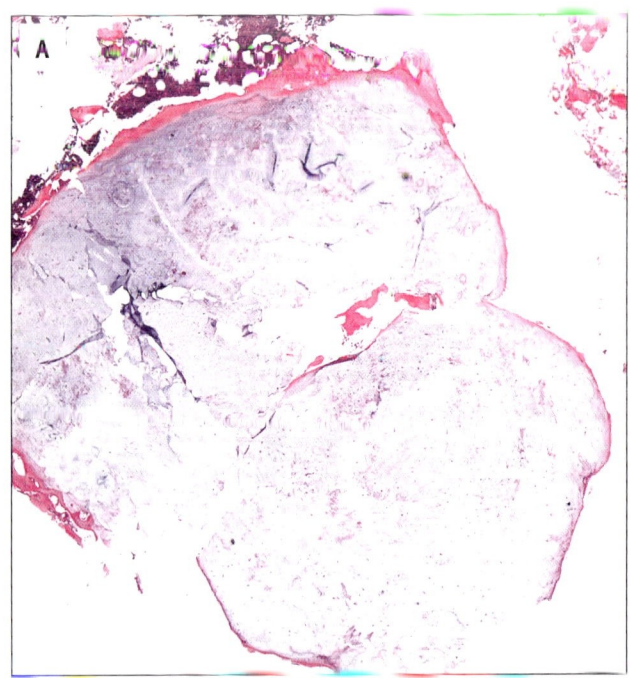

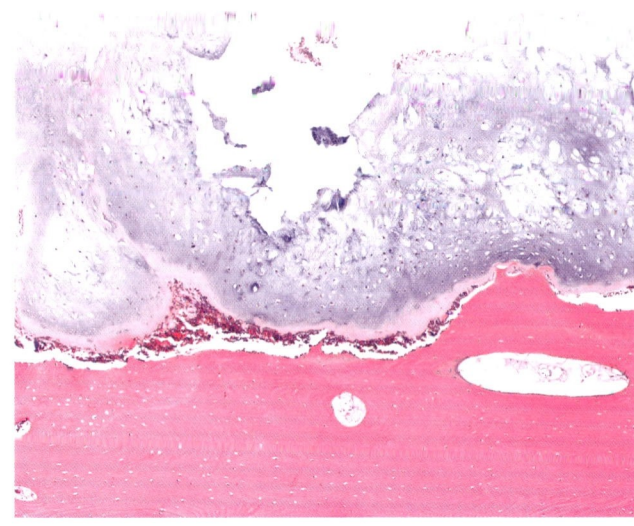

FIGURE 15-19
The border of an enchondroma with the surrounding cortex is sharp.

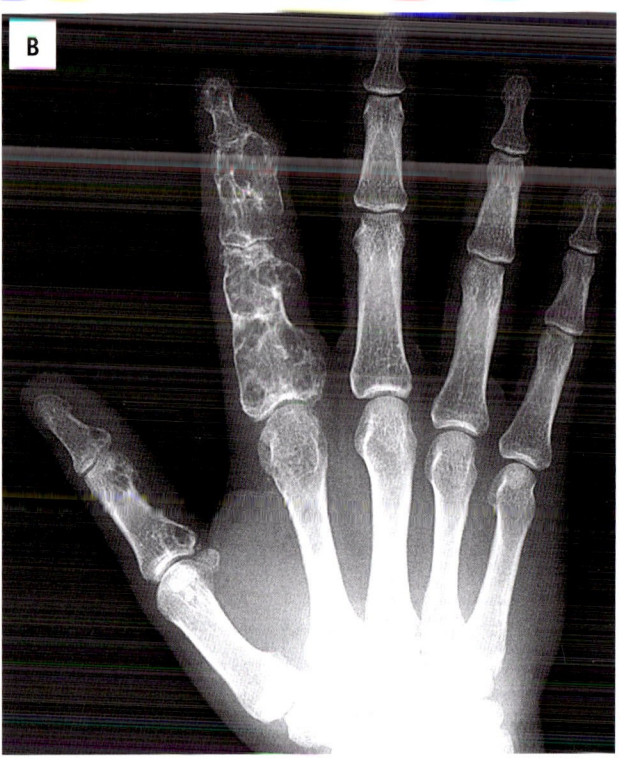

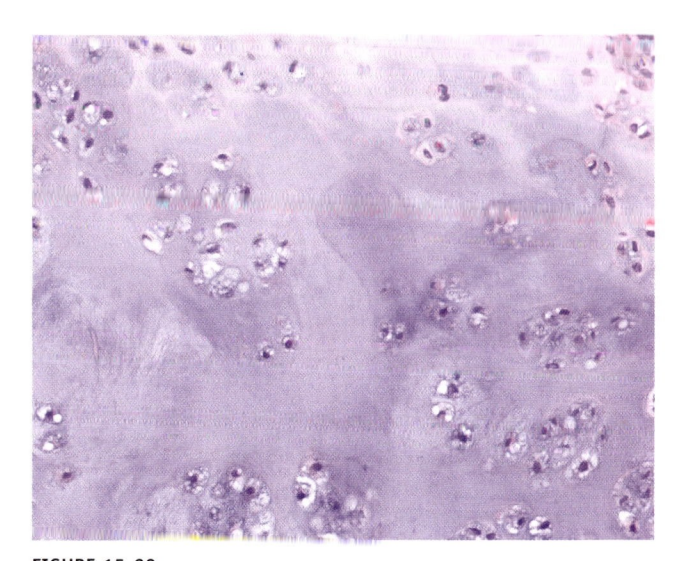

FIGURE 15-20
Enchondromas may demonstrate increased cellularity, but nuclear detail is not visible at intermediate power (200X).

FIGURE 15-18
A, Lobules of cartilage can undergo peripheral endochondral ossification. B, Calcification of the osteoid correlates with the characteristic *ring* calcifications of enchondromas observed on plain films.

or radiology, have been proposed to distinguish these entities. Radiographically, the features that have been most reproducibly associated with chondrosarcoma are pathologic fracture, soft tissue mass, periosteal reaction, and cortical disruption or thickening. The presence of permeation of viable, lamellar bone by the cartilage tumor represents the best histologic criterion to separate enchondroma from grade 1 chondrosarcoma. More specifically, enchondroma demonstrates islands of cartilage separated by marrow or endochondral ossification that conforms to the cartilage (Figure 15-23A). Conversely, chondrosarcoma circumferentially entraps the preexisting lamellar bone (see Figure 15-23B) or *seeps* through Haversian canals. In fragmented curettage specimens and especially in small needle biopsies, architecture is difficult to discern. The histology is sufficient only to recognize the presence of a cartilage-forming tumor. Some tumors contain a less overt degree of hypercellularity and cytologic atypia than grade 1 chondrosarcoma in combination with borderline radiographic features of

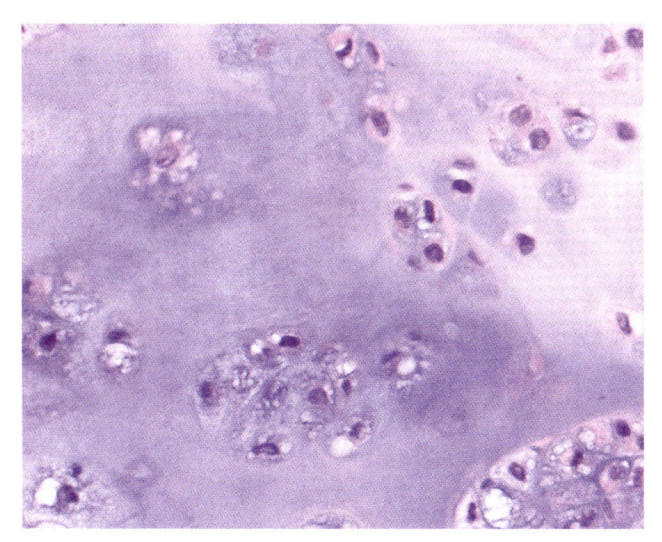

CHAPTER 15 Cartilage-Forming Tumors

FIGURE 15-21
Enchondroma at high magnification (400X). Nuclear detail is visible, but chondrocytes demonstrate small, usually dark nuclei with sharp nuclear contours and ample cytoplasm.

malignancy. These have been called *aggressive* or *active enchondromas*. The distinction between enchondroma and chondrosarcoma of the small bones of the hands and feet is further discussed later in the Chondrosarcoma section.

ANCILLARY STUDIES

The diagnostic utility of molecular techniques in separating enchondroma from chondrosarcoma is evolving. Karyotypic analysis has demonstrated that enchondromas and borderline lesions are karyotypically normal in contrast with grade 1 chondrosarcomas, which harbor both numeric and structural aberrations. In contrast, recent work by using more sensitive comparative genomic hybridization suggests similar numbers of aberrations (an average of seven) between enchondromas and chondrosarcomas, although some aberrations are specific to either chondrosarcoma or enchondroma. It also appears that peripheral chondrosarcomas (those arising in association with osteochondromas) show more

---

ENCHONDROMA—FACT SHEET

Definition
- Benign, intramedullary tumor of hyaline cartilage

Incidence and Location
- Common, exact incidence is unknown because many cases are undetected
- Estimated 5% of all bone tumors and 16% of cartilage tumors

Sex, Race, and Age Distribution
- Approximately equal sex distribution
- Wide age range (10-80 years), with most cases in their 20s to 50s

Clinical Features
- Large bone examples are asymptomatic
- Small bones of hands and feet present with slow-growing mass and pain

Prognosis and Treatment
- Asymptomatic tumors with benign radiographic findings can be observed
- In symptomatic tumors, curettage is curative

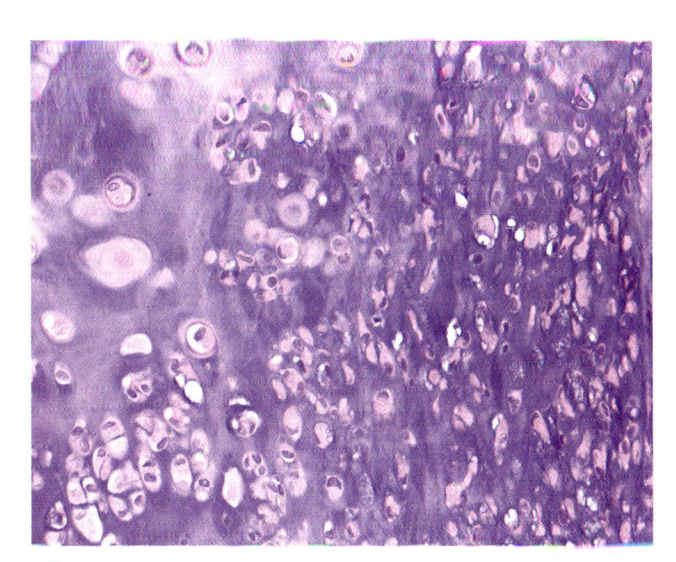

FIGURE 15-22
Enchondromas of the small bones of the hands and feet often demonstrate increased cellularity and nuclear atypia.

ENCHONDROMA—PATHOLOGIC FEATURES

Gross Findings
- Curettage specimens composed of firm, pale blue hyaline cartilage with occasional gritty calcifications
- Resection specimens are well circumscribed

Microscopic Findings
- Pale-blue cartilage matrix
- Low cellularity of round chondrocytes in lacunae
- Minimal nuclear atypia: small, dark nuclei with nuclear detail visible only at high magnification
- Examples in small bones of hands and feet can display more cellularity and atypia

Differential Diagnosis
- Low-grade chondrosarcoma
- Chondroblastic osteosarcoma

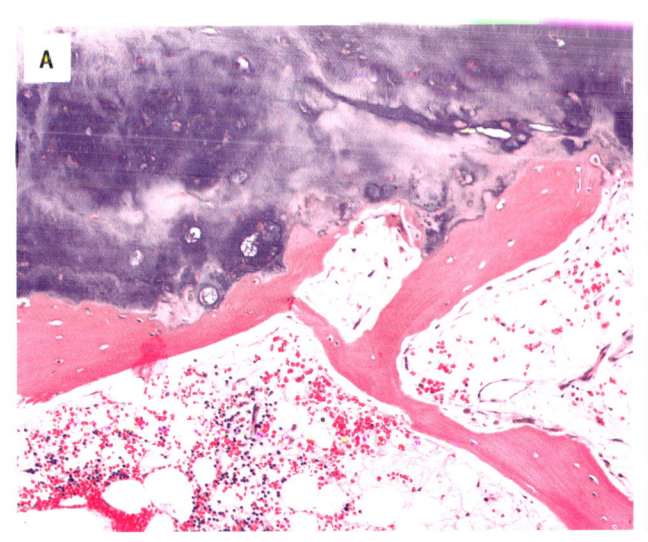

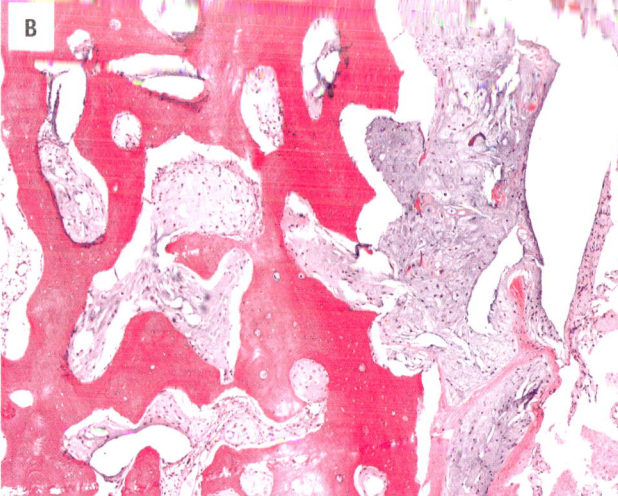

FIGURE 15-23
Endochondral ossification should not be confused with permeative growth of cartilage tumors. **A,** Endochondral ossification in an enchondroma is a gradual transformation from cartilage to lamellar bone that conforms to the shape of the cartilage lobule. **B,** Permeation of a chondrosarcoma characterized by a single mass of cartilage that entraps host lamellar bone with an abrupt transition between bone and cartilage.

loss of heterozygosity and wider variation in ploidy status than intramedullary, or *central*, chondrosarcomas.

MALIGNANT

CONVENTIONAL CHONDROSARCOMA

CLINICAL FEATURES

Chondrosarcoma arising in an intramedullary location has also been termed *central* chondrosarcoma to contrast with *peripheral* chondrosarcoma arising in association with osteochondroma. Chondrosarcoma is primarily a tumor of adulthood with a wide age distribution (20s to 80s) and a peak in the fourth to sixth decades of life. Unlike most enchondromas, chondrosarcomas commonly affect the proximal appendicular skeleton and axial skeleton, especially the pelvic and shoulder girdles and ribs. The pelvis is the single-most common location. Most patients have pain, sometimes slowly increasing for years or even decades. Pain may be referred if the tumor affects the spinal nerve roots. A palpable, firm, tender mass is often present.

RADIOGRAPHIC FEATURES

In long bones, the tumors are metadiaphyseal. The matrix demonstrates the typical calcifications suggesting a cartilage tumor (Figure 15-24). However, the tumor is poorly marginated with infiltration of the medullary cavity and erosion of the cortex. Other general features that have been most reproducibly associated with chondrosarcoma are pathologic fracture, soft tissue mass, periosteal reaction, and cortical disruption or thickening. Periosteal reaction is uncommon. In the small bones of the hands and feet, cortical erosion without soft tissue extension may be observed in enchondromas and, therefore, does not constitute a diagnosis of chondrosarcoma.

PATHOLOGIC FEATURES

GROSS FINDINGS

The matrix consists of translucent pale blue hyaline cartilage with scattered gritty calcifications. However, prominent myxoid change to a viscous, transparent liquid may be prominent and suggests malignancy. High-grade examples may demonstrate necrosis, cysts, and hemorrhage. Resection specimens show poor circumscription and infiltrative growth within the medullary cavity into soft tissue or both (Figure 15-25).

MICROSCOPIC FINDINGS

The matrix consists of pale, basophilic, hyaline cartilage, but areas of cystic change to myxoid matrix can be prominent (Figure 15-20). On average, chondrosarcomas display more cellularity and cytologic atypia than enchondromas. However, field for field, overlap can exist. Therefore, it is important to take into consideration the overall picture. The single-best histologic diagnostic criterion supporting chondrosarcoma is the presence of permeation of existing trabecular bone (Figure 15-27).

CHAPTER 15 Cartilage-Forming Tumors

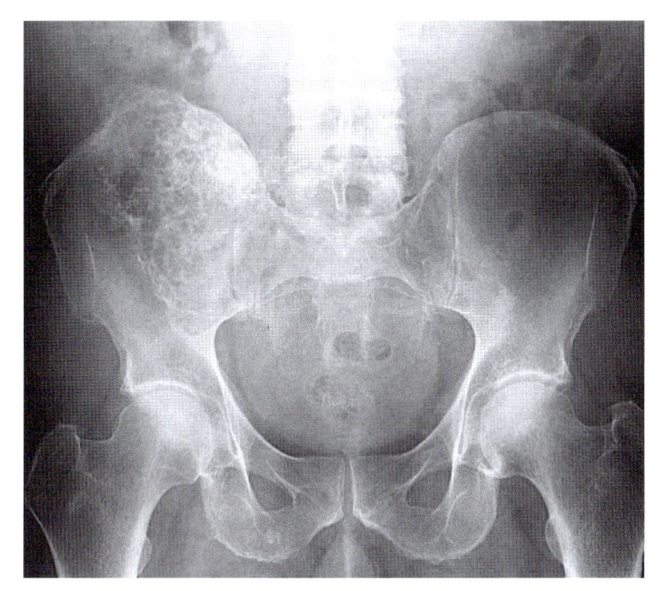

FIGURE 15-24
Chondrosarcoma involving the ilium. Radiographically, the tumor is large, lytic, and mineralized.

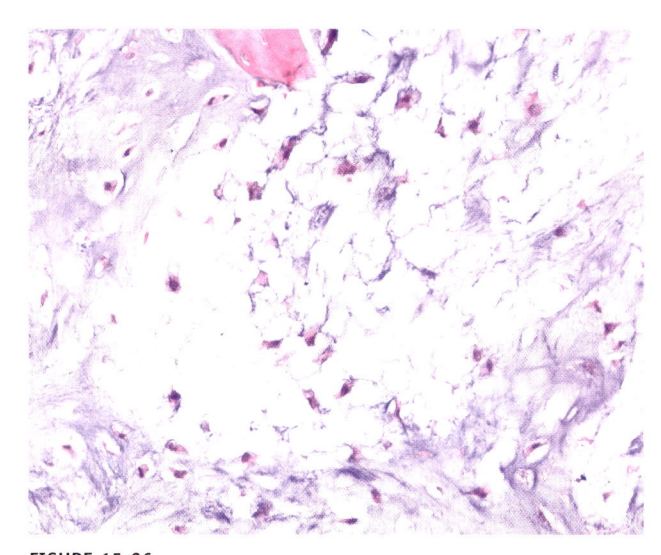

FIGURE 15-26
Myxoid change in chondrosarcoma results in a paler blue, stringy quality to the matrix.

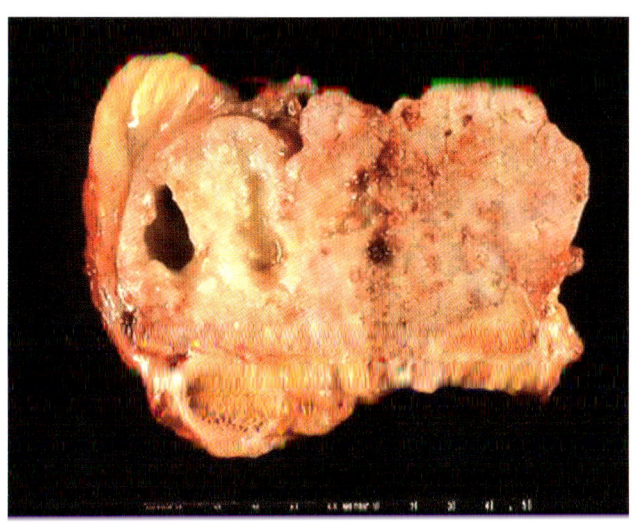

FIGURE 15-25
Chondrosarcoma forming a large, destructive mass arising from the right acetabulum. Some areas have the gray-white color of hyaline cartilage, whereas other show cystic myxoid change typically seen in chondrosarcoma 001.

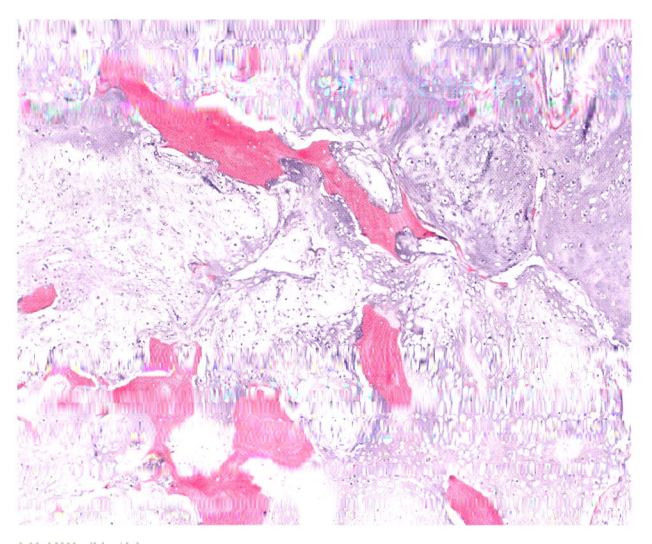

FIGURE 15-27
Chondrosarcoma permeates bone as a single, confluent mass entrapping existing bony trabeculae.

Permeation can also take the form of growth of the tumor through the Haversian canals of the cortex (Figure 15-28). Endochondral ossification should not be mistaken for true permeation. Both benign and malignant cartilage can undergo endochondral ossification in which one sees a *gradual* transition from cartilage to *woven* bone. This is in contrast with the *abrupt* transition of cartilage to *lamellar* bone characteristic of permeation.

Cytomorphologically, the chondrocytes demonstrate increased nuclear-to-cytoplasmic ratios, irregular nuclear membranes, and nucleoli. The nuclei are usually sufficiently large to make out detail at intermediate magnification (200X) (Figure 15-29). Binucleation of chondrocytes is relatively insensitive in distinguishing benign from malignant cartilage tumors. Spindling of chondrocytes, however, does point to chondrosarcoma (Figure 15-30). Mitotic activity is rare, except in high-grade tumors.

Of note, benign cartilage tumors of the small bones of the hands and feet can demonstrate many of the features described earlier. Histologically, enchondromas of small bones are often hypercellular and contain nuclear enlargement, features that would suggest chondrosarcoma in larger bones. Thus, in the small bones, cortical destruction and soft tissue extension radiographically

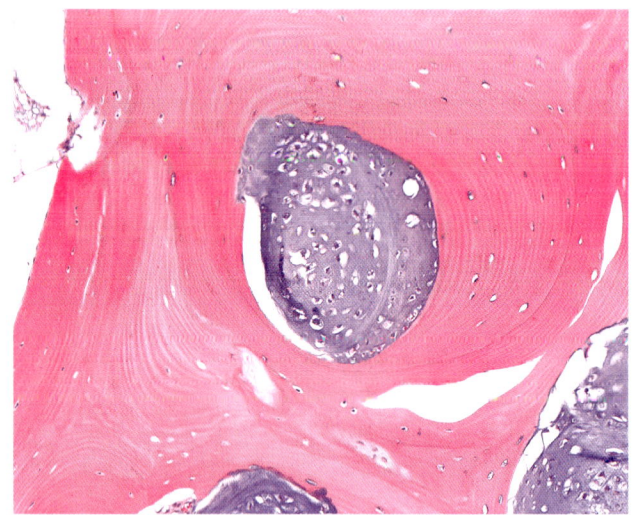

FIGURE 15-28
Permeation in chondrosarcoma may also extend through the Haversian canals of the cortex.

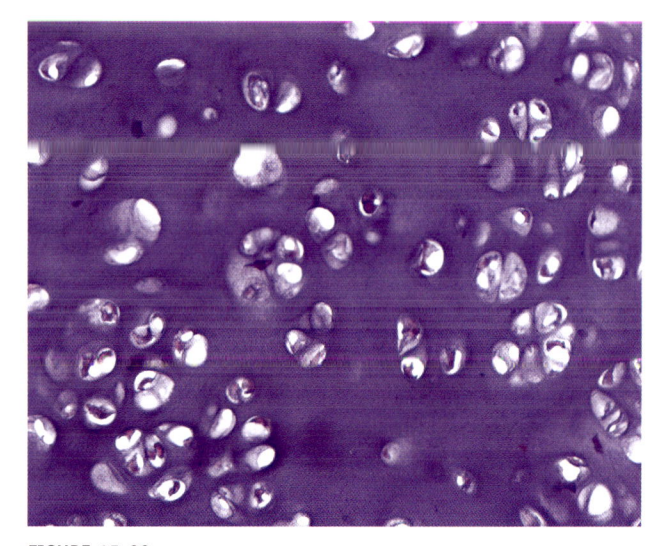

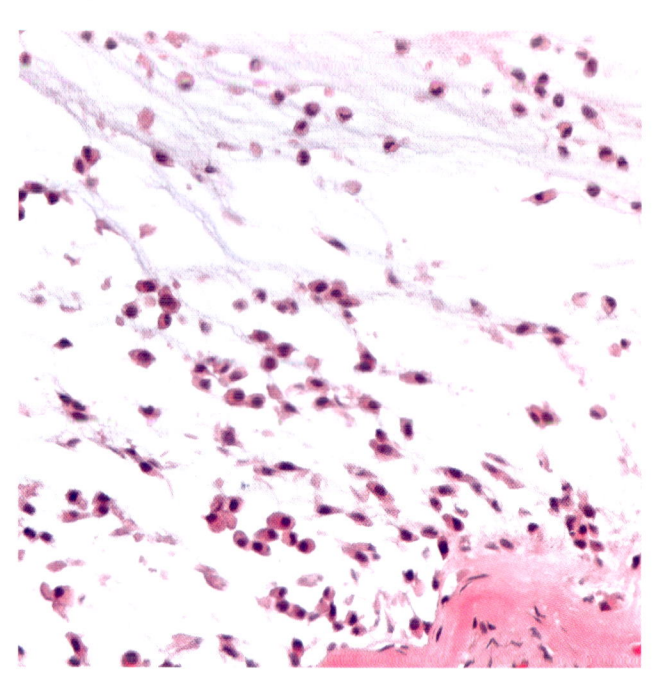

FIGURE 15-30
Spindling of chondrocytes is a feature of chondrosarcoma.

FIGURE 15-29
Nuclei of low-grade chondrosarcomas may show only slightly more atypia than enchondroma at intermediate magnification.

or histologically, or permeation through cortex into soft tissues (Figure 15-31), are required for the diagnosis of chondrosarcoma. Not all authors agree that the diagnosis can be made on cytologic features, but the presence of grade 3 findings should be viewed with high suspicion as chondrosarcoma.

Chondrosarcoma Grading

Although no strict scoring system is universally accepted, the general features of cellularity, nuclear size and detail, and mitotic activity are the variables associated with grade. Figures 15-32, 15-33, and 15-34 are examples of Grades 1, 2, and 3, respectively. It should be noted that decalcification can obscure nuclear detail, and interobserver variability can be high. Nevertheless, grade does correlate with prognosis.

Differential Diagnosis

The distinction between enchondroma and low-grade chondrosarcoma can be challenging. Clinically, chondrosarcomas present in the proximal skeleton as large masses in late adulthood. Radiographically, malignancy should be suspected if destructive cortical changes, permeative growth or soft tissue extension, and cortical thickening and expansion are observed. Individual tumors may have some or all of the worrisome radiographic features for malignancy. As described earlier, histologic evidence of permeation of viable, trabecular bone substantiates a diagnosis of chondrosarcoma. Myxoid change, increased cellularity, nuclear atypia, and mitotic activity all point to chondrosarcoma.

Chondroblastic osteosarcoma typically affects a younger age group but can resemble chondrosarcoma because of hypercellular cartilage and atypical chondrocytes. Although atypia of the chondrocytes can be present, growth of atypical tumor cells in sheets should suggest osteosarcoma. The presence of osteoid associated with malignant cells and zones of atypical spindle cells that

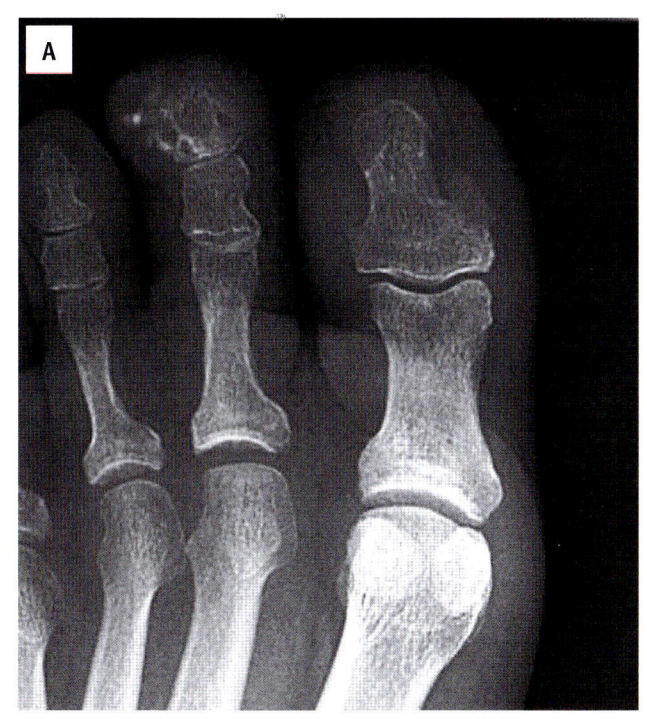

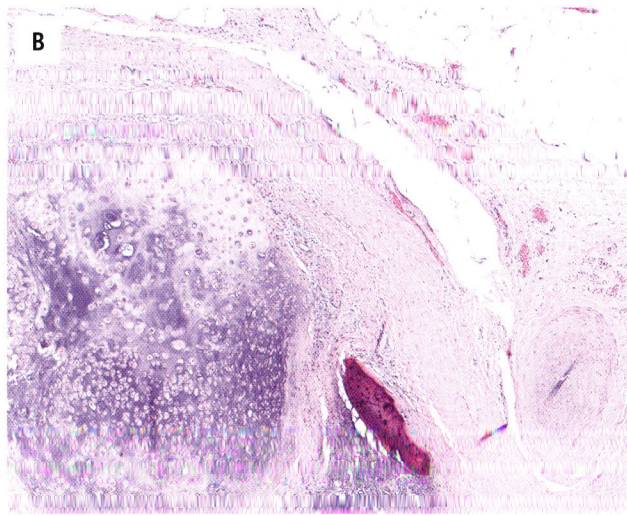

CONVENTIONAL CHONDROSARCOMA—FACT SHEET

Definition
- Malignant tumor of hyaline cartilage

Incidence and Location
- Rare, representing 10% of bone tumors and 15% of malignant bone tumors

Sex, Race, and Age Distribution
- Slight male sex predominance (1.1:1)
- Majority of patients in fourth through sixth decades of life

Clinical Features
- Pain is invariably present
- Pain may be referred if tumor affects vertebral or sacral nerve roots
- A hard, tender mass is often present

Prognosis and Treatment
- Prognosis related to grade: 5-year survival rate ranges from 90% for grade 1 tumors to 40% for grade 3 chondrosarcomas
- Significant mortality from local recurrence without metastasis even decades after diagnosis, therefore requiring long follow-up
- Resection with wide margins is preferred, limb sparing or amputation depending on reconstruction options

FIGURE 15-31
Chondrosarcomas of the small bones of the hands and feet are rare. The diagnosis requires demonstration of transcortical spread and soft tissue growth as suggested on this plain radiograph **(A)** or histologically **(B)**.

frequently surround the cartilage establishes the diagnosis of osteosarcoma.

CONVENTIONAL CHONDROSARCOMA—PATHOLOGIC FEATURES

Gross Findings
- Pale blue, firm cartilage with myxoid, viscous liquid change in matrix
- Gritty calcifications may be present
- Resection specimens show permeation through medulla or cortex into soft tissue

Microscopic Findings
- Permeation through viable, lamellar bone or Haversian canals
- Increased cellularity
- Spindling of chondrocytes, increased nuclear atypia
- Mitotic activity is rare
- A diagnosis of chondrosarcoma in the small bones of hands and feet requires permeation through cortex or soft tissue extension, or both

Differential Diagnosis
- Enchondroma
- Chondromyxoid fibroma
- Chondroblastic osteosarcoma

PROGNOSIS AND TREATMENT

Chondrosarcomas are treated by surgical resection with wide margins. They do not respond to radiation or chemotherapy. Some have suggested that chondrosarcomas of the phalanges may be treated by intralesional excision and close follow-up, with amputation as a last resort.

CHONDROSARCOMA VARIANTS

Most chondrosarcomas are of the conventional hyaline cartilage type. However, less common variants of dedifferentiated, clear cell, and mesenchymal types (representing 10%, 1%, and 1% of cartilage tumors,

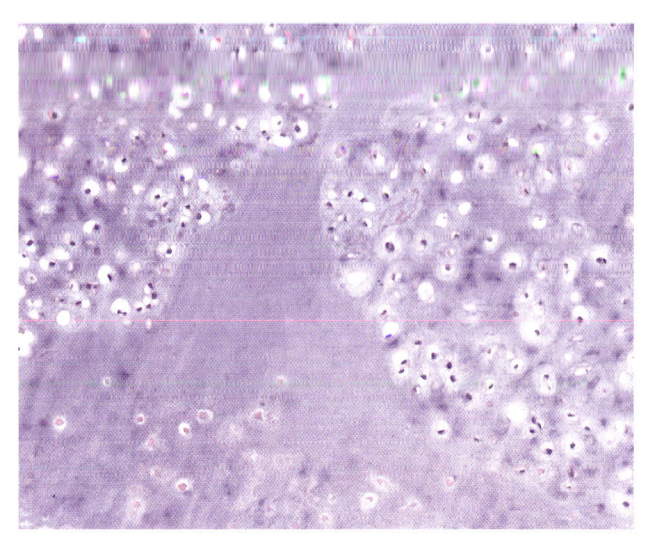

FIGURE 15-32
Grade 1 chondrosarcoma shows only mildly increased cellularity and minimal atypia compared with normal cartilage. The morphology overlaps substantially with enchondroma.

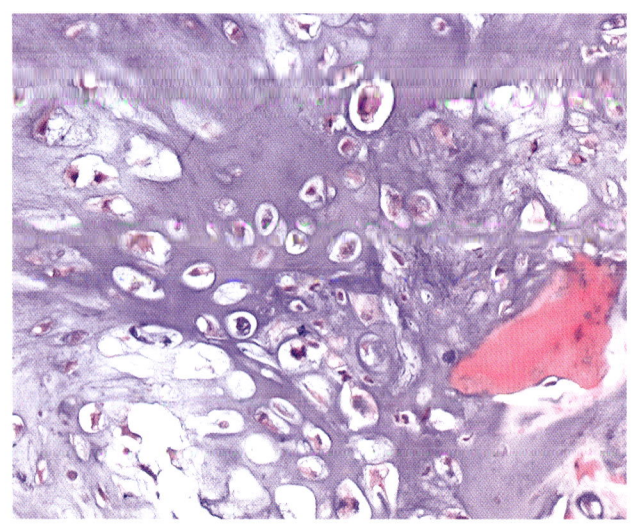

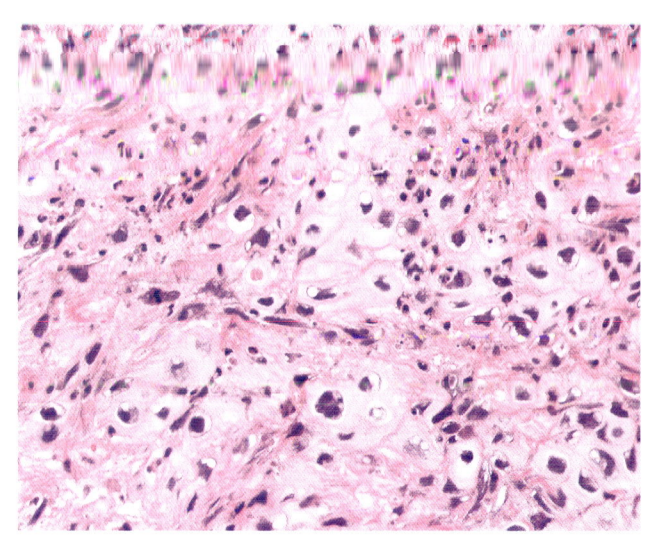

FIGURE 15-34
Grade 3 chondrosarcoma demonstrates diffuse hypercellularity, pleomorphic chondrocytes with nuclear hyperchromasia, irregular nuclear membranes, and necrosis. Mitotic activity is present in this case, but mitoses may be rare even in grade 3 tumors.

FIGURE 15-33
Grade 2 chondrosarcoma is visible with increased cellularity and cytologic atypia (note nuclear detail is visible even at intermediate magnification). Permeation of viable lamellar bone is also present on the right.

respectively) form distinct clinicopathologic entities that are described in the following sections.

CLEAR CELL CHONDROSARCOMA

CLINICAL FEATURES

Clear cell chondrosarcoma is probably the rarest variant of chondrosarcoma, representing 1% to 2% of chondrosarcomas, and is unusual in that it affects a younger age group than conventional chondrosarcoma (peak in third decade). The male-to-female ratio is approximately 2:1. Most patients have pain of several years duration and a tender mass. More than half of clear cell chondrosarcomas involve the proximal femur, with the proximal humerus and distal femur other common sites. However, examples involving the spine, calvarium, and distal extremities have been reported.

RADIOLOGIC FEATURES

Unlike other chondrosarcomas, the clear cell type is usually epiphyseal. The tumors can be osteolytic or sclerotic (Figure 15-35) but often circumscribed, sometimes even marginated, leading to a radiographic differential diagnosis of chondroblastoma. Calcifications indicative of cartilage matrix may be present in a quarter of cases. However, larger tumors may demonstrate features of malignancy including permeative growth and soft tissue destruction.

PATHOLOGIC FEATURES

GROSS FINDINGS

Curettage specimens demonstrate gritty calcifications, cyst formation, and variable amounts of pale blue matrix that is usually softer than normal hyaline cartilage.

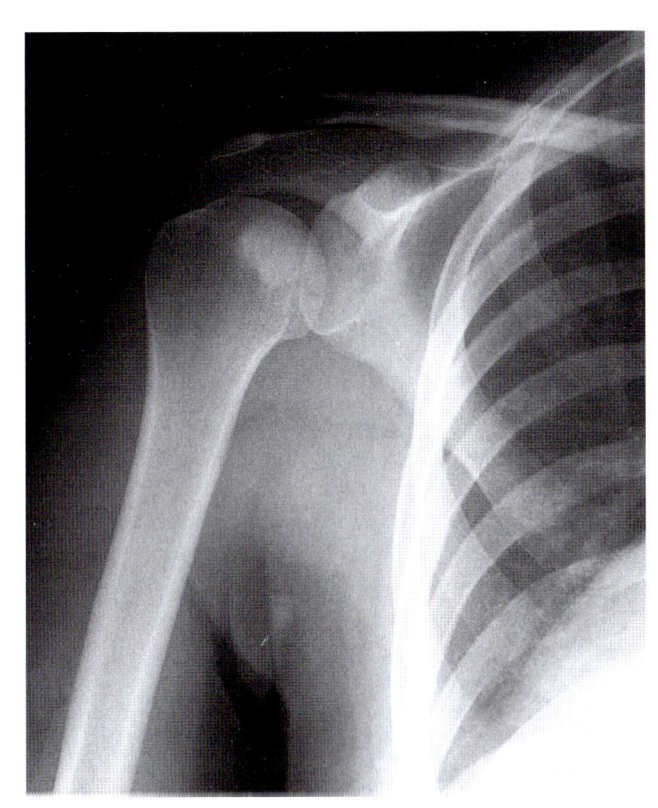

FIGURE 15-35
Radiographically, clear cell chondrosarcoma presents as a sclerotic, epiphyseal lesion with relatively good circumscription. The radiographic differential diagnosis includes chondroblastoma.

FIGURE 15-36
Clear cell chondrosarcoma typically contains delicate trabeculae of osteoid and multinucleated giant cells.

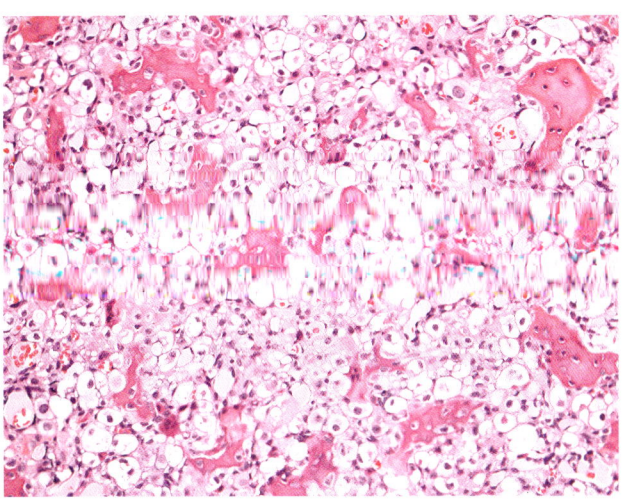

FIGURE 15-37
The cells of clear cell chondrosarcoma show ample pale to clear cytoplasm, well-defined nuclear membranes, and centrally placed round to ovoid nuclei with prominent nucleoli. Nuclear atypia is typically not marked.

MICROSCOPIC FINDINGS

Histologically, the tumor consists of plump cells with well-defined cytoplasmic borders, clear-to-pale eosinophilic cytoplasm, and round nuclei with prominent nucleoli and vesicular chromatin (Figure 15-36). The growth pattern is at least focally permeative. Hyaline cartilage is not prominent and can be completely absent. Variable amounts of woven bone are typically present (Figure 15-37). Osteoclast-like giant cells are common, a finding that is unusual in conventional chondrosarcoma. Mitotic activity is usually low. Approximately half of cases demonstrate areas resembling conventional chondrosarcoma. By immunohistochemistry, the clear cells are strongly S-100 protein–positive. Rare examples of dedifferentiated clear cell chondrosarcoma have been described.

DIFFERENTIAL DIAGNOSIS

The histologic differential diagnosis of clear cell chondrosarcoma includes chondroblastic osteosarcoma and osteoblastoma. The unique clear cells and the radiographic features of a well-marginated epiphyseal lesion help exclude these possibilities. The degree of pleomorphism, nuclear hyperchromasia, and mitotic activity of osteosarcoma is not present in clear cell chondrosarcoma.

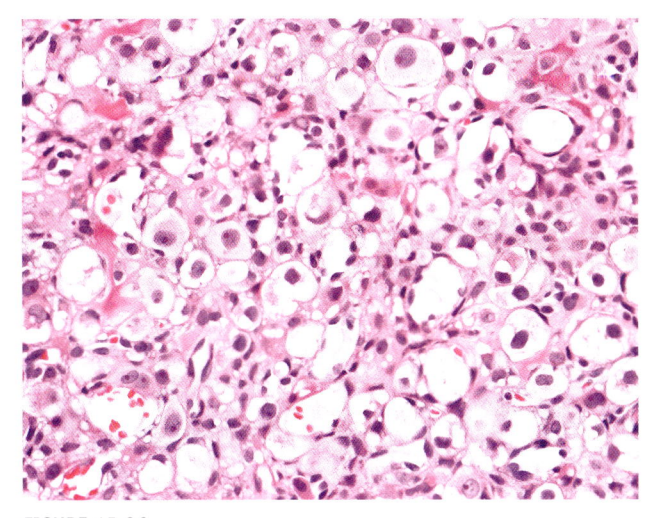

Radiographically, chondroblastoma can be difficult to distinguish from clear cell chondrosarcoma, especially in a skeletally immature patient. The cytomorphology of the clear cells, the hyaline cartilage (when present), and the presence of delicate woven bone trabeculae help distinguish clear cell chondrosarcoma from chondroblastoma.

PROGNOSIS AND TREATMENT

In general, clear cell chondrosarcoma is treated as a low-grade sarcoma with en bloc resection whenever possible. If insufficiently eradicated, for example, with intralesional curettage, patients may progress with destructive or local recurrence. Pulmonary or other metastases lead to mortality in 15% of cases.

CLEAR CELL CHONDROSARCOMA—FACT SHEET

Definition
- Low grade malignant neoplasm of cartilage with characteristic large, clear cells

Incidence and Location
- Rare, 1% to 2% of all cartilage tumors
- Most commonly affects proximal femoral epiphysis, less common in proximal humerus and distal femur

Sex, Race, and Age Distribution
- 2:1 male-to-female ratio
- Affects younger patients (peak in third decade of life) than does conventional chondrosarcoma but with wide age range (20-70 years)

Clinical Features
- Pain of several years' duration
- Tender mass

Radiographic Features
- Variable, most present as well-circumscribed, lytic lesion involving the epiphysis
- Sclerotic rim may be present suggesting a benign lesion including chondroblastoma
- Stippled calcifications in 25% of cases
- Larger examples are permeative with soft tissue destruction

Prognosis and Treatment
- En bloc resection results in cure as a rule
- Incomplete eradication by curettage may result in metastases and mortality in 15% of such cases

---

CLEAR CELL CHONDROSARCOMA—PATHOLOGIC FEATURES

Gross Findings
- Curettage specimens have gritty calcifications, pale blue cartilage softer than normal hyaline cartilage, cysts

Microscopic Findings
- Large, clear cells with prominent cytoplasmic borders, round-to-oval nuclei with vesicular chromatin, and prominent nucleoli
- Matrix including variable amounts of woven bone and hyaline cartilage
- Multinucleated, osteoclast-like giant cells may be present

Differential Diagnosis
- Chondroblastic osteosarcoma
- Osteoblastoma

DEDIFFERENTIATED CHONDROSARCOMA

Dedifferentiated chondrosarcoma is defined by the presence of a biphasic tumor composed of a conventional chondrosarcoma (usually grade 1) and a high-grade sarcoma. The term *dedifferentiated* chondrosarcoma may not accurately describe the pathogenesis of the tumor. That is, dedifferentiated chondrosarcoma probably does not represent true *dedifferentiation* of a well-differentiated chondrosarcoma into a high-grade sarcoma but diversion of a common progenitor cell down chondrogenic and nonchondrogenic differentiation pathways.

CLINICAL FEATURES

Dedifferentiated chondrosarcomas represent about 10% of all chondrosarcomas and tend to occur in the same locations as conventional chondrosarcomas (pelvis and proximal humerus) but with a far worse prognosis (5-year survival rate of < 10% in some series). The peak incidence is in the sixth decade, and the sexes are equally affected. Pain is invariably present, and a mass is common. Some patients have rapid increase in pain and/or size of a mass that may have been asymptomatic for years.

RADIOLOGIC FEATURES

The tumors are large and contain: (1) a mineralized chondroid-containing tumor with evidence of permeation or cortical erosion; and (2) a second component that is lytic, destructive, and oftentimes associated with a soft tissue mass (Figure 15-38). Usually the transition between the two components is sharp.

PATHOLOGIC FEATURES

GROSS FINDINGS

Typically, the dedifferentiated chondrosarcoma lesion is centered in the medullary cavity and consists of pale blue hyaline cartilage, possibly with cystic or liquefied myxoid areas. Peripherally, or at times within the cartilage component, the tumor is composed of fleshy, soft tumor with necrosis and hemorrhage that extends into the soft tissues (Figure 15-39).

MICROSCOPIC FINDINGS

Microscopic findings of dedifferentiated chondrosarcoma include a biphasic pattern with an abrupt transition between hyaline cartilage tumor and a high-grade sarcoma (Figure 15-40). The well-differentiated component typically consists of grade 1 chondrosarcoma. The high-grade component demonstrates sheets of pleomorphic cells with large, hyperchromatic, sometimes

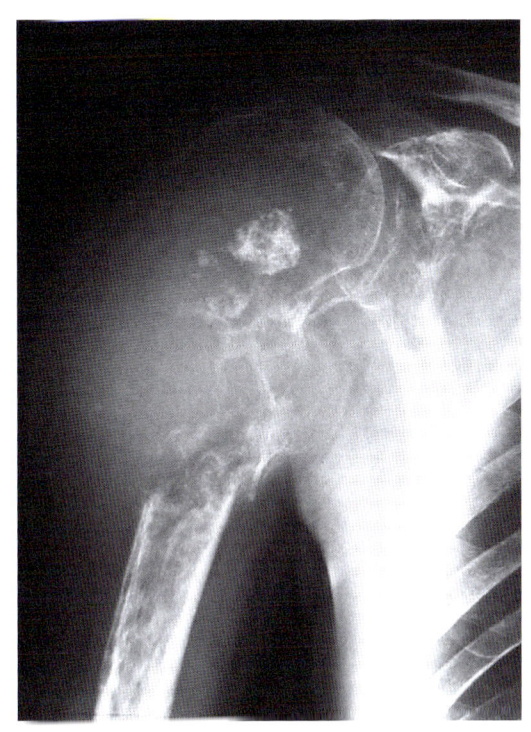

CHAPTER 15 Cartilage-Forming Tumors 349

FIGURE 15-38
Radiograph shows a dedifferentiated chondrosarcoma involving the proximal humerus. The pattern of central mineralization is typical for chondrosarcoma. However, the aggressive appearance with a large soft tissue mass suggests dedifferentiated chondrosarcoma.

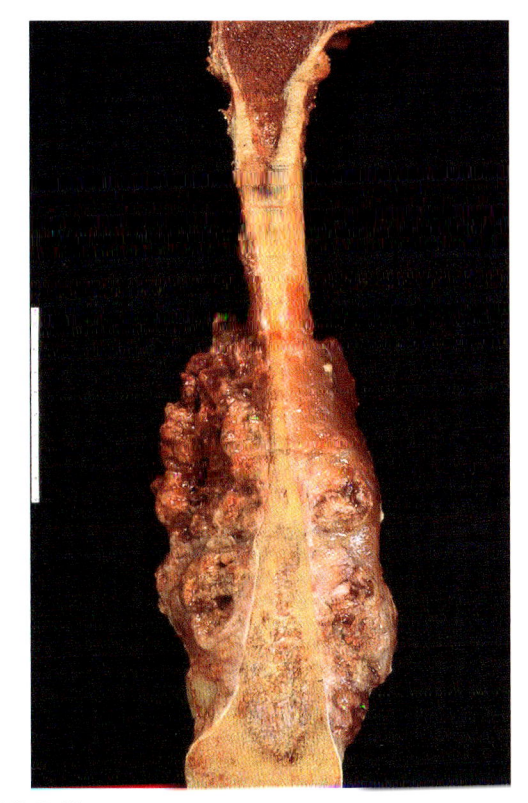

FIGURE 15-39
Dedifferentiated chondrosarcoma.
The medullary part of the tumor is composed of gray-white cartilage. The tan-brown extraosseous portion represents the high-grade sarcoma component.

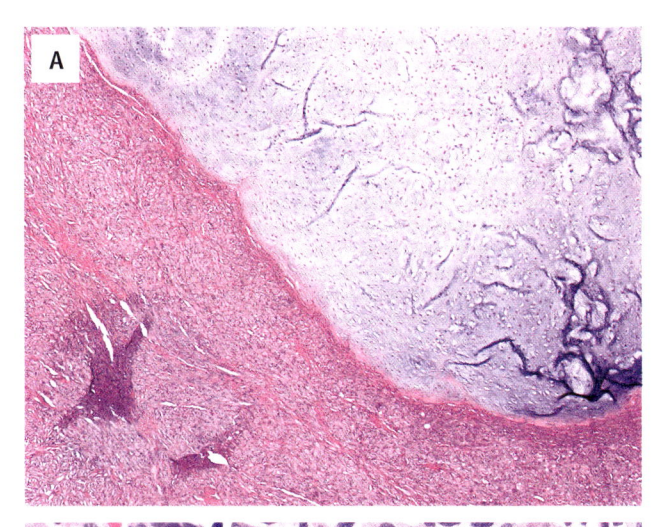

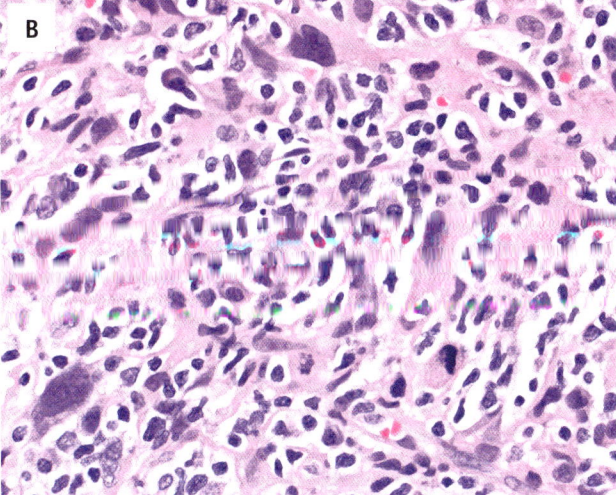

FIGURE 15-40
A, Dedifferentiated chondrosarcoma is characteristically a biphasic tumor with broad zones of hyaline cartilage juxtaposed with a second high grade sarcoma. B, The dedifferentiated component consists of a high-grade sarcoma such as malignant fibrous histiocytoma, as in this example, or osteosarcoma.

bizarre nuclei. The latter cells can grow in various patterns including storiform to fascicular and may produce osteoid. Mitotic figures, including atypical forms, are common.

DIFFERENTIAL DIAGNOSIS

The presence of a malignant tumor producing both cartilage and bone raises the possibility of chondroblastic osteosarcoma. However, in the latter tumor, cartilage- and osteoid-forming areas merge and are intermixed without the abrupt transition seen radiographically, grossly, and microscopically in dedifferentiated chondrosarcoma.

Conventional chondrosarcoma can be distinguished by the absence of the high-grade component. Conversely, malignant fibrous histiocytoma and fibrosarcoma may

DEDIFFERENTIATED CHONDROSARCOMA—FACT SHEET

Definition
- Malignant tumor of cartilage with a second, high-grade, noncartilaginous component

Incidence and Location
- Rare, 10% of all chondrosarcomas
- Most commonly affects pelvis and proximal femur epiphysis

Sex, Race, and Age Distribution
- Male-to-female ratio is 1:1
- Affects same age range as conventional chondrosarcoma, with peak in sixth decade of life

Clinical Features
- Pain, sometimes with recent increase in severity
- Tender mass

Radiographic Features
- Biphasic tumor
- Intramedullary component with ring or stippled calcifications suggesting cartilage
- Second component is aggressive, permeative, usually with a large soft tissue mass

Prognosis and Treatment
- Wide excision, usually with amputation and adjuvant chemotherapy
- Long-term survival rate is < 10%

DEDIFFERENTIATED CHONDROSARCOMA—PATHOLOGIC FEATURES

Gross Findings
- Biphasic tumor
- Central zone of pale blue hyaline cartilage with rubbery to liquid myxoid consistency
- Peripheral tumor and soft tissue component fleshy, soft with necrosis and hemorrhage

Microscopic Findings
- The two components are sharply demarcated
- Central area of conventional chondrosarcoma (usually grade 1)
- High-grade component of osteosarcoma, fibrosarcoma, or malignant fibrous histiocytoma; pleomorphic nuclei, necrosis, abundant mitoses

Differential Diagnosis
- Chondroblastic osteosarcoma
- Chondrosarcoma
- Malignant fibrous histiocytoma
- Fibrosarcoma

be indistinguishable from the high-grade component of a dedifferentiated chondrosarcoma microscopically, especially if the biopsy is from the periphery of the lesion. Radiologic evidence of a pre-existing cartilaginous lesion is helpful in such cases.

PROGNOSIS AND TREATMENT

Unfortunately, the prognosis of dedifferentiated chondrosarcoma is poor with a 5-year survival rate of less than 10%. Standard management consists of wide resection of the tumor, although limb salvage is often impossible given the large soft tissue component of these tumors. The response to adjuvant chemotherapy has been unsatisfactory.

MESENCHYMAL CHONDROSARCOMA

CLINICAL FEATURES

Mesenchymal chondrosarcoma is a rare variant of chondrosarcoma, representing 1% to 3% of chondrosarcomas. Like clear cell chondrosarcoma, the mesenchymal variant peaks during the second and third decades of life. Most patients have pain and swelling. The sexes are equally affected. These tumors often involve the pelvis, ribs, and jaw. Unlike the other malignant cartilage tumors, mesenchymal chondrosarcomas may frequently occur primarily in extraosseous sites (approximately 30%).

RADIOLOGIC FEATURES

Mesenchymal chondrosarcoma is infiltrative with cortical destruction and soft tissue extension. Most examples are primarily lytic with matrix calcifications. However, the findings are not specific and may suggest conventional chondrosarcoma or osteosarcoma (Figure 15-41). Rare examples may demonstrate margination and a rim of sclerotic bone belying their malignant nature.

PATHOLOGIC FEATURES

GROSS FINDINGS

The most common finding in mesenchymal chondrosarcoma is a haphazard admixture of pale blue, firm cartilage, and fleshy pink, soft tumor tissue. Gritty calcifications may be present. Cystic change, necrosis, and hemorrhage are common.

MICROSCOPIC FINDINGS

Mesenchymal chondrosarcoma demonstrates a biphasic pattern composed of a hyaline cartilage component and a small blue cell malignancy (Figure 15-42) in

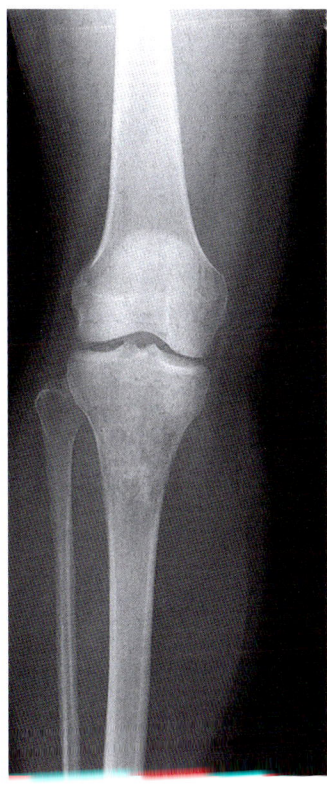

FIGURE 15-41
Radiograph of mesenchymal chondrosarcoma involving the proximal tibia. It is a permeative metaphyseal lesion with calcifications.

MESENCHYMAL CHONDROSARCOMA—FACT SHEET

Definition
- High-grade malignant biphasic neoplasm of benign cartilage and primitive small round blue cells

Incidence and Location
- Rare, 1% to 3% of all cartilage tumors
- Most commonly affects pelvis, ribs, and jaw, 30% are extraosseous

Sex, Race, and Age Distribution
- Equal sex ratio
- Affects younger patients than conventional chondrosarcoma; peak in second and third decades of life

Clinical Features
- Pain with tender mass

Radiographic features
- Permeative, lytic mass with cortical destruction and soft tissue destruction
- Calcifications suggesting cartilage are common

Prognosis and Treatment
- Recurrence and metastases can be observed decades after initial diagnosis
- Wide local excision with adjuvant chemotherapy is warranted in most cases

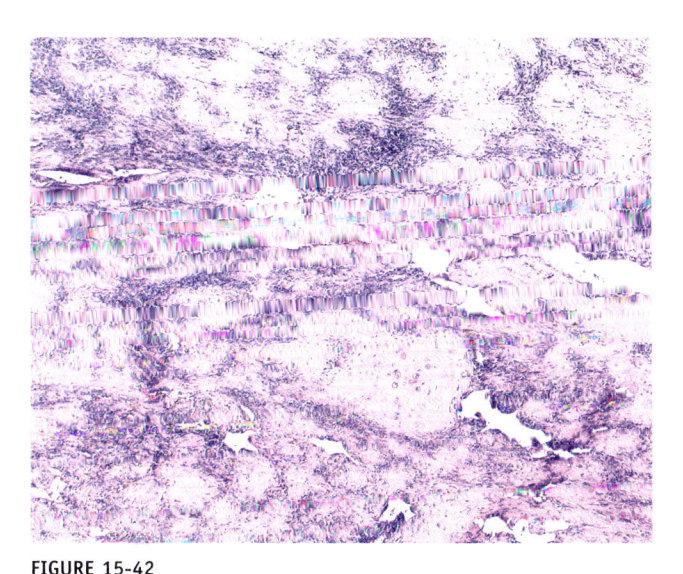

FIGURE 15-42
At low power, mesenchymal chondrosarcoma is a biphasic tumor composed of hyaline cartilage and small round blue cells. Hemangiopericytoma-like vessels may be prominent.

MESENCHYMAL CHONDROSARCOMA—PATHOLOGIC FEATURES

Gross Findings
- Admixture of firm, pale blue cartilage and soft, fleshy, pink tissue; gritty calcifications may be present

Microscopic Findings
- Biphasic, composed of cytomorphologically well-differentiated hyaline cartilage and a small round blue cell neoplasm
- Haphazard arrangement of two components, interface may be gradual or abrupt
- Small-cell component contains spindled areas and demonstrates hemangiopericytoma-like vascular pattern, necrosis, and hemorrhage

Differential Diagnosis
- Chondroblastic osteosarcoma
- Ewing sarcoma
- Dedifferentiated chondrosarcoma

variable amounts. The two components are oftentimes abruptly adjacent to one another, however, occasionally, the interface is more gradual. The cartilage component is well differentiated cytologically and may demonstrate areas of endochondral ossification (Figure 15-43A). In contrast, the small cell component is hypercellular with a high nuclear-to-cytoplasmic ratio, raising the possibility of Ewing sarcoma or lymphoma (see Figure 15-43B). Spindling in the small-cell component can be seen as a "hemangiopericytomatous" pattern of vasculature.

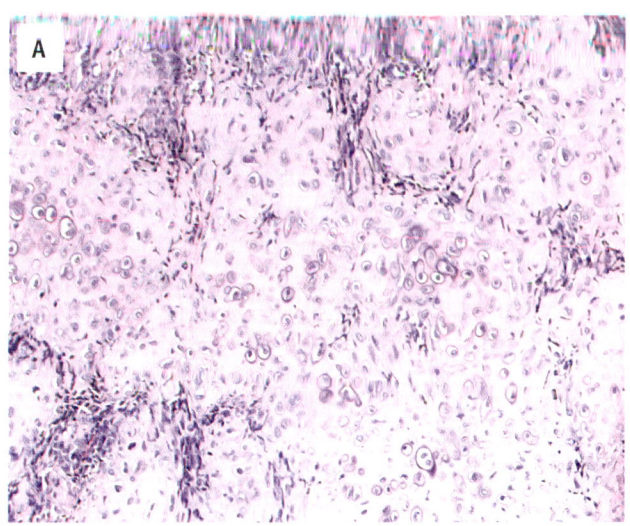

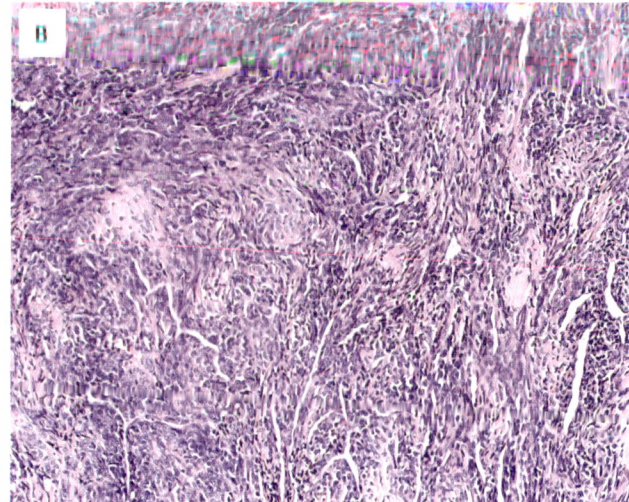

FIGURE 15-43
A, The cellularity of the cartilage areas of mesenchymal chondrosarcoma is lower than the round cell areas and typically displays low grade features. **B,** The round cell component of mesenchymal chondrosarcoma shows hemangiopericytoma-like vasculature and dense sheets of monomorphic round to oval cells.

ANCILLARY STUDIES

Specific immunohistochemical stains do not establish the diagnosis of mesenchymal chondrosarcoma. The cartilage component is typically S-100 positive, and importantly, the small-cell component can express CD99. However, the t(11;22) EWS:FLI1 translocation of Ewing sarcoma has not been detected in mesenchymal chondrosarcoma.

DIFFERENTIAL DIAGNOSIS

The presence of matrix production by the tumor should exclude Ewing sarcoma and lymphoma, although confirmation by cytogenetic or molecular genetic means (confirming an absence of the EWS translocation) may be necessary on small biopsies. Dedifferentiated chondrosarcoma may be a consideration because of the biphasic pattern. However, the high-grade component in dedifferentiated component is typically not a small round blue cell tumor but rather an osteosarcoma or malignant fibrous histiocytoma. Dedifferentiated chondrosarcoma also typically affects an older age group. The diagnosis of chondroblastic osteosarcoma should be considered in the differential but can be distinguished by the presence of cytologically malignant cells in the cartilage component, which blend gradually, rather than abruptly, into the spindle cell proliferation.

PROGNOSIS AND TREATMENT

Mesenchymal chondrosarcoma typically has an extended clinical course with recurrence and pulmonary metastasis, sometimes after a long interval. Primary treatment consists of wide excision and reconstruction. Extensive soft tissue involvement may negate the possibility of limb-sparing surgery. Adjuvant chemotherapy may be useful, but established protocols do not exist for this rare tumor. Unresectable tumors may be treated with definitive chemoradiation.

SUGGESTED READINGS

Osteochondroma

1. Ahmed AR, Tan TS, Unni KK, et al: Secondary chondrosarcoma in osteochondroma; report of 107 patients.. Clin Orthop Relat Res 2003;411:193-206.
2. Bovee JV, Cleton-Jansen AM, Wuyts W, et al: EXT-mutation analysis and loss of heterozygosity in sporadic and hereditary osteochondromas and secondary chondrosarcomas. Am J Hum Genet 1999;65: 689-698.
3. Fletcher CDM, Unni KK, Mertens F: Pathology and genetics of tumours of soft tissue and bone. Lyon, IARC Press, 2002.
4. Hameetman L, Szuhai K, Yavas A, et al: The role of EXT1 in nonhereditary osteochondroma: identification of homozygous deletions. J Natl Cancer Inst 2007;99:396-406.
5. Horvai A, Unni KK: Premalignant conditions of bone. J Orthop Sci 2006;11:412-423.
6. Kronenberg HM: Developmental regulation of the growth plate. Nature 2003;423:332-336.
7. Schmale GA, Conrad EU 3rd, Raskind WH: The natural history of hereditary multiple exostoses. J Bone Joint Surg Am 1994;76:986-992.
8. Unni KK: Cartilaginous lesions of bone. J Orthop Sci 2001;6:457-472.
9. Vink GR, White SJ, Gabelic S, et al: Mutation screening of EXT1 and EXT2 by direct sequence analysis and MLPA in patients with multiple osteochondromas: splice site mutations and exonic deletions account for more than half of the mutations. Eur J Hum Genet 2005;13:470-474.

Periosteal Chondroma

1. Bauer TW, Dorfman HD, Latham JI Jr: Periosteal chondroma. A clinicopathologic study of 23 cases. Am J Surg Pathol 1982;6(7):631-637.
2. Bertoni F, Boriani S, Laus M, Campanacci M: Periosteal chondrosarcoma and periosteal osteosarcoma. Two distinct entities. J Bone Joint Surg Br 1982;64(3):370-376.

3. Lewis MM, Kenan S, Yabut SM, et al: Periosteal chondroma. A report of ten cases and review of the literature. Clin Orthop Relat Res 1990;256:185–192.
4. Nojima T, Unni KK, McLeod RA, et al: Periosteal chondroma and periosteal chondrosarcoma. Am J Surg Pathol 1985;9:666–677.
5. Schajowicz F: Juxtacortical chondrosarcoma. J Bone Joint Surg Br 1977;59-B(4):473–480.

Conventional Chondroblastoma

1. Aigner T, Loos S, Inwards C, et al: Chondroblastoma is an osteoid-forming, but not cartilage-forming neoplasm. J Pathol 1999;189(4):463–469.
2. Dahlin DC, Ivins JC: Benign chondroblastoma. A study of 125 cases. Cancer 1972;30(2):401–413.
3. de Silva MV, Reid R: Chondroblastoma: varied histologic appearance, potential diagnostic pitfalls, and clinicopathologic features associated with local recurrence. Ann Diagn Pathol 2003;7(4):205–213.
4. Kurt AM, Unni KK, Sim F, et al: Chondroblastoma of bone. Hum Pathol 1989;20(10):965–976.
5. Ramappa AJ, Lee FY, Tang P, et al: Chondroblastoma of bone. J Bone Joint Surg Am 2000;82-A(8):1140–1145.

Chondromyxoid Fibroma

1. Rahimi A, Beabout JW, Ivins JC, et al: Chondromyxoid fibroma: a clinicopathologic study of 76 cases. Cancer 1972;30(3):726–736.
2. White PG, Saunders L, Orr W, et al: Chondromyxoid fibroma. Skeletal Radiol 1996;25(1):79–81.
3. Wu CT, Inwards CY, O'Laughlin S, et al: Chondromyxoid fibroma of bone: a clinicopathologic review of 278 cases. Hum Pathol 1998;29:438–446.
4. Zillmer DA, Dorfman HD: Chondromyxoid fibroma of bone: thirty-six cases with clinicopathologic correlation. Hum Pathol 1989;20(10):952–964.

Enchondroma

1. Giudici MA, Moser RP Jr., Kransdorf MJ: Cartilaginous bone tumors. Radiol Clin North Am 1993;31(2):237–259.
2. Hopyan S, Gokgoz N, Poon R, et al: A mutant PTH/PTHrP type I receptor in enchondromatosis. Nat Genet 2002;30(3):306–310.
3. Rozeman LB, Sangiorgi L, Briaire-de Bruijn IH, et al: Enchondromatosis (Ollier disease, Maffucci syndrome) is not caused by the PTHR1 mutation p.R150C. Hum Mutat 2004;24(6):466–473.
4. Tallini G, Dorfman HD, Brys P, et al: Correlation between clinicopathological features and karyotype in 100 cartilaginous and chordoid tumours. A report from the Chromosomes and Morphology (CHAMP) Collaborative Study Group. J Pathol 2002;196(2):194–203.
5. Wold LE, Adler C P, Sim FH, et al: Atlas of orthopedic pathology. Philadelphia: Saunders, 2003, pp 225–231.

Chondrosarcoma

1. Bjornsson J, McLeod RA, Unni KK, et al: Primary chondrosarcoma of long bones and limb girdles. Cancer 1998;83(10):2105–2119.
2. Bovee JV, van der Heul RO, Taminiau AH, et al: Chondrosarcoma of the phalanx: a locally aggressive lesion with minimal metastatic potential: a report of 35 cases and a review of the literature. Cancer 1999;86(9):1724–1732.
3. Evans HL, Ayala AG, Romsdahl MM: Prognostic factors in chondrosarcoma of bone: a clinicopathologic analysis with emphasis on histologic grading. Cancer 1977;40(2):818–831.
4. Geirnaerdt MJ, Hermans J, Bloem JL, et al: Usefulness of radiography in differentiating enchondroma from central grade 1 chondrosarcoma. AJR Am J Roentgenol 1997;169(4):1097–1104.
5. Gitelis S, Bertoni F, Picci P, et al: Chondrosarcoma of bone. The experience at the Istituto Ortopedico Rizzoli. J Bone Joint Surg Am 1981;63(8):1248–1257.
6. Lee FY, Mankin HJ, Fondren G, et al: Chondrosarcoma of bone: an assessment of outcome. J Bone Joint Surg Am 1999;81(3):326–338.
7. Mirra JM, Gold R, Downs J, et al: A new histologic approach to the differentiation of enchondroma and chondrosarcoma of the bones. A clinicopathologic analysis of 51 cases. Clin Orthop Relat Res 1985;201:214–237.
8. Murphey MD, Walker EA, Wilson AJ, et al: From the archives of the AFIP: imaging of primary chondrosarcoma: Radiologic-pathologic correlation. Radiographics 2003;23(5):1245–1247.
9. Ozaki T, Wai D, Schafer KL, et al: Comparative genomic hybridization in cartilaginous tumors. Anticancer Res 2004;24(3a):1721–1725.
10. Ogose A, Unni KK, Swee RG, et al: Chondrosarcoma of small bones of the hands and feet. Cancer 1997;80(1):50–59.
11. Pritchard DJ, Lunke RJ, Taylor WF, et al: Chondrosarcoma: a clinicopathologic and statistical analysis. Cancer 1980;45(1):149–157.
12. Rosenthal DI, Schiller AL, Mankin HJ: Chondrosarcoma: correlation of radiological and histological grade. Radiology 1984;150(1):21–26.

Clear Cell Chondrosarcoma

1. Bjornsson J, Unni KK, Dahlin DC, et al: Clear cell chondrosarcoma of bone. Observations in 47 cases. Am J Surg Pathol 1984;8(3):223–230.
2. Collins MS, Koyama T, Swee RG, et al: Clear cell chondrosarcoma: radiographic, computed tomographic, and magnetic resonance findings in 34 patients with pathologic correlation. Skeletal Radiol 2003;32(12):687–694.
3. Itala A, Leerapun T, Inwards C, et al: An institutional review of clear cell chondrosarcoma. Clin Orthop Relat Res 2005;440:209–212.
4. Kalil RK, Inwards CY, Unni KK, et al: Dedifferentiated clear cell chondrosarcoma. Am J Surg Pathol 2000;24:1079–1086.
5. Lichtenstein L, Bernstein D: Unusual benign and malignant chondroid tumors of bone. A survey of some mesenchymal cartilage tumors and malignant chondroblastic tumors, including a few multicentric ones, as well as many atypical benign chondroblastomas and chondromyxoid fibromas. Cancer 1959;12:1142–1157.
6. Unni KK, Dahlin DC, Beabout JW, et al: Chondrosarcoma: clear-cell variant. A report of sixteen cases. J Bone Joint Surg Am 1976;58(5):676–683.

Dedifferentiated Chondrosarcoma

1. Dahlin DC, Beabout JW: Dedifferentiation of low-grade chondrosarcomas. Cancer 1971;28(2):461–466.
2. Dickey ID, Rose PS, Fuchs B, et al: Dedifferentiated chondrosarcoma: the role of chemotherapy with updated outcomes. J Bone Joint Surg Am 2004;86A(11):2412–2418.
3. Frassica FJ, Unni KK, Beabout JW, et al: Dedifferentiated chondrosarcoma. A report of the clinicopathological features and treatment of seventy-eight cases. J Bone Joint Surg Am 1986;68:1197–1205.
4. Littrell LA, Wenger DE, Wold LE, et al: Radiographic, CT, and MR imaging features of dedifferentiated chondrosarcomas: a retrospective review of 174 de novo cases. Radiographics 2004;24(5):1397–1409.
5. McCarthy FF, Dorfman HD: Chondrosarcoma of bone with dedifferentiation: a study of eighteen cases. Hum Pathol 1982;13(1):36–40.
6. Mirra JM, Marcove RC: Fibrosarcomatous dedifferentiation of primary and secondary chondrosarcoma. Review of five cases. J Bone Joint Surg Am 1974;56(2):285–296.
7. Staals EL, Bacchini P, Bertoni F: Dedifferentiated central chondrosarcoma. Cancer 2006;106(12):2682–2691.

Mesenchymal Chondrosarcoma

1. Bertoni F, Picci P, Bacchini P, et al: Mesenchymal chondrosarcoma of bone and soft tissues. Cancer 1983;52(3):533–541.
2. Huvos AG, Rosen G, Dabska M, et al: Mesenchymal chondrosarcoma. A clinicopathologic analysis of 35 patients with emphasis on treatment. Cancer 1983;51:1230–1237.
3. Nakashima Y, Unni KK, Shives TC, et al: Mesenchymal chondrosarcoma of bone and soft tissue. A review of 111 cases. Cancer 1986;57(12):2444–2453.
4. Naumann S, Krallman PA, Unni KK, et al: Translocation der(13;21)(q10;q10) in skeletal and extraskeletal mesenchymal chondrosarcoma. Mod Pathol 2002;15(5):572–576.
5. Salvador AH, Beabout JW, Dahlin DC: Mesenchymal chondrosarcoma—observations on 30 new cases. Cancer 1971;28(3):605–615.

6. Swanson PE, Lillemoe TJ, Manivel JC, et al: Mesenchymal chondrosarcoma. An immunohistochemical study. Arch Pathol Lab Med 1990;114(9):943–948.
7. Vencio EF, Reeve CM, Unni KK, et al: Mesenchymal chondrosarcoma of the jaw bones. Clinicopathologic study of 19 cases. Cancer 1988;82:2350–2355.
8. Wehrli BM, Huang W, De Crombrugghe B, et al: Sox9, a master regulator of chondrogenesis, distinguishes mesenchymal chondrosarcoma from other small blue round cell tumors. Hum Pathol 2003;34(3):263–269.

16 Fibroblastic and Fibrohistiocytic Tumors

Edward F. McCarthy

FIBROUS LESIONS
- Nonossifying Fibroma (Metaphysical Fibrous Defect, Fibrous Cortical Defect)
- Desmoplastic Fibroma
- Fibrosarcoma of Bone

FIBROHISTIOCYTIC LESIONS
- Benign Fibrous Histiocytoma of Bone
- Malignant Fibrous Histiocytoma of Bone

The four principle fibrous tumors of bone differ from one another and cover the entire spectrum of clinical behavior. They can be entirely benign, or they can behave in an aggressive, malignant fashion. At the benign end of the spectrum is nonossifying fibroma. This is a self-limited developmental lesion that oftentimes does not require treatment. At the aggressive end of the spectrum are high-grade malignant fibrous histiocytoma and fibrosarcoma, both of which can be lethal tumors. Between these extremes of clinical behavior are two other fibrous lesions that carry more moderate prognoses: desmoplastic fibroma, a locally aggressive lesion that does not metastasize, and low-grade fibrosarcoma, a low-grade malignancy that is often curable.

FIBROUS LESIONS

NONOSSIFYING FIBROMA (Metaphysical Fibrous Defect, Fibrous Cortical Defect)

Nonossifying fibromas are common benign proliferations of fibrous tissue that occur in the metaphyseal region of long bones. They form during skeletal growth and most probably are caused by exaggerated subperiosteal osteoclastic resorption during metaphyseal modeling. This exaggerated resorptive process often begins at the site of tendon insertions. Small lesions, known as fibrous cortical defects, result from the same process. Although nonossifying fibromas form in the metaphyseal region, they migrate into the diaphysis during bone growth. Although they are lytic processes initially, lesions often fill in with reparative new bone.

CLINICAL FEATURES

Nonossifying fibromas most commonly involve the distal femur and the proximal tibia, sites that account for 80% of lesions. The distal tibia, both ends of the fibula, and the distal radius may also be involved. The flat bones, the small bones of the hands and foot, the spine, and the craniofacial skeleton are not affected. Lesions in these locations with similar histologic features are best regarded as benign fibrous histiocytomas. Many nonossifying fibromas are asymptomatic and are discovered incidentally on radiographs taken for other lesions. Undoubtedly, many are never diagnosed. Large nonossifying fibromas may cause pain, and some present with pathologic fracture. Symptoms, when present, usually develop when patients are in their midteens. The development of a nonossifying fibroma before age 5 is rare. Occasionally, patients have multiple nonossifying fibromas in the same bone. A syndrome of nonossifying fibromas in multiple bones and café-au-lait spots on the skin is known as the Jaffe–Campanacci syndrome.

RADIOLOGIC FEATURES

Nonossifying fibromas are lytic metaphyseal lesions. Characteristically, lesions are eccentric in the medullary canal and are juxtaposed to one cortex. In addition, the margins are scalloped, and a sclerotic rim is present (Figure 16-1). Nonossifying fibromas in older patients often have intralesional radiodensity, a manifestation of healing (Figure 16-2). Small lesions, from 1 to 2 cm, are regarded as fibrous cortical defects (Figure 16-3). Alternatively, some lesions reach 7 cm in maximum diameter and cause cortical expansion, and some present with pathologic fracture (Figure 16-4).

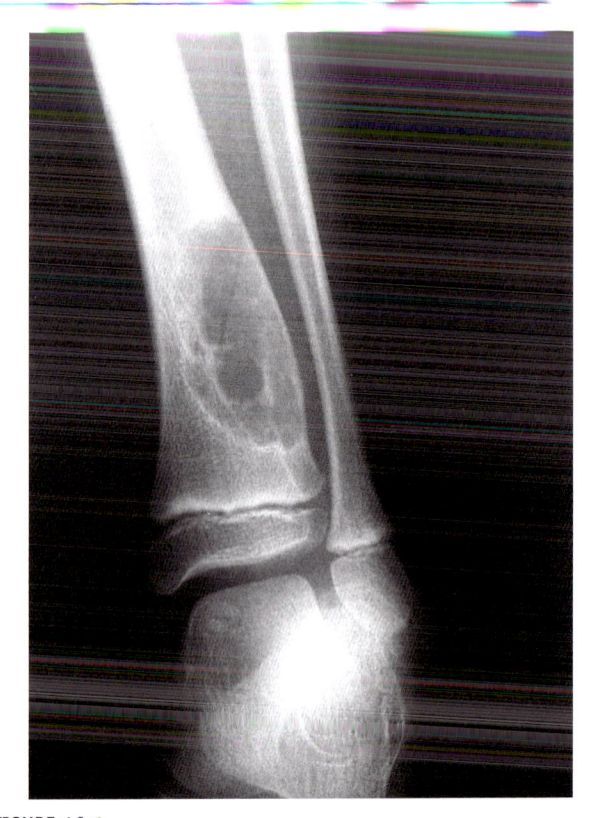

FIGURE 16-1
Nonossifying fibroma: radiographic appearance.
Lesions show a well-defined lytic area in the metaphyseal portion of a long bone. A sclerotic rim is present, and the lesion is based on the cortex.

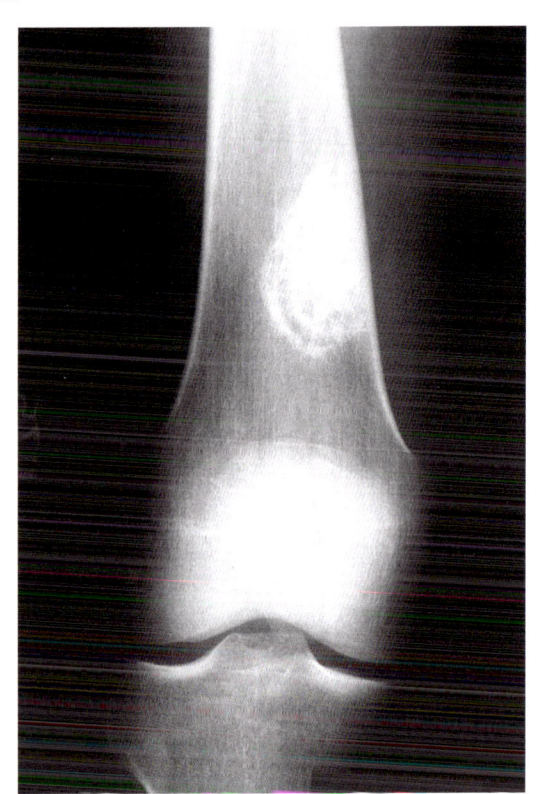

FIGURE 16-2
Nonossifying fibroma: radiographic appearance.
Lesions in older patients show features of healing. Well-defined radiodensity is in the metaphysis adjacent to the cortex.

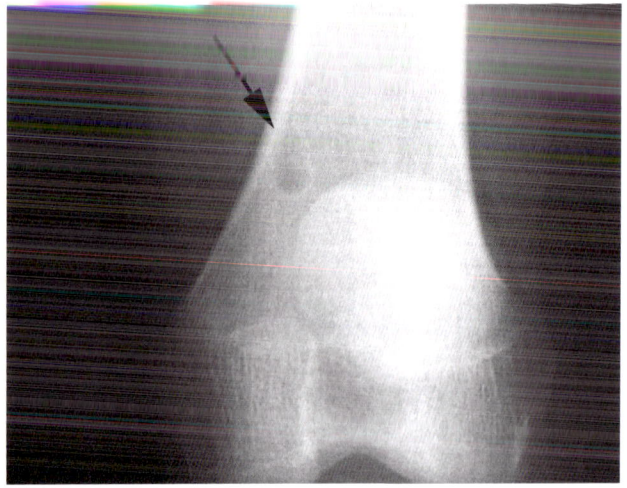

FIGURE 16-3
Nonossifying fibroma: radiographic appearance.
Small radiolytic lesions in the metaphysis are known as fibrous cortical defects *(arrow)*.

Pathologic Features

Gross Findings

Curettings from a nonossifying fibroma are portions of friable, yellow–brown soft tissue.

Microscopic Findings

Nonossifying fibromas consist of a spindle cell stroma with scattered small multinucleated giant cells, although the giant cells may be scarce. Characteristically, the spindle cells are arranged in a whorled or storiform pattern (Figure 16-5). Occasionally, the stroma is cellular, and the spindle cells often have plump uniform nuclei (Figure 16-6). In some larger lesions, a moderate number of typical mitotic figures are present. In addition to the giant cells and the stromal cells, foam cells and occasional hemosiderin-laden macrophages are present (Figure 16-7). Reactive bone is common, especially in older lesions.

Differential Diagnosis

Because nonossifying fibromas consist of spindle cells admixed with many giant cells, giant cell tumor of bone may be considered as a diagnosis. However, giant cell tumor of bone always involves both the epiphyseal and metaphyseal portions of a bone, whereas nonossifying fibromas are confined to the metaphases.

The fibrous stroma of a nonossifying fibroma frequently contains reactive new bone. This combination of new bone and a fibrous stroma may lead to the misdiagnosis of fibrous dysplasia. However, the radiographic pattern of nonossifying fibroma is characteristically an

CHAPTER 16 Fibroblastic and Fibrohistiocytic Tumors

NONOSSIFYING FIBROMA—FACT SHEET

Definition
- Nonossifying fibromas are benign spindle cell proliferations that occur in the metaphyseal portion of long bones

Incidence and location
- 80% of lesions occur in the distal femur or proximal tibia; the exact incidence is unknown, but they are relatively common

Morbidity and Mortality
- Occasionally, lesions present with pathologic fracture

Sex, Race, and Age Distribution
- Lesions form in childhood during skeletal growth

Clinical Features
- Most lesions are asymptomatic; rarely, larger lesions cause pain
- Lesions may present with pathologic fracture

Radiologic Features
- A well-defined eccentric lytic lesion in the metaphyseal portion of a long bone
- A sclerotic rim is present

Prognosis and Treatment
- Most lesions can be left untreated. Larger lesions or lesions with pathologic fracture may need to be curetted

NONOSSIFYING FIBROMA—PATHOLOGIC FEATURES

Gross Findings
- Lesions consist of friable, yellow-brown tissue

Microscopic Findings
- Cellular but uniform spindle cells arranged in a storiform pattern; often, multinucleated giant cells, foam cells, and hemosiderin-laden macrophages are present

Differential Diagnosis
- Giant cell tumor
- Malignant fibrous histiocytoma
- Fibrous dysplasia

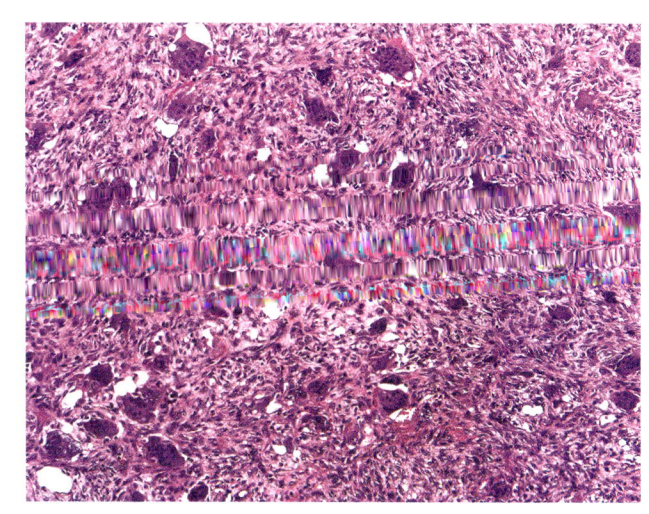

FIGURE 16-5
Nonossifying fibroma: histologic appearance
Low-power view photomicrograph showing bland spindle cells admixed with multinucleated giant cells. The spindle cells assume a storiform pattern.

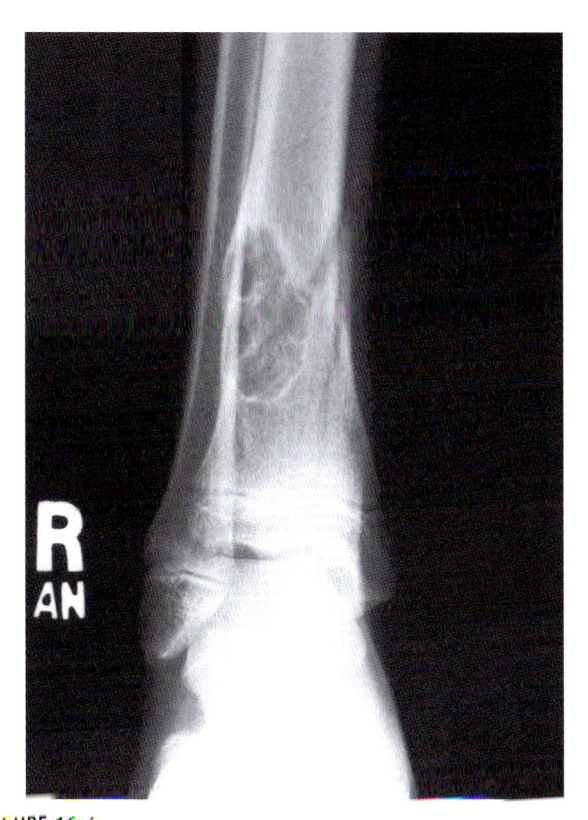

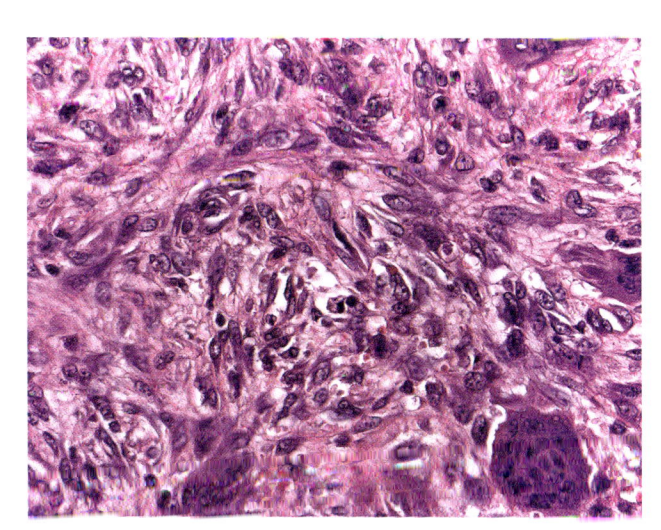

FIGURE 16-4
Nonossifying fibroma: radiographic appearance.
Lesions may occasionally present with a pathologic fracture.

FIGURE 16-6
Nonossifying fibroma: histologic features.
The spindle cells are often numerous and contain plump vesicular nuclei.

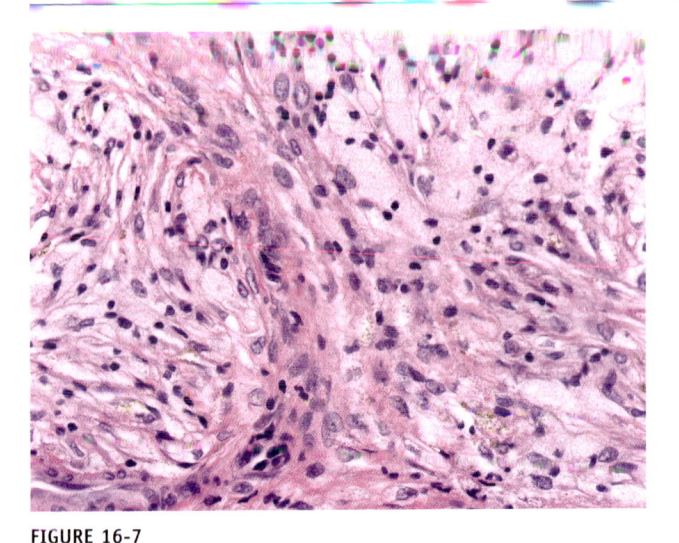

FIGURE 16-7
Nonossifying fibroma: histologic appearance.
Lesions often contain large numbers of hemosiderin-laden macrophages and foam cells. These features have led some pathologists to the name *fibroxanthoma*.

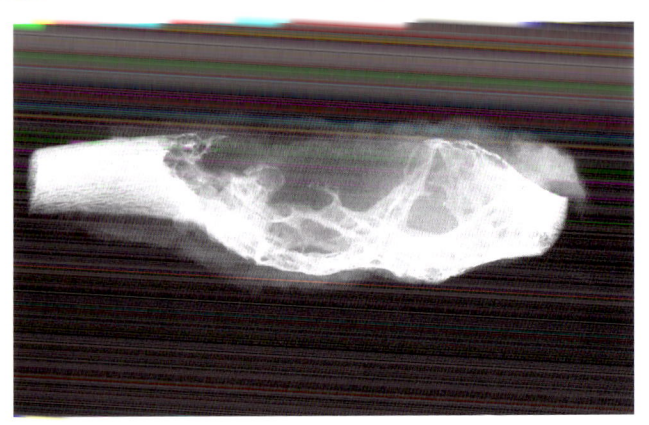

FIGURE 16-8
Desmoplastic fibroma of bone: radiographic appearance.
This specimen radiograph of a lesion in a rib shows a multicystic, expansile pattern.

eccentric lucency with a sclerotic rim, a pattern almost never seen in fibrous dysplasia.

Some nonossifying fibromas may show extreme cellularity and contain numerous mitotic figures. These features may lead to the misdiagnosis of a malignant fibrous histiocytoma. However, nuclear pleomorphism and atypical mitotic figures are never present in a nonossifying fibroma. Moreover, the radiographic features are those of a benign, well-circumscribed lesion with a sclerotic rim, features not seen in malignant neoplasms.

PROGNOSIS AND TREATMENT

Nonossifying fibromas are self-limited lesions. Although a rare lesion may reach 7 cm in maximum diameter, lesions are usually from 2 to 4 cm. Small, asymptomatic, nonossifying fibromas need no therapy; most heal spontaneously over several years. Larger lesions, particularly those that expand the cortex or those that present with pathologic fracture, should be treated with curettage and bone grafting. Recurrence after treatment is rare. Because nonossifying fibromas are almost never discovered in older adults, asymptomatic lesions must have healed spontaneously.

DESMOPLASTIC FIBROMA

Desmoplastic fibroma is an extremely rare bone tumor. This lesion is the interosseous counterpart of soft tissue fibromatosis. Like fibromatosis of soft tissue, desmoplastic fibroma of bone does not metastasize. However, it is extremely aggressive locally, and incomplete removal often leads to a recurrence.

CLINICAL FEATURES

Desmoplastic fibroma has occurred in patients between ages 20 months and 60 years. However, most lesions occur in adolescents and young adults, the peak incidence being between ages 15 and 25 years. Patients have pain, often for several years, which suggests slow growth. On rare occasions, a desmoplastic fibroma may be an incidental finding. Any bone may be affected by desmoplastic fibroma. However, most lesions occur in the long bones, particularly the distal femur and proximal tibia. The pelvis is frequently involved. Desmoplastic fibroma also shows a predilection for the mandible.

RADIOLOGIC FEATURES

Desmoplastic fibromas are radiolytic lesions that characteristically show a multicystic, expansile pattern (Figure 16-8). Lesions are usually well defined and often have a bubbly appearance (Figure 16-9). When they occur in a long bone, they are centered in the metaphysis (Figure 16-10). Occasionally, the epiphyseal portion may also be involved. The cortex is often focally destroyed, and a soft tissue mass, best visualized on magnetic resonance imaging (MRI), may be present. Twelve percent of patients present with pathologic fracture. A helpful clue to the diagnosis of desmoplastic fibroma on MRI is that most lesions have a low to intermediate signal on T2-weighted images.

CHAPTER 16 Fibroblastic and Fibrohistiocytic Tumors

FIGURE 16-9
Desmoplastic fibroma of bone: radiographic appearance.
This lesion in the calcaneus shows a well-defined, bubbly area of bone destruction.

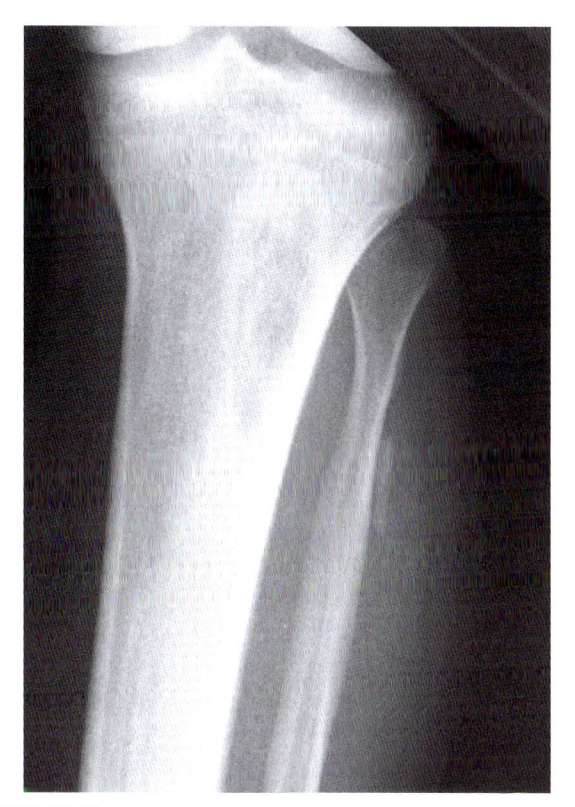

FIGURE 16-10
Desmoplastic fibroma of bone: radiographic appearance.
This lesion in the proximal tibia is well-defined and involves the metaphyseal portion of bone.

DESMOPLASTIC FIBROMA—FACT SHEET

Definition
- Desmoplastic fibroma of bone is a benign but locally aggressive interosseous proliferation of fibroblasts; it is the intraosseous equivalent to soft tissue fibromatosis

Incidence and Location
- Desmoplastic fibroma is rare; it most commonly occurs in the long bones; the mandible is also a frequently involved site

Morbidity and Mortality
- Desmoplastic fibroma is a benign tumor; morbidity results from local recurrence of incompletely removed lesions

Sex, Race, and Age Distribution
- Desmoplastic fibroma usually occurs in adolescents and young adults; however, cases have been reported between the ages of 20 months and 60 years

Clinical Features
- Pain is the most frequent presenting complaint; often, the pain has been present for many years

Radiologic Features
- Lesions are lytic with a multicystic appearance; the tumor is often in longest; with MRI, lesions are low to intermediate signal on T2 weighted images

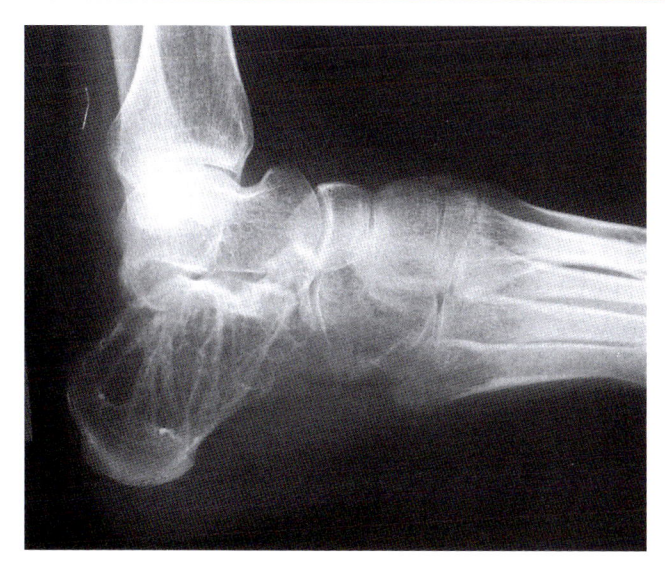

Prognosis and Treatment
- Resection with clear margins is the treatment of choice; a curettage results in a recurrence rate of 50%

DESMOPLASTIC FIBROMA—PATHOLOGIC FEATURES

Gross Findings
- Lesions are shiny, gray, firm tissue that range from 3 to 10 cm in maximum diameter

Microscopic Findings
- Bland spindle-shaped fibroblasts in a collagenized extracellular matrix; atypia is absent, and mitotic figures are rare

Immunohistochemical Features
- Vimentin stains are usually positive

Differential Diagnosis
- Low-grade fibrosarcoma
- Fibrous dysplasia
- Nonossifying fibroma

PATHOLOGIC FEATURES

GROSS FINDINGS

Desmoplastic fibromas are extremely dense fibrous lesions. They are gray-white and range in size from 3 to 10 cm, although lesions as large as 20 cm have been reported.

MICROSCOPIC FINDINGS

Desmoplastic fibromas are histologically identical to the fibromatoses of soft tissue. They show a patternless proliferation of benign-appearing myofibroblasts with a densely collagenized stroma (Figure 16-11). The fibroblasts have bland, oval, or elongated nuclei,

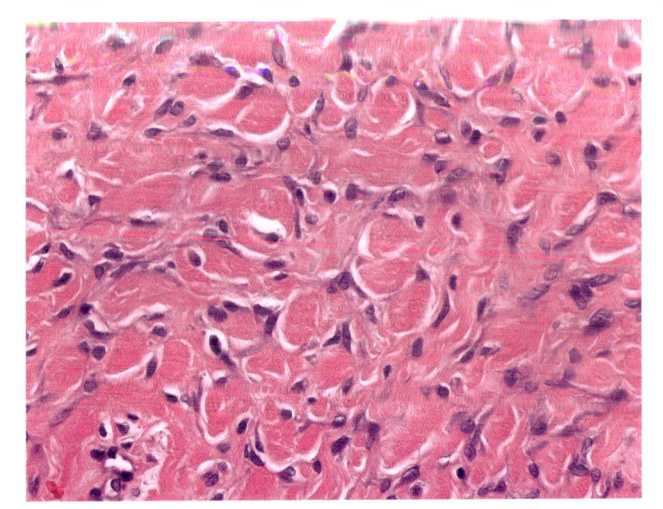

FIGURE 16-11
Desmoplastic fibroma of bone: histologic features. Bland spindle cells are present in a heavy collagenized matrix.

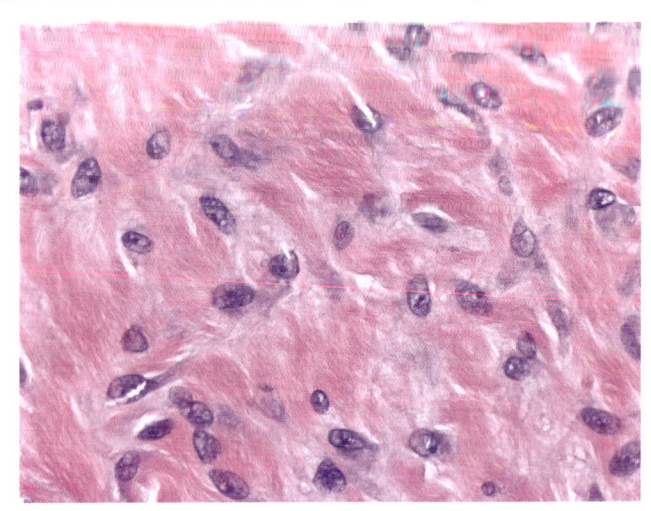

FIGURE 16-12
Desmoplastic fibroma of bone: histologic features. The spindle cells show no atypia, and mitotic figures are extremely rare.

usually without a nucleolus (Figure 16-12). Mitotic figures are rare. The fibroblastic proliferation has an infiltrative growth pattern, often entrapping native trabeculae.

ANCILLARY STUDIES

IMMUNOHISTOCHEMISTRY

Immunohistochemistry is not helpful in the diagnosis of desmoplastic fibroma of bone. Lesions are usually positive for vimentin and negative for other markers. This finding is nonspecific and nondiagnostic.

DIFFERENTIAL DIAGNOSIS

Desmoplastic fibroma of bone may be extremely difficult to distinguish from low-grade fibrosarcoma of bone. Fibrosarcoma, however, will have cellular atypia, occasional mitotic figures, and a "herringbone" arrangement of cells.

Lesions of fibrous dysplasia that show little woven bone may also be confused with desmoplastic fibroma. However, careful attention to radiographic features typical of fibrous dysplasia, as well as thoroughly searching the neoplastic tissue for woven bone, will help diagnose fibrous dysplasia.

Desmoplastic fibroma may also be misdiagnosed as a nonossifying fibroma. However, the radiographic features of nonossifying fibroma are characteristic. Lesions are well demarcated with a sclerotic rim and based on the cortex. By contrast, desmoplastic fibroma has an expansile destructive pattern. In addition, nonossifying fibroma has a storiform pattern of spindle cells admixed with multinucleated giant cells and foam cells pattern. These features are not present in desmoplastic fibroma.

PROGNOSIS AND TREATMENT

Wide local excision with tumor-free margins is the treatment of choice for desmoplastic fibroma. A simple curettage has a recurrence rate of close to 50%. Patients with huge lesions or patients who have had recurrences may require an amputation. Desmoplastic fibroma does not metastasize.

FIBROSARCOMA OF BONE

Fibrosarcoma of bone is a spindle cell neoplasm that is usually of low- to intermediate-grade malignancy. Since the 1970s, when the concept of malignant fibrous histiocytoma was formulated, the diagnosis of fibrosarcoma in bone has become rare. This is because lesions formally classified as high-grade spindle cell neoplasms are now regarded as malignant fibrous histiocytomas or fibroblastic osteosarcomas.

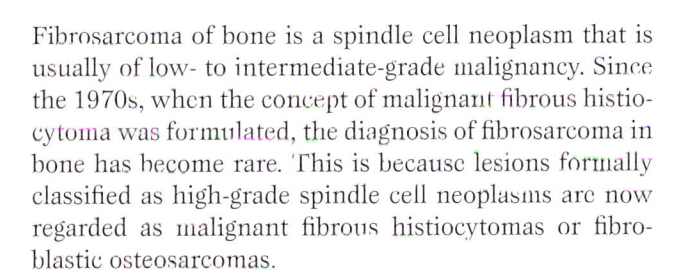

CLINICAL FEATURES

Although rare cases of fibrosarcoma of bone have been reported in infancy, this neoplasm usually occurs in adults, the peak incidence being in the fifth decade of life. Patients have pain, usually long standing, or they

CHAPTER 16 Fibroblastic and Fibrohistiocytic Tumors

FIBROSARCOMA OF BONE—FACT SHEET

Definition
- Spindle cell neoplasm of low- to intermediate-grade malignancy

Incident and Location
- Fibrosarcoma of bone is rare; most commonly, lesions affect the distal femur and proximal tibia

Sex, Race, and Age Distribution
- Most patients are adults, the peak incidence being between ages 40 and 50

Clinical Features
- Patients present with pain

Radiologic Features
- Lesions are poorly defined radiolytic lesions, often with a permeative pattern of bone destruction; a soft tissue mass may also be present

Prognosis and Treatment
- Treatment is surgical ablation with disease-free margins; low-grade fibrosarcomas have a 10-year survival rate of 80%; high-grade lesions have a lower survival rate

FIBROSARCOMA OF BONE—PATHOLOGIC FEATURES

Gross Findings
- Shiny, white, firm soft tissue replacing bone

Microscopic Findings
- Cellular spindle cell neoplasm with mild nuclear atypia
- Spindle cells are arranged in a "herringbone" pattern
- Varying amount of collagen may be present

Immunohistochemical Features
- Lesions are positive for vimentin
- A few tumor cells may be weakly positive with smooth muscle actin

Differential Diagnosis
- Desmoplastic fibroma
- Malignant fibrous histiocytoma

---

may present with pathologic fracture. This neoplasm usually occurs in the long bones, and more than half the cases occur in either the distal femur or proximal tibia.

RADIOLOGIC FEATURES

Fibrosarcomas are poorly defined radiolucent lesions (Figure 16-13). The lytic process typically involves the central portion of the medullary canal, although occasional lesions may be centered on the cortex (Figure 16-14) and have a significant soft tissue mass. Many lesions have a permeative or "moth-eaten" pattern of bone destruction. Pathologic fracture may be present.

PATHOLOGIC FEATURES

GROSS FINDINGS

Fibrosarcoma of bone is a firm, white soft tissue mass that shows extensive replacement of the cancellous and cortical bone.

MICROSCOPIC FINDINGS

Fibrosarcoma of bone is composed of spindle cells arranged in a fascicular or "herringbone" pattern (Figure 16-15). In low-grade tumors, the spindle cells are uniform and mild-to-moderate nuclear atypia is present (Figure 16-16). High-grade tumors are highly cellular and contain obvious cytologic atypia with numerous mitotic figures. Some lesions have large amounts of extracellular collagen (Figure 16-17). Occasionally lesions have a myxoid appearance.

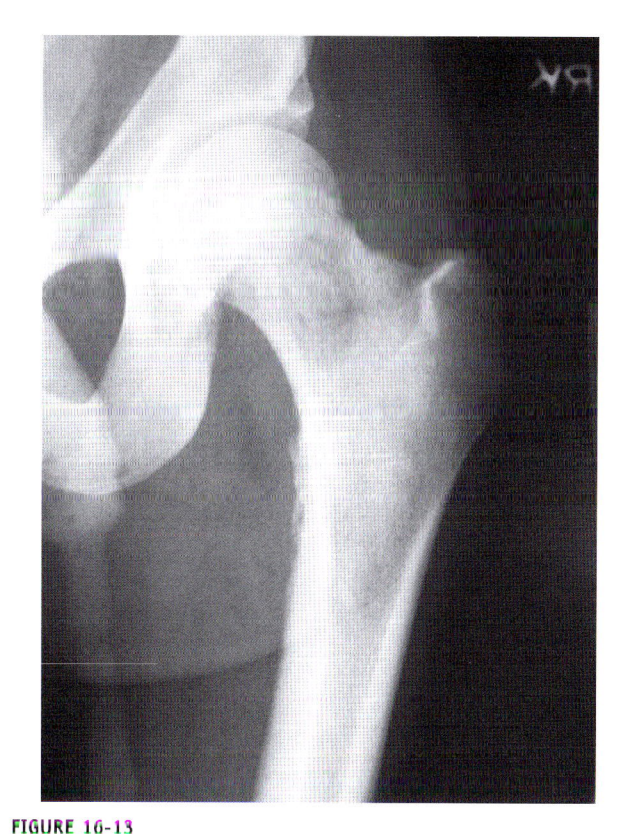

FIGURE 16-13
Fibrosarcoma of bone: radiographic features.
This fibrosarcoma in the neck of the femur exhibits a poorly defined area of bone destruction.

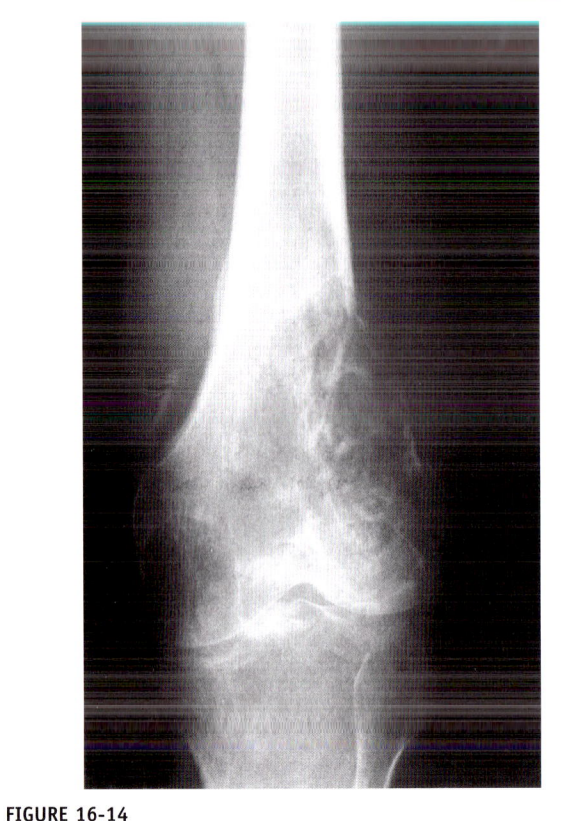

FIGURE 16-14
Fibrosarcoma of bone: radiographic features.
This fibrosarcoma in the distal femur shows a poorly defined lytic lesion centered on the cortex with an associated soft tissue mass.

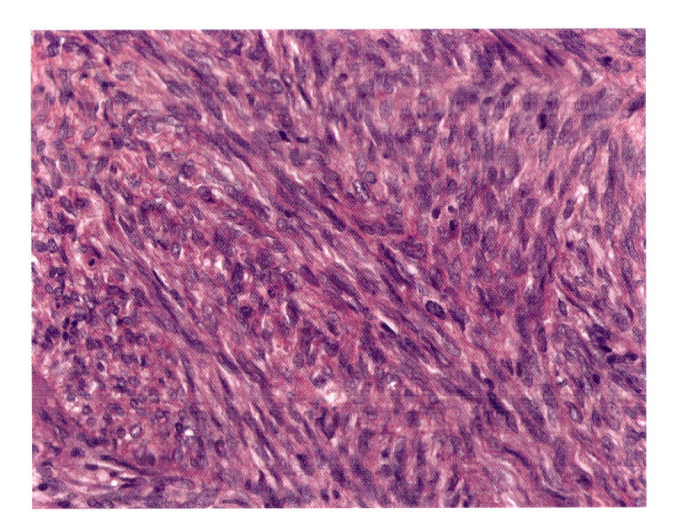

FIGURE 16-15
Fibrosarcoma of bone: histologic features.
Lesions consist of a cellular population of spindle cells that often assumes a "herringbone" pattern.

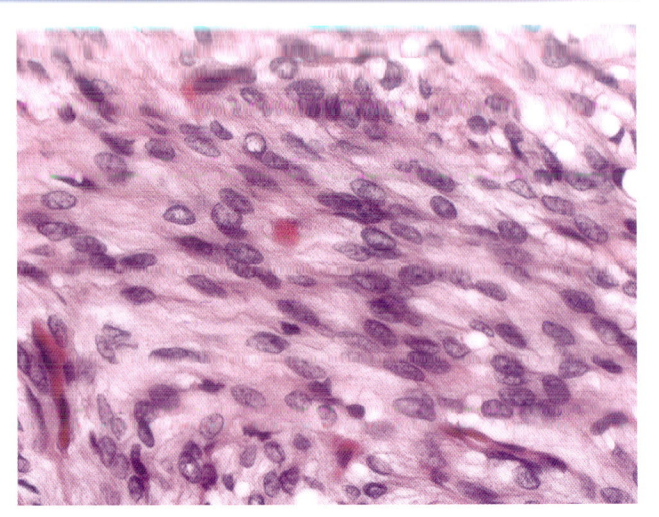

FIGURE 16-16
Fibrosarcoma of bone: histologic features.
The spindle cells usually show mild nuclear atypia.

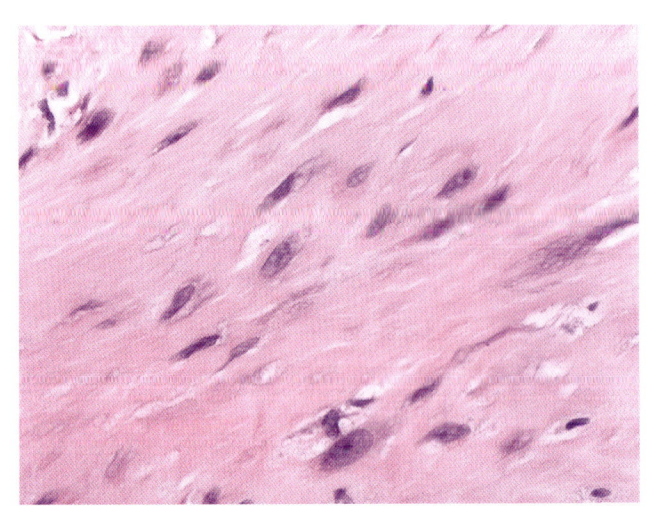

FIGURE 16-17
Fibrosarcoma of bone: histologic features.
Some low-grade lesions are heavily collagenized. The spindle cells, however, show some mild nuclear atypia.

ANCILLARY STUDIES

IMMUNOHISTOCHEMISTRY

Fibrosarcoma of bone is positive for vimentin. These tumors typically are also mildly or focally positive with smooth muscle actin.

DIFFERENTIAL DIAGNOSIS

Histologically, a low-grade fibrosarcoma may be difficult to distinguish from a desmoplastic fibroma. However, two important histologic differences exist. First, unlike the spindle cells of a desmoplastic fibroma, which are haphazardly arranged, the spindle cells of fibrosarcoma are usually arranged in bundles. Sometimes the bundles interlace to form the "herringbone" pattern. Second, fibrosarcoma of bone has mild-to-moderate nuclear atypia, a feature that is missing in desmoplastic fibroma.

High-grade fibrosarcoma of bone may also be confused with malignant fibrous histiocytoma. However, malignant fibrous histiocytoma generally contains a storiform, rather than a herringbone, pattern and more nuclear pleomorphic. A diagnosis of fibroblastic osteosarcoma should be made whenever any amount of osteoid production is identified.

PROGNOSIS AND TREATMENT

Fibrosarcoma of bone is treated with ablative surgery. Chemotherapy may also be considered for high-grade tumors.

Prognosis depends on histologic grade. Low-grade (grade 1) lesions have a 10-year survival rate of about 80%. In higher-grade tumors, the survival approaches that of malignant fibrous histiocytoma. These higher-grade fibrosarcomas may have a 10-year survival closer to 34%.

FIBROHISTIOCYTIC LESIONS

BENIGN FIBROUS HISTIOCYTOMA OF BONE

Some pathologists recognize an entity called *benign fibrous histiocytoma of bone*. This lesion is histologically characterized by a storiform arrangement of spindle cells, scattered foam cells, and giant cells. When a lesion of this histologic pattern is seen in the metaphysis, it is more properly regarded as a nonossifying fibroma. The term *benign fibrous histiocytoma* should be used for tumors with similar histologic features that occur in other locations, such as the flat bones and vertebrae. In the epiphysis, where most cases have been reported, this histologic pattern most probably represents involutional change in a conventional giant cell tumor.

MALIGNANT FIBROUS HISTIOCYTOMA OF BONE

The concept of malignant fibrous histiocytoma was formulated in the 1960s to describe a pleomorphic spindle cell sarcoma with a storiform pattern. This neoplasm was believed to be a proliferation of facultative fibroblasts that could either have a spindle cell or histiocytic morphology. This sarcoma could be primary in any organ, including bone.

With the increasing use of immunohistochemical stains, the idea of malignant fibrous histiocytoma has become blurred. Lesions may exhibit a wide variety of antigens, including actin, desmin, S-100, epithelial membrane antigen (EMA), and even keratin. This finding has led some pathologists to postulate that malignant fibrous histiocytoma should not be regarded as a distinct entity. However, a large proportion of these neoplasms lack these specific immunohistochemical markers, and because they usually have a significant population of spindle cells, they may be regarded as pleomorphic fibrosarcomas. In addition, many contain desmin and may be regarded as pleomorphic myofibroblastic sarcomas. Alternatively, this entity may be thought of as undifferentiated sarcoma, the connective tissue counterpart of undifferentiated carcinomas of parenchymal organs. For convenience, however, we will continue to regard this neoplasm as a malignant fibrous histiocytoma in this chapter.

CLINICAL FEATURES

Malignant fibrous histiocytoma may occur in bone as a primary lesion. However, it can also arise secondarily in preexisting osseous lesions such as radiation damage, Paget disease, and cartilaginous neoplasms. In addition, malignant fibrous histiocytoma may, on rare occasions, occur as a complication of a bone infarct.

Primary malignant fibrous histiocytoma may involve any bone. However, the femur is the most common site (one-third of cases), followed by the tibia and humerus. Patients range in age from 6 to 81 years, but more than 50% of cases occur in patients older than 40 years. Patients present with pain, and 67% have swelling or a mass. Some patients have a pathologic fracture.

RADIOLOGIC FEATURES

Malignant fibrous histiocytomas are poorly circumscribed lytic lesions (Figure 16-18). Often, a permeative or moth-eaten pattern of bone destruction is present. Destruction of the cortex is common. Most commonly, malignant fibrous histiocytoma involves the metaphyseal portion of bone. However, secondary involvement of the epiphysis is common. A periosteal new bone reaction is usually absent, and no evidence of matrix mineralization exists. An MRI scan shows a high signal on T2-weighted images, and often an adjacent soft tissue mass is apparent. Because malignant fibrous histiocytoma is a complication of preexisting bone diseases, radiographic evidence of Paget disease, radiation osteodysplasia, and a cartilaginous lesion may be adjacent to or within the lytic lesion.

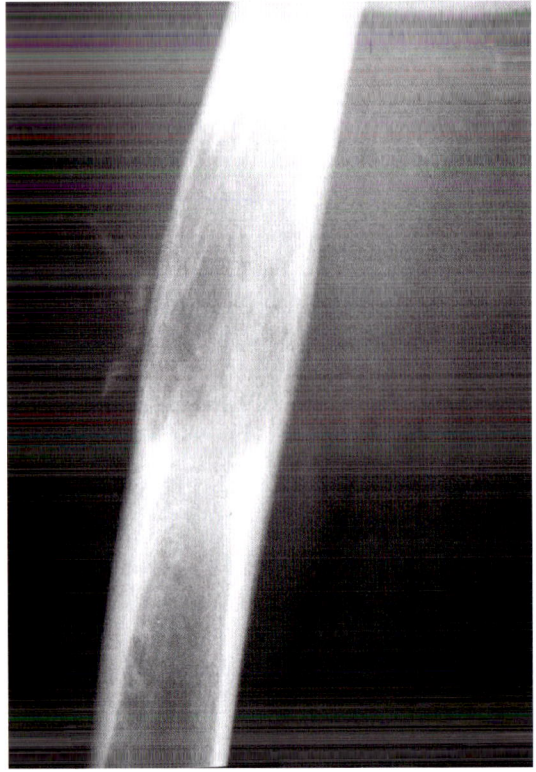

FIGURE 16-18
Malignant fibrous histiocytoma: Radiographic features.
Lesions are poorly defined areas of radiolucency. Often a "moth-eaten" pattern is present.

FIGURE 16-19
Malignant fibrous histiocytoma: histologic features.
Most commonly, lesions show pleomorphic, spindle cells in a storiform pattern.

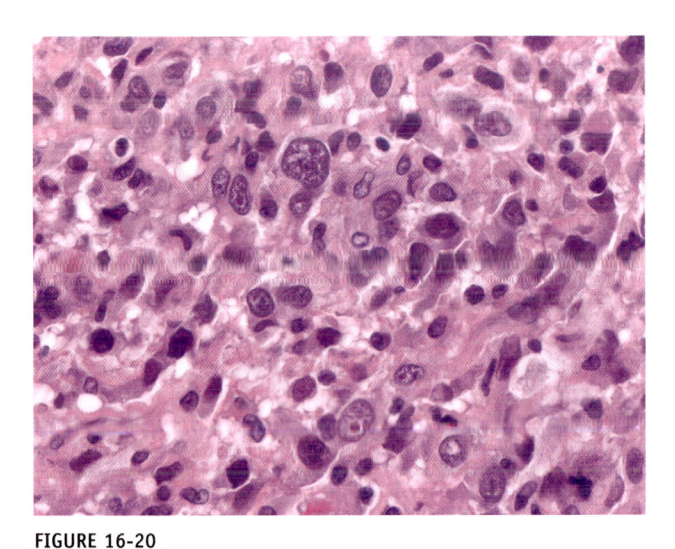

FIGURE 16-20
Malignant fibrous histiocytoma: histologic features.
Other lesions show a predominately histiocytic-like pattern with bizarre round cells and highly pleomorphic nuclei.

PATHOLOGIC FEATURES

GROSS FINDINGS

Malignant fibrous histiocytoma is a pink–tan, fleshy, soft tissue. Frequently, large areas of necrosis are present.

MICROSCOPIC FINDINGS

Malignant fibrous histiocytoma is composed of spindle cells, rounded histiocyte-like cells, or a combination of the two in varying proportions. The spindle cells are arranged in a storiform pattern, the most characteristic feature of malignant fibrous histiocytoma (Figure 16-19). The nuclei are oval and fascicular, with mild-to-moderate pleomorphism. Occasionally, broad bands of osteoid-like collagens separate the stroma cells, a feature that may lead to the misdiagnosis of osteosarcoma. In contrast with the spindle cell/storiform pattern, some malignant fibrous histiocytomas exhibit a histiocyte-like differentiation (Figure 16-20). The cells of these tumors are rounded and have a large oval or lobulated nucleus, often with a prominent eosinophilic nucleolus. Some of the histiocytic cells contain hemosiderin or lipid, an expression of histiocyte-like activity. Large, bizarre, multinucleated giant cells may also be present.

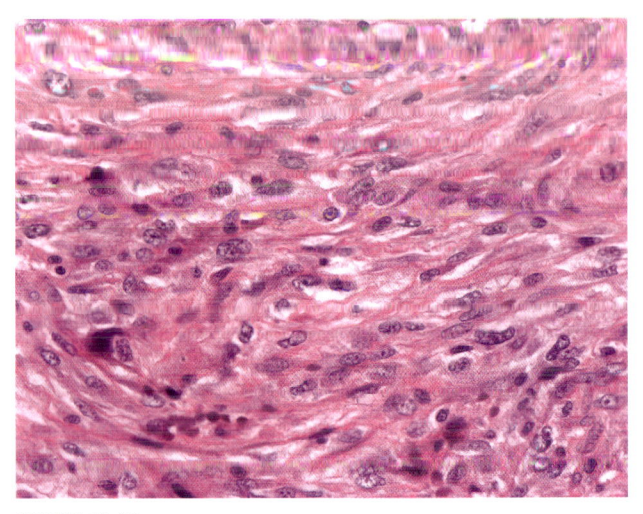

Malignant fibrous histiocytomas may have a variety of secondary histopathologic features. First, some may have a heavy inflammatory cell infiltrate, a feature that may lead to the misdiagnosis of Hodgkin's disease. Second, large areas of myxoid stroma may be present, a change that is also seen in malignant fibrous histiocytomas of soft tissue (Figure 16-21). Some have a collagenized stroma. Finally, neoplastic cells may be arranged in an organoid pattern around branching of vascular spaces, a pattern reminiscent of hemangiopericytoma. As in analyzing the radiographs, histologic evaluation should include the search for underlying pre-existing bone diseases such as Paget disease and radiation osteodysplasia.

CHAPTER 16 Fibroblastic and Fibrohistiocytic Tumors

MALIGNANT FIBROUS HISTIOCYTOMA OF BONE—FACT SHEET

Definition
▸▸ A high-grade, pleomorphic spindle cell sarcoma with a storiform pattern; matrix calcification or ossification is not present

Incident and Location
▸▸ Malignant fibrous histiocytoma usually involves the appendicular skeleton, most commonly the femur; the humerus and tibia are also frequent sites of involvement

Morbidity and Mortality
▸▸ Patients usually require ablative surgery

Sex, Race, and Age Distribution
▸▸ Patients range from age 6 to 80 years; however, 50% of cases occur in patients older than 40

Clinical Features
▸▸ Patients most commonly present with pain and swelling; a pathologic fracture sometimes occurs

Radiologic Features
▸▸ Lesions are poorly circumscribed lytic lesions with a permeative pattern of bone destruction; the cortex is frequently destroyed

Prognosis and Treatment
▸▸ Patients usually undergo surgical ablation with disease-free margins; chemotherapy is often a helpful adjuvant; the 5-year survival rate is 34% to 50%

MALIGNANT FIBROUS HISTIOCYTOMA OF BONE—PATHOLOGIC FEATURES

Gross Findings
▸▸ Lesions consist of gray–tan, fleshy, soft tissue; necrosis is frequent

Microscopic Findings
▸▸ Cells have either a spindle cell or histiocyte-like morphology, or they may have a mixture of both; the spindle cells are elongated pleomorphic cells that assume a storiform pattern; the histiocyte-like cells are large, bizarre, rounded cells; multinucleated giant cells are often present

Immunohistochemical Features
▸▸ Vimentin is almost always positive; occasional lesions will be positive for S-100, smooth muscle markers, keratin, and EMA

ANCILLARY STUDIES

IMMUNOHISTOCHEMISTRY

The immunohistochemical profile of malignant fibrous histiocytomas is varied. Most commonly, the cells are positive only with vimentin, a nonspecific marker. Lesions with significant histiocyte-like differentiation may be positive with antitrypsin or antichymotrypsin stains. In addition, occasional malignant fibrous histiocytomas will exhibit muscle markers such as desmin or smooth muscle actin. Also, S-100 may be positive occasionally. Keratin stains and stains for EMA may be focally positive.

DIFFERENTIAL DIAGNOSIS

In patients older than 40 years, malignant fibrous histiocytoma must be distinguished from metastatic carcinoma with a sarcomatoid growth pattern, particularly sarcomatoid renal cell carcinoma. Most sarcomatoid renal cell carcinomas will have more extensive keratin immunoreactivity than seen in malignant fibrous histiocytoma. Rarely, malignant fibrous histiocytoma may

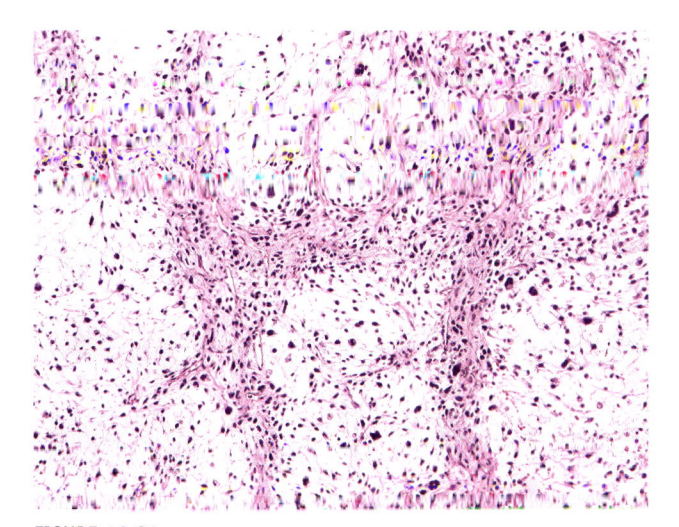

FIGURE 16-21
Malignant fibrous histiocytoma: histologic features.
Occasionally, lesions show extensive extracellular mucoid material, a pattern similar to myxoid variant of malignant fibrous histiocytoma of soft tissue.

contain some cells that are positive with keratin markers. Sometimes, the final diagnosis may require a chest and abdominal computed tomographic scan in order to rule out a primary carcinoma.

Occasionally, malignant fibrous histiocytomas will be confused with osteogenic sarcomas that have little osteoid production. This differentiation may, at times, be extremely difficult. But it may also be unnecessary because both are high-grade lesions that require the same treatment and have the same prognosis. Reactive bone formation is sometimes present in malignant fibrous histiocytomas, but this bone has a zonal pattern. To be regarded as a true malignant fibrous histiocytoma, tumor osteoid production must be absent.

Prognosis and Treatment

Malignant fibrous histiocytoma is best treated by wide surgical excision. A high risk for local failure exists unless the entire tumor and a cuff of normal tissue are removed. Sometimes amputation may be necessary to remove the whole lesion. Pulmonary metastasis developed in 30% to 40% of patients. The 5-year survival rate of malignant fibrous histiocytoma is from 34% to 50%. Survival can be prolonged with adjuvant chemotherapy.

SUGGESTED READINGS

Nonossifying Fibroma

1. Betsy M, Kupersmith LM, Springfield DS: Metaphyseal fibrous defects. J Am Acad Orthop Surg 2004;12:89–95.
2. Levine SM, Lambiase RE, Petchprapa CN: Cortical lesions of the tibia: characteristic appearances at conventional radiography. Radiographics 2003;23:157–177.
3. Mirra JM, Gold RH, Rand F: Disseminated non ossifying fibromas in association with café-au-lait spots (Jaffe-Campanacci syndrome). Clin Orthop 1982;168:192–205.

Desmoplastic Fibroma

1. Böhm P, Kröber S, Greschniok A, et al: Desmoplastic fibroma of the bone. A report of two patients, review of the literature, and therapeutic implications. Cancer 1996;78:1011–1023.
2. Inwards CY, Unni KK, Beabout JW, et al: Desmoplastic fibroma of bone. Cancer 1991;68:1978–1983.
3. Taconis WK, Schutte HE, van der Heul RO: Desmoplastic fibroma of bone: A report of 18 cases. Skeletal Radiol 1994;23:283–288.
4. Vanhoenacker FM, Hauben E, De Beuckeleer LH, et al: Desmoplastic fibroma of bone: MRI features. Skeletal Radiol 2000;29:171–175.

Fibrosarcoma of Bone

1. Papagelopoulos PJ, Galanis E, Frassica FJ, et al: Primary fibrosarcoma of bone. Outcome after primary surgical treatment. Clin Orthop 2000;373:88–103.
2. Papagelopoulos PJ, Galanis EC, Trantafyllidis P, et al: Clinicopathologic features, diagnosis, and treatment of fibrosarcoma of bone. Am J Orthop 2002;31:253–257.
3. Smith SE, Kransdorf MJ: Primary musculoskeletal tumors of fibrous origin. Semin Musculoskelet Radiol 2000;4:73–88.

Malignant Fibrous Histiocytoma of Bone

1. Bielack SS, Schroeders A, Fuchs N, et al: Malignant fibrous histiocytoma of bone. A retrospective EMSOS study of 125 cases. Acta Orthop Scand 1999;70:353–360.
2. Link TM, Haeussler MD, Poppek S, et al: Malignant fibrous histiocytoma of bone: Conventional x-ray and MR imaging features. Skeletal Radiol 1998;27:552–558.
3. Nishida J, Sim FH, Wenger DE, et al: Malignant fibrous histiocytoma of bone. A clinicopathologic study of 81 patients. Cancer 1997;79:482–493.
4. Rosenberg AE: Malignant fibrous histiocytoma: past, present, and future. Skeletal Radiol 2003;32:613–618.

17

Ewing Sarcoma

Michael J. Klein

In 1921, James Ewing described a highly lethal, undifferentiated tumor of bone he termed *diffuse endothelioma*. The origins of this tumor were hotly debated over the next several decades by some of the world's most prominent pathologists but remained obscure. Although its origins would wait many years for clarification, Ewing sarcoma has the distinction of being the only eponymic tumor of bone without a universally accepted pathologic synonym. It is currently used to describe a tumor composed of small, round cells lacking extracellular matrix, containing variable amounts of glycogen, and showing scant evidence of neuroectodermal derivation histologically, ultrastructurally, and immunohistochemically. In 1979, a histologically similar tumor involving the thoracopulmonary region of young individuals was described by Askin and colleagues. The concept of primitive neuroectodermal tumor (PNET) of bone was introduced in 1984 by Jaffe and coworkers based on their reclassification of four Ewing sarcomas that were sparse in glycogen, contained Homer Wright rosettes, and exhibited neural differentiation in tissue culture. In the same year, the presence of a unique reciprocal translocation of the long arms of chromosomes 11 and 22 in Ewing sarcomas was independently confirmed. Whang-Peng, Triche, and Knutsen and researchers soon described the same translocation in PNET and in Askin tumors. Most pathologists now believe that based on their common cytogenetic and molecular features, Ewing sarcoma, PNET, and small-cell thoracopulmonary tumors comprise a single family of tumors that show varying degrees of neural differentiation. Those tumors at the least differentiated end of the spectrum are still classified as Ewing sarcomas; those with the most neural differentiation are referred to as PNETs.

Clinical Features

The Ewing sarcoma family is the most malignant of all primary bone tumors of childhood. At an estimated incidence of 1 case per 1.5 million individuals, Ewing sarcoma is about one-third as common as osteosarcoma, with an estimated frequency of about 200 new cases per year in a U.S.-sized population. Like most malignant bone tumors, a slight male predilection exists. It is exceptionally rare in African Americans. Although there have been cases reported in infancy and even in octogenarians, more than 80% of cases arise between the ages of 8 and 20. Ewing sarcoma tends to originate in skeletal sites populated by hematopoietic marrow, so a tendency exists for younger individuals to have more distal tumors than older individuals. It is extremely uncommon in the phalanges. When long bones are affected, the tumor tends to arise in the metadiaphyseal regions.

Patients with Ewing sarcoma have signs and symptoms that are not specific. As with any malignant bone tumor, a history of pain, often beginning as pain noticed on exertion, is usually present, and it may cause loss of normal function. The pain is usually present at rest by the time patients present, and it is sometimes severe enough to wake the patient from sleep. On physical examination, localized tenderness is demonstrable, and an associated fullness or even a mass may be present. Approximately 10% of patients present with pathologic fracture. Other clinical findings include nonspecific systemic symptoms such as intermittent low-grade fever, easy fatigability, and weight loss. Laboratory findings are nonspecific and occasionally include leukocytosis, increased erythrocyte sedimentation rate, and anemia.

Radiologic Features

The radiographic appearance of Ewing sarcoma is the result of its rapid expansion and its characteristic interaction with the host bone. The pattern of radiographic destruction associated with Ewing sarcoma is often described as permeative, implying that radiographs do not demonstrate obvious defined lesional margins. This is because Ewing sarcoma will often grow and spread within the confines of the bone at a more rapid rate than the capacity of the bone to react to the tumor. Where the lesion is oldest, there may be small, poorly delimited areas of bone destruction, but occasionally, unless a significant soft tissue mass is present, permeative lesions may be almost invisible on routine roentgenograms.

The radiodensity of bone in conventional roentgenographs is primarily dependent on the integrity of the cortex in the metadiaphysis and more on the integrity of cancellous bone in the bone ends. Replacement of the intertrabecular spaces by tumor without osseous destruction is insignificant on a routine x-ray film. This is because tumor cells, having the radiodensity of water, replace the marrow, which has the radiodensity of fat. Both radiodensities are minuscule when contained to the radiodensity of an intact cortex (Figure 17-1).

Because the tumor cells of Ewing sarcoma have the ability to percolate through the Haversian and Volkmann canals, and thereby gain access to the less confining periosteal connective tissues of the outer cortex, there is often a large soft tissue mass outside the bone even without obvious radiographic evidence of cortical destruction. Should the bulk of this mass be confined between the periosteum and the cortex, a concave pressure erosion of the cortex by osteoclasts on its outer surface will develop over time. This is sometimes referred to radiographically as cortical *saucerization* (Figure 17-2).

Alternately, and sometimes simultaneously, rapid and repeated periosteal elevation and irritation by the expanding tumor mass results in a multilayered, discontinuous periosteal reaction resembling *onion skin* (Figure 17-3). In general, the greater the discontinuity of the periosteal new bone, the more rapid is the growth of the underlying process. Less commonly, the periosteal reaction in Ewing sarcoma is vertically oriented with respect to the underlying cortex, and a discontinuous *hair-on-end* or *sunburst* periosteal reaction is generated (Figure 17-4). Finally, periosteal new bone discontinuous only at the edge of a soft tissue extension of tumor will result in an open periosteal reaction, or Codman's angle (Figure 17-5).

Complementary imaging studies are good for demonstrating the extent of osseous and soft tissue involvement in Ewing sarcoma when this is not obvious by conventional radiography. One of the best ways to accomplish this is by technetium99 radionuclide scanning. Because this technique demonstrates early osteoblast activity, reactive changes at the interface of bone and lesional tissue are demonstrable long before actual anatomic changes in the bone can be seen on a conventional roentgenogram (Figure 17-6A, B). Magnetic resonance imaging (MRI) is useful in demonstrating the extent of both intraosseous tumor and any tumor mass in the overlying soft tissues before there is any evidence of osseous abnormality on conventional radiographs (see Figure 17-6C). Computerized tomographic scanning may also be used to demonstrate the presence and extent of intramedullary and soft tissue tumor. Because computed tomography (CT) has higher resolution than MRI and is an x-ray technique, it is particularly valuable in demonstrating cortical destruction too subtle to be seen on conventional radiography

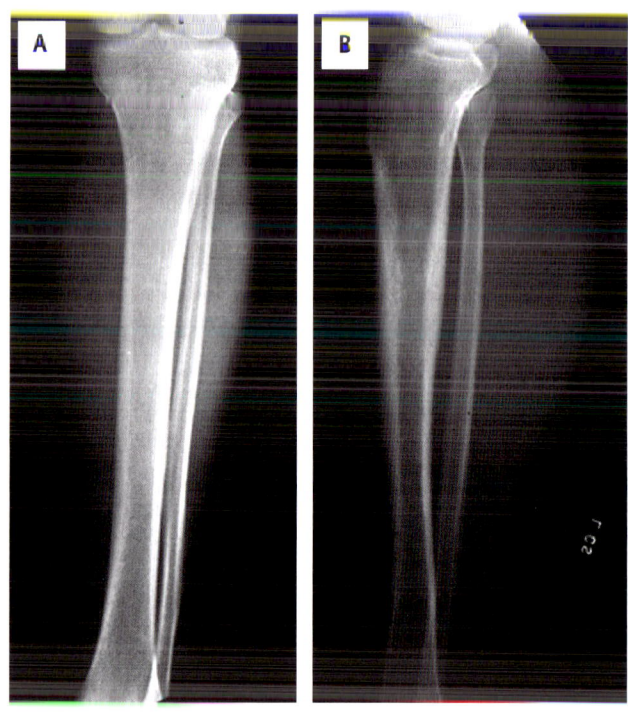

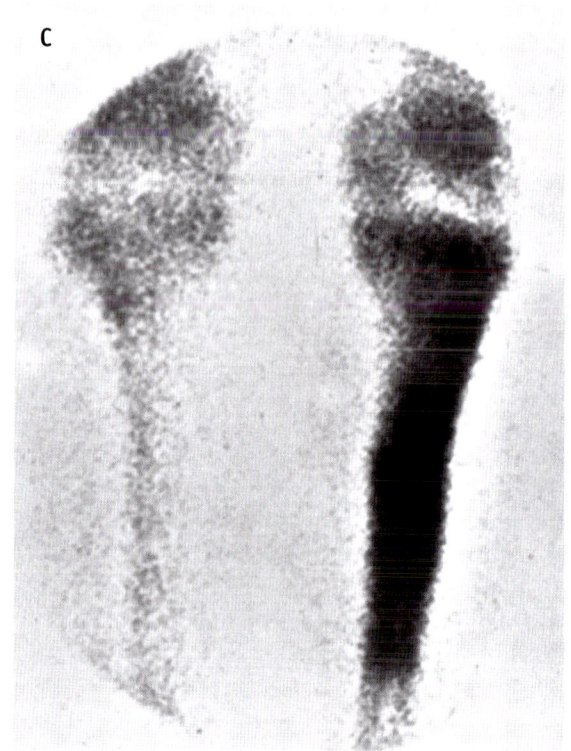

FIGURE 17-1
Ewing sarcoma.
A, B, Anteroposterior and lateral views of the left lower leg in an 18-year-old high-school football player who complained of lower leg pain persisting on exercise 3 months after football season but now present at rest. A slight increase in tibial metadiaphyseal radiodensity visible only in the lateral view is present. This is not due to the tumor permeating the medullary cavity, but because the tumor has caused the periosteum to form reactive new cortical bone. No visible soft tissue mass is present. The tumor is otherwise invisible on these conventional roentgenographs. **C,** The technetium bone scan shows markedly increased uptake from the proximal tibia to the mid-diaphysis, corresponding to the areas in which the bone reacts to the tumor. These cannot be seen in the conventional views.

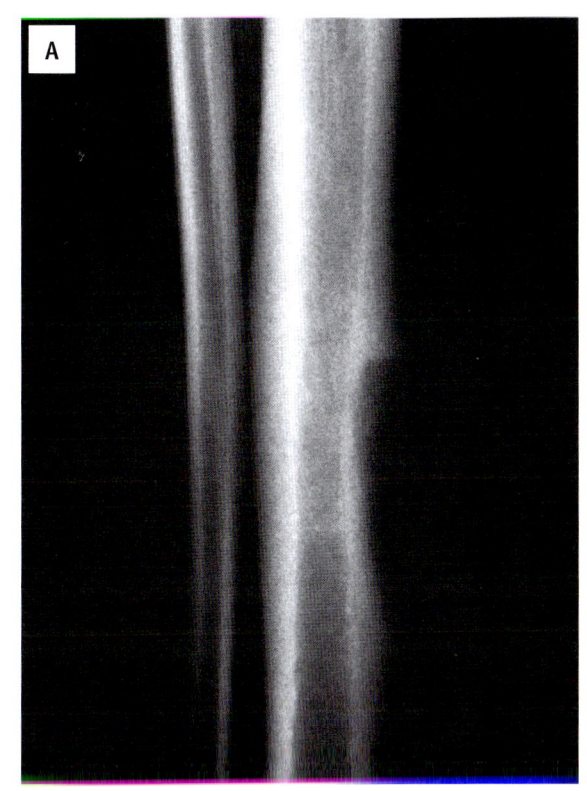

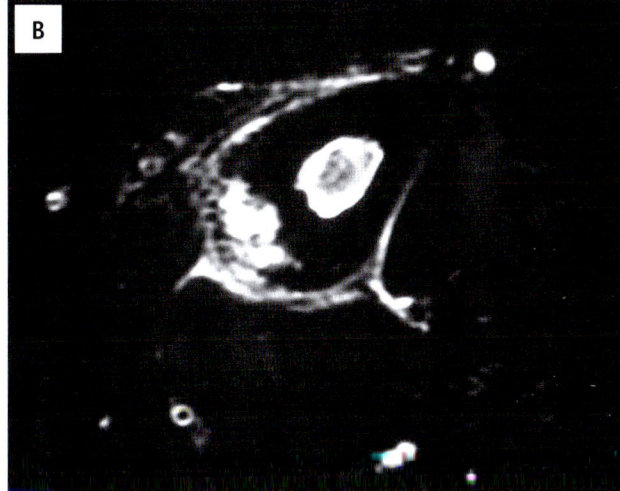

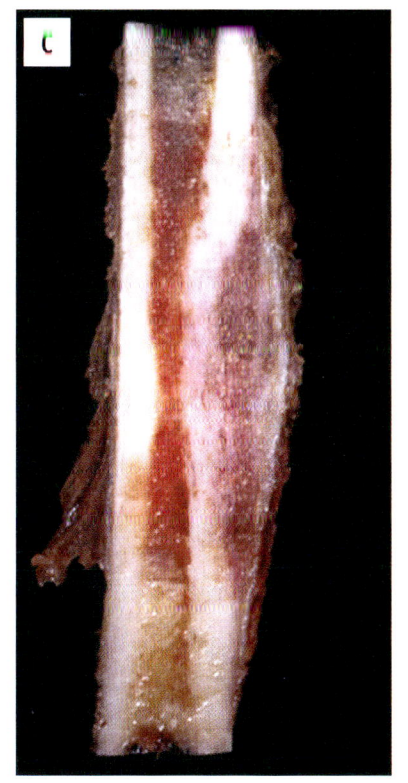

FIGURE 17-2

A, Saucerization of the tibial cortex in Ewing sarcoma. A concavity of the outer tibial cortex is present. The soft tissue mass is poorly visible, and no periosteal reaction is visible. **B,** T2-weighted magnetic resonance imaging demonstrates increased marrow signal and increased signal in extraosseous soft tissue mass with underlying pressure erosion of cortex. **C,** Resected tibial specimen demonstrating a subperiosteal mass eroding the underlying cortex. Tumor necrosis with associated organized periosteal reaction after neoadjuvant chemotherapy.

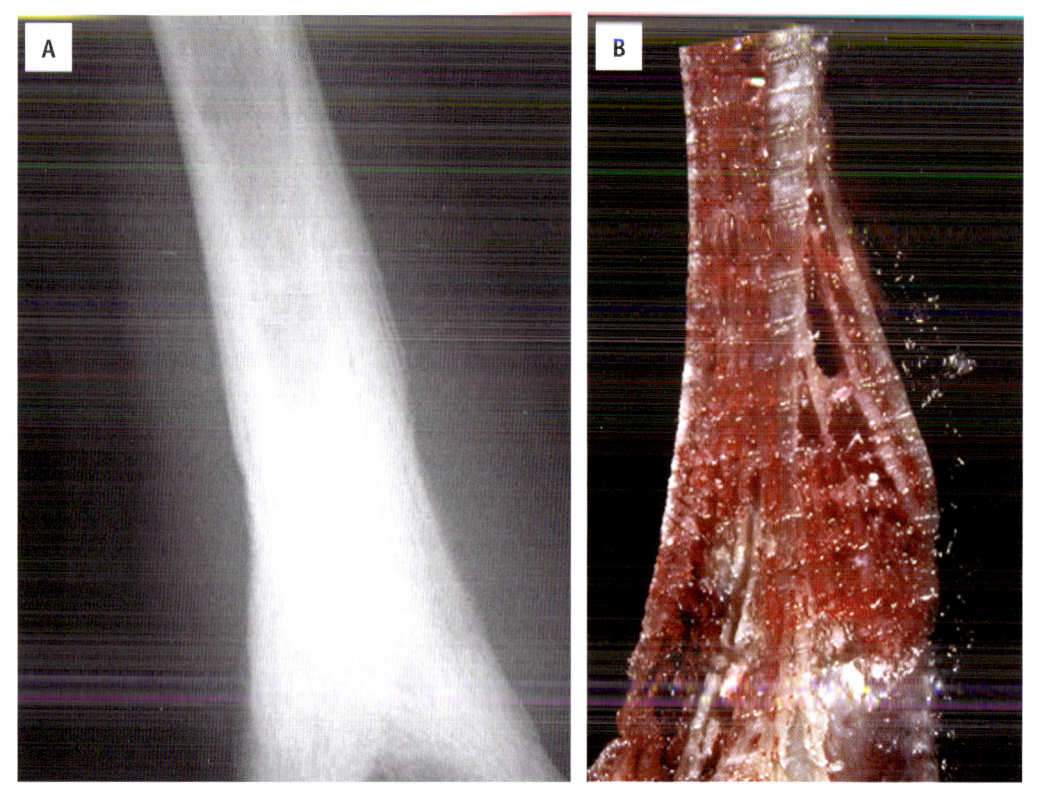

FIGURE 17-3

A, Onion-skin periosteal reaction of Ewing sarcoma showing multiple delicate layers of periosteal reaction surrounding the distal humerus, which are discontinuous distally. Note slight saucerization of the humeral surface because of soft tissue extension of tumor external to the metadiaphysis. **B,** Gross illustration of duplicated subperiosteal bone layers having an onion-skin configuration in a chemotherapy-treated resection specimen.

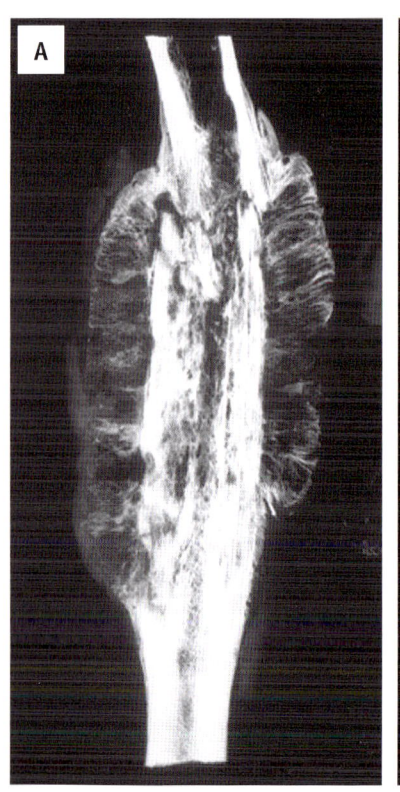

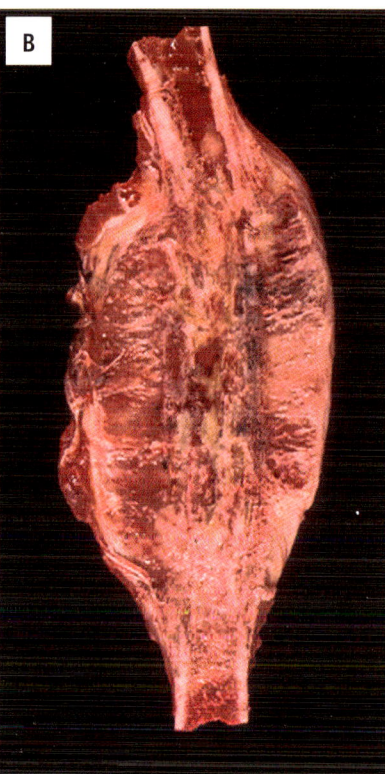

FIGURE 17-4

A, Specimen radiograph of resected midfemur specimen containing Ewing sarcoma. Cortical and medullary permeation are plainly visible, and the soft tissue extensions of tumor contain vertically oriented periosteal new bone streamers that are discontinuous and resemble hairs-on-end. A fracture is in the proximal specimen, but this occurred intraoperatively and does not constitute true pathologic fracture. **B,** Gross specimen demonstrates nontumorous new bone beneath the periosteum and within the tumor mass external to the bone on both sides.

CHAPTER 17 Ewing Sarcoma 371

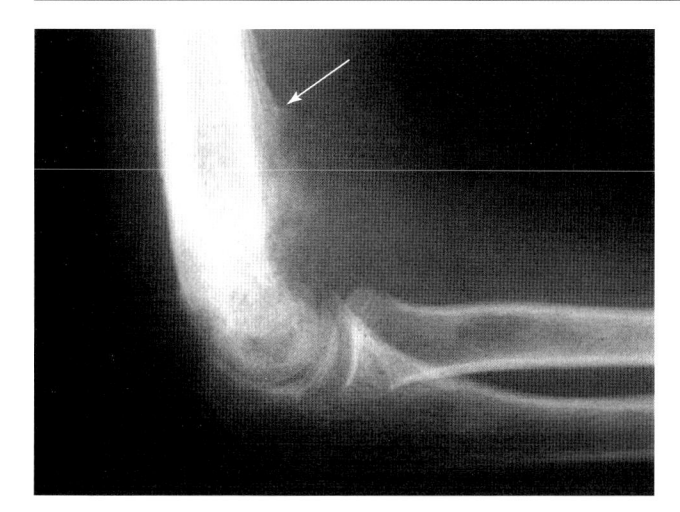

FIGURE 17-5
So-called Codman's angle (or triangle, *arrow*) is unusual in Ewing sarcoma. It reflects periosteal new bone that abruptly stops at the extension of the soft tissue mass out of the cortex. Reactive overlapping of periosteal new bone associated with the periosteal separation from the cortex is responsible for the apparent sclerosis of the distal humerus.

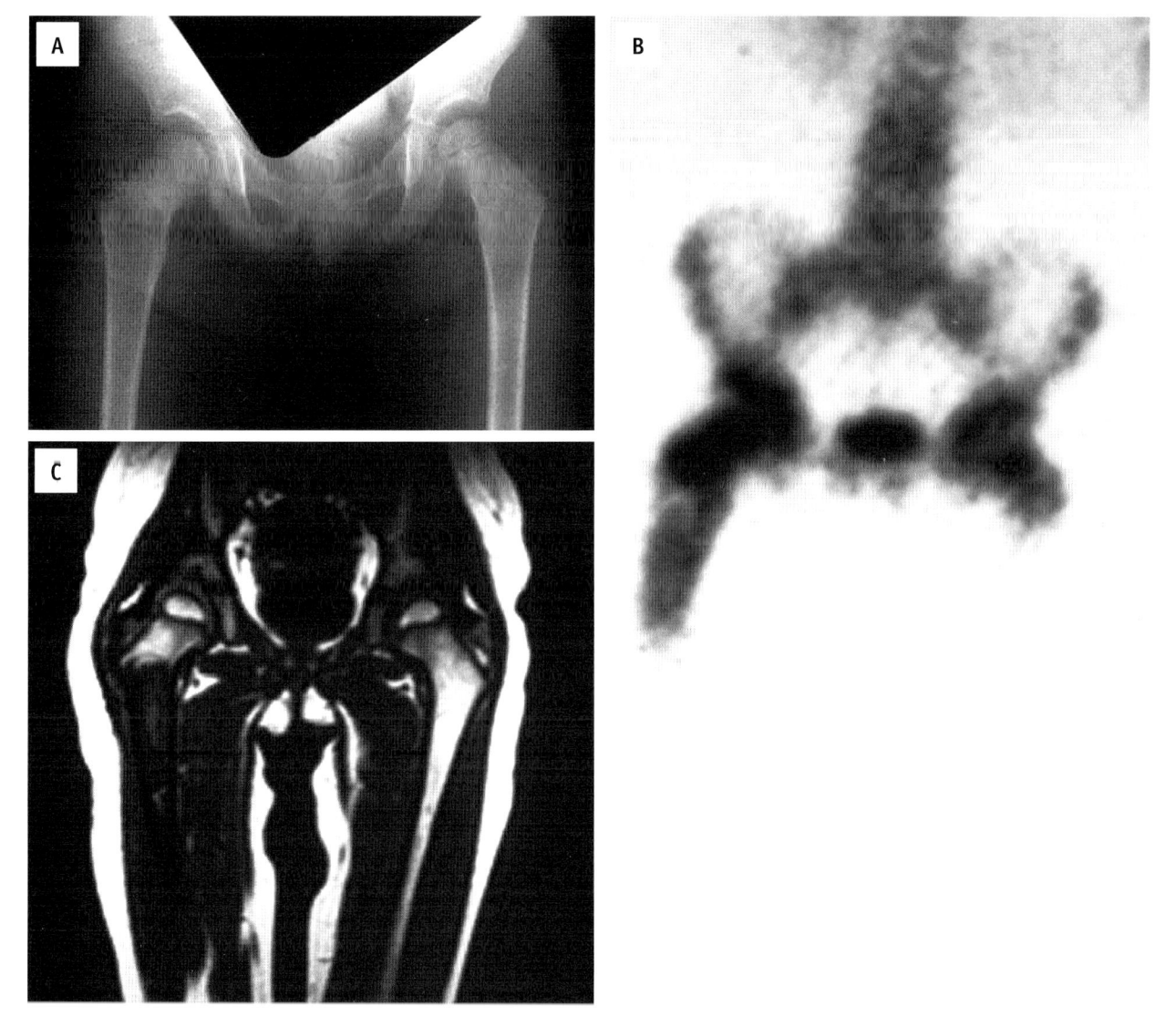

FIGURE 17-6
A, Ewing sarcoma, causing a slight expansion and relative area of poorly circumscribed lucency in the intertrochanteric region of the right femur. B, Technetium-99 radionuclide scan of the pelvis reveals increased uptake not only in the right femoral metaphysis compared with the left, but extension of the increased uptake well into the diaphysis, indicating distal permeation invisible on the radiograph. C, Corresponding T1-weighted coronal magnetic resonance imaging demonstrates a lengthy area of replacement of normal bright marrow signal (seen in the patient's left femur) compared with that on the right.

(Figure 17-7). On the other hand, because it is a lower-contrast technique than MRI, the extent of medullary and soft tissue tumor is more difficult to visualize on CT than in MRI.

PATHOLOGIC FEATURES

GROSS FINDINGS

In the age of neoadjuvant chemotherapy, it is unusual to examine intact specimens from patients with Ewing sarcoma. When whole specimens are examined, the areas of tumor are yellow to gray–pink. In the areas in which the tumor is oldest, the bone is replaced by tumor, which is soft to liquid in consistency, and may even resemble pus. Places where the tumor has been present for a shorter time show less bone destruction, and tumor may be seen between intact trabeculae or even within vascular canals in the cortex that are normally not visible to the unaided eye (Figure 17-8A). Depending on the rate of spread through the cortex and the type of external reaction, periosteal new bone may be visible in a multilayered onion-skin distribution, in a hair-on-end distribution, as an open-ended Codman's angle, or as no reaction at all. In specimens from patients who did not receive chemotherapy, or when there has been poor response to neoadjuvant chemotherapy, there is often an associated soft tissue mass outside the bone, which may be larger than the entire intraosseous tumor component (see Figure 17-8B).

MICROSCOPIC FINDINGS

Histologically, Ewing sarcoma is uniform and dark blue at low power. Areas that stain pink at low power usually contain fibrous tissue or have some degree of

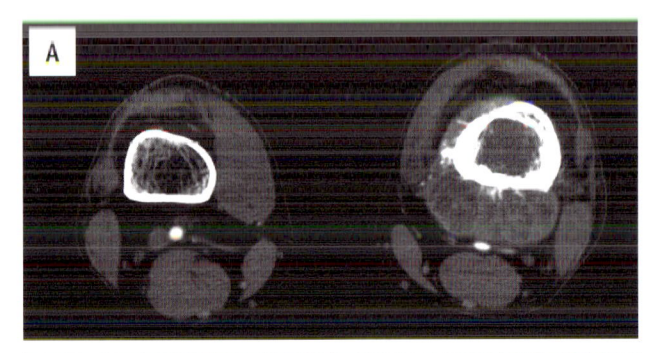

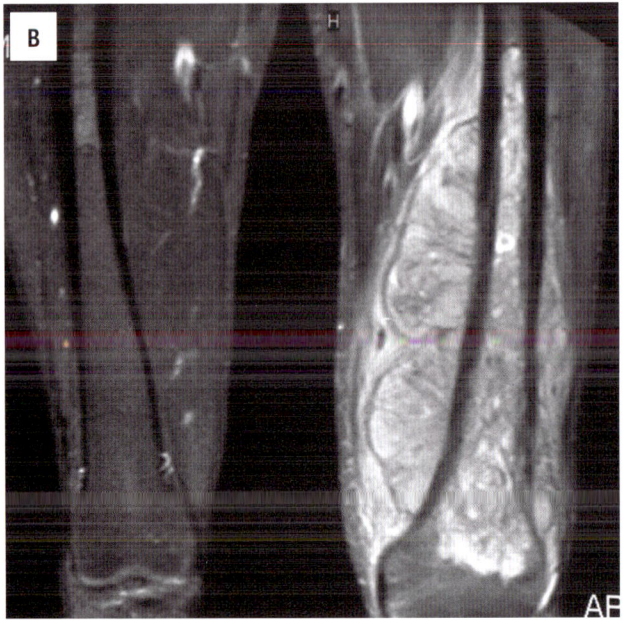

FIGURE 17-7

A, Ewing sarcoma. Computed tomographic scan demonstrating cortical thickening with subtle internal erosion and posteromedial soft tissue mass involving the left femur. At this level, some cancellous bone destruction is visible. **B,** Coronal T2-weighted magnetic resonance imaging of same patient demonstrates extensive intramedullary and extraosseous bright signal corresponding to tumor. Compare with normal hypointense medullary signal in right femur.

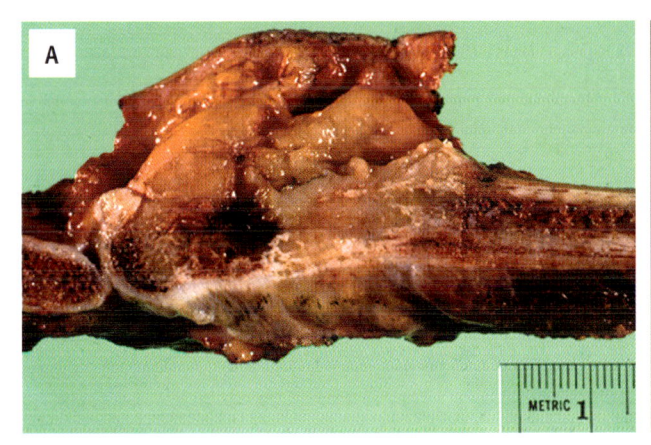

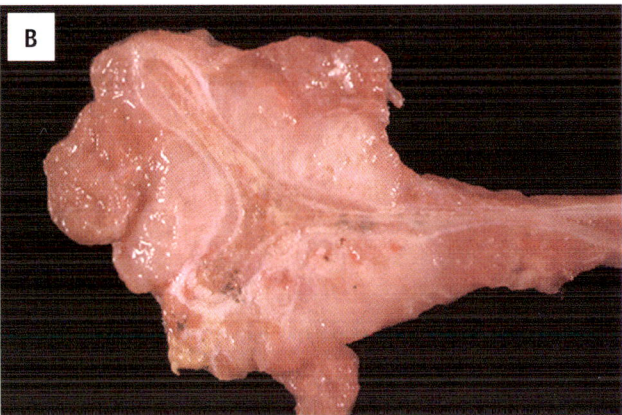

FIGURE 17-8

A, Ewing sarcoma of the clavicle. The gross specimen demonstrates cystic destruction of the proximal clavicle and yellow–gray tumor destroying the adjacent cortex with extension into the superior soft tissues. Note that the tumor replaces much of the normal red marrow between trabeculae and causes linear defects in the adjacent cortex. These correspond to expanded Haversian systems. **B,** Ewing sarcoma of the scapula. The red marrow has been completely replaced by tumor, but the associated soft tissue mass of tumor infiltrating the periscapular muscles is much larger than the intraosseous tumor.

CHAPTER 17 Ewing Sarcoma

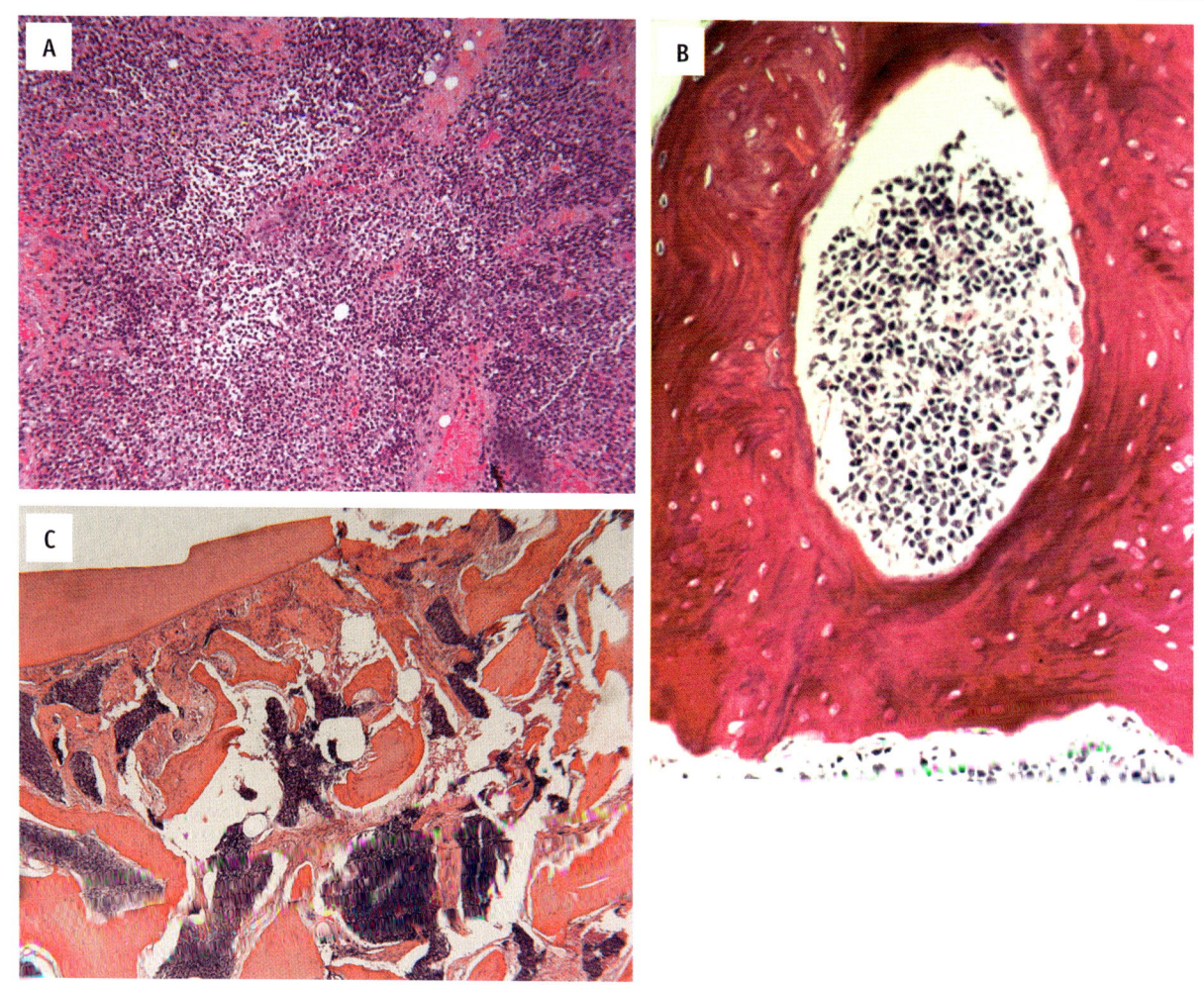

FIGURE 17-9
A, At low-power magnification, Ewing sarcoma appears to be a sea of blue nuclei. The pink areas correspond to spontaneous necrosis. **B,** At medium power, the permeation of preexisting Haversian canals by the tumor cells is easily appreciated. **C,** At low power, the permeation of intertrabecular spaces with displacement of normal marrow fat demonstrates the local invasive potential of the tumor.

necrosis, but extracellular matrix is characteristically lacking in the tumor (Figure 17-9A). At low magnification, the spread of the tumor throughout the intertrabecular marrow spaces and in the Haversian canals when cortex is present in the biopsy is usually striking (see Figure 17-9B, C). The tumor cells themselves are monomorphic with cytoplasmic borders that are inconspicuous (Figure 17-10). Because their large, spherical nuclei with finely divided chromatin are their dominant characteristic, the cells appear round at almost all magnifications. The typical low mitotic activity and rather inconspicuous nucleoli in fairly uniform hyperchromatic nuclei further contribute to the impression of tumor monomorphism. Some tumors, regardless of whether neural differentiation is demonstrable by other techniques, contain structures that resemble rosettes. In most instances, rosette-like structures are due to the presence of either spotty tumor necrosis or of tumor cells surrounding small blood vessels or collagen bands, particularly when viewed on end. It is the presence of true Homer Wright rosettes, particularly when they predominate in a small round cell tumor of bone, that first led to the use of the term *primitive neuroectodermal tumor (PNET)* (Figure 17-11). These structures are characterized by the grouping of tumor cells about a central space containing cytoplasmic processes from the cells bordering the space. The term *PNET* was first used for a tumor otherwise identical to Ewing sarcoma that had identifiable rosettes in 20% or more of the section volume. Currently, it is generally accepted that Ewing sarcoma and PNET are histologic variants of the same tumor spectrum. Because almost all the tumors in this group share a common cytogenetic and molecular abnormality, and in general have the same prognosis, the designation of a particular tumor as Ewing sarcoma or as PNET may be relatively unimportant.

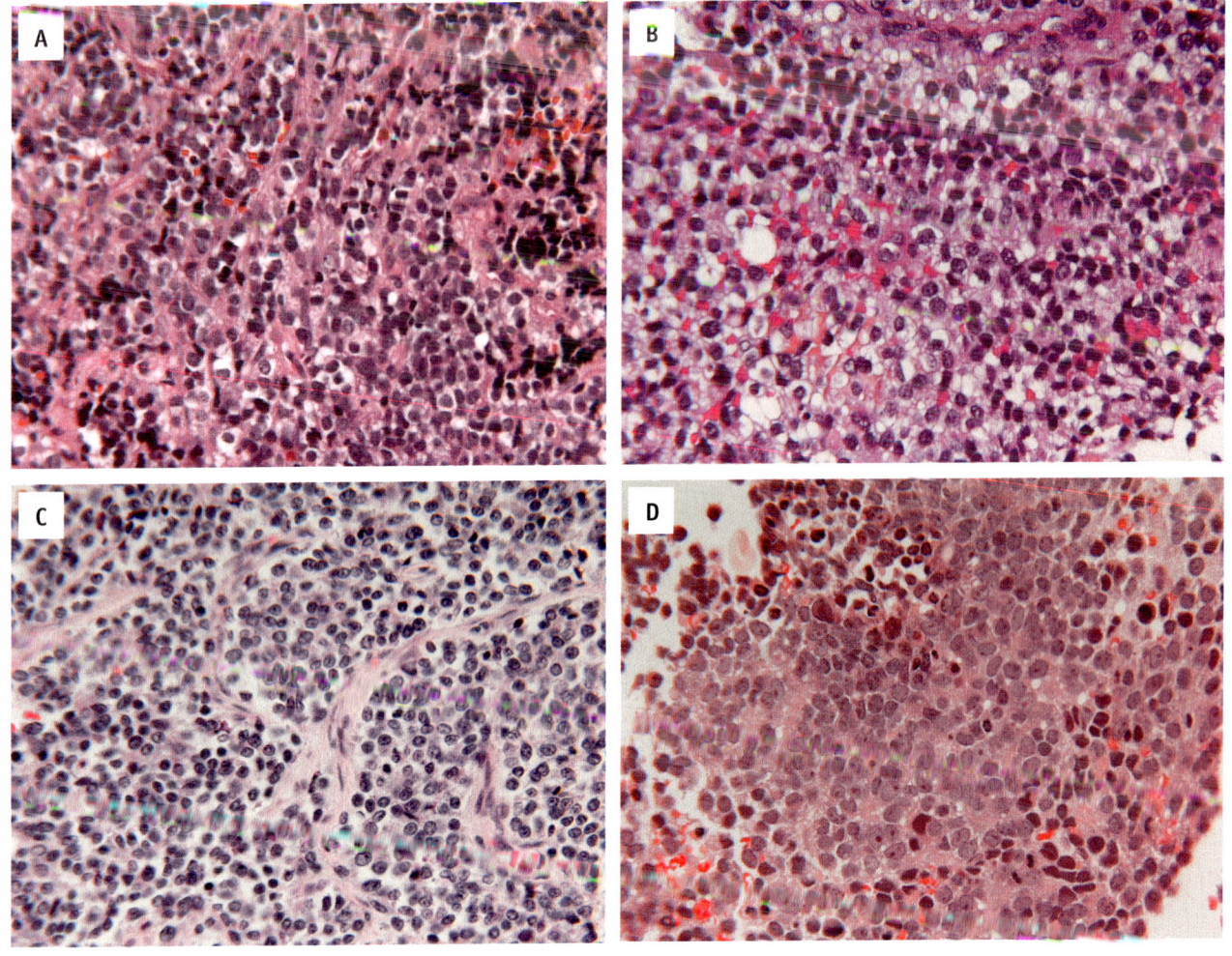

FIGURE 17-10

A, Ewing sarcoma at high magnification demonstrates prominent large blue nuclei with amphophilic cytoplasm. Note that a few nuclei at the periphery appear darker and more condensed; this may be because of early apoptosis. **B,** Ewing sarcoma. A different high-power field demonstrates tumor cells with clear to amphophilic cytoplasm. A population of cells with round nuclei and finely divided chromatin and a subpopulation of cells with condensed chromatin that may be undergoing apoptosis are present. **C,** Ewing sarcoma. Another high-power field demonstrates monotonous and uniformly appearing nuclei with solid groupings of viable tumor cells in an alveolar arrangement created by delicate vasculature. **D,** Ewing sarcoma. A very-high-power photograph demonstrates that in the nonapoptotic tumor cells, nucleoli, when present, are single and not prominent. Note the lack of mitotic activity and poor cellular demarcations.

ANCILLARY STUDIES

IMMUNOHISTOCHEMISTRY

Although no immunohistochemical marker is pathognomonic for Ewing sarcoma, some markers are more specific for classes of other tumors that have a similar histology. The most important of these other tumors are hematologic malignancies, because lymphoma and leukemia may affect patients at the youngest and oldest ends of the Ewing sarcoma age spectrum. Because Ewing sarcoma and PNET are tumors of nonhematologic origin, positivity for CD45 (leukocyte common antigen) is important because it eliminates the Ewing sarcoma family as a consideration. On the other hand, negativity for CD45 does not disprove a primitive tumor of hematopoietic/lymphoid origin.

An additional antigen of importance is CD99 or O-13, a marker for the expression of the *MIC2* gene product. Although it is not specific for the Ewing sarcoma group of tumors, it is identifiable in about 90% of the tumors of this group. Because the antigen it detects is associated with T-cell adhesion, it may be seen in some types of lymphoma, so it is best interpreted in concert with leukocyte markers (Figure 17-12). It is also a useful marker because small, round cell tumors of bone in very young children must be differentiated from metastatic neuroblastoma, which does not express CD99. In tumors that are positive for this antigen, the staining is localized on the cell membrane. FLI-1 is another sensitive, but not specific, marker for Ewing sarcoma.

Immunohistochemistry for neural markers occasionally may also be useful. The expression of neuron-specific

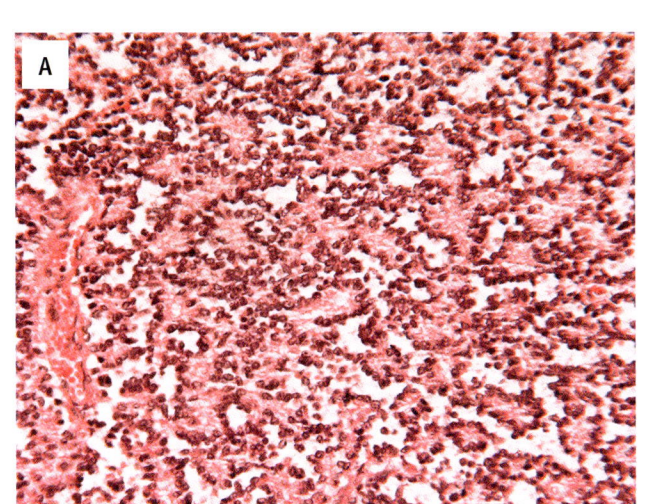

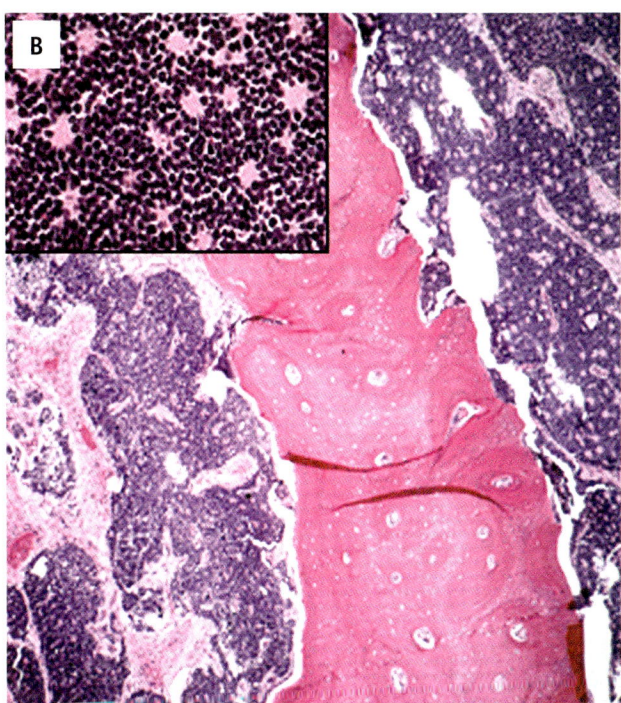

FIGURE 17-11

A, Ewing sarcoma demonstrating rosette-like organization of tumor cells. **B,** Ewing sarcoma low-power view of tumor demonstrating Homer Wright rosettes in both intramedullary (bottom left) and soft tissue portions (right). Inset demonstrates detail of rosettes composed of small cells arranged about neural processes.

enolase is usually regarded as a nonspecific finding. Other markers such as synaptophysin, neuron triplet filament protein, glial fibrillar acid protein, and even S-100 protein are considered more specific of neural differentiation when they are positive in the presence of neuron specific enolase staining.

CYTOGENETICS/MOLECULAR PATHOLOGY

The unifying feature of the Ewing sarcoma tumor family is a fixed reciprocal translocation involving the long arm of chromosome 22 and the long arm of another chromosome. The first and most common such translocation is a reciprocal translocation between bands q24 and q12 of chromosomes 11 and 22, respectively (Figure 17-13). The revelation that the identical chromosomal abnormality was present not only in 90% of Ewing sarcomas but also in the same percentage of Askin tumors and PNETs of bone more than anything else has led to the unifying hypothesis that the entire group of small, round cell tumors of bone should be considered a spectrum of the same disease.

Molecular cloning of the Ewing sarcoma family has revealed that the chromosomal translocation creates new chimeric genes that encode for proteins having major secondary effects on cell regulation. The first of these described was the *EWS/FLI 1* gene associated with the t(11;22) (q24; q12) translocation. The *EWS* gene is located on chromosome 22 at band q12. The latter *(FLI-1)* gene is a member of a family of oncogenes related to avian leukemia retrovirus E26 that was originally designated v-ETS, standing for E 26 specific.

Other, less common variant translocations all involving the EWS locus on chromosome 22 have been

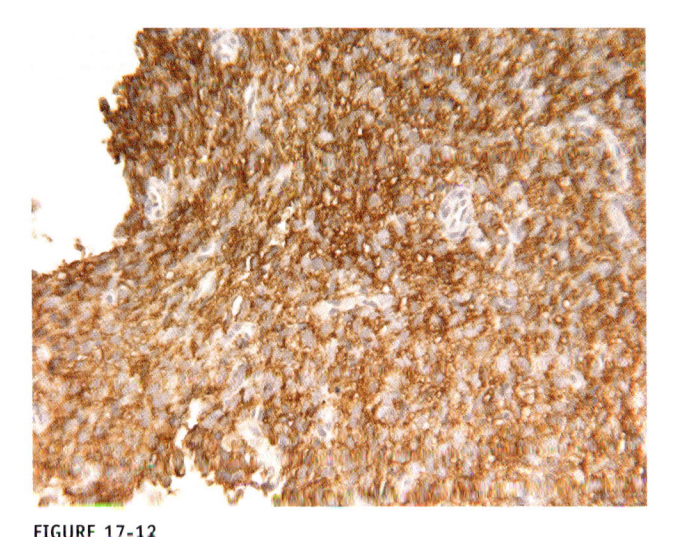

FIGURE 17-12

Ewing sarcoma cells demonstrate diffuse membrane distribution staining with CD99 (O-13).

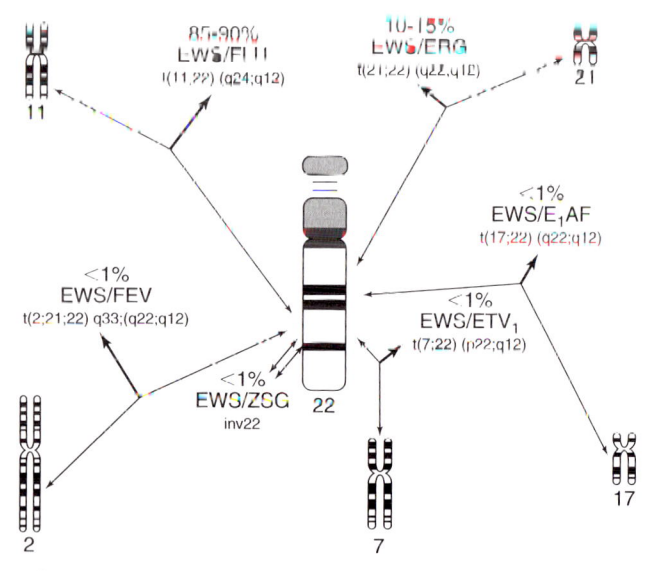

FIGURE 17-13
Schematic diagram of chromosomal translocations and fusion transcripts described for EWS.

elucidated that conjoin EWS to at least four additional transcription factors in the ETS family. Translocations between chromosomes 21 and 22 fuse the *EWS* gene on chromosome 22 with the *ERG* gene on chromosome 21 (see Figure 17-13). Translocations between chromosomes 7 and 22 fuse the *EWS* gene with ETV-1 on chromosome 7.

Translocations between chromosomes 17 and 22 fuse the *EWS* gene with E1AF on chromosome 17, whereas those between chromosomes 2 and 22 fuse the *EWS* gene with FEV on chromosome 2. Although they are not usually necessary for diagnosis, the actual translocations may be demonstrated by interphase fluorescence in situ hybridization on cytologic suspensions, as well as by short-term cell cultures. The chimeric sequences may be amplified and demonstrated with reverse transcriptase-polymerase chain reaction.

DIFFERENTIAL DIAGNOSIS

Ewing sarcoma may be confused with other tumors composed of small cells in which the nuclei predominate. The entities in the differential diagnoses have changed somewhat over the years. From the time Ewing described the tumor until the 1970s, the major differential diagnosis was metastatic neuroblastoma and malignant lymphoma of bone. The differentiation was often made by age, because neuroblastoma tended to arise early in the first decade of life, Ewing sarcoma in the late first decade and second decade of life, and lymphoma after the second or third decades of life. Even though there is no immunohistochemical profile specific for Ewing sarcoma, the use of leukocyte antigenic markers can almost always be used to distinguish lymphomas and leukemias from Ewing sarcoma. The necessity for distinguishing Ewing sarcoma from PNET was a short lived problem once cytogenetic techniques and molecular cloning demonstrated that they were spectral ends of the same neoplastic transformation.

The remaining tumors in the differential diagnosis of Ewing sarcoma are mesenchymal chondrosarcoma, round cell variants of rhabdomyosarcoma that may metastasize to bone or rarely arise as primary lesions in bone, and small-cell osteosarcoma.

Mesenchymal chondrosarcoma has a small-cell, undifferentiated component, as well as a cartilaginous component. Particularly in small biopsies, no cartilage may be visible, and if the undifferentiated component is not perceived as a spindle cell lesion, the diagnosis of Ewing sarcoma might otherwise be rendered. The usual immunohistochemistry battery may not aid in the distinction because both tumors are usually positive for CD99 and vimentin, and negative for leukocyte common antigen. Stains for S-100 protein are positive in the cartilaginous areas of mesenchymal chondrosarcoma but are negative in the small-cell component. If the cartilage component is present histologically, the diagnosis can be made without the differentiating immunohistochemistry.

Rhabdomyosarcomas resembling Ewing sarcoma are usually of alveolar or so-called *solid alveolar* morphology. They almost always represent tumors metastatic to bone, although a few have been ascribed to be primary lesions. If they are carefully sectioned, some of their small, round cells have distinctly eosinophilic cytoplasm and are larger than the smaller background cells in Ewing sarcoma. Immunohistochemistry will usually demonstrate the presence of muscle antigens absent in Ewing sarcoma, and negativity for CD99 more than 80% of the time.

Small-cell osteosarcoma is a tumor that has a small, round cell stromal component resembling Ewing sarcoma, but because it produces variable amounts of bone or osteoid matrix, it is classified as an osteosarcoma. Interestingly, some of the cells in this tumor have shown positivity for glycogen, and its immunohistochemistry is essentially the same as that for Ewing sarcoma. A few cases defined histologically as small-cell osteosarcoma have demonstrated the same chromosomal translocation on cytogenetic analysis. Because osteosarcoma is defined as a malignant connective tissue tumor producing bone or osteoid, the problem in differentiating small-cell osteosarcoma from Ewing sarcoma is whether the histologic definition of osteosarcoma applies to small-cell osteosarcoma having the typical Ewing sarcoma translocation or whether its apparent production of bone merely represents divergent differentiation in a tumor that is otherwise phenotypically and genotypically Ewing sarcoma.

CHAPTER 17 Ewing Sarcoma

EWING SARCOMA/PRIMITIVE NEUROECTODERMAL TUMOR—FACT SHEET

Definition
- A group of primitive sarcomas composed of small cells with uniform, round, hyperchromatic nuclei that demonstrate differing degrees of neuroectodermal differentiation
- Ewing sarcoma is the name applied when the tumors are devoid of neural differentiation by conventional means
- PNET is applied when some degree of neuroendocrine differentiation can be demonstrated

Incidence and Location
- Rare, with an estimated annual incidence of 1 per 1.5 million persons per year
- Usually affects the metadiaphyseal regions of long bones in children
- In adolescents and young adults, it may be seen in the axial bones
- Rare in the short tubular bones.

Sex, Race, and Age Distribution
- Male predominance (male/female ratio, 1.4:1)
- Extremely uncommon in black individuals of African ancestry
- Peak incidence is in the second decade of life; only 20% of patients are younger than 8 years or older than 20 years

Clinical Features
- Pain severe enough to wake patients from sleep is the most common symptom
- Pain may be associated with a mass
- Systemic symptoms include intermittent low grade fever, easily fatigued, and weight loss
- Laboratory findings are nonspecific and include leukocytosis, increase of the erythrocyte sedimentation rate, and anemia

Radiological Features
- No absolute radiographic appearance for Ewing sarcoma exists
- Tumor is often radiolucent and ill-defined
- Lesions are usually in the metadiaphysis or diaphysis of long bones
- The degree of periosteal reaction may be disproportionate to the amount of bone destruction
- A large soft tissue mass may be present
- The outer cortex may be indented or "saucerized" from the outside, even when the soft tissue mass originates in the bone
- CT may demonstrate cortical destruction more readily
- Radionuclide scanning demonstrates intramedullary spread better than conventional radiographs
- MRI best demonstrates associated extraosseous soft tissue masses

Prognosis and Treatment
- Overall survival rate in long-term studies is about 60% to 75%
- Current studies show an approximately 65% survival rate at 5 years
- In general, the more proximal the lesion, the worse the prognosis, especially for lesions of the trunk
- The larger the lesion at presentation, the worse the prognosis
- Patients with systemic symptoms or fractures often have a poorer prognosis
- Surgery (with a wide margin) and chemotherapy are the mainstays of therapy
- Local radiation may be part of treatment plan
- An increased incidence of post-treatment osteosarcomas in long-term survivors who have received both local radiation and chemotherapy exists

EWING SARCOMA/PRIMITIVE NEUROECTODERMAL TUMOR—PATHOLOGIC FEATURES

Gross Findings
- Grayish yellow and soft
- Areas of spontaneous necrosis may resemble chyle or pus
- Gross specimens not altered by prior chemotherapy demonstrate permeative destruction
- There is often but not always an overlying soft tissue tumor mass connected to the intraosseous tumor histologically even though their gross continuity is not always obvious

Microscopic Findings
- Tumor is monomorphous at low magnification
- No extracellular matrix is present
- Tumor cells are small and contain round, dark nuclei with scant mitoses and small nucleoli
- The cytoplasm is fairly scant and clear to amphophilic with poorly visualized cell borders
- A few tumors contain larger cells with prominent nucleoli and increased mitotic activity
- Aggregates of cells may be arranged along delicate fibrous septae or around small blood vessels
- Rosettes or pseudorosettes may be present
- Necrosis is a regular feature, even in the absence of prior therapy

Immunohistochemical Findings
- CD99 (O-13, HBA-74) stains the cells in a characteristic membranous distribution
- FLI-1 is a sensitive but not specific marker for Ewing sarcoma
- Neuron-specific enolase, synaptophysin, and neuron triplet filament protein are expressed in tumors with neural differentiation
- Tumor cells are negative with CD45 (leukocyte common antigen)

Genetics and Molecular Findings
- A characteristic reciprocal translocation between chromosomes 11 and 22 is found in about 85% of cases
- A second variant of reciprocal translocation between chromosomes 21 and 22 is found in 10% to 15% of cases
- The remaining tumors have shown translocations of chromosomes 7 and 22, 17 and 22, 2 and 22, and inversions of chromosome 22; the resulting chimeric proteins function as abnormal transcription factors

Differential Diagnosis
- Lymphoma
- Leukemia
- Osteomyelitis
- Metastatic neuroblastoma
- Mesenchymal chondrosarcoma
- Small-cell osteosarcoma
- Embryonal rhabdomyosarcoma

PROGNOSIS AND TREATMENT

The prognosis for patients with Ewing sarcoma has changed dramatically. Up to 25% of patients with these tumors have demonstrable metastatic disease at the time of presentation. Before the advent of effective systemic chemotherapy, the 5-year survival rate of patients regardless of clinical presentation was less than 5%. With the advent of multimodality therapy, patients with localized tumors have reported 5- and 10-year survival rates of 57% and 49%, respectively. The overall survival rates have been reported as ranging from 61% to 72%. Patients who present with metastatic tumors have survival rates of about 20%. The most important clinical prognostic factors other than whether the disease is localized at the time of presentation include anatomic location and tumor size. Tumors arising in axial locations, particularly in the pelvis and spine, impart a poor prognosis. In addition, an inverse relation exists between tumor size and survival. It has also been reported that patients having tumors with the most common type of fusion transcript (EWS/FLI1) have better prognoses than those with EWS/ERG and other less common fusion transcripts. More recent reports have suggested a strong positive correlation between telomerase activity and negative outcome in patients with nonmetastatic Ewing sarcoma tumors. Complications including local recurrence, metastatic disease, the development of other malignancies, pathologic fractures, and the comorbidities of radiation and chemotherapy thus develop in a majority of patients. The implications are that patients with Ewing sarcoma require longer-term follow-up than the standard 5 years.

SUGGESTED READING

1. Arvand A, Denny CT: Biology of EWS/ETS fusions in Ewing's family tumors. Oncogene 2001;20:5747-5754.
2. Aurias A, Rimbaut C, Buffe D, et al: Translocation involving chromosome 22 in Ewing's sarcoma. Cancer Genet Cytogenet 1984;12:21-25.
3. Bacci G, Forni C, Longhi A, et al: Long-term outcome for patients with non-metastatic Ewing's sarcoma treated with adjuvant and neoadjuvant chemotherapies: 402 patients treated at Rizzoli between 1972 and 1992. Eur J Cancer 2004;40:73-83.
4. Bacci G, Longhi Al, Ferrari S, et al: Prognostic factors in non-metastatic Ewing's sarcoma tumor of bone: an analysis of 579 patients treated at a single institution with adjuvant or neoadjuvant chemotherapy between 1972 and 1998. Acta Oncol 2006;45:469-475.
5. Cotterill SJ, Wright CM, Pearce MS, Craft AW: Stature of young people with malignant bone tumors. Pediatr Blood Cancer 2004;42:59-63.
6. de Alava E, Kawai A, Healy JH, et al: EWS/FLI1 fusion transcript structure is an independent determinant of prognosis in Ewing's sarcoma. J Clin Oncol 1998;16:1248-1255.
7. Dorfman HD, Czerniak B: Bone Tumors. St. Louis, Mosby, 1998, p 658.
8. Ewing J: Diffuse endothelioma of bone. Proc N Y Pathol Soc 1921;21:17-24.
9. Ewing J: Further report on endothelial myeloma of bone. Proc N Y Pathol Soc 1924;24:93-101.
10. Folpe AL, Goldblum JR, Rubin BP, et al: Morphologic and immunophenotypic diversity in Ewing family tumors: A study of 66 genetically confirmed cases. Am J Surg Pathol 2005;29:1025-1033.
11. Foote FW, Anderson HR: Histogenesis of Ewing's tumor. Am J Pathol 1941;17:497-502.
12. Fuchs B, Valenzuela RG, Inwards C, et al: Complications in long-term survivors of Ewing sarcoma. Cancer 2003;98:2687-2692.
13. Grier HE, Krailo MD, Tarbell NJ, et al: Addition of ifosfamide and etoposide to standard chemotherapy for Ewing's sarcoma and primitive neuroectodermal tumor of bone. N Engl J Med 2003;348:694-701.
14. Jaffe HL: The problem of Ewing sarcoma of bone. Bull Hosp Joint Dis 1945;6:82-85.
15. Jaffe R, Santamaria M, Yunis EJ, et al: The neuroectodermal tumor of bone. Am J Surg Pathol 1984;8:885-898.
16. Leprince D, Gegonne A, Coll J: A putative second cell-derived oncogene of the avian leukaemia retrovirus E26. Nature 1983;306:395-397.
17. Lichtenstein L, Jaffe HL: Ewing sarcoma of bone. Am J Pathol 1947;23:43.
18. Mastrangeo T, Modena P, Tornielli S, et al: A novel zinc finger gene is fused to EWS in small round cell tumor. Oncogene 2000;19:3799-3804.
19. Ohali A, Avigad S, Cohen IJ, et al: Association between telomerase activity and outcome in patients with nonmetastatic Ewing family tumors. J Clin Oncol 2003;21:3836-3843.
20. Parham DM, Hijazi Y, Steinber SM, et al: Neuroectodermal differentiation in Ewing's sarcoma family of tumors does not predict tumor behavior. Hum Pathol 1999;30:911-918.
21. Rodriguez-Galindo C, Liu T, Krasin MJ, et al: Analysis of prognostic factors in Ewing sarcoma family of tumors: review of St. Jude Children's Research Hospital studies. Cancer 2007;110(2):375-384.
22. Rodriguez-Galindo C, Spunt SL, Pappo AS: Treatment of Ewing sarcoma family of tumors: Current status and outlook for the future. Med Pediatr Oncol 2003;40:276-287.
23. Schmidt D, Herrmann C, Jurgens H, et al: Malignant peripheral neuroectodermal tumor and its necessary distinction from Ewing's sarcoma: a report from the Kiel Pediatric Tumor Registry. Cancer 1991;68:2251-2259.
24. Teitell MA, Thompson AD, Sorensen PH, et al: EWS/ETS fusion genes induce epithelial and neuroectodermal differentiation in NIH 3T3 fibroblasts. Lab Invest 1999;79:1535-1543.
25. Thompson AD, Teitell MA, Arvand A, et al: Divergent Ewing's sarcoma EWS/ETS fusions confer a common tumorigenic phenotype on NIH 3T3 cells. Oncogene 1999;18:5506-5513.
26. Turc-Carel C, Philip T, Berger M-P, et al: Chromosome study of Ewing's sarcoma (ES) cell lines. Consistency of a reciprocal translocation t (11;22) (q24;q12). Cancer Genet Cytogenet 1984;12:1-19.
27. Wehrli BM, Huang W, DeCrombrugghe B, et al: Sox-9, a master regulator of chondrogenesis, distinguishes mesenchymal chondrosarcoma from other small blue round cell tumors. Hum Pathol 2003;34:263-269.
28. Whang-Peng J, Triche TJ, Knutsen T, et al: Cytogenetic characterization of selected small round cell tumors of childhood. Cancer Genet Cytogenet 1986;21:185-208.
29. Willis R: Metastatic neuroblastoma in bone presenting the Ewing syndrome, with a discussion of "Ewing sarcoma." Am J Pathol 1940;16:317-333.

18 Hematopoietic Tumors
Edward F. McCarthy

- Multiple Myeloma
- Lymphoma of Bone
- Hodgkin Lymphoma of Bone

Lymphocytes and plasma cells often reside in company with the hematopoietic elements of the bone marrow. Therefore, malignant proliferations of lymphocytes and plasma cells are often centered in the bone marrow and destroy bone secondarily. When these neoplasms are confined to a finite area of a single bone, they respond well to radiation therapy and chemotherapy, and the prognosis may be excellent. However, these neoplasms can spread rapidly, and a delay in diagnosis leads to dissemination. In this event, there is a poorer prognosis. Although some lymphomas occur in children, hematopoietic neoplasms in bone usually affect older adults.

MULTIPLE MYELOMA

Multiple myeloma is a neoplastic proliferation of monoclonal plasma cells involving multiple sites in the skeleton. This disease is part of a spectrum of disorders called the *plasma cell dyscrasias*. These disorders are all characterized by a monoclonal plasma cell proliferation, but they vary in clinical severity. The plasma cells in these disorders preserve their function—they secrete immunoglobulins. Because these immunoglobulins are monoclonal, these disorders can be recognized by a monoclonal immunoglobulin spike in the patient's serum. The monoclonal immunoglobulin, known as an M protein, is usually an IgG. In addition to a serum M protein, the light chains released from the breakdown of the immunoglobulins are excreted in the urine. These urinary light chains, known as Bence–Jones proteins, can be identified by urinary immunoelectrophoresis.

There are several well-defined syndromes in the spectrum of plasma cell dyscrasia. One syndrome, known as monoclonal gammopathy of undetermined significance, is an indolent disorder. It occurs in more than 3% of individuals older than 50 and progresses to myeloma or related malignancy at a rate of 1% per year. Patients are asymptomatic and have no bone lesions. They do have a serum M protein, but marrow histology shows less than 10% plasma cells.

Solitary plasmacytoma is another disease in the spectrum of plasma cell dyscrasia. In this disorder, a single skeletal lesion caused by a neoplastic plasma cell proliferation is present. The histologic and immunohistochemical features of tissue from a solitary plasmacytoma of bone are indistinguishable from those of multiple myeloma. Widespread involvement is ruled out by bone marrow biopsies showing less than 5% plasma cells in the marrow and no radiographic evidence of additional lesions. The prevalence of an M protein in the serum or urine of patients with solitary plasmacytoma varies from 24% to 72%, and the levels of the M protein tend to be low. Although some patients are cured with radiation therapy or surgery, almost 50% experience development of multiple myeloma, typically after a median duration of 2 to 3 years.

Multiple myeloma, the most aggressive manifestation of plasma cell dyscrasia, is the principal topic of this chapter section. The diagnosis of this disorder rests on meeting specific criteria, including 10% or more plasma cells in the bone marrow (or plasmacytoma of bone), M protein in the serum and/or urine, and evidence of end-organ damage (hypercalcemia, renal insufficiency, anemia, or bone lesions).

CLINICAL FEATURES

Although multiple myeloma is a hematologic malignancy, it almost always confines itself to the skeleton. It is the most common primary malignancy to involve bone. Each year about 15,000 new cases are diagnosed in the United States. This disease is twice as common in African Americans, and is slightly more common in male than in female individuals (1.62:1.0). Multiple myeloma is a disease of older adults and is generally discovered between the ages of 50 and 80 with a median age at onset of 66 years. Therefore, it should be considered in the differential diagnosis of all lytic bone lesions in patients in this age range. Less than 2% of cases occur in patients younger than 40 years.

Multiple myeloma often has a nonspecific presentation. Pain, present in two-thirds of patients, is the most common symptom. Back and chest pain (secondary to rib fractures) commonly occur. Although the onset of pain is usually insidious, it may be sudden, especially when pathologic fracture occurs. This is particularly true when compression fractures of the vertebra occur.

Other presenting symptoms in patients with myeloma include bacterial infections, gross bleeding (most commonly, epistaxis), and fever. Weakness and fatigue may occur secondary to anemia and may be found in up to two-thirds of patients.

Patients may experience development of systemic complications from the myeloma protein. Renal insufficiency, hypercalcemia, and amyloid deposition often complicate the late stages of the disease. Light chains are often deposited in tissue as amyloid and may cause congestive heart failure, hypercalcemia, nephrotic syndrome, peripheral neuropathy, or increased bleeding tendency.

The most important laboratory studies in the diagnosis of multiple myeloma are the serum and urine immunoelectrophoresis and immunofixation. Almost 99% of patients will have a serum immunoglobulin spike, Bence–Jones proteinuria, or both. Other laboratory tests may provide helpful clues. Anemia and an increased erythrocyte sedimentation rate occur in 62% and 76% of patients, respectively. Hypercalcemia and hyperuricemia are also common.

RADIOLOGIC FEATURES

Multiple myeloma is characterized by a wide spectrum of radiographic changes. In keeping with the insidious evolution of this disorder, some patients present only with diffuse osteopenia. This change may mimic senile or postmenopausal osteoporosis, especially if there is significant spinal involvement. As in osteoporosis, there may be a loss of height and biconcave deformities of the vertebrae. Single or multiple compressions fractures may occur. As the disease progresses, subtle, moth-eaten radiolucencies appear (Figure 18-1). A misdiagnosis of diffuse osteoporosis is common in this radiographic presentation.

The most common radiographic change of myeloma, however, is multiple, discrete, punched-out lytic bone lesions (Figure 18-2). They are most commonly seen in the skull, spine, pelvis, and proximal femurs or humeri. Lesions may vary in size from 3 to 4 mm to 5 to 10 cm. They have well-defined borders and lack a sclerotic rim. In the long bones, a circular or elliptical lytic area may be seen on the endosteal bone surface.

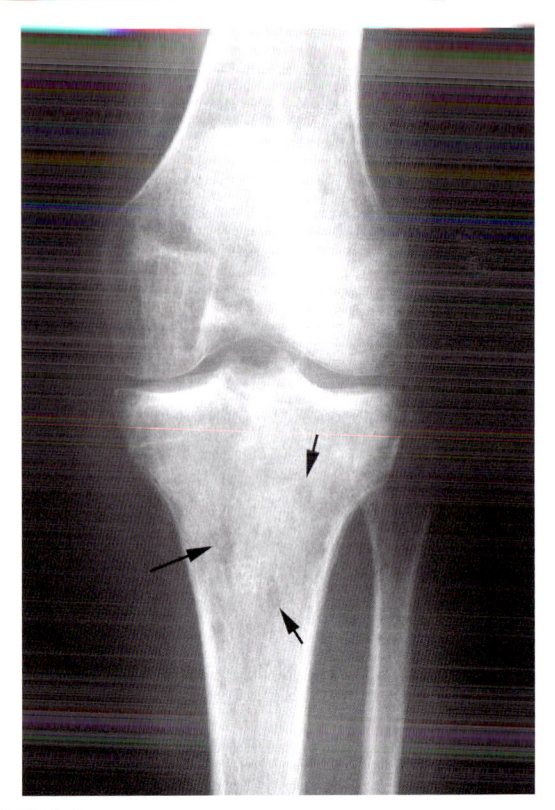

FIGURE 18-1
Early multiple myeloma involving the proximal femur. Arrows highlight faint, ill-defined radiolucencies.

Larger lesions cause extensive cortical destruction (Figure 18-3). In other bone diseases, such as metastatic carcinoma, the technetium bone scan is useful to quantify the extent of skeletal involvement. However, in multiple myeloma, the bone scan often fails to

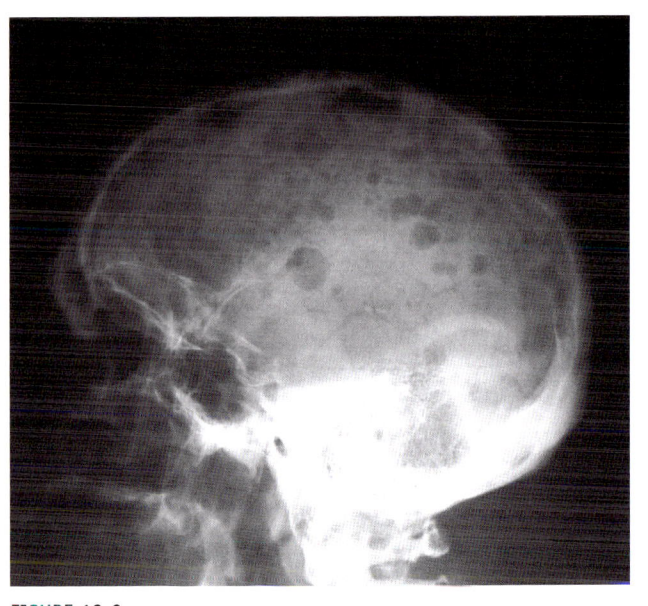

FIGURE 18-2
Classic pattern of lytic bone lesions of multiple myeloma. The skull is involved with multiple, discrete, punched-out lytic lesions characteristic of advanced multiple myeloma.

identify all the lesions. This is because many lytic myeloma foci lack a secondary osteoblastic response and, therefore, do not concentrate radioactive tracer. But because many myeloma lesions do accumulate tracer, a positive bone scan does not rule out this disease.

On rare occasions (about 3% of cases), patients have radiodense lesions (Figure 18-4). This presentation, known as osteosclerotic myeloma, occurs in a slightly younger age group (median age, 56 years) and more likely affects male individuals. Many patients with this presentation have disorders in other organ systems that are not related to plasma cells. The most common associated disorder, affecting 30% to 50% of patients, is polyneuropathy. However, numerous other organ systems may be involved and result in a disorder known as POEM syndrome (polyneuropathy, organomegaly, endocrinopathy, M protein).

PATHOLOGIC FEATURES

GROSS FINDINGS

In the early phases of myeloma, cancellous bone may be intact. The marrow, however, is deeply red or hemorrhagic. In advanced disease, bone is replaced by hemorrhagic, friable soft tissue. When tumor masses are large, pathologic fractures may occur.

MICROSCOPIC FINDINGS

Bone biopsies in multiple myeloma show marrow replacement by diffuse sheets of plasma cells. From case to case, the plasma cells exhibit a spectrum of differentiation. Some patients have well-differentiated myeloma with mature plasma cells that are not dissimilar from normal plasma cells (Figure 18-5). The cells are characterized by an eccentric nucleus with a clock-faced chromatin pattern. Adjacent to nucleus is an amphophilic area, the hallmark of a plasma cell, which corresponds to the Golgi apparatus on electromicroscopy. This is the zone where the immunoglobulin is packaged for secretion. Other patients may have a poorly differentiated plasma cell neoplasm. Plasma cells in these cases are barely recognizable as plasma cells. Considerable nuclear pleomorphism, a prominent nucleolus, and numerous mitotic figures are present (Figure 18-6). The perinuclear clear zone is much less prominent. In about 10% of cases, the bone marrow and visceral sites will show infiltration by amyloid deposits. The amyloid deposited is AL amyloid—the light chains deposited by the immunoglobulin molecule. On rare occasions, a single deposit of amyloid in bone will be the only presentation of plasma cell dyscrasia (Figure 18-7). Patients with these lesions almost always experience a progression to multiple myeloma.

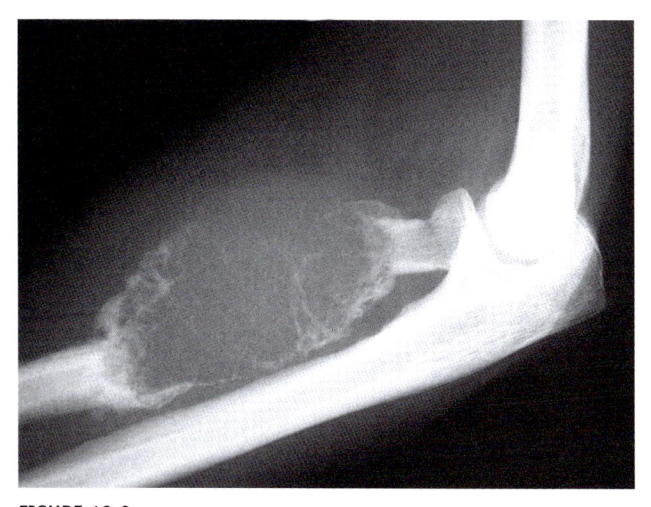

FIGURE 18-3
Larger lesions of multiple myeloma cause significant bone destruction and cortical expansion as present in this radius lesion.

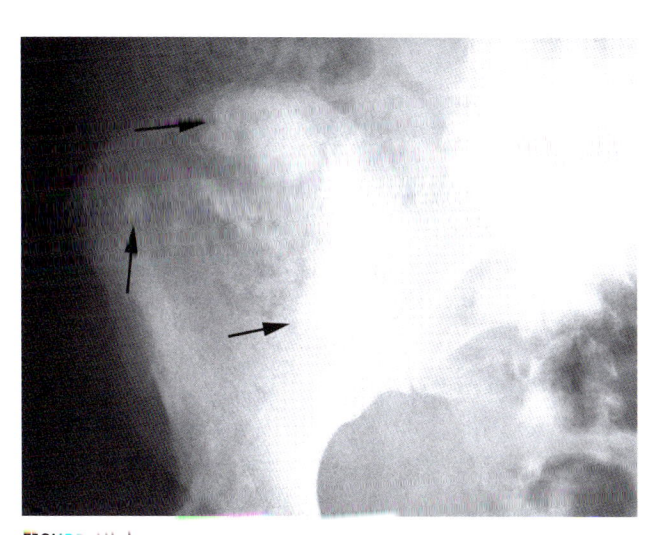

FIGURE 18-4
Osteosclerotic myeloma is characterized by poorly defined radiodensities (arrows).

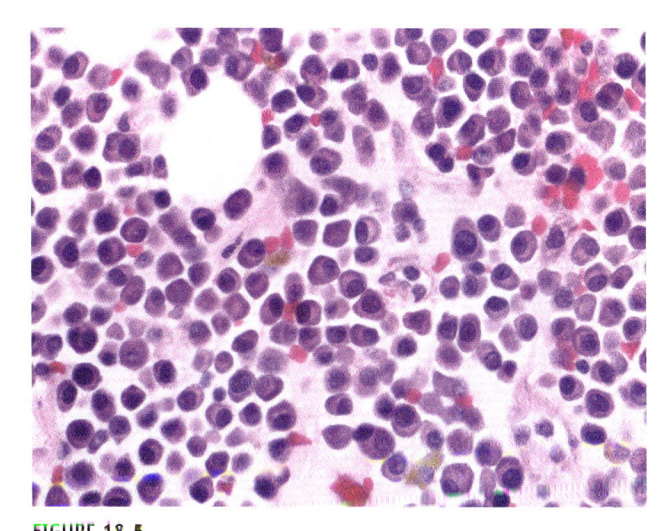

FIGURE 18-5
Histologic features of well-differentiated myeloma are characterized by cells easily recognizable as plasma cells.

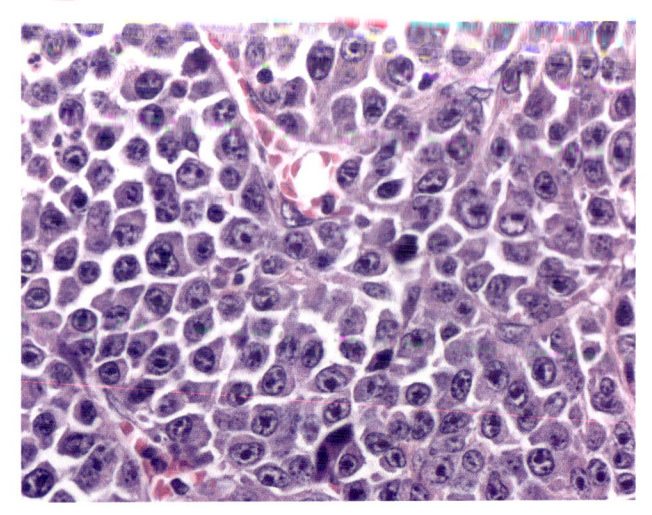

FIGURE 18-6
Poorly differentiated myeloma is occasionally difficult to recognize. Cells show significant pleomorphism. Nuclear features of plasma cells are absent, and a large nucleus is prominent.

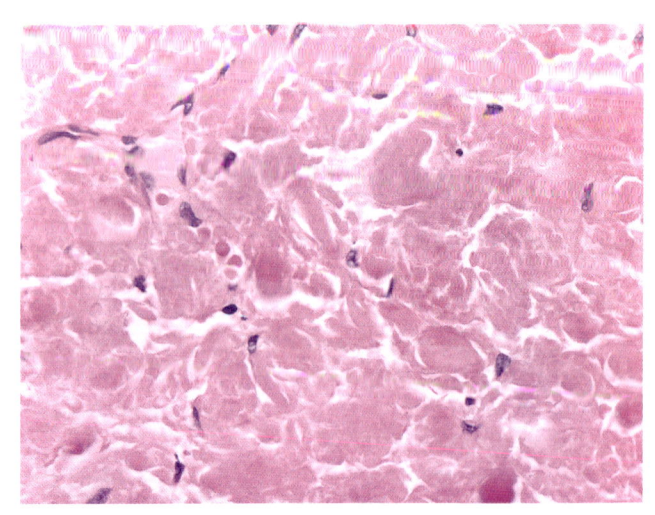

FIGURE 18-7
Characteristic lesion of amyloid in a patient with plasma cell dyscrasia. This is AL amyloid and will show the characteristic apple green birefringence in polarized light.

ANCILLARY STUDIES

IMMUNOHISTOCHEMISTRY

Immunohistochemistry is often necessary to firmly establish the diagnosis of myeloma. Although plasma cells are in the B-cell lineage of lymphocytes, they usually do not express the typical B-cell markers such as CD20 or CD19. However, plasma cells express CD138. CD138 is a reliable marker of both normal and neoplastic plasma cells (Figure 18-8). The monoclonal nature of the myeloma neoplasm is best identified by staining with kappa and lambda light chains. Plasma cells in inflammatory lesions will exhibit both kappa and lambda light chains, whereas multiple myeloma will exhibit only one or the other.

DIFFERENTIAL DIAGNOSIS

Metastatic carcinoma to bone and multiple myeloma may have identical clinical and radiographic presentations. Fortunately, virtually all patients with multiple myeloma have an M-protein spike, and this is an important tool to differentiate these diseases. Problems may arise differentiating a solitary plasmacytoma from a focus of metastatic cancer because solitary plasmacytoma may not cause an M-protein spike. Therefore, in destructive bone lesions in adults, cytokeratin stains may be used to differentiate myeloma from metastatic carcinoma. Plasmacytomas are positive with CD138, but alone not necessarily diagnostic because occasionally carcinomas are immunoreactive with this marker.

Myeloma must sometimes be differentiated from malignant lymphoma in bone. Both processes present with diffuse populations of small, rounded cells. Malignant lymphoma of bone will show an immunophenotypic profile of B cells, or less often, T cells. These markers are typically absent in myeloma.

Occasionally, chronic osteomyelitis with a heavy plasma cell infiltration can be mistaken for multiple myeloma. However, the radiographic appearance of chronic osteomyelitis is almost always a sclerotic lesion, whereas multiple myeloma causes punched-out lytic areas. Also, the plasma cells of chronic osteomyelitis will be polyclonal for both kappa and lambda light chains. By contrast, myeloma plasma cells are monoclonal for either kappa or lambda lights chains.

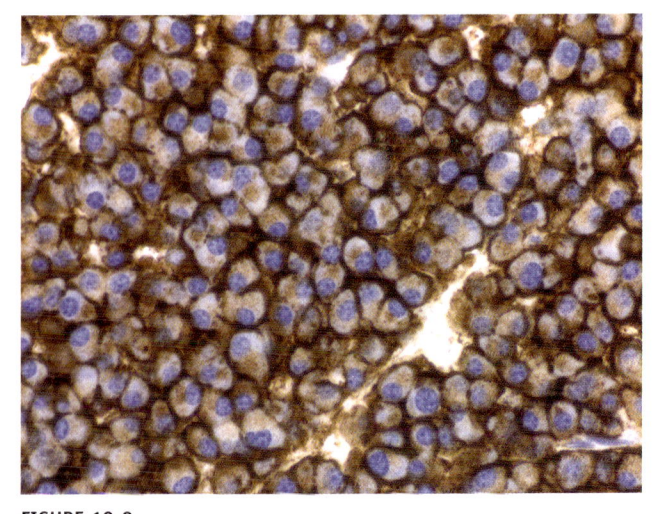

FIGURE 18-8
Immunohistochemical stain for CD138 highlights plasma cells with a uniform membrane positivity.

MULTIPLE MYELOMA—FACT SHEET

Definition
- A monoclonal neoplastic proliferation of plasma cells that is usually confined to the skeleton; the malignant plasma cells almost always secrete an immunoglobulin that can be detected in the urine or serum

Incidence and Location
- 15,000 new cases per year are reported in the United States
- Can involve any area of the skeleton but is most common in the skull, spine, and pelvis

Sex, Race, and Age Distribution
- African Americans are affected twice as often as Caucasian Americans
- Most cases occur between the ages of 50 and 80 years (median, 66 years)
- Less than 2% of cases occur in patients younger than 40 years

Clinical Features
- Pain is the most common presentation; some patients present with pathologic fracture, usually in the spine
- Weakness and fatigue are often secondary to anemia
- 99% of patients have a serum immunoglobulin spike, Bence–Jones proteinuria, or both

Radiologic Features
- Early involvement may show only osteoporosis; developed lesions are usually multiple and show punched-out, discrete radiolucencies
- The bone scan is not as sensitive as a skeletal survey for defining all lesions
- Rarely lesions may be osteoblastic

Prognosis and Treatment
- Chemotherapy oftentimes is associated with autologous stem-cell transplantation
- Radiation therapy may be necessary for individual lesions that threaten skeletal integrity
- Median survival of all patients with multiple myeloma is 3 years
- 50% of patients with solitary plasmacytoma of bone experience development of multiple myeloma after a median duration of 2 to 3 years

MULTIPLE MYELOMA—PATHOLOGIC FEATURES

Gross Findings
- Early lesions may show only deep red marrow without bone destruction
- Well-developed lesions are soft and friable

Microscopic Findings
- Solid sheets of plasma cells are present
- Often the plasma cells are well differentiated; sometimes they are poorly differentiated with large nuclei and prominent nucleoli

Immunohistochemical Findings
- Neoplastic cells consistently stain with CD138, the marker for plasma cells
- Monoclonal staining for either kappa or lambda light chains will be present

Differential Diagnosis
- Malignant lymphoma
- Metastatic carcinoma
- Chronic osteomyelitis

PROGNOSIS AND TREATMENT

Chemotherapy, most commonly consisting of melphalan and prednisone, is the mainstay of treatment for patients with multiple myeloma. In addition, high-dose therapy with autologous stem-cell transplantation is also incorporated routinely into the treatment strategy.

Although chemotherapy is the mainstay of treatment, radiation therapy is often used in specific clinical situations. These would include impending cord compression caused by spinal lesions or impending long-bone fractures. Occasionally, radiation therapy is useful to control pain related to bone lesions. Surgery may be necessary to prevent pathologic fracture, and in the spine, vertebroplasty is frequently used.

Currently, no cure for multiple myeloma exists. Standard therapy affords a median survival time of about 3 years. However, some patients can live longer than 10 years.

LYMPHOMA OF BONE

Malignant lymphomas primarily involve lymph nodes. The classification of these neoplasms is complex and in a constant state of flux. They are divided into two major groups: Hodgkin lymphomas and the non-Hodgkin lymphomas. The non-Hodgkin lymphomas, the main topic of this section, may be generally classified according whether they are of B-cell, T-cell, or natural killer cell lineage. As malignant lymphomas progress, they spread from lymph nodes to other visceral organs. The skeletal system is frequently involved secondarily as malignant lymphomas progress to extranodal sites.

Approximately one-third of lymphomas originate in tissues other than lymph nodes. These tissues have native population of lymphoid cells, such as lung, gastrointestinal tract, and bone. Lymphomas of these extranodal sites are regarded as primary extranodal lymphomas. Approximately 5% of extranodal lymphomas are primary in bone. This entity is known as primary lymphoma of bone, and it accounts for 7% of all malignant bone tumors.

CLINICAL FEATURES

Primary lymphoma of bone occurs at any age. However, 50% of patients are older than 40 years. Rarely, children may experience development of primary lymphoma of bone. In a child, a variant of this neoplasm may be the precursor B-cell (lymphoblastic) lymphoma.

The femur and pelvis are the most common bones to be involved. The spine and other long bones are also frequently affected. In about 25% of cases, multiple bones are involved. Pain is the most common presenting symptom, although some patients present with a pathologic fracture.

RADIOLOGIC FEATURES

The radiologic features of primary lymphoma of bone are nonspecific and are typical of any aggressive bone-destroying process. The femur, pelvis, and spine are the most common locations. In the long bones, the metadiaphyseal region is favored, and there is often a long segment of involvement. Lymphoma of bone is usually a poorly defined, permeative lytic lesion (Figure 18-9). Some lesions have varying amounts of intraosseous reactive bone that imparts a mottled appearance. Occasionally, a lesion may have extensive osteosclerosis, a feature that often leads lymphoma of bone to be misdiagnosed as other lesions, particularly Paget disease (Figure 18-10).

Occasionally, the permeative pattern of bone destruction is subtle and difficult to appreciate on plain radiographs (Figure 18-11A). However, an MRI may show a strikingly strong signal on T2-weighted images. Therefore, the amount of the magnetic resonance signal may be out of proportion to the subtle changes seen on plain radiographs (see Figure 18-11B).

Primary lymphoma of bone easily penetrates the cortex such that an adjacent soft tissue mass is present in about half of cases (Figure 18-12). Although an aggressive periosteal reaction occurs in 60% of the cases, the amount of periosteal reaction is not proportional to the amount of bone destruction. About 25% of patients have a pathologic fracture.

PATHOLOGIC FEATURES

MICROSCOPIC FINDINGS

Almost all primary lymphomas of bone are diffuse large B-cell lymphomas (DLBCLs). The malignant cells diffusely infiltrate the bone marrow, often leaving

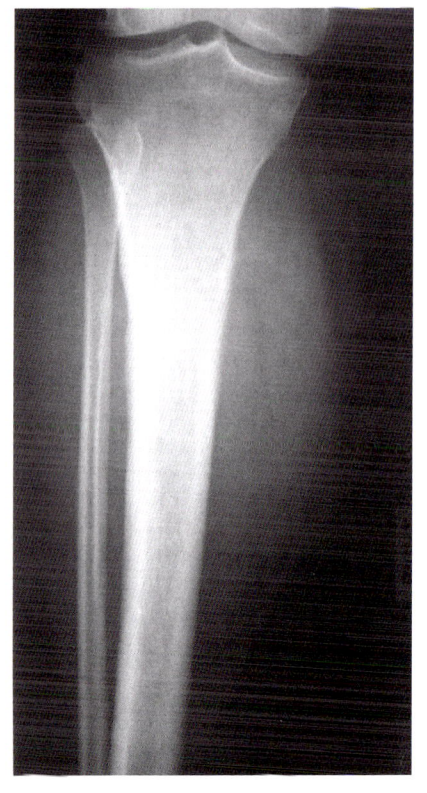

FIGURE 18-9
Typical plain radiographic lesion of a primary lymphoma of bone showing a poorly defined area of radiolucency in the tibia.

FIGURE 18-10
Occasionally, radiodensity is present diffusely throughout the lesion as a result of reactive bone formation. The radiodense variant may be mistaken for Paget disease.

CHAPTER 18 Hematopoietic Tumors

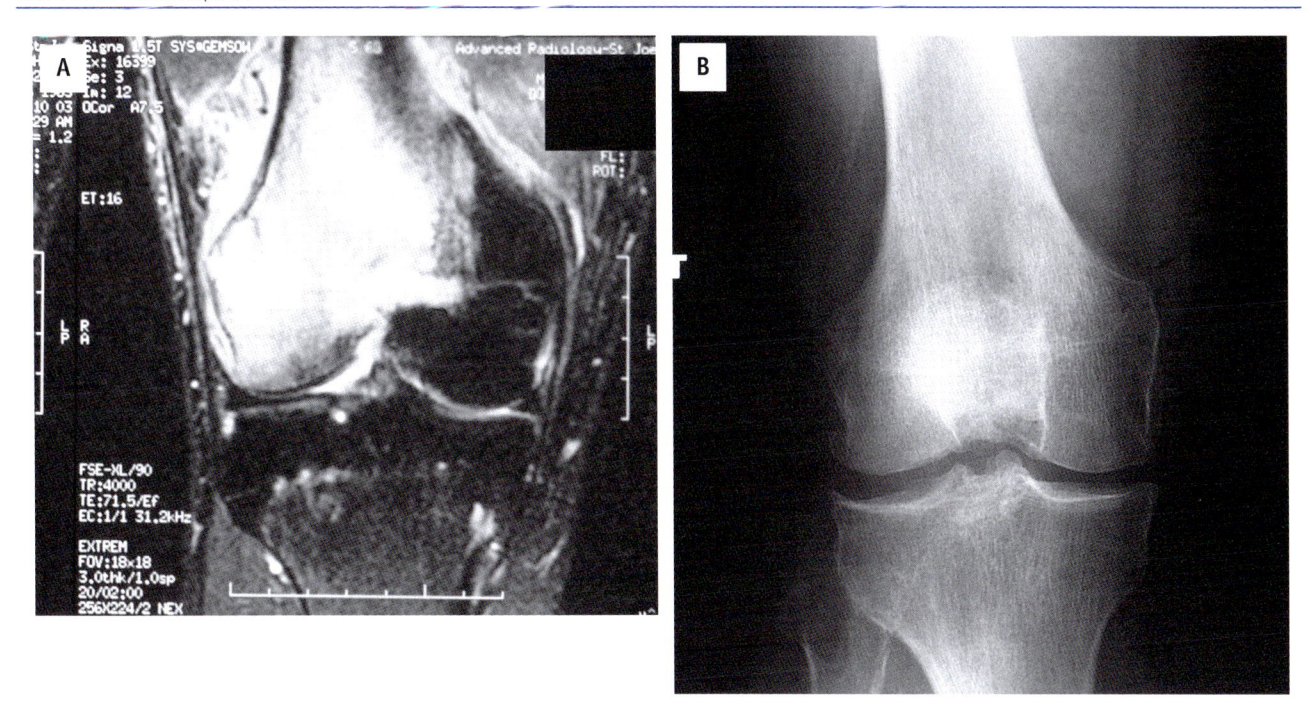

FIGURE 18-11

A, T2-weighted magnetic resonance imaging of a lymphoma in the distal femur shows diffuse involvement of the bone marrow. **B,** The plain radiograph shows almost no changes.

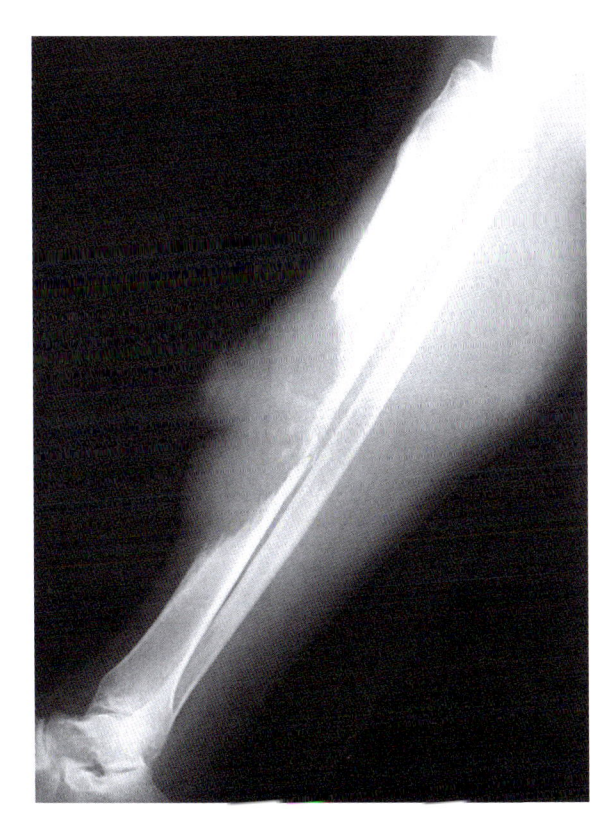

FIGURE 18-12

Malignant lymphoma of the tibia with extensive cortical destruction and a soft tissue mass.

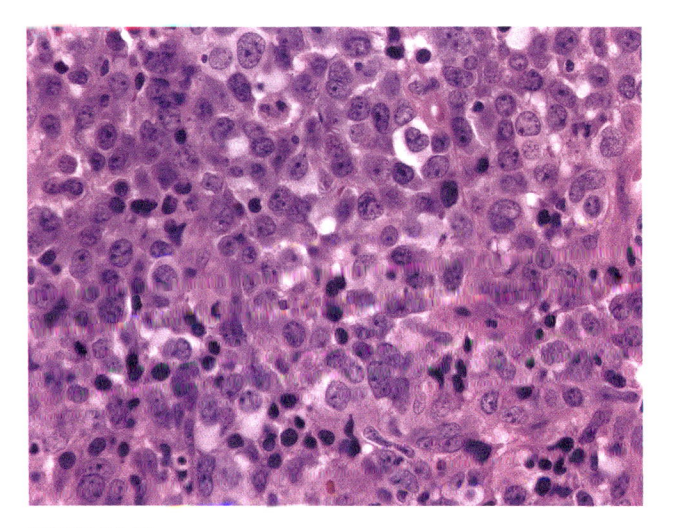

FIGURE 18-13

Almost all lymphomas of bone are diffuse large B-cell lymphomas. The cells have a large, round, noncleaved nucleus with clumped chromatin. Cytoplasm is scant.

trabeculae intact. Most often the tumor cells display a centroblastic morphology with scant cytoplasm, significant nuclear pleomorphism, finely clumped chromatin, and two or three membrane-bound nucleoli (Figure 18-13). An immunoblastic morphology with round nuclei, a single prominent nucleoli, and abundant amphophilic cytoplasm is seen in some tumors.

In addition to DLBCLs, occasionally other lymphoid malignancies including precursor B-cell lymphoblastic

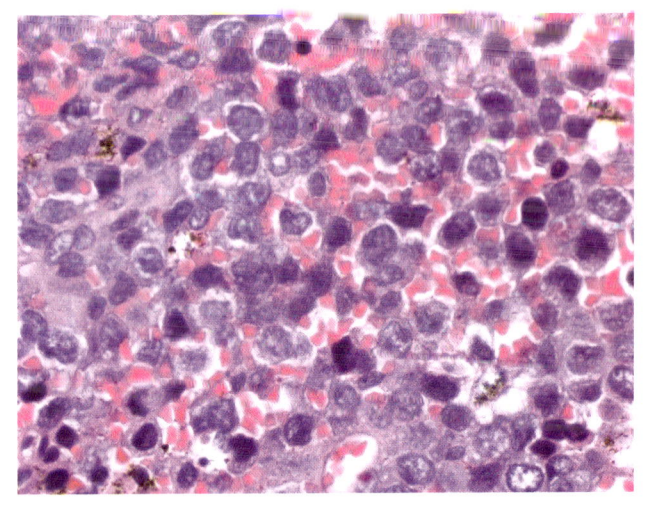

FIGURE 18-14
Anaplastic large-cell lymphoma shows considerable nuclear pleomorphism. These cells are almost always T cells.

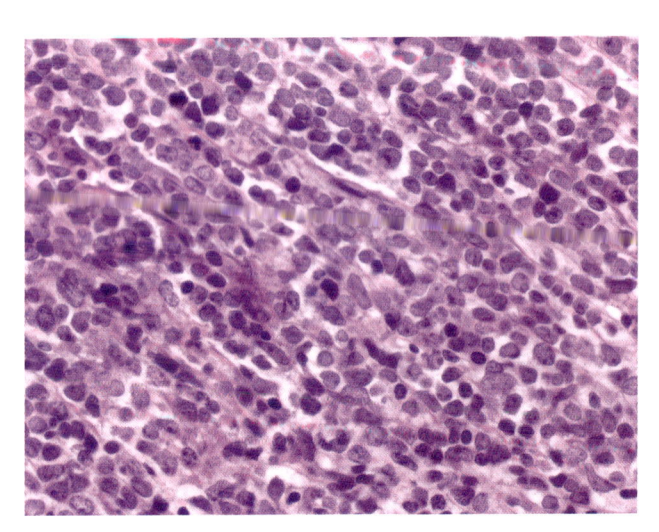

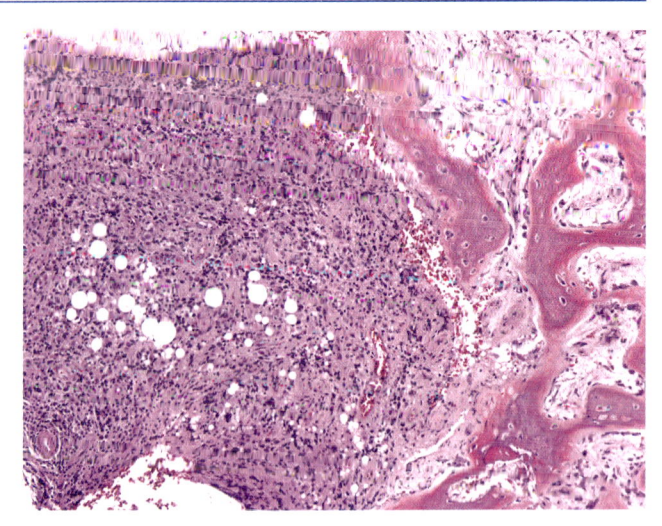

FIGURE 18-16
Many primary lymphomas of bone have areas of fibrosis and reactive bone formation.

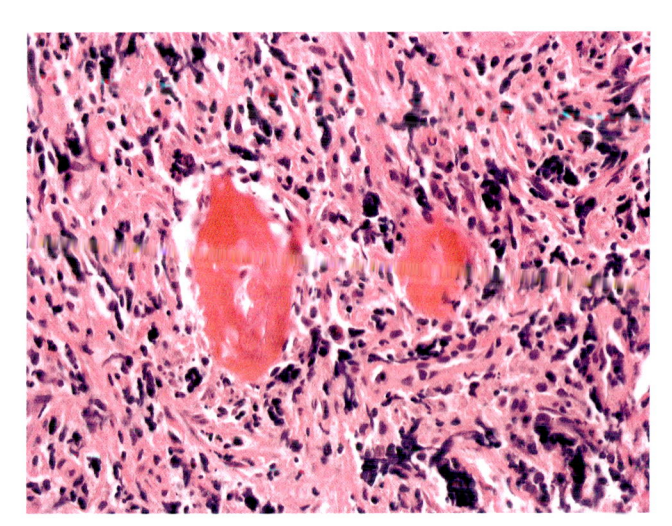

FIGURE 18-15
Lymphoblastic variant.
Lymphoblastic lymphoma typically shows uniform rounded nuclei with almost no cytoplasm. The chromatin of the nuclei shows a fine granularity typical of primitive cells.

FIGURE 18-17
Extensive crush artifact oftentimes obscures the cytologic features of the lymphoid cells in malignant lymphomas of bone.

lymphoma, T-cell lymphoma, and anaplastic large-cell lymphoma present as primary lymphoma of bone. Anaplastic large-cell lymphomas show nuclei of markedly varying sizes and shapes (Figure 18-14). Horseshoe nuclei are common. Lymphoblastic lymphoma, which is usually restricted to children, contains sheets of tumor cells with rounded nuclei, and a fine, stippled chromatin pattern infiltrates the marrow spaces (Figure 18-15).

Many lymphomas of bone have associated histologic features that make a diagnosis difficult. First, many contain a dense population of inflammatory cells, most of which are T lymphocytes; neutrophils may also be present. These inflammatory infiltrates may obscure the lymphoma cells and lead to the incorrect diagnosis of osteomyelitis. Second, lymphoma of bone may contain loose or dense fibrous tissue, which entraps the neoplastic cells in a pseudo-organoid pattern. This pattern may lead to the misdiagnosis of metastatic carcinoma. Lesions with extensive fibrosis also have abundant reactive bone (Figure 18-16). These cells may be arranged in a storiform pattern and masquerade as a sarcoma. Third, decalcification, and in particular crush artifact, can also hinder accurate histologic interpretation of surgical biopsies (Figure 18-17).

ANCILLARY STUDIES

IMMUNOHISTOCHEMISTRY

Immunohistochemical studies are required to establish an accurate histologic diagnosis of primary lymphoma of bone. The panel should include markers against B cells (CD20 and CD79a), T cells (CD3), and leucocyte common antigen (CD45). Because anaplastic large-cell lymphoma cells express CD30, this marker should be added to the panel when large pleomorphic lymphoid cells are the predominate finding. Most anaplastic large-cell lymphomas are of T lineage and, therefore, are generally positive for T-cell markers such as CD3 and CD4. When precursor B-cell lymphoblastic lymphoma of bone is in the differential diagnosis, additional immunostains including CD10, CD43, CD79a, and Tdt are required.

Differential Diagnosis

The differential diagnosis depends on the age of the patient. In children, primary lymphoma of bone must be differentiated from other round blue cells tumors, particularly Ewing sarcoma. Ewing sarcomas will be positive with CD99 and negative with CD45. However, precursor B-cell lymphoblastic lymphomas can also be positive with CD99, and negative with CD45 and CD20. Therefore, it may be easy to misdiagnose a lymphoblastic lymphoma as a Ewing sarcoma. Additional markers such as Tdt, CD43, and CD79a that are expressed by lymphoblastic lymphoma but not Ewing sarcoma are helpful in sorting through the differential diagnosis.

In adults, primary lymphoma of bone may be confused with multiple myeloma. In some poorly differentiated myelomas, the plasma cell features are not apparent. In this setting, clinicopathologic and radiographic findings will solve the problem in most instances. Immunostains can also be helpful because myeloma cells show strong cytoplasmic immunoglobulin light-chain stain restriction, whereas they are weakly positive or negative for CD45 and CD20. In contrast, most B-cell lymphomas show the converse staining pattern, with strong positivity for CD45 and CD20, and little reactivity for CD138 and immunoglobulin light chains.

Metastatic carcinoma must also be included in the differential diagnosis in adults. Some lymphomas are anaplastic and may be confused with metastatic epithelial neoplasms. Therefore, cytokeratin stains should be performed to rule out metastatic carcinoma.

Some primary lymphomas of bone have a secondary population of inflammatory cells, particularly lymphocytes. These lymphocytes are most often T lymphocytes. Therefore, it is important to recognize that the

---

LYMPHOMA OF BONE—FACT SHEET

Definition
- A neoplastic proliferation of lymphocytes involving a bone without evidence of systemic or nodal disease

Incidence and Location
- Primary lymphoma of bone accounts for 7% of all malignant bone tumors
- Femur and pelvis are the most common bones to be involved

Sex, Race, and Age Distribution
- Lymphoma of bone affects both children and adults, but 50% of patients are older than 40 years
- No significant age or racial variation

Clinical Features
- Pain is the most common symptom
- Some patients present with pathologic fracture
- Some patients also have a soft tissue mass

Radiologic Features
- Lesions are usually poorly defined with a permeative pattern of bone destruction
- Some lesions have interosseous reactive bone that causes focal radiodensity
- MRI shows long segments of increased signal on T2-weighted images, often larger than the lytic area
- Periosteal reactive bone is frequently present

Prognosis and Treatment
- Treatment includes radiation and chemotherapy
- Five-year survival rate ranges from 50% to 90%
- Patients older than 60 years have a worse prognosis

LYMPHOMA OF BONE—PATHOLOGIC FEATURES

Gross Findings
- Areas of bone destruction are replaced by soft hemorrhagic or fleshy tissue

Microscopic Findings
- Diffuse sheets of lymphoid cells
- Most often, centroblastic morphology with multilobated nuclei
- Occasionally, immunoblastic morphology with round nuclei and abundant amphophilic cytoplasm
- Rarely, anaplastic large-cell lymphoma with large pleomorphic nuclei
- May contain dense fibrosis associated with crush artifact of tumor cells or sarcomatoid appearance
- Reed-Sternberg cells in Hodgkin lymphoma

Immunohistochemical Findings
- Most commonly DLBCL; cells will be positive for CD45 and CD20
- Anaplastic large-cell lymphomas are positive with CD30
- Precursor B-cell lymphoblastic lymphomas may be positive for CD99, and negative for CD20 and CD3; Tdt, CD43, and CD79a will be positive

Differential Diagnosis
- Ewing sarcoma
- Metastatic carcinoma
- Sarcoma in tumors with extensive fibrosis
- Myeloma

neoplastic cells stain with B-cell markers and the smaller, non-neoplastic lymphocytes stain for T cells. Similarly, chronic osteomyelitis with an abundant population of lymphocytes can be excluded by the polyclonal nature of the lymphocytes. Inflammatory lesions in bone will consist mainly of T lymphocytes with an admixture of a smaller number of B lymphocytes.

Prognosis and Treatment

Unlike most primary bone malignancies, surgical resection is not the treatment of choice for primary lymphoma of bone. This disease is best treated with radiation and chemotherapy. Lymphomas of bone without visceral or nodal disease have a good prognosis with this therapy. In patients with lymphoma confined to the bone, reported 5-year survival rates range from 60% to 90%. Tumor location is not a factor in prognosis. In general, patients older than 60 have a somewhat worse prognosis. Surgery may be used in the event of local recurrence.

HODGKIN LYMPHOMA OF BONE

As with non-Hodgkin lymphomas, bones may be secondarily involved in disseminated Hodgkin lymphoma in the late stages. In Hodgkin lymphoma, radiologic evidence of bone involvement is present in 13% of advanced cases, although the incidence at autopsy is much greater. Bone marrow involvement without radiologic change may occur in 15% of advanced cases. In disseminated (stage IV) disease, bone involvement is due to hematogenous spread.

On rare occasions, Hodgkin lymphoma presents primary in bone without obvious lymph-node involvement. To date, only 21 cases of this presentation have been documented. After close clinical and radiologic study, however, many of these cases also had adjacent nodal disease, a finding that suggests that bones were secondarily involved by contiguous spread from nodal disease. The bones most frequently involved were the sternum, femur, vertebrae, tibia, and humerus. The bone lesions were usually lytic, and the age range was 5 to 83 years, with the average age being 31 years.

In most cases, the Hodgkin lymphoma associated with bone involvement is the nodular sclerosing or mixed cellularity type. Histologically, Reed-Sternberg cells and mononuclear variants are present in a polymorphous background that includes lymphocytes, plasma cells, eosinophils, and fibrous tissue. Reed–Sternberg cells stain with CD15, CD30, and PAX 5. They are negative with CD45 and T cell and B-cell markers.

Hodgkin lymphoma in bone with only limited nodal disease responds to combine aggressive radiotherapy and chemotherapy. Most patients survive at least 3 years. By contrast, patients with bone involvement secondary to disseminated Hodgkin disease have a poorer prognosis.

SUGGESTED READINGS

Multiple Myeloma

1. Anderson KC, Shaughnessy JD, Barlogie B, et al: Multiple myeloma. Hematology 2002;1:214–240.
2. Angtuaco EJC, Fassas ABT, Walker R, et al: Multiple myeloma: clinical review and diagnostic imaging. Radiology 2004;231:11–23.
3. Dingli D, Kyle RA, Rajkumar SV, et al: Immunoglobulin free light chains and solitary plasmacytoma of bone. Blood 2006;108(6):1979–1983.
4. Kyle RA, Gertz MA, Witzig TE, et al: Review of 1027 patients with newly diagnosed multiple myeloma. Mayo Clin Proc 2003;78:21–33.
5. Larson RS, Sukpanichnant S, Greer JP, et al: The spectrum of multiple myeloma: diagnostic and biological implications. Hum Pathol 1997;28:1336–1347.
6. Rajkumar SV, Kyle RA: Multiple myeloma: diagnosis and treatment. Mayo Clin Proc 2005;80(10):1371–1382.
7. Seidl S, Kaufmann H, Drach J: New insights into the pathophysiology of multiple myeloma. Lancet 2003;4:557–564.
8. Terpos E, Politou M, Rahemtulla A: New insights into the pathophysiology and management of bone disease in multiple myeloma. Br J Haematol 2003;123:758–769.

Lymphoma of Bone

1. Gianelli U, Patriarca C, Moro A, et al: Lymphomas of the bone: a pathological and clinical study of 54 cases. Int J Surg Pathol 2002;10:257–266.
2. Huebner-Chan D, Fernandes B, Yang G, et al: An immunophenotypic and molecular study of primary large B-cell lymphoma of bone. Mod Pathol 2001;14:1000–1007.
3. Jones D, Kraus MD, Dorfman HD: Lymphoma presenting as a solitary bone lesion. Am J Clin Pathol 1999;111:171–178.
4. Mulligan ME, McRae GA, Murphey MD: Imaging features of primary lymphoma of bone. Am J Roentgenol 1999;173:1691–1697.
5. Nagasaka T, Nakamura S, Medeiros LJ, et al: Anaplastic large cell lymphomas presented as bone lesions: A clinicopathologic study of six cases and review of the literature [Review]. Mod Pathol 2000;13(10):1143–1149.
6. Ozdemirli M, Fanburg-Smith JC, Hartmann DP, et al: Precursor B-lymphoblastic lymphoma presenting as a solitary bone tumor and mimicking Ewing's sarcoma. A report of four cases and review of the literature. Am J Surg Pathol 1998;22:795–804.
7. Pettit CK, Zukerberg LR, Gray MH, et al: Primary lymphoma of bone. A B-cell neoplasm with a high frequency of multilobated cells. Am J Surg Pathol 1990;14(4):329–334.
8. Ruzek KA, Wenger DE: The multiple faces of lymphoma of the musculoskeletal system. Skeletal Radiol 2004;33:1–8.
9. Zhao XF, Young KH, Frank D, et al: Pediatric primary bone lymphoma-diffuse large B-cell lymphoma: morphologic and immunohistochemical characteristics of 10 cases. Am J Clin Pathol 2007;127(1):47–54.

Hodgkin Lymphoma of Bone

1. Ostrowski ML, Inwards CY, Strickler JG, et al: Osseous Hodgkin disease. Cancer 1999;85:1166–1178.

19 Vascular Tumors of Bone
Andrew Horvai

- Hemangioma
- Epithelioid Hemangioendothelioma
- Angiosarcoma

Vascular tumors of bone range from common, and usually asymptomatic, benign hemangiomas to rare malignant angiosarcomas. Multifocality is common in both benign and malignant vascular tumors. Syndromes such as Klippel–Trenaunay and Sturge–Weber can predispose patients to vasoformative bone tumors, but most tumors are sporadic.

Some controversy exists in the nomenclature of lesions with intermediate grade histology: The term *hemangioendothelioma* has historically been used to describe both benign and malignant lesions. Currently, most authors agree that *epithelioid hemangioendothelioma (EHE)* straddles the clinical spectrum between hemangioma and angiosarcoma; that is, it represents a low grade malignancy with a more favorable prognosis than angiosarcoma. To avoid confusion, we recommend the diagnoses of angiosarcoma and hemangioma be used to identify malignant and benign vascular tumors, respectively, whereas the term *hemangioendothelioma* be reserved for the specific diagnosis of *EHE* only. For practical purposes, assignment of a vascular tumor into one of these three categories is clinically relevant in predicting outcome.

HEMANGIOMA

CLINICAL FEATURES

Hemangioma is a benign proliferation of blood vessels that is most often asymptomatic. It commonly affects the spine, specifically the vertebral bodies, and can be multifocal, involving multiple bones or adjacent soft tissue sites, or both. Autopsy studies suggest that asymptomatic hemangiomas of the spine are quite common, with an incidence rate of 12% in adults. The age range is broad (first to eighth decades of life), but the majority of cases present in middle age (peak during fifth decade of life). Men are affected about twice as often as women. Although mostly asymptomatic, hemangiomas may come to clinical attention through local mass effect (particularly in the skull), or pain from spinal cord compression or pathologic fracture. In congenital examples, hemangiomas can produce limb hyperplasia or hypoplasia. The distinction between hemangioma and arteriovenous malformation is best made clinically or angiographically insofar as the latter demonstrates direct continuity between arterial and venous channels without an interposed capillary bed. Consequently, arteriovenous malformations may present with hemodynamic sequelae of a left-to-right shunt.

RADIOLOGIC FEATURES

The classic spinal hemangioma often affects multiple adjacent vertebral bodies and may include pathologic fracture (Figure 19-1). Plain films demonstrate a *corduroy* appearance, and computed tomography (CT) scans show a *polka-dot* pattern (Figure 19-2). The above terms correspond to hyperintense, coarsened, vertical trabeculae interposed between hypointense fat and are sufficiently specific that, in asymptomatic cases, the diagnosis can be made without tissue confirmation. The findings in the skull and long bones are less specific, and include sharp margins and a variegated density.

PATHOLOGIC FEATURES

GROSS FINDINGS

If resected intact, a hemangioma shows sclerotic trabeculae radiating between soft, bloody clefts. More often, however, hemangiomas are curetted, resulting in soft, friable clot, rare spicules of bone, and firm pink connective tissue.

390　BONE AND SOFT TISSUE PATHOLOGY

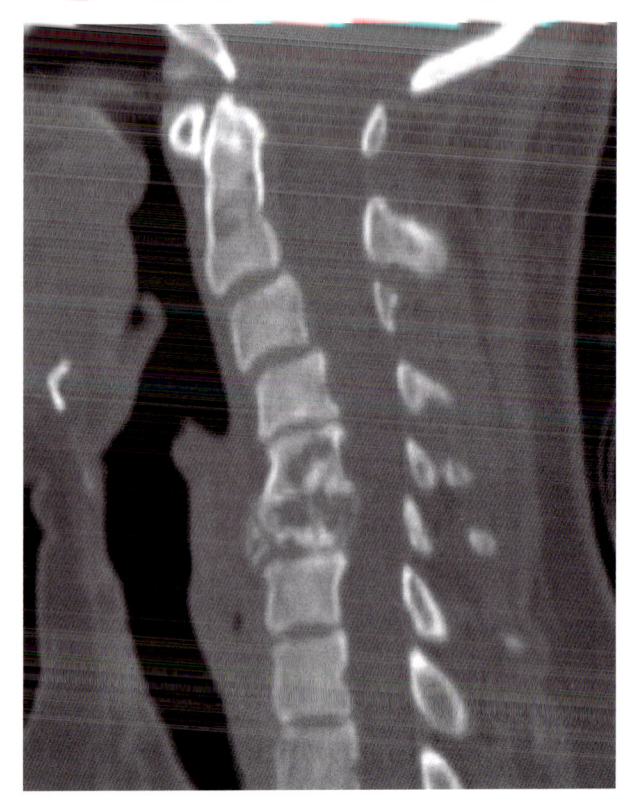

FIGURE 19-1
Reformatted sagittal computed tomographic scan of a hemangioma involving C5 and C6 vertebrae with a compression fracture of C6.

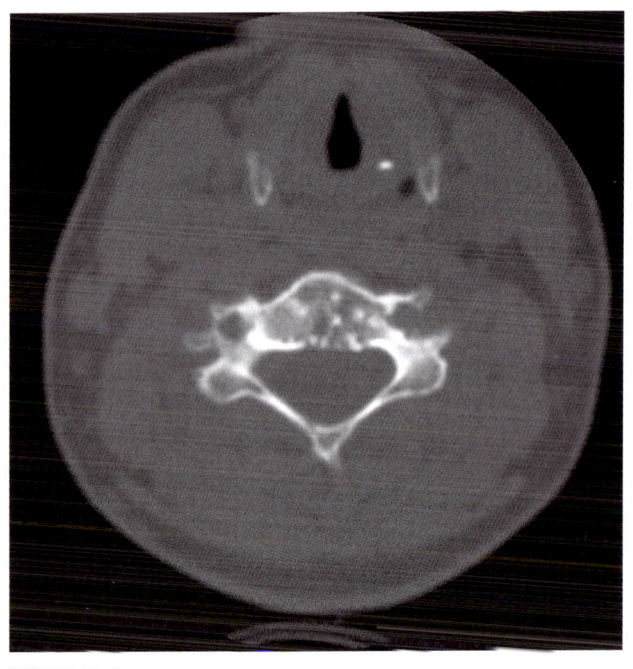

FIGURE 19-2
Axial computed tomographic scan of a hemangioma affecting C5 vertebral body shows characteristic polka-dot pattern. The pattern corresponds to dense vertical trabeculae interposed between adipose tissue and vascular spaces.

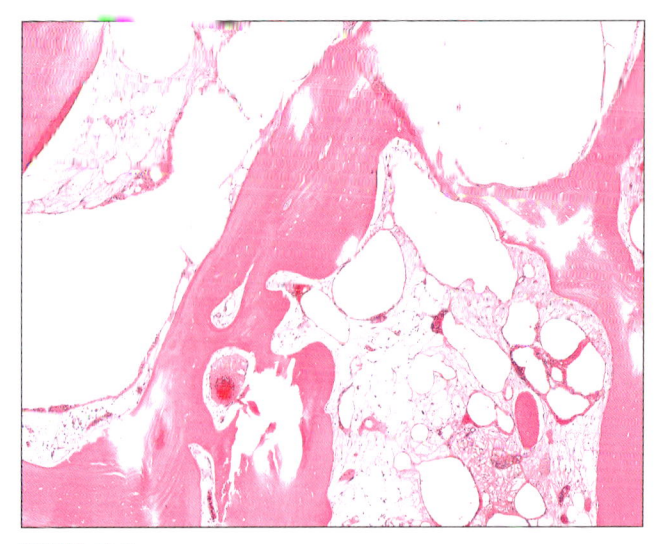

FIGURE 19-3
Low-power view of cavernous hemangioma demonstrates growth pattern with gaping vascular spaces replacing marrow cavity between trabeculae.

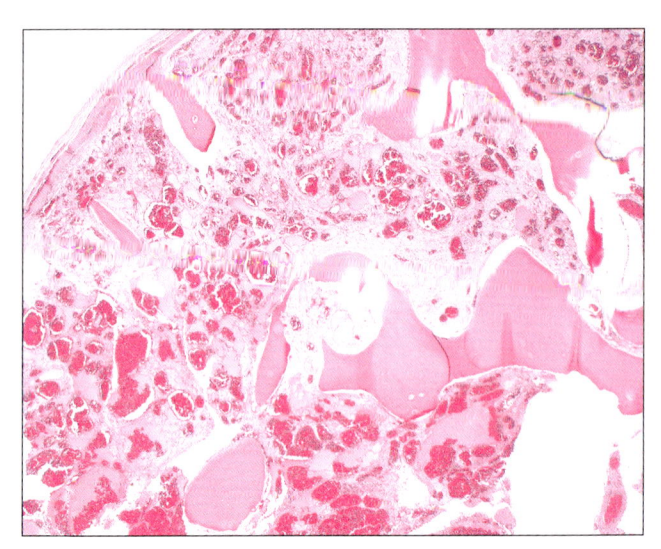

FIGURE 19-4
Low-power view of cavernous hemangioma with erosion of cortical bone (top left).

MICROSCOPIC FINDINGS

Hemangiomas may be subdivided based on the predominant type of vessel, analogous to their soft tissue counterparts. However, most examples consist of vessels of a variety of sizes. Cavernous hemangiomas consist of large, gaping vascular lakes that replace the marrow space (Figure 19-3) and may erode the cortex (Figure 19-4). The vascular structures are lined by flattened, cytologic bland endothelial cells (Figure 19-5). Capillary hemangiomas consist predominantly of small vascular spaces lined by a single layer of endothelial cells (Figure 19-6). By definition, the endothelial cells lack atypia, and in the stroma between individual capillaries is hypocellular with little to no inflammation. Occasionally, the endothelial cells may be plump and cuboidal, producing an epithelioid appearance (Figure 19-7). Focal areas of

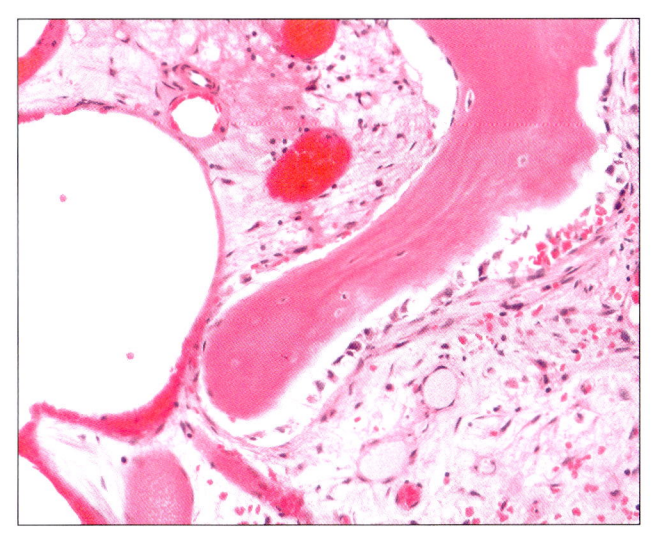

FIGURE 19-5
High-power view of cavernous hemangioma showing a dilated vascular space is lined by a single layer of attenuated, cytologically bland endothelial cells.

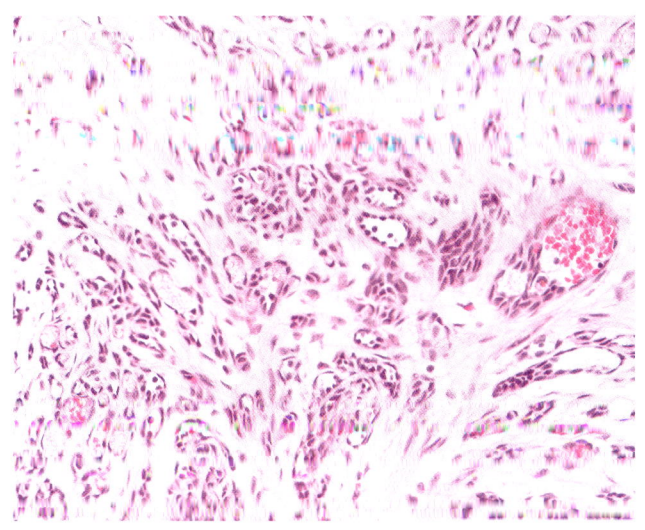

FIGURE 19-7
Epithelioid hemangiomas demonstrate predominantly cuboidal endothelial cells but still confined to a single layer around well-formed vascular channels. Cytologic atypia and mitotic activity are not prominent.

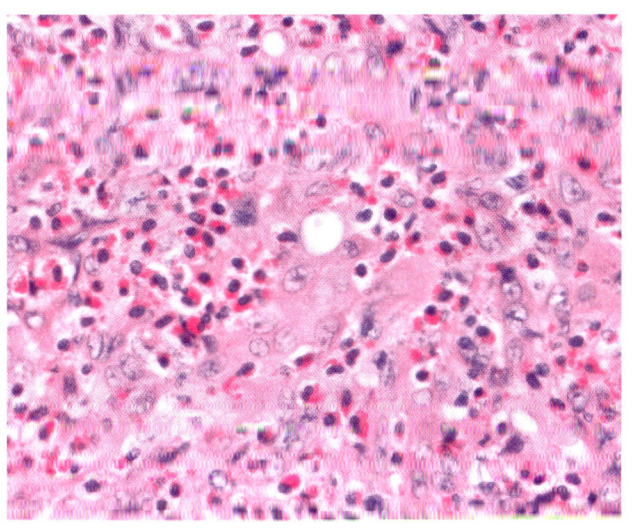

FIGURE 19-6
High-power view of capillary hemangioma with a predominance of small vascular spaces, still lined by a single layer of endothelial cells without atypia.

FIGURE 19-8
Some examples of epithelioid hemangioma of bone may show a prominent lymphoeosinophilic infiltrate between vascular channels in a pattern similar to the analogous lesion in soft tissue (angiolymphoid hyperplasia with eosinophilia).

such epithelioid endothelial cells may be a component in many hemangiomas. However, if this finding is diffuse, such lesions have been classified as epithelioid hemangioma, especially if they also demonstrate the prominent lymphoeosinophilic infiltrate analogous to the soft tissue epithelioid hemangioma (angiolymphoid hyperplasia with eosinophilia) (Figure 19-8).

ANCILLARY STUDIES

The endothelial cells of hemangioma stain for antibodies against CD31, CD34, factor VIII antigen, and Fli-1, although immunohistochemistry is seldom required to diagnose these lesions.

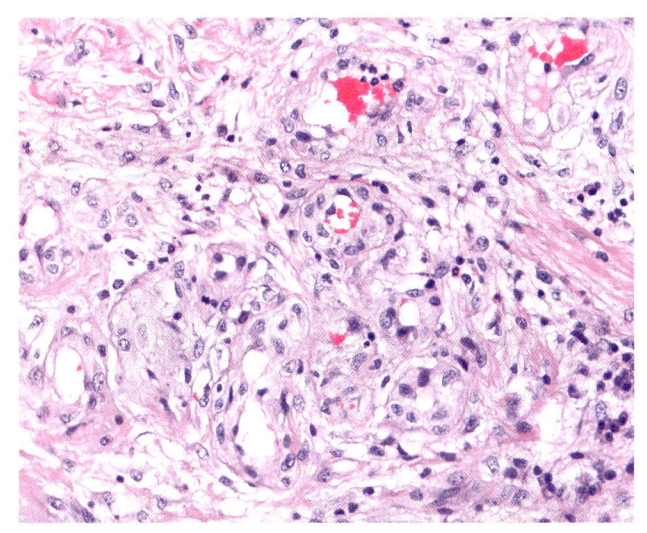

DIFFERENTIAL DIAGNOSIS

Radiographically, the presence of multiple lytic lesions of the long bones or calvarium may suggest Langerhans histiocytosis in young patients or metastatic carcinoma in adults. Reactive vascular proliferations, such as granulation tissue from a fracture callus, may mimic vasoformative neoplasms. Reactive proliferations often demonstrate a proliferation of benign mesenchymal cells between the vascular spaces, as well as mixed inflammation including neutrophils. Angiosarcoma may enter the differential if the radiographic appearance is particularly aggressive. The distinction is based on the presence

HEMANGIOMA—FACT SHEET

Definition
- Benign vascular proliferation of bone

Incidence and Location
- Incidence rate of up to 12% of autopsy cases
- Wide skeletal distribution
- Most commonly affects the spine (vertebral body) and calvarium

Sex, Race, and Age Distribution
- Male-to-female ratio of 2:1, peak in fifth decade of life

Clinical Features
- Mostly asymptomatic
- Pain associated with spinal cord compression and mass in tumors of calvarium

Radiographic Features
- Plain films of spine show corduroy pattern
- CT demonstrates polka-dot pattern

Prognosis and Treatment
- Incidental cases require no treatment
- Curettage and cement is usually curative
- Other options include external beam radiation

HEMANGIOMA—PATHOLOGIC FEATURES

Gross Findings
- Predominantly hemorrhage, scattered spicules of bone, and soft pink vascular tissue

Microscopic Findings
- Vasoformative nature is evident at low power
- Size of predominant vessels determines subtype (cavernous, capillary), although most examples are mixed
- Epithelioid endothelial cells may be focal or diffuse
- Cytologic atypia and mitotic activity absent

Differential Diagnosis
- Reactive vascular proliferation
- Angiosarcoma
- Epithelioid hemangioendothelioma

---

of cytologic atypia, mitotic activity, and a diffuse, rather than lobular, growth pattern.

The presence of epithelioid endothelial cells in a vascular lesion raises the differential of EHE. This differential diagnosis is further confused by nonuniformity in nomenclature. Some authors have used the terms *hemangioendothelioma* (without the *epithelioid* qualifier) interchangeably with *epithelioid hemangioma*. It is best to consider *epithelioid hemangioma* as a completely benign vascular proliferation in which the endothelial cells are plump and cuboidal but line well-formed vessels throughout the lesion; in other words, the tumor is uniformly vasoformative. *EHE* (described in more detail in the next section) shows at least focal presence of endothelial cells in clusters, cords, or singly without well-formed vessels but with intracytoplasmic lumina.

Prognosis and Treatment

The prognosis for hemangioma is excellent. Incidental hemangiomas require no treatment. Symptomatic cases may be treated with curettage and cement with a low rate of local recurrence. Tumors that may not be amenable to surgical eradication (i.e., multiple bones involved in a limb) may occasionally be treated with radiation therapy.

EPITHELIOID HEMANGIOENDOTHELIOMA

Clinical Features

EHE represents a vascular neoplasm intermediate between hemangioma and angiosarcoma in terms of recurrence and metastatic potential. The tumor, especially in bone, is often multicentric, and most patients have pain, a mass, or both. A slight predilection for the spine and pelvis has been reported, but these tumors have a widespread distribution throughout the axial and appendicular skeleton. EHE can present simultaneously in somatic soft tissue and viscera including the liver. The sexes are affected equally with a slight peak in the third decade but with a wide age range (20–80 years). For solitary bone lesions, the treatment of choice is wide local excision, with possible regional lymph-node dissection, but without adjuvant radiotherapy or chemotherapy. Patients with multicentric, monomelic tumors can be offered radiation therapy, with or without surgery. Novel techniques such as radiofrequency thermal ablation are most often necessary in cases of multifocal bone involvement.

Radiologic Features

The radiographic features of EHE are relatively nonspecific and may mimic a number of other entities. In long bones, EHE most commonly affects the metaphysis. The plain radiographic appearance of EHE of bone is typically osteolytic but may be either poorly demarcated or show a sclerotic rim. Periosteal reaction is usually absent. CT (Figures 19-9 and 19-10) and magnetic resonance scans are not entirely specific in this setting either; the radiographic differential diagnosis will likely include entities such as lymphoma, metastatic carcinoma, and fibrous dysplasia. The presence of multiple lesions clustering in a single bone or anatomic region may imply a vascular neoplasm including EHE.

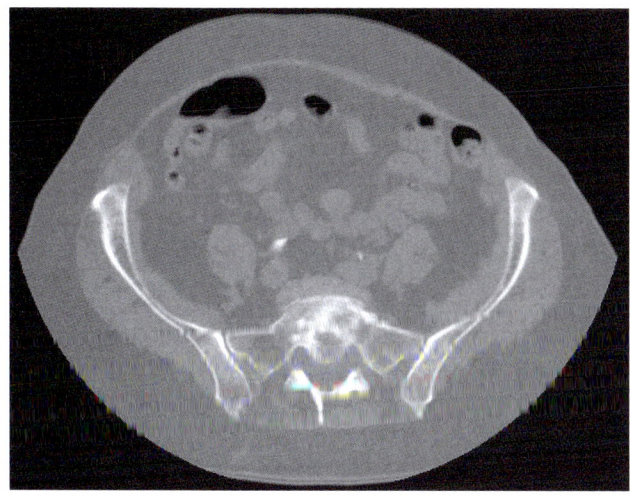

Pathologic Features

Gross Findings

Curettage specimens show bloody, soft red tissue with a few intact spicules of bone. Higher-grade lesions may have necrosis and little to no residual bone. Soft tissue extension may be present.

Microscopic Findings

EHE demonstrates a vaguely lobulated growth pattern. The predominant matrix is myxoid (Figure 19-11) to hyalinized (Figure 19-12). At low power, a distinct vasoformative growth pattern is typically *absent*. Rather, the tumor cells grow in nests

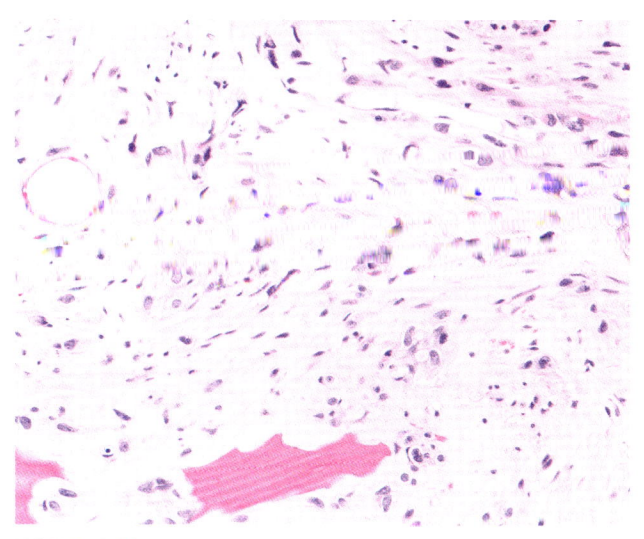

FIGURE 19-9
Axial computed tomographic image of sacral epithelioid hemangioendothelioma (EHE). The presence of multiple lesions, in this case, lytic with sclerotic margins, suggests a vascular lesion but is not entirely specific for EHE.

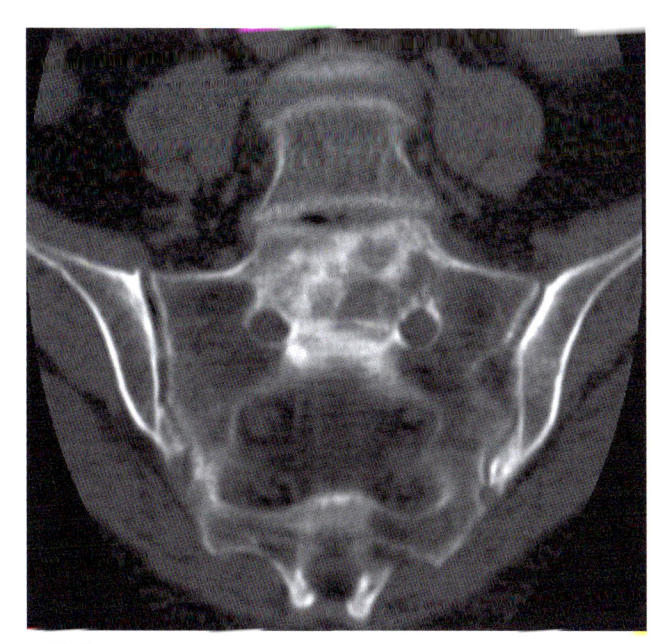

FIGURE 19-11
Epithelioid hemangioendothelioma usually contains myxoid stroma and epithelioid cells in nests.

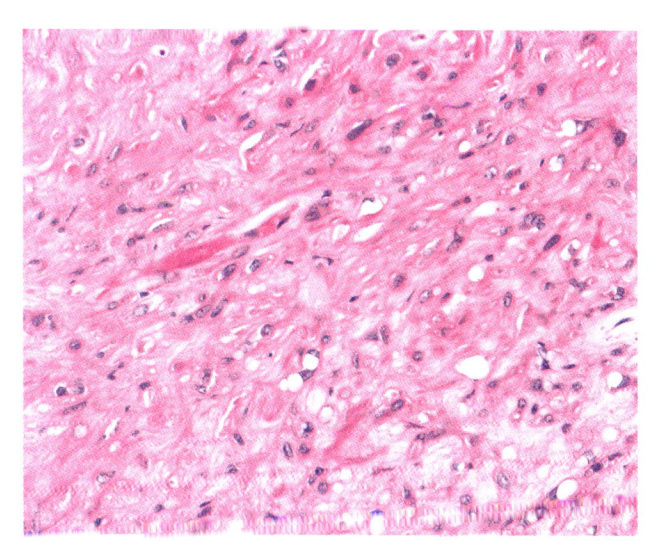

FIGURE 19-10
Coronal reformatted computed tomographic image of sacral epithelioid hemangioendothelioma shows multiple lytic lesions.

FIGURE 19-12
In some examples of epithelioid hemangioendothelioma, the stroma may be focally or diffusely hyalinized.

or anastomosing cords (Figure 19-13). Individual tumor cells are plump, and have ample pale eosinophilic cytoplasm and round nuclei with prominent central nucleoli imparting a distinctly epithelioid cytomorphology at high power. A characteristic feature of this tumor is the presence of a single intracytoplasmic vacuole in occasional tumor cells (Figure 19-14). Such cells have been termed *blister cells*. Some authors have divided EHE into conventional and high-grade forms. The latter shows more nuclear pleomorphism (Figure 19-15), necrosis, and mitotic activity, essentially resembling conventional angiosarcoma.

ANCILLARY STUDIES

A variety of proteins, with varying degrees of specificity for endothelial cells, may be useful to identify EHE, including factor VIII–related antigen, CD34, and CD31. Generally, a panel of CD31 (Figure 19-16), CD34 (Figure 19-17), and Fli-1 (Figure 19-18) can achieve high sensitivity and specificity. Importantly, like other epithelioid vascular tumors, EHE can express cytokeratins (Figure 19-19) and epithelial membrane antigen.

Only small numbers of EHE cases have been analyzed for genetic abnormalities. Of these, two have demonstrated a t(1;3)(p36.3;q25) translocation, although the specificity of this finding remains to be determined.

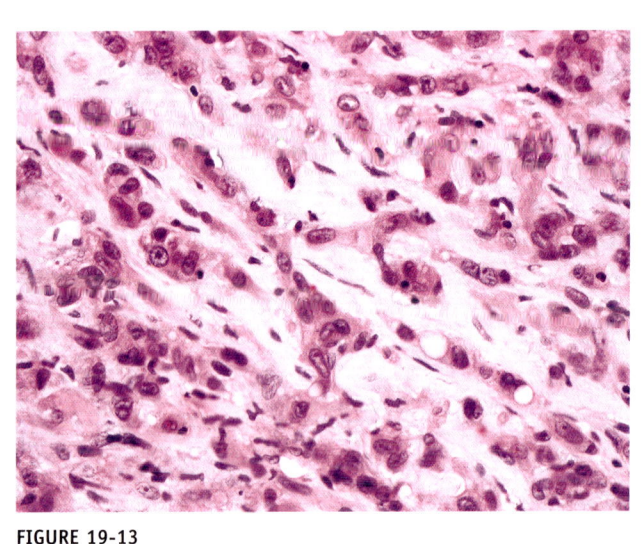

FIGURE 19-13
The neoplastic cells of epithelioid hemangioendothelioma may grow in anastomosing cords.

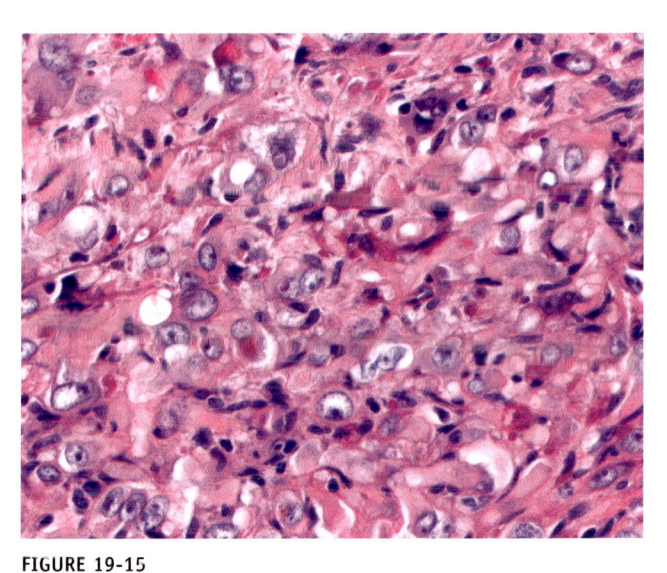

FIGURE 19-15
Example of a high-grade epithelioid hemangioendothelioma with more striking nuclear pleomorphism and increased cellularity.

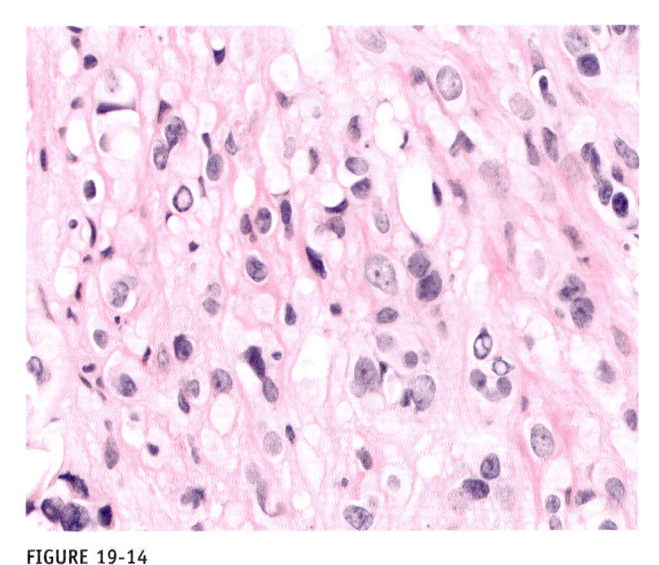

FIGURE 19-14
Occasional cells of epithelioid hemangioendothelioma contain intracytoplasmic lumina (so-called blister cells) that may mimic adenocarcinoma.

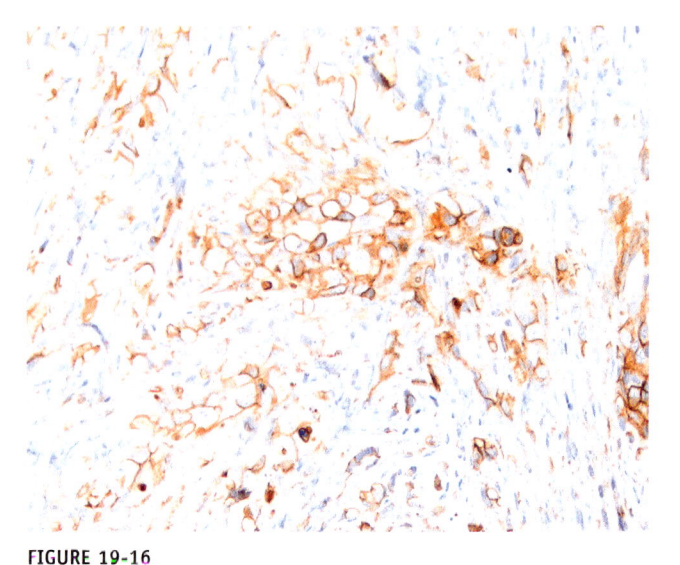

FIGURE 19-16
Immunohistochemical stain for CD31 shows membrane positivity in epithelioid hemangioendothelioma.

DIFFERENTIAL DIAGNOSIS

The combination of multifocal lesions and nonspecific radiographic findings may suggest the diagnosis of metastatic carcinoma in an adult. The epithelioid cytomorphology, intracytoplasmic vacuoles, and expression of epithelial makers in EHE can cause further confusion. Although the lobular growth pattern, at low power, and relative lack of nuclear anaplasia may suggest EHE over carcinoma, resolution of this differential diagnosis will usually require immunohistochemical confirmation of expression of vascular markers. As mentioned earlier, the panel of CD34, CD31, and Fli-1 achieves high specificity in establishing a diagnosis of EHE and excluding carcinoma, particularly in keratin- or EMA-positive cases. Based on clinical history, specific markers for a site of origin (prostate, breast, among others) may be useful to confirm the diagnosis of carcinoma.

Because EHE straddles a continuum between benign epithelioid hemangioma and epithelioid angiosarcoma, these two entities may enter into the differential diagnosis. As mentioned earlier, epithelioid hemangioma is uniformly vasoformative and lacks nests and cords of cells with intracytoplasmic vacuoles. It may be difficult to distinguish between an EHE with increased nuclear atypia and an epithelioid angiosarcoma. In fact, the distinction between such a *malignant EHE* and frank angiosarcoma is somewhat subjective and without much practical clinical utility. In any event, most epithelioid angiosarcomas (discussed later in more detail) are high grade and are composed of sheets of anaplastic cells with abundant mitotic activity, occasional atypical mitotic figures, and necrosis. A vasoformative growth pattern may not be evident.

The lobular growth pattern and myxoid to hyaline stroma may suggest chondromyxoid fibroma. However, chondromyxoid fibroma demonstrates spindled and stellate cells rather than nests of epithelioid or histiocytic cells. Furthermore, chondromyxoid fibroma tends not to be multifocal. Finally, immunohistochemistry for endothelial differentiation can help confirm the diagnosis.

A tibial or fibular EHE may raise the possibility of adamantinoma given keratin positivity and a pattern of anastomosing cords. The stroma of adamantinoma is typically fibrous rather than myxoid or hyaline. Adamantinoma lacks expression of endothelial markers.

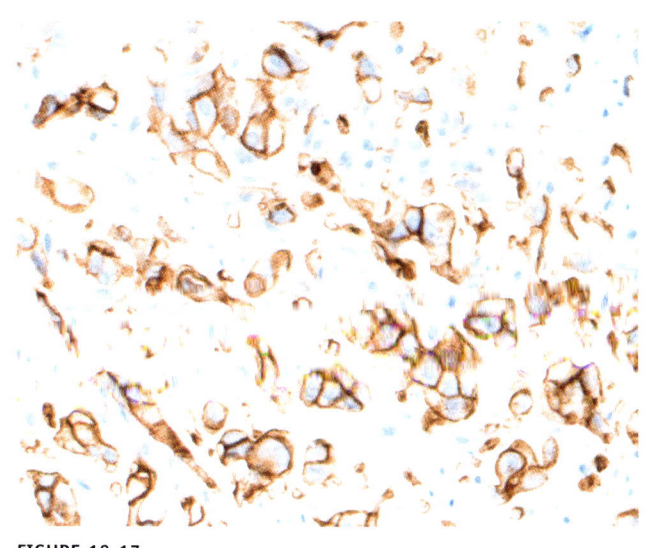

FIGURE 19-17
CD34 stains the cell membrane and, to a lesser extent, the cytoplasm of epithelioid hemangioendothelioma but is less specific than CD31.

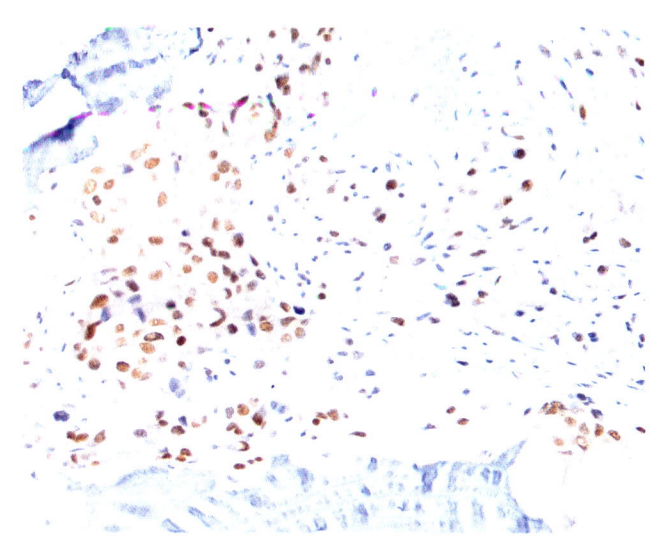

FIGURE 19-18
Fli-1 transcription factor is a sensitive marker for endothelial cells. It is useful in the diagnosis of epithelioid hemangioendothelioma, and the nuclear staining may be easier to interpret than some membrane or cytoplasmic antigens.

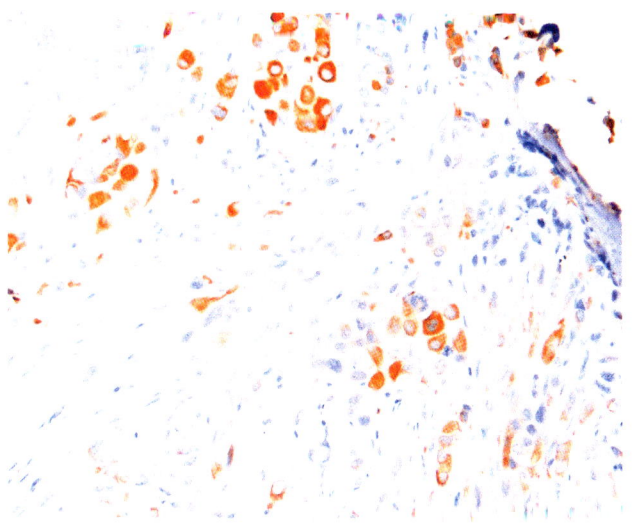

FIGURE 19-19
Focal keratin expression is common in epithelioid hemangioendothelioma, so vascular markers (CD34, CD31, and Fli-1) are required to differentiate this tumor from metastatic carcinoma.

> **EPITHELIOID HEMANGIOENDOTHELIOMA—FACT SHEET**
>
> **Definition**
> ▸ A neoplasm of endothelial cells of intermediate malignancy
>
> **Incidence and Location**
> ▸ Rare; < 1% of malignant bone tumors
>
> **Sex, Race, and Age Distribution**
> ▸ Male-to-female ratio is 1:1
> ▸ Wide age distribution from third to eighth decades of life
>
> **Clinical Features**
> ▸ Pain at site, mass if tumor is in a superficial bone
>
> **Radiographic Features**
> ▸ Findings are nonspecific; many are lytic with a sclerotic rim
> ▸ Multifocality in an anatomic region suggests vascular neoplasm but not specifically EHE
>
> **Prognosis and Treatment**
> ▸ Prognosis is generally good for tumors limited to the skeleton
> ▸ Mortality increases with visceral involvement
> ▸ Wide local excision for localized tumors
> ▸ Radiotherapy or radiofrequency thermal ablation considered for multifocal disease

> **EPITHELIOID HEMANGIOENDOTHELIOMA—PATHOLOGIC FEATURES**
>
> **Gross Findings**
> ▸ Predominantly bloody, scattered spicules of bone and soft pink vascular tissue
>
> **Microscopic Findings**
> ▸ Lobular growth at low power
> ▸ Myxoid to hyalinized matrix
> ▸ Cells in nests or anastomosing cords
> ▸ Epithelioid cells with pale eosinophilic cytoplasm, prominent nucleoli, and occasional intracytoplasmic vacuoles (blister cells)
>
> **Differential Diagnosis**
> ▸ Metastatic carcinoma
> ▸ Epithelioid hemangioma
> ▸ Epithelioid angiosarcoma
> ▸ Chondromyxoid fibroma
> ▸ Adamantinoma

PROGNOSIS AND TREATMENT

The most important predictor of outcome for EHE is the presence of visceral (especially liver and lung) involvement. Patients who have localized bone disease have a good survival rate. The mainstay of treatment is wide local excision with negative margins for localized tumors. Additional options for multifocal disease include radiation therapy or radiofrequency ablation.

ANGIOSARCOMA

CLINICAL FEATURES

Angiosarcoma of bone is rare, representing less than 1% of malignant bone tumors. Patients typically report bone pain and a mass if the tumor is in a superficial site. Vertebral tumors may produce spinal cord compression symptoms. The sex predilection is approximately equal. The age distribution is fairly even from the second through seventh decades of life. Similar to their soft tissue counterparts, angiosarcomas can arise as postradiation sarcomas. The tumors are slightly more prevalent in the spine and pelvic bones (each approximately 15% of cases, respectively), but the entire skeleton can be affected. Like other vascular tumors, multicentricity in a given anatomic region is common.

RADIOLOGIC FEATURES

Angiosarcoma lesions are predominantly lytic without periosteal reaction. A sclerotic rim may be present in grade 1 angiosarcomas and is less common with increasing grade. Cortical destruction with a soft tissue mass is also more common with high-grade tumors. Multifocality involving a single bone or limb is frequent (Figure 19-20).

PATHOLOGIC FEATURES

GROSS FINDINGS

Curettage specimens consist of soft, reddish, bloody tissue usually without bone. Resection specimens have infiltrative borders, more so in grade 3 lesions, that replace the medullary space with reddish clot. Cortical destruction and soft tissue extension may be present (Figure 19-21).

MICROSCOPIC FINDINGS

At low power, the growth pattern of angiosarcoma is vasoformative with irregular, anastomosing channels permeating and destroying native bone (Figure 19-22).

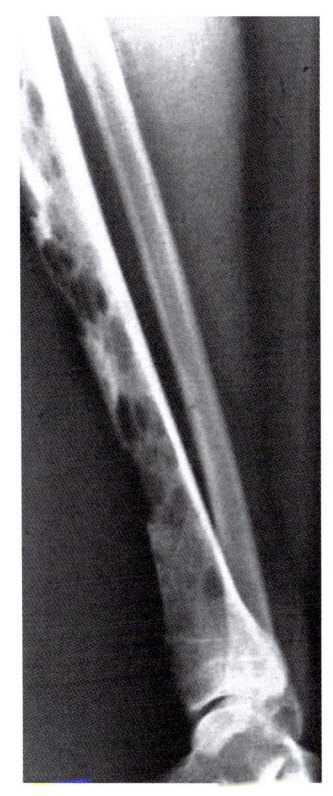

CHAPTER 19 Vascular Tumors of Bone

FIGURE 19-20
Radiograph of angiosarcoma showing multiple lytic lesions involving the tibia. Angiosarcoma should be in the differential diagnosis with other malignant tumors such as metastatic carcinoma and lymphoma that can present as a multicentric process.

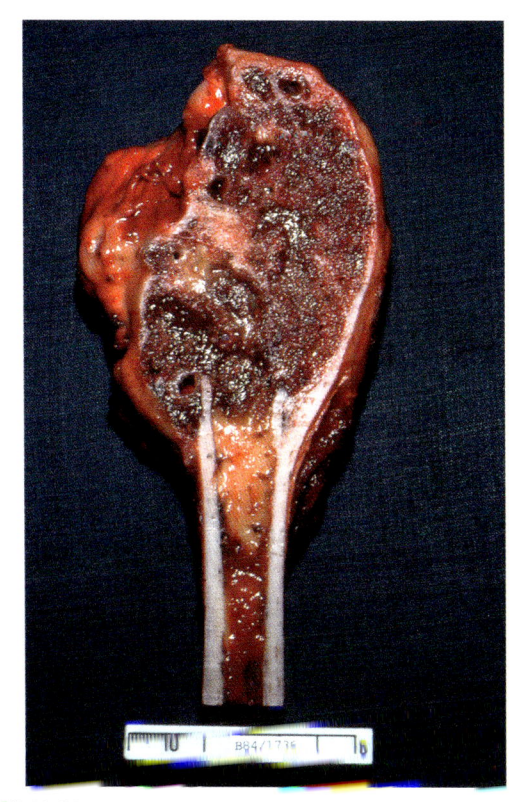

FIGURE 19-21
Gross photo of angiosarcoma involving the proximal fibula. The tumor is red-brown and extending into soft tissue.

ANCILLARY STUDIES

If a definitive vasoformative growth pattern is present, additional studies are generally not necessary. In grade 3 angiosarcomas, and especially epithelioid angiosarcomas, immunohistochemical staining for

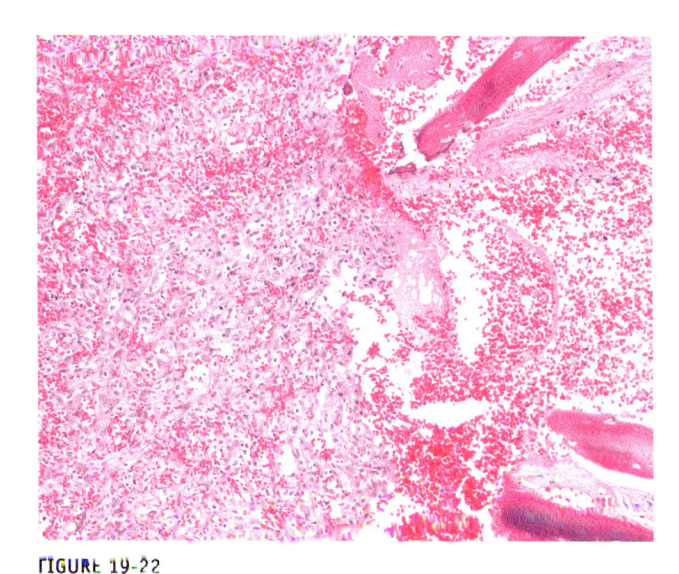

Extensive hemorrhage may obscure the vasoformative pattern at scanning magnification. Collagenous or bony matrix is usually absent. The defining feature of angiosarcoma is the presence of cytologic atypia in the endothelial cells lining the vascular channels. In grade 1 angiosarcomas, mitotic activity and necrosis may not be prominent, but nuclear hyperchromasia, nuclear membrane irregularity, and intravascular budding are present (Figure 19-23). Grade 2 angiosarcomas demonstrate increased nuclear atypia but still retain a vasoformative growth pattern. Grade 3 angiosarcomas show more marked nuclear anaplasia, necrosis, and mitotic activity, including atypical mitotic figures (Figure 19-24).

Some grade 3 angiosarcomas may present with sheet-like growth and plump cells with abundant eosinophilic cytoplasm and marked nuclear atypia, whereas the vasoformative nature may be subtle or essentially absent. These tumors have been classified as epithelioid angiosarcomas if the plump cells dominate the histologic picture (Figure 19-25). In such cases, the diagnosis of angiosarcoma may require immunohistochemical confirmation of endothelial cell differentiation.

FIGURE 19-22
At low-power view, angiosarcoma has a destructive, vasoformative growth pattern of anastomosing channels and extensive hemorrhage.

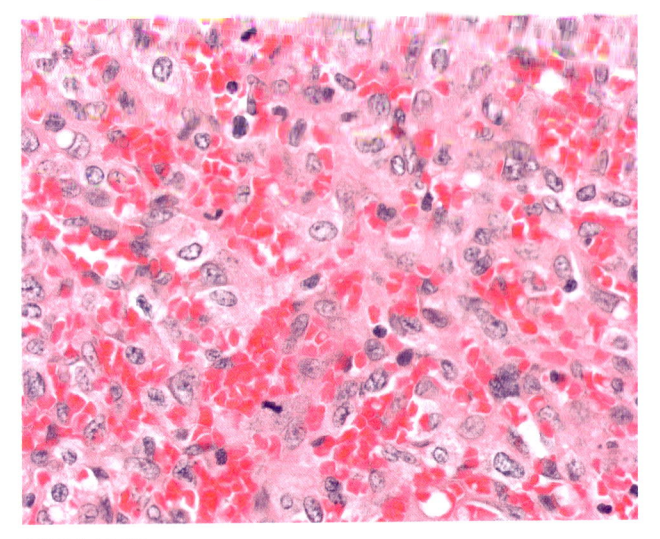

FIGURE 19-23
Grade 1 angiosarcoma typically shows only mild cytologic atypia. Mitotic activity, though present in this case, may be relatively low.

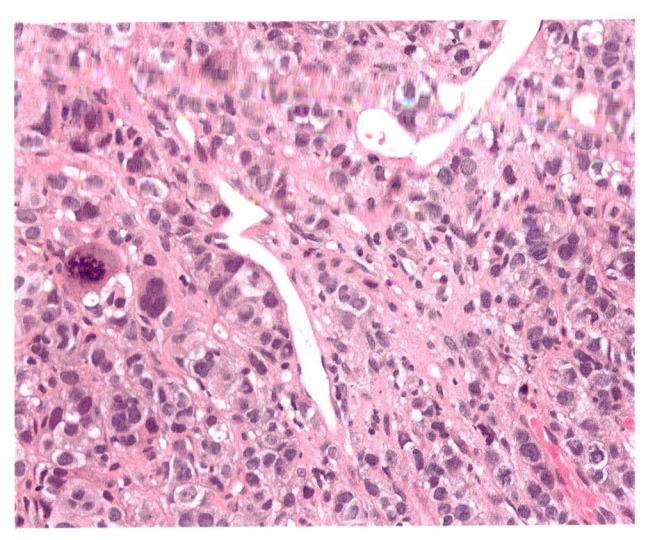

FIGURE 19-25
Epithelioid angiosarcoma (by definition grade 3) is composed of sheets of highly pleomorphic cells with atypical mitotic figures. A vasoformative growth pattern may not be obvious, raising the differential of other high-grade malignancies.

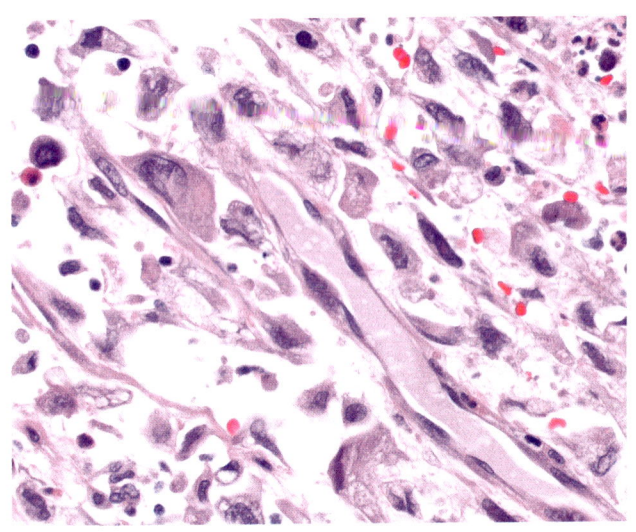

FIGURE 19-24
Grade 3 angiosarcoma demonstrates more marked cytologic atypia with at least some cells lining vascular spaces.

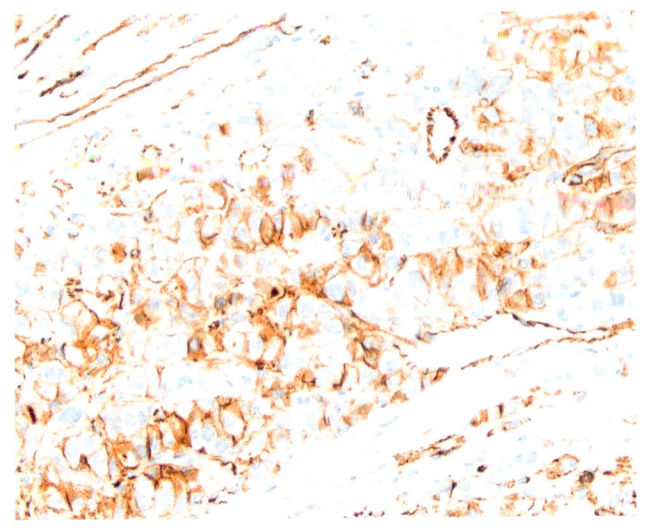

FIGURE 19-26
CD34 immunostaining is positive in most angiosarcomas but may be variable such as in this epithelioid angiosarcoma.

CD34 (Figure 19-26) and CD31 (Figure 19-27) is usually positive. Of note, keratin and epithelial membrane antigen may be positive in a subset of epithelioid angiosarcomas.

Differential Diagnosis

The distinction between grade 1 angiosarcomas and hemangiomas may be difficult. However, angiosarcomas should demonstrate cytologic atypia and an anastomosing network of capillary-sized vessels. The vessels of angiosarcoma never demonstrate a muscular media but consist exclusively of endothelial cells.

An epithelioid angiosarcoma, typically composed of sheets of anaplastic cells without a defined vasoformative growth pattern, raises the differential diagnosis of a variety of high-grade epithelioid malignancies including metastatic carcinoma, melanoma, or pleomorphic undifferentiated sarcoma. A panel of immunohistochemical stains including CD31 and CD34 to confirm endothelial differentiation may be necessary to establish the diagnosis. Immunostaining for keratin

ANGIOSARCOMA—FACT SHEET

Definition
▸▸ A malignant neoplasm of endothelial cells

Incidence and Location
▸▸ Rare; < 1% of malignant bone tumors

Sex, Race, and Age Distribution
▸▸ Male-to-female ratio is approximately 1:1
▸▸ Wide age distribution from second to seventh decades of life

Clinical Features
▸▸ Pain at site
▸▸ Mass if tumor is in a superficial bone

Radiographic Features
▸▸ Lytic usually without periosteal reaction
▸▸ Sclerotic rim may be present in grade 1 tumors, absent in higher-grade angiosarcomas
▸▸ Multifocality in an anatomic region suggests vascular neoplasm but not necessarily malignancy

Prognosis and Treatment
▸▸ Prognosis correlates with histologic grade (some controversy exists); survival rate ranges from 95% for grade 1 to < 20% for grade 3 angiosarcomas
▸▸ Wide local excision for localized tumors
▸▸ Radiation therapy for positive margins or multifocal disease

ANGIOSARCOMA—PATHOLOGIC FEATURES

Gross Findings
▸▸ Predominantly bloody, scattered spicules of bone and soft pink tissue

Microscopic Findings
▸▸ Anastomosing vascular channels permeating and destroying native structures, lined by endothelial cells with cytologic atypia
▸▸ Extensive hemorrhage may obscure vasoformative growth pattern
▸▸ Cytologic atypia of endothelial cells ranges from mild (grade 1) to marked anaplasia (grade 3)
▸▸ Necrosis and atypical mitotic figures in grade 3 angiosarcomas
▸▸ Epithelioid angiosarcomas may show sheets of pleomorphic cells without obvious vasoformative growth

Differential Diagnosis
▸▸ Hemangioma
▸▸ Metastatic carcinoma (especially for epithelioid angiosarcoma)
▸▸ Epithelioid hemangioendothelioma

---

and epithelial membrane antigen may be positive in epithelioid angiosarcomas (and, focally, even in conventional angiosarcomas). However, CD31 is usually negative in carcinomas. Additional immunostains tailored to exclude melanoma and other high-grade malignancies may be necessary.

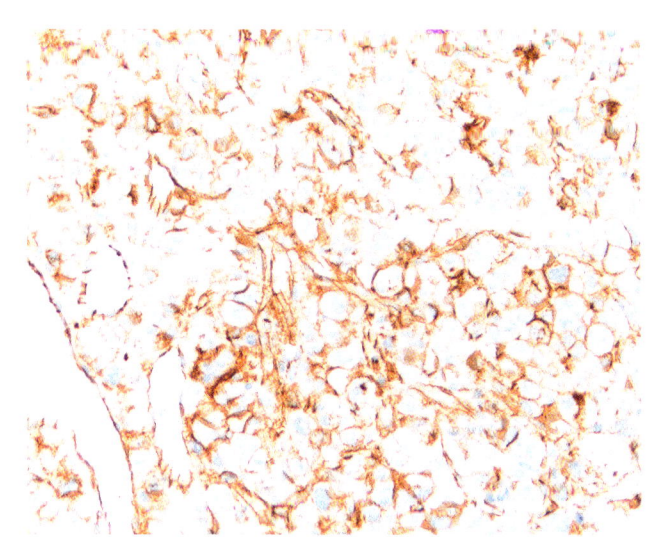

EHE and epithelioid angiosarcoma, as discussed earlier, probably exist on a continuum such that EHEs with sheet-like growth and marked cytologic atypia should probably be classified as angiosarcomas outright. EHEs can be distinguished from conventional angiosarcomas by the presence of myxoid to hyaline stroma, nests and cords of cells, and blister cells.

PROGNOSIS AND TREATMENT

Treatment of angiosarcoma involves complete resection of the tumor with wide margins and adjuvant radiotherapy for close or positive margins. Multifocal lesions not amenable to surgery may be treated with primary radiation therapy. Most studies indicate that prognosis is related to grade, with an up to 95% survival rate in grade 1 lesions as opposed to a less than 20% survival rate in grade 3 tumors. Notably, conflicting prognostic data from other studies suggest poor survival rates even in grade 1 angiosarcomas.

SUGGESTED READINGS

Hemangioma

1. Dorfman HD, Steiner GC, Jaffe HL: Vascular tumors of bone. Hum Pathol 1971;2:349–376.
2. Evans HL, Raymond AK, Ayala AG: Vascular tumors of bone: a study of 17 cases other than ordinary hemangioma, with an evaluation of the relationship of hemangioendothelioma of bone to epithelioid hemangioma, epithelioid hemangioendothelioma, and high-grade angiosarcoma. Hum Pathol 2003;34:680–689.
3. Jacob AG, Driscoll DJ, Shaughnessy WJ, et al: Klippel-Trenaunay syndrome: spectrum and management. Mayo Clin Proc 1998;73:28–36.
4. O'Connell JX, Kattapuram SV, Mankin HJ, et al: Epithelioid hemangioma of bone. A tumor often mistaken for low-grade angiosarcoma or malignant hemangioendothelioma. Am J Surg Pathol 1993;17:610–617.

FIGURE 19-27
CD31 immunostaining is a relatively sensitive and specific marker for endothelial cells, and is useful in the diagnosis of high-grade angiosarcomas.

5. Robbins LR, Fondren FTM: Hemangiomas of bone associated with spinal-cord compression. N Engl J Med 1958;258:685-687.
6. Stout AP: Hemangio-endothelioma: a tumor of blood vessels featuring vascular endothelial cells. Ann Surg 1943;118:445-464.
7. Unni KK: Dahlin's Bone Tumors: General Aspects and Data on 11,087 Cases, 5th ed. Philadelphia, Lippincott-Raven, 1996.
8. Wenger DE, Wold LE: Benign vascular lesions of bone: radiologic and pathologic features. Skeletal Radiol 2000;29:63-74.
9. Wold LE, Swee RG, Sim FH: Vascular lesions of bone. Pathol Annu 1985;20(pt 2):101-137.

Epithelioid Hemangioendothelioma

1. Evans HL, Raymond AK, Ayala AG: Vascular tumors of bone: a study of 17 cases other than ordinary hemangioma, with an evaluation of the relationship of hemangioendothelioma of bone to epithelioid hemangioma, epithelioid hemangioendothelioma, and high-grade angiosarcoma. Hum Pathol 2003;34:680-689.
2. Gill RM, O'Donnell RJ, Horvai AE: Utility of immunohistochemistry for endothelial markers in distinguishing epithelioid hemangioendothelioma from carcinoma metastatic to bone. Arch Pathol Lab Med (in press).
3. Gray MH, Rosenberg AE, Dickersin GR, et al: Cytokeratin expression in epithelioid vascular neoplasms. Hum Pathol 1990;21:212-217.
4. Kleer CG, Unni KK, McLeod RA: Epithelioid hemangioendothelioma of bone. Am J Surg Pathol 1996;20:1301-1311.
5. Mendlick MR, Nelson M, Pickering D, et al: Translocation t(1;3)(p36.3;q25) is a nonrandom aberration in epithelioid hemangioendothelioma. Am J Surg Pathol 2001;25:684-687.
6. Miettinen M, Fetsch JF: Distribution of keratins in normal endothelial cells and a spectrum of vascular tumors: implications in tumor diagnosis. Hum Pathol 2000;31:1062-1067.
7. Rosenthal DI, Treat ME, Mankin HJ, et al: Treatment of epithelioid hemangioendothelioma of bone using a novel combined approach. Skeletal Radiol 2001;30:219-222.
8. Tsuneyoshi M, Dorfman HD, Bauer TW: Epithelioid hemangioendothelioma of bone. A clinicopathologic, ultrastructural, and immunohistochemical study. Am J Surg Pathol 1986;10:754-764.
9. Unni KK: Dahlin's Bone Tumors: General Aspects and Data on 11,087 Cases, 5th ed. Philadelphia, Lippincott-Raven, 1996.
10. Weiss SW, Ishak KG, Dail DH, et al: Epithelioid hemangioendothelioma and related lesions. Semin Diagn Pathol 1986;3:259-287.

Angiosarcoma

1. Campanacci M, Boriani S, Giunti A: Hemangioendothelioma of bone: a study of 29 cases. Cancer 1980;46:804-814.
2. Deshpande V, Rosenberg AE, O'Connell JX, et al: Epithelioid angiosarcoma of the bone: a series of 10 cases. Am J Surg Pathol 2003;27:709-716.
3. Dorfman HD, Steiner GC, Jaffe HL: Vascular tumors of bone. Hum Pathol 1971;2:349-376.
4. Unni KK: Dahlin's Bone Tumors: General Aspects and Data on 11,087 Cases, 5th ed. Philadelphia, Lippincott-Raven, 1996.
5. Volpe R, Mazabraud A: Hemangioendothelioma (angiosarcoma) of bone: a distinct pathologic entity with an unpredictable course? Cancer 1982;49:727-736.
6. Wold LE, Unni KK, Beabout JW, et al: Hemangioendothelial sarcoma of bone. Am J Surg Pathol 1982;6:59-70.

20 Giant Cell Tumor of Bone
Patrizia Bacchini · Franco Bertoni

GIANT CELL TUMOR OF BONE

Giant cell tumor of bone consists of a mononuclear cell proliferation intermixed with numerous multinucleated, osteoclast-like giant cells (Figure 20-1). It has been referred to as *osteoclastoma* and *benign giant cell tumor*. However, because of the slightly unpredictable behavior of the lesion, the adjective *benign* is better dropped. The mononuclear cells are considered to be reactive and non-neoplastic in nature. However, they may also be present in distant metastases.

CLINICAL FEATURES

Most giant cell tumors occur in skeletally mature persons, principally young adults; they are rare in children (less than 2% of cases). Women are more commonly affected than men and may be affected at a slightly younger age (late adolescence) because of earlier closure of the epiphyseal plates. These tumors are rare in the elderly.

The most common locations are the ends of long bones, principally around the knee, distal femur and proximal tibia, which are the two most common sites of involvement in the Mayo Clinic files, followed by the distal radius and sacrum (Figure 20-2). The lesion is always epiphyseal or metaepiphyseal; only in rare cases that occur before closure of the growth plate may it be purely metaphyseal. The spine is less frequently involved; in this setting, the vertebral body is more often involved than the posterior elements (which tend to be affected more by osteoblastoma and aneurysmal bone cyst). Almost any bone may be affected, but lesions in the ribs, scapula, skull, long-bone diaphysis, and small bones of the hands and feet are extremely rare. Multicentric lesions are likewise exceptional, and hyperparathyroidism or Paget disease has to be ruled out in these cases. Giant cell tumor usually presents with swelling, pain, or both, rarely with pathologic fracture.

RADIOLOGIC FEATURES

Plain radiographs will show a purely lucent, destructive lesion that extends to the end of the bone—at least into the epiphysis, if not up to the articular cartilage (Figure 20-3). The margins may be well-defined but without sclerosis (puddle on the sand) in lesions considered latent or inactive. In aggressive cases, margins are poorly demarcated and the cortex may be thinned, expanded, or destroyed with soft tissue extension, but little or no periosteal reaction occurs. Marginal sclerosis may be present in old or inactive lesions, and peripheral ossification around a soft tissue recurrence or a lung metastasis (egg-shell appearance) (Figure 20-4). The tumor will appear solid on computed tomography and with a nonhomogenous signal on magnetic resonance imaging: low in T1 and high in T2. An isotope scan will show a focus with a cooler center and hotter rim (donut sign).

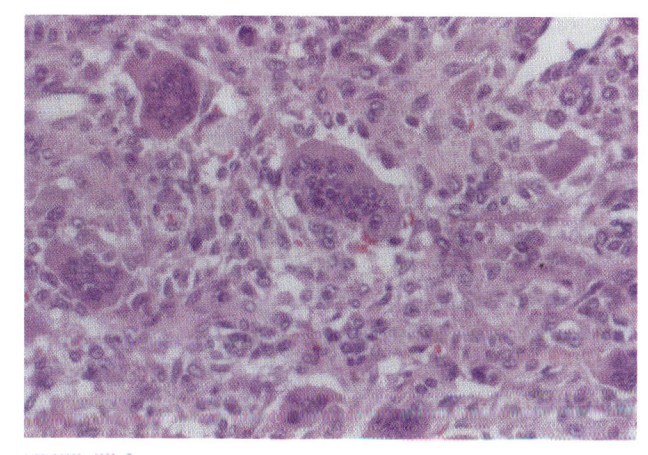

FIGURE 20-1
Giant cell tumor of bone.
High-power view showing the two typical cell populations.

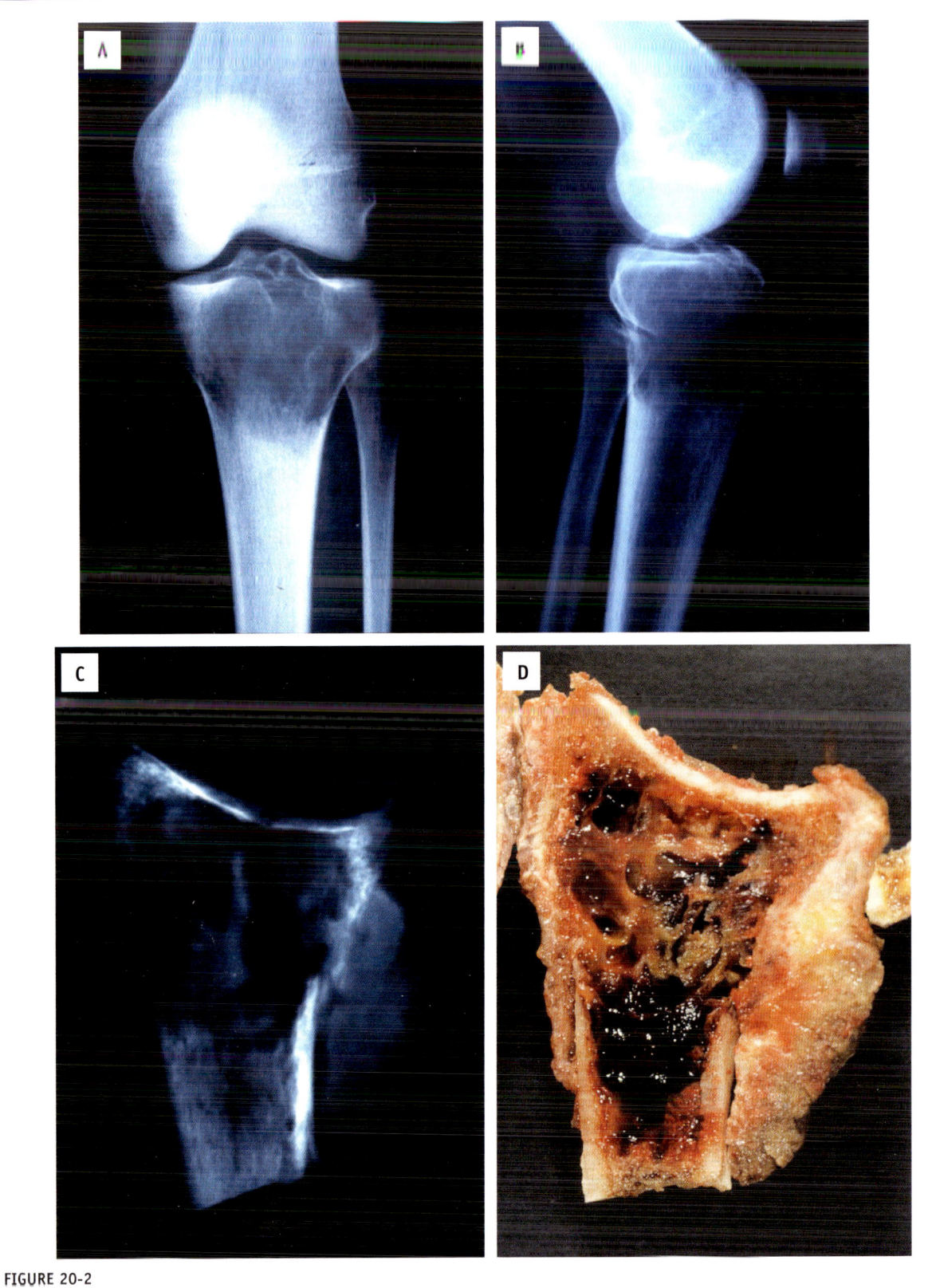

FIGURE 20-2
Typical locations of giant cell tumor.
Proximal tibia: Plain radiograph, **(A)** anteroposterior view, and **(B)** lateral view. Distal radius: **(C)** radiograph of specimen and **(D)** corresponding gross appearance.

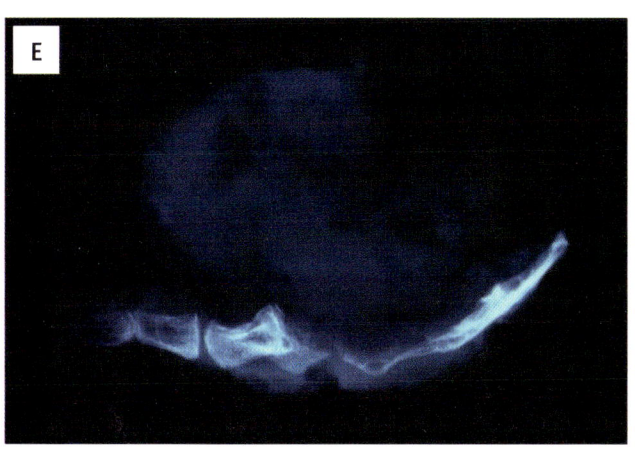

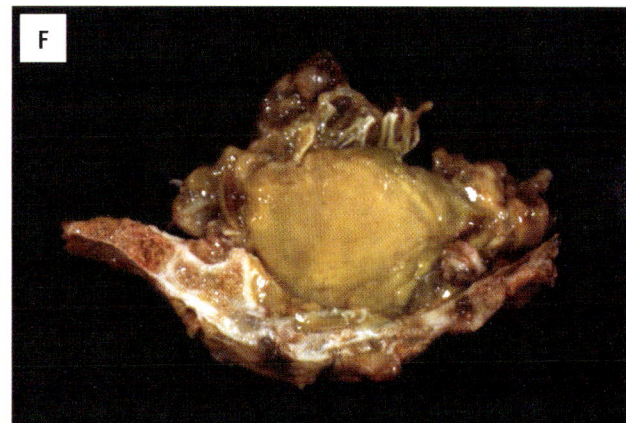

FIGURE 20-2—CONT'D
Sacrum: **(E)** radiograph of specimen and **(F)** corresponding gross appearance.

PATHOLOGIC FEATURES

GROSS FINDINGS

Giant cell tumor of bone has a variable gross appearance. It is usually meaty, soft, purple-red to brown, and may be uniform or variegated in aspect, with small, squishy yellow foci or extensive areas of cystic change. Extension into soft tissues, or soft tissue recurrence, will appear as a well-defined mass with peripheral calcification.

MICROSCOPIC FINDINGS

Microscopically, giant cell tumors of bone consist of two cell populations: a fairly dense mononucleated cell population, among which the multinucleated giant cells are uniformly distributed. The nuclei of the mononuclear cells are round to oval with granular chromatin and one or two nucleoli. The nuclei of the giant cells are identical, to such an extent that it may be difficult to pick out the limits of a giant cell against a mononuclear cell background. The giant cells have abundant eosinophilic cytoplasm and may contain dozens of nuclei (Figure 20-5A, B). Mitotic figures may be numerous in the mononuclear cell population but not atypical. The mononuclear cells are irregular in contour and tend to form sheets but may be spindled, and storiform areas can often be identified, as can aggregates of foam cells (the yellow areas grossly visible). Also present can be foci of infarct-type necrosis, usually small, but which can, on occasion, comprise almost the entire tumor (see Figure 20-5C). Little or no cellular reaction to this necrosis occurs. Occasionally, tumor plugs can be identified in vessels at the periphery of the lesion, but these do not affect the prognosis adversely. Other features found more rarely include the formation of osteoid or bone, usually focal (see Figure 20-5D, E) or aneurysmal bone cyst–like changes. Exceptionally, there may be areas within a lesion or even entire lesions in which few or no giant cells can be seen. A purely histologic diagnosis in these cases in impossible, and correlation with clinical and radiographic features becomes paramount. Rarely, nuclear hyperchromasia or degenerative atypia may also complicate the diagnosis.

DIFFERENTIAL DIAGNOSIS

As with all bone tumors, radiographic correlation is essential when diagnosing giant cell tumor. Virtually any tumor of bone may contain multinucleated giant cells in varying numbers, but most do not show the characteristic resemblance between the ovoid cell nuclei and the giant cell nuclei. The main sources of confusion are aneurysmal bone cyst, benign fibrous histiocytoma, chondroblastoma, and giant-cell-rich osteosarcoma. Pure *aneurysmal bone cysts* usually occur at a younger age and in metaphyseal locations, so much so that if a lesion with the appearance of an aneurysmal bone cyst occurs in an epiphyseal location, microscopic foci of giant cell tumor must be sought. *Benign fibrous histiocytoma* is usually more storiform in appearance and contains more foam cells; an inactive giant cell tumor may present this pattern, but small foci of typical giant cell tumor will also be identifiable. The diagnosis of *chondroblastoma* requires the identification of chondroid matrix or mineralization, at least focally. The nuclei of the principal cell population are often grooved (coffee-bean appearance) and do not resemble the nuclei of the giant cells. Clinically, chondroblastomas usually appear in skeletally immature patients and predominate in male individuals. Finally, *giant cell–rich osteosarcoma*, albeit rare, must not be mistaken for giant cell tumor. The former is a histologic variant of conventional osteosarcoma and may, therefore, be found in the same locations (long-bone metaphyses or metaepiphyses,

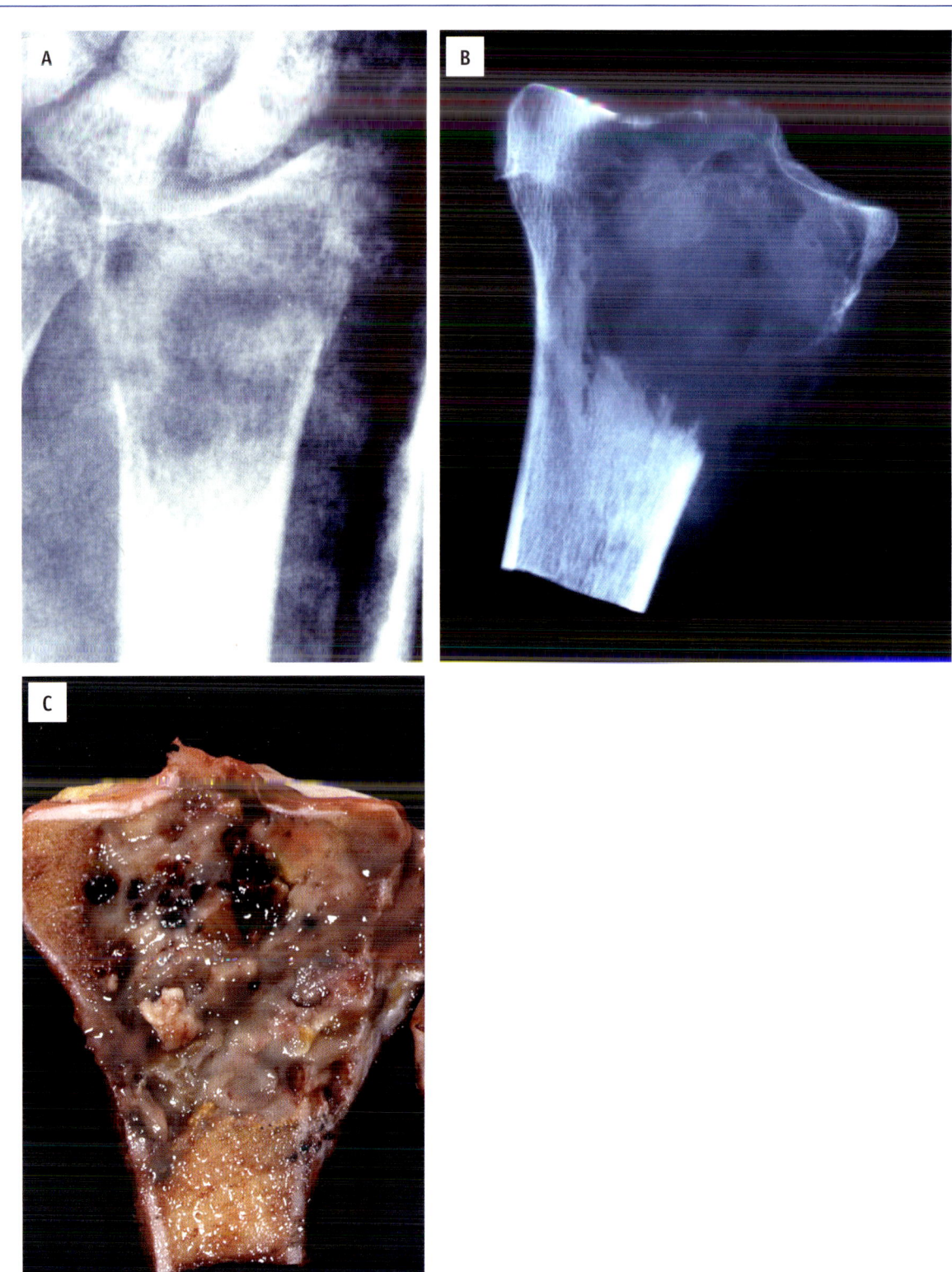

FIGURE 20-3
Radiologic features of giant cell tumor.
A large, purely lytic lesion involving the metaepiphyseal region of the radius, with thinning and focal destruction of the cortex, soft tissue extension, and extension to the articular cartilage. **(A)** Plain radiograph, anteroposterior view; **(B)** radiograph of specimen; and **(C)** corresponding gross appearance.

CHAPTER 20 Giant Cell Tumor of Bone 405

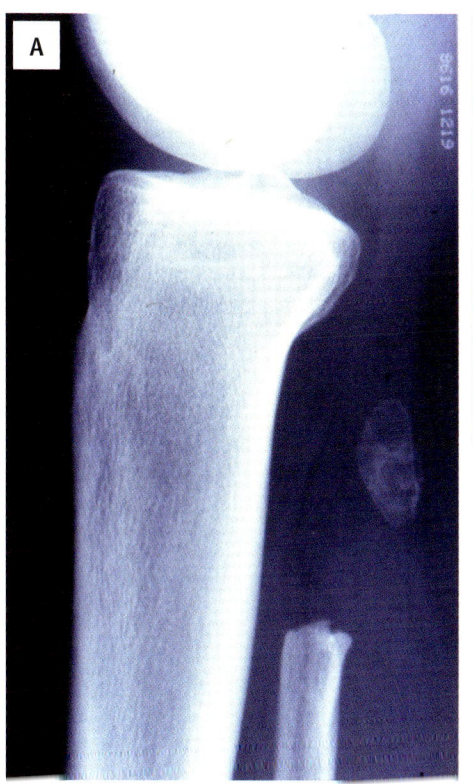

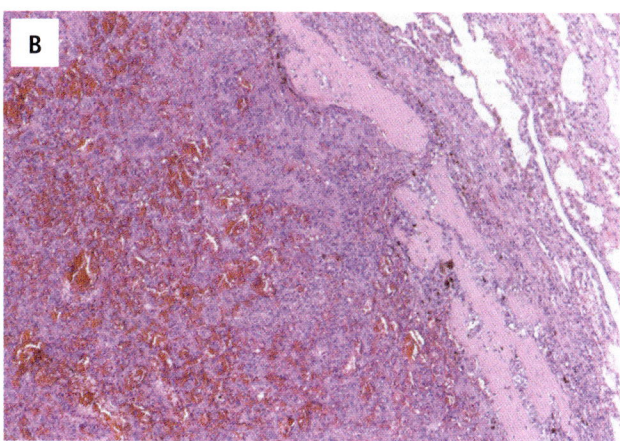

FIGURE 20-4
Giant cell tumor.
A, Peripheral ossification around a soft tissue recurrence giving an egg-shell appearance on plain X-ray. **B,** Low-power histologic view of a lung metastasis with peripheral ossification.

around the knee) and in the same age group as giant cell tumor. However, histologically, the degree of cellular atypia in the stromal cells is greater, and atypical mitotic figures may be found. Formation of osteoid and bone is also more apparent. Historically, an important differential diagnosis was with brown tumor of hyperparathyroidism, which is histologically similar in appearance, but this rarely poses a clinical problem nowadays.

PROGNOSIS AND TREATMENT

Most giant cell tumors of bone are benign, but they may be locally aggressive—in long bones, up to 25% recur after surgery. The surgical approach chosen depends on the desired result: Wide resection reduces the risk for recurrence but may have a significant impact on limb function, depending on the site of the tumor; a thorough curettage, followed or not by phenol/alcohol injection or cement, may better preserve function but is at greater risk for recurrence. Recurrences are likewise treated surgically. Radiotherapy may be administered in surgically difficult locations (e.g., vertebral body). Chemotherapy is not used in the treatment of giant cell tumor.

A small minority of giant cell tumors (2%) metastasizes to the lungs, but these metastases are slow growing and may regress spontaneously. No histologic criteria exist to identify which lesions have metastatic potential. Conventional giant cell tumors are locally aggressive but progress slowly, and lead to the death of the patient only in exceptional cases; they are not considered malignant.

A different problem is posed by the rare cases of malignancy in giant cell tumor, sometimes called *dedifferentiated giant cell tumor* or *malignant giant cell tumor*. This means a high-grade sarcoma that develops at the site of a previously excised or irradiated giant cell tumor (secondary malignancy in giant cell tumor). More rarely, a sarcoma may develop adjacent to, or juxtaposed on, an untreated giant cell tumor (primary malignancy in giant cell tumor). In this case, both the benign and the sarcomatous components are visible histologically, and the limits between the two are abrupt. The sarcoma is usually of spindle-cell type (fibrosarcoma, malignant fibrous histiocytoma) and may produce osteoid. The prognosis in malignant giant cell tumor is that of a high-grade spindle cell sarcoma. These cases account for less than 1% of all cases of giant cell tumor.

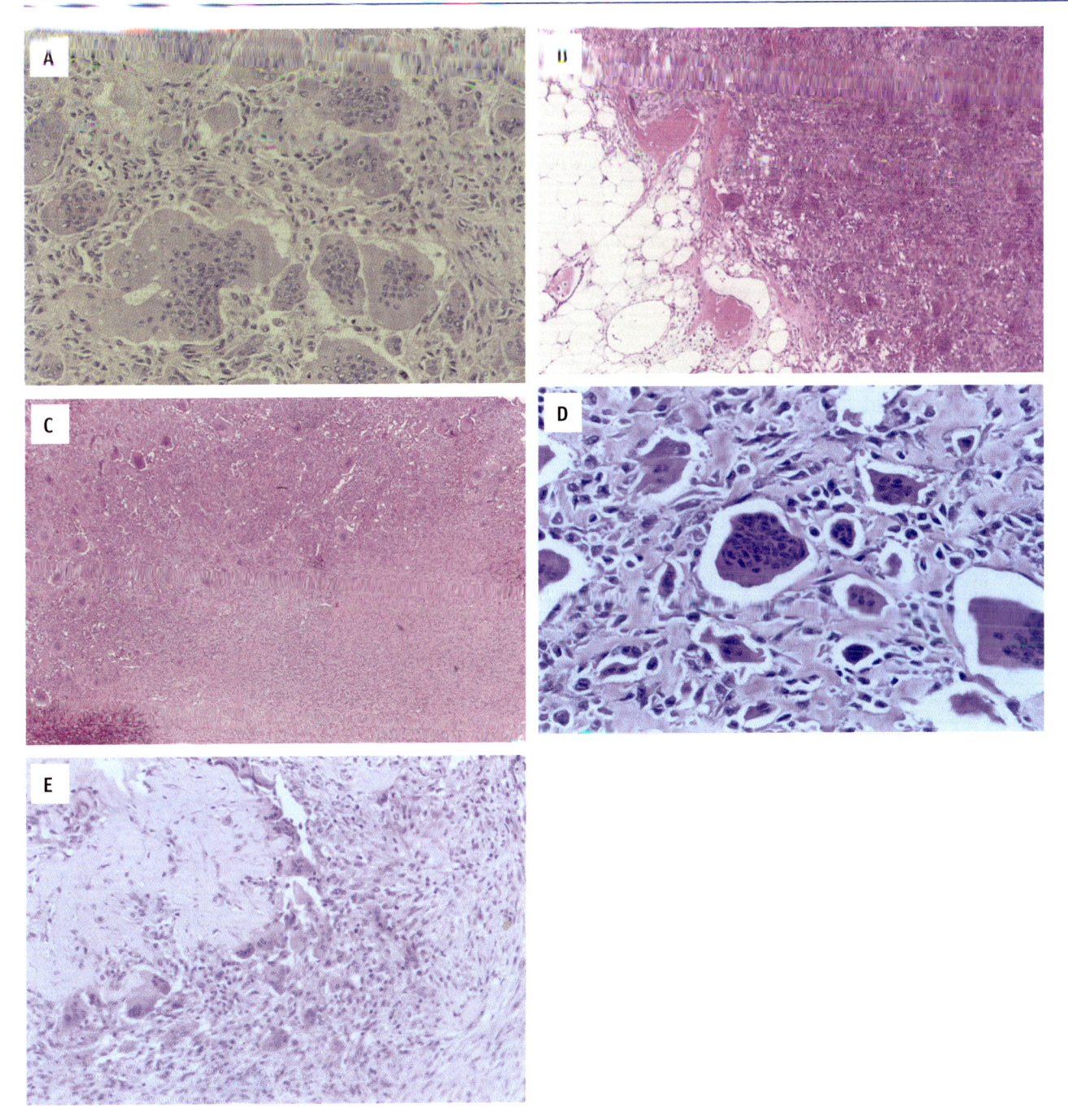

FIGURE 20-5
Microscopic appearance of giant cell tumor.
A, High-power view showing sheets of spindled or ovoid cells interspersed with multinucleated giant cells. Both cell populations have eosinophilic cytoplasm and the same fairly regular, oval nuclei with a distinct membrane and one or two small nucleoli. Note large numbers of nuclei in some of the giant cells. **B,** Low-power view showing dense cellularity and peripheral ossification. **C,** Low-power view of an area of infarct-type necrosis. **D, E,** High-power views of small foci of osteoid production within the tumor.

GIANT CELL TUMOR OF BONE—FACT SHEET

Definition
- Benign neoplasm composed of sheets of ovoid or spindled mononuclear cells interspersed with numerous osteoclast-like multinucleated giant cells

Incidence and Location
- 20% of benign bone tumors (5% of all bone tumors)
- Metaepiphyseal or epiphyseal, long bones: distal femur, proximal tibia, distal radius; sacrum; also rarely occurs in spine, typically in the vertebral body
- Multicentric forms exceptional

Morbidity and Mortality
- Benign but locally aggressive: extension into soft tissues common; overall 20% to 25% recurrence rate
- Distant metastases rare (< 2%)

Sex, Race, and Age Distribution
- Slight female predominance
- Mature skeleton, mainly young adults (third to fourth decades of life); rare in childhood and old age.

Clinical Features
- Pain, swelling, pathologic fracture

Radiologic Features
- Purely lytic lesion with either well-defined, but not sclerotic, margins or poorly defined margins
- Aggressive cases may show cortical destruction and occasionally periosteal reaction
- Soft tissue extension or recurrence has marginal calcification (egg-shell appearance)

Prognosis and Treatment
- Surgical excision or curettage; radiotherapy for inaccessible lesions
- Recurrences usually appear within 2 years and are treated surgically
- Lung metastases rare (2%), usually slow growing
- Malignancy in giant cell tumor: < 1% of cases overall; prognosis is that of a high grade spindle-cell sarcoma

GIANT CELL TUMOR OF BONE—PATHOLOGIC FEATURES

Gross Findings
- Red-brown, fleshy, well-demarcated mass
- May be yellow areas and/or cystic areas

Microscopic Findings
- Sheets of ovoid, mononuclear cells interspersed with numerous osteoclast-like, multinucleated giant cells
- The nuclei of the giant cells and the mononuclear cells look similar
- Mitotic figures common in mononuclear cells, not atypical
- May also be aggregates of foam cells; focal osteoid or bone production; aneurysmal bone cyst-like changes; storiform areas; necrosis, often small foci with little or no cellular reaction

Pathologic Differential Diagnosis
- Aneurysmal bone cyst
- Benign fibrous histiocytoma
- Chondroblastoma
- Giant cell-rich osteosarcoma

SUGGESTED READING

1. Bertoni F, Bacchini P, Staals EL: Malignancy in giant cell tumor of bone. Cancer 2003;97:2520-2529.
2. Bullough PG, Bansal M: Malignancy in giant cell tumor. World Health Organization Classification of Tumors: Pathology and Genetics of Tumors of Soft tissue and Bone. Lyon, France, IARC Press, 2002.
3. Reid R, Banerjee SS, Sciot R: Giant cell tumor. World Health Organization Classification of Tumors: Pathology and Genetics of Tumors of Soft tissue and Bone. Lyon, France, IARC Press, 2002.
4. Szendroi M: Giant-cell tumor of bone. J Bone Joint Surg [Br] 2004;86:5-12.
5. Unni KK: Giant cell tumor. Dahlin's Bone Tumors: General Aspects and Data on 11,087 Cases, 5th ed. Philadelphia, Lippincott-Raven, 1996.
6. Unni KK: Malignancy in giant cell tumor. Dahlin's Bone Tumors: General Aspects and Data on 11,087 Cases, 5th ed. Philadelphia, Lippincott-Raven, 1996.
7. Vetrani A, Fulciniti F, Boschi R, et al: Fine needle aspiration biopsy diagnosis of giant cell tumor of bone: an experience with nine cases. Acta Cytol 1990;34:863-867.
8. Wulling M, Delling G, Kaiser E: The origin of the neoplastic stromal cell in giant cell tumor of bone. Hum Pathol 2004;34:983-993.

21 Notochordal Tumors
Andrew Horvai

- Chordoma

CHORDOMA

The notochord is a midline, ectoderm-derived structure that defines the phylum of chordates. In humans, the degeneration of the notochord begins during fetal development and is complete by the second decade of life. However, asymptomatic vestigial rests can occasionally be found in the nucleus pulposus of intervertebral disks in adults. Some controversy exists as to the origin of chordomas from these cells because chordomas arise from bone (clivus, sacrum, and coccyx), not intervertebral disks. Furthermore, histochemical differences have been reported between fetal notochord and chordoma cells. Nevertheless, chordoma represents a low-grade malignant mesenchymal neoplasm with distinct clinical and pathologic features and histologic similarities to the notochord. It represents approximately 4% of malignant bone tumors.

CLINICAL FEATURES

Most patients have pain. The majority of chordomas are located in the sacrococcygeal region (35-50%) or the base of the skull (30%-40%). Approximately 20% to 30% are located in the vertebrae of the mobile spine. Sacrococcygeal tumors produce lower back pain, oftentimes of long duration. A mass may be palpable on rectal examination. Patients with clivus tumors may report visual impairment (from abducens nerve involvement) in addition to headache. Male individuals are affected about twice as frequently as female individuals, with a peak incidence in the fifth and sixth decades of life, though clivus tumors present slightly earlier. Rare examples may recur as a high-grade spindle cell sarcoma, an entity known as *dedifferentiated chordoma,* although some of these examples may represent postradiation sarcomas.

RADIOLOGIC FEATURES

Chordoma presents as a midline, lytic, destructive lesion with soft tissue involvement in the majority of cases. Plain radiographs may be difficult to interpret because of overlying structures in the pelvis and cranium; therefore, computed tomography (CT) and especially magnetic resonance imaging studies are particularly useful for diagnosis and treatment planning (Figure 21-1). Matrix calcification may be present in some cases but most likely represents residual native bone rather than

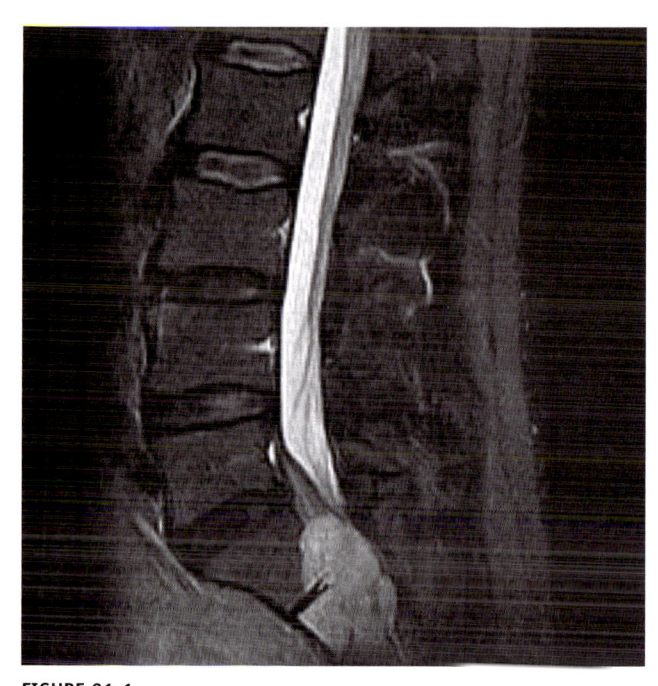

FIGURE 21-1
Sagittal T2-weighted magnetic resonance image of sacral chordoma. Chordomas may show extension into soft tissue anteriorly or, as in this case, posteriorly.

CHAPTER 21 Notochordal Tumors 409

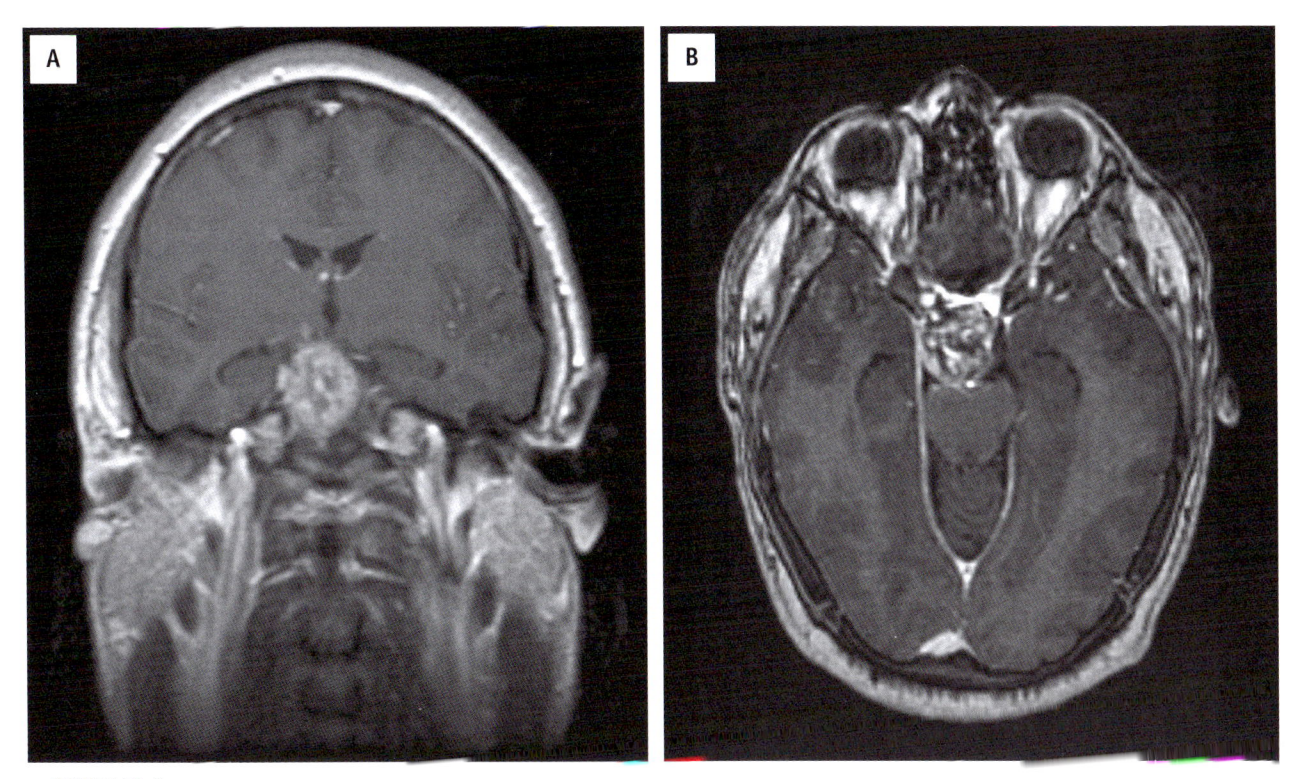

FIGURE 21-2
A, Coronal and **(B)** axial T1-weighted magnetic resonance images of chordoma involving clivus. Note that the tumor is well circumscribed with a pushing border that may involve the optic nerves and sella turcica.

neoplastic bone. Clivus tumors may extend to the sella turcica (Figure 21-2), whereas sacral tumors commonly involve the soft tissues anteriorly. Vertebral chordomas often cross intervertebral disks to involve more than one vertebral body.

PATHOLOGIC FEATURES

GROSS FINDINGS

Chordomas have a characteristic lobular architecture. Tumor lobules are shiny, translucent blue–gray and separated by thin, white fibrous septae (Figure 21-3). Gross resections demonstrate soft tissue extension and a pushing border. Recurrences may be multifocal.

MICROSCOPIC FINDINGS

At low magnification, chordomas invariably show a lobular growth pattern (Figure 21-4). Abundant basophilic myxoid stroma comprises the majority of the tumor volume. Thin, collagenous septae divide lobules. The cells of chordoma are round to ovoid with pale eosinophilic cytoplasm growing in strands, cords, and clusters (Figure 21-5). Variable amounts of the so-called *physaliphorous* tumor cells may be present. The latter cells contain one or several intracytoplasmic vacuoles, creating a bubbly appearance (Figure 21-6). Nuclei are generally small and central, although occasional tumors may demonstrate focal areas of enlarged, pleomorphic, and hyperchromatic nuclei (Figure 21-7). In the latter case, the nuclear-to-cytoplasmic ratio is retained, and this finding does not predict a worse prognosis. Rare tumors may be highly cellular with sheet-like growth of round to ovoid cells and scant stroma. Necrosis is seen

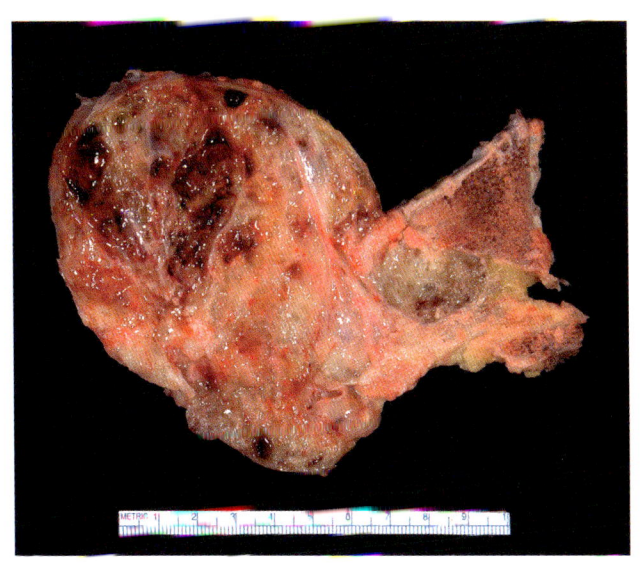

FIGURE 21-3
Gross image of chordoma showing a lobulated and destructive tumor.

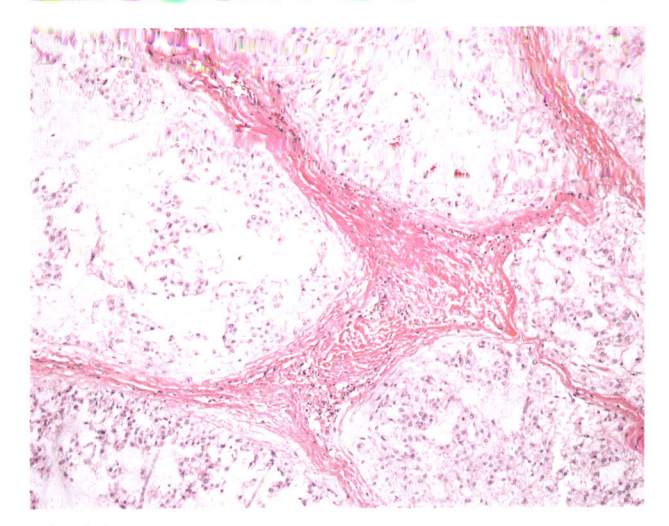

FIGURE 21-4
Low-power view of a lobular growth pattern in a chordoma.

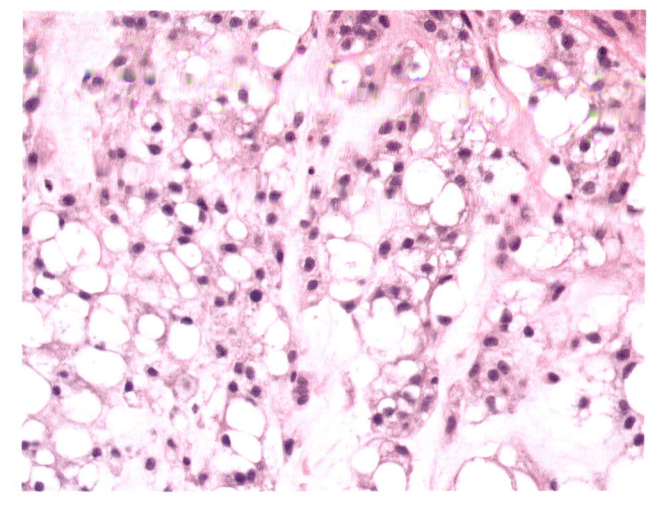

FIGURE 21-6
The cells of chordoma demonstrate pale eosinophilic to somewhat foamy cytoplasm with central ovoid to round and cytologically bland nuclei.

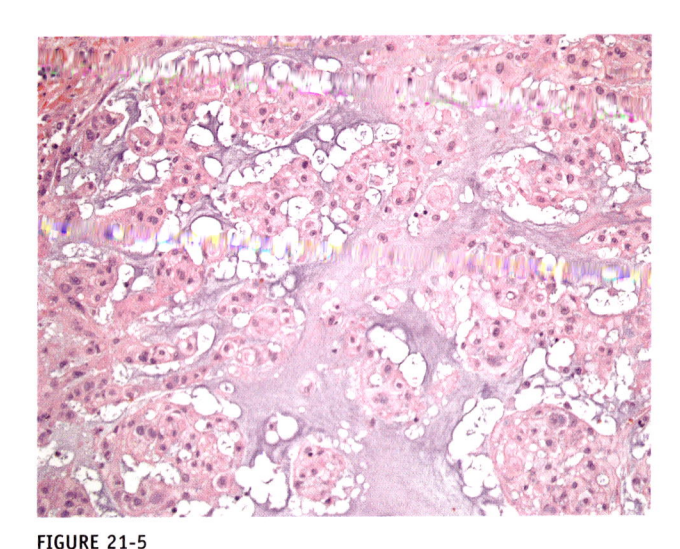

FIGURE 21-5
At intermediate magnification, the cells in chordoma grow in cords, strands, and clusters amid a loose myxoid stroma.

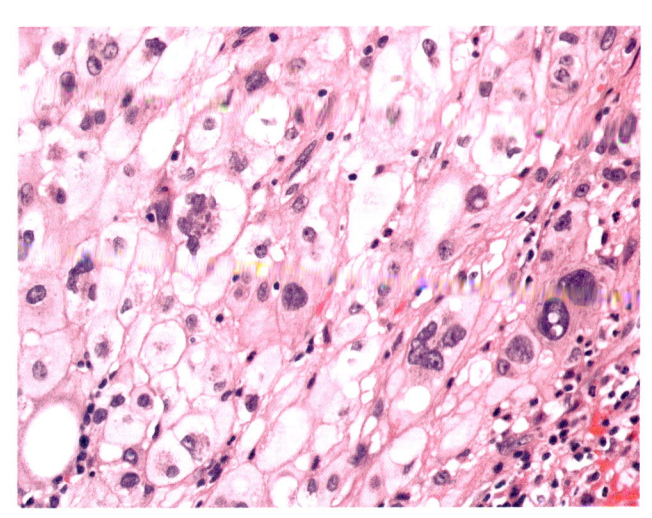

FIGURE 21-7
Chordoma containing pseudomalignant cells.

in approximately 35% of sacral tumors. Mitotic activity is rare in chordomas.

Chondroid chordoma occurs almost exclusively in the base of the skull. Histologically, chondroid chordoma contains chondroid tissue in addition to conventional chordoma. Both components stain positive with epithelial markers. Highly cellular histologic variants of chordoma have recently been described in the skull base of children and adolescents. These tumors have a solid growth pattern and lack the myxoid matrix of classic chordoma. A subset within this group that lacks the typical cytologic features of chordoma has been termed *poorly differentiated chordoma*. The poorly differentiated variant has been associated with a poorer prognosis when compared with the other variants.

ANCILLARY STUDIES

Chordomas express cytokeratins, specifically CK8, CK18, and CK19, and epithelial membrane antigen (EMA). S-100 protein expression is variable. Chordomas also express a relatively new marker, brachyury, that can be useful in the differential diagnosis.

DIFFERENTIAL DIAGNOSIS

The myxoid matrix, lobular growth pattern, and cytomorphology of chordoma may suggest chondrosarcoma. The diagnosis can be particularly challenging for base of

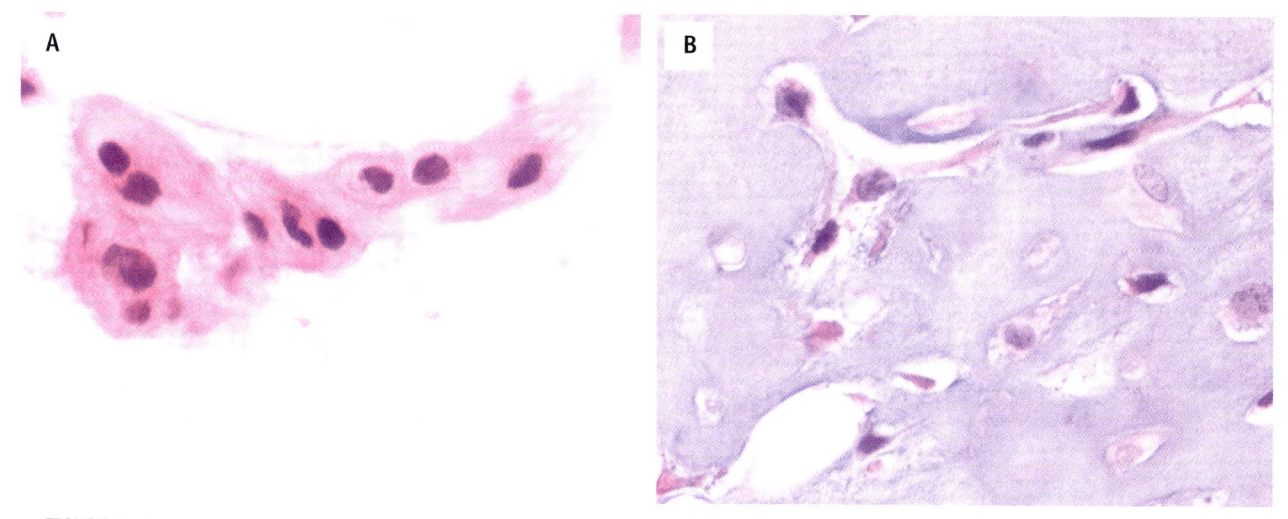

FIGURE 21-8

A, Chordoma shows broad attachment of cells. **B,** In contrast, spindle cells in a conventional intraosseous chondrosarcoma extend delicate processes to establish intercellular contact.

skull tumors if hyaline cartilage is present (chondroid chordoma) and on small biopsies. The distinction may have prognostic implications in that chondrosarcoma of the skull base tends to have a better prognosis than does chordoma. Although the cells of chondrosarcoma may grow in cords, the cell-cell contact consists of delicate processes projecting between cells as opposed to the broad contact between the chains of cells in chordoma (Figure 21-8). Both chondrosarcoma and chordoma may stain for S-100 protein. However, positive immunoreactivity with EMA, keratin, and brachyury supports the diagnosis of chordoma.

Extraskeletal myxoid chondrosarcoma shares some gross and histologic features with chordoma but is almost exclusively a soft tissue tumor that does not stain for keratins. If necessary, molecular or genetic techniques to detect the t(9;22) (*EWS;NR4A3*) translocation can help confirm the diagnosis of extraskeletal myxoid chondrosarcoma and exclude chordoma.

Metastatic adenocarcinoma usually lacks a lobular growth pattern but may be confused with chordoma on a small biopsy. The presence of keratin and EMA staining in both chordoma and carcinoma can also cause diagnostic confusion. Metastatic adenocarcinoma, however, shows diffuse nuclear atypia, necrosis, and mitotic activity. Additional immunohistochemical stains, including brachyury (supporting a diagnosis of chordoma) or lineage-specific markers (e.g., CDX-2 for colorectal, TTF-1 for thyroid and lung, estrogen and progesterone receptors for breast) may be necessary in difficult cases.

Giant notochordal rest (GNR) is a recently described entity of notochordal origin that has also been termed *giant notochordal hamartoma* and *intraosseous benign notochord cell tumor*. Conventional radiograph and CT images of GNR are normal or show minimal sclerosis. This differs from the lytic and destructive findings seen with chordomas. GNR is usually detected in magnetic resonance images as a homogeneous mass that occupies some or nearly all of a vertebra. However, it does not show aggressive features of a soft tissue mass. Histologically, at low magnification, GNR lacks the lobulated growth pattern of conventional chordoma. In contrast, it fills the marrow spaces without destroying the medullary or cortical bone. The cells do not display the degree of cytologic atypia seen in chordoma. They contain small, round nuclei containing fine nuclear chromatin surrounded by clear to faintly eosinophilic cytoplasm with varying amounts of vacuolization. The tumor may be overlooked because of its resemblance to marrow fat. Immunostains can be helpful because GNR shows strong immunoreactivity with keratin markers. So far, it appears that the biologic behavior of GNR is that of a benign or indolent lesion (Figure 21-9).

PROGNOSIS AND TREATMENT

Chordomas involving the sacrum and mobile spine are treated with surgery, preferably with a wide surgical margin. Cranial base chordomas are treated with surgery and various types of high-dose radiation therapy (stereotactic radiosurgery, proton beam, heavy particle). Chordomas are difficult to excise because of their location and intimate relation to critical structures. Thus, they are associated with a high incidence of local recurrence. Five- and 10-year survival rates of 45% to 77% and 28% to 52%, respectively, have been reported for sacral chordomas. Distant metastases, most commonly to the lung, occur late in disease in approximately 30% of cases, but mortality is most often related to recurrence and progression with local effects.

CHORDOMA—FACT SHEET

Definition
- Low-grade malignant neoplasm of notochord origin

Incidence and Location
- 4% of malignant bone tumors
- 35–50% located in sacrococcygeal region
- 30–40% located in base of skull
- 20–30% located in the mobile spine

Sex, Race, and Age Distribution
- Male-to-female ratio is 2:1; peak incidence in fifth and sixth decades of life

Clinical Features
- Lower back pain from sacrococcygeal tumors; headache and visual disturbances from cranial tumors

Prognosis and Treatment
- Complete surgical resection with negative margins
- Adjuvant radiation therapy or radiosurgery for cranial base chordomas
- Morbidity and mortality from local destructive recurrence
- Metastasis in ~30% of cases

CHORDOMA—PATHOLOGIC FEATURES

Gross Findings
- Lobules of glistening blue-gray tumor separated by white, fibrous septae
- Cortical destruction and soft tissue extension usually anteriorly

Microscopic Findings
- Fibrovascular bands separate lobules of tumor
- Tumor cells grow in cords and small nests
- Tumor cells set in a blue myxoid background
- Small, round uniform nuclei with abundant cytoplasm
- Bubbly cytoplasm (physaliphorous cells)

Differential Diagnosis
- Chondrosarcoma
- Metastatic adenocarcinoma
- Giant notochordal rest
- Extraskeletal myxoid chondrosarcoma

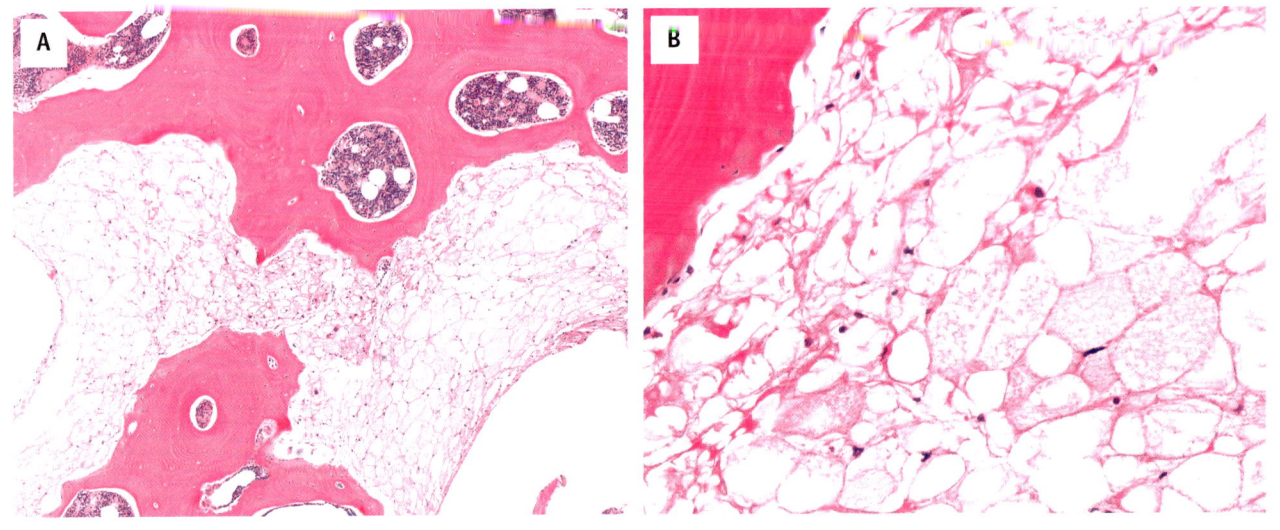

FIGURE 21-9
Giant notochordal rest.
A, Rather than lobular growth, the tumor is composed of a single mass amid trabeculae of lamellar bone. **B,** The physaliphorous cells predominate with an appearance that can mimic fat necrosis.

SUGGESTED READINGS

1. Almefty K, Pravdenkova S, Colli BO, et al: Chordoma and chondrosarcoma: similar, but quite different, skull base tumors. Cancer 2007;110(11):2457–2467.
2. Bottles K, Beckstead JH: Enzyme histochemical characterization of chordomas. Am J Surg Pathol 1984;8(6):443–447.
3. Brooks JJ, Trojanowski JQ, LiVolsi VA: Chondroid chordoma: A low-grade chondrosarcoma and its differential diagnosis. Curr Top Pathol 1989;80:165–181.
4. Eriksson B, Gunterberg B, Kindblom LG: Chordoma. A clinicopathologic and prognostic study of a Swedish national series. Acta Orthop Scand 1981;52(1):49–58.
5. Fuchs B, Dickey ID, Yaszemski MJ, et al: Operative management of sacral chordoma. J Bone Joint Surg Am 2005;87(10):2211–2216.
6. Hoch BL, Nielsen GP, Liebsch NG, et al: Base of skull chordomas in children and adolescents; a clinicopathologic study of 73 cases. Am J Surg Pathol 2006;30(70):811–818.
7. Hruban RH, Traganos F, Reuter VF, et al: Chordomas with malignant spindle cell components. A DNA flow cytometric and immunohistochemical study with histogenetic implications. Am J Pathol 1990;137(2):435–447.
8. Huvos AG: Bone Tumors: Diagnosis, Treatment and Prognosis. 2nd ed. Philadelphia, Saunders, 1991, pp 591–624.

9. Kaiser TE, Pritchard DJ, Unni KK: Clinicopathologic study of sacrococcygeal chordoma. Cancer 1984;53(11):2574–2578.
10. Kyriakos M, Totty WG, Lenke LG: Giant vertebral notochordal rest: a lesion distinct from chordoma: Discussion of an evolving concept. Am J Surg Pathol 2003;27(3):396–406.
11. Meis JM, Raymond AK, Evans HL, et al: "Dedifferentiated" chordoma. A clinicopathologic and immunohistochemical study of three cases. Am J Surg Pathol 1987;11(7):516–525.
12. Mirra JM, Brien EW: Giant notochordal hamartoma of intraosseous origin: a newly reported benign entity to be distinguished from chordoma. Report of two cases. Skeletal Radiol 2001;30:698–709.
13. Mitchell A, Scheithauer BW, Unni KK, et al: Chordoma and chondroid neoplasms of the spheno-occiput. An immunohistochemical study of 41 cases with prognostic and nosologic implications. Cancer 1993;72(10):2943–2949.
14. Rosenberg AE, Brown GA, Bhan AK, et al: Chondroid chordoma—a variant of chordoma. A morphologic and immunohistochemical study. Am J Clin Pathol 1994;101:36–41.
15. Rosenberg AE, Nielsen GP, Keel SB, et al: Chondrosarcoma of the base of the skull. A clinicopathological study of 200 cases with emphasis on its distinction from chordoma. Am J Surg Pathol 1999;23:1370–1378.
16. Tirabosco R, Mangham DC, Rosenberg AE, et al: Brachyury expression in extra-axial skeletal and soft tissue chordomas: a marker that distinguishes chordoma from mixed tumor/myoepithelioma/parachordoma in soft tissue. Am J Surg Pathol 2008;32(4):572–580.
17. Utne JR, Pugh DG: The roentgenologic aspects of chordoma. Am J Roentgenol Radium Ther Nucl Med 1955;74(4):593–608.
18. Volpe R, Mazabraud A: A clinicopathologic review of 25 cases of chordoma (a pleomorphic and metastasizing neoplasm). Am J Surg Pathol 1983;7(2):161–170.
19. Vujovic S, Henderson S, Presneau N, et al: Brachyury, a crucial regulator of notochordal development, is a novel biomarker for chordomas. J Pathol 2006;209(2):157–165.
20. Yamaguchi T, Iwata J, Sugihara S, et al: Distinguishing benign notochordal cell tumors from vertebral chordoma. Skeletal Radiol 2008;37(4):291–299.
21. Yamaguchi T, Suzuki S, Ishiiwa H, et al: Benign notochordal cell tumors: a comparative histological study of benign notochordal cell tumors, classic chordomas, and notochordal vestiges of fetal intervertebral discs. Am J Surg Pathol 2004;28:756–761.

22 Adamantinoma

Leonard B. Kahn

- Adamantinoma
- Differentiated Adamantinoma

ADAMANTINOMA

CLINICAL FEATURES

Adamantinoma is a low-grade malignant epithelial neoplasm of uncertain embryogenesis with a strong predilection for involvement of the midshaft of the tibia with or without involvement of the fibula. A stromal component with a fibrous dysplasia-like appearance is present in many cases. A close histogenetic relation to osteofibrous dysplasia (OFD) and differentiated adamantinoma is suggested by clinical, histologic, immunohistochemical, and cytogenetics features.

Adamantinomas constitute between 0.1% to 0.5% of all malignant bone tumors. A wide age spectrum exists, but young adults are most frequently affected. The mean age at presentation is about 30 years with only about 3% of patients younger than 10 years. Some series report a slight male preponderance. A striking feature of this neoplasm is its predilection for involvement of the midshaft of the tibia, which accounts for about 85% of all cases. Synchronous involvement of tibia and fibula occurs in about 10% of all cases. Isolated case reports document involvement of ulna, femur, humerus, radius, rib, ischium, tarsal, metatarsal, and capitate. Reports also exist of extraskeletal pretibial soft tissue involvement. Swelling with or without pain is the usual presenting feature. The lesion may cause a pathologic fracture. A history of significant trauma has been noted in some cases. Adamantinoma exhibits a tendency to both long recurrence and metastasis, predominantly to the lung. The mean duration to local recurrence may be as long as 7 years, and metastases have been documented more than two decades after diagnosis.

RADIOLOGIC FEATURES

The typical mid-diaphyseal tibial lesion is osteolytic, eccentric, expansile, and medullary in location. It is composed of multifocal radiolucencies surrounded by ring-shaped densities producing the characteristic *soap-bubble* appearance (Figure 22-1). The entire lesion may have a prominent sclerotic margin indicative of slow growth. The lesion is longitudinally oriented with an average length in one series of 11 cm. The expansile element tends to involve the anterior tibial surface, and the lesion may produce a bowing deformity of the tibia. The periosteal reaction is variable from minimal to prominent. In about 15% of cases, extracortical extension into soft tissues occurs. Additional computed tomography (CT) and magnetic resonance imaging (MRI) studies are of limited diagnostic value but are helpful in assessing the extent and invasiveness of the lesion.

PATHOLOGIC FEATURES

The neoplasm is composed of epithelial cells surrounded by a fibrous stroma. In some cases, the stroma contains woven bone spicules rimmed by osteoblasts resembling OFD. Based on the pattern of the epithelial cell component and the presence or absence of the OFD-like element, several histologic variants have been described. The most frequent is the *tubular* variant in which narrow cords of epithelial cells form branching and anastomosing structures. A central gland-like space produces the tubular appearance and probably results from loss of cellular cohesion rather than true gland formation (Figure 22-2). A *basaloid* variant resembles basal cell carcinoma with palisading of its peripheral layer (Figure 22-3). The *squamous* variant resembles a well-differentiated squamous carcinoma and may exhibit keratinization, or cell separation may result in formation of the stellate reticulum pattern seen commonly in gnathic ameloblastoma (Figure 22-4). Frequently, overlapping patterns are present between these variants in individual cases. The *spindle cell* variant is the most complicated to recognize because the spindle-shaped

CHAPTER 22 Adamantinoma 415

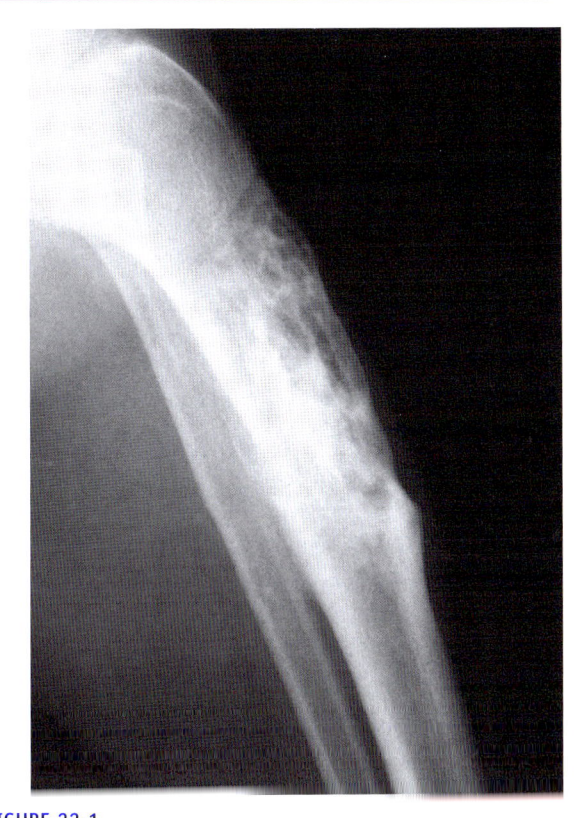

FIGURE 22-1
Adamantinoma.
Osteolytic, eccentric, expansile lesion involving the cortex and medulla of the proximal third of the diaphysis of the tibia. Note the multiple radiolucencies surrounded by ring-shaped densities producing the characteristic *soap-bubble* appearance.

cleft-like or tubule-like spaces. The *OFD-like* variant is usually composed of scant strands and single epithelial cells within a lesion otherwise indistinguishable from OFD. The relation between this variant and OFD will be elaborated on in the sections dealing with OFD and differentiated adamantinoma. The least common variant has been described as *Ewing's-like adamantinoma* or *adamantinoma-like Ewing's sarcoma* and is composed of anastomosing cords of small, uniform, round cells set in a myxoid stroma. However, the demonstration of a t(11:22) translocation in this variant favors a closer pathogenetic relation to Ewing's sarcoma than to adamantinoma.

ANCILLARY STUDIES

GENETICS

Cytogenetic studies have demonstrated trisomies in chromosomes 7, 8, 12, 19, and 21 in classic and differentiated adamantinoma.

IMMUNOHISTOCHEMISTRY

Initial immunohistochemical studies showed strong positive staining of the neoplastic cells with pan-cytokeratin antibody, confirming the epithelial histogenesis. It has been demonstrated utilizing antibodies to cytokeratin subtypes that the immunoprofile differs from that of other bone and soft tissue neoplasms with known epithelial characteristics, namely, synovial sarcoma, chordoma, and epithelioid sarcoma, which exhibit immunoreactivity for keratins 8 and 18. By contrast, all adamantinomas studied, irrespective of histologic subtype, showed uniform positivity for keratins

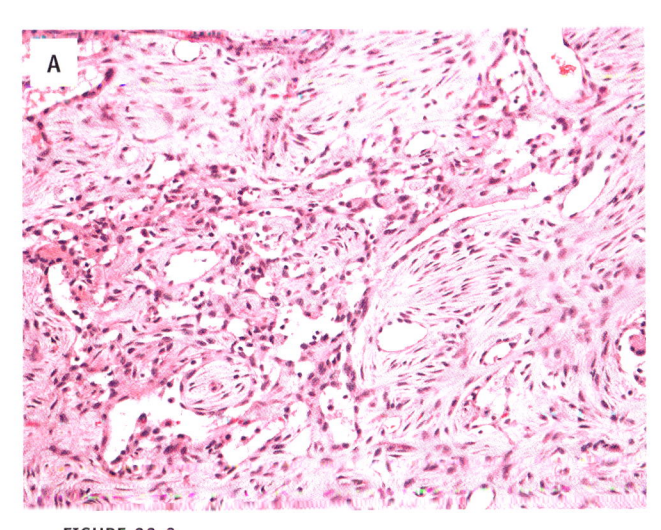

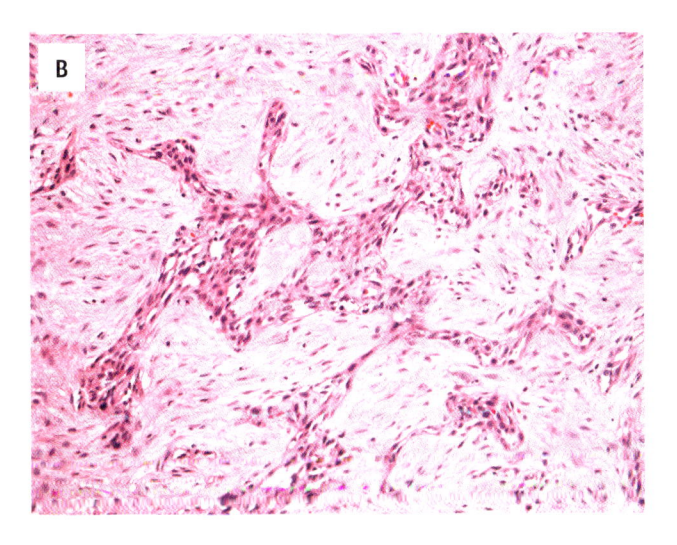

neoplastic epithelial cells may be difficult to distinguish from the mesenchymal cells and may produce patterns resembling those of mesenchymal neoplasms, namely, storiform, fascicular, and herringbone (Figure 22-5). A clue to their identification is their tendency to outline

FIGURE 22-2
Adamantinoma.
Tubular variant. **A,** Small, tubular spaces lined by cuboidal cells embedded in a spindle cell stroma. The central gland-like spaces result from loss of cellular cohesion. **B,** The spaces are nearly filled with the cuboidal cells in this area of the same tumor.

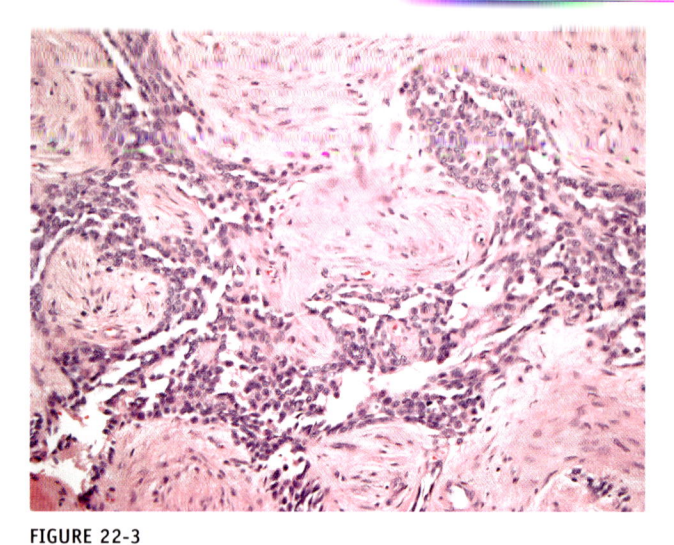

FIGURE 22-3
Adamantinoma.
Basaloid variant. Nests of epithelial cells resembling those of a basaloid cell carcinoma.

14 and 19, 74% showed positivity for keratin 5, and 50% positivity for keratin 17. These findings suggest a histogenesis from basal epithelial–type cells. The proliferation marker Ki-67, epidermal growth factor receptor, and fibroblast growth factor type 2 have been identified either exclusively or predominantly in the epithelial component, suggesting that this component constitutes the primary proliferating neoplastic cell population that is able to stimulate a reactive fibrous growth. DNA flow cytometry and p53 immunohistochemistry have demonstrated aneuploidy and significant p53 immunoreactivity only in nuclei of cells of epithelial phenotype. Furthermore, in several cases, with pulmonary metastasis, only cytokeratin-positive epithelial cells and not the osteofibrous stromal component were detected in the metastatic lesions.

DIFFERENTIAL DIAGNOSIS

Adamantinoma of the usual variety should be distinguished from the closely related histiogenic entities, OFD (see Chapter 23) and differentiated adamantinoma (see later discussion), in view of the more indolent behavior of these latter two diseases. OFD occurs in a younger age group and histologically is composed of only a fibro-osseous lesion devoid of recognizable epithelial cells in hematoxylin-and-eosin–stained sections. Likewise, differentiated adamantinoma affects a younger age group and exhibits a fibro-osseous lesion with a paucity of epithelial cells forming small nests or strands. The typical location and radiologic features will usually serve to distinguish adamantinoma from metastatic carcinoma. In addition, one or more of the typical histologic patterns of adamantinoma in the lesion are usually fairly diagnostic. The trabecular pattern of adamantinoma may be misconstrued as indicative of a vascular histogenesis and the diagnosis of an epithelioid hemangioendothelioma (low-grade angiosarcoma) rendered. The presence of foci with a more obvious epithelial configuration and immunohistochemical studies for endothelial and epithelial markers will aid in this distinction. The biphasic epithelial-mesenchymal pattern in adamantinoma may be mistaken for a synovial sarcoma especially if the lesion has extended into adjacent soft tissue mimicking a soft tissue tumor with secondary bone involvement. The mesenchymal component in adamantinoma

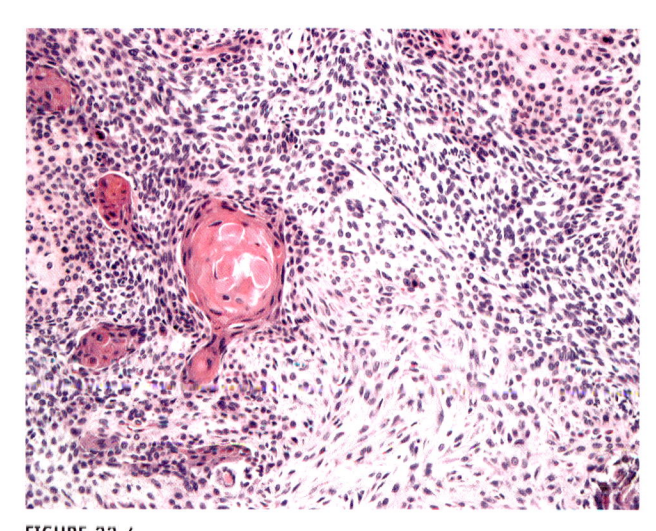

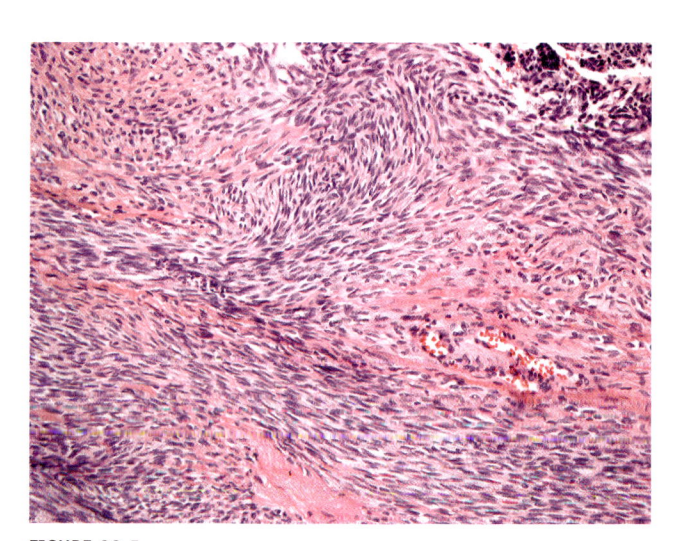

FIGURE 22-4
Adamantinoma.
Squamous variant. Nests of epithelial cells with squamous differentiation within a spindle cell stroma.

FIGURE 22-5
Adamantinoma.
Spindle cell variant. Histologically, the broad solid nests of tumor cells resemble other types of spindle-cell sarcomas and may be so misdiagnosed.

lacks the hypercellularity, nuclear atypia, and mitotic activity seen in the spindle cell component of a synovial sarcoma. The distinction of a monophasic synovial sarcoma from a pure spindle cell variant of adamantinoma may be more problematic and require careful clinical and radiologic correlation. Immunohistochemical analysis is not helpful in making this distinction.

PROGNOSIS AND TREATMENT

Adamantinomas have a propensity to both local recurrence and metastatic disease, predominantly to the lung. The mean duration to local recurrence may be as long as 7 years, and metastases have been documented as occurring up to 27 years after diagnosis. A relatively large series studied 70 patients with adamantinoma who were treated at 23 different cancer centers in Europe and North America between 1982 and 1992 with a median follow-up period of 7 years. More than 90% of these patients were treated by wide, local, limb-sparing resections. The local recurrence rate was 19%, and the mortality rate was 13%. These results indicate that wide local resection with reconstructive surgery is the treatment of choice, with results at least as good as those after amputation. Radiotherapy and chemotherapy have not been shown to be effective modalities of treatment.

DIFFERENTIATED ADAMANTINOMA

In a number of reported cases otherwise resembling OFD in young children, the presence of epithelial cells forming small nests or strands recognizable in routine hematoxylin-stained sections has been identified (Figures 22-6 and 22-7). These lesions have been designated as *differentiated, regressive, juvenile intracortical,* or

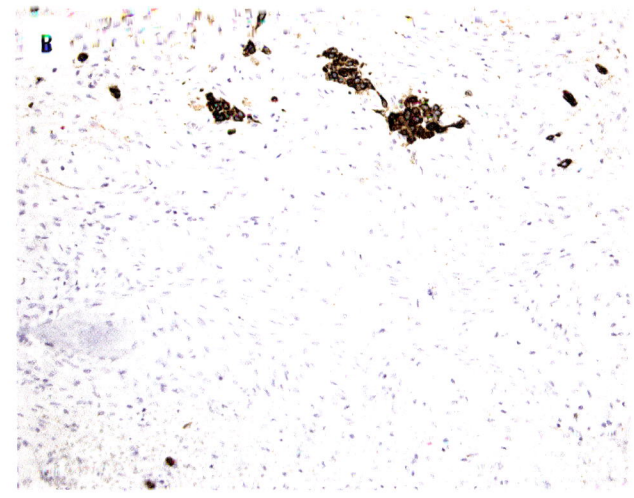

FIGURE 22-6
Differentiated adamantinoma.
Plain radiograph showing an intracortical radiolucent lesion involving the midshaft of the tibia. *(Courtesy of Dr. Michael Klein.)*

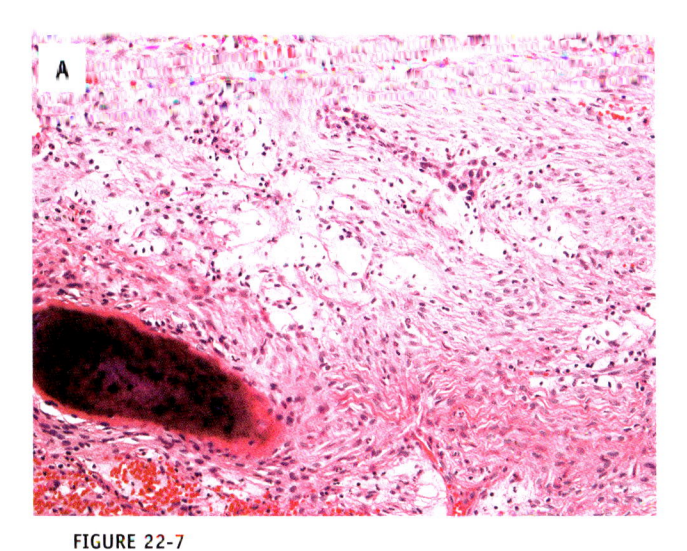

FIGURE 22-7
Differentiated adamantinoma.
A, At low magnification of this fibro-osseous lesion from the tibia, the stromal element contains numbers foamy histiocytes. It would be easy to overlook the epithelial nest in the top right of the photo. **B,** A keratin immunostain highlights the epithelial nest together with additional cells that were not visible in the hematoxylin and eosin stained slide.

ADAMANTINOMA—FACT SHEET

Definition
▸▸ Low-grade malignant epithelial neoplasm involving predominantly midshaft of tibia with or without involvement of fibula

Incidence and Location
▸▸ Constitute between 0.1% to 0.5% of malignant bone tumors
▸▸ Most common: tibia (85% of cases); tibia and fibula (10% of all cases); other bones (ulna, femur, humerus, radius, rib, ischium, tarsal, metatarsal, capitate)

Morbidity and Mortality
▸▸ Tendency to local recurrence and metastases, especially lung with long mean duration from diagnosis
▸▸ Current local recurrence rate of about 19% and mortality rate of 13% after wide local limb-sparing resection

Sex, Race, and Age Distribution
▸▸ Slight male preponderance
▸▸ Racial distribution unknown
▸▸ Mean age at presentation is 30 years

Clinical Features
▸▸ Swelling with or without pain
▸▸ Pathologic fracture in some cases

Radiologic Features
▸▸ Osteolytic, eccentric, expansile, and medullary in location; characteristic *soap-bubble* appearance
▸▸ Sclerotic margin indicative of slow growth
▸▸ Longitudinally oriented with average length of 11.0 cm
▸▸ CT and MRI helpful in assessing extent and invasiveness of lesion
▸▸ Extracortical extension into soft tissue in 15% of cases

ADAMANTINOMA—PATHOLOGIC FEATURES

Gross Findings
▸▸ Well-demarcated lesion with peripheral lobulated contours
▸▸ Eccentric involving cortex and medulla

Microscopic Findings
▸▸ Nests of epithelial cells within a fibrous or fibro-osseous stroma
▸▸ Epithelial cells arranged in tubular, basaloid, squamous with stellate reticulum, or spindle cell patterns

Immunohistochemical Findings
▸▸ Epithelial cells positive for pan-cytokeratin
▸▸ Exhibit a more specific subset profile (CK14 and CK19, CK5 and CK17)

Differential Diagnosis
▸▸ OFD
▸▸ Differentiated adamantinoma
▸▸ Epithelial hemangioendothelioma (low-grade angiosarcoma)
▸▸ Synovial sarcoma
▸▸ Metastatic carcinoma

Prognosis and Treatment
▸▸ Wide, local, limb-sparing resection is treatment of choice
▸▸ Radiotherapy and chemotherapy ineffective
▸▸ Exhibits local recurrence and metastatic disease, predominantly to lungs

---

OFD-like adamantinomas. The follow-up information on these cases is limited, but the overwhelming majority has pursued a benign course. However, a few well-documented cases have been reported in which patients initially diagnosed with OFD or juvenile adamantinoma have experienced development of full-blown classic adamantinoma. In some instances, this apparent evolution may be explained by inadequate curettage or sampling of the curetted material so that the more classic pattern of adamantinoma was missed. As with OFD, these examples of juvenile adamantinoma have also exhibited immunohistochemical homology of cytokeratin subsets with the classic form of adamantinoma. They also share the same cytogenetic abnormalities (extra copies of chromosomes 7, 8, 12, 19, and 21) seen in classic adamantinoma. With a few notable exceptions, as mentioned earlier, juvenile adamantinomas have exhibited a relatively indolent course comparable with that of OFD. The therapeutic recommendations parallel those for OFD.

SUGGESTED READINGS

Adamantinoma

1. Hazelbag HM, Fleuren JG, van den Broek LJ, et al: Adamantinoma of the long bones: keratin subclass immunoreactivity pattern with reference to its histogenesis. Am J Surg Pathol 1993;17:1225-1233.
2. Jain D, Jain VK, Vasishta RK, et al: Adamantinoma: a clinicopathological review and update. Diagn Pathol 2008;3:8.
3. Jundt G, Remberger K, Roessner A, et al: Adamantinoma of long bones. A histopathological and immunohistochemical study of 23 cases. Pathol Res Pract 1995;191:112-120.
4. Keeney GL, Unni KK, Beabout JW, et al: Adamantinoma of long bones. A clinicopathologic study of 85 cases. Cancer 1989;64:730-737.
5. Qureshi AA, Shott S, Mallin BA, et al: Current trends in the management of adamantinoma of long bones. An international study. J Bone Joint Surg Am 2000;82:1122-1131.

Differentiated Adamantinoma

1. Czerniak B, Rojas-Corona RR, Dorfman HD: Morphologic diversity of long bone adamantinoma. The concept of differentiated (regressing) adamantinoma and its relationship to osteofibrous dysplasia. Cancer 1989;64:19-34.
2. Gleason BC, Leigl-Atzwanger B, Kozakewich HP, et al: Osteofibrous dysplasia and adamantinoma in children and adolescents: a clinicopathologic reappraisal. Am J Surg Pathol 2008;32:363-376.
3. Ishida J, Iijima T, Kikuchi F, et al: A Clinicopathologic and immunohistochemical study of osteofibrous dysplasia, differentiated adamantinoma and adamantinoma of long bones. Skeletal Radiol 1992;21:493-502.
4. Ueda Y, Roessner A, Bosse A, et al: Juvenile intracortical adamantinoma of the tibia with predominant osteofibrous dysplasia-like features. Pathol Res Pract 1991;187:1039-1043.

23 Bone Tumors of Miscellaneous Type or Uncertain Lineage

S. Fiona Bonar

FIBROUS LESIONS
- Fibrous Dysplasia
- Osteofibrous Dysplasia

CYSTIC LESIONS
- Aneurysmal Bone Cyst
- Simple (Unicameral/Solitary) Bone Cyst
- Intraosseous Ganglion
- Langerhans Cell Histiocytosis
- Erdheim–Chester Disease

FIBROUS LESIONS

FIBROUS DYSPLASIA

Fibrous dysplasia represents a noninherited *dysplastic* disorder of bone characterized by a solitary or multifocal intraosseous proliferation of fibrous stroma within which trabeculae of woven immature bone are formed. The defective bone maturation is related to postzygotic point mutation of the *GNAS1* gene, which encodes the α subunit of the Gs α-stimulatory protein.

CLINICAL FEATURES

Fibrous dysplasia most commonly occurs as an isolated skeletal lesion (monostotic, 70%) and less frequently affects multiple sites (polyostotic, 30%). In a small proportion of patients (3%), predominantly those with polyostotic disease, McCune–Albright syndrome occurs. This is characterized by associated endocrine abnormalities and cutaneous pigmentation. Approximately 50% of patients with McCune–Albright syndrome experience development of renal phosphate wasting. Soft tissue myxomas occurring in conjunction with fibrous dysplasia form the basis of Mazabraud syndrome, a rare phenomenon. Polyostotic fibrous dysplasia is most often monomelic in distribution, although the more severe cases may be polymelic. All forms occur most often in the long bones (in particular, the proximal femur and the tibia), the craniofacial bones (in particular, the maxilla), and the ribs. The monomelic variant of polyostotic fibrous dysplasia usually affects the lower limbs and homolateral pelvis. Involvement of the vertebrae is rare, but documented. The disease is slightly more common in male individuals, although the female sex predominates in cases involving the jaws and long bones, and the male sex is more frequently represented in those involving the ribs and skull. The disease may present at any age, but the majority of cases manifest in the first three decades of life. Those with rib lesions alone tend to be older and are often asymptomatic. Symptoms vary depending on the location and extent of the abnormality. Fracture and deformity of the weight-bearing bones is not uncommon, and large craniofacial lesions are characterized by asymmetry and deformity. Cases with polyostotic fibrous dysplasia usually present in the first decade, often with symptoms related to endocrine hyperactivity, in particular, sexual precocity, hyperthyroidism, acromegaly, hyperprolactinemia, and adrenal hyperplasia. Fracture and deformity are more frequent in these patients, both of which may result in crippling disease, compounded by the effects of phosphate wasting.

RADIOLOGIC FEATURES

The lesions of fibrous dysplasia are centered in the medulla of the metaphysis or diaphysis, or both, of long bones. They are usually well circumscribed, bordered by a sclerotic rim that may be quite thick, forming a *rind* (Figure 23-1A). The density of the lesion varies depending on the relative proportions of bone and fibrous tissue. Those with abundant immature bone, as seen in the craniofacial skeleton, may be dense, whereas those with sparse trabeculae are relatively lucent. The classic appearance is that of *ground glass* (see Figure 23-1B). Expansion of the contour of the bone may occur particularly in smaller tubular bones and in flat bones (fibula, rib, pelvis). Bone deformity is most common in the weight-bearing long bones resulting in the classic *shepherd's crook deformity*. If cartilaginous metaplasia is

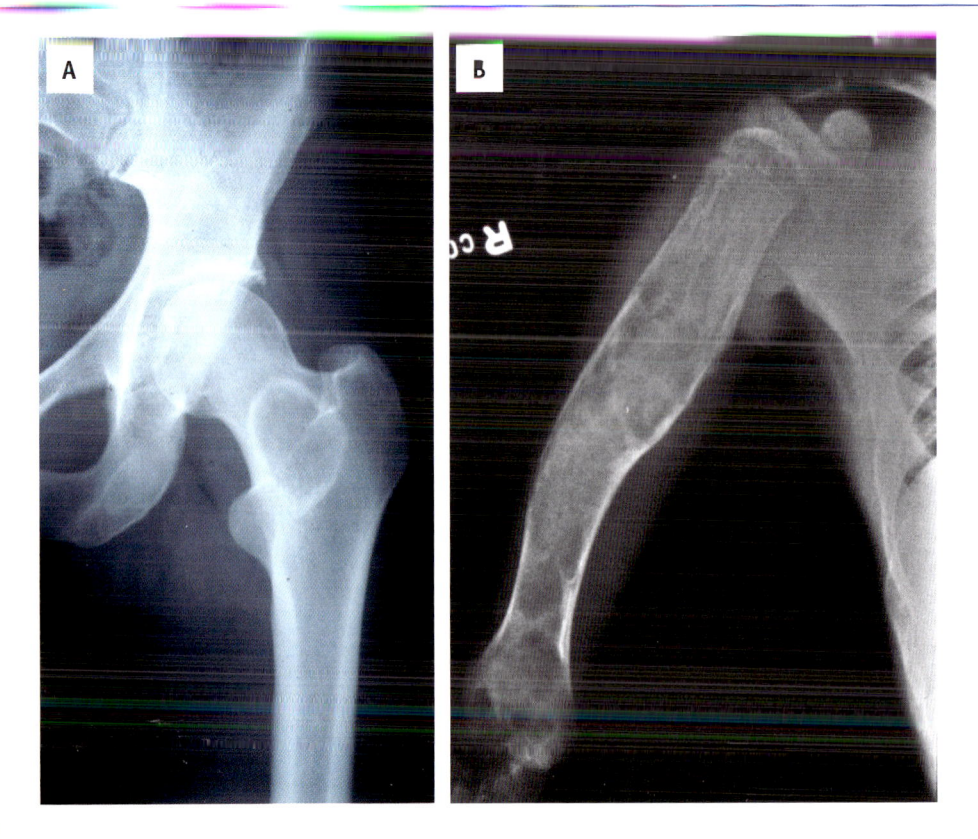

FIGURE 23-1

A, Characteristic appearance of fibrous dysplasia comprising a centrally located, well-circumscribed lesion with a thick sclerotic rim forming a rind, located in the metaphysis of the femur. **B,** Extensive involvement of humerus by intramedullary lesion with a ground-glass appearance of variable texture. Associated bone deformity is present.

prominent, ring-like and dot-like calcifications may be present, mimicking a chondroid tumor.

Pathologic Features

Gross Findings

The lesions are clearly defined and centrally located, with an expanded bony contour and thinned cortex. They have a tan-to-gray appearance and a gritty consistency because of the presence of small bone spicules (Figure 23-2A). The bone is rarely sufficiently sclerotic to warrant decalcification, but if so, areas with a more yellow-to-white appearance may be seen. Cyst formation, including blood filled, spongy cysts caused by aneurysmal bone cyst (ABC) formation, may be present, xanthogranulomatous areas may have a yellow appearance, and chondroid foci may be represented by bluish white opalescent nodules (see Figure 23-2B).

Microscopic Findings

Fibrous dysplasia is characterized by the presence of plump spindle cells in a fibrous stroma arranged in a vague whorled or storiform pattern in which admixed variably distributed trabeculae of immature woven bone that lacks osteoblastic rimming are present. Osteogenic cells associated with the trabecular surfaces are inconspicuous in nature with a retracted stellate morphology. The stromal cells are cytologically bland without atypia, nuclear pleomorphism, or hyperchromatism. Mitoses are rare, and atypical mitoses are not seen. The bony trabeculae are widely spaced within the stroma, and they most often have a distinct curvilinear or branching appearance, so-called *Chinese character, hockey stick,* or *C, S,* and *Y* shapes (Figure 23-3A, B).

The amount of bone within lesions varies considerably from sparse to abundant, the latter often seen in craniofacial lesions where the trabeculae may have a rounded concentric and laminated appearance, so-called *cementoid bodies*. These rounded cementoid bodies may rarely be the exclusive component of lesions elsewhere. In addition, in the craniofacial skeleton, the bone may have a dense sclerotic nature reminiscent of Paget disease, and occasionally the trabeculae have a parallel arrangement (see Figure 23-3C, D). The bony trabeculae in fibrous dysplasia are consistently immature with a disordered, woven appearance on polarization microscopy, the collagen fibers being arranged like threads in a fabric. Direct continuity of collagen between the fibrous stroma and the immature trabeculae may be seen on hematoxylin and eosin (H&E), and on polarization microscopy, so-called *combed* bone

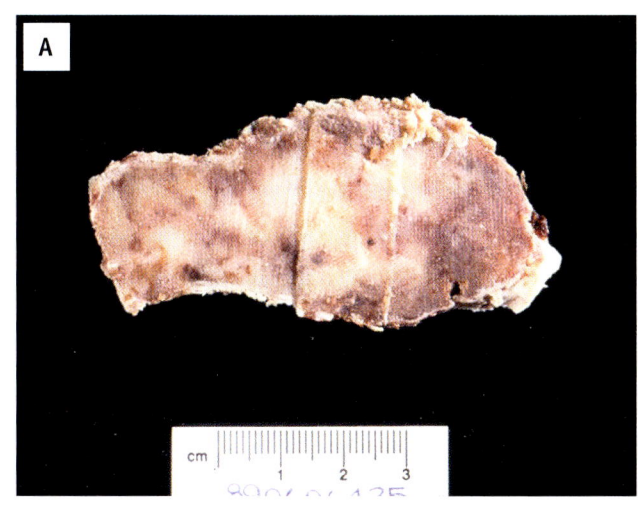

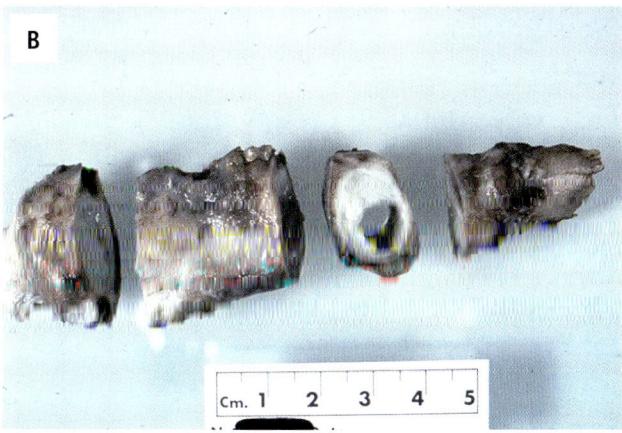

FIGURE 23-2

A, Macroscopically, fibrous dysplasia within a rib causes an expanded contour clearly demarcated at one edge, comprising tan and gray tissue with markedly thinned cortex. **B,** Expanded lesion of rib comprising solid pale fibrous component and exhibiting cystic change. The margins of the lesion are well defined. *(A: Courtesy of Dr. Stan McCarthy, NSW Tumour Registry.)*

or *Sharpey's fibers* may be seen (see Figure 23-3E, F). Secondary changes such as hemorrhage, admixed foamy histiocytes, fibrohistiocytic proliferation, and giant cell reaction are frequent. Osteoclasts may be found sometimes in clusters and occasionally forming tunnels within the immature trabeculae, the latter having recently been recognized as participating in active bone turnover in these lesions. Myxoid change within the stroma is well documented, and fatty change may also occur. Microscopic foci of chondroid metaplasia may be present, although massive cartilaginous differentiation that can occur and mimic cartilaginous tumors is rare but well recognized (see Figure 23-3G, H). Cystic change with accumulation of serous fluid is common. ABC formation is well documented, and reactive new bone formation with osteoblastic rimming may occur with fracture, confusing the histologic findings. Malignant change is extremely rare, manifest as high-grade osteosarcoma or malignant fibrous histiocytoma.

ANCILLARY STUDIES

Ancillary studies are usually not helpful for diagnostic purposes.

Careful radiological correlation may support any concerns, a lack of clear margination of the tumor lending support to the diagnosis of a low grade malignancy.

DIFFERENTIAL DIAGNOSIS

The differential diagnosis includes a number of other fibrous or fibro-osseous lesions. *Osteofibrous dysplasia* bears a strong histologic resemblance to fibrous dysplasia because it is composed of a mixture of woven and lamellar bone embedded in bland fibrous tissue. However, it also contains prominent osteoblastic rimming, which is a feature not typically seen in fibrous dysplasia. In addition, osteofibrous dysplasia is a cortically based lesion that predominately affects the tibia of young patients. *Cementifying fibroma* is a fibro-osseous lesion located in the jaw bones. In contrast with fibrous dysplasia, which merges with the bony cortex, cemento-ossifying fibroma is clearly demarcated and can be shelled out rather than removed piecemeal; hence, radiographic studies are usually necessary to make the distinction. If numerous foamy histiocytes are present in the stroma, the possibility of *nonossifying fibroma* must be considered. This lacks metaplastic bone, and any reactive bone that is present is usually related to a pathologic fracture. Radiologically are eccentric lesions centered in the cortex in contrast with that of fibrous dysplasia, which is located in the medulla. If the fibrous component is prominent, *desmoplastic fibroma* may be considered. This is usually associated with cortical disruption radiologically. *Chondrosarcoma* may be considered in tumors with massive cartilaginous differentiation. However, in fibrocartilaginous fibrous dysplasia, the cartilage contains no cytologic atypia, a bone infiltration pattern is not expected, and the lobules of cartilage will show a bone encasement pattern with endochondral ossification at their margins. *Parosteal osteosarcoma* may closely mimic fibrous dysplasia, but this is a surface lesion, not central, so with radiologic correlation, confusion should not occur. The most difficult differential diagnosis is that of *low grade intraosseous fibrous dysplasia-like osteosarcoma*. In the latter, there is usually some, albeit subtle, cytologic atypia of the stromal cells with variability in size and shape and hyperchromatism. Most importantly, low-grade osteosarcoma typically permeates the surrounding pre-existing normal lamellar bone, soft tissue, or both.

In recent years the molecular basis of all forms of fibrous dysplasia has been clarified. All have post zygotic activating mutation of the Gs alpha protein encoded by the GNAS1 locus on the distal long arm of chromosome 20. The affected individuals are somatic mosaics and

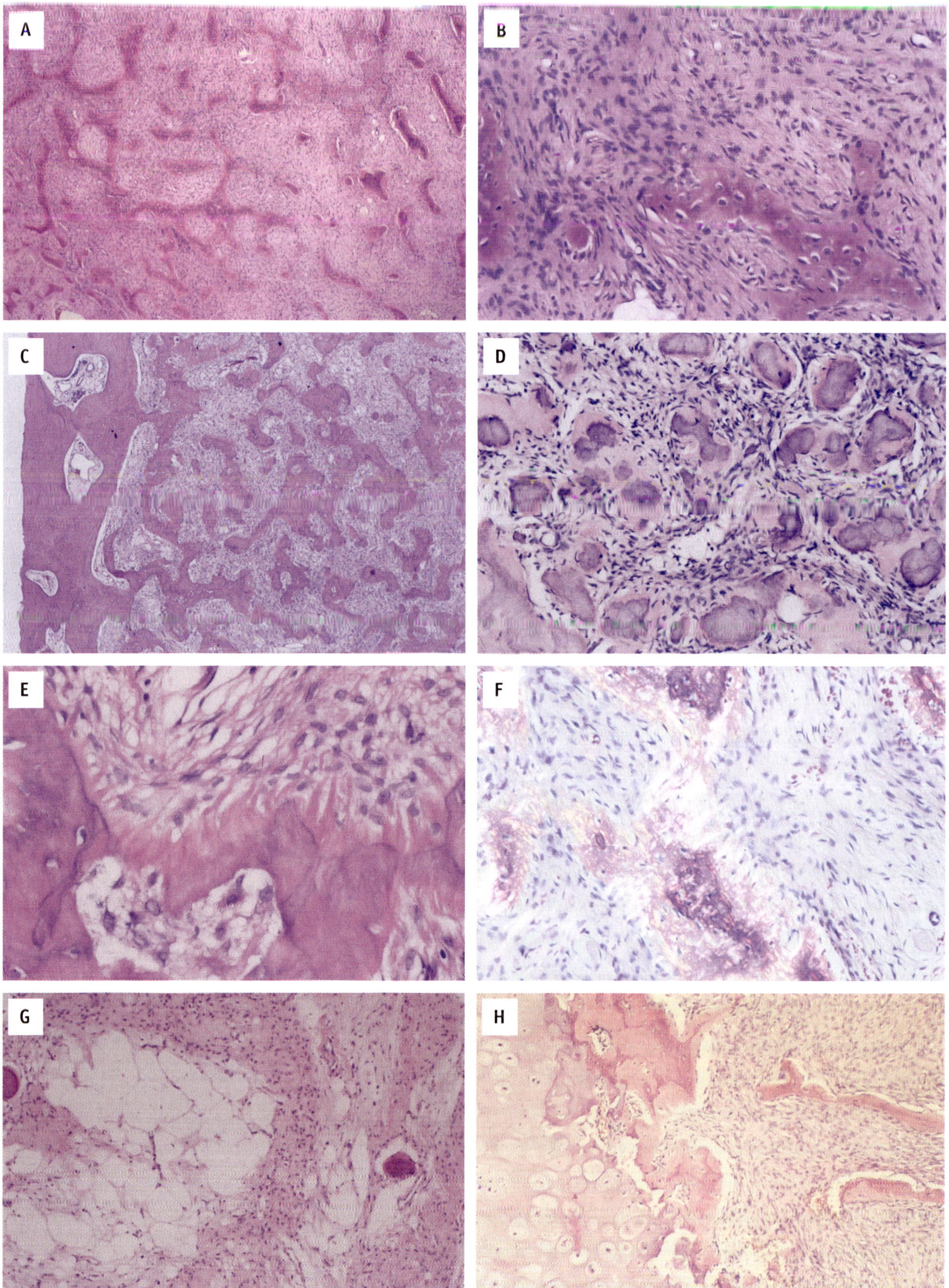
A
B
C
D
E
F
G
H

FIGURE 23-3
Fibrous dysplasia.
A, Low-power view shows bony trabeculae with a curvilinear branching appearance, so-called *Chinese* characters, *hockey stick,* or *C, S,* and *Y* shapes, within a fibrous stroma. **B,** At higher power, trabeculae of immature woven bone are devoid of a plump lining osteoblast layer and lie within a fibrous stroma comprising bland stromal cells arranged in a whorled or storiform manner. **C,** Trabeculae of immature bone merge with mature cortical bone. The trabeculae are somewhat thick in this example from the craniofacial skeleton. **D,** Rounded *cementoid* bodies occur occasionally, most frequently in the craniofacial skeleton. **E,** At high power, immature bony trabeculae are bordered by somewhat retracted osteoblast/stromal cells and exhibit continuity of collagen fibers between stroma and trabeculae, so-called *combed bone* or *Sharpey's fibers*. **F,** Polarization microscopy accentuates the woven nature of trabeculae and Sharpey's fibers. **G,** Focal fatty change within the stroma may be seen. **H,** Areas of chondroid metaplasia may occur and may be extensive. *(Courtesy of Dr. Stan McCarthy, NSW Tumour Registry.)*

FIBROUS DYSPLASIA—FACT SHEET

Definition
- Noninherited dysplastic disorder characterized by fibrous stroma with trabeculae of immature woven bone, reflecting defective bone maturation, due to somatic mutation of GNAS 1 gene

Incidence and Location
- Approximately 1% of bone tumors for which biopsy was performed
- Long bones (neck of femur, tibia), craniofacial bones, and ribs
- Rare in spine

Sex, Race, and Age Distribution
- Slight male predominance (1.2:1)
- Racial distribution equal
- Age range from infant to adult, majority younger than 30 years
  - Polyostotic form presents in the first decade of life
  - Monostotic form presents in the second and third decades of life
  - Rib lesions present often in fourth and fifth decades of life

Clinical Features
- Monostotic
  - Often asymptomatic/incidental finding
  - Fracture
  - Deformity/asymmetry (craniofacial bones particularly)
- Polyostotic
  - Effects of endocrine hyperplasia
    - Sexual precocity, hyperthyroidism, acromegaly, hyperprolactinemia, adrenal hyperplasia
  - Fracture, deformity

Radiologic Features
- Centrally located medullary lesions
- Metadiaphyseal in long bones
- Well circumscribed with sclerotic rim *rind*
- Variable density with *ground glass* appearance
- Expansion of smaller bones in particular
- Deformity of long bones: *shepherd's crook deformity* of proximal femur

Prognosis and Treatment
- Conservative treatment recommended
- Monostotic has excellent outcome
- Often stabilize after puberty
- May progress within an individual bone
- In polyostotic forms, the outlook depends on extent and severity of both bone lesions and endocrine abnormalities in McCune-Albright syndrome
- Some evidence of beneficial effect of bisphosphonate in all forms

---

FIBROUS DYSPLASIA—PATHOLOGIC FEATURES

Gross Findings
- Centrally located, clearly defined
- Thin cortex, expanded contour
- Tan–gray fibrous tissue, gritty consistency
- With or without cysts and hemorrhage

Microscopic Findings
- Bland fibrous stroma with vague storiform appearance
- Trabeculae of immature woven bone without osteoblastic rimming
  - Chinese character, C, Y, and S shapes
- May contain foam cells
- Occasional stromal myxoid and/or cystic change
- Continuity of collagen from stroma to bone
- Sarcomatous transformation is rare

Immunohistochemistry
- Generally not useful for diagnosis

Differential Diagnosis
- Osteofibrous dysplasia
- Cemento-ossifying fibroma of gnathic bones
- Desmoplastic fibroma
- Parosteal and low-grade intraosseous osteosarcoma
- Chondrosarcoma if prominent chondroid component

---

represent a heterogeneous patient population, depending on the pattern of mutated cells throughout the body. It is believed that mutations early in embryogenesis induce more severe abnormalities as seen in McCune Albright syndrome, whereas those occurring later induce the more restricted form of monostotic disease. The mutations inhibit intrinsic GTPase of the Gs alpha such that it remains active in stimulating adenylyl cyclase and leads to overproduction of cyclic AMP (cAMP). In osteoblastic cells, overproduction of cAMP results in cell retraction from the surface of forming bone with abnormally organized collagen fibres resulting in immature woven bone. Cyclic AMP overactivity in endocrine tissues leads to increased cellular proliferation and secretion in these tissues, characteristic of McCune Albright syndrome. Elevation in cAMP also leads to alteration in the expression of downstream genes resulting in altered osteoblastic and osteoclastic recruitment and function. It is thought that the increased osteoclastogenesis and bone resorption seen in some cases of fibrous dysplasia may be a reflection of interleukin 6 activity in particular. Point mutation of the Gs alpha proteins has also been documented in liposclerosing myxofibrous tumor, supporting the general impression that rather than being a separate distinct entity, it represents a variant of fibrous dysplasia. The mutation has also been characterized in the myxomas present in patients with Mazzabraud's syndrome. In the dysplastic bone lesions Gs alpha mutations are expressed in osteoprogenitor cells in the marrow and can be identified by RT PCR analysis.

PROGNOSIS AND TREATMENT

The distribution of disease within individuals is stable in that progression from monostotic to polyostotic forms does not occur; however, an individual lesion may show enlargement and progression. This is most likely to occur during skeletal growth, often stabilizing after puberty. Surgical treatment depends on the extent and site of disease, but in general is conservative. The goal of treatment is aimed at correction of deformity and prevention of fracture. Radiation therapy is no longer recommended. In recent years, some suggestion has been made that bisphosphonates, which decrease bone remodeling, may be of benefit in McCune–Albright syndrome in particular. Management of renal phosphate wasting may also alter the fracture risk in these patients. Malignant transformation is extremely rare. It can be spontaneous or, more frequently, associated with prior radiotherapy. The risk is greater for the more severely affected polyostotic variant, and it usually develops in the third and fourth decades of life.

OSTEOFIBROUS DYSPLASIA

Osteofibrous dysplasia is a benign fibro-osseous lesion of childhood characteristically occurring in an intracortical location in the anterior aspect of the midshaft of the tibia with or without involvement of the fibula. It is a distinctly separate entity from fibrous dysplasia.

CLINICAL FEATURES

Osteofibrous dysplasia occurs predominantly in children younger than 10 years with an age range from newborn to 39 years, and most cases (95%) being younger than 15. Male and female sexes are equally affected. Characteristically, these lesions occur in the diaphysis of the tibia, a small proportion exhibiting synchronous fibular involvement. Involvement of the fibula alone is rare, and involvement of other bones including the ulna and radius, although documented, is rare. The majority of patients have pain, swelling, and deformity. It may present as congenital pseudoarthrosis.

RADIOLOGIC FEATURES

Osteofibrous dysplasia affects the cortex of the diaphysis of the tibia as an intracortical radiolucency, which is well marginated with surrounding sclerosis (Figure 23-4 A, B). It may have a *ground-glass* texture. Multiple lucencies with intervening sclerosis are frequent. The lesions are elongated and can vary in size from several centimeters to involvement of most of the bone, some being circumferential (see Figure 23-4C, D). Although medullary involvement may occur, the medullary margin is sclerotic and well defined with narrowing of the medullary canal. The cortex is usually thickened or expanded, or both. Periosteal reaction is rare, and is thick and solid when present. Soft tissue extension is not seen. Bowing is common and is most often anterior.

PATHOLOGIC FEATURES

GROSS FINDINGS

The lesion is confined to the cortex and is white to yellow–brown with a firm fibrous, sometimes gritty consistency (Figure 23-5).

MICROSCOPIC FINDINGS

Histologically, osteofibrous dysplasia has a distinct *zonal* architecture, the central portions composed predominantly of fibrous tissue that may have a loose somewhat myxoid appearance and usually storiform pattern (Figure 23-6A). Within this are relatively sparse, irregularly distributed bony trabeculae that are predominantly immature and woven in nature (see Figure 23-6B). Peripherally, these gradually become larger and more numerous, composed of a mixture of immature woven and mature lamellar bone, the latter predominating at the edges of the lesion, where they merge with either the cortical bone or reactive sclerotic bone at the medullary aspect (see Figure 23-6C–E). In contrast with fibrous dysplasia, the bony trabeculae throughout most of the lesion are rimmed, in part, by a layer of plump osteoblasts. Scattered osteoclasts are present, sometimes clustered. Foamy histiocytes are rare, and ABC formation is not seen. In occasional foci the changes may simulate fibrous dysplasia. Groups of epithelial cells are not identifiable on H&E.

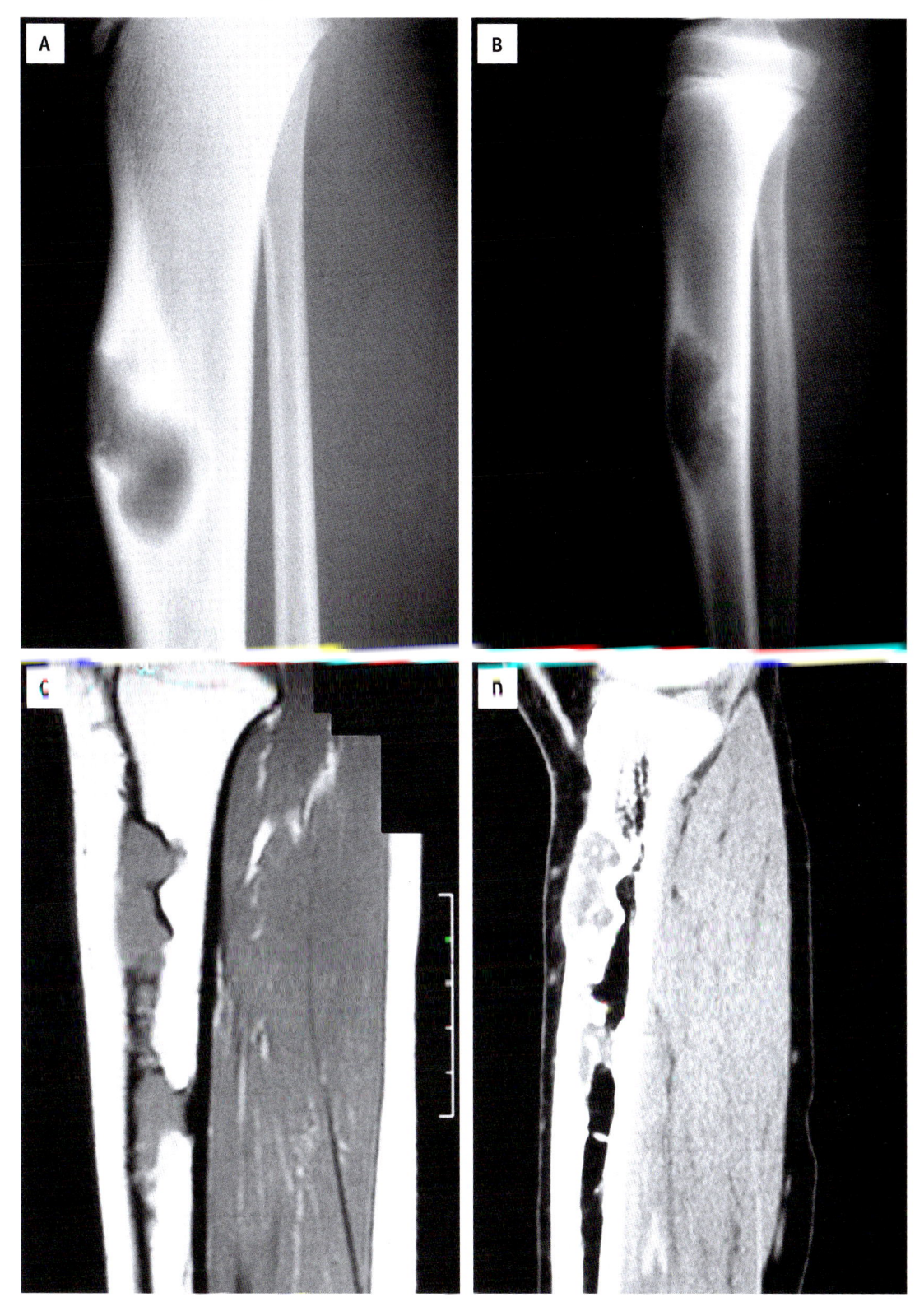

FIGURE 23-4
A, B, Plain radiographs of cases of osteofibrous dysplasia. They are predominantly or exclusively cortical-based radiolucent lesions. The lesions are well marginated. **C, D,** Magnetic resonance imaging and computed tomographic scan of osteofibrous dysplasia demonstrating a lesion confined to the cortex but involving a considerable length of the diaphysis.

OSTEOFIBROUS DYSPLASIA—FACT SHEET

Definition
- Benign fibro-osseous lesion of childhood occurring in an intracortical location predominantly in the midshaft of the tibia with or without involvement of the fibula

Incidence and Location
- Rare, less than 1% of all primary bone tumors
- Diaphysis of tibia, predominantly anterior cortex
- Occasional involvement of fibula
- Rare documented cases in radius and ulna

Morbidity and Mortality
- Most undergo spontaneous regression after puberty

Sex, Race, and Age Distribution
- Roughly equal sex distribution
- Racial distribution unknown
- Majority (95%) of patients are younger than 15 years

Clinical Features
- Pain
- Swelling
- Deformity

Radiologic Features
- Centered in cortex of tibial diaphysis
- Lucent, possibly ground glass
- Multiple lucencies frequent
- Surrounding mature sclerosis with thickened cortex
- Bowing
- No soft tissue mass

Prognosis and Treatment
- Majority of cases regress spontaneously after puberty
- Conservative treatment
- 25% of cases recur after biopsy/excision
- Surgery only for extensive disease or severe deformity

OSTEOFIBROUS DYSPLASIA—PATHOLOGIC FEATURES

Gross Findings
- Confined to cortex
- Firm, fibrous, pale-to-light-brown tissue with gritty texture

Microscopic Findings
- Zonal architecture
- Central loose fibrous tissue with storiform architecture
- Admixed immature woven bony trabeculae
- Peripheral, more abundant, larger trabeculae of mixed immature woven and mature lamellar bone
- Prominent osteoblastic rimming

Immunohistochemical Findings
- Cytokeratin (AE1/3, pankeratin) positive in 80% as single isolated cells
- CAM5.2 (cytokeratins 8 and 18) negative

Differential Diagnosis
- Fibrous dysplasia
- Osteofibrous dysplasia-like (differentiated) adamantinoma
- Classic adamantinoma with focal osteofibrous dysplasia-like areas

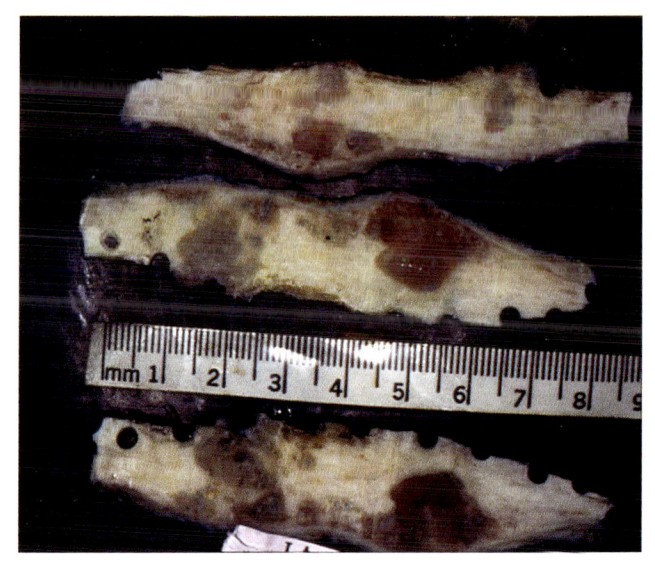

ANCILLARY STUDIES

IMMUNOHISTOCHEMISTRY

In approximately 80% of cases with characteristic H&E histologic features of osteofibrous dysplasia on H&E, without recognizable epithelial cells, positivity for cytokeratin AE1/3 in scattered largely isolated cells within the fibrous stroma is identified (Figure 23-7). The keratin profile is that of a basal cell phenotype with expression of cytokeratins 14 and 19 in particular, with lesser numbers also expressing cytokeratins 1 and 5. Cytokeratins 8 and 18 are negative. This pattern of expression is also seen in adamantinoma.

GENETIC STUDIES

In a small number of cases tested, clonal chromosomal abnormalities have been identified, including trisomy 7, 8, 12, and 21. Extra copies of one or more of these chromosomes have also been found in osteofibrous dysplasia-like (differentiated) adamantinoma (with recognizable epithelial cells on H&E) and classic adamantinoma. Mutations for Gs α protein and *NF1* gene have not been detected. Expression of epidermal and fibroblastic growth factors and their receptors (EGF, EGFR, and FGF-2) expression have been identified in osteofibrous dysplasia.

The constellation of shared histologic, immunophenotypical, and chromosomal characteristics, together

FIGURE 23-5
Osteofibrous dysplasia.
Macroscopically, multiple areas of soft tissue are present within the cortex with associated surrounding sclerosis. They vary in texture and color from white to brown.

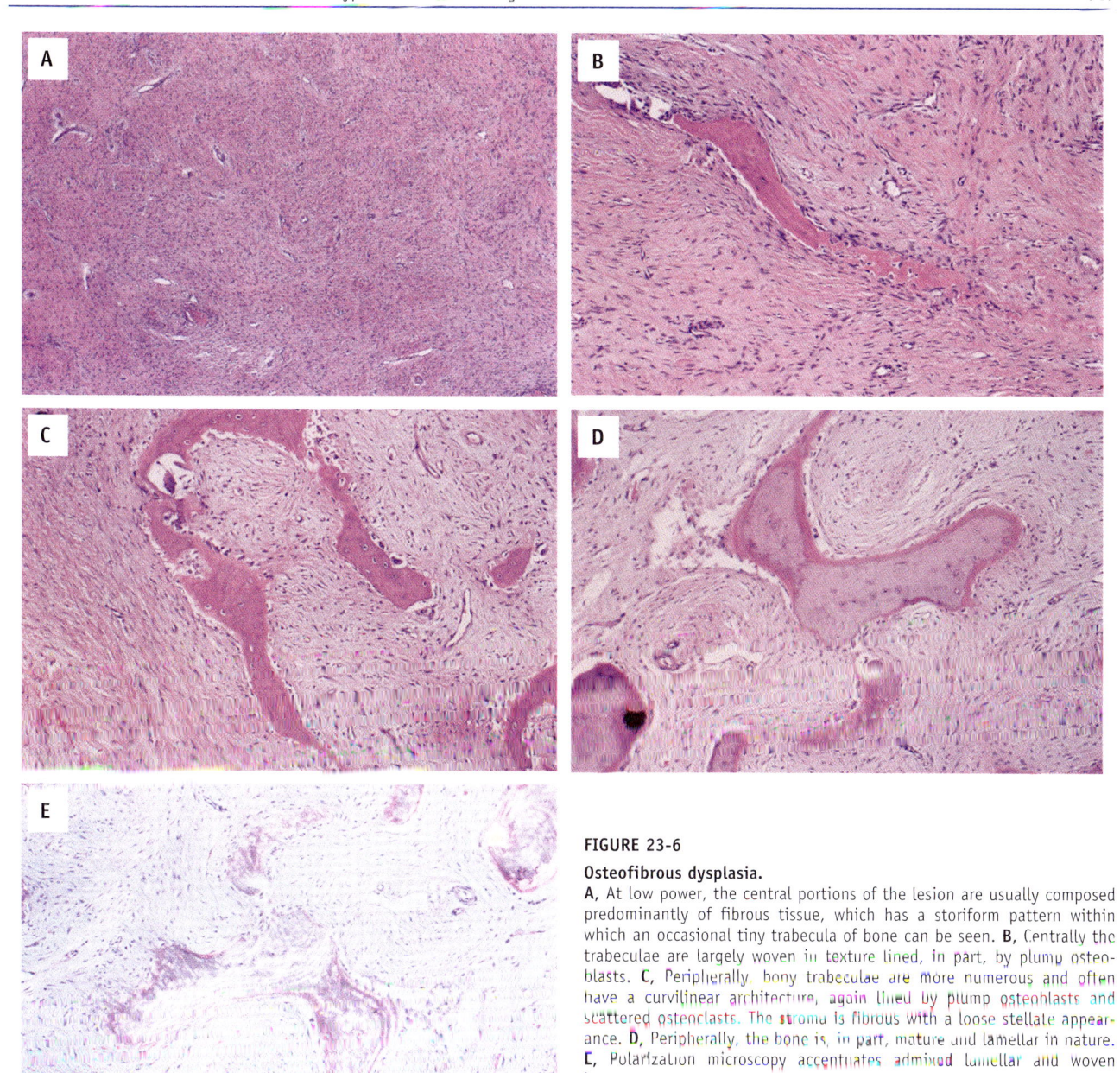

FIGURE 23-6
Osteofibrous dysplasia.
A, At low power, the central portions of the lesion are usually composed predominantly of fibrous tissue, which has a storiform pattern within which an occasional tiny trabecula of bone can be seen. **B,** Centrally the trabeculae are largely woven in texture lined, in part, by plump osteoblasts. **C,** Peripherally, bony trabeculae are more numerous and often have a curvilinear architecture, again lined by plump osteoblasts and scattered osteoclasts. The stroma is fibrous with a loose stellate appearance. **D,** Peripherally, the bone is, in part, mature and lamellar in nature. **E,** Polarization microscopy accentuates admixed lamellar and woven bone.

with occasional rare cases of progression clinically from osteofibrous dysplasia to osteofibrous dysplasia-like adamantinoma and classical adamantinoma, support the supposition that these three entities reflect a spectrum of disease.

DIFFERENTIAL DIAGNOSIS

Osteofibrous dysplasia must be distinguished from fibrous dysplasia and both classic and osteofibrous dysplasia-like adamantinoma. Fibrous dysplasia is centered in the medulla, not the cortex. The bony trabeculae are all immature and woven in nature, and plump osteoblastic rimming is not seen. Differentiation may be difficult with fracture in fibrous dysplasia when reactive bony trabeculae may be present. In this case, hemorrhage, hemosiderin deposition, and xanthomatous change with inflammatory cells are usual findings, all of which are unusual in osteofibrous dysplasia. Cytokeratin expression is not seen in fibrous dysplasia. A diagnosis of osteofibrous dysplasia like adamantinoma (juvenile or differentiated adamantinoma) should be made when scattered epithelial cell groups are identified on H&E, usually centrally located. Categorization of those cases in which groups of epithelial cells are identified on

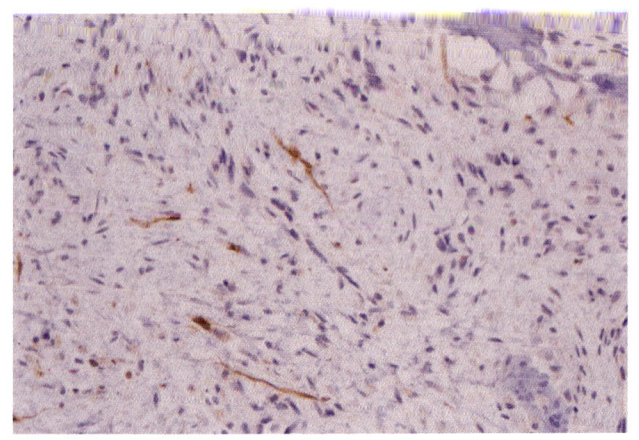

FIGURE 23-7
Osteofibrous dysplasia containing scattered single stromal cells that exhibit positivity for cytokeratin.

cytokeratin staining only is contentious as yet. This finding has led some authors to designate these lesions are *osteofibrous dysplasia-like adamantinoma*, whereas others require that groups of epithelial cells be identifiable on H&E alone, admixed with otherwise characteristic features of osteofibrous dysplasia. To date, no evidence suggests any difference in behavior for these lesions; thus, nomenclature remains speculative. In classic adamantinoma, the epithelial component is predominant with focal osteofibrous dysplasia-like areas only, noted particularly at the periphery. Because the epithelial component of these latter lesions is irregularly distributed and is sparse in osteofibrous dysplasia-like adamantinoma, complete curettage of the lesions and complete sampling of the curetted material is paramount for accurate diagnosis.

Prognosis and Treatment

Based on the two largest series of cases, osteofibrous dysplasia appears to undergo spontaneous regression at puberty in the majority of cases. The local recurrence rate after curettage or local resection is approximately 25%. It is therefore recommended that surgery be delayed until after puberty unless dictated by the presence of extensive disease with associated deformity and fracture. In these cases, stabilization procedures without actual excision may be indicated. The overwhelming majority of patients with a diagnosis of osteofibrous dysplasia-like adamantinoma have followed a benign course. Rare cases exist where full-blown classic adamantinoma ensued even with complete and adequate sampling of the original lesion. The rate of evolution has varied from 5 to 17 years. Excision of lesions after puberty is indicated if increasing growth of the lesion, deformity, or both occur.

CYSTIC LESIONS

ANEURYSMAL BONE CYST

Aneurysmal bone cyst (ABC) is a benign, usually intraosseous or subperiosteal, multiloculated, blood-filled cystic lesion that most frequently causes a blowout distension of the contour of bone. In some instances, blood-filled spaces are lacking and the lesion is solid in nature with histologic features essentially the same as giant cell reparative granuloma. It can occur de novo, as a primary phenomenon (50–70% of cases), or as a secondary phenomenon in a preexisting condition (30-50% of cases). It accounts for approximately 2% of all primary bone tumors. Rare soft tissue variants have been described. Until recently, the exact nature of ABC was unclear. However, recent studies have confirmed its clonal neoplastic nature.

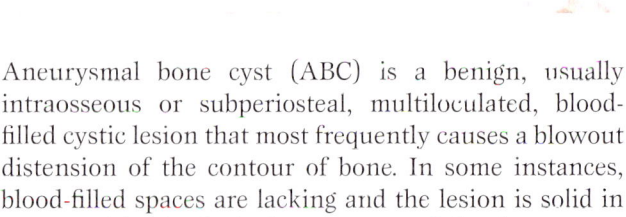

Clinical Features

The majority (80%) of patients are skeletally immature individuals, the peak incidence being in the second decade of life with rare cases younger than 5 years. The sex ratio is equal, and although any bone may be affected, the majority (>80%) is seen in either the metaphysis of long bones, mostly around the knee, or in the vertebral column. The craniofacial skeleton and tarsal bones are also well represented. Multifocal involvement is rare, except in the spine. Most patients describe pain and swelling of variable duration, often having a rapid evolution over several weeks. Vertebral involvement may induce rapidly progressive spinal cord compression. Secondary ABC occurs predominantly in the weight-bearing bones, its location and clinical presentation reflecting that of the original tumor. It most commonly arises in association with benign lesions, in particular, chondroblastoma, giant cell tumor, and osteoblastoma.

Radiologic Features

The characteristic feature of ABC is that of an eccentric metaphyseal expansile lucency with cortical destruction and a paper-thin peripheral *eggshell* of periosteal bone. The intramedullary component is usually well marginated. It often has a multiloculated appearance (Figure 23-8). Computed tomography (CT) scan and magnetic resonance imaging (MRI) confirm its expansile nature, and fluid levels are usually present. It may cross joints

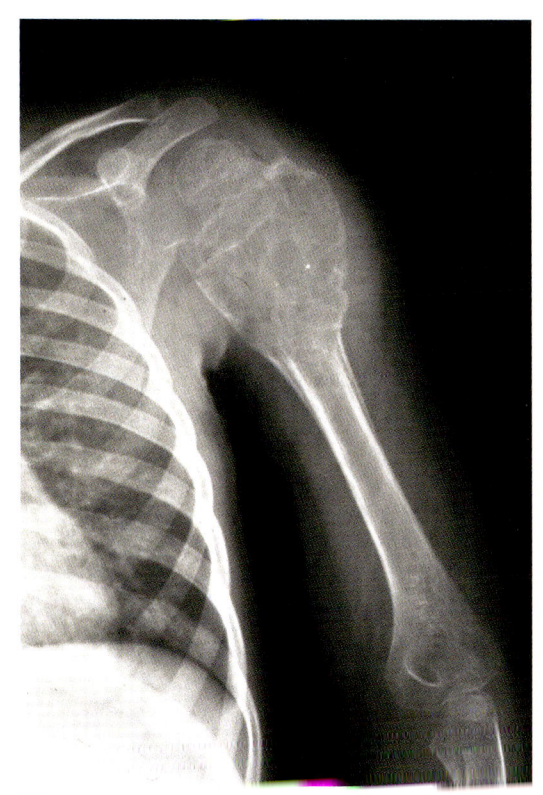

CHAPTER 23 Bone Tumors of Miscellaneous Type or Uncertain Lineage

FIGURE 23-8
Radiographically, aneurysmal bone cyst is characterized by an expansile radiolucency with associated cortical destruction and a peripheral eggshell of bone. The intramedullary component is well marginated, and the lesion has a multiloculated appearance.

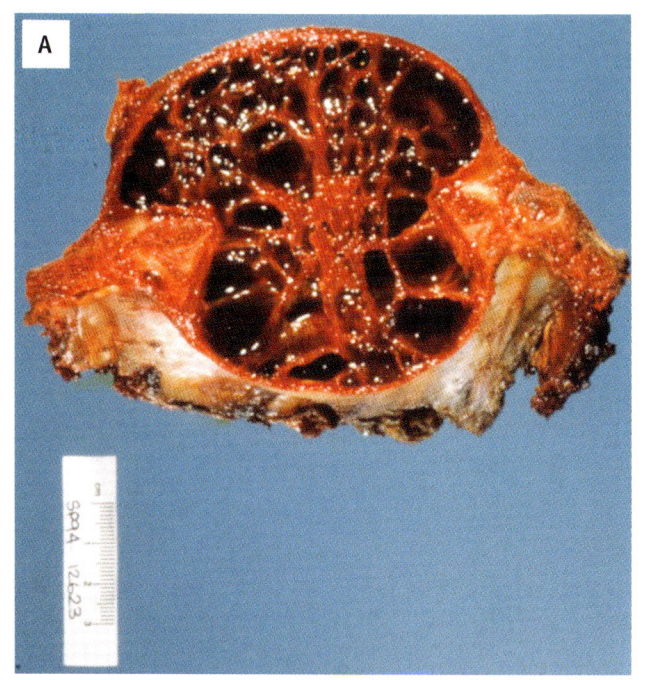

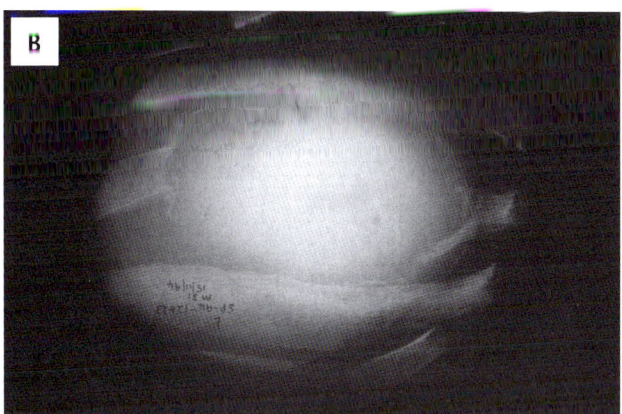

and involve multiple adjacent bones, most often noted in the vertebrae. In secondary ABC, the characteristics of the original lesion may or may not be retained, and the location of the lesion (e.g., epiphyseal) may be the only indication of its existence.

FIGURE 23-9
Aneurysmal bone cyst.
A, Macroscopically, a well-demarcated markedly expansile lesion in rib is present, comprising variably sized blood-filled vessels traversed by fibrous membranes. The lesion is separated from the surrounding soft tissue by a layer of fibrous tissue. **B,** A radiograph of the specimen from **(A)** shows its markedly expansile appearance with a thin peripheral shell of bone. *(Courtesy of Dr. Stan McCarthy, NSW Tumour Registry.)*

PATHOLOGIC FEATURES

GROSS FINDINGS

Because these lesions are rarely removed intact, the curettage tissue comprises red–brown granular tissue, which may have a spongy consistency. The amount of curetted material is small in comparison with the size of the lesion clinically and radiologically. If excision has been performed (e.g., rib or fibula), the lesion is well demarcated, often with cortical destruction and a shell of bone clearly delineating it from the surrounding soft tissue. It contains variably sized blood-filled spaces traversed by thin septae, often more numerous peripherally (Figure 23-9). Solid components are noncystic, gray, and white, and may represent the primary lesion in a secondary ABC.

MICROSCOPIC FINDINGS

Characteristically, ABC is composed of blood-filled spaces lined by thin membranous septae composed of loose fibrous tissue within which capillaries, chronic inflammatory cells, and osteoclast-like giant cells are present. The margin of the lesion in soft tissue is delineated by a layer of fibrous tissue in which reactive bony trabeculae occur (Figure 23-10A-C). Trabeculae of reactive bone comprising immature osteoid lined by plump osteoblasts are evident (see Figure 23-10D). Osteoid with a more fibrillary character is also often present, deposited in a linear manner (see Figure 23-10E). An endothelial lining is not present.

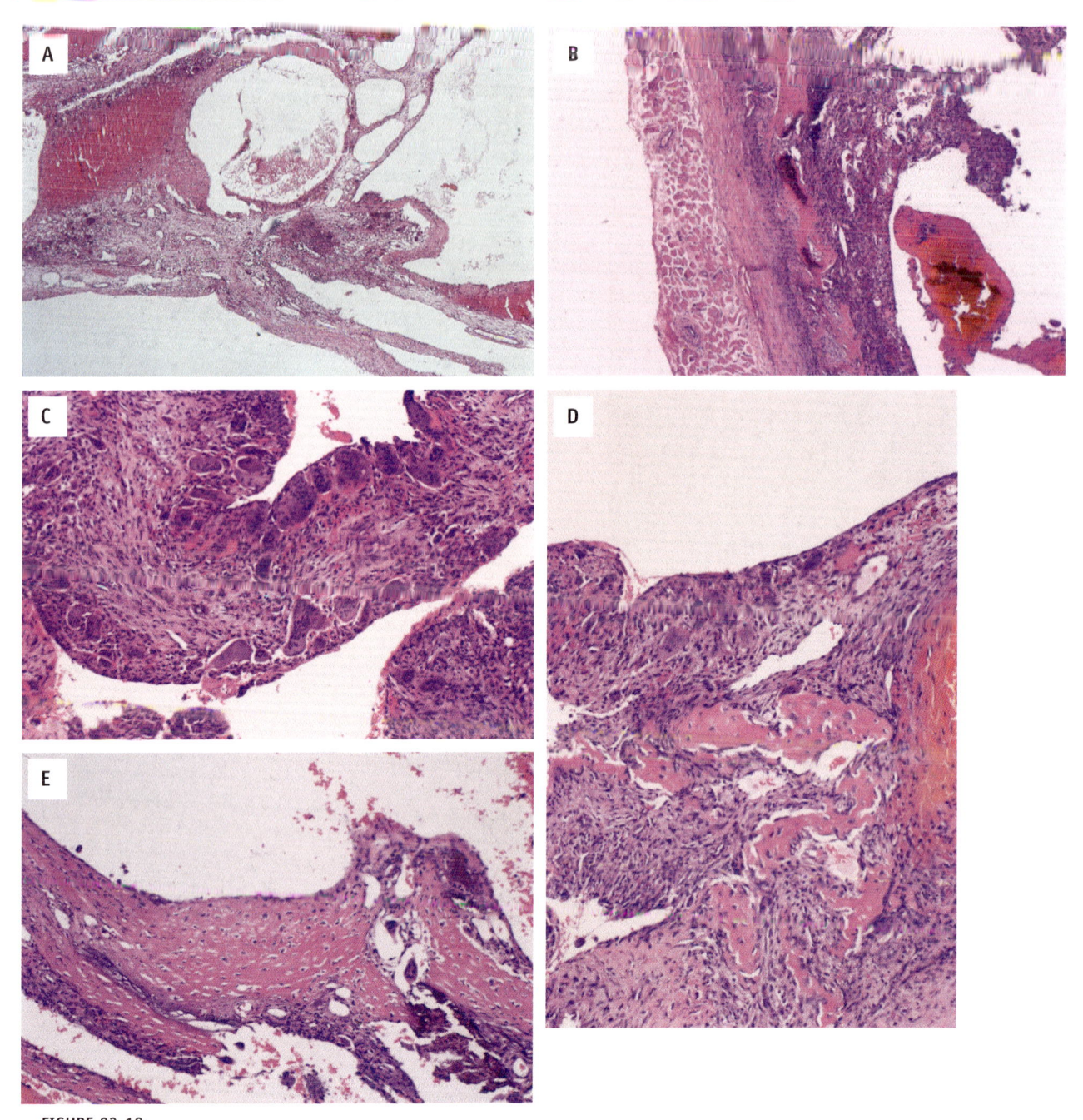

FIGURE 23-10
Aneurysmal bone cyst.
A, At low power, multiple variably sized spaces are present, traversed by thin fibrous membranes with a peripheral shell of bone. **B,** The lesion is separated from the surrounding muscle by a layer of reactive bone, which, in turn, is covered by a layer of fibrous tissue. **C,** At high power, osteoclast-like giant cells are often numerous. **D,** Reactive bony trabeculae bordered by plump osteoblasts are common and usually arranged parallel to the surface of the membranes. **E,** Immature osteoid with a linear arrangement is frequent, again organized parallel to the membrane surface, sometimes having a buckled appearance.

Irregular calcification may be seen in areas that have a fibrochondroid appearance, the calcification having a basophilic blue appearance (see Figure 23-10F, G). In solid variants, clusters of osteoclast giant cells with hemorrhage are present admixed with collections of foamy histiocytes and trabeculae of reactive osteoid lying in a fibrohistiocytic stroma, often with storiform architecture, similar to that of giant cell reparative granuloma (see Figure 23-10H, I). Cellular atypia, hyperchromatism, and pleomorphism are not identified, and although mitotic activity may be brisk, atypical mitoses are not seen.

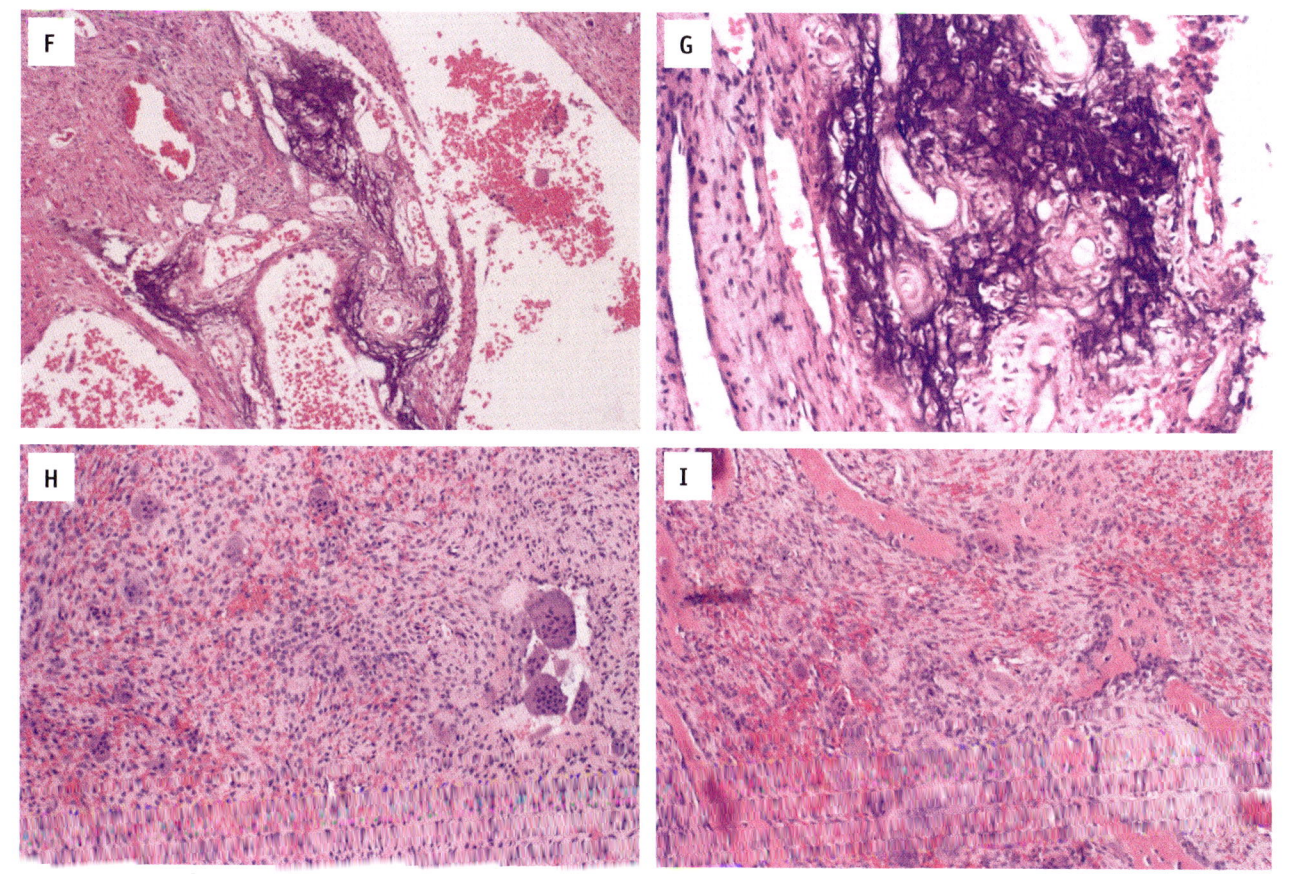

CHAPTER 23 Bone Tumors of Miscellaneous Type or Uncertain Lineage   431

F, Irregular calcification within stroma that has a fibrochondroid and basophilic blue appearance is frequently seen and considered to be characteristic of aneurysmal bone cyst. **G,** Calcification of this immature fibrochondroid material may be prominent. **H,** In solid aneurysmal bone cyst/giant cell reparative granuloma, clusters of osteoclast-like giant cells with hemorrhage are frequently seen within a fibrohistiocytic stroma. Small spaces with osteoclasts are frequent. **I,** Intermingled trabeculae of reactive bone bordered by plump osteoblasts are evident.

ANCILLARY STUDIES

IMMUNOHISTOCHEMISTRY

Immunohistochemistry is not useful for diagnostic purposes in ABC.

GENETIC STUDIES

Cytogenetic and molecular genetic studies have shown that approximately 70% of ABCs contain *USP6* fusion genes. The most common is *CDH11-USP6*, but several others have been described. However, *USP6* fusion genes have not been found in secondary ABC.

DIFFERENTIAL DIAGNOSIS

The most important differential is telangiectatic osteosarcoma because this may have overlapping clinical and radiologic features. Histologically, telangiectatic osteosarcoma and ABC share an almost identical low-power appearance. However, on higher magnification, the tumor cells within the septae of telangiectatic osteosarcoma show marked cytologic atypia, whereas in ABC they are bland and devoid of anaplastic features. Because ABC may contain numerous giant cells, differentiation from giant cell tumor may be difficult. Reactive new bone formation is not a common finding in giant cell tumor, and the component giant cells are usually, although not exclusively, bigger with more centrally located nuclei. In addition, ABC has a more consistently fibrous stroma. Differentiation between the secondary lesions may have to be made from clinical and radiologic features in some instances, for example, skeletally mature patients with lesions at the end of bone.

Extensive sampling to exclude a background lesion is important, particularly when ABC occurs in unusual locations. Occasionally, the ABC will predominate and obscure an underlying lesion such as chondroblastoma or osteoblastoma. *Giant cell reparative granuloma* shares many features with ABC, in particular, the solid variant. These lesions are less expansile, lacking the blown-out appearance radiographically, and large blood-filled spaces are not present. Lesions located in the small bones and acral bones are the most challenging, and

ANEURYSMAL BONE CYST—FACT SHEET

Definition
- Benign, multiloculated, blood-filled cystic lesion of bone that is locally destructive and may arise de novo (primary) or on a background of a preexisting lesion (secondary)

Incidence and Location
- 2% of primary bone tumors
- Annual incidence of 0.14 per 10^5 people
- Predominantly affects metaphysis of long bones and vertebral column

Sex, Race, and Age Distribution
- Equal sex distribution
- No race predilection
- Majority (80%) of cases in skeletally immature individuals, ages 5 to 20

Clinical Features
- Most common complaints are of pain and swelling
- Symptoms of spinal cord compression in vertebral lesions

Radiologic Features
- Eccentric metaphyseal, lytic lesion with soap-bubble appearance
- Balloon distension with cortical destruction
- Periosteal eggshell of bone
- Multiloculated, often times with fluid levels on CT and MRI
- Vertebral collapse

Prognosis and Treatment
- 90% of cases have good outcome with treatment
- Recurrence common, 20% to 70%, most within 6 months, rare after 2 years
- Treated occasionally by resection, mostly by curettage and bone grafting with adjuvant preoperative embolization, cryotherapy, or both
- Radiotherapy reserved for unresectable lesions only
- Postradiation and spontaneous malignant transformation documented, but rare

ANEURYSMAL BONE CYST—PATHOLOGIC FEATURES

Gross Findings
- Red-brown soft curettage fragments (scanty)
- Well-demarcated lesion with blood-filled cystic spaces of variable size with spongy consistency (resection specimen)
- Well-defined margins with peripheral shell of bone

Microscopic Findings
- Variably sized blood-filled spaces
- Lined by thin membranous septae of loose fibrous tissue
- Admixed osteoclast-like giant cells, which may be numerous
- Reactive bony trabeculae lined by osteoblasts
- Immature osteoid arranged in a linear manner along septae
- Irregular immature chondroid with calcification
- Cellular atypia/pleomorphism/hyperchromatism not seen
- Mitosis frequent, atypical mitoses not present
- Solid areas with xanthogranulomatous appearance admixed with reactive bony trabeculae
- Areas reminiscent of giant cell reparative granuloma

Differential Diagnosis
- Telangiectatic osteosarcoma
- Giant cell tumor
- Chondroblastoma
- Osteoblastoma
- Simple bone cyst
- Giant cell reparative granuloma

differentiation may be impossible. Solitary bone cysts may be challenging, especially after fracture, when reactive changes including new bone formation and numerous osteoclast-like giant cells may be identified in the cyst lining associated with hemorrhage. A careful search will usually yield a simple bland fibrous lining with or without cementum-like material. Radiologically, simple bone cysts also do not expand the bone more than the epiphyseal plate. In contrast with ABC, at surgery, they contain serous or serosanguineous fluid.

PROGNOSIS AND TREATMENT

Despite their rapid evolution and destructive behavior, the overall prognosis is good, with 90% having cosmetic and functional resolution. Most lesions require intervention, some urgently, particularly those in the spine. Complete excision is the most effective treatment, although this is reserved for *expendable* bones, for example, the fibula and ribs. Curettage and bone grafting is associated with a recurrence rate of 20% to 70%, usually within 2 years and the majority within 6 months, with a suggestion that recurrence is most common in the very young. Adjuvant treatment including preoperative embolization, sclerotherapy, and cryotherapy are sometimes used. Sclerotherapy alone and low-dose radiotherapy are effective; however, the latter in particular is reserved for those cases for whom surgical intervention is risky, because of the risk for postradiation sarcoma, a rare but documented event. Occasional cases of spontaneous malignant transformation have also been documented. The treatment of secondary ABC is guided by the nature of the primary lesion.

SIMPLE (UNICAMERAL/SOLITARY) BONE CYST

Simple bone cyst represents a central, intramedullary unilocular cystic cavity filled with serous or serosanguineous fluid and lined by a thin fibrovascular connective tissue membrane. It characteristically occurs in the metaphyseal position of the major long bones, most commonly in the proximal humerus and femur, in skeletally immature patients. The pathogenesis is unknown, but it is considered likely to be reactive or developmental in nature, probably related to a disturbance in growth at the epiphyseal plate.

CLINICAL FEATURES

Simple bone cyst is identified in approximately 3% of bone lesion biopsies. It typically presents in the first two decades of life with a peak incidence between 3 and 14 years and an age range from 2 to 69. It is more common in male individuals (more than 2:1), and more than 80% of cysts affect the proximal humerus and femur. Its occurrence in the gnathic bones is well documented. In older patients, involvement of the ilium, talus, and calcaneus may occur. Involvement of other bones is rare. The majority of cysts are identified as incidental findings on radiographs. In those who are symptomatic, pain, swelling, and pathologic fracture may occur.

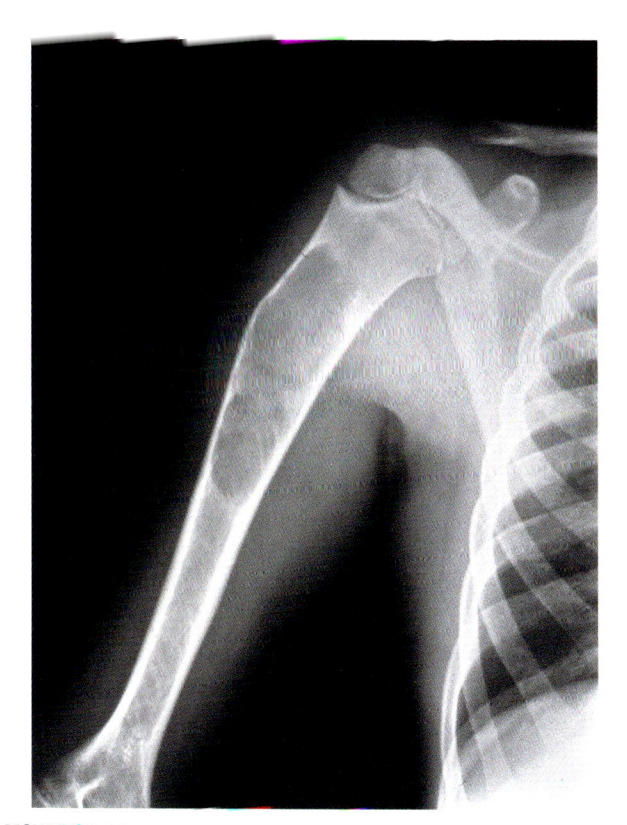

RADIOLOGIC FEATURES

Characteristically, a central intramedullary metaphyseal well-circumscribed lucency with fine trabeculation and scalloped borders is present, associated with cortical thinning, but without disruption, unless fracture has occurred (Figure 23-11). In younger patients, it abuts the epiphysis and with increasing age becomes increasingly separate from the epiphyseal plate. In contrast with ABC, it is never wider than the epiphysis. Fracture will result in cortical disruption, and in some instances, a bony fragment may be identified within the cyst lumen, so-called *fallen fragment*.

PATHOLOGIC FEATURES

GROSS FINDINGS

The majority of tumors are submitted as sparse curettage fragments representing only the thin fibrous membrane, which is usually translucent and less than 1 mm in thickness. In some instances, the cyst may be described as communicating *directly* with the medullary shaft. Those rare intact cases have a cavity filled with clear to yellowish fluid with or without internal septations and internal mural ridges (Figure 23-12). Hemorrhagic fluid may reflect prior fracture.

MICROSCOPIC FINDINGS

The lining of a simple bond cyst is often composed of a thin layer of fibrous tissue only (Figure 23-13A). Amorphous pink material in keeping with fibrin deposition in the wall is common, often forming large conglomerations that may have a concentric appearance giving them a

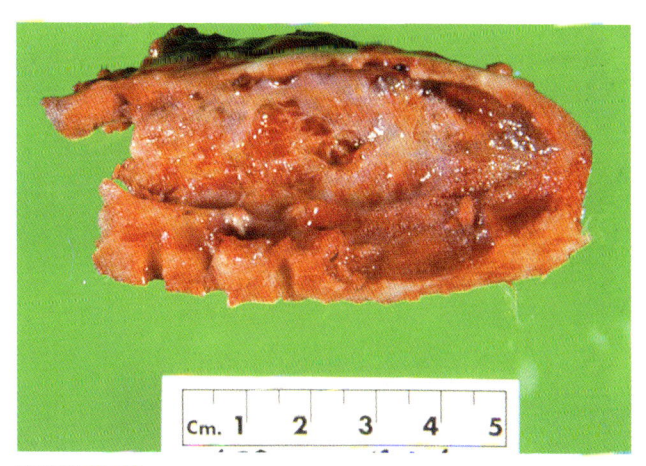

FIGURE 23-11
Radiologically, simple bone cyst is characterized by a central intramedullary metaphyseal well-circumscribed lucency with fine trabeculation and scalloped borders. The cortex is thinned. With increasing age, the lesion extends increasingly farther from the epiphyseal plate.

FIGURE 23-12
Macroscopically, this simple bone cyst is characterized by a single cystic space with cortical thinning lined by a thin fibrous membrane. *(Courtesy of Dr. Stan McCarthy, NSW Tumour Registry.)*

434　　BONE AND SOFT TISSUE PATHOLOGY

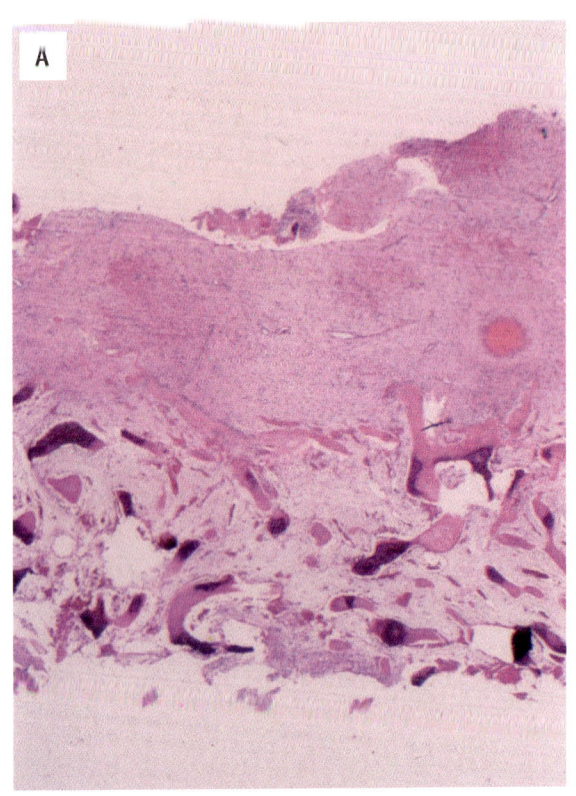

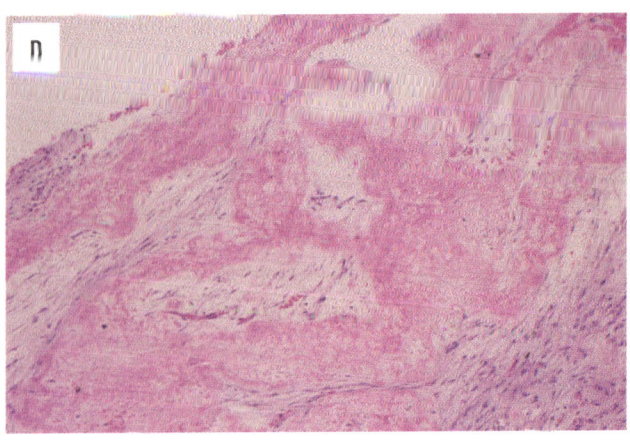

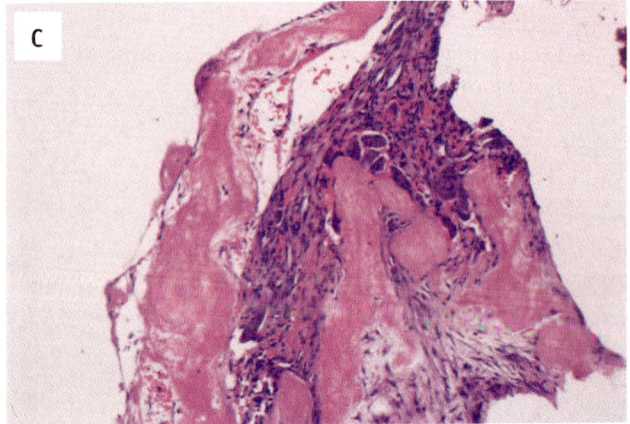

FIGURE 23-13
A, Histologically, the cyst wall of this simple bone cyst is composed of a fibrous membrane with a flat inconspicuous lining layer, bordered in this instance by bony trabeculae. **B,** In many simple bone cysts, pink *cementum*-like material probably representing fibrin can be seen, a characteristic finding. **C,** Extravasated red cells and scattered osteoclast-like giant cells can be seen, suggestive of associated fracture.

SIMPLE BONE CYST— FACT SHEET

Definition
- Central intramedullary unilocular cystic cavity containing serous or serosanguineous fluid, lined by a thin fibrous membrane

Incidence and Location
- 3% of all bone lesions for which a biopsy was performed
- Proximal metaphysis of humerus and femur most common

Sex, Race, and Age Distribution
- Greater incidence in male than female sex, 2/3:1
- Majority (80%) of cases are skeletally immature, ages 3 to 15
- No race predilection

Clinical Features
- Many cases are symptomatic
- Pain and swelling
- Pathologic fracture

Radiologic Features
- Central intramedullary metaphyseal radiolucency
- Well marginated with scalloped borders

SIMPLE BONE CYST— FACT SHEET—CONT'D

- Cortex thin, but intact
- May have "fallen fragment" sign
- Never wider than epiphyseal plate

Prognosis and Treatment
- Good
- Majority involute or respond to intralesional steroid injection
- 20% recur in patients younger than 10 years
- May require curettage and bone grafting
- Recent treatment modalities include trephination and bone marrow injections

---

cementum-like appearance (see Figure 23-13B). Ossification of these structures may occur. Scattered osteoclast giant cells may be admixed with inflammatory cells and hemosiderin-laden macrophages, especially if there has been a pathologic fracture, in which case the changes may simulate ABC, especially if internal septations are present (see Figure 23-13C). Reactive bone formation is common, especially after fracture.

CHAPTER 23 Bone Tumors of Miscellaneous Type or Uncertain Lineage

SIMPLE BONE CYST—PATHOLOGIC FEATURES

Gross Findings
- Minimal curettage material
- Thin translucent fibrous membrane
- Simple cystic structure with serous or serosanguineous fluid

Microscopic Findings
- Thin fibrous membrane
- Scattered osteoclast-like giant cells, reactive bony trabeculae, and hemosiderin-laden macrophages, particularly after fracture
- Pink cementum-like material in some

Differential Diagnosis
- ABC
- Intraosseous ganglion

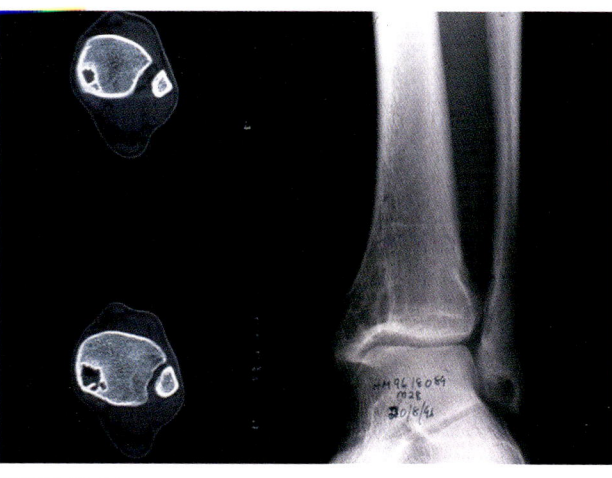

FIGURE 23-14
Radiologically, intraosseous ganglion characteristically comprises a well-defined lucency with sclerotic margins in the direct subchondral bone. This lesion is in the region of the lateral malleolus of the distal tibia. The accompanying computed tomographic scan confirms its clearly defined sclerotic edges.

DIFFERENTIAL DIAGNOSIS

The main differential diagnoses of simple bone cyst include ABC and intraosseous ganglion. In the absence of adequate clinical and radiologic data, the cystic nature of the tissue may not be appreciated and the changes in the wall misinterpreted as a preexisting lesion of fibrous dysplasia or giant cell tumor depending on the character of the mural changes. Cementum-like material is not seen in ABC. Variably sized blood-filled spaces are not expected, and giant cell accumulation with reactive osteoid is sparse; the majority of the tissue represents thin fibrous membrane. Radiologic correlation usually resolves the issue. Intraosseous ganglion is not seen in the metaphysis, usually being subchondral in location and containing mucoid viscous fluid. It may be associated with osteoarthritis. Myxoid change is common and not expected in simple bone cyst.

PROGNOSIS AND TREATMENT

Recurrence of simple bone cyst lesions is documented in up to 20% of patients, usually in children younger than 10. Aspiration of the cyst combined with intralesional injections of methylprednisolone is a highly effective treatment in most instances, although occasional cases may require combined curettage with bone grafting. Recently, success with trephination and injection of allogeneic demineralized bone matrix and autogenous bone marrow has been reported. Resection is rarely necessary. Rare cases of sarcomatous transformation of simple bone cyst have been documented.

INTRAOSSEOUS GANGLION

Intraosseous ganglia are intramedullary, non-neoplastic, subchondral cystic lesions containing mucoid fluid. They are lined by fibrous tissue with myxoid change and are not associated with osteoarthritis in the adjacent joint. They are the equivalent of soft tissue ganglia. If osteoarthritis is present, the lesion represents a degenerative subchondral cyst.

CLINICAL FEATURES

Intraosseous ganglia are common lesions (present in 10% of cadaveric wrists in a recent study), with most being incidental findings. They usually occur in skeletally mature patients, most often in late middle age, with a slight male predominance. The hip, knee, and ankle are most frequently affected, followed by the shoulder and wrist. Pain is the most frequent complaint, often related to motion. At surgery, the cyst contains gelatinous mucoid material.

RADIOLOGIC FEATURES

Characteristically, intraosseous ganglia are associated with a well-defined lucency with sclerotic margins present in subchondral bone, usually measuring less than 2 cm, rarely more than 5 cm (Figure 23-14). Some of these lesions, particularly those in the wrist, occur at the site of ligamentous insertion and are considered to be the result of degeneration of these ligaments.

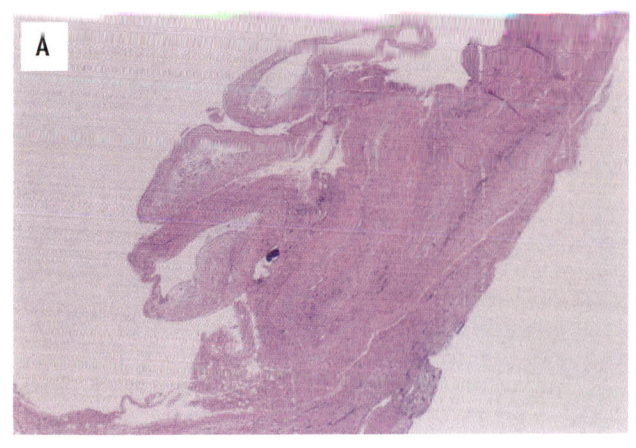

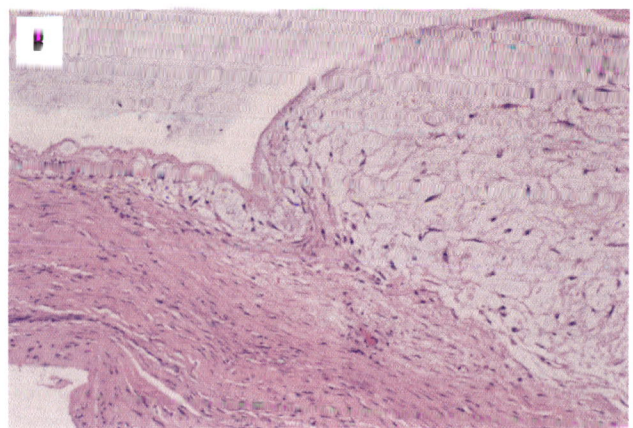

FIGURE 23-15
Intraosseous ganglion. **A**, At low power, a fibrous membrane is present within which areas of myxoid change can be seen. Fragmented bony debris may be present, related to curettage effect. **B**, At high power, the lining is flat and inconspicuous with variable myxoid change within the fibrous stroma. The lumen contains mucoid material.

INTRAOSSEOUS GANGLION—FACT SHEET

Definition
- Non-neoplastic intramedullary cyst lined by fibrous tissue with myxoid change and containing viscous mucous fluid, usually subchondral in location

Incidence and Location
- Common, usually incidental finding (10% of wrists)
- Hip, knee, ankle, shoulder, and wrist most often affected

Sex, Age, and Race Distribution
- Slight male sex predominance
- Skeletally mature, late middle age
- No racial predominance

Clinical Features
- Often asymptomatic
- Pain often aggravated by standing or exercise

Radiologic Features
- Small, well-demarcated, subchondral lucency with surrounding sclerosis
- Often related to ligamentous insertions, in wrist in particular

Prognosis and Treatment
- Curettage with or without bone graft
- Rarely recurs

INTRAOSSEOUS GANGLION—PATHOLOGIC FEATURES

Gross Findings
- Mucoid viscous contents
- Fibrous lining with mucoid areas

Microscopic Findings
- Fibrous wall with myxoid change
- Scattered admixed inflammatory cells

Differential Diagnosis
- Chondromyxoid fibroma
- Simple bone cyst

PATHOLOGIC FEATURES

GROSS FINDINGS

The curetted material of intraosseous ganglion is sparse. The cyst contains glairy viscous mucoid material, and small fragments of thin fibrous wall may be included.

MICROSCOPIC FINDINGS

The wall of intraosseous ganglion is fibrous with myxoid change and stellate fibroblasts. An admixed, mild, nonspecific chronic inflammatory infiltrate including foamy macrophages may or may not be present. The appearances are similar to those of soft tissue ganglia (Figure 23-15).

DIFFERENTIAL DIAGNOSIS

Without knowledge of the clinical or radiologic features, the possibility of chondromyxoid fibroma may be considered; however, a lobulated pattern is not present, and admixed cellular areas with giant cells are not found. In the presence of adjacent osteoarthritis, the lesion represents a subchondral cyst. Myxoid change is rare in simple bone cyst, cementum-like material may be present, and the clinical and radiologic features, in particular the location, will help differentiate these lesions.

Prognosis and Treatment

Recurrence is rare in the absence of osteoarthritis. Curettage and bone grafting, if necessary, is usually curative and can be repeated in the rare event of recurrence.

LANGERHANS CELL HISTIOCYTOSIS

Langerhans cell histiocytosis (LCH) is an encompassing term for a spectrum of clinical syndromes characterized by a proliferation of Langerhans histiocytes. It includes the group of disorders previously known as histiocytosis X, including eosinophilic granuloma, *Hand–Schüller–Christian* disease, and *Letterer–Siwe* disease. Langerhans cells are antigen-presenting peripheral dendritic cells derived from CD34-positive stem cells in bone marrow. They express major histocompatibility complex class II, bear Fc and C3 receptors, consistently express CD1A, and contain Birbeck granules ultrastructurally. They have poorly developed phagocytic properties. The disorder is classified clinically according to the extent of involvement. The localized, nonsystemic form includes those with single organ involvement, either skeletal (eosinophilic granuloma) or extraskeletal (lymph node, skin, lung), in all of which Langerhans cells normally reside. Multifocal or systemic forms reflect involvement of multiple bones, organs, or both, the severity of involvement reflecting outcome. Multifocal involvement is characteristic of the clinical entities in childhood, previously known as Hand–Schüller–Christian disease and Letterer–Siwe disease.

Clinical Features

The localized form of LCH accounts for most cases and usually occurs in the first three decades of life, mostly between the ages of 5 and 15 years. In the systemic form, patients are typically younger than 5, the most severe cases occurring before the age of 2. A male sex predominance exists, with a male-to-female ratio of at least 2:1, except in pulmonary disease where female smokers prevail. The commonest skeletal sites of involvement are the craniofacial bones, mandible and ribs (in adults in particular), pelvis, diaphyseal and metaphyseal locations in long bones, especially the femur, and vertebral bodies. Involvement of the small bones of the hands and feet is rare. Presenting symptoms typically are pain, swelling, and tenderness. An associated mass is rare. Back pain, stiffness, and scoliosis may occur with vertebral involvement and mastoiditis, and otitis media–like symptoms may be seen with skull involvement. Loosening of the teeth may occur in mandibular lesions. In systemic LCH, the clinical presentation varies depending on the severity and extent of disease. Skeletal lesions are frequent, and in Hand–Schüller–Christian disease, these are associated with diabetes insipidus, exophthalmos, and proptosis. In Letterer–Siwe disease, skin rashes, hepatosplenomegaly, fever, and multiple organ failure occurs. Peripheral eosinophilia is rare.

Radiologic Features

Radiologic features of LCH are variable but generally reflect a geographic lytic process in the medulla. In the skull, lesions are usually round or ovoid with well-defined, nonsclerotic margins, often with a beveled edge because of the uneven lysis of the outer and inner tables (Figure 23-16A). Variations in tumor margin and periosteal reaction occurs, some having ill-defined margins with laminated periosteal reaction and some being well-defined with sclerosis and a solid continuous periosteal reaction (see Figure 23-16B). The lesions generally measure between 1 and 2 cm, but may become large, particularly in the long bones, up to 6 cm. Soft tissue involvement is well documented, and occasionally the lesions have a cortical location, most often in the long bones. Lysis in the mandible may result in "floating teeth" (see Figure 23-16C). Involvement of the vertebral body may result in vertebra plana. The radiologic differential diagnosis includes chronic osteomyelitis and Ewing sarcoma in particular.

Pathologic Features

Gross Findings

Most LCH lesions are curetted, yielding small fragments of tan–gray tissue with or without yellow areas and hemorrhage depending on the proportions of component cells. The tissue often has a soft, *runny* consistency. Occasionally, these lesions are excised in toto in expendable bones. They are usually well circumscribed and vary in color from gray to yellow to red. Cortical destruction is common, and soft tissue extension may be seen.

Microscopic Findings

The pathognomonic cell is the Langerhans cell, which is present in variable distribution and numbers, lying in a background rich in other inflammatory cells. The Langerhans cells may be largely obscured by the inflammatory component or they may be present in large sheets. They usually have abundant lightly

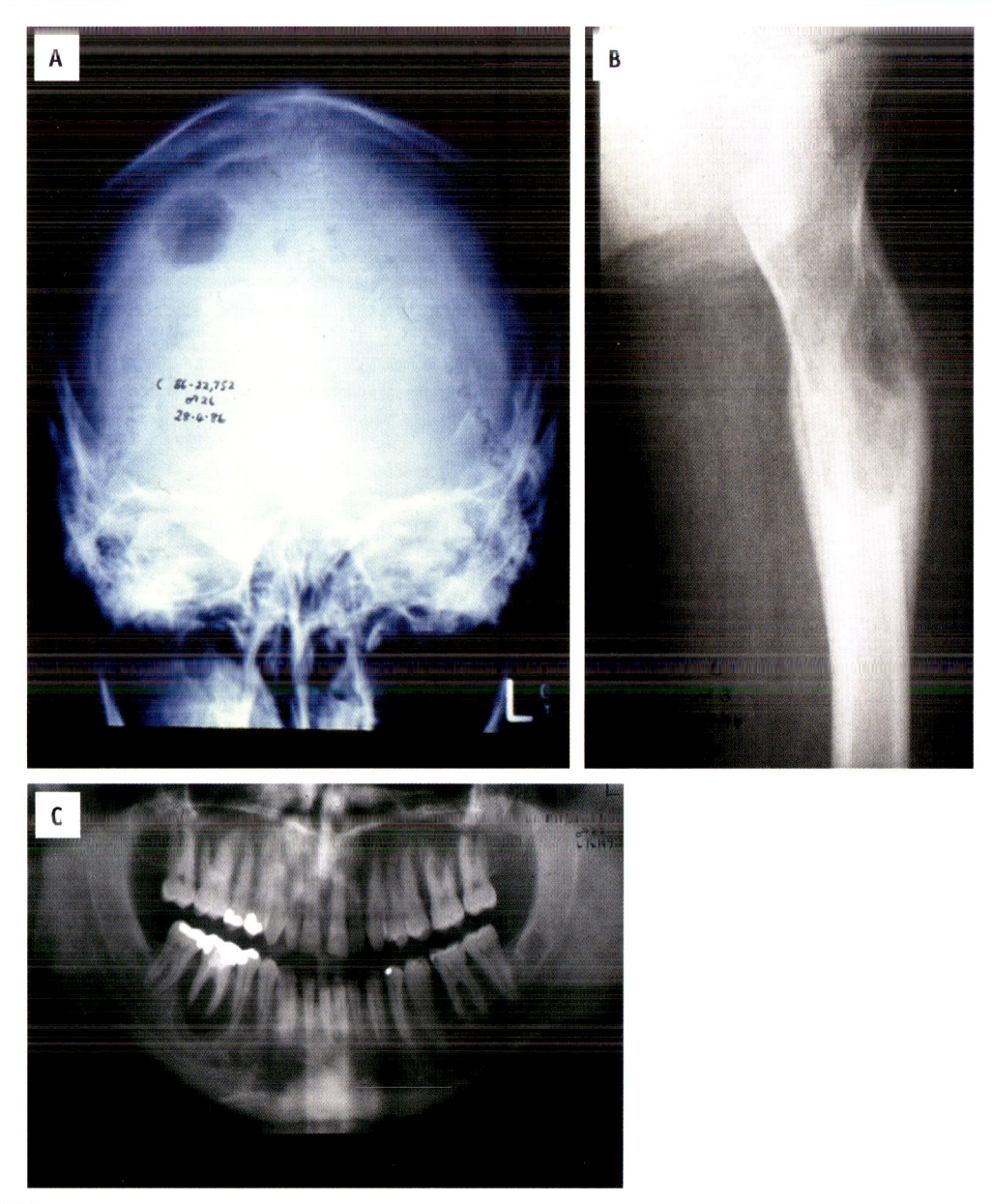

FIGURE 23-16

A, The lesions of Langerhans cell histiocytosis are usually round to ovoid lucencies with well-defined, nonsclerotic margins. In the skull, they characteristically have a beveled edge. **B,** In the long bones, in particular, the tumor margin may be ill defined and variable periosteal reaction may be present, in this instance, having a somewhat immature lamellated appearance. **C,** In the mandible, the lesion is lytic and well defined. Loosening of teeth is frequent. *(A, Courtesy of Dr. Stan McCarthy, NSW Tumour Registry.)*

eosinophilic, somewhat powdery vacuolated cytoplasm that can be well or poorly demarcated. Nuclei characteristically are vesicular in nature with dispersed chromatin nuclear indentations often giving them a reniform or *coffee-bean* shape. Multinucleated forms are frequent, exhibiting similar nuclear features (Figure 23-17A-F). Some variation in shape and size is common; however, significant pleomorphism is not a feature, and mitoses, which usually number less than 5 per 10 high power fields, are never atypical. Scattered admixed osteoclast-like giant cells may also be present. The inflammatory component often includes abundant eosinophils, at times forming small eosinophilic abscesses with necrosis. Admixed histiocytes with round or ovoid nuclei and phagocytosed cellular debris are frequent, as are foamy histiocytes, lymphocytes, plasma cells, and neutrophils. In some instances, eosinophils may be inconspicuous, mimicking osteomyelitis. Extension of the accompanying inflammatory infiltrate between and around the bony trabeculae may be present, simulating osteomyelitis (see Figure 23-17F).

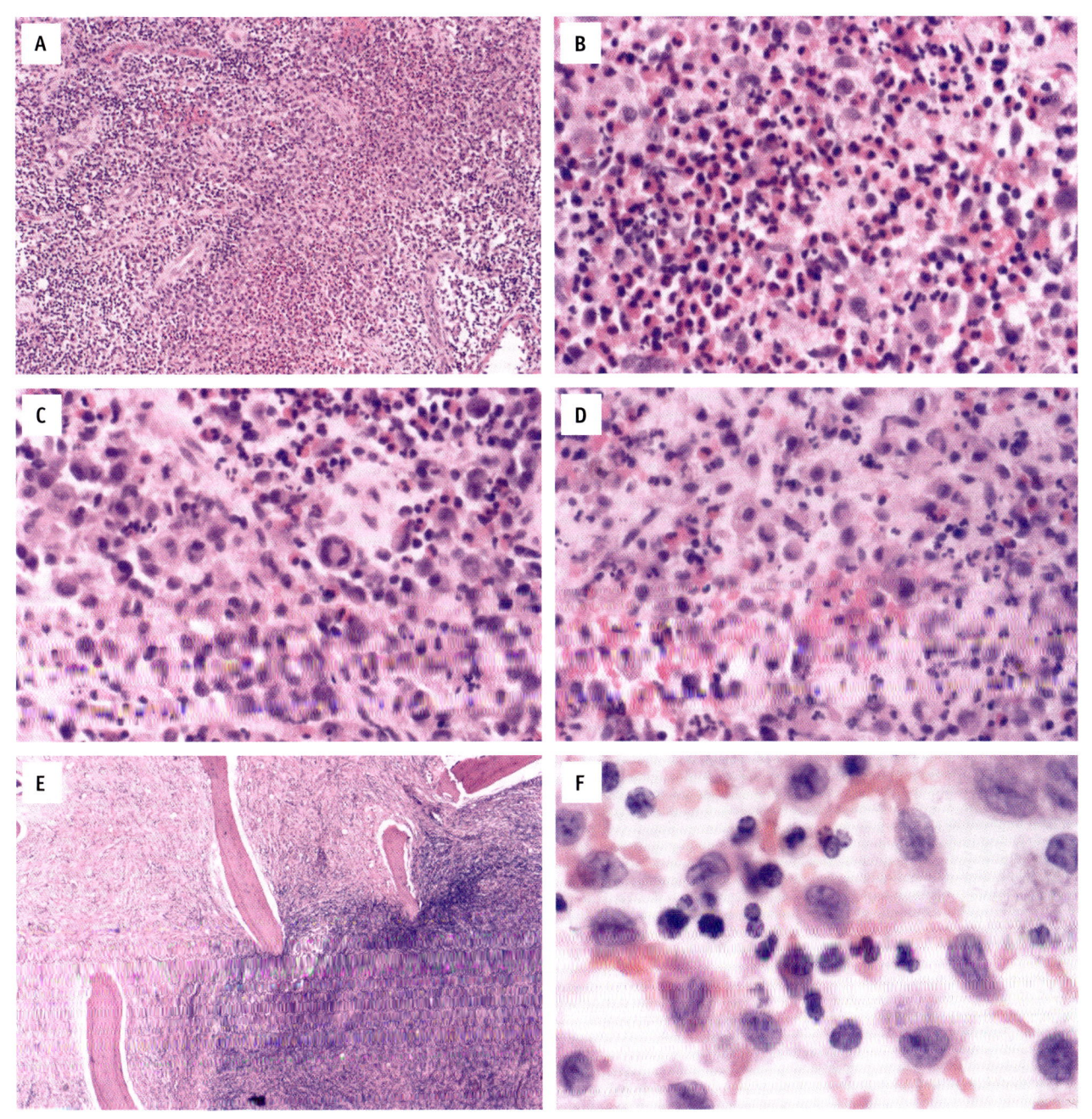

CHAPTER 23 Bone Tumors of Miscellaneous Type or Uncertain Lineage

FIGURE 23-17
Langerhans cell histiocytosis.
A, At low power, an intense inflammatory cell infiltrate is usually lying within loose granulation tissue. Abundant eosinophils are present. **B,** Eosinophils may obscure the Langerhans cells present in the background. **C,** At high power, the Langerhans cells have irregular, indented nuclei with somewhat poorly demarcated eosinophilic cytoplasm. A single binucleated form and admixed eosinophils and neutrophils are present. **D,** Langerhans cells have abundant lightly eosinophilic powdery and lightly vacuolated cytoplasm. **E,** At the margins of the more cellular area, organizing fibrosis with admixed inflammatory cells is seen extending between and around the adjacent trabeculae. **F,** Wet fixed smears confirm the presence of numerous irregular nuclear indentations (hematoxylin and eosin).

ANCILLARY STUDIES

IMMUNOHISTOCHEMISTRY

Langerhans cells are characteristically decorated by S-100 protein. However, CD1a and Langerin (CD207) are more specific markers of Langerhans cells (Figure 23-18). CD68 and peanut agglutinin positivity may also be identified. CD45 is not demonstrable in paraffin-embedded tissue. CD15, CD30, epithelial membrane antigen, and cytokeratin are negative, enabling distinction from Hodgkin disease and epithelial neoplasms.

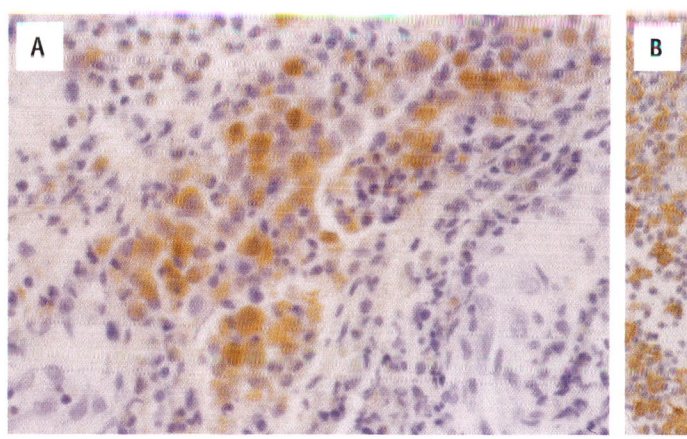

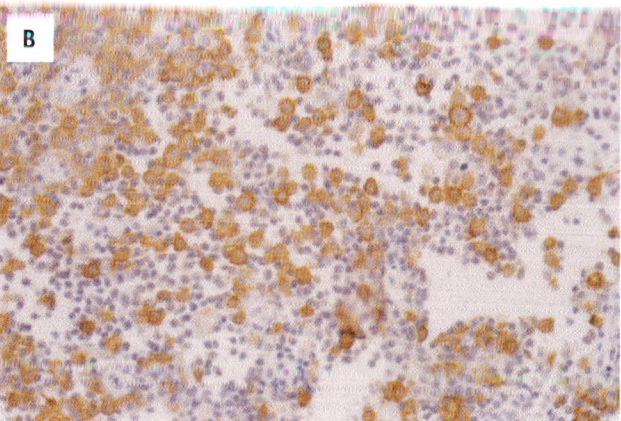

FIGURE 23-18
A, The Langerhans cells are positive for S-100 protein. **B,** CD1a positivity is characteristic of Langerhans cells.

LANGERHANS CELL HISTIOCYTOSIS—FACT SHEET

Definition
- Group of disorders of unknown cause characterized by a proliferation of Langerhans cells, the distribution of which may be localized or disseminated

Incidence and Location
- Rare, incidence from 3 to 4 per million
- Less than 1% of all bone tumors
- Craniofacial bones affected predominantly, lesser numbers in long bones, ribs, pelvis, and vertebral body

Morbidity and Mortality
- Localized form usually benign, self-limited
- High mortality in disseminated form, mostly in children younger than 2 years

Sex, Race, and Age Distribution
- Male sex predominance (more than 2:1)
- No definite racial predilection
- Majority present in the first three decades of life
  - Localized form aged 5 to 15
  - Severe systemic disease aged 0 to 2
  - Multifocal form aged 2 to 10

Clinical Features
- Depends on clinical extent and location of disease
- Localized skeletal forms
  - Pain and tenderness common
  - Swelling less frequent
- Disseminated forms
  - Diabetes insipidus
  - Exophthalmos/proptosis
  - Skin rashes
  - Hepatosplenomegaly
  - Marrow dysfunction

Radiologic Features
- Usually intraosseous, lytic, well-defined lesion 1 to 2 cm
- Often beveled margins in skull
- Often associated cortical destruction
- Possible soft tissue mass

LANGERHANS CELL HISTIOCYTOSIS—FACT SHEET—CONT'D
- Possible button sequestrum
- Possible mature or immature periosteal reaction

Prognosis and Treatment
- Dependent on site and extent of lesion
- Localized bone lesions
  - May resolve spontaneously
  - Usually cured by simple curettage or intralesional steroids
- Multifocal systemic disease has guarded prognosis
  - Poor prognostic factors
    - Hepatosplenomegaly
    - Anaemia
    - Thrombocytopenia
    - Polyostotic disease
    - Age younger than 3 at diagnosis
    - Multiagent chemotherapy has some success

GENETIC STUDIES

In recent years it has emerged that LCH represents a clonal expansion of Langerhans cells detected with HUMARA assay. Recurrent abnormalities of chromosomal loci 9p and 22q have been found, and recently, frequent loss of chromosomes in the region of 1p in particular has been identified. These findings have led to the suggestion that LCH represents a neoplasm rather than a reactive lesion; however, reactive abnormalities may exhibit chromosomal abnormalities, and thus far, the exact nature of LCH is unresolved.

DIFFERENTIAL DIAGNOSIS

The main alternative diagnoses of LCH to be considered are osteomyelitis, granulomatous inflammation, Hodgkin lymphoma and non-Hodgkin lymphoma,

> **LANGERHANS CELL HISTIOCYTOSIS—PATHOLOGIC FEATURES**
>
> **Gross Findings**
> - Variable color tan, gray, yellow, or hemorrhagic
> - Variable consistency, runny or firm
> - May have soft tissue extension
>
> **Microscopic Findings**
> - Cells with abundant, lightly eosinophilic, powdery, vacuolated cytoplasm that may or may not be well demarcated
> - Vesicular nuclei with well-defined nuclear borders and prominent indentations; *coffee-bean*, reniform appearance
> - Binucleated, trinucleated, and multinucleated forms common
> - Background mixed inflammatory infiltrate
>   - Usually including abundant eosinophils
>   - Lymphocytes, plasma cells, and neutrophils in variable quantities
>   - Phagocytic and foamy macrophages
>   - Scattered osteoclast-like giant cells
>   - Scattered mitoses, never atypical
>   - Variably fibrous background
>
> **Immunohistochemical Findings**
> - S-100 protein positive
> - CD1a positive
> - Langerin positive
> - Often CD68 positive
> - Negative CD45, AE1/3, CD15 and CD30
>
> **Differential Diagnosis**
> - Osteomyelitis
> - Granulomatous inflammation
> - Hodgkin lymphoma
> - Non-Hodgkin lymphoma
> - Rosai–Dorfman disease
> - Erdheim–Chester disease
> - Fibrohistiocytic lesions of bone, for example, nonossifying fibroma

Rosai–Dorfman disease, Erdheim–Chester disease, and in resolving cases, fibrohistiocytic proliferations of bones, particularly nonossifying fibroma. Osteomyelitis is characterized by a mixed inflammatory infiltrate; however, eosinophils are usually not prominent, and Langerhans cell proliferation is not found. Radiologic overlap may occur, particularly in the long bones. Granulomatous inflammatory processes may cause confusion, although caseating granulomata are not a feature of LCH, and clusters of S-100 protein and CD1a-positive cells would not be expected. Although the presence of eosinophils and binucleate and trinucleate Langerhans cells may mimic Reed–Sternberg cells, nuclear indentation would not be expected and they usually have large prominent eosinophilic nucleoli, not seen in Langerhans cells. In addition, Reed–Sternberg cells are negative for CD1a, Langerin, and S-100 protein, and are decorated by CD15 and CD30. In Rosai–Dorfman disease, the histiocytes have round, ovoid, non-indented nuclei and emperipolesis is evident. They express S-100 protein but are CD1a negative. In Chester–Erdheim disease, a xanthogranulomatous inflammatory infiltrate predominates, and S-100 protein and CD1a are not expressed. In the resolving phase of LCH, stromal fibrosis with admixed foamy histiocytes and lymphocytes may simulate benign fibrohistiocytic lesions of bone, in particular, nonossifying fibroma. A careful search for Langerhans cells with S-100 protein and CD1a will usually resolve the issue. Radiologically, these lesions are usually distinctive.

PROGNOSIS AND TREATMENT

In general, the outcome of LCH is related to the degree of involvement of various organ systems at the time of diagnosis. Those with localized disease often spontaneously resolve and are usually cured by simple curettage or intralesional steroid injection. Low-dose radiotherapy is less frequently used. Recurrences are rare, although an occasional individual does go on to acquire further lesions. In general, adults with more than three osseous lesions are apt to have visceral involvement; however, death caused by disease is rare in this age group. Progressive disease tends to occur in the first 2 years of life predominantly, the outcome reflecting the extent of multiorgan involvement. Multiagent chemotherapy gives a high rate of initial response (70–87%); however, a third of patients with disseminated disease die.

ERDHEIM–CHESTER DISEASE

Erdheim–Chester disease is a rare, distinctive, disseminated, infiltrative disorder of histiocytes of unknown cause. It is characterized by intraosseous and systemic xanthogranulomatous change and has distinct radiologic features.

CLINICAL FEATURES

Erdheim–Chester disease has a slight male predominance with age range from 7 to 84 years. The majority of cases presenting in the fifth, sixth, and seventh decades of life. Symptoms depend on the extent of disease, but bone pain is the commonest complaint, usually affecting the lower limbs in particular. Because extraosseous deposition can occur at many sites and in many organs, the symptomology is protean. Orbital

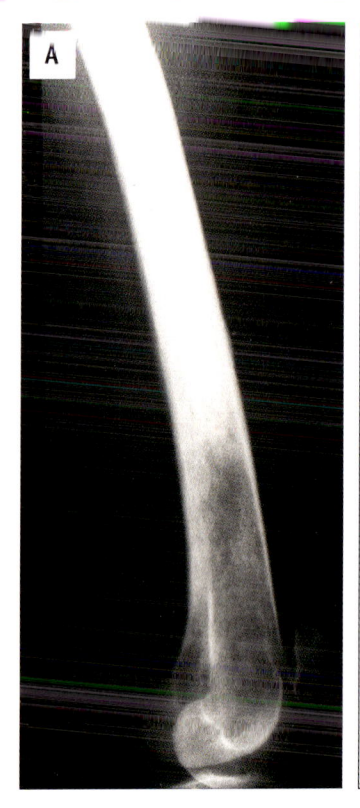

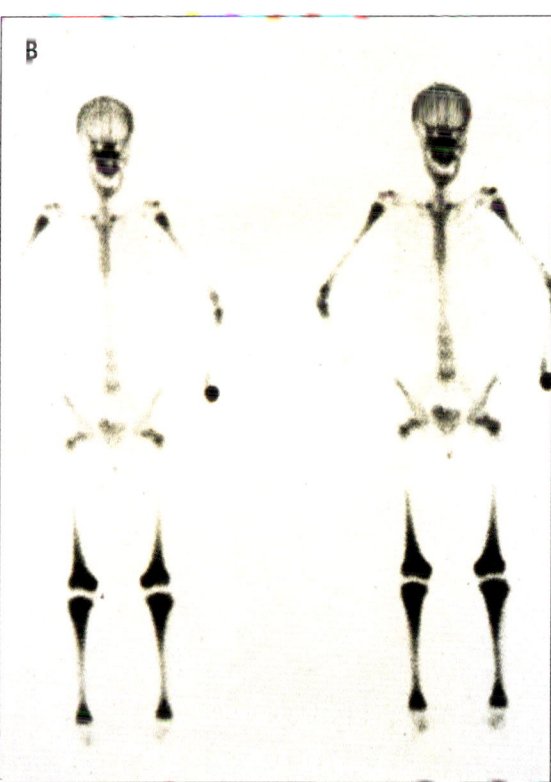

FIGURE 23-19

Erdheim-Chester disease.
A, Prominent osteosclerosis of the diaphysis of the femur extends into the metaphysis. Characteristically, this is bilateral and symmetrical. **B,** The bone scan shows marked increased uptake in the metaphyseal regions of the distal femur, and proximal and distal tibiae in a bilateral symmetrical distribution. *(Courtesy of Dr. Stan McCarthy, NSW Tumour Registry.)*

deposits produce proptosis and exophthalmos; pituitary deposits cause pituitary dysfunction, for example, diabetes insipidus; cerebral and cerebellar deposits elicit a multiple sclerosis–like syndrome; myocardial and pericardial deposits lead to cardiac failure; and pulmonary deposits cause advanced interstitial lung disease. Soft tissue masses have also been described in the retroperitoneum causing urinary obstruction. In the skeleton, involvement of the bone marrow is characteristically seen in the appendicular long bones bilaterally, most specifically in the metaphysis of the femur and tibia.

Radiologic Features

Typical findings of Erdheim–Chester disease are those of bilateral symmetrical osteosclerosis of the metaphysis and diaphysis of the appendicular skeleton, particularly involving the lower limbs, specifically the distal femur and proximal tibia and fibula. The epiphyses are usually spared (Figure 23-19). Osteolytic lesions have been described in the skull and ribs, and occasionally the lesions in the long bones may have a mixed lytic and sclerotic character.

Pathologic Features

Gross Findings

Macroscopically, biopsy fragments comprise tan-brown tissue with yellow areas corresponding to xanthogranulomatous change.

Microscopic Findings

Histologically, the osseous lesions in Erdheim–Chester disease contain numerous foamy histiocytes admixed with multinucleated giant cells, many of which represent Touton giant cells, lying in a variably fibrous stroma with admixed chronic inflammatory cells, including lymphocytes, histiocytes, and plasma cells (Figure 23-20). The accompanying bone is thickened woven and lamellar bone that may have a pagetoid appearance.

Ancillary Studies

Immunohistochemistry

The histiocytes in Erdheim–Chester disease are CD68- and CD163- positive, in keeping with their

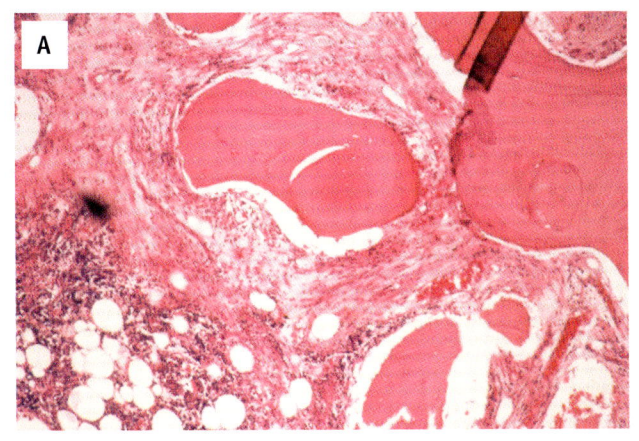

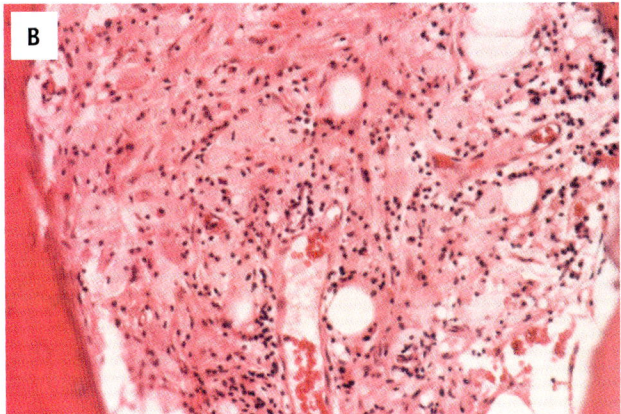

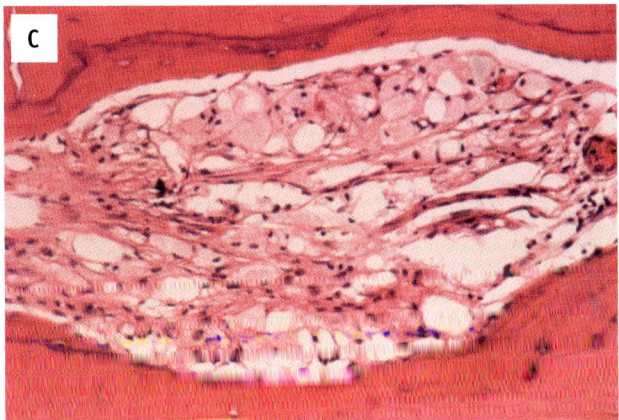

CHAPTER 23 Bone Tumors of Miscellaneous Type or Uncertain Lineage 443

FIGURE 23-20
Erdheim-Chester disease.
A, At medium power, thick sclerotic bony trabeculae lie within marrow in which there is extensive fibrovascular stroma. **B**, At higher power, a mixed inflammatory infiltrate comprising lymphocytes, plasma cells, and numerous foamy histiocytes is present. **C**, Abundant foamy histiocytes lie between the sclerotic bony trabeculae. *(Courtesy of Dr. Sian McCarthy, NSW Tumour Registry.)*

ERDHEIM–CHESTER DISEASE—FACT SHEET

Definition
- A rare, disseminated, xanthogranulomatous, infiltrative disease of unknown cause that affects many organs including bone and exhibits characteristic radiologic features

Incidence and Location
- Extremely rare, less than 100 cases documented in the literature
- Most often affects the distal femur, proximal tibia, and fibula bilaterally

Sex, Race, and Age Distribution
- Slight male sex predominance
- Ages 7 to 84, majority in fifth, sixth, and seventh decades of life
- Racial distribution unknown

Clinical Features
- Depends on extent and severity of involvement
- Bone pain for months or years, usually in the lower limb

Systemic Effects
- Exophthalmos, diabetes insipidus, general symptoms including fever, weight loss, xanthomas, cerebral symptoms, cardiac failure, pulmonary fibrosis

Radiologic Features
- Bilateral symmetrical metadiaphyseal sclerosis

ERDHEIM–CHESTER DISEASE—FACT SHEET—CONT'D

- Predominantly affecting long bones in particular distal femur, proximal tibia, and fibula
- Epiphyseal sparing
- Occasional lytic lesions in skull and ribs

Prognosis and Treatment
- Depends on extent of systemic involvement
- Majority have a prolonged indolent course
- Approximately one third die within 10 years from various systemic effects
- No distinctive useful treatment, although chemotherapy and corticosteroids are most often used

---

monocyte/macrophage lineage. CD1a is consistently negative, and S-100 protein is usually negative (a single case with S-100 positivity has been reported).

GENETIC STUDIES

Recent cytogenetic and HUMARA-based studies of a few cases have shown clonal abnormalities, thus supporting the idea that Erdheim–Chester disease is a neoplastic disorder rather than a reactive process.

ERDHEIM–CHESTER DISEASE—PATHOLOGIC FEATURES

Gross Findings
- Tan tissue with yellow areas representing xanthogranulomatous change

Microscopic Findings
- Xanthogranulomatous change, numerous vacuolated foamy histiocytes with round oval nuclei without nuclear grooves, admixed with multinucleated giant cells often of Touton type
- Variably fibrous stroma with admixed lymphocytes, plasma cells, and histiocytes
- Thickened bony trabeculae with remodeling representing sclerosis

Immunohistochemical Findings
- CD68 and CD163 positive
- S-100 negative
- CD1a negative

Differential Diagnosis
- Chronic osteomyelitis
- LCH
- Rosai–Dorfman disease/sinus histiocytosis with massive lymphadenopathy

DIFFERENTIAL DIAGNOSIS

Erdheim–Chester disease must be distinguished particularly from chronic inflammatory processes and other histiocytic disorders. LCH is characterized by histiocytes with indented grooved nuclei and eosinophilic cytoplasm rather than foamy histiocytes seen in Erdheim–Chester disease. In *Rosai–Dorfman* disease (sinus histiocytosis with massive lymphadenopathy), the component histiocytes exhibit emperipolesis, and are also positive for S-100 protein. In addition, both LCH and Rosai–Dorfman disease are lytic radiologically and sclerotic bone would not be expected. In Gaucher disease, the histiocytes have a characteristic tissue-paper appearance and are Periodic Acid Schiff positive. Chronic osteomyelitis is the main differential diagnosis, and clear distinction depends on the constellation of clinical, microbiologic, histologic, and radiologic data.

PROGNOSIS AND TREATMENT

Although many cases of Erdheim–Chester disease have a prolonged indolent course, the outcome is dependent on the extent of systemic involvement and, in a recent review, more than a third of patients died after a mean follow-up of 3 years with a range from 3 months to 10 years. Clinical trials for efficacy of treatment regimens have not been conducted, and treatment is based on anecdotal experience. It has included steroids, chemotherapy, radiation therapy, immunotherapy, and no therapy, all with variable success.

SUGGESTED READINGS

Fibrous Dysplasia

1. Dorfman HD, Czerniak B: Bone Tumors. St. Louis, Mosby, 1998, pp 441–481.
2. Ippolito E, Bray EW, Corsi A, et al: Natural history and treatment of fibrous dysplasia of bone: a multicentric clinicopathological study promoted by the European Paediatric Orthopaedic Society. J Paediatr Orthop B 2003;12:155–177.
3. Lumbroso S, Paris F, Sultan C: McCune Albright syndrome: molecular genetics. J Paediatr Endocrinol Metab 2002;15:875–882.
4. Marie PJ: Cellular and molecular basis of fibrous dysplasia: review. Histol Histopathol 2001;16:981–988.
5. Matsuba A, Ogose A, Tokunaga K, et al: Activating Gs alpha mutation at the ARG 201 codon in liposclerosing myxofibrous tumor. Hum Pathol 2003;34:1204–1209.
6. Riminucci M, Liu B, Corsi A, et al: Histopathology of fibrous dysplasia of bone in patients with activating mutations of the Gs alpha gene: sites-specific patterns and recurrent histological hallmarks. J Pathol 1999;187:249–258.
7. Ruggieri P, Sim FH, Bond RJ, et al: Malignancies in fibrous dysplasia. Cancer 1994;73:1411–1424.
8. Shidham VB, Chavan A, Rao RN, et al: Fatty metamorphosis and other patterns of fibrous dysplasia. BMC Musculoskel Disord 2003;4:20–28.

Osteofibrous Dysplasia

1. Bovee JV, van den Broek LJ, de Boer WI, et al: Expression of growth factors and their receptors in adamantinoma of long bones and the implications for its histogenesis. J Pathol 1998;184:24–30.
2. Bridge JA, Dembinski A, De Boer J, et al: Clonal chromosomal abnormalities in osteofibrous dysplasia: implications for histopathogenesis and its relationship to adamantinoma. Cancer 1994;73:1746–1752.
3. Dorfman HD, Czerniak B: Bone Tumors. St. Louis, Mosby, 1998, pp 481–491.
4. Gleason BC, Leigl-Atzwanger B, Kozakewich HP, et al: Osteofibrous dysplasia and adamantinoma in children and adolescents: a clinicopathologic reappraisal. Am J Surg Pathol 2008;32:363–376.
5. Hazelbag HM, Wessels JW, Mollevangers P, et al: Cytogenetic analysis of adamantinoma of long bones: further indications for a common histogenesis with osteofibrous dysplasia. Cancer Genet Cytogenet 1997;97:5–11.
6. Khan LB: Adamantinoma, osteofibrous dysplasia and differentiated adamantinoma. Skeletal Radiol 2003;32:245–258.
7. Kuruvilla G, Steiner GC: Osteofibrous dysplasia like adamantinoma of bone: a report of five cases with immunohistochemical and ultrastructural studies. Hum Pathol 1998;29:808–814.
8. Maki M, Saitoh K, Kaneko Y, et al: Expression of cytokeratin 1, 5, 14, 19 and transforming growth factors (beta) 1, (beta) 2, (beta) 3 in osteofibrous dysplasia and adamantinoma: a possible association of transforming growth factor (beta) with basal cell phenotype promotion. Pathol Int 2000;50:801–807.
9. McCaffrey M, Letts M, Carpenter B, et al: Osteofibrous dysplasia: a review of the literature and presentation of an additional three cases. Am J Orthop 2003;32:479–486.
10. Park YK, Unni KK, McLeod RA, et al: Osteofibrous dysplasia: clinicopathological study of 80 cases. Hum Pathol 1993;24:1339–1347.
11. Sweet DE, Vinh TN, Devaney K: Cortical osteofibrous dysplasia of long bone and its relationship to adamantinoma. Am J Surg Pathol 1992;16:282–290.

Aneurysmal Bone Cyst

1. Dorfman HD, Czerniak B: Bone Tumors. St. Louis, Mosby, 1998, pp 855–879.
2. Ilaslan H, Sundaram M, Unni KK: Solid variant of aneurysmal bone cyst in long tubular bones: giant cell reparative granuloma. Am J Roentgenol 2003;180:1681–1687.

3. Kransdorf MJ, Sweet DE: aneurysmal bone cyst: concept, controversy, clinical presentation and imaging. Am J Roentgenol 1995;164:573–580.
4. Martinez V, Sissons HA: Aneurysmal bone cyst: a review of 123 cases including primary lesions and those secondary to other bone pathology. Cancer 1988;61:2291–2304.
5. Oliveira AM, Perez-Atayde AR, Dal Cin P, et al: Aneurysmal bone cyst variant translocations upregulate USP6 transcription by promoter swapping with the ZNF9, COL1A1, TRAP150, and OMD genes. Oncogene 2005;24:3419–3426.
6. Oliveira AM, Perez-Atayde AR, Inwards CY, et al: USP6 and CDH11 oncogenes identify the neoplastic cell in primary aneurysmal bone cysts and are absent in so-called secondary aneurysmal bone cysts. Am J Pathol 2004;165:1773–1780.
7. Schreuder HW, Veth RP, Pruszczynski M, et al: Aneurysmal bone cyst treated by curettage, cryotherapy and bone grafting. J Bone Joint Surg Br 1997;79:20–25.
8. Sciot R, Dorfman H, Brys P, et al: Cytogenetic-morphologic correlations in aneurysmal bone cyst, giant cell tumor of bone and combined lesions. A report from the CHAMP study group. Mod Pathol 2000;13:1206–1210.
9. Vergel De Dios AM, Bond JR, Shives TC, et al: Aneurysmal bone cyst: a clinicopathologic study of 238 cases. Cancer 1992;69:2921–2931.

Simple Bone Cyst

1. Dorfman HD, Czerniak B: Bone Tumors. St. Louis, Mosby, 1998, pp 879–891.
2. Lokiec F, Wientroub S: Simple bone cyst: aetiology, classification, pathology and treatment modalities. J Pediatr Orthop (B) 1998;7:262–273.
3. Matsumara S, Murakami S, Kakimoto N, et al: Histopathological and radiographic findings of simple bone cyst. Oral Surg Med Oral Pathol Oral Radiol Endod 1998;85:619–625.
4. Mylle J, Burssens A, Fabry G: Simple bone cyst: a review of 59 cases with special reference to their treatment. Arch Orthop Trauma Surg 1992;111:297–300.
5. Rougraff BT, Kling TJ: Treatment of active unicameral bone cyst with percutaneous injection of demineralised bone matrix and autogenuos bone marrow. J Bone Joint Surg Am 2002;84A:921–929.

Intraosseous Ganglion

1. Dorfman HD, Czerniak B: Bone Tumors. St. Louis, Mosby, 1998, 891–901.
2. Murff R, Ashry HR: Intraosseous ganglia of the foot. J Foot Ankle Surg 1994;33:396–401.
3. Schajowicz F, Clavel Sainz M, Slullitel JA: Juxta-articular bone cysts (intra-osseous ganglia): a clinicopathological study of 88 cases. J Bone Joint Surg Br 1979;61(B):107–116.
4. Schrank C, Meirer R, Stabler A, et al: Morphology and topography of intraosseous ganglion cyst in the carpus: an anatomic, histopathologic and magnetic resonance imaging correlation study. J Hand Surg [Am] 2003;28(A):52–61.

Langerhans Cell Histiocytosis

1. Dacic S, Trusky C, Bakker A, et al: Genotypic wanalysis of pulmonary Langerhan's cell histiocytosis. Hum Pathol 2003;34:1345–1349.
2. Dorfman HD, Czerniak B: Bone Tumors. St. Louis, Mosby, 1998, 689–701.
3. Kilpatrick SE, Wenger DE, Gilchrist GS, et al: Langerhans' cell histiocytosis (histiocytosis X) of bone. A clinicopathologic analysis of 263 pediatric and adult cases. Cancer 1995;76:2471–2484.
4. Kransdorf MJ, Smith SE: Lesions of unknown histogenesis: Langerhan's cell histiocytosis and Ewing's sarcoma. Semin Musculoskel Radiol 2000;4:113–125.
5. Ladisch S: Langerhan's cell histiocytosis. Curr Opin Haematol 1998;5:54–58.
6. Lau SK, Chu PG, Weiss LM: Immunohistochemical expression of Langerin in Langerhans cell histiocytosis and non-Langerhans cell histiocytic disorders. Am J Surg Pathol 2008;32:615–619.
7. Lieberman PH, Jones CR, Steinman RN, et al: Langerhans' cell (eosinophilic) granulomatosis: a clinicopathological study encompassing fifty years. Am J Surg Pathol 1996;20:519–552.
8. Murakami I, Gogusev J, Fournet JC, et al: Detection of molecular cytogenetic aberrations in Langerhan's cell histiocytosis of bone. Hum Pathol 2000;33:555–560.
9. Nezelof C, Basset F: Langerhan's cell histiocytosis research: past, present, future. Haematol Oncol Clin North Am 1998;12:385–405.

Erdheim–Chester Disease

1. Chetritt J, Paradis V, Dargere D, et al: Chester-Erdheim disease: a neoplastic disorder. Hum Pathol 1999;30:1093–1096.
2. Dickson BC, Pethe V, Chung CT, et al: Systemic Erdheim-Chester disease. Virchows Arch 2008;452:221–227.
3. Egan MAJ, Boardman LA, Tazelaar HD, et al: Erdheim-Chester disease: clinical, radiological and histopathologic findings in five patients with interstitial lung disease. Am J Surg Pathol 1999;23:17–26.
4. Kenn W, Eck M, Allolio B, et al: Erdheim-Chester disease: evidence for a disease entity different from Langerhan's cell histiocytosis? Three cases with detailed radiological and immunohistochemical analysis. Hum Pathol 2000;31:734–739.
5. Vencio EF, Jenkins RB, Schiller JL, et al: Clonal cytogenetic abnormalities in Erdheim-Chester disease. Am J Surg Pathol 2007;31:319–321.
6. Veyssier-Belot C, Cacoub P, Caparros-Lefebvre D, et al: Erdheim-Chester disease. Clinical and radiological characteristics of 59 cases. Medicine 1996;75:157–169.

24 Metastases Involving Bone

Yasuaki Nakashima

Metastatic tumor of bone is the secondary skeletal deposit of a neoplasm from another primary site and is the most common form of all malignant tumors involving bone. The metastatic lesions are multiple or, less frequently, solitary. Most of the primary malignant tumors are carcinomas. Rarely, neoplasms showing benign histology can metastasize to bone. If the histology of a primary site is known, fine-needle aspiration biopsy (cytology) or core needle biopsies of metastatic lesions may determine the diagnosis. Primary malignancies can invade bone by direct extension or through lymphatic and vascular channels including vertebral Batson plexus of veins. Bony change seen in metastatic tumors is osteolytic or, less frequently, osteoblastic or mixed. They may be modulated by the postulated effects of humoral factors or cytokines, including transforming growth factor-β (TGF-β), fibroblast growth factor, bone morphogenetic proteins, prostaglandins, interleukin-1, parathormone-related protein, among others, secreted by neoplastic cells. Activity of osteoclasts transformed from macrophages may also induce the structural change of bones affected by metastasis.

CLINICAL FEATURES

Because the incidence of primary sarcomas of bone is substantially less than that of carcinomas in other organs, metastatic carcinomas are the most common malignant tumor involving the bone, and after the lungs and liver, the skeleton is the third most frequent site of metastatic disease. According to several reports, approximately 30% to 90% of the patients with common carcinomas are estimated to have skeletal metastases in their course of the disease. As is often the case with the secondary malignancy, bone metastases tend to affect older patients, and more than 60% of patients are in their sixth to seventh decade of life. Osseous metastatic disease in children is rare and most commonly originates from neuroblastoma, clear cell sarcoma of kidney, osteosarcoma, Ewing sarcoma/primitive neuroectodermal tumor (PNET) group, and rhabdomyosarcoma. It is difficult to determine significant sex predilection.

Metastases can affect any bone containing red marrow. Nearly 70% occur in axial skeleton, including the cranium, vertebrae, rib, sternum, sacrum, and pelvis. Approximately 30% of bone metastases involve the appendicular skeleton, but rarely distal to the knee and elbow. Metastatic tumor involving the small bones of the hands and feet is rare, and usually originates from the lung or kidney.

In more than 80% of patients, a pertinent clinical search, including physical examination, laboratory studies, and radiological investigations, usually identifies the primary site. Lung, breast, prostate, kidney, and thyroid gland account for more than 80% of all skeletal metastases. Carcinomas of the kidney and thyroid gland frequently involve the skull, sternum, pelvis, bones of the shoulder girdle, and pelvic flat bones. These locations comprise more than 70% of all sites for metastatic deposits. Skeletal metastasis of sarcoma is relatively rare and more frequently seen in children. Examples of skip metastasis or even bone-to-bone metastasis of osteosarcoma are reported.

Symptoms of patients with metastatic carcinoma are generally nonspecific. Pain, with or without swelling, pathologic fracture, and neurological symptoms when the lesion affects spine are common findings. Systemic symptoms, including hypercalcemia secondary to osteolysis and Collet–Sicard syndrome in skull base metastases, may occur. Hypercalcemia and increased serum alkaline phosphatase may be seen due to extensive osteolytic activity of metastatic tumor. Prominent osteoblastic metastases of prostate carcinoma may cause osteomalacia secondary to the high calcium demand for new bone formation.

RADIOLOGIC FEATURES

Radiographically, most metastases produce osteolytic and destructive changes predominantly located in the marrow cavity (Figures 24-1 and 24-2). Osteoblastic or mixed lytic and blastic change can also occur (Figure 24-3). In the long bones, metastatic deposits tend to involve the metaphysis, and a solitary lesion can mimic a primary bone sarcoma. Metastatic renal cell

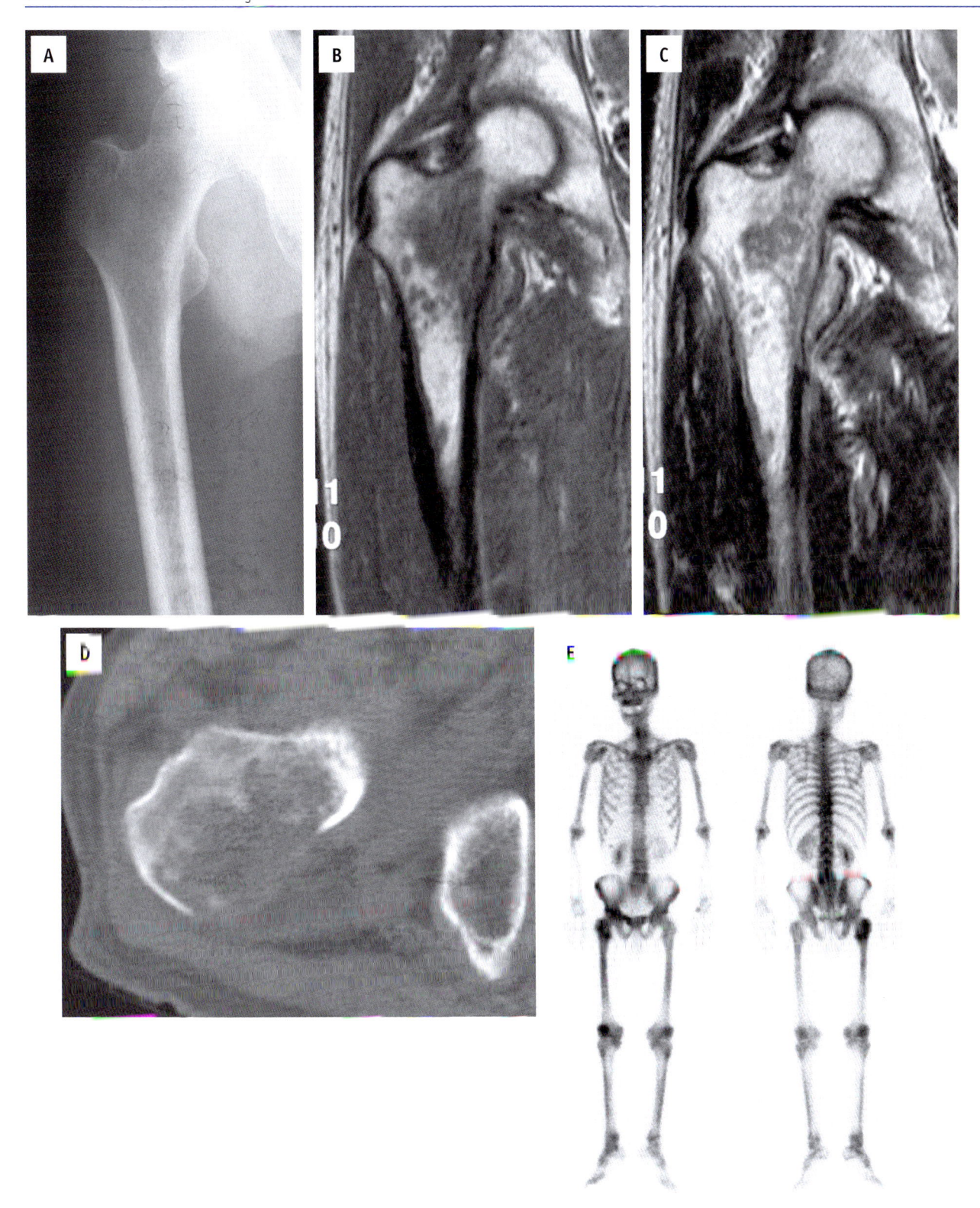

FIGURE 24-1

Metastatic carcinoma involving the proximal femur.
A, Anteroposterior view shows osteolytic lesions in the proximal femur. **B,** T1-weighted and **C,** T2-weighted coronal magnetic resonance images and **D,** an axial computed tomographic image demonstrate osteolytic and destructive lesions with ill-defined margins. **E,** Radioisotope scintigram using technetium-99m is positive in the proximal femur.

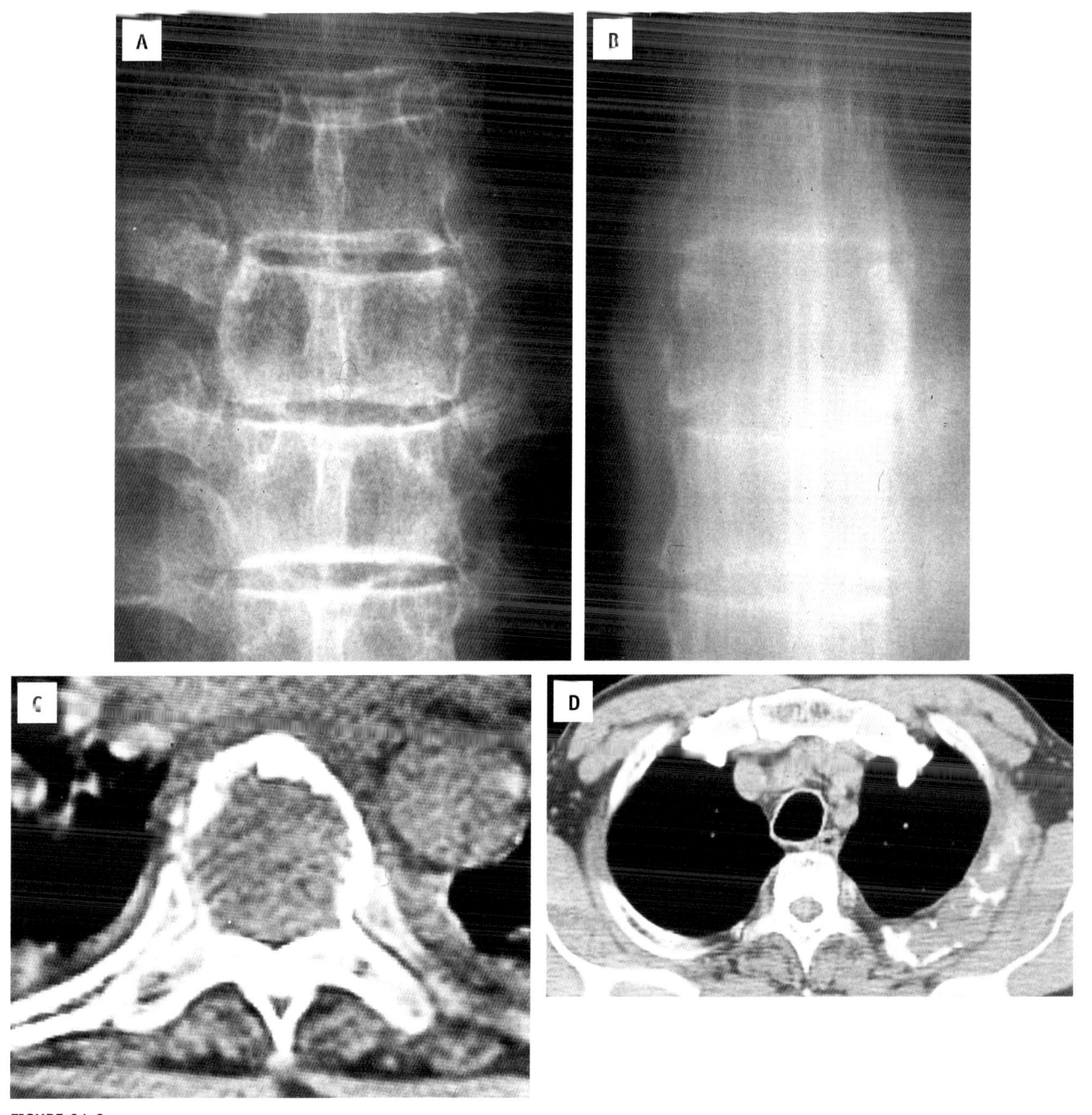

FIGURE 24-2
Metastatic renal cell carcinoma involving the spine and rib.
A, Anteroposterior view of radiograph, **B,** anteroposterior tomographic view, and **C,** an axial computed tomographic (CT) image visualize medullary osteolysis and destruction of vertebral body. **D,** An axial CT image shows osteolytic and destructive change of the rib.

carcinoma frequently produces purely lytic destruction with aneurysmal bone cyst-like change. Similar radiographic features are occasionally seen in metastases from carcinoma of the gastrointestinal tract, thyroid carcinoma, or malignant melanoma. Metastases from lung or breast can show mixed lytic and blastic change. Prostatic adenocarcinoma is one of the well-known examples frequently presenting with purely osteoblastic metastasis. When such a sclerotic metastatic lesion is solitary and associated with periosteal reaction, differentiation from a primary bone sarcoma may be difficult. Florid ossification due to pathologic fracture of a metastatic tumor may even simulate the roentgenologic features of osteosarcoma. Computed tomography (CT) scan and magnetic resonance imaging (MRI) have the advantage of detecting metastatic lesions in the vertebrae where only about a quarter of metastases are identified by conventional plain radiographs. Radioisotope scintigram bone scan of metastatic carcinoma is almost invariably positive and thus useful for detecting multiple skeletal metastases (see Figure 24-3C).

CHAPTER 24 Metastases Involving Bone

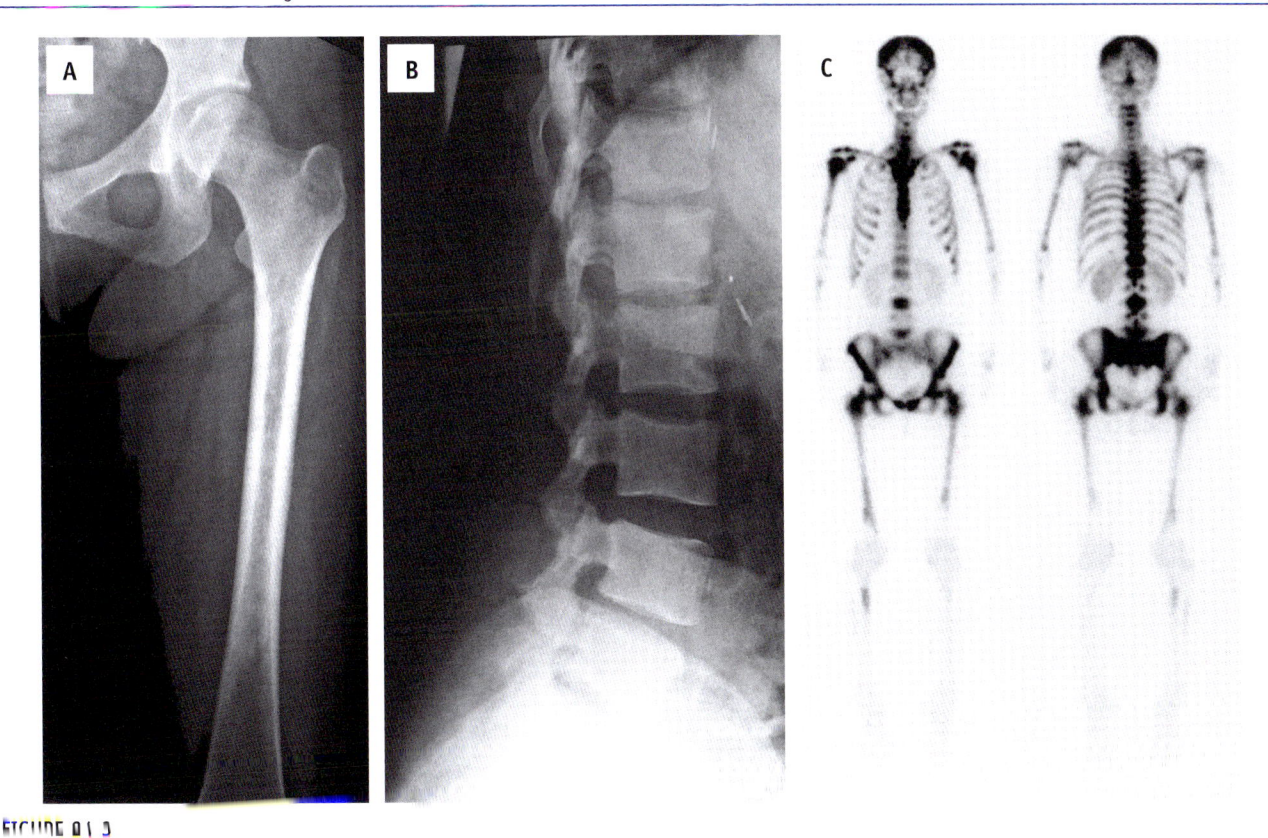

FIGURE 24-3
Multiple skeletal metastases of adenocarcinoma from the stomach
A, Anteroposterior view of the femur and **B**, lateral view of the spine show diffuse sclerotic change. **C**, Radioisotope scintigram using technetium-99m is positive in multiple bones of the axial skeleton.

PATHOLOGIC FEATURES

GROSS FINDINGS

The gross appearance of metastatic carcinoma involving bone is nonspecific and oftentimes not too dissimilar from that of primary bone sarcomas (Figure 24-4) Osteoblastic metastases can be particularly dense and hard, simulating osteosarcoma. Extraosseous extension of metastatic deposits can also produce a soft tissue mass.

MICROSCOPIC FINDINGS

Osseous metastatic carcinoma tends to resemble the histology of the primary tumor, and in most cases, its metastatic nature is histologically evident. Metastatic adenocarcinomas or squamous cell carcinomas from the most common primary sites, including the lung, breast, kidney, prostate, and thyroid gland, usually retain their inherent morphologic features and cause practically no diagnostic problems (Figure 24-5). Reactive stromal changes, including fibroblastic spindle cell proliferation, vascular proliferation, and infiltration of osteoclastic multinucleated giant cells are relatively common. In the case of poorly differentiated or undifferentiated carcinomas, it may be difficult to determine the primary site.

Sarcomatoid carcinomas, especially from the kidney, lung, or thyroid gland, sometimes lack apparent epithelial differentiation and therefore simulate primary spindle cell sarcomas of bone (Figure 24-6). Osteoblastic metastases such as prostate, neuroendocrine, and breast carcinomas are occasionally associated with reactive bone formation and therefore simulate osteosarcoma with epithelioid features (Figure 24-7). When the proliferation of osteoclastic multinucleated giant cells is prominent, metastatic tumors can even be confused with giant cell tumor of bone.

IMMUNOHISTOCHEMISTRY

Immunostains for epithelial membrane antigen (EMA) and keratins (CAM 5.2, AE1/3, CK7, CK20, among others) are frequently positive in epithelial tumors and negative in most mesenchymal lesions. Therefore, they may be useful for differentiating between metastatic carcinomas and primary bone sarcomas. Since rare keratin positive cells can be seen in some sarcomas, caution should be taken when interpreting results. In some cases, immunohistochemical markers may be helpful in identifying the primary site and histologic type

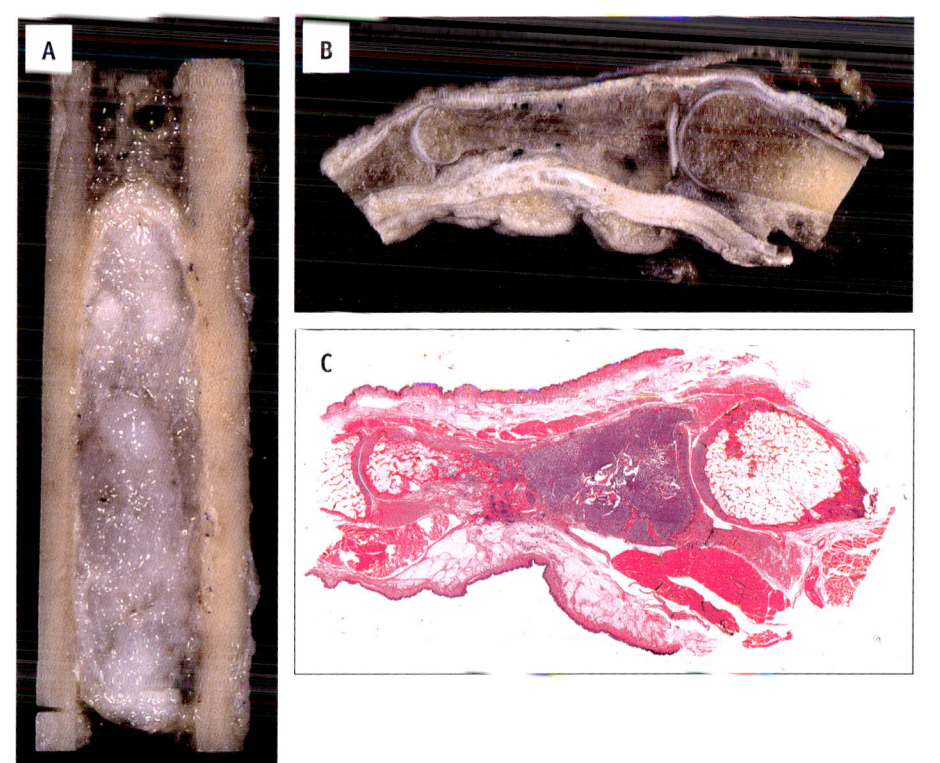

FIGURE 24-4
A, Gross photograph of a mid femur with metastatic gastric adenocarcinoma, showing a well-circumscribed pale mass with focal myxoid change. **B**, Gross appearance of an amputated proximal phalanx of the finger with metastatic renal cell carcinoma. **C**, Microscopically, the tumor is composed of clear cells expanding the bone. Kidney and lung are the most common primary sites of acral metastasis.

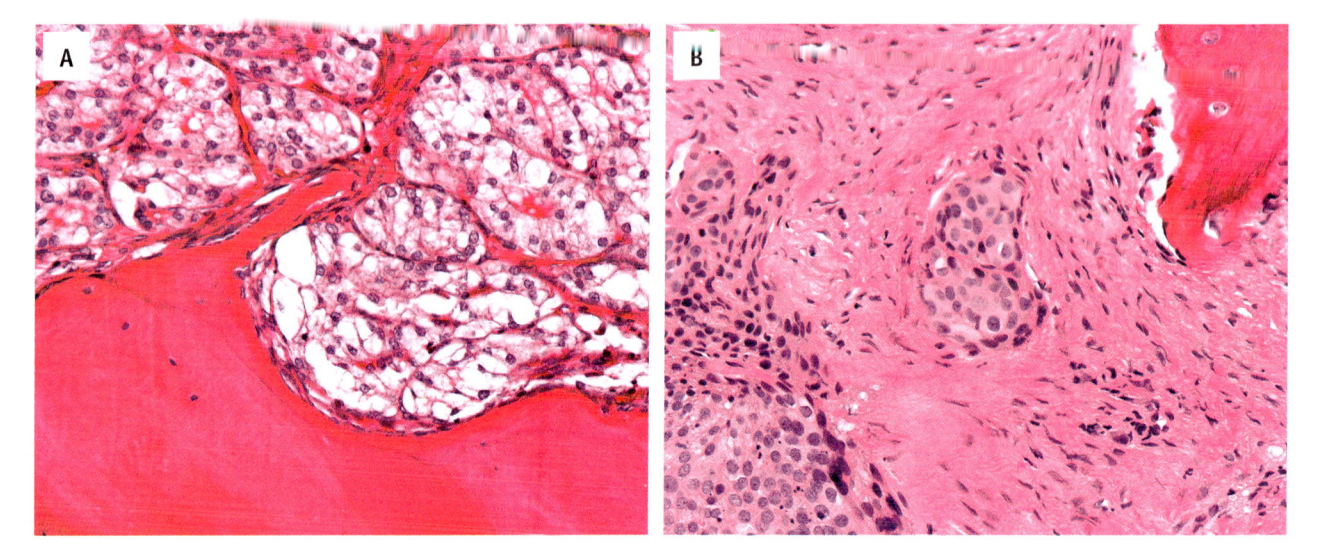

FIGURE 24-5
A, Histology of metastatic renal cell carcinoma with clear cell features. **B**, Metastatic squamous cell carcinoma from the cervix shows epithelial nests associated with dense fibrosis.

of the metastatic tumor. Some examples include thyroid transcription factor-1 (TTF-1) for lung or thyroid cancer, prostatic-specific antigen (PSA) for carcinoma of the prostate, estrogen and progesterone receptors for breast cancer, S-100 protein, HMB-45, or Melan-A for malignant melanoma, and chromogranin A for neuroendocrine tumors. Immunohistochemical studies tend to be positive more often in well-to moderately-differentiated tumors. They are of more limited value in poorly differentiated tumors.

DIFFERENTIAL DIAGNOSIS

For any bone malignant tumor in patients older than 60 years, whether histologically showing epithelioid spindle cell or round cell features, one should always be concerned about the possibility of metastatic carcinoma. Meticulous clinical and imaging evaluations are mandatory for patients with a bone lesion suggestive of metastasis. Nevertheless, even with immunohistochemical

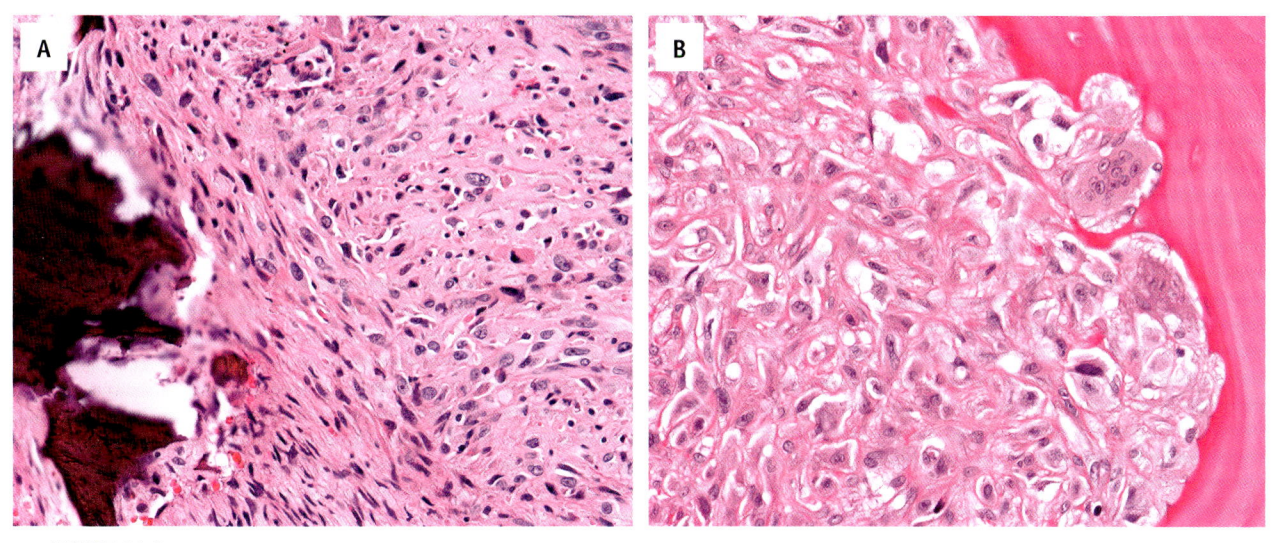

CHAPTER 24 Metastases Involving Bone   451

FIGURE 24-6
A, Metastatic sarcomatoid carcinoma from papillary thyroid carcinoma, closely simulating primary spindle cell sarcoma of bone. **B,** Metastatic sarcomatoid renal cell carcinoma from the kidney.

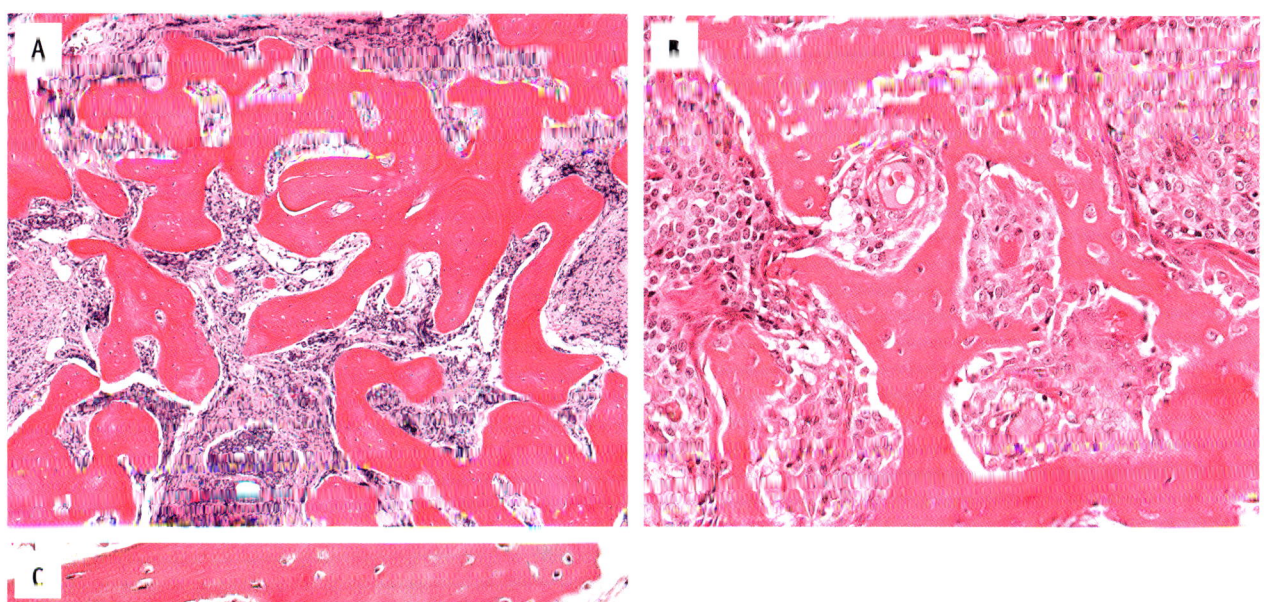

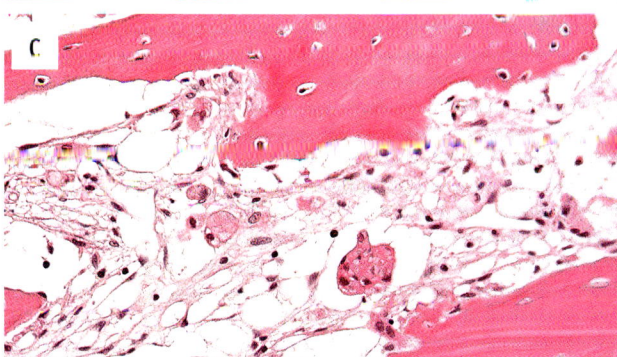

FIGURE 24-7
A, Low-power view of a metastatic adenocarcinoma from the prostate with osteosclerotic change. **B,** Osteoblastic metastasis of carcinoma from the breast. **C,** Metastatic adenocarcinoma from the stomach. Only a few malignant cells are scattered in the intertrabecular fibrous stroma.

METASTASES INVOLVING BONE—FACT SHEET

Definition
▸▸ Secondary bone involvement of tumor originating from another primary site

Incidence and Location
▸▸ Most common malignant tumor involving bone
▸▸ Predominantly occurs in cranium, vertebrae, rib, sternum, sacrum, pelvis, pelvic girdles including proximal femur
▸▸ Frequently multiple
▸▸ In the long bones, tends to involve the metaphysis
▸▸ Rare in small bones of the hands and feet

Morbidity and Mortality
▸▸ Up to 90% of the patients with common carcinomas may have skeletal metastasis
▸▸ Metastatic carcinoma from lung, breast, prostate, kidney, and thyroid glands accounts for more than 80%
▸▸ Skeletal metastasis of sarcoma is rare and most frequently seen in children
▸▸ Mortality depends on histologic type and site of the primary tumor

Sex, Race, and Age Distribution
▸▸ No significant sex predilection
▸▸ Peak incidence at 40 to 60 years

Clinical Features
▸▸ Symptoms are nonspecific and simulate those of a primary bone sarcoma
▸▸ Pain, with or without swelling, and pathologic fracture are main symptoms
▸▸ Neurologic symptoms may be noted with the lesion of the spine
▸▸ Hypercalcemia and increased serum alkaline phosphatase secondary to osteolysis may be demonstrated.
▸▸ Collet–Sicard syndrome in skull base metastasis may occur
▸▸ Prominent osteoblastic metastases may cause osteomalacia secondary to the high calcium demand

Radiologic Features
▸▸ Usually suggests a malignant tumor
▸▸ Osteolytic and destructive change mainly located in marrow cavity
▸▸ Osteoblastic or mixed lytic and blastic change may occur
▸▸ Prostatic adenocarcinoma frequently shows purely osteoblastic metastasis
▸▸ Periosteal reaction and florid ossification with pathologic fracture may simulate osteosarcoma
▸▸ CT scan and MRI particularly useful for detecting metastatic lesions in the vertebrae
▸▸ Radioisotope scintigram bone scan is positive for metastatic carcinoma

Prognosis and Treatment
▸▸ Prognosis depends on the primary site of the tumor, histologic type of neoplasm, and extent of disease
▸▸ Relief of pain and prevention of fracture are goals of treatment
▸▸ A localized single deposit may be surgically resected
▸▸ Radiation and chemotherapy may be effective in controlling the symptoms
▸▸ Specific therapies, including hormonal treatment for breast and prostate carcinoma, may be indicated

---

studies confusion between metastatic sarcomatoid carcinoma and primary skeletal spindle cell sarcoma may be inevitable.

Multiple myeloma commonly presents as multiple osteolytic lesions in older patients and thus may simulate metastatic carcinoma. Radioisotope bone scan is generally negative, and demonstration of monoclonal protein in the serum and urine is practically diagnostic. Angiosarcoma of bone can also involve multiple skeletal sites similar to metastatic carcinoma. The histologic features of angiosarcoma, particularly epithelioid angiosarcoma, can mimic metastatic carcinoma. Immunostains for CD31 and CD34 are, however, generally positive in angiosarcomas and negative in carcinoma. However, both malignancies can be positive with keratin. Since osteosarcomas occasionally show epithelial features and, on the other hand, reactive bone production may be prominent in some osteoblastic metastases, differentiation between osteosarcoma and metastatic carcinoma may sometimes be difficult. The age of the patient, location of the lesion, and immunohistochemical studies may help solve the problem. Adamantinoma of long bones usually have an epithelial component and therefore mimic metastatic carcinoma. Characteristic involvement of the tibia or, less frequently, the fibula may be a clue in making the correct diagnosis. Primary leiomyosarcoma of bone is extremely rare, and therefore the possibility of metastasis from uterine leiomyosarcoma should be completely excluded before establishing this unusual diagnosis. Melanocytic malignancy involving bone is almost always metastatic tumor from another primary site. Squamous cell carcinoma, usually well differentiated, can occur in association with draining sinus in longstanding osteomyelitis. Clinical history of the patient and roentgenologic study are of great help in the differential diagnosis of secondary squamous cell carcinoma in chronic osteomyelitis from metastatic carcinoma.

Prognosis and Treatment

Metastatic tumors of bone always represent advanced disease, generally associated with a poor outcome. The prognosis of patients may depend on the primary site of the tumor, histologic type of neoplasm, and extent of disease. Palliative therapies for relief of pain and for prevention of fracture are the most common treatments of choice. A localized single deposit may be surgically resected. Radiation and chemotherapy may be effective in diminishing the symptoms and in detaining progression of the disease. Radioactive iodine is used for controlling some thyroid cancers. Carcinomas from breast and prostate may be treated by hormonal medication. Immunostains for HER2/neu protein and estrogen and progesterone receptors help guide treatment of metastatic breast carcinoma.

MESTASTASES INVOLVING BONE—PATHOLOGIC FEATURES

Gross Findings
- Usually nonspecific and simulate primary bone sarcomas
- Frequently osteolytic, soft, and hemorrhagic
- Grayish white, firm, and fibrotic by desmoplastic reaction of the stroma
- Dense and hard osteoblastic metastases, particularly in metastatic prostatic carcinoma
- Periosteal new bone formation is infrequent
- Extraosseous extension with a soft tissue mass may occur

Microscopic Findings
- Tend to retain the morphologic features of the primary tumor
- Adenocarcinomas or squamous cell carcinomas from the lung, breast, kidney, prostate, and thyroid gland are common
- Fibroblastic proliferation, vascular proliferation, and osteoclastic multinucleated giant cells in the stroma are frequent
- Sarcomatoid carcinomas may simulate primary or secondary spindle cell sarcomas
- Metastases from the prostate, breast, or neuroendocrine tumor, among others, are occasionally associated with reactive bone formation or production of osteoid

Immunohistochemical Findings
- EMA or keratins (CAM 5.2, AE1/3, CK7, CK20, among others) are frequently positive in metastatic carcinomas
- Sarcomatoid carcinomas tend to be positive for vimentin and negative or focally positive for keratins
- Immunohistochemical markers frequently used are TTF-1 for lung or thyroid cancer, PSA for carcinoma of the prostate, estrogen and progesterone receptors for breast cancer, S-100 protein, HMB-45, or Melan-A for malignant melanoma, and chromogranin A or CD56 for neuroendocrine tumors

Differential Diagnosis
- Plasmacytoma
- Angiosarcoma
- Osteosarcomas with epithelioid features
- Adamantinoma of long bones
- Fibrosarcoma or malignant fibrous histiocytoma of bone
- Squamous cell carcinoma arising in longstanding osteomyelitis

SUGGESTED READINGS

1. Aebi M: Spinal metastasis in the elderly. Eur Spine J 2003;12(suppl 2):S202–S213.
2. Ali SM, Harvey HA, Lipton A: Metastatic breast cancer: overview of treatment. Clin Orthop 2003;(415 suppl):S132–S137.
3. Bendre M, Gaddy D, Nicholas RW, et al: Breast cancer metastasis to bone: it is not all about PTHrP. Clin Orthop 2003;(415 suppl):S39–S45.
4. Brage ME, Simon MA: Evaluation, prognosis, and medical treatment considerations of metastatic bone tumors. Orthopedics 1992;15(5):589–596.
5. Campanacci M: Bone and Soft Tissue Tumors. Berlin, Germany: Springer-Verlag, 1999, pp 756–787.
6. Carlin BI, Andriole GL: The natural history, skeletal complications, and management of bone metastases in patients with prostate carcinoma. Cancer 2000;88(12 suppl):2989–2994.
7. Cheville JC, Tindall D, Boelter C, et al: Metastatic prostate carcinoma to bone: clinical and pathologic features associated with cancer-specific survival. Cancer 2002;95(5):1028–1036.
8. Choong PF: The molecular basis of skeletal metastases. Clin Orthop 2003;(415 suppl):S19–S31.
9. Dorfman HD: Czerniak B: Bone Tumors. St. Louis, MO: Mosby, 1998, 1009–1040.
10. Falkmer U, Jarhult J, Wersall P, et al: A systematic overview of radiation therapy effects in skeletal metastases. Acta Oncol 2003;42:620–633.
11. Goltzman D, Karaplis AC, Kremer R, et al: Molecular basis of the spectrum of skeletal complications of neoplasia. Cancer 2000;88(12 suppl):2903–2908.
12. Guise TA: Molecular mechanisms of osteolytic bone metastases. Cancer 2000;88(12 suppl):2892–2898.
13. Healey JH, Turnbull AD, Miedema B, et al: Acrometastases. A study of twenty-nine patients with osseous involvement of the hands and feet. J Bone Joint Surg Am 1986;68:743–746.
14. James JJ, Evans AJ, Pinder SE, et al: Bone metastases from breast carcinoma: histopathological-radiological correlations and prognostic features. Br J Cancer 2003;89:660–665.
15. Kager L, Zoubek A, Potschger U, et al: Primary metastatic osteosarcoma: presentation and outcome of patients treated on neoadjuvant Cooperative Osteosarcoma Study Group protocols. J Clin Oncol 2003;21:2011–2018.
16. Kakonen SM, Mundy GR: Mechanisms of osteolytic bone metastases in breast carcinoma. Cancer 2003;97(3 suppl):834–839.
17. Mundy GR: Mechanisms of bone metastasis. Cancer 1997;80(8 suppl):1546–1556.
18. Peterson JJ, Kransdorf MJ, O'Connor MI: Diagnosis of occult bone metastases: Positron emission tomography. Clin Orthop 2003;(415 suppl):S120–S128.
19. Resnick D: Bone and Joint Imaging. Philadelphia, Saunders, 1996, pp 1076–1091.
20. Rodan GA: The development and function of the skeleton and bone metastases. Cancer 2003;97(3 suppl):726–732.
21. Rougraff BT: Evaluation of the patient with carcinoma of unknown origin metastatic to bone. Clin Orthop 2003;(415 suppl):S105–S109.
22. San-Julian M, Diaz-de-Rada P, Noain E, et al: Bone metastases from osteosarcoma. Int Orthop 2003;27:117–120.
23. Simon MA, Bartucci EJ: The search for the primary tumor in patients with skeletal metastases of unknown origin. Cancer 1986;58:1088–1095.
24. Troncoso A, Ro JY, Grignon DJ, et al: Renal cell carcinoma with acrometastasis: report of two cases and review of the literature. Mod Pathol 1991;4:66–69.
25. Unni KK: Dahlin's Bone Tumors: General Aspects and Data on 11,087 Cases. Philadelphia: Lippincott-Raven, 1996, pp 355–360.
26. Weber MH, Goltzman D, Kostenuik P, et al: Mechanisms of tumor metastasis to bone. Crit Rev Eukaryot Gene Expr 2000;10:281–302.
27. Wilner D: Radiology of Bone Tumors and Allied Disorders, vol. 4. Philadelphia, Saunders, 1982, pp 3641–3908.

Index

A
Abdominal desmoid tumors, 54–55
Adamantinoma
　clinical features, 414
　differential diagnosis, 416–417
　differentiated, 417–418
　fact sheet, 418b
　genetics, 415
　immunohistochemistry, 415–416
　pathologic features, 414–415, 418b
　prognosis/treatment, 417
　radiologic features, 414
Adipocytic tumors
　angiolipoma, 100–101
　chondroid lipoma, 107–108
　dedifferentiated liposarcoma, 111–113
　hibernoma, 104–105
　lipoblastoma, 103–104
　lipoma, 97–99
　lipomatosis of nerve, 99–100
　myolipoma, 105–106
　myxoid liposarcoma, 113–115
　pleomorphic liposarcoma, 115–117
　spindle cell and pleomorphic lipoma, 101–103
　well-differentiated liposarcoma, 108–110
Adult fibrosarcoma and variants
　clinical features, 63
　differential diagnosis, 66–67
　fact sheet, 67b
　genetics, 66
　immunohistochemistry, 66
　pathologic features, 63–66, 68b
　prognosis/treatment, 67–69
Adult rhabdomyoma, 131–132
Adult sclerosing rhabdomyosarcoma, 144
Aggressive angiomyxoma, 283–284
Aggressive rhabdomyoma, 144
AJCC system of staging, 15, 15t
Alveolar rhabdomyosarcoma, 33t, 139–142
Alveolar soft part sarcoma, 20t, 33t, 295–296
American Joint Committee of Cancer (AJCC) system of staging, 15t
Amplification, 32
Anaplastic large-cell lymphoma, 385–386
Aneurysmal bone cyst, 33t, 36, 403–405, 428–432
Aneurysmal cyst of soft tissue (ACST), 252–254
Angiectid spaces, 80–81
Angioleiomyoma, 122–123
Angiolipoma, 100–101
Angiolymphiod hyperplasia with eosinophilia, 177–179
Angiomatoid (malignant) fibrous histiocytoma, 20t, 33t, 83–86
Angiomatosis, 175–177
Angiomyofibroblastoma, 281–283
Angiosarcoma, 20t, 186–188, 396–400
Atypical decubital fibroplasia, 45–46
Atypical fibroxanthoma, 78–79
Atypical glomus tumors, 154–156
Atypical lipomatous tumor, 108–110
Autophosphorylation, 37–38

B
Bacillary angiomatosis, 167–168
Bednar tumor, 79–83
Bence-Jones protein, 379
Benign fibrous histiocytoma, 72–75, 363
Benign fibrous histiocytoma (BFH), 120, 403–405
Benign giant cell tumor, 401
Benign vascular tumors, 169–179. *See also* Benign vascular tumors
Bilateral retinoblastoma, 321t
Biopsy, 10–13
Biphasic synovial sarcoma (BSS), 298–300
Bloom syndrome, 321t
Blue rubber bleb nevus syndrome, 172
Bone island, 309–311
Bone sarcoma staging, 15t
Bone tumor grades, summary, 14–15
Bone tumors of miscellaneous type/uncertain lineage
　ABC, 428–432
　cystic lesions, 428–445
　Erdheim Chester disease, 441–445
　fibrous dysplasia, 419–424
　fibrous lesions, 419–428
　intraosseous ganglion, 435–437
　LCH, 437–441
　osteofibrous dysplasia, 424–428
　simple bone cyst, 432–435
Bone-forming tumors
　bone island, 309–311
　osteoblastoma, 316–320
　osteoid osteoma, 313–316
　osteoma, 311–313
　osteosarcoma, 320–328
　overview, 309
Brachyury, 170
Breakapart probe, 28–30
Buschke-Ollendorff, 309

C
C-kit, 25t
C-kit mutations in GIST, 37–38
Calcifying aponeurotic fibroma (CAF), 51–52
Caldesmon, 19t
Capillary hemangioma, 169–172
Carboxy-terminus, 19t
Carney's complex, 211–213
Cartilage-forming tumors
　benign tumors, 330–342
　chondroblastoma, 334–336
　chondromyxoid fibroma, 337–339
　chondrosarcoma variants, 345–354
　clear cell chondrosarcoma, 346–348
　conventional chondrosarcoma, 342–345
　dedifferentiated chondrosarcoma, 348–350
　enchondroma, 339–342

Page numbers followed by f indicate figures; t, tables, and b, box.

455

Cartilage-forming tumors *(Continued)*
   malignant tumors, 342–345
     mesenchymal chondrosarcoma, 350–354
     osteochondroma, 330–333
     overview, 330
     periosteal chondroma, 333–334
Cavernous hemangioma, 172–173
CD30, 19t, 29t, 31t
CD31, 19t, 29t
CD34, 19t, 25t
CD45, 19t–20t, 29t
CD68, 19t
CD99, 19t–20t
CD117, 25t, 160
CD163, 19t
CDK4, 19t
Cellular angiofibroma, 281
Cellular myxoma, 276–277
Cellular neurothekeoma, 88, 225
Cellular schwannoma, 22
Cementifying fibroma, 421
Cementoid bodies, 420–421
Chondroblastic osteosarcoma, 324
Chondroblastoma, 334–336, 403–405
Chondroid lipoma, 107–108
Chondrolipoma, 97
Chondroma, 339
Chondromyxoid fibroma, 337–339
Chondrosarcoma, 20t, 270, 342–345
Chondrosarcoma variants, 345–354
Chordoma, 23
   ancillary studies, 410
   clinical features, 408
   differential diagnosis, 410–411
   fact sheet, 412b
   pathologic features, 409–410, 412b
   prognosis/treatment, 411–412
   radiologic features, 408–409
Claudin-1, 19t
Clear cell chondrosarcoma, 346–348
Clear cell sarcoma, 33t, 35
   clinical features, 231
   differential diagnosis, 232–235
   fact sheet, 235b
   immunohistochemistry, 232
   pathologic features, 232, 236b
   prognosis/treatment, 235
   radiologic features, 231
Codman's triangle, 322–323
COL1A1-PDGEB, 33–34
Computed tomography (CT), 9
Congenital (infantile) fibrosarcoma, 36, 69
Conventional chondrosarcoma, 342–345
Conventional fibrosarcoma, 63–64. *See also* Adult fibrosarcoma and variants
Conventional osteosarcoma, 320–329
Core biopsy, 13
Cranial fasciitis, 45
Craniofacial osteoma, 311
CT-guided needle biopsy, 13
Cultures, 13
Cutaneous angiosarcoma, 186
Cutaneous leiomyosarcoma, 124–126
Cutaneous myxoma, 279–280
Cystic osteoblastoma, 318–320
Cytogenetic alterations, 33t
Cytokeratin, 19t, 29t, 31t

D

Dabska-type and retiform hemangioendothelioma, 181–183
Dedifferentiated chondrosarcoma, 348–350
Dedifferentiated giant cell tumor, 405
Dedifferentiated liposarcoma, 33t, 111–113
Deep fibromatosis
   clinical features, 54–55
   differential diagnosis, 58
   fact sheet, 55b
   genetics, 57
   immunohistochemistry, 57
   pathologic features, 55–57, 55b
   prognosis/treatment, 58
Deeply located hemangioma, 173–177
Dermatofibroma, 72
Dermatofibrosarcoma protuberans, 33t, 36, 79–83
Desmin, 19–20t, 31t
Desmoid tumors, 54–58
Desmoplastic fibroblastoma, 58
Desmoplastic fibroma, 358–360
Desmoplastic small round cell tumor (DSRCT), 20t, 21, 301–305
Detritic synovitis, 271–275
Diagnostic imaging. *See* Imaging studies
Differentiated adamantinoma, 417–418
Diffuse large B-cell lymphoma (DLBCL), 384–385
Diffuse neurofibroma, 200
Dupuytren disease, 53

E

Elastofibroma, 48–50
Embryonal rhabdomyosarcoma
   anaplastic variant, 139
   botryoid variant, 139
   clinical features, 135
   differential diagnosis, 137–139
   fact sheet, 138b
   genetics, 137
   immunohistochemistry, 140
   pathologic features, 135–137, 139b
   prognosis/treatment, 139
   spindle cell variant, 139
Enchondroma, 339–342
Endoneurium, 193
Enneking System, 15–16
Enostosis, 309–311
Eosinophilic granuloma, 437
Epithelial membrane antigen, 19t
Epithelioid angiosarcoma, 397–399, 398f
Epithelioid hemangioendothelioma (EHE), 183–186, 392–396
Epithelioid hemangioma, 177–179
Epithelioid malignant peripheral nerve sheath tumor, 23
Epithelioid sarcoma, 20t, 23, 293–295
Epstein-Barr virus-associated smooth muscle tumor (EBV-SMT), 129–130
Erdheim-Chester disease, 441–445
ETV6-NTRK3, 33–34
Evaluation of tumors
   biopsy, 10–13
   cultures, 13
   history, 3–4
   imaging studies, 3–7
   laboratory studies, 10–13
   location of tumor, 7t
   physical exam, 3–4
   questions to ask, 4b
Ewing family of tumors (EFT), 296

Ewing sarcoma
   CD99, 23f
   clinical features, 296, 367
   cytogenetic alterations, 33t
   cytogenetics/molecular pathology, 375–376
   differential diagnosis, 297–298, 376–377
   embryonal rhabdomyosarcoma, contrasted, 137–139
   fact sheet, 298b, 377b
   genetic findings, 297
   immunohistochemistry, 297, 374–375
   overview, 367
   pathologic features, 296–297, 298b, 372–373, 377b
   prognosis/treatment, 377–378
   radiologic features, 367–372
EWS-CHN, 35
EWS-WT1, 34–35
Excisional biopsy, 13
Extra-abdominal desmoid tumors, 54–55
Extrarenal rhabdoid tumor, 33t
Extraskeletal chondroma with lipoblast-like cells, 107
Extraskeletal myxoid chondrosarcoma, 35, 247–249
Extraskeletal myxoid liposarcoma, 33t

F

Factor VIII-related protein, 19t
Fallen fragment, 433
Familial syndromes, 32
Fasciitis ossificans, 45
FDG-PET, 9
Fetal rhabdomyoma, 132–133
FGF23, 318–320
Fibroblastic and fibrohistiocytic tumors
   benign fibrous histiocytoma, 363
   desmoplastic fibroma, 358–360
   fibrosarcoma of bone, 360–363
   malignant fibrous histiocytoma, 363–366
   nonossifying fibroma, 355–358
Fibroblastic/myofibroblastic tumors
   adult fibrosarcoma and variants, 63–69
   CAF, 51–53
   deep fibromatoses, 54–58
   elastofibroma, 48–50
   fibroma of tendon sheath, 47–48
   fibrous hamartoma of infancy, 50–51
   IMT, 58–61
   infantile fibrosarcoma, 69–71
   MIFS, 61–63
   nodular fasciitis, 43–47
   superficial fibromatoses, 53–54
Fibroblastic osteosarcoma, 324
Fibrohistiocytic lesions, 363–366
Fibrohistiocytic tumors
   AMFH, 83–86
   atypical fibroxanthoma, 78–79
   benign fibrous histiocytoma, 72–75
   DFSP, 79–83
   juvenile xanthogranuloma, 75–77
   PFHT, 86–88
   soft tissue giant cell tumor, 88–90
   undifferentiated pleomorphic sarcoma, 90–96
   xanthoma, 77–78
Fibrolipoma, 97
Fibrolipomatous hamartoma of nerve, 99
Fibroma of tendon sheath, 47–48
Fibroma of tendon sheath (FTS), 264–266
Fibromatosis, 86b
Fibro-osseous pseudotumor of digits (FOPD), 242–243

Fibrosarcoma, 22. *See also* Adult fibrosarcoma and variants. Infantile fibrosarcoma
Fibrosarcoma of bone, 360–363
Fibrous cortical defect, 355–358
Fibrous dysplasia, 319–320, 419–424
Fibrous hamartoma of infancy, 50–51
Fibrous lesions, 355–363, 419–428. *See also* Bone tumors of miscellaneous type/uncertain lineage; Fibroblastic and fibrohistiocytic tumors
FISH, 28–32
Fluorescent in situ hybridization (FISH), 28–32

G

Ganglioneuroblastoma, 226–227
Ganglioneuroma, 226–227
Gardner syndrome, 57, 311
Gastrointestinal stromal tumor (GIST), 20t, 33t, 208b
   clinical features, 158
   cytogenetics, 160
   differential diagnosis, 161
   DNA sequencing, 160
   fact sheet, 163b
   fine-needle aspiration biopsy, 161
   immunohistochemistry, 160
   pathologic features, 158–159, 163b
   prognosis/treatment, 161–163
   radiologic features, 158
   risk, 162t
   ultrastructural features, 159
Genital leiomyoma, 120–121
Genital rhabdomyoma, 133–135
Germline mutations of RB, 32
Giant cell angiofibroma, 146–150
Giant cell fibroblastoma, 33t, 36, 79–83
Giant cell malignant fibrous histiocytoma, 91
Giant cell reparative granuloma, 431–432
Giant cell-rich osteosarcoma, 324–325, 403–405
Giant cell tumor of bone
   clinical features, 401
   differential diagnosis, 403–405
   fact sheet, 407b
   pathologic features, 403, 407b
   prognosis/treatment, 405–407
   radiologic features, 401
Giant cell tumor of low malignant potential, 88
Giant cell tumor of tendon sheath (GCTTS), 259–261
Giant notochordal hamartoma, 411
Giant notochordal rest (GNR), 411
GIST familial syndrome, 32
Glial fibrillary acidic protein, 19t
Glomangioma, 153–154
Glomangiomyoma, 153–154
Glomangiopericytoma, 150–152
Glomangiosarcoma, 153–157
Glomeruloid hemangioma, 168–169
Glomus tumor, 20t
   clinical features, 153
   differential diagnosis, 156
   fact sheet, 156b
   genetics, 155–156
   immunohistochemistry, 155
   pathologic features, 153–154, 156b
   prognosis/treatment, 156
Glomus tumors of uncertain malignant potential, 154–155
Glomuvenous malformation, 153–154
Glut-1, 19t
Grading of soft tissue and bone sarcomes, 13–15

Granular cell tumor
    clinical features, 217–222
    differential diagnosis, 220–221
    fact sheet, 220b
    immunohistochemistry, 219
    pathologic features, 219, 220b
    prognosis/treatment, 222

H

Hand-Schuller-Christian disease, 437
Hemangioendothelioma, 179–186, 389. *See also* Vascular tumors of soft tissue
Hemangioma, 389–392. *See also* Vascular tumors of soft tissue
Hemangiopericytoma, 20t, 146–150
Hematopoietic tumors
    Hodgkin lymphoma, 388
    lymphoma of bone, 383–388
    multiple myeloma, 379–383
    non-Hodgkin lymphoma, 383–388
Hemosiderotic fibrohistiocytic lipomatous lesions, 288
Hemosiderotic synovitis, 261–263
Hereditary multiple exostoses, 331
Hibernoma, 104–105
High-grade myxofibrosarcoma, 67
High-grade osteoblastic osteosarcoma, 320–329
High-grade surface osteosarcoma, 320–329
Histiocytosis X, 76, 437
HMB-45, 19t
Hobnail hemangioma, 182–183
Hodgkin lymphoma, 388
HPC/SFT
    clinical features, 146
    differential diagnosis, 148–150
    fact sheet, 149b
    genetic studies, 148
    immunohistochemistry, 147–148
    pathologic features, 146–147, 149b
Hyalinizing spindle cell tumor with giant rosettes, 64–65

I

Imaging studies
    CT, 9
    isotope scanning, 7–8
    MRI, 9
    radiography, 4, 6
    ultrasound, 6
Immunohistochemistry
    differential diagnosis, 18–21
    monomorphic spindle cell neoplasms, 21–22
    overview, 18
    pleomorphic spindle cell tumors, 23–24
    poorly differentiated epithelioid tumors, 22–23
Infantile fibrosarcoma, 33t, 36, 69–71
Infantile hemangiopericytoma, 150–152
Infantile myofibromatosis, 150–152
Inflammatory fibrosarcoma, 58–61
Inflammatory malignant fibrous histiocytoma, 91
Inflammatory myofibroblastic tumor, 33t, 58–61
Inflammatory pseudotumor, 58–61
INI1, 19t
Interzonal mesenchyme, 255
Intra-abdominal desmoid tumors, 55, 56f, 57f
Intramedullary well-differentiated osteosarcoma, 320–329
Intramuscular myxoma, 276–277
Intraneural hemangioma, 175
Intraneural perineurioma, 225
Intraosseous benign notochord cell tumor, 411
Intraosseous ganglion, 435–437

Intra-synovial hemangioma, 262
Intravascular fasciitis, 45
Ischemic fasciitis, 45–46
Isotope scanning, 7–8

J

Jaffe-Campanacci syndrome, 355
Joint mice, 268
Juvenile hemangioma, 169–170
Juvenile intracortical adamantinoma, 417–418
Juvenile xanthogranuloma, 75–77
Juxta-articular myxoma, 277–279
Juxtacortical intermediate-grade chondroblastic osteosarcoma, 320–329
Juxtacortical well-differentiated osteosarcoma, 320–329

K

Kaposi sarcoma, 20t, 188–191
Kaposiform hemangioendothelioma (KHE), 179–181
Ki-1, 19t
KIT (CD117), 160
Klippel-Trenaunay syndrome, 186, 389

L

Laboratory studies, 10–13
Landscape effect, 255–256
Langerhans cell histiocytosis (LCH), 437–441
Large joint detritic synovitis, 271–273
Ledderhose disease, 53
Leiomyoma
    fact sheet, 123b
    leiomyoma of deep soft tissue, 121–122
    leiomyoma of external genitalia, 120–121
    leiomyoma of the retroperitoneum, 123–124
    pilar leiomyoma, 119–120
    vascular leiomyoma, 122–123
Leiomyoma of deep soft tissue, 121–122
Leiomyoma of external genitalia, 120–121
Leiomyoma of the retroperitoneum, 123–124
Leiomyosarcoma, 20t, 24
    cutaneous leiomyosarcoma, 124–126
    EPV-SMT, 129–130
    fact sheet, 126b
    leiomyosarcoma of deep soft tissue, 126–127
    pathologic features, 126b
    retroperitoneal leiomyosarcoma, 128–129
    vascular leiomyosarcoma, 127–128
Leiomyosarcoma of deep soft tissue, 126–127
Letterer-Siwe disease, 437
Leukocyte common antigen, 19t
Li-Fraumeni syndrome, 32, 321t
Lipoblastoma, 103
Lipoblastomatosis, 103
Lipoleiomyoma, 105
Lipoma, 97–99
Lipoma arborescens, 263–264
Lipomatosis of nerve, 99
Lipomatous hemangiopericytoma, 146–150
Liposarcoma, 20t
Lobular capillary hemangioma, 166–167
Localized GCTTS, 259–261
Location of tumor, 7b
Loose bodies, 268–269
Loosened joint arthroplasties, 271–274
Low-grade fibromyxoid sarcoma, 33t, 58, 63. *See also* Adult fibrosarcoma and variants
Low-grade intraosseous fibrous dysplasia-like osteosarcoma, 421

Low-grade MPNST, 58
Low grade myxofibrosarcoma, 67
Lymphoblastic lymphoma, 385–386
Lymphoma, 18–21, 23
Lymphoma of bone, 383–388

M

M protein, 379
Magnetic resonance imaging (MRI), 9
Malignant fibrous histiocytoma, 91, 363–366
Malignant giant cell tumor, 405
Malignant glomus tumor, 153–156
Malignant perineurioma, 223
Malignant peripheral nerve sheath tumor (MPNST), 20t, 214–217
Malignant tenosynovial giant cell tumor, 270–275
Malignant Triton tumor, 214
Malignant tumors of the joint, 270
Masson's lesion, 262
Maturing ganglioneuroma, 227–228
Mazabraud syndrome, 276, 419
McCune-Albright syndrome, 419, 421–424
Melanoma, 18, 23–24
Melanosome-specific antigens, 19t
Melorheostosis, 309, 313
Mesenchymal chondrosarcoma, 350–352
Mesenchymal chondrosarcoma (MC), 250–252
Metal debris, 271–272
Metallosis, 262
Metaphyseal fibrous defect, 355–358
Metastases involving bone, 440–447
Metastatic renal cell carcinoma, 449f, 451f
Metastatic spindle cell carcinoma, 451f
Metastatic squamous cell carcinoma, 451f
Metastatic tumor of bone
　clinical features, 446–447
　differential diagnosis, 447–452
　fact sheet, 452b–453b
　immunohistochemistry, 447
　pathologic features, 447, 453b
　prognosis/treatment, 452–454
　radiologic features, 447
Methyl methacrylate, 271–272
MIC2 gene product, 101
Microphthalmia transcription factor, 19t
Molecular pathology
　familial syndromes, 32
　FISH, 28–29
　overview, 24–39
　point mutations, 37
　practical significance of mutation detection, 37–39
　RT-PCR, 26–28
　somatically acquired alterations, 32
　translocation, 33–34
Monomorphic spindle cell neoplasms, 21–22
Monophasic synovial sarcoma (MSS), 298–300
Mucosal neuroma, 195–197
Multiple myeloma
　clinical features, 379–380
　differential diagnosis, 382
　fact sheet, 383b
　immunohistochemistry, 381–382
　pathologic features, 381, 383b
　prognosis/treatment, 383
　radiologic features, 380–381
Multiple osteochondroma, 331
Multiple skeletal metastases of adenocarcinoma, 450f
MyoD1, 19t

Myoepithelial tumor, 20t
Myoepithelioma, 23
Myofibroblastic lesions, 20t
Myofibroblastic tumors. *See* Fibroblastic/myofibroblastic tumors
Myofibroma, 150–152
Myogenic nuclear regulatory proteins, 19t
Myolipoma, 105–106
Myopericytoma, 150–152
Myositis ossificans (MO), 239–241
Myxofibrosarcoma, 63f. *See also* Adult fibrosarcoma and variants
Myxoid liposarcoma, 113–115
Myxoid malignant fibrous histiocytoma, 63
Myxoid neurothekeoma, 225–226
Myxoid-round cell liposarcoma, 33t
Myxoinflammatory fibroblastic sarcoma (MIFS), 61–63, 67
Myxolipoma, 97
Myxoma, 276. *See also* Tumors of miscellaneous type/uncertain lineage

N

Needle biopsy, 13
Nerve sheath and neuroectodermal tumors
　clear cell sarcoma, 231–238
　ganglioneuroblastoma, 226–227
　ganglioneuroma, 226–227
　granular cell tumor, 217–222
　MPNST, 214–217
　mucosal neuroma, 195–197
　neuroblastoma, 226–227
　neurofibroma, 199–206
　neurothekeoma, 225–226
　PEN, 197–199
　perineurioma, 222–225
　psammomatous melanotic schwannoma, 211–213
　schwannoma, 206–211
　traumatic neuroma, 193–195
Nerve sheath myxoma, 225–226
Neuroblastoma, 226–237
Neuroectodermal tumors, 193. *See also* Nerve sheath and neuroectodermal tumors
Neurofibroma, 58
　clinical features, 199–200
　differential diagnosis, 205–206
　fact sheet, 202b
　immunohistochemistry, 205
　pathologic features, 200–203, 202b
　prognosis/treatment, 206
　radiologic features, 200
Neurofibromatosis Type 1, 199–206
Neurofibromatosis Type 2, 206–211
Neurofilaments, 19t
Neurothekeoma, 225–226
NF1, 199–206
NF2, 206–211
Nodular fasciitis, 20t
　clinical features, 43
　differential diagnosis, 47
　fact sheet, 45b
　genetics, 47
　immunohistochemistry, 46–47
　pathologic features, 44–45, 45b
　prognosis/treatment, 47
　variants, 45–46
Non-Hodgkin lymphoma, 383–388
Nonossifying fibroma, 355–358, 421
Normal nerve, 193

Normalization, 309
Notochordal tumors. *See* Chordoma

O

Ochronosis, 262
OFD-like adamantinoma, 417–418
Oligomerization, 37–38
Ollier disease, 330
Orbital osteoma, 311
Ossifying fasciitis, 45
Ossifying fibromyxoid tumor of soft parts (OFMT), 285
Osteoblastic osteosarcoma, 324
Osteoblastic rimming, 240f
Osteoblastoma, 316–320
Osteocalcin, 19t
Osteochondroma, 330–333
Osteoclastoma, 401
Osteofibrous dysplasia, 424–428
Osteofibrous dysplasia (OFD), 414, 417–418, 421
Osteogenic sarcoma, 20t
Osteoid osteoma, 313–316
Osteolipoma, 97
Osteoma, 311–313
Osteopoikilosis, 309
Osteosarcoma
 ancillary studies, 315, 326
 categorization/variants, 320
 clinical features, 321
 cytogenetic abnormalities, 321
 differential diagnosis, 327b–328b
 fact sheet, 327b–328b
 genetic syndrome, 320–321
 pathologic features, 322–326, 328b
 prognosis/treatment, 327–329
 radiologic features, 321–322
Osteosclerotic myeloma, 381

P

Paget disease, 321
Palisaded encapsulated neuroma (PEN), 197–199
Palmar fibromatosis, 53
Pan-cytokeratin, 20t, 25t
Pan-muscle actin, 19t
Papillary endothelial hyperplasia (PEH), 164–166
Papillary intralymphatic angioendothelioma, 181–183
Parosteal osteosarcoma, 320–329, 421
PAX3-FKHR, 36
PAX7-FKHR, 36
PDSS, 21, 298–300
PEComa, 290–292
Perineurial MPNST, 223
Perineurioma, 222–225
Periosteal chondroma, 333–334
Periosteal osteosarcoma, 320–329
Perivascular cells. *See* Tumor of perivascular cells
Perivascular epithelioid cell neoplasm, 20t, 290–292
Permeative, 4, 6
Phosphaturic mesenchymal tumor, 288–290
Phosphaturic mesenchymal tumor, mixed connective tissue (PMTMCT), 288–290
Pigmented villonodular synovitis (PVNS), 256–258
Pilar leiomyoma, 119–120
Plantar lesions, 53
Plasma cell dyscrasia, 379
Plasma cell granuloma, 58–61
Pleomorphic hyalinizing angiectatic tumor (PHAT), 287
Pleomorphic liposarcoma, 115–117
Pleomorphic malignant fibrous histiocytoma, 90–91
Pleomorphic rhabdomyosarcoma, 142–144
Pleomorphic spindle cell tumors, 23–24
Plexiform fibrohistiocytic tumor (PFHT), 86–88
Plexiform neurofibroma, 200
PNET. *See* ES/PNET
POEMS syndrome, 381
Point mutation, 32, 37
Polyethylene, 271–273
Polyostotic fibrous dysplasia, 419
Poorly differentiated chordoma, 410
Poorly differentiated epithelioid tumors, 22–23
Poorly differentiated synovial sarcoma (PDSS), 298–300
Precursor B-cell lymphoblastic lymphoma, 385–386
Primary synovial chondromatosis, 266–268
Primitive neuroectodermal tumor. *See* ES/PNET
Proliferative fasciitis, 45–46
Proliferative myositis, 45–46
Protein kinase c-θ, 19t
Proximal type epithelioid sarcoma, 33t
Psammomatous melanotic schwannoma, 211–214
Pseudomalignant osteoblastoma, 318
Pyogenic granuloma, 166–167

R

Radiography
Reactive vascular proliferations
 bacillary angiomatosis, 167–168
 fact sheet, 168b
 glomeruloid hemangioma, 168–169
 pathologic features, 169b
 PEH, 164–166
 pyogenic granuloma, 166–167
Regressive adamantinoma, 417–418
Reticulohistiocytosis, 75
Retroperitoneal leiomyoma, 123–124
Retroperitoneal leiomyosarcoma, 128–129
Reverse transcripase-polymerase chain reaction (RT-PCR), 26–28
Rhabdomyoma
 adult, 131–132
 fact sheet, 134b
 fetal, 132–133
 genital, 133–135
 pathologic features, 134b
Rhabdomyosarcoma, 20t
 adult sclerosing, 144–145
 alveolar, 139–141
 embryonal, 135–139
 pleomorphic, 142–144
Rothmund-Thompson syndrome, 321t
Round cell liposarcoma, 113

S

S-100 protein, 20t, 25t, 29t, 31t
Saucerization, 368
Schwannoma
 clinical features, 206–207
 differential diagnosis, 210–211
 fact sheet, 208b
 immunohistochemistry, 209
 NF2, 208f
 pathologic features, 207–208, 208b
 prognosis/treatment, 211
 radiologic features, 207
Sclerosing epithelioid fibrosarcoma, 63–69. *See also* Adult fibrosarcoma and variants
Sclerosing liposarcoma, 108

INDEX

Sclerosing perineuroma, 223f
Sclerosing pseudovascular rhabdomyosarcoma in adults, 144
Sclerosing rhabdomyosarcoma in adults, 144
Scrotal leiomyoma, 121
Secondary chondrosarcoma, 332
SFT, 146–150
Sharpey's fibers, 421
Shepherd's crook deformity, 419–420
Simple bone cyst, 432–435
Skeletal muscle tumors. *See* Rhabdomyoma; Rhabdomyosarcoma
Small-cell carcinoma, 18
Small-cell osteosarcoma, 324–325
Small joint detritic synovitis, 273–275
Smooth muscle actin, 25t, 35t
Smooth muscle hyperplasia in the scrotum, 121
Smooth muscle tumor (SMT)
   leiomyoma, 119–124
   leiomyosarcoma, 124–130
Soft tissue chondroma (STC), 245–247
Soft tissue giant cell tumor, 88–90
Soft tissue osteosarcoma (STO), 243–245
Soft tissue perineurioma, 223, 224f
Soft tissue sarcoma staging, 15t
Solid glomus tumor, 153–154
Solitary bone cyst, 432–435
Solitary circumscribed neuroma, 197–199
Solitary fibrous tumor, 20t, 22, 146–150
Solitary myofibroma, 150–153
Solitary neurofibroma, 200
Solitary plasmacytoma, 379
Solitary reticulohistiocytoma, 75
Somatically acquired alterations, 32
Spindle cell and pleomorphic lipoma, 101–103
Spindle cell hemangioma (SCH), 173–175
Spindle cell liposarcoma, 108–110
SSX1, 34
SSX2, 34
Staging systems, 15–16
Stewart-Treves angiosarcoma, 186
Stress fracture, 327
Sturge-Weber syndrome, 389
Superficial angiomyxoma, 279
Superficial fibromatosis, 50–51
Superficial myxoma, 279
Surface osteosarcoma, 320–328
Symplastic glomus tumors, 153–154, 156
Synovial hemangioma, 175
Synovial osteochondromatosis, 266–267
Synovial sarcoma, 20t, 21–22, 33t, 34, 298–300
Synovial tissue. *See* Tumors of synovial tissue
Synovioma, 255–256
Synovium, 255, 257–258
System of the American Musculoskeletal Tumor Society, 15–16
SYT-SSX1, 34
SYT-SSX2, 34

T
Target sign, 200
Targetoid hemosiderotic hemangioma, 182–183
Tc-99 scan, 7
T-cell lymphoma, 385–386
TdT, 19, 20t
Technetium (Tc)-99 scan, 7
Telangiectatic osteosarcoma, 324–325

Tenosynovial giant cell tumor, 255–270. *See also* Tumors of synovial tissue
Terminal deoxynucleotide transferase (TdT), 19t
TFE3, 19t
Thallium scan, 7
TLE1, 19t
TLS/FUS-CHOP, 35–36
Translocation, 32–34
Traumatic neuroma, 193–195
Tumors of miscellaneous type/uncertain lineage
   aggressive angiomyxoma, 283–284
   angiomyofibroblastoma, 281–283
   ASPS, 295–296
   cutaneous myxoma, 279–280
   DSRCT, 301–305
   epithelioid sarcoma, 293–295
   ES/PNET. *See* ES/PNET
   intramuscular myxoma, 276–277
   juxta-articular myxoma, 277–279
   OSFMT, 285–286
   PEComa, 290–292
   PHAT, 287
   PMTMCT, 288–290
   synovial sarcoma, 298–300
Tumors of perivascular cells
   atypical glomus tumors, 154–157
   glomus tumors, 153–157
   HPC/SFT, 146–150
   myopericytoma, 150–153
Tumors of synovial tissue
   detritic synovitis, 271–275
   FTS, 264–266
   hemosiderotic synovitis, 261–262
   lipoma arborescens, 263–264
   localized GCTTS, 259–261
   loose bodies, 268–270
   malignant tenosynovial giant cell tumor, 270–274
   malignant tumors of the joint, 270
   normal anatomy, 255
   primary synovial chondromatosis, 266–268
   PVNS, 256–258
Tyrosinase, 19t

U
Ultrasound, 6–7
Undifferentiated pleomorphic sarcoma, 24, 90–96
Unicameral bone cyst, 432–435

V
Vascular leiomyoma, 122–123
Vascular leiomyosarcoma, 127–128
Vascular tumors of bone
   angiosarcoma, 396–400
   EHE, 392–396
   hemangioma, 389–392. *See also* Vascular tumors of soft tissue
Vascular tumors of intermediate malignancy, 179–186. *See also* Vascular tumors of soft tissue
Vascular tumors of soft tissue
   angiosarcoma, 186–188
   benign vascular tumors, 169–179
   capillary hemangioma, 169–172
   cavernous hemangioma, 172–173
   Dabska-type and retiform hemangioendothelioma, 181–183
   deeply located hemangioma, 175–177
   EHE, 183–186
   epithelioid hemangioma, 177–179
   fully malignant vascular tumors, 186–192

Vascular tumors of soft tissue *(Continued)*
    KHE, 179–181
    KS, 188–192
    reactive vascular proliferations. *See* Reactive vascular proliferations
    SCH, 173–175
    vascular tumors of intermediate malignancy, 179–186
Villous lipomatous proliferation of synovial membrane, 263–264
Vimentin, 19t
von Recklinghausen disease, 199
Von Willebrand factor, 19t
Vulvar leiomyoma, 120–121

W

Wagner-Meissner bodies, 200–203
Well-differentiated juxtacortical osteosarcoma, 320–329
Well-differentiated liposarcoma, 33t, 108–110
Well-differentiated myeloma, 381
Werner syndrome, 321t
WT1, 19t, 34–35

X

Xanthoma, 77–78